MARY IMOGENE BASSETT HOSPITAL

69972

26

AE037041

BULLETIN

OF THE NEW YORK ACADEMY OF MEDICINE

EDITORIAL BOARD

Charles A. Ragan, Jr., *Chairman*
Ralph W. Gause
Frank L. Horsfall, Jr.
J. Lawrence Pool
Robert J. Slater
Frank C. Spencer
Stuart S. Stevenson
Frederick G. Zak

Saul Jarcho, *Editor in Chief*

Volume 46

1970

THE NEW YORK ACADEMY OF MEDICINE
NEW YORK, N. Y. 10029

SECOND SERIES JANUARY 1970 VOL. 46, NO. 1

BULLETIN OF THE NEW YORK ACADEMY OF MEDICINE

CONTENTS

Paulus Zacchias on Mental Deficiency and on Deafness
Paul F. Cranefield and Walter Federn 3

The Effects of Anesthesia and Cardiac Bypass on Pulmonary Compliance in Man
Bernard R. Hand, James R. Malm, Frederick O. Bowman, Jr., and Stuart F. Sullivan 22

Christianus Helwich on Difficulty of Respiration (Augsburg, 1722)
Saul Jarcho 34

On Clinical Medicine: With Notes from the Diary of a Part-Time Researcher
Alfred Vogl 39

Statement by The New York Academy of Medicine on Methadone Management of Heroin Addiction 61

Astérix the Gaul 62

Unpublished Papers of Thomas Hodgkin 67

A Few Comments by Aristotle . . . . , ... 70

AUTHORS ALONE ARE RESPONSIBLE FOR OPINIONS EXPRESSED IN THEIR CONTRIBUTIONS

SAUL JARCHO, *Editor in Chief*

Published monthly by THE NEW YORK ACADEMY OF MEDICINE
2 East 103 Street, New York, N. Y. 10029

SUBSCRIPTION OFFICE: S-H SERVICE AGENCY, INC., 31 E. 10TH ST., NEW YORK, N. Y. 10003
Annual Subscription United States $10.00. Canada $11.00. All other countries $12.00. Single copies $2.00.
ADVERTISING OFFICE • 421 HUDSON STREET, NEW YORK, N. Y. 10014 • CIrcle 7-7706

Copyright 1970 by The New York Academy of Medicine

MARY IMOGENE BASSETT HOSPITAL
18910

OFFICERS AND STAFF OF THE ACADEMY: 1970

JOHN L. POOL, *President*

Vice Presidents

ARTHUR A. FISCHL — EDWARD E. FISCHEL — ALBERT C. SANTY

JAMES E. THOMPSON, *Treasurer*

HANS H. ZINSSER, *Recording Secretary*

Trustees

GORDON M. BRUCE
HOWARD REID CRAIG
JOSE M. FERRER, JR.
MILTON J. GOODFRIEND
WILLIAM J. GRACE
LOUIS M. HELLMAN
ROBERT L. LEVY
JOHN L. MADDEN
AUBRE DE L. MAYNARD
JOHN P. WEST

Council

The President
The Vice Presidents
The Trustees
The Treasurer
The Recording Secretary

Chairmen of the Standing Committees on:

Admission
Medical Education
Library
Public Health
Medicine in Society

JAMES E. McCORMACK, *Director*

GERTRUDE L. ANNAN, *Librarian*

Executive Secretaries of the Standing Committees

ARTHUR J. LEWIS, *Public Health*

ROBERT S. GOODHART, *Medical Education*

MARVIN LIEBERMAN, *Medicine in Society*

SAUL JARCHO, *Publications*

Business Manager

ROBERT BRERETON

Library Consultants

JANET DOE — CURT PROSKAUER

Legal Counsel

DAVIS POLK AND WARDWELL

EDITORIAL BOARD

CHARLES A. RAGAN, JR., *Chairman*
RALPH W. GAUSE
FRANK L. HORSFALL, JR.
J. LAWRENCE POOL
ROBERT J. SLATER
FRANK C. SPENCER
STUART S. STEVENSON
FREDERICK G. ZAK

SAUL JARCHO, *Editor in Chief*

SECOND SERIES FERBUARY 1970 VOL. 46, NO. 2

BULLETIN OF THE NEW YORK ACADEMY OF MEDICINE

CONTENTS

Urban Ecology, Geography, and Health Problems
George W. Carey 73

The Problem of Pain in Paraplegia and Tetraplegia
L. S. Michaelis 88

Mount Sinai's Approach to the East Harlem Community
Charles H. Goodrich, Margaret Olendzki, and Kurt W. Deuschle . 97

Group Practice Development: A Service of the Department of Health, New York City
Louis L. Feldman 113

The India Office Records: A Source for Historians of Psychiatry . . 124

AUTHORS ALONE ARE RESPONSIBLE FOR OPINIONS EXPRESSED IN THEIR CONTRIBUTIONS

SAUL JARCHO, *Editor in Chief*

Published monthly by THE NEW YORK ACADEMY OF MEDICINE
2 East 103 Street, New York, N. Y. 10029

SUBSCRIPTION OFFICE: S-H SERVICE AGENCY, INC., 31 E. 10TH ST., NEW YORK, N. Y. 10003
Annual Subscription United States $15.00. Canada $16.00. All other countries $17.00. Single copies $3.00.
ADVERTISING OFFICE • 421 HUDSON STREET, NEW YORK, N. Y. 10014 • CIrcle 7-7706

Copyright 1970 by The New York Academy of Medicine

OFFICERS AND STAFF OF THE ACADEMY: 1970

JOHN L. POOL, *President*

Vice Presidents

ARTHUR A. FISCHL — EDWARD E. FISCHEL — ALBERT C. SANTY

JAMES E. THOMPSON, *Treasurer*
HANS H. ZINSSER, *Recording Secretary*

Trustees

GORDON M. BRUCE
HOWARD REID CRAIG
JOSE M. FERRER, JR.
MILTON J. GOODFRIEND
WILLIAM J. GRACE
LOUIS M. HELLMAN
ROBERT L. LEVY
JOHN L. MADDEN
AUBRE DE L. MAYNARD
JOHN P. WEST

Council

The President — The Vice Presidents — The Trustees
The Treasurer — The Recording Secretary

Chairmen of the Standing Committees on:

Admission
Medical Education
Library
Public Health
Medicine in Society

JAMES E. MCCORMACK, *Director*
GERTRUDE L. ANNAN, *Librarian*
Executive Secretaries of the Standing Committees
ARTHUR J. LEWIS, *Public Health*
ROBERT S. GOODHART, *Medical Education*
MARVIN LIEBERMAN, *Medicine in Society*
SAUL JARCHO, *Publications*

Business Manager
ROBERT BRERETON

Library Consultants
JANET DOE — CURT PROSKAUER

Legal Counsel
DAVIS POLK AND WARDELL

EDITORIAL BOARD

CHARLES A. RAGAN, JR., *Chairman*
RALPH W. GAUSE
FRANK L. HORSFALL, JR.
J. LAWRENCE POOL
ROBERT J. SLATER
FRANK C. SPENCER
STUART S. STEVENSON
FREDERICK G. ZAK

SAUL JARCHO, *Editor in Chief*

SECOND SERIES MARCH 1970 VOL. 46, NO. 3

BULLETIN OF THE NEW YORK ACADEMY OF MEDICINE

CONTENTS

Radiation Carcinogenesis
Shields Warren 131

American Medicine: Technology Outruns Social Usefulness
George A. Silver 148

Discussion of Paper by Dr. George A. Silver:
"American Medicine: Technology Outruns Social Usefulness"
Mack Lipkin 161

Richard Wiseman: His Contributions to English Surgery
Alan DeForest Smith 167

The Use of an Authority for Hospitals
Harvey Sherman 183

The Chelsea Physic Garden 189

The Anthropological Writings of Theophil Mitchell Prudden
(1849-1924) 194

The Effects of Albuminuria upon Vision 197

Smallpox in New York City, 1868-1870 199

AUTHORS ALONE ARE RESPONSIBLE FOR OPINIONS EXPRESSED IN THEIR CONTRIBUTIONS

SAUL JARCHO, *Editor in Chief*

Published monthly by THE NEW YORK ACADEMY OF MEDICINE
2 East 103 Street, New York, N. Y. 10029

SUBSCRIPTION OFFICE: S-H SERVICE AGENCY, INC., 31 E. 10TH ST., NEW YORK, N. Y. 10003
Annual Subscription United States $15.00. Canada $16.00. All other countries $17.00. Single copies $3.00.
ADVERTISING OFFICE • 421 HUDSON STREET, NEW YORK, N. Y. 10014 • CIrcle 7-7706

Copyright 1970 by the New York Academy of Medicine

OFFICERS AND STAFF OF THE ACADEMY: 1970

John L. Pool, *President*

Vice Presidents

Arthur A. Fischl — Edward E. Fischel — Albert C. Santy

James E. Thompson, *Treasurer*

Hans H. Zinsser, *Recording Secretary*

Trustees

Gordon M. Bruce
Howard Reid Craig
Jose M. Ferrer, Jr.
Milton J. Goodfriend
William J. Grace
Louis M. Hellman
Robert L. Levy
John L. Madden
Aubre de L. Maynard
John P. West

Council

The President — The Vice Presidents — The Trustees

The Treasurer — The Recording Secretary

Chairmen of the Standing Committees on:

Admission — Medical Education

Library — Public Health

Medicine in Society

James E. McCormack, *Director*

Gertrude L. Annan, *Librarian*

Executive Secretaries of the Standing Committees

Arthur J. Lewis, *Public Health*

Robert S. Goodhart, *Medical Education*

Marvin Lieberman, *Medicine in Society*

Saul Jarcho, *Publications*

Business Manager

Robert Brereton

Library Consultants

Janet Doe — Curt Proskauer

Legal Counsel

Davis Polk and Wardell

EDITORIAL BOARD

Charles A. Ragan, Jr., *Chairman*
Ralph W. Gause
Frank L. Horsfall, Jr.
J. Lawrence Pool
Robert J. Slater
Frank C. Spencer
Stuart S. Stevenson
Frederick G. Zak

Saul Jarcho, *Editor in Chief*

SECOND SERIES APRIL 1970 VOL. 46, NO. 4

BULLETIN OF THE NEW YORK
ACADEMY OF MEDICINE

CONTENTS

Madness and Poetry: A Note on Collins, Cowper, and Smart
William B. Ober 203

Mozart: His Tragic Life and Controversial Death
Louis Carp 267

The Present Status of Abortion Laws:
A Statement by the New York Academy of Medicine 281

Lepers, Pariahs, and Churches 287

Lord Bryce on Intellectual Productivity 290

The Condition of Agricultural Laborers in England 293

AUTHORS ALONE ARE RESPONSIBLE FOR OPINIONS EXPRESSED IN THEIR CONTRIBUTIONS

SAUL JARCHO, *Editor in Chief*

Published monthly by the NEW YORK ACADEMY OF MEDICINE
2 East 103 Street, New York, N. Y. 10029

SUBSCRIPTION OFFICE: S-H SERVICE AGENCY, INC., 31 E. 10TH ST., NEW YORK, N. Y. 10003
Annual Subscription United States $15.00. Canada $16.00. All other countries $17.00. Single copies $3.00.
ADVERTISING OFFICE • 421 HUDSON STREET, NEW YORK, N. Y. 10014 • CIrcle 7-7706

Copyright 1970 by the New York Academy of Medicine

OFFICERS AND STAFF OF THE ACADEMY: 1970

John L. Pool, *President*

Vice Presidents

Arthur A. Fischl — Edward E. Fischel — Albert C. Santy

James E. Thompson, *Treasurer*

Hans H. Zinsser, *Recording Secretary*

Trustees

Gordon M. Bruce
Howard Reid Craig
Jose M. Ferrer, Jr.
Milton J. Goodfriend
William J. Grace
Louis M. Hellman
Robert L. Levy
John L. Madden
Aubre de L. Maynard
John P. West

Council

The President
The Treasurer
The Vice Presidents
The Recording Secretary
The Trustees

Chairmen of the Standing Committees on:

Admission
Library
Medical Education
Public Health
Medicine in Society

James E. McCormack, *Director*

Gertrude L. Annan, *Librarian*

Executive Secretaries of the Standing Committees

Arthur J. Lewis, *Public Health*

Robert S. Goodhart, *Medical Education*

Marvin Lieberman, *Medicine in Society*

Saul Jarcho, *Publications*

Business Manager

Robert Brereton

Library Consultants

Janet Doe — Curt Proskauer

Legal Counsel

Davis Polk and Wardell

EDITORIAL BOARD

Charles A. Ragan, Jr., *Chairman*
Ralph W. Gause
Frank L. Horsfall, Jr.
J. Lawrence Pool
Robert J. Slater
Frank C. Spencer
Stuart S. Stevenson
Frederick G. Zak

Saul Jarcho, *Editor in Chief*

SECOND SERIES MAY 1970 VOL. 46, NO. 5

BULLETIN OF THE NEW YORK ACADEMY OF MEDICINE

CONTENTS

SYMPOSIUM ON MEDICINE AND DIPLOMACY IN THE TROPICS

Opening Statement
Angie Brooks 299

Introduction
Kevin M. Cahill 300

Diplomacy and Medicine
John S. Badeau 303

Health Problems and Goals of a Recipient Nation
Abdulrahim Abby Farah 313

The Evolution and Delivery of Medical Programs in Developing Lands
Edward E. Swanstrom 324

A War We Can Win: Health as a Vector of Foreign Policy
Hugh L. Carey 334

Medical Research Activities Overseas
Gustave J. Dammin 351

Observations on America's International Medical Programs
George I. Lythcott 361

Empyema or Hydrothorax in the Ninety-Fifth Doge of Venice
Saul Jarcho 378

The *Jackdaw* Series on the History of Medicine and Science 386

AUTHORS ALONE ARE RESPONSIBLE FOR OPINIONS EXPRESSED IN THEIR CONTRIBUTIONS

SAUL JARCHO, *Editor*

Published monthly by the NEW YORK ACADEMY OF MEDICINE
2 East 103 Street, New York, N. Y. 10029

SUBSCRIPTION OFFICE: S-H SERVICE AGENCY, INC., 31 EAST 10TH ST., NEW YORK, N. Y. 10003
Annual Subscription United States $15.00. Canada $16.00. All otehr countries $17.00. Single copies $3.00.
ADVERTISING OFFICE • 421 HUDSON STREET, NEW YORK, N. Y. 10014 • CIrcle 7-7706

Copyright 1970 by The New York Academy of Medicine

OFFICERS AND STAFF OF THE ACADEMY: 1970

JOHN L. POOL, *President*

Vice Presidents

ARTHUR A. FISCHL — EDWARD E. FISCHEL — ALBERT C. SANTY

JAMES E. THOMPSON, *Treasurer*
HANS H. ZINSSER, *Recording Secretary*

Trustees

GORDON M. BRUCE
HOWARD REID CRAIG
JOSE M. FERRER, JR.
MILTON J. GOODFRIEND
WILLIAM J. GRACE
LOUIS M. HELLMAN
ROBERT L. LEVY
JOHN L. MADDEN
AUBRE DE L. MAYNARD
JOHN P. WEST

Council

The President — The Vice Presidents — The Trustees
The Treasurer — The Recording Secretary

Chairmen of the Standing Committees on:

Admission
Medical Education
Library
Public Health
Medicine in Society

JAMES E. MCCORMACK, *Director*
GERTRUDE L. ANNAN, *Librarian*
Executive Secretaries of the Standing Committees
ARTHUR J. LEWIS, *Public Health*
ROBERT S. GOODHART, *Medical Education*
MARVIN LIEBERMAN, *Medicine in Society*
SAUL JARCHO, *Publications*

Business Manager
ROBERT BRERETON

Library Consultants
JANET DOE — CURT PROSKAUER

Legal Counsel
DAVIS POLK AND WARDELL

EDITORIAL BOARD

CHARLES A. RAGAN, JR., *Chairman*
RALPH W. GAUSE
FRANK L. HORSFALL, JR.
J. LAWRENCE POOL
ROBERT J. SLATER
FRANK C. SPENCER
STUART S. STEVENSON
FREDERICK G. ZAK

SAUL JARCHO, *Editor in Chief*

SECOND SERIES JUNE 1970 VOL. 46, NO. 6

BULLETIN OF THE NEW YORK ACADEMY OF MEDICINE

CONTENTS

Methadone Management of Heroin Addiction 391

Symposium on Hemolytic Anemia

Hereditary Hemolytic Disorders
Ernst R. Jaffé 397

Disease-Associated Autoimmune Hemolytic Anemia
Arthur Sawitsky and Panfilo B. Ozaeta, Jr. 411

Drug-Associated Hemolytic Anemia
Ralph Zalusky 427

Teen-Age Out-of-Wedlock Pregnancy
W. Godfrey Cobliner 438

Medical Numismatics: A Denarius Commemorating Rome's First Doctor, Arcagathus (219 B.C.)
Adrian W. Zorgniotti 448

Career Scientists of the Health Research Council of the City of New York

Proceedings 451

Officers and Members 452

Program 453

Two Health Problems: One Solution / *Mary C. McLaughlin* 454

Abstracts of Presentations by Career Scientists 457

Career Scientists of The Health Research Council 463

The Doctor Travels with Karl Baedeker
Bruno Gebhard 469

Medical and Nonmedical Items in Baedeker's Description of New York 479

Climatic Treatment of Hypochondriasis 482

Disease in Nepal, 1819 484

Daniel Drake on Geographic Variations of Disease 486

AUTHORS ALONE ARE RESPONSIBLE FOR OPINIONS EXPRESSED IN THEIR CONTRIBUTIONS

SAUL JARCHO, *Editor in Chief*

Published monthly by the NEW YORK ACADEMY OF MEDICINE
2 East 103 Street, New York, N. Y. 10029

SUBSCRIPTION OFFICE: S-H SERVICE AGENCY, INC., P.O. Box 2000
260 Heights Road, Darien, Conn. 06820

Annual Subscription United States $15.00. Canada $16.00. All other countries $17.00. Single copies $3.00.

ADVERTISING OFFICE • 421 HUDSON STREET, NEW YORK, N. Y. 10014 • CIrcle 7-7706

Copyright 1970 by the New York Academy of Medicine

OFFICERS AND STAFF OF THE ACADEMY: 1970

John L. Pool, *President*

Vice Presidents

Arthur A. Fischl — Edward E. Fischel — Albert C. Santy

James E. Thompson, *Treasurer*

Hans H. Zinsser, *Recording Secretary*

Trustees

Gordon M. Bruce
Howard Reid Craig
Jose M. Ferrer, Jr.
Milton J. Goodfriend
William J. Grace
Louis M. Hellman
Robert L. Levy
John L. Madden
Aubre de L. Maynard
John P. West

Council

The President — The Vice Presidents — The Trustees

The Treasurer — The Recording Secretary

Chairmen of the Standing Committees on:

Admission — Medical Education

Library — Public Health

Medicine in Society

James E. McCormack, *Director*

Gertrude L. Annan, *Librarian*

Executive Secretaries of the Standing Committees

Arthur J. Lewis, *Public Health*

Robert S. Goodhart, *Medical Education*

Marvin Lieberman, *Medicine in Society*

Saul Jarcho, *Publications*

Business Manager

Robert Brereton

Library Consultants

Janet Doe — Curt Proskauer

Legal Counsel

Davis Polk and Wardell

EDITORIAL BOARD

Charles A. Ragan, Jr., *Chairman*
Ralph W. Gause
Frank L. Horsfall, Jr.
J. Lawrence Pool
Robert J. Slater
Frank C. Spencer
Stuart S. Stevenson
Frederick G. Zak

Saul Jarcho, *Editor in Chief*

SECOND SERIES JULY 1970 VOL. 46, NO. 7

BULLETIN OF THE NEW YORK ACADEMY OF MEDICINE

CONTENTS

The Physician and the Community
Lamar Soutter 489

Resistance to Salmonella Infections in Inbred Mouse Strains
Diethelm H. Boehme 499

Statement on the Controlled Dangerous Substances Act of 1969 (S. 3246)
The New York Academy of Medicine 509

Treatment of Malignant Tumors of the Salivary Glands
John Conley 511

The New Role of the Autopsy in the Community Hospital
Alfred Angrist 523

Needed: A Health Consumers' Organization
Greer Williams 532

Tollund Man and Other Bog Burials 554

Effects of the American Revolution 558

AUTHORS ALONE ARE RESPONSIBLE FOR OPINIONS EXPRESSED IN THEIR CONTRIBUTIONS

SAUL JARCHO, M.D., *Editor in Chief*

Published monthly by the NEW YORK ACADEMY OF MEDICINE
2 East 103 Street, New York, N. Y. 10029

SUBSCRIPTION OFFICE: S-H SERVICE AGENCY, INC., P.O. Box 2000
260 Heights Road, Darien, Conn. 06820
Annual Subscription United States $15.00. Canada $16.00. All other countries $17.00. Single copies $3.00.
ADVERTISING OFFICE • 421 HUDSON STREET, NEW YORK, N. Y. 10014 • CIrcle 7-7706

Copyright 1970 by the New York Academy of Medicine

OFFICERS AND STAFF OF THE ACADEMY: 1970

JOHN L. POOL, *President*

Vice Presidents

ARTHUR A. FISCHL   EDWARD E. FISCHEL   ALBERT C. SANTY

JAMES E. THOMPSON, *Treasurer*
HANS H. ZINSSER, *Recording Secretary*

Trustees

GORDON M. BRUCE
HOWARD REID CRAIG
JOSE M. FERRER, JR.
MILTON J. GOODFRIEND
WILLIAM J. GRACE
LOUIS M. HELLMAN
ROBERT L. LEVY
JOHN L. MADDEN
AUBRE DE L. MAYNARD
JOHN P. WEST

Council

The President   The Vice Presidents   The Trustees
The Treasurer   The Recording Secretary

Chairmen of the Standing Committees on:

Admission   Medical Education
Library   Public Health
Medicine in Society

JAMES E. MCCORMACK, *Director*
GERTRUDE L. ANNAN, *Librarian*
Executive Secretaries of the Standing Committees
ARTHUR J. LEWIS, *Public Health*
ROBERT S. GOODHART, *Medical Education*
MARVIN LIEBERMAN, *Medicine in Society*
SAUL JARCHO, *Publications*

Business Manager
ROBERT BRERETON

Library Consultants
JANET DOE   CURT PROSKAUER

Legal Counsel
DAVIS POLK AND WARDELL

EDITORIAL BOARD

CHARLES A. RAGAN, JR., *Chairman*
RALPH W. GAUSE
FRANK L. HORSFALL, JR.
J. LAWRENCE POOL
ROBERT J. SLATER
FRANK C. SPENCER
STUART S. STEVENSON
FREDERICK G. ZAK

SAUL JARCHO, *Editor in Chief*

SECOND SERIES AUGUST 1970 VOL. 46, NO. 8

BULLETIN OF THE NEW YORK ACADEMY OF MEDICINE

CONTENTS

Nineteenth Century Wound Management of the Parturient Uterus and Compound Fracture: The Semmelweis-Lister Priority Controversy
Owen H. Wangensteen 565

Current Concepts of the Pathogenesis and Management of Asthma
Michael H. Grieco 597

The Origins of Modern Scientific Thinking
Gregory I. Altschuller 611

Statement on the Federal Drug Abuse and Drug Dependence, Prevention, Treatment, and Rehabilitation Act of 1970 (S. 3562)
The New York Academy of Medicine 642

The Mouth as an Instrument Holder 643

The Phrenologist Discusses Friendship 646

AUTHORS ALONE ARE RESPONSIBLE FOR OPINIONS EXPRESSED IN THEIR CONTRIBUTIONS
SAUL JARCHO, M.D., *Editor in Chief*

Published monthly by the NEW YORK ACADEMY OF MEDICINE
2 East 103 Street, New York, N. Y. 10029

SUBSCRIPTION OFFICE: S-H SERVICE AGENCY, INC., P.O. Box 2000
260 Heights Road, Darien, Conn. 06820
Annual Subscription United States $15.00. Canada $16.00. All other countries $17.00. Single copies $3.00.
ADVERTISING OFFICE • 421 HUDSON STREET, NEW YORK, N. Y. 10014 • CIrcle 7-7706
Copyright 1970 by the New York Academy of Medicine

OFFICERS AND STAFF OF THE ACADEMY: 1970

John L. Pool, *President*

Vice Presidents

Arthur A. Fischl — Edward E. Fischel — Albert C. Santy

James E. Thompson, *Treasurer*

Hans H. Zinsser, *Recording Secretary*

Trustees

Gordon M. Bruce
Howard Reid Craig
Jose M. Ferrer, Jr.
Milton J. Goodfriend
William J. Grace
Louis M. Hellman
Robert L. Levy
John L. Madden
Aubre de L. Maynard
John P. West

Council

The President — The Vice Presidents — The Trustees
The Treasurer — The Recording Secretary

Chairmen of the Standing Committees on:

Admission — Medical Education
Library — Public Health
Medicine in Society

James E. McCormack, *Director*

Gertrude L. Annan, *Librarian*

Executive Secretaries of the Standing Committees

Arthur J. Lewis, *Public Health*

Robert S. Goodhart, *Medical Education*

Marvin Lieberman, *Medicine in Society*

Saul Jarcho, *Publications*

Business Manager

Robert Brereton

Library Consultants

Janet Doe — Curt Proskauer

Legal Counsel

Davis Polk and Wardwell

EDITORIAL BOARD

Charles A. Ragan, Jr., *Chairman*
Ralph W. Gause
Frank L. Horsfall, Jr.
J. Lawrence Pool
Robert J. Slater
Frank C. Spencer
Stuart S. Stevenson
Frederick G. Zak

Saul Jarcho, *Editor in Chief*

SECOND SERIES SEPTEMBER 1970 VOL. 46, NO. 9

BULLETIN OF THE NEW YORK ACADEMY OF MEDICINE

CONTENTS

Annual Meeting of the New York Academy of Medicine

The Responsibility of the New York Academy of Medicine in the Community
John L. Pool 649

Universal Health Insurance
Nelson A. Rockefeller 657

Presentation of the Academy Plaque to James Burns Amberson, M.D.
Dickinson W. Richards 663

Presentation of the Academy Medal to Harry Eagle, M.D.
Alfred Gilman 666

Standing Committees and Officers of Sections of the Academy 1970 . . 670

Statement on Implementation of the New York State Abortion Law
The New York Academy of Medicine 674

The Battered-Child Syndrome: Parental Motivation, Clinical Aspects
Gabriel V. Laury 676

Defunct and Dying Diseases
Bernard Straus 686

The Relevance of the Kaiser-Permanente Experience to the Health Services of the Eastern United States
Ernest W. Saward 707

Assuring Stable and Effective Financing of Local Health Services: The Role of Intergovernmental Grants-in-Aid
James F. Kelly 718

Discussion of the Paper by James F. Kelly
Alanson Willcox 732

Hospitals Depicted in Old Maps and Panoramas (I) 737

Opinions of the American Aborigines 742

AUTHORS ALONE ARE RESPONSIBLE FOR OPINIONS EXPRESSED IN THEIR CONTRIBUTIONS

SAUL JARCHO, M.D., *Editor in Chief*

Published monthly by the NEW YORK ACADEMY OF MEDICINE
2 East 103 Street, New York, N. Y. 10029

ALL SUBSCRIPTIONS AND ORDERS FOR BACK NUMBERS SHOULD BE SENT TO:
S-H SERVICE AGENCY, INC., P.O. Box 2000
260 Heights Road, Darien, Conn. 06820
Annual Subscription United States $15.00. Canada $16.00. All other countries $17.00. Single copies $3.00.
ADVERTISING OFFICE • 421 HUDSON STREET, NEW YORK, N. Y. 10014 • CIrcle 7-7706

Copyright 1970 by the New York Academy of Medicine

OFFICERS AND STAFF OF THE ACADEMY: 1970

JOHN L. POOL, *President*

Vice Presidents

ARTHUR A. FISCHL — EDWARD E. FISCHEL — ALBERT C. SANTY

JAMES E. THOMPSON, *Treasurer*

HANS H. ZINSSER, *Recording Secretary*

Trustees

GORDON M. BRUCE
HOWARD REID CRAIG
JOSE M. FERRER, JR.
MILTON J. GOODFRIEND
WILLIAM J. GRACE
LOUIS M. HELLMAN
ROBERT L. LEVY
JOHN L. MADDEN
AUBRE DE L. MAYNARD
JOHN P. WEST

Council

The President — The Vice Presidents — The Trustees
The Treasurer — The Recording Secretary

Chairmen of the Standing Committees on:

Admission — Medical Education
Library — Public Health
Medicine in Society

JAMES E. MCCORMACK, *Director*

THOMAS BASSLER, *Librarian*

Executive Secretaries of the Standing Committees

ARTHUR J. LEWIS, *Public Health*

ROBERT S. GOODHART, *Medical Education*

MARVIN LIEBERMAN, *Medicine in Society*

SAUL JARCHO, *Publications*

Business Manager

ROBERT BRERETON

Library Consultants

JANET DOE — CURT PROSKAUER

Legal Counsel

DAVIS POLK AND WARDWELL

EDITORIAL BOARD

CHARLES A. RAGAN, JR., *Chairman*
RALPH W. GAUSE
FRANK L. HORSFALL, JR.
J. LAWRENCE POOL
ROBERT J. SLATER
FRANK C. SPENCER
STUART S. STEVENSON
FREDERICK G. ZAK

SAUL JARCHO, *Editor in Chief*

SECOND SERIES OCTOBER 1970 VOL. 46, NO. 10

BULLETIN OF THE NEW YORK
ACADEMY OF MEDICINE

CONTENTS

NEW YORK HEART ASSOCIATION
CONFERENCE ON GLOMERULONEPHRITIS

Introduction
E. Lovell Becker 747

Glomerulonephritis: Clinical Aspects
David P. Earle 749

Pathology of Glomerulonephritis
Jacob Churg 761

[CONTINUED ON FOLLOWING PAGE]

AUTHORS ALONE ARE RESPONSIBLE FOR OPINIONS EXPRESSED IN THEIR CONTRIBUTIONS

SAUL JARCHO, M.D., *Editor in Chief*

Published monthly by the NEW YORK ACADEMY OF MEDICINE
2 East 103 Street, New York, N. Y. 10029

ALL SUBSCRIPTIONS AND ORDERS FOR BACK NUMBERS SHOULD BE SENT TO:
S-H SERVICE AGENCY, INC., P.O. Box 2000
260 Heights Road, Darien, Conn. 06820
Annual Subscription United States $15.00. Canada $16.00. All other countries $17.00. Single copies $3.00.
ADVERTISING OFFICE • 421 HUDSON STREET, NEW YORK, N. Y. 10014 • CIrcle 7-7706

Copyright 1970 by the New York Academy of Medicine

CONTENTS (Continued)

Evidence for Immunologic Mechanisms in Several Forms of Human Glomerular Diseases
Robert T. McCluskey 769

Glomerulonephritis: Pediatric Aspects
Wallace W. McCrory 789

Closing Morning Discussion
David P. Earle, David S. Baldwin, and Chester M. Edelmann, Jr. . . 797

An Overview of Nephritis
John P. Merrill 806

The Renal Regulation of Sodium Transport
Norman Bank 818

Proteinuria in Renal Disease
E. Lovell Becker 830

[CONTINUED ON FOLLOWING PAGE]

CONTENTS (Concluded)

Management of End-State Nephritis: Biochemical Alterations
George E. Schreiner 838

Dietary Management of End-Stage Uremia
Milton E. Rubini and Joel D. Kopple 850

Renal Transplantation: Present Status
Albert L. Rubin, John C. Whitsell, Robert R. Riggio, Gabriel H. Schwartz, David S. David, and Kurt H. Stenzel . . 869

Panel Discussion, Afternoon Session
Jerome Lowenstein, Norman Bank, Milton E. Rubini, George E. Schreiner 884

An Anthropological Essay by Thomas Hodgkin 889

OFFICERS AND STAFF OF THE ACADEMY: 1970

JOHN L. POOL, *President*

Vice Presidents

ARTHUR A. FISCHL   EDWARD E. FISCHEL   ALBERT C. SANTY

JAMES E. THOMPSON, *Treasurer*

HANS H. ZINSSER, *Recording Secretary*

Trustees

GORDON M. BRUCE
HOWARD REID CRAIG
JOSE M. FERRER, JR.
MILTON J. GOODFRIEND
WILLIAM J. GRACE
LOUIS M. HELLMAN
ROBERT L. LEVY
JOHN L. MADDEN
AUBRE DE L. MAYNARD
JOHN P. WEST

Council

The President   The Vice Presidents   The Trustees
The Treasurer   The Recording Secretary

Chairmen of the Standing Committees on:

Admission   Medical Education
Library   Public Health
Medicine in Society

JAMES E. MCCORMACK, *Director*

THOMAS BASLER, *Librarian*

Executive Secretaries of the Standing Committees

ARTHUR J. LEWIS, *Public Health*

ROBERT S. GOODHART, *Medical Education*

MARVIN LIEBERMAN, *Medicine in Society*

SAUL JARCHO, *Publications*

Business Manager

ROBERT BRERETON

Library Consultants

JANET DOE   CURT PROSKAUER

Legal Counsel

DAVIS POLK AND WARDWELL

EDITORIAL BOARD

CHARLES A. RAGAN, JR., *Chairman*
RALPH W. GAUSE
FRANK L. HORSFALL, JR.
J. LAWRENCE POOL
ROBERT J. SLATER
FRANK C. SPENCER
STUART S. STEVENSON
FREDERICK G. ZAK

SAUL JARCHO, *Editor in Chief*

SECOND SERIES NOVEMBER 1970 VOL. 46, NO. 11

BULLETIN OF THE NEW YORK ACADEMY OF MEDICINE

CONTENTS

Continuing Education of the Practicing Physician
The New York Academy of Medicine 893

A Critique of the Conflict Between Mission-Oriented and Clinical Research
Louis M. Rousselot 906

The Use of Amniocentesis for Prenatal Genetic Counseling
Melvin Gertner, Lillian Y. F. Hsu, Joan Martin, and Kurt Hirschhorn 916

Nasal Reconstruction by Scalping Flap in a Case of Malignant Melanoma of the Nasal Tip
Robert Hoehn 922

Application of Electrotherapy to Noncardiac Disorders
David Charles Schechter 932

Utilizing Computers in Evaluating Health Data
John C. Duffy 952

Infibulation, Population Control, and the Medical Profession
Gerhart S. Schwarz 964

New York Heart Association: Abstracts, Scientific Session on Research 997

Hospitals Depicted in Old Maps and Panoramas (II) 1013

Government and Welfare in Nineteenth Century England 1018

AUTHORS ALONE ARE RESPONSIBLE FOR OPINIONS EXPRESSED IN THEIR CONTRIBUTIONS

SAUL JARCHO, M.D., *Editor in Chief*

Published monthly by the NEW YORK ACADEMY OF MEDICINE
2 East 103 Street, New York, N. Y. 10029

ALL SUBSCRIPTIONS AND ORDERS FOR BACK NUMBERS SHOULD BE SENT TO:
S-H SERVICE AGENCY, INC., 866 Third Avenue, New York, N. Y. 10022

Annual Subscription United States $15.00. Canada $16.00. All other countries $17.00. Single copies $3.00.
ADVERTISING OFFICE • 421 HUDSON STREET, NEW YORK, N. Y. 10014 • CIrcle 7-7706

Copyright 1970 by the New York Academy of Medicine

OFFICERS AND STAFF OF THE ACADEMY: 1970

John L. Pool, *President*

Vice Presidents

Arthur A. Fischl
Edward E. Fischel
Albert C. Santy

James E. Thompson, *Treasurer*
Hans H. Zinsser, *Recording Secretary*

Trustees

Gordon M. Bruce
Howard Reid Craig
Jose M. Ferrer, Jr.
Milton J. Goodfriend
William J. Grace
Louis M. Hellman
Robert L. Levy
John L. Madden
Aubre de L. Maynard
John P. West

Council

The President
The Vice Presidents
The Trustees
The Treasurer
The Recording Secretary

Chairmen of the Standing Committees on:

Admission
Library
Medical Education
Public Health
Medicine in Society

James E. McCormack, *Director*
Thomas Basler, *Librarian*

Executive Secretaries of the Standing Committees

Arthur J. Lewis, *Public Health*
Robert S. Goodhart, *Medical Education*
Marvin Lieberman, *Medicine in Society*
Saul Jarcho, *Publications*

Business Manager

Robert Brereton

Library Consultants

Janet Doe
Curt Proskauer

Legal Counsel

Davis Polk and Wardwell

EDITORIAL BOARD

Charles A. Ragan, Jr., *Chairman*
Ralph W. Gause
Frank L. Horsfall, Jr.
J. Lawrence Pool
Robert J. Slater
Frank C. Spencer
Stuart S. Stevenson
Frederick G. Zak

Saul Jarcho, *Editor in Chief*

SECOND SERIES DECEMBER 1970 VOL. 46, NO. 12

BULLETIN OF THE NEW YORK ACADEMY OF MEDICINE

CONTENTS

The 1970 Health Conference
The New York Academy of Medicine
JOHN W. V. CORDICE, JR., *conference chairman*

COMMUNITY PARTICIPATION FOR EQUITY AND EXCELLENCE IN HEALTH CARE

Community Participation and National Health Policy
John W. V. Cordice, Jr. 1025

Role of the Community in Developing Improved Health Care

Discussions:
Herman Badillo 1028
Edgar Cahn 1031
Theodore O. Cron 1038
Lloyd Wescott 1042

GENERAL DISCUSSION I 1048

Role of the Health Profession in Achieving Effective Consumer Participation

Discussions:
Thomas E. Bryant 1054
Robert C. Long 1057
Paul Lowinger 1059
P. Walton Purdom 1063
Stephen R. Smith 1067
Walter Waldron 1071

[CONTINUED ON FOLLOWING PAGE]

AUTHORS ALONE ARE RESPONSIBLE FOR OPINIONS EXPRESSED IN THEIR CONTRIBUTIONS

SAUL JARCHO, M.D., *Editor in Chief*

Published monthly by the NEW YORK ACADEMY OF MEDICINE
2 East 103 Street, New York, N. Y. 10029

ALL SUBSCRIPTIONS AND ORDERS FOR BACK NUMBERS SHOULD BE SENT TO:
S-H SERVICE AGENCY, INC., 866 Third Avenue, New York, N. Y. 10022

Annual Subscription United States $15.00. Canada $16.00. All other countries $17.00. Single copies $3.00.
ADVERTISING OFFICE • 421 HUDSON STREET, NEW YORK, N. Y. 10014 • CIrcle 7-7706

Copyright 1970 by the New York Academy of Medicine

CONTENTS (Continued)

GENERAL DISCUSSION II 1077

The "How" of Community Participation in Delivering Health Care

Discussions:

Miguel F. Barragan 1080

John W. Hatch 1084

Olly Neal, Jr. 1091

Missing Links in Achieving Effective Services

1) ABSENCE OF A NATIONAL HEALTH POLICY IN TRAINING AND UTILIZATION OF MANPOWER

Discussions:

Stanley S. Bergen, Harold Nierenberg, Arnold M. Lewis, and Dominick Firriolo 1099

Michael M. Dacso 1107

Tom Levin 1112

2) ABSENCE OF A NATIONAL HEALTH POLICY IN MATTERS OF FINANCING

Discussions:

Howard Ennes 1120

David French 1129

Bennett J. McCarthy 1136

GENERAL DISCUSSION III 1141

Concluding Remarks

Community Health and Community Participation

Shirley Chisholm 1144

GENERAL DISCUSSION IV 1149

Demography in Early America 1152

Indexes: Volume 46, 1970

General Index 1155

Author Index 1163

BULLETIN OF
THE NEW YORK ACADEMY
OF MEDICINE

VOL. 46, NO. 1 JANUARY 1970

PAULUS ZACCHIAS ON MENTAL DEFICIENCY AND ON DEAFNESS*

PAUL F. CRANEFIELD AND WALTER FEDERN

The Rockefeller University
and
The New York Academy of Medicine
New York, N. Y.

PAULUS ZACCHIAS (1584-1659) was a papal physician and the author of the first extensive modern treatise devoted to medicolegal problems. The treatise contains a chapter that deals with mental deficiency which is followed by a chapter dealing with deafness. These chapters are offered in translation because they form a very useful summary of the opinions about mental deficiency held by the classical authorities upon whom Zacchias relied. The translation follows the first edition: Paulus Zacchias, *Quaestiones Medico-legales* [Rome, 1621], Tomus Primus, Liber II, Titulus I, Quaestio VII (De Ignorantibus, Fatuis, Stolidis, Obliviosis & Memoria Orbatis) and Quaestio VIII (De Mutis and Surdis).

The footnotes to the text of the translation require special explanation. The two chapters which we have translated contain very condensed references to Zacchias's sources. These references have been

*This article is based upon research supported by a grant from the National Institute for Child Health and Human Development (HD-01198). The article is based on a first draft written by the authors prior to the death of Dr. Federn in 1967; much of the article was written while Dr. Cranefield was executive secretary of the Committee on Publications and Medical Information of The New York Academy of Medicine. Dr. Cranefield is now associate professor at The Rockefeller University, New York, N. Y.

expanded and appear as footnotes to the translation. Even in their present form they fall short of a high standard of bibliographical detail. Nevertheless they will lead the reader to the source of the material more readily than the original citations. The first footnote may be taken as an example. Zacchias had "Card. comm. 6. Aphor. 51." We have changed the text to read "Cardanus"[1] and have added a footnote which reads "Cardanus (Girolamo Cardano, 1501-1576), *Commentarius in Hippocratis Aphorismos*, Liber 6. Aphorismus 51, *Opera*, 1663, vol. 8, 523, 1st ed, 1564." This expanded citation more fully identifies the author, gives the exact location of the passage, gives the date of the first edition of the work referred to, and also notes where the passage may be found in the 1663 edition of the *Opera* of Cardanus. To give full details would make the annotations excessively long but the present annotations are much more useful than the original citations given by Zacchias. An occasional footnote identified by a number and a letter (e.g., 3*a*) is used to add a citation or comment which does not appear in the original text. In those footnotes which have been designated by numbers only, all material is essentially an expansion of Zacchias's citation, with the occasional addition of the source of a modern translation of a quotation. All of the text has been translated but we have not translated the summaries which precede each chapter since they add little if anything to the text.

The text is straightforward and does not require extensive commentary. There are some aspects of it which are nevertheless of special interest. References to mental retardation are not at all common in the medical literature prior to the time of Zacchias; nor can one say with certainty that the condition was regarded as a clinical entity prior to that time. It thus seems worthy of mention that Zacchias is in fact discussing the phenomenon which we would call mental deficiency or mental retardation. Apart from some passages about those who have suffered from a failure of memory, the text deals with persons of inferior ability to learn. Zacchias is explicit, for example, in saying that those about whom he writes ought not be called crazed. Many of the earlier authors who mention diminution of intelligence lump together congenital mental deficiency with a great variety of acquired conditions including senility, postpsychotic apathy, and deterioration following prolonged and severe epilepsy. The fairly clearcut limitation of the condition by Zacchias is thus important in itself.

Zacchias offers a rather simple and unsophisticated classification of mental deficiency according to the severity of the defect. The least severe degree he suggests calling obtuseness; he later indicates that the obtuse may be taken as having no more judgment than a child of 14 years. These "slow learners" may be allowed to marry; interestingly he supports this opinion by a ruling of the Rota. He also holds that the obtuse cannot be held wholly free from responsibility if they commit crimes. A more severe grade of mental deficiency is illustrated by "those who are properly called fools by all." These, Zacchias says, seem to exist below the condition of human nature. They cannot be instructed in anything but trifles, but they can speak, even though their speech may be foolish and childish. The most extreme form of the condition is represented by persons Zacchias describes as mindless. Such persons are excused from the penalties of the law if they commit crimes and they are also debarred from civil actions, including, by implication, marriage. Those of the second grade ("properly called fools by all") may perhaps marry, but this must be left to the discretion of a judge.

It would be an exaggeration to say that the classification given by Zacchias corresponds in any precise way to the later classification into moron, imbecile, and idiot, but a rough comparison of those classes with the *obtuse*, the *foolish*, and the *mindless* is not entirely inappropriate. While Zacchias uses his classification largely in the interests of deciding legal questions, he also makes it clear that he was aware of the possibility of alleviating the condition of the obtuse by education.

Zacchias's chapter on the dumb and the deaf offers some curious and interesting ideas. That congenital deafness leads to defective intelligence has been known since the time of Aristotle; even today it affects intelligence unfavorably unless special educational procedures are applied early and skillfully. The congenitally deaf are to be treated as being in the class of the most severely retarded and "regarded in all things like as infants and madmen." They cannot be allowed to make a will even if they wish to make a pious bequest!

By far the most important statements in the two chapters are those concerning the reasons why the congenitally deaf ought not to be allowed to marry. Quite apart from various religious objections, Zacchias says that the congenitally deaf should not be allowed to marry because "there is evidence that they beget children like themselves, and now it profits the commonwealth that sound and in every respect perfect people are born, not so strikingly impaired ones." This statement is peculiarly important. It means that Zacchias was aware of the hereditary factor in congenital deafness and it means that he was willing to adopt a "eugenic" position. In the interest of the commonwealth, he says explicitly that those whose children may be imperfect should not have children. This is not, of course, a particularly early statement of a eugenic point of view. What is interesting and important is that Zacchias, holding this view, did not apply it to the mentally retarded of *any* degree. He did debar from marriage the severely retarded, but he did so on religious grounds (inability to understand the sacraments), not on eugenic grounds. It seems clear that Zacchias, who did recognize a hereditary factor in deafness and who did believe in the application of eugenic concepts, did not believe that heredity plays a major role in the transmission of mental deficiency.

Without granting Zacchias any extraordinary sophistication we may well note that there is no doubt or difference of opinion among modern geneticists about the existence of hereditary factors in deafness while there is a great deal of doubt and controversy about the role, if any, played by heredity in mental retardation.

Question VII
On the Ignorant, Foolish, Stupid, Forgetful, and Bereft of Memory

The impairments of reason with which we have dealt before are not properly numbered among the dementias. Among the dementias proper (or among those persons who do not possess the sound reason required by the human condition) the first place is taken by those persons commonly called fools. There are several kinds of fools, however, according to the greater or lesser slowness and indolence of the mind and intellect. Cardanus[1] set up only two kinds of folly, in one of which the victim does not recognize the things which should be recognized. Such persons may be those whom the jurists call witless (Ripa)[2]; according to Cardanus they are called rude because everything they do or say is done or said without grace or wit. For that reason the ancients called people of this sort by the term blite because it is a herb of dull and insipid taste and has no pungency (as Pierius Valerianus[3] reports). Hence this herb is rightly termed foolish by Martial[3a] in this poem: "That insipid beet, the noon meal of artisans, may acquire flavor."

The other kind of folly according to Cardanus is that kind in which the victims do not reason correctly from things which they have recognized, and he would limit the term folly to this sort. But the kinds of folly and of fools are far more differentiated. In some persons one merely discerns some laziness and indolence of intelligence which renders them unfit to obtain by the use of their intellect things which other people obtain easily (either on their own, or with nature dictating or by a little application). Those things include the first beginnings of education, some mechanical skills, manners, some civic regulations, the civil care of one's own body, the natural cunning common to all, and alacrity in domestic affairs. Such persons we call ignorant and unlearned, not because they are the opposite of persons whose knowledge comes from a skillfully acquired education, but because (as I have said) they are incapable of arriving at a natural and less than mediocre knowledge of things. Persons like these formerly were called Boeotians, which was the origin of the proverb, "a Boeotian intelligence," for a man of gross and dull intelligence; whence Horace:[4] "You would swear he was born a Boeotian in thick air."

Such persons might better be called obtuse, and this kind of folly might better be called obtuseness, as Cardanus[1] calls it. Among the jurists, the Rota[5] calls these undiscerning and witless. This ignorance or obtuseness is the rudiment and beginning of folly, but it is not truly folly and, as Galen[6] asserted, people should not be called fools on account of it. Plato[7] said that ignorance is dementia of the soul, and if we say that he spoke of this ignorance then I should say that Plato meant nothing but what we have said above.

Persons afflicted with obtuseness of this sort are reckoned among those whom we ordinarily term simpletons or people of a coarse grain or gross mind; in addition we call them slow, dolts, buffoons, clowns (and about these see Budaeus[8]), and by comparison blocks, etc. Plautus[9] reviews terms of this sort very nicely:

> Of all the silly, stupid, fatuous, fungus-grown, doddering, drivelling dolts anywhere, past or future, I alone am far and away ahead of the whole lot of 'em in silliness and absurd behavior!

In imitation of which Terrence[10] says:

> Any one of the terms used for a fool is a cap for my head, block-

head, wooden-pate, ass, leaden-wit—not one of them fits him, for his folly is in size too large for any of 'em.

But while we are dealing with terms, it should be called to mind that the word crazed is by no means appropriate to describe a fool, even though it is used by a number of jurists (Decius,[11, 11a] Thesaurus[12]) unless the term is understood in a broad manner or applied to fools of the third kind. Neither should fools be called insane, as Bartolus[13] declares. A number of jurists divide fools into those who have as much judgment as a child of 14 years and those who in judgment hardly equal a 10-year-old child (Thesaurus,[14] and of the physicians, Aetius[15]). It is the former group to which the first class of folly, termed by us ignorance and obtuseness, belongs. Ripa[2] meant the same when he said that among fools there are some who are only rude and obtuse while others are entirely mindless and without sense. But of the jurists, Menochius[16] distinguished more diligently between the kinds of fools. He does not proceed by our method, though, but by one which seemed to him to serve his cause better.

The first kind of folly does have its signs: for ignorant persons of this sort or (to use the word of the jurists) macaroons, are known by the fact that they are of slow intellect in all things, whence they are quite incapable of learning even childish elements of education. They are also devoid of natural courage, wherefore they stand in awe of their elders' frowns and threats even after attaining manhood. This vain awe of their elders causes them to dread to execute things which are not only permitted by their greater age but are for that reason exceedingly becoming to them to do. For instance, Melitides, having taken a wife did not touch her lest she accuse him before his mother, as related in the Adagia.[16a] Anything whatever is palmed off on them quite easily, and they are persuaded of vain and infeasible things by what sometimes deceiving friends have said. Persons kept down by this ignorance also, as I have said, give witless answers to questions. To say it in a word, where an effort of the intellect is needed, they perform everything slowly and without measure, and not at the proper occasion or time. On the other hand, they excel in an exquisite memory of things, as Fracastorius[17] reports. This as a rule happens naturally so that those who are slow of intellect are most retentive of memory, as is known to the philosophers, and noted among the jurists by Tiraquellus.[18] Though on the whole they are of moderate judgment, at times they have in certain things a not mediocre judgment as, among the jurists, Corsettus[19] notes.

It should be noted, however, that this defect as a rule is innate, while the other kinds of folly usually spring from both old age and disease. Though this kind of folly, called ignorance or obtuseness, can occur in old age and in disease, in such instances it always tends toward the worse, that is, toward perfect folly or toward death, as in cold diseases, whenever the sick already are close to death.

Besides, since folly is nothing but a coldness of the brain, having its origin in paucity and lack of heat and spirits (Galen[20] and Aetius[15]), it is clear that the brain's cooling or lack of heat can have many grades, whence a greater or a lesser faculty will arise. In the first grade of folly, therefore, it should be believed that there is in the brain a moderate cooling compared with the others (in whom however the coldness always increases, while the heat itself dwindles). To those, therefore, who attain this grade only, many of the sanctions of the laws and many decrees of the jurists ought not to apply. Indeed, though these do not obtain perfect use of reason, they are not alien from it [reason] to such a degree that they cannot apprehend by long use some things familiar to normal people. Thus in certain cases I do not see why they ought to be restrained from testifying, especially about those things which they have seen since, as I have said elsewhere, they may have an exquisite memory. About things which they have heard, some doubt could be allowed, since a greater soundness of reason is required in signifying the latter than in signifying the former, for the sense of sight is more direct and moves the imagination even more than the sense of hearing does, as has been said earlier.

I think they are rightly allowed to make a will, for of these I deem that Decius[21] correctly understands the teachers, moreover, the Rota[22] makes it plain by what follows that it speaks of this sort of fool. No less does it seem to me in accordance with the law that such persons are by no means prohibited from entering into religion and from making profession, because whatever use of reason there is in them can be adequate to these things, for a dementia that hinders profession has to be such as to take away every use of reason. (The same Rota.[23])

Nor do I believe that marriage should be forbidden to these persons, because even with such obtuseness of intelligence continuing unchanged they can obtain the power of the sacrament and the goal of marriage. This also is the view of the same Rota.[24] Nay, in my opinion, they can more easily be admitted to marry than to enter into religion, for in marriage nature itself cooperates somewhat and teaches ignorant persons also. Now from other things which require soundness and perfection of the intellect (for instance ordination, succession to fiefs, administration of a guardianship or of a public office) they should be debarred by right, it seems.

Furthermore, whether they should be excused for crimes can be difficult to decide. It is a fact that these persons can easily apprehend the nature of crimes at least from habit, even if they cannot do so from intellective cognition, since these children, especially those close to puberty, with whose intelligence we said the intelligence of these persons should be put on a par, easily recognize that crimes are bad by their own nature and therefore should be shunned. Yet it would seem that it should be said that just as children of this sort are excused for most things, so fools of this sort ought to be excused, since we stated that they have no greater judgment than the aforesaid children.

I hold the opinion that for a few crimes fools should not be excused the same way as children are; I am speaking of these fools only, not of the others. The reason is that though we like to compare these fools to children of fourteen years with respect to the use of reason, fools can advance in some things through habit since the power of habit is very great and it is capable of instructing not only these fools but even animals devoid of a rational soul. Well, then, if children close to puberty are able to deceive (lex Pupillum, i.e., Corpus Juris, Digesta, Liber I, Tit. XVII,[25] Num. CXI; Zabarellus)[26] much more should these persons be considered able to deceive. Now where deceit is present, and malice, guilt takes effect. Guilt, however, ought to be accompanied by punishment, by an argument opposite to that which states that where there is no guilt, there is no punishment (Angelus a Gambellionibus, quoted by Zilettus).[27] In the same way, where there is no deceit no crime deserving of punishment is thought to exist either (Menochius).[28]

There follow in the second grade those persons who are properly called fools by all, both by the jurists and by physicians (for extremely few or, rather, none I know of has expressly mentioned the first sort). These persons not only have indolent and slow intellect, but seem to exist below the condition of human nature with respect to the use of reason. They are hardly taught to speak and are known to be incapable of those things which human nature itself is wont to dictate on its own. Neither do they advance in reasoning with age, but they are distinguished from seven-year-old infants by nothing but their speech, in which they seem for a while to be prompter. But by their very speech they make plain that they are fools, whence they have therefore been called fools *(fatui)*, because by talking *(fando)* they show their imperfection (Bartolus).[29] This sort are of an altogether childish intelligence and delight in childish things, as for instance: "To play at odd or even, to ride on a long reed [hobby-horse]."[29a]

Otherwise they are thought to be incapable of anything and can not be instructed in anything save some trifles; for they have very little intellect and are also devoid of memory. That is because the brain's coldness, and its lack of spirits, is both greater and more constant in these persons: for folly is nothing else but either diminution or loss of memory at the same time as of reason, as Paulus[30] holds. Consequently it is of these that the dictum of the jurists should be understood, viz., that a person who has a disordered memory should be presumed to be a fool (Alexander;[31] Grammaticus;[32] Caevalus[33]). For in these persons the natural heat of the brain is so modest that it cannot serve any function of the brain. Hence we say correctly in common speech that a fool has no brain, as Galen[34] attests. Plautus[35] says facetiously: "Oh, no! You cleaned out all the brain from my cranium!"

In worse condition, though, are those persons in the next class, in whom neither any reason nor any memory at all is found. They reveal their folly both by words and by deeds, do not learn anything at all, nor advance in anything by civil habit, and in sum do not tell good from bad, appropriate from inappropriate, vice from virtue. (This does not take place in the same way as it does in the others about whom we spoke above). Therefore they are properly called stupid and mindless, and metaphorically stones, inasmuch as they seem to be devoid of all sense like stones. This term we use whenever we charge somebody with stupidity, as Plautus[36] did facetiously: ". . . for no flint's as foolish as you, that love her," and:[37] "My master is circumcompassed with an elephant's hide, not a human being's and he has no more sense than a stone. *P.* I know that, myself."

This affection was called by the Greeks *anonia*, just as the one mentioned earlier was called by them *morosis*, though in the authors both terms are accepted for the same affection. However, to the same extent as those mentioned earlier, these persons—though both classes are at times affected by greater or lesser folly, since some gradations of both ailments according to severity are allowed—are altogether rightfully debarred from all civil actions and are entirely excused for crimes.

About the former, though, it should be seen whether they can marry, since they preserve some shadow or rudiment of human intellect and are not entirely devoid of memory. Nor do they entirely lack human sense and passions like those whom we reviewed before. And because, as I have said repeatedly, the range of folly of this sort is great, I deem it correct to leave these decisions to the discretion of a judge, along with many other problems that can arise concerning this class of fool.

Now there can be doubt whether such persons ought to be permitted to draw a will. The reason for the doubt is that in him who disposes of his property an entirely sound mind is not required, but rather it is required that he should not be deranged. (Joseph Ludovicus;[38] and the Rota.[39]) This very matter though, like the things mentioned earlier, I remit to the discretion of the judge, for he will easily discern whether a fool is so devoid of sense and human passions that he by no means recognizes those who are closely connected with him, and who are his benefactors, or contrariwise; and so the judge will easily state a just opinion.

After the fools there are persons who are called forgetful, and wanting in memory. Between them, however, it is meet to make an important distinction. Let us say, then, that by "forgetful persons" we understand those who retain the memory of things with difficulty. By "persons wanting in memory," however, we mean those who do not retain any memory at all of things that have passed, either a long time or a short time ago, at least while they suffer from this condition. I prefer to distinguish them even though they seem not to differ except in degree, because to the latter group many things apply that by no means apply to the former. The latter should be regarded in every way as nothing less than fools of the second grade of folly. The reason is that as soon as the affection by which memory is impaired intensifies greatly, reason is also ruined (Galen;[40] Forestus[41]). It is from a dwindling of memory at the same time as of reason that folly arises, as I have already said.[30]

Now this affection as a rule arises from long and severe diseases, as Pliny[42] relates of Messala Corvinus. Pestilential diseases also provoke this illness; Lucretius relates that it occurred in a severe plague:[43] "And there were others who fell into oblivion of all things, so that they could not even tell who they were." Among the jurists, Menochius[44] has noticed this.

Besides, since in the former group memory has not been impaired in a manner that also impairs reason it should be said that many things may be allowed them that cannot be allowed the latter. The former ought not to be prevented from drawing a will; the latter contrariwise. The former should not be prohibited from entering into religion and making profession, the latter very much so. The former should be permitted to marry, to contract, to obligate themselves, to administer their property, and other things of this kind; the latter by no means. In some other things, though, the former perhaps should not be admitted (for about the latter there should be no question). These things I would lay before the jurists, who are to see whether such persons can be ordained licitly, since because of this defect they are not equal to many things to which a person who is to be ordained ought to be equal. The jurist may also determine whether these persons ought to be admitted to the exercise of public offices, since in public office both prudence and an exquisite memory of things are needed. Finally, the jurists may determine whether these are capable of testifying; for how would they be capable of doing so, who remember the things they have seen and heard either not at all or with the greatest difficulty? Wherefore, since it is mostly old people who are subject to this defect, may they notice how cautiously old people are admitted to testify, especially of things that have passed a long time since. Furthermore, since we have been talking of forgetfulness, let us discuss that question of the jurists in which they inquire how much time it takes for forgetfulness to be induced. Although a number of jurists (quoted by Menochius[45]) have tried to define the limit of forgetfulness on this point, it is plain that they have exerted themselves in vain. The reason is that there are a great many things that make people more and less forgetful, namely the temperament of the body and especially of the back of the head, sex, age, the constitution of the parts, the quality and the regulation of one's life, the exercise of memory itself, and other things of this sort. For with respect to sex it is clear, for example, that women are more forgetful than men, as the same Menochius[46] notes. This should be regarded as happening in consequence of the moister temperament of the former, which is fluid and less capable of retention; hence forgetfulness will be more easily induced in a woman than in a man. With regard to age, it is known that old people have very little memory of things; for this is first encroached upon by old age, as shown by experience and as Seneca notices,[47] and before him Aristotle.[48] But for these things he who wants more may read Mascardus.[49] As for temperament, persons who have a dry one have a more retentive memory, persons who have a moist one have a less retentive memory (Aristotle[48] and Averroes[50]); as a result of which it can hardly, if at all come to pass that people are strong in judgment and memory at the same time (Plato,[51] Forestus[52] and, of the jurists, Caevalus[53]). Regarding the conformation of the parts, those who have larger upper parts than lower parts are less strong in memory, as Aristotle[48] testifies. Finally, with respect to the quality of one's life, those who attend to affairs are easily forgetful, as the same Menochius witnesses.[54] Forgetfulness, then, can be induced more easily or with more difficulty, according to the diversity of these and similar things, to which the condition of the deed and of the event is to be added, since extraordinary deeds and great things are not presumed to be readily forgotten (the same Menochius);[55] and forgetfulness is more easily induced in the case of a strange deed (Verallus);[56] consequently the same Menochius prudently determines that this part of the question is remitted to the discretion of the judge, who must however take into consideration both these and many other things.

Question VIII
On the Dumb and the Deaf

We must consider the dumb and deaf separately, for it seems that we cannot correctly include them among the mindless or among the fools, and yet it cannot be truly affirmed that they are of sound judgment. For the present we speak of the dumb and deaf who are such from birth. About the others it is wrong to have doubts: for in my judgment no distinction should be made between them and those persons who both are of a sound mind and hear well and speak (provided you make one little bit of exception, as you will find at the end of this *Question*).

Besides, everybody knows that those who are deaf from birth are at the same time dumb. However, it has never come to my knowledge that one dumb from birth hears, so that conversely he who is dumb from birth at the same time is also deaf. My opinion is seconded by the lex Discretis[57] and the gloss there on the word raro.[58] Now the cause of both facts should be believed to have its origin in a dwindling of the nerves that are common to both senses. So Andreas Laurentius[59] judges after having denied the cause adduced by others, which is that the deaf are also dumb because they cannot learn a language or speak. Though if one concedes another cause of deafness from birth (about which Hieronymus Fabritius[60] writes), it would seem that this cause adduced by others [and denied by Laurentius] could act. That cause, about which Fabritius writes, is some thick extra tunic which has grown in the ear in front of the membrane that is called the tympanum; perhaps such deafness need not hinder speech. Consequently, I have not been greatly astonished at what Vallesius[61] relates about a friend of his, a monk, who taught those deaf from birth to speak. I do not believe that this could succeed with all the deaf, but with those about whom Fabritius writes, I believe it could.

Now while it should by no means be questioned that all the dumb and deaf from birth are deficient in prudence and vigor of mind, yet there are among them those of greater or lesser judgment, prudence, and vigor of mind, as of the jurists, Bartolus[62] maintains. But speaking of them as a whole, the same jurists, for instance Bartolus,[63] Cujacius,[64] Vantius,[65] Farinacius,[66] assert absolutely that one who is dumb and at the same time deaf from birth is put on a par with an infant and a madman, and is treated as absent. The distinction made by a few, however, that those who understand by nods do not lack prudence (Bartolus),[67] should not be understood to mean a prudence sufficient to render them fit for all things, but only for a few things of minor moment. Not without an evident reason, however, such a person is put on a par with a madman, which is double, one sensory, the other physical [physical here seems to be equivalent to our psychological]. The sensory one is the dwindling of the nerves, on account of which they are hindered both in hearing and in speaking. Now this dwindling presupposes a dwindling of the brain, which is the instrument of the intellect, whence without doubt intellection deteriorates, as it happens in madmen and in the mindless.

For that dwindling of the nerves is the true cause of both defects (rather than that the hindered hearing takes away speaking) is demonstrated by the very babes who hear most exquisitely yet do not speak, since they are hindered by the softness of the nerves that serve speech, which owing to their softness are not capable of being moved in order to articulate the voice. On the other hand, if you let a child that hears well hear nobody speak, as long as he can articulate and speak on his own, he will speak in his own manner when he has grown older. It is not necessary, then, that he who hears well also speaks. Nor, on the other hand, is it necessarily true that he who hears nobody speak does not speak because he cannot learn to speak.

The other cause, which is physical, I deem to be the fact that human intellect is perfected from day to day. On its own, the intellect is rude. It can be perfected only by habit and by learning, which is obtained from hearing. As a result, deprivation of hearing makes the intellect ruder; and if the deprivation of hearing is innate, it prevents instruction of the intellect.

It should be noted that this imperfection of the intellect in those who are dumb and deaf from birth is entirely irreparable. It cannot be hoped under any circumstances that they will obtain a sounder mind. According to their age, though, they can be said to have greater or lesser intellect, so that a number of things ought to apply to them when they are younger which perhaps will not apply when they grow in years. Yet they should be regarded in all things as infants and madmen, as I said above; for the perfection of intellect which they require on account of their age is not so great that they can ever be equal to anything.

Since, then, the imperfection of their intellect is irreparable to such a degree: just as infants and children, as long as they are of that age, and madmen, as long as they persist in their madness, are prohibited from all actions, the same opinion should be held about the dumb and the deaf (the lex Discretis, i.e., Corpus Juris, Codex, Liber VI, Tit. XXII, Num. X).[68] In particular they are not permitted to make a will, as is found in the same law and in the lex Qui in potestate, (i.e., Corpus Digesta Liber XXVIII, Tit. I,[69] Num. VI) surdus[70] (Decius;[71] Nepos a Motalbano);[72] which fact the teachers amplify to make it the procedure even in the case of pious bequests (Baldus).[73] They cannot contract a marriage (Abbas,[74] Jason[75]) and much less enter into religion;

(Brunellus[76] and others quoted by him; he himself, however, maintains the opposite).[77] It seems troublesome, though, to advocate his opinion, since such persons (even those who are of a more vivacious nature and endowed with some prudence) except for a rude and gross understanding of things which they have by nature, cannot obtain the power of marriage and the end and the purpose of that sacrament, to wit, the procreation of children for the glory of God. Now nature by itself does not dictate this, unless implicitly, but merely the enjoyment of coitus and of the expulsion of semen. Therefore animals, to which these persons are akin with respect to their understanding, copulate to no other purpose but in order to excrete semen, just as they also urinate and defecate, goaded by the quantity of urine and of feces, as Galen[78] teaches. Since, however, in my opinion a person who contracts a marriage, or whatever else, ought to recognize the true and real purpose of this action or contract, and since these persons do not recognize this purpose, but rather another, feigned one, which is insinuated to them by nature, I do not see how they ought to be permitted to contract a marriage; for one does not contract unless he wants to do so, and with the dwindling of the will the assent ceases. With the purpose not being recognized it cannot be said that one acts by choice and voluntarily; it is by chance, then, that he will contract, since his action lacks an end. Not to mention the fact that the deaf and dumb ought to abstain from marriage not only because they do not understand the end of marriage, but also for the good of the commonwealth, because there is evidence that they beget children like themselves, and it profits the commonwealth that people sound and in every respect perfect are born, not such strikingly impaired ones. Now apart from these things they are restrained from testifying, as is evidenced by Mascardus.[79]

Next, about those whose dumbness and deafness is acquired, one could hesitate whether they should be regarded as fit for all things. First about the merely dumb, who have lost their speech by accident, in my judgment one need have no doubts whatever about their abilities; this opinion is supported by the same lex Discretis,[68] Ubi autem. Their dumbness does not prevent them from doing whatever things other people can do. This has been asserted in the case of the limits of donation by the text in the law Qui id quod, (i.e., Corpus Juris, Digesta, Liber XXXIX, Tit. V,[80] Num. XXXIII), Mutis,[81] and by the gloss there which Maranta[82] adduces. One chance, though, you are to except, namely when the dumbness results from a defect of the brain; for such dumbness is always attended by some folly and diminution of intellect or at least ignorance; these persons, then, should be dealt with more cautiously,

Now about the deaf, doubts are occasioned by what the philosopher has said, from whom Valescus[83] borrows it. This is that hearing is the gate of the mind; thus, complete deafness without diminution of mind and intellect seems hardly to occur. In my judgment, in people of rude intelligence and a base condition, the intellect suffers greatly on account of their complete deafness; of others, inasmuch as they were very much in their right minds before their deafness, though on account of their deafness henceforth it [the intellect] is injured, I would say that it is not injured to such a degree that they need to be forbidden anything on account of this cause; the same lex Discretis[68] favors this view.

REFERENCES

1. Cardanus (Girolamo Cardano, 1501-1576). *Commentarius in Hippocratis Aphorismos,* Liber 6, Aphorismus 51, *Opera,* 1663, vol. 8, 1st ed., 1564.
2. Ripa (Giovanni Francesco de Santo Nazario de la Ripa, 14??-1534). In legem ex facto. *Digesta,* Liber 28, tit. 6. De vulgari & pupillari substitutione, lex 43, Num. 82.
3. Pierius Valerianus (born as Giovan Pietro della Fosse, 1477-1560). *Hieroglyphica,* Liber 58. Fol. 423vo of the ed. of 1567, 1st ed. 1556.

3a. Martialis. *Epigrammata,* Liber 13 (Xenia), 13. Ker, Walter R. A., transl. Loeb Classical Library.

4. Horatius, *Epistalarum,* Liber secundus, Epistula 1, line 244.
5. Decisiones Sacrae Rotae Romanae, Melitensis Testamenti, Friday, February 17, 1612, coram Manzanedo. *D. Prosperi Farinacii I.C. Romani Sacrae Romanae Rotae Decisionum ab ipso selectarum, nec unquam alias impressarum Tomi quatuor.* Aurelianae 1621, vol. 1, pp. 440-41. Reverendissimo P.D. Manzanedo. Meliten. Testamenti. Veneris 17 Februarij 1612. (Argumentum. Testamentum a demente conditum non valet, & qualis debeat esse ista dementia, de quo tempore, & quomodo probanda.) P. 441, Num. 5. [This decision is also found, as Decisio XXXIV, in the *Decisiones S. Rotae Romanae, ad praedictas materias spectantes,* a Cl.D. Lanfranco Zacchia collectae, which form an appendix to Horst's folio-editions of the *Quaestiones Medico-legales.* Lanfranco Zacchias (16??-1685) was a grandson of Paolo Zacchias. Unfortunately, his collection is not comprehensive.]
6. Galenus. *Commentarius 2. in Hippocratis Prorrheticum I,* textus 60(?) (In Kuehn's ed. it is 94, in Kuehn's ed. of Hippocrates, it is 92; see Kuehn, XVI, 696.)
7. Plato. *Sophistes,* cap. 15.
8. Budaeus (Guillaume Budé, 1467-1540). *Annotationes in XXIV pandectarum libros* (1508), in *Digesta,* Liber. 21, tit. 1: de Aedilitio Edicto, et redhibitione, et quanti minoris, lex. 4.
9. Plautus. *Bacchides* ("The Two Bacchises"), Act V, scene 1, Nixon, P., transl. Loeb Classical Library.
10. Terentius. *Heautontimorumenos* ("The Self-Tormentor"), Act 5, Scene 1. Sargeaunt, J., transl., Loeb Classical Li-

brary.
11. Decius (Filippo Decio, 1454-1536). *In legum Humanitatis,* Codex. Liber 6, Tit. 26. De Impuberum & aliis substitutionibus, lex 9, Num. 1, Gloss in Institutiones, Liber 2, tit. 12: Quibus est permissum facere testamentum, Praeterea, on the word Furiosi.
11*a*. Cf. Zacchias, II, 1, 9 De melancholicis, Num. 13/14.
12. Thesaurus (Gasparo Antonio Tesauro, 15??-16??). *Decisiones Pedimontanae,* 1610. Decisio 92, Num. 2.
13. Bartolus (Bartolo da Sassoferrato, 1314-1357). *Tractatus de testimoniis,* Num. 98. *Opera,* 1552, vol. 3, p. 178.
14. Thesaurus (as in note 12). Num. 4.
15. Aetius. Sermo 6, cap. 22. *Tetrabiblos,* 1535, vol. 1, p. 249.
16. Menochius (Giacomo Menochio, 1532-1607). *De Arbitrariis Judicum Quaestionibus et Causis, Centuriae sex,* 1569. Liber 2, cas. 529, Num. 2 ff.; pp. 920-21, ed. of 1691.
16*a*. Erasmus of Rotterdam. *Adagia,* 1515. Chil. IIII, Cent. IIII, 69, pp. 976-77, ed. of 1612.
17. Fracastorius (Girolamo Fracastoro, 1483-1553). *Turrius sive de intellectione dialogus,* Liber 1. Opera omnia 1573 & 1584, fol. 127ro; *Opera,* 1555, fol. 173ro.
18. Tiraquellus (Andre Tiraqueau, 1488-1558). *De Legibus Connublialibus,* 1513; after 1524 the title continues: *et jure maritali,* Gloss. 5, Num. 24.
19. Corsettus (Antonio Corsettus, 14??-1503). *Singularia,* Num. 2, on the word Testamentum, 1477.
20. Galenus, Liber 4, de praesagitione ex pulsibus, cap. 8; IX, 407 Kuehn.
20*a*. Galenus, Liber 2. De symptomatum causis, cap. 7; VII, 200-01, Kuehn.
21. Decius (cf. note 11). *In legem Furiosum.* Codex, Liber 6, tit. 22. De his qui testamenta facere possunt, vel. non, lex 9, Num. 8 & 11.
22. *Sacrae Rotae Romanae decisiones novissimae,* decisio 384, Num. 5, pars 1, tom. 1. Decisio XI in Lanfranco Zacchia's collection, which is not necessarily identical with the Decisio 384 here mentioned, in any case says the same thing: Romana Haereditatis, Veneris 15. Novembris 1592. Coram R. P. D. Penia. Num. 5.
22*a*. The above is found also in *Melitensis Testamenti* (see note 5).
23. *Rota,* as in note 22, dec. 134, Num. 1, pars 2.
24. *Rota,* as above, decis. 107, Num. 29, pars 2.
25. *Lex Pupillum, Digesta,* Liber 50, tit. 17. De (diversis) regulis juris antiqui, lex 111.
26. Zabarellus (probably Francesco Zabarella, 1360-1417). *De homicidiis casualibus & voluntariis,* cap. si furiosis, Num. 3.
27. Angelus a Gambellionibus (Angelo Gambiglioni, 15th cent.). Quoted by Zilettus, (Giovanni Battista Ziletti, 16th cent.). *Consilia,* cons. 95, Num. 1.
28. Menochius (cf. note 16). *Consiliorum sive Responsorum,* liber primus, consilium 28, Num. 13, vol. 1, p. 146, ed. of 1628; 1st ed., 1572.
29. Bartolus (cf. note 13). *Tractatus de Testimoniis,* Num. 98.
29*a*. Horatius. *Sermonum,* Liber secundus, sermo 3, line 248.
30. Paulus Aegineta. *Medicina,* Liber 3, cap. 11, p. 146, ed. of 1551.
31. Alexander (Alessandro Tartagna, 1424-1477). *In legem Cum servus,* para. constat, Digesta, Liber 30. Liber 1: De legatis et fidei commissis, lex 39, para. 7. See also *In legem si cum dotem,* para. si maritus. *Digesta,* Liber 24, tit. 3: soluto matrimonio, lex 3, para. 7.
32. Grammaticus (Tommaso Grammatico, 1473-1556). *Decisiones,* 1547, Decisio 2, Num. 1.
33. Caevalus (Geronimo de Cevallos, 16th? cent.). *Quaestiones Communes contra Communes* (Speculum aureum opinionum communium contra communes?), in the preface, Num. 98 (1602).
34. Galenus. Liber 3, de locis affectis, cap. 4.
34*a*. Galenus, Liber 3, de Placitis Hippocratis & Platonis, cap. 4 (V, 310-11, Kuehn).
35. Plautus. *Mostellaria* ("The Haunted House"). Act V, scene 1, line 1110. Nixon, P., transl. Loeb Classical Library.

36. Plautus, *Poenulus* ("The Little Carthaginian"), Act I, scene 2, lines 291-2. Nixon, P., transl. Loeb Classical Library.
37. Plautus. *Miles Gloriosus* ("The Braggart Warrior"), Act II, scene 2, lines 235-36.
38. Joseph Ludovicus (Giuseppe Ludovisi, 15??-16??). *Decisio Perusina prima,* Num. 14, pars I. In: *Decisionem seu Diffinitionum causarum perusinarum et provinciae Umbriae pars prima,* 1572.
39. *Decisiones Sacrae Rotae Romanae coram J. Cavalerio,* 1629. Romana Donatio de Gualteruciis, 1622, Monday, December 12, coram Cavalerio [Decisio 50 in Lanfranco Zacchias's collection, Num. 5].
40. Galenus, *De locis affectis,* Liber 3, cap. 4 (VIII, 460, Kuehn).
41. Forestus (Pieter van Foreest, 1521-1597). *Observationum et curiationum medicinalium libri tres,* 1590, Liber 10, observ. 1, p. 13.
42. Plinius. *Naturalis historia,* Liber 7, cap. 24. Loeb edition, vol. 2, p. 564. Actually, Zacchias is not quoting Pliny, but rather Caius Iulius Solinus, *Polyhistor,* cap. 1, para. 104, ed. of 1777, p. 34. The reason for his mistake was that he took the quotation at second hand from Menochius; see note 44.
43. Lucretius. *De rerum natura,* Liber 6, lines 1213-14. Rouse, W. H. D., transl., Loeb Classical Library.
44. Menochius (as in note 16), Liber 2, cas. 26, Num. 5, p. 170 of ed. of 1691.
45. Menochius, as above. This refers to note 44, but not merely to Num. 5 but to the entire Casus 26, the title of which is: Tempus quod sit, quo causatur oblivio, & quid in ea re a judice observandum sit.
46. Menochius. Ibid., Num. 3.
47. Seneca ("Rhetor"). In the preface to his book of Declamations, i.e., *Controversiae,* Liber 1, p. 51 in vol. of the Elzevir ed., 1639, of the work of his son, the philosopher Seneca.
48. Aristoteles. *Liber de Memoria & Reminiscentis,* cap. 2.
49. Mascardus (Guiseppe Mascardi, 15??-1588). *De Probationibus.* Conclusiones probationum omnium, quae in utroque Foro quotidie versantur, 4th ed. 1619; 1st ed., 1584-1588, Conclusio 1122, vol. 3.
50. Averroes. *Ibidem,* i.e., as in note 48: *De Memoria et Reminiscentia,* last chapter (Compendia librorum Aristotelis qui Parva Naturalia vocantur).
51. Plato. *Theaetetus,* cap. 34.
52. Forestus. As in note 41, Liber 10, Observ. 1 in the Scholion, p. 15.
53. Caevalus. Cf. note 33, preface to *Practicae Quaestiones Communes* (probably the same work as that quoted in note 33), Num. 94.
54. Menochius. As in note 16; as above (notes 44, 45, 46), same case (26), Num. 4.
55. Menochius. Ibid., Num. 6.
56. Verallus (Paolo Emilio Verallo, 16th cent.). *Decisiones Aureae Causarum sacri Palatii apostolici,* 1589, decisio 279, Num. 7, pars 3.
57. *Lex Discretis.* Codex, Liber 6, tit. 22: qui testamenta facere possunt, vel non (the text says wrongly: de testamentis, that is: tit. 23) lex 10. para. 1 Sin autem.
58. As in note 57, gloss there on the word "raro."
59. Andreas Laurentius (Andre Du Laurens, 1558-1609). *Historia Anatomica Humani Corporis,* Liber 11, cap. 13: De aure interna, quae verum auditus est organum Controversiae, quaestio 11, De mira aurium & palati, linguae ac laryngis sympathia (1600, p. 430). (In the 1st ed., 1593, *Opera anatomica . . . .* it is Liber 4, cap. 18, q. 26, pp. 745-46.)
60. Hieronymus Fabricius (Girolamo Fabrici d'Acquapendente, 1533-1619). *De aure, Auditus Organo,* pars 1: De dissectione et historia auris, cap. 4: De Membrana Tympano appellata (1600, pp. 4-5, p. 142 in ed. of 1614).
61. Vallesius (Francisco Valles Covarrubias, 1524-1592). *Liber de sacra philosophia sive de iis quae scripta sunt physice in libris sanctis,* 1558, cap. 3.
62. Bartolus. Cf. note 13. *Tractatus de Testimoniis,* Num. 93, *Opera,* 1552, vol. 2, p. 177.
63. Bartolus. *Ibid.,* Num. 97.

64. Cujacius (Jacques de Cujas, 1522-1590). *Notationes ad Justiniani libros IV Institutionum,* Liber 2, tit. 10: de Testamentis ordinandis, vol. 1 of his *Opera* of 1577. Or p. 96 in vol. 1 of his *Opera omnia* of 1658: Notae in Librum 2. Institutionum Justiniani. De testamentis ordinandis, cap. 10, para. 6.
65. Vantius (Sebastiano Vanti, 16. Cent.) *Tractatus de nullitatibus processuum ac sententiarum* . . . 1554. Tit. de nullitatibus ex defectu inhabilitatis Num. 25.
66. Farinacius (Prospero Farinacci, 1544-1618). *Praxis et Theorica Criminalis,* 1597-1610, pars 2, vol. 1, q. 98.
67. See note 63.
68. *Lex Discretis.* Cf. note 57.
69. *Lex Qui in Potestate,* Digesta, Liber. 28, tit. 1: (de Testamentis &) qui testamenta facere possunt, et quemadmodum testamenta fiant, lex 6.
70. As in note 69, para. I, surdus.
71. Decius. Cf. note 11. *In legem Discretis* (quoted in notes 69 and 57), Num. 1.
72. Nepos a Montalbano (Nepos de Montauban, 13th cent.). *Tractatus exceptionum qui dicitur, liber fugitivus,* 1512, artic. 20, Num. 10.
73. Baldus (Baldo degli Ubaldi, 1319 or 1327-1400). *In lege prima,* in 2 col. Codex, Liber 1, tit. 2: de Sacrosantis Ecclesiis et de rebus et privilegii earum, in repetitionibus (i.e., in his Repetiones).
74. Abbas (Panormitanus or Niccolo de Tedeschi, 1389-1466). In cap. cum apud. Num. 6, de sponsalibus(?).
75. Jason (Jason Mainus, 1435-1519). *In legem Mutum,* Digesta, Liber 29, tit. 2. De adquirenda vel omittenda haereditate, lex 5, Num. 4.
76. Brunellus (Jean Bruneau or Brunel, 14??-15??). *Tractatus de matrimoniis & sponsalibus,* 1521, conclus. 14, Num. 6.
77. Ibid. Num. 8.
78. Galenus. Liber 6, de locis affectis, cap. 5; VIII, 419-20, Kuehn.
79. Mascardus. As in note 49, conclusio 1358, Num. 24, vol. 3.
80. *Lex qui id quod. Digesta,* Liber 39, tit. 5. De donationius, lex 33.
81. As in note 80, para 2, mutus.
82. Maranta (Roberto Maranta, 14??-1530). *Singularia et iuris notabilia* (1616), on the word Mutus.
83. Valescus (Valesco de Taranta, 13??-14??). *Philonium* (begun 1418), lib. 2, cap. 50. De nocumentis aurium: et primo de surditate. Clarificatio. Fol. 69ro, ed. of "1401" (1501); fol. 44ro ed. of 1521; fol. 87ro ed. of 1535; 1st printed., 1478.

THE EFFECTS OF ANESTHESIA AND CARDIAC BYPASS ON PULMONARY COMPLIANCE IN MAN*

BERNARD R. HAND†

National Institutes of Health Postdoctoral
Research Fellow

JAMES R. MALM

Professor of Surgery

FREDERICK O. BOWMAN, JR.

Associate Professor of Surgery

STUART F. SULLIVAN

Associate Professor of Anesthesiology

Presbyterian Hospital in the City of New York
New York, N. Y.

PULMONARY compliance has been shown to be decreased for a period of several weeks following anesthesia and open-heart operations.[1, 2] This postoperative decrease in compliance is a further change from the low preoperative values seen in patients with heart disease and pulmonary hypertension.[3,4] The prolonged postoperative decrease in pulmonary compliance has not been correlated with changes in lung volumes or in pulmonary gas exchange. The purpose of this study is to relate changes in compliance to other pulmonary functions in the postcardiotomy patient an an attempt to simplify the study of pulmonary function in patients who undergo operations on the heart.

METHODS

Patients with mitral stenosis were studied before and after cardiac bypass. The subjects were studied in the supine position on four occasions: preoperatively, 1 to 2 days prior to operation; in the recovery room immediately after operation while breathing continued spon-

*Presented at a meeting of the Section on Anesthesia and Resuscitation, May 7, 1969.
†Now at the U.S. Naval Hospital, National Naval Medical Center, Bethesda, Md.
This study was supported in part by Public Health Service Research Grants 2T 1-GM-00056, GM-09069, and GM-14419 from the National Institute of General Medical Sciences and 5K3-HE-11,900 from the National Heart Institute, Bethesda, Md.

GLOSSARY

C_L	lung compliance in ml/cm H_2O
W_T	total work of breathing in gram-cm/ml
Wel	elastic work of breathing in gram-cm/ml
Wres	resistive work of breathing in gram-cm/ml
VC	vital capacity
FRC	functional residual capacity
RV	residual volume
TLC	total lung capacity
$FE_{V_{1.0}}$	forced expiratory volume in one second
FVC	forced vital capacity
V_D/V_T	dead space-tidal volume ratio
P_{aO_2}	arterial oxygen tension in mm Hg
(A-a) D_{O_2}	alveolar-arterial oxygen tension difference in mm Hg
$\dot{Q}_{V_A}/\dot{Q}_T$	venous admixture in per cent (breathing air)
$\dot{Q}_S/\dot{Q}_T$	right to left shunt on 100% O_2
%	per cent of predicted value
Shunt component	shunt portion of the (A-a)D_{O_2} (breathing air)
Nonshunt component	nonshunt portion of the (A-a) D_{O_2} (breathing air)

taneously; and approximately 1 week (6 to 10 days) and 3 weeks (14 to 21 days) after operation. Anesthesia was maintained with halothane and oxygen before, during, and after the bypass procedure. Pulmonary compliance was measured by means of a water-filled esophageal catheter placed in the lower esophagus and a Statham PR-23-2D-300 manometer, calibrated with a water manometer.[5, 6, 7] A Fleisch pneumotachograph, dead space 15 ml. linear over the flow rates used, heated with an external voltage source to prevent condensation of water was used with a Starham PM 5-0.2-300 manometer measuring the differential pressure across the penumotachograph. Volume (V) was determined by electronic integration of the flow signal. Calibration was made with a 1-liter super syringe. A photographic X-Y recorder was used for the pressure-volume loop. Dynamic pulmonary compliance, the ratio of tidal volume to change in pressure between the points of zero flow at the extremes of the tidal volume, is expressed in ml.BPTS/cm.H_2O. Per cent predicted pulmonary compliance was derived for each patient based on the relation to compliance as developed by Frank and his co-workers.[8] The areas in the pressure-volume record representing elastic work (W_{el}) and flow-resistive work (W_{res}) were measured with a self-compensating polar planimeter, and are expressed in gram-cm./ ml.BTPS. All measurements of the mechanics of breathing were made with subjects supine and breathing spontaneously. Lung volumes are reported at BTPS. Vital capacity (VC) and forced expiratory volume in one second ($FEV_{1.0}$) were measured with a Collins 13.5-l spirometer. Functional residual capacity (FRC) was measured with an open circuit technique while the patient breathed oxygen for seven minutes.[9] Nitrogen was measured with a nitrogen analyzer (Model 305AR, Med-Science). The per cent of predicted values for lung volumes are based on the relation: $\frac{\text{measured value}}{\text{predicted value}} \times 100 = \%$ predicted value. The predicted values are based on a compilation of currently available norms.[10] Arterial blood samples were collected through an indwelling teflon catheter and were iced immediately. Arterial oxygen (P_aO_2) and carbon dioxide (P_aCO_2) tensions and *p*H were measured with modified Clark O_2 electrode,[11] a modified Severinghaus CO_2 electrode,[12] and a modified capillary glass electrode respectively in a water bath at 37°C. The O_2 electrode was calibrated with blood of known PO_2 obtained by tonometry at 37°C. using 5 ml. of the original arterial sample.[13]

Alveolar oxygen tension (P_AO_2) is derived from the following reactions:

(breathing air) $$P_AO_2 = P_IO_2 + \frac{P_ACO_2 \times F_IO_2 \times (1\text{-}R)}{R} - \frac{P_ACO_2}{R}$$

(breathing 100% oxygen) $$P_AO_2 = P_IO_2 - P_ACO_2 - P_AN_2$$

where P_ACO_2 was assumed equal to P_aCO_2. Alveolar nitrogen tension (P_AN_2) was measured with the nitrogen analyzer. Respiratory quotient (R) was determined from measurements of the O_2 consumption ($\dot{V}O_2$) and CO_2 production ($\dot{V}CO_2$).

TABLE I. CHARACTERISTICS OF PATIENTS

Subject No.	Age	Sex	BSA M^2	PA mm. Hg.	Cardiac catheterization Mean PA mm. Hg.	Wedge mm. Hg.	C.I. l/min./m.²	Diagnosis
1	54	M	1.9	50/19	43	18	2.1	MS & MI
2	17	M	1.7	88/38	53	40	1.5	MS & MI
3	49	M	1.9	102/46	72	33	1.9	MS
4	53	F	1.48	70/15	—	13	—	MS
5	36	F	1.56	41/17	29	16	—	MS & AS & AI
6	57	M	1.98	52/30	36	24	—	MS
7	70	M	1.86	73/21	44	31	1.8	MS & MI
8	64	F	1.31	—	—	—	—	MS
9	51	M	1.76	—	—	—	—	MS
10	50	F	1.64	—	—	—	—	MS & MI
11	58	F	1.48	—	—	—	—	MS
12	50	F	1.48	—	—	—	—	MS

M=mitral; A=aortic; S=stenosis; I=insufficiency.

The shunt and nonshunt components of the (A-a) D_{O_2} breathing air were calculated using the value of Q_S/Q_T obtained during oxygen breathing.[14]

$$\text{Venous admixture } (Q_{VA}/Q_T) = \frac{C_c'O_2 - C_aO_2}{C_c'O_2 - C_{\bar{v}}O_2}$$

where $C_c'O_2$ C_aO_2 and $C_{\bar{v}}O_2$ are oxygen contents in end capillary, arterial, and mixed venous blood samples, respectively. $C_c'O_2$ was estimated from $P_c'O_2$ which is assumed to equal alveolar arterial tension (P_{AO_2}). Also assumed was an arteriovenous oxygen content difference of 5 volumes per cent.[15] Q_S/Q_T, the fraction of cardiac output that passed through right to left shunts during 100% oxygen breathing, is based on the same relation as the venous admixture equation.

Results

Characteristics of the 12 patients studied are listed in Table I. All were patients with mitral stenosis. In the 7 patients who underwent cardiac catheterization the pressures in the pulmonary artery varied from 102/46 to 41/17. The preoperative lung function studies included determinations of pulmonary mechanics, lung volumes, and arterial blood gases.

In Table II are the values of mechanics of breathing studied preoperatively. Pulmonary compliance is reduced to 52% of the predicted value preoperatively.

TABLE II. PREOPERATIVE PULMONARY MECHANICS*

	Mean	*± SE*
C_L (ml.BTPS/cm. H_2O)	76.3	9.2
C_L (per cent)	51.6	6.4
W_T (gram-cm./ml.)	6.3	0.8
Wel (gram-cm./ml.)	3.4	0.3
Wres (gram-cm./ml.)	2.9	0.6

*Eleven patients.

TABLE III. PREOPERATIVE PULMONARY VOLUME*

	Measured values		*Per cent predicted values*	
	Mean	*± SE*	*Mean*	*± SE*
VC (L_{BTPS})	2.5	0.2	72.8	6.3
FRC (L_{BTPS})	2.4	0.2	78.7	7.4
TLC (L_{BTPS})	4.4	0.3	79.8	4.8
RV/TLC (%)	44.8	3.8	129.8	8.9
$FEV_{1.0}$ (L_{BTPS})	1.7	0.2	61.5	5.3
$FEV_{1.0}$/FVC (%)	75.6	2.9	97	3.7
RV (L_{BTPS})	1.9	0.2	105.4	10.2

*Twelve patients.

TABLE IV. PREOPERATIVE ARTERIAL BLOOD GASES*

	Breathing air	
	Mean	*± SE*
Pa_{O_2} (mm. Hg)	77.8	4.6
(A-a) D_{O_2} (mm. Hg)		
Total	32.6	3.2
Shunt	12.6	2.7
Nonshunt	20.0	4.3
$Q_{VA}/Q_T \times 100$ (%)	10.3	1.7
$V_D/V_T \times 100$ (%)	42.2	2.4
	Breathing 100% O_2	
	Mean	*± SE*
Pa_{O_2} (mm. Hg)	589.9	15.6
(A-a) D_{O_2} (mm. Hg)	81.8	14.3
$Q_S/Q_T \times 100$ (%)	4.7	0.8

*Eleven patients.

TABLE V. POSTOPERATIVE STUDIES OF PULMONARY FUNCTION

	Preoperative			Postoperative								
				Intermediate			6 to 10 Days			14 to 21 Days		
	Mean	± SE	n	Mean	± SE	n	Mean	± SE	n	Mean	± SE	n
CL (ml.BTPS/cm. H_2O)	76.3	9.2	11	***40.1	7.8	6	64.8	11.2	5	76.3	13.7	6
CL % (per cent)	51.6	6.4	11	***26	3.6	6	44.4	5.4	5	49.9	6.6	6
WT (gram-cm./ml.)	6.3	0.8	11	*8.5	0.5	5	8	0.7	5	6	0.9	5
Wel (gram-cm./ml.)	3.4	0.3	11	3.8	0.7	5	4	0.5	5	3.9	0.5	5
Wres (gram-cm./ml.)	2.9	0.6	11	4.7	1.0	5	4	0.7	5	2.1	0.7	5
Pa_{O_2} (AIR) (mm. Hg)	77.8	4.6	11	*55.9	3.3	6	N. D.		–	70.8	4.8	6
Pa_{O_2} (100% O_2) (mm. Hg)	589.9	15.6	11	**389	65.9	6	N. D.		–	572.6	19.2	6
VC (LBTPS)	2.5	0.2	12	N. D.		–	N. D.		–	***1.8	0.4	5
VC% (per cent)	72.8	6.8	12	N. D.		–	N. D.		–	***54	4.9	5

N.D.—not done.
Paired comparison.[16] Significant differences from preoperative values are noted as follows:
*$P < 0.05$.
**$P < 0.02$.
***$P < 0.01$.

Preoperative lung volumes listed in Table III show the following to be reduced: vital capacity (VC), functional residual capacity (FRC), total lung capacity (TLC), and forced expiratory volume in one second ($FEV_{1.0}$). The ratio of residual volume/total lung capacity (RV/TLC) is increased while the residual volume (RV) and $FEV_{1.0}$/FVC ratio are within normal limits.

Listed in Table IV are the preoperative values for arterial blood gases. The values of P_aO_2 while the patient breathed air or 100% O_2 are reduced; while (A-a) D_{O_2}, venous admixture (Q_{VA}/Q_T), Q_S/Q_T, dead space/tidal volume ratio (V_D/V_T) are increased from expected values.

In Table V and Figure 1 are the mean values (±SE) of pulmonary compliance, per cent predicted pulmonary compliance, total work of breathing, and elastic and resistive components of the work of breathing P_aO_2 while the patient breathed air and 100% O_2, vital capacity, and per cent predicted vital capacity at each of the four periods of measurement. In the immediate postoperative period the functions to show a significant difference ($P<0.05$) from the preoperative values were pulmonary compliance ($P<0.01$), total work ($P<0.05$) and P_aO_2 breathing air ($P<0.05$) and 100% O_2 ($P<0.02$). Total work of breathing was still significantly elevated ($P<0.05$) at 6 to 10 days postoperatively. The only measurement that still showed a significant change at 14 to 21

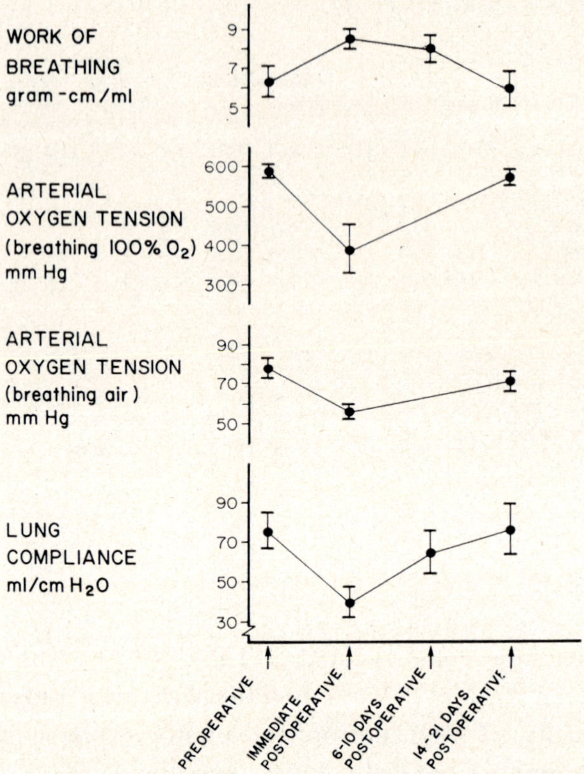

Fig. 1. Work of breathing, arterial oxygen tension breathing air and oxygen, and pulmonary compliance before and after cardiac bypass.

days into the postoperative period was vital capacity and per cent predicted vital capacity ($P<0.01$).

Data from all four study periods were used for correlation analysis. In Figure 2 are plotted the values of lung compliance versus per cent of predicted vital capacity, where the correlation coefficient (r) = 0.622 ($P<0.02$). In Figure 3 is the plot of P_aO_2 breathing air versus pulmonary compliance where $r = 0.558$ ($P<0.02$). P_aO_2 on 100% O_2 had a correlation coefficient of 0.453 ($P<0.05$) when plotted versus pulmonary compliance. Per cent predicted vital capacity had the same degree of correlation with P_aO_2 breathing air ($r = 0.785$; $P<0.001$) and 100% O_2 ($r = 0.748$; $P<0.005$) as pulmonary compliance. Figure 4 represents the correlation of the residual volume/total lung capacity ratio to pulmonary compliance where $r= -0.603$ ($P<0.02$); a similar degree of association was present when RV/TLC was plotted against per cent predicted vital capacity.

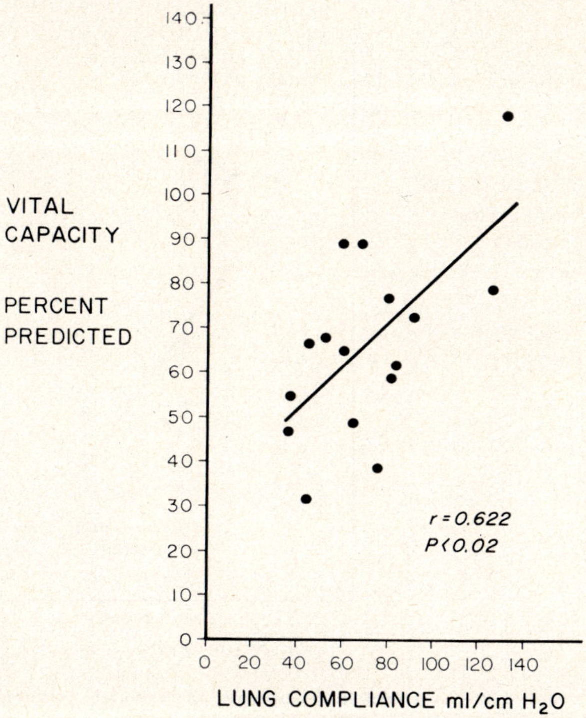

Fig. 2. Plot of vital capacity, per cent of predicted value, versus pulmonary compliance.

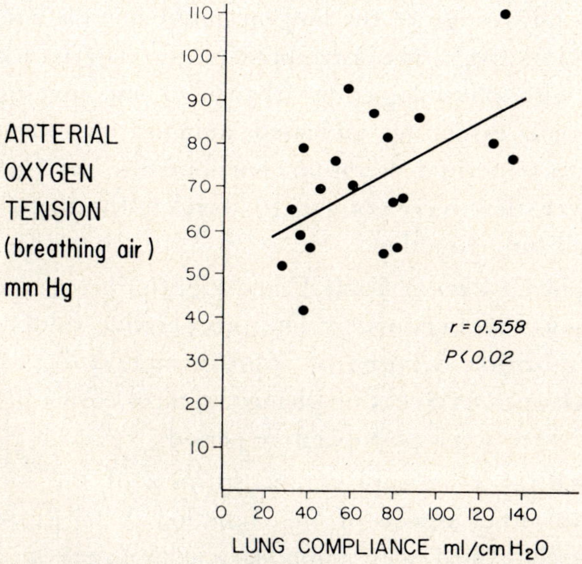

Fig. 3. Plot of arterial oxygen tension while patient is breathing air versus lung compliance.

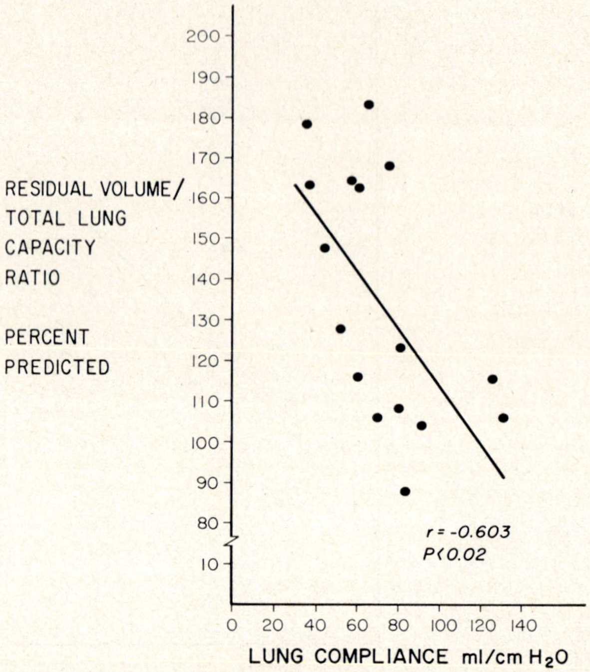

Fig. 4. Plot of residual volume/total lung capacity ratio versus pulmonary compliance.

Discussion

The pathophysiology of the lung in mitral stenosis has been studied by Parker and Weiss,[17] who attempted to correlate structural changes in the lung with physiologic disturbance. These investigators found thickened alveoli exhibiting increased amounts of collagen and considered that this structural alteration contributed to the "stiffness" of the lungs. However, they were not able to correlate the anatomical changes with disturbed lung function.

The compliance data in Table V and Figure 1 are in agreement with data of previous investigators.[1, 2] The preoperative values are less than normal and a further decrease of approximately 50% was noted immediately postoperatively. Compliance returns toward preoperative values over a three-week postoperative period.

Compliance, as a measure of the stiffness of the lung, has been correlated with other aspects of lung function. Vital capacity has been found to correlate well with pulmonary compliance in a number of studies in which different techniques were used.[4, 5, 18-20] This correlation was observed in the present study ($r = 0.585$, $P<0.02$). When per cent predicted vital capacity was correlated with pulmonary compliance (Figure 2) this association was also of a high degree ($r = 0.622$, $P<0.02$).

In some instances the location of the esophageal catheter has been found to influence the measured value of pulmonary compliance. Mead and Whittenberger[21] demonstrated a marked variation with differing lengths of esophageal catheters whereas other workers[4, 5] have concluded that the location of the catheter was not critical. The present studies were performed with the catheter tip located in the lower third of the esophagus.

In some studies functional residual capacity has been found to have a high degree of correlation with compliance,[7, 18, 22] whereas in others no correlation was found.[4, 20] In the present study we found a poor and statistically insignificant correlation between functional residual capacity and pulmonary compliance.

Frank et al.[4] and Cherniack and Brown[20] found a significant correlation between TLC and pulmonary compliance. We did not demonstrate this, but found RV/TLC per cent of predicted to have a high degree of association with compliance ($r = -0.603$, $P<0.02$). See Figure 4.

The values of work of breathing plotted in Figure 1 are in agreement with previous studies, which demonstrated the marked increase in the work of breathing immediately after operation on the heart and a return toward preoperative control values over several postoperative weeks.[1, 23, 24]

There seem to have been no previous attempts to correlate arterial oxygen tension with compliance. As shown in Figure 3, the value of P_{aO_2} while the patient breathed air has a high degree of association with pulmonary compliance. This magnitude of association is also present for the (A-a) D_{O_2} and venous admixture when breathing air, and for the P_{aO_2}, (A-a) D_{O_2}, and Q_S/Q_T when he is breathing 100% O_2.

Vital capacity measured at the 14- to 21-day postoperative period was the single measurement which remained significantly different from the preoperative value. Compliance is one of numerous factors that influence the measurement of vital capacity.[25] Measurements of lung volumes in the preoperative period (Table III) show a pattern consistent with restrictive pulmonary disease but not of obstructive pulmonary disease. Values for arterial blood gases at 14 to 21 days are not significantly different from the preoperative values; therefore it is likely that there has been no loss in lung tissue available for gas exchange. It is most improbable that neuromuscular or respiratory center depression persists this late in the postoperative period. The most reasonable explanation for the failure of vital capacity to return to preoperative values as other functions studied had done at 14 to 21 days is limitation of thoracic expansion secondary to the surgical incision. As a single test, vital capacity appears to yield reliable information about over-all pulmonary function in patients undergoing operation for the relief of mitral stenosis.

Summary

Measurement of pulmonary function before and after cardiac bypass in 12 patients with mitral stenosis was undertaken in an attempt to simplify the study of pulmonary function in these patients. Correlations between pulmonary compliance and vital capacity, arterial oxygen tension, and residual volume/total lung capacity ratio are of such a degree that measurement of vital capacity has a 95% or better probability of reflecting the disturbed lung function present in these patients. As a single measurement, vital capacity provides reliable information regarding over-all lung function in the surgical patient who is suffering from acquired valvular heart disease.

REFERENCES

1. Garzon, A. A., Seltzer, B. and Karlson, K. E. Respiratory mechanics following open-heart surgery for acquired valvular disease. *Circulation* (Suppl. 1) *33:* 57, 1966.
2. Ellison, L. T., Duke, J. F. and Ellison, R. G. Pulmonary compliance following open heart surgery and its relationship to ventilation and gas exchange. *Circulation* (Suppl. 1) *35:*217, 1967.
3. Marshall, R., McIlroy, M. B. and Christie, R. V. The work of breathing in mitral stenosis. *Clin. Sci. 13:*137, 1954.
4. Frank, N. R., Lyons, H. A., Siebens, A. A. and Nealson, T. F. Pulmonary compliance in patients with cardiac disease. *Amer. J. Med. 22:*516, 1957.
5. Banchero, N., Schwartz, P. and Wood, E. Intraesophageal pressure gradient in man. *J. Appl. Physiol. 22:*1066, 1967.
6. Fry, D., Stead, W., Ebert, R., Lubin, R. and Wells, H. The measurement of intraesophageal pressure and its relationship to intrathoracic pressure. *J. Lab. Clin. Med. 40:*664, 1952.
7. Lim, T. P. K. and Luft, U. C. Alterations in lung compliance and functional residual capacity with posture. *J. Appl. Physiol. 14:*164, 1959.
8. Frank, N. R., Mead, J., Siebens, A. A. and Storey, C. F. Measurements of pulmonary compliance in seventy healthy young adults. *J. Appl. Physiol. 9:*38, 1956.
9. Darling, R. C., Cournand, A. and Richards, D. W., Jr. Studies on the intra-

pulmonary mixture of gases: III. An open circuit for measuring residual air. *J. Clin. Invest. 19*:609, 1940.
10. Sullivan, S. F., Patterson, R. W. and Papper, E. M. Evaluation of pulmonary function data using computer time-sharing. *Proc. I.E.E.E.* 1969. In press.
11. Clark, L. C.: Monitor and control of blood and tissue oxygen tensions. *Trans. Amer. Soc. Artif. Intern. Organs 2*:41, 1956.
12. Severinghaus, J. W. and Bradley, A. F. Electrodes for blood Po_2 and Pco_2 determination. *J. Appl. Physiol. 13*:515, 1958.
13. Finley, T. N., Lenfant, C., Haab, P., Piiper, J. and Rahn, H. Venous admixture in the pulmonary circulation of anesthetized dogs. *J. Appl. Physiol. 15*: 418, 1960.
14. Ayres, S. M., Criscitiello, A. and Grabovsky, E. Components of alveolar-arterial O_2 difference in normal man. *J. Appl. Physiol. 19*:43, 1964.
15. Carroll, D., Cohn, J. E. and Riley, R. L. Pulmonary function in mitral valvular disease: Distribution and diffusion characteristics in resting patients. *J. Clin. Invest. 32*:510, 1953.
16. Hill, A. B. *Principles of medical statistics.* New York, Oxford Univ. Press, 1961.
17. Parker, F., Jr. and Weiss, S. The nature and significance of the structural changes in the lungs in mitral stenosis. *Amer. J. Pathol. 12*:573, 1936.
18. Cook, C. D., Helliesen, P. J. and Agathon, S. Relation between mechanics of respiration, lung size and body size from birth to young adulthood. *J. Appl. Physiol. 13*:349, 1958.
19. Frank, N. R., Mead, J. and Ferris, B. G., Jr. The mechanical behavior of the lungs in healthy elderly persons. *J. Clin. Invest. 36*:1680, 1957.
20. Cherniack, R. M. and Brown, E. A simple method for measuring total respiratory compliance: Normal values for males. *J. Appl. Physiol. 20*:87, 1965.
21. Mead, J. and Whittenberger, J. Physical properties of human lungs measured during spontaneous respiration. *J. Appl. Physiol. 5*:779, 1953.
22. Marshall, R. The physical properties of the lungs in relation to the subdivisions of lung volume. *Clin. Sci. 16*:507, 1957.
23. Larmi, T. K. I. and Karvonen, M. J. Work of breathing after cardiovascular surgery in cases of mitral stenosis and of a patent ductus arteriosis. *Ann. Med. Int. Fenn 51*:99, 1962.
24. Garzon, A. A., Seltzer, B., Lightenstein, S. and Karlson, K. E. Influence of open-heart surgery on respiratory work. *Dis. Chest 52*: 392, 1967.
25. Comroe, J. H., Jr., Forster, R. E., Dubois, A. B., Briscoe, W. A. and Carlsen, E. *The Lung.* Chicago Year Book Med. Pub., 1965, p. 12.

CHRISTIANUS HELWICH ON DIFFICULTY OF RESPIRATION (AUGSBURG, 1722)*

SAUL JARCHO

DURING recent investigations of our concepts of heart failure—investigations which originated ultimately at the bedside—it became necessary to study a number of clinical writings that reflect conceptions discarded, superseded, or radically modified long ago. A few of these writings have been translated and edited for publication.[1-5]

To this series I have elected to add a contribution by Christianus Helwich, since it is not only the work of an eminent physician but it was quoted widely during the 18th century and it describes in relatively small compass the opinions that were then held concerning the nature, diagnosis, and treatment of hydrothorax.

Christianus Helwich (1666-1740) was councillor and personal physician to several of the dukes of Silesia and *Stadtarzt* at Breslau.[6] He was an eminent member of the Imperial Leopoldo-Caroline Academy and the probable author of its official essay on pectoral dropsy,[5] which appeared in 1706.

The article which is here reproduced *in toto* in English translation is titled *Observata quaedam ex anatome matronae difficiliori respiratione per totum vitae spatium laborantis* (Observations made at the autopsy of a woman who had suffered from lifelong difficulty of respiration). It was published in *Academiae Caesareae Leopoldino-Carolinae Naturae Curiosorum Ephemerides*, centuria 10, observatio 32, pp. 307-10. Augustae Vindelicorum [Augsburg], Kühtz, 1722.

* * * *

*Based on research assisted by the National Institutes of Health (HE-10948).

1. Jarcho, S.: *Morgagni, Vicarius, and the Difficulty of Clinical Diagnosis.* In Stevenson, L. G. and Multhauf, R. B., editors: *Medicine, Science, and Culture; Historical Essays in Honor of Owsei Temkin.* Baltimore, Johns Hopkins Press, 1968, pp. 87-95.
2. Büchner, A. E.: De Hydrope Pectoris Ejusque Signis. *Acta Physico-Medica Academiae Caesareae Leopoldino-Carolinae Naturae Curiosorum Exhibentia Ephemerides,* vol. 6, observatio 50, pp. 191-98. Nuremberg, Endter, 1742.
3. Jarcho, S.: An Eighteenth-Century Treatise on Dropsy of the Chest (Büchner, 1742). *Bull. N.Y. Acad. Med.* 45:799-806, 1969; errata 45:993, 1969.
4. Jarcho, S.: *Roderigo de Fonseca and His Consultation on Dropsy of the Lung.* In press.
5. Academia Leopoldina Naturae Curiosorum Vratislaviae. *Observationes Practicae de Hydrope Pectoris.* Vratislaviae, Bauchius, 1706. English translation by S. Jarcho in preparation.
6. Grätzer, J.: *Lebensbilder Hervorragender Schlesischer Aertze.* Breslau, Schottlaender, 1889, p. 209.

During her entire lifetime a certain fat and hunchbacked woman had rather severe difficulty in breathing during bodily movement. As long as she lived she spent most of the day sitting. Toward the close of her mortal lifetime the distress in her chest was greatly increased. Moreover, having called me three days before her death, she indicated, in words frequently interrupted,[7] that the symptoms which she now suffered seemed to her to be of a different kind from those with which she had been afflicted since early life and which were caused by bad conformation of her chest and by conspicuous obesity, the concomitant of highly luxurious food and sedentary life. She said that her present difficulty of respiration not only was greater and was accompanied by more insistent rapidity, urgency, and heaviness than that which she had suffered since infancy, but that most of all the symptoms disturbed her at the time of the first sleep, when the most urgent danger of suffocation threatened and excited her. These attacks of strangulation she so greatly dreaded that she had spent many sleepless nights. Unless she was relieved she preferred to be consumed by perpetual vigils rather than to compose herself for sleep.

I carefully considered these and all other details, and I turned to my colleagues, one of whom had taken care of the patient for many years; the other had had the responsibility for two weeks. I discreetly hinted to them that I did not doubt she had an extravasation of serum in the thoracic cavity as well as irreparable disease of the internal organs. Morever, it was impossible to dispute the truth of the pathognomonic sign which was established by Carolus Piso in *Selected Observations on Diseases thus far Overlooked Originating from Serous Effusion*, Book 3, chapter 7[8] and which is repeated by me in *Practical Observations on Hydrops of the Chest*,[5] published in the name of the Academy of Sciences of Breslau. Thus far my guiding star in the recognition of pectoral dropsy had been the difficulty and frequency in breathing which afflicts the patient suddenly in the first period of sleep. And so when my patient, as she herself related, fell into that difficulty of breathing in the first hours of her sleep, I concluded that there remained no doubt of the presence of serous material in the cavity of the chest.

Never shall I forget Morstinia, a lady famous for her ancestry and

7. Presumably by dyspnea.
8. Piso, Carolus: *Selectiorum Observationum et consiliorum de Praetervisis hactenus morbis affectibusque praeter naturam ab acqua, seu serosa colluvie et diluvie ortis.* Pont-à-Mousson, 1617, also 1618; also Leyden, 1650, 1714, and 1733.

character, from the neighboring kingdom of Poland, who had remained for many months at Breslau and quite often was imperilled by nocturnal suffocation at about the 12th hour at night. She feared these terrible attacks more than death itself and therefore she persistently requested the opinion of many physicians concerning this very serious symptom. Often, indeed, after a consultation on the causes and treatment of her sickness, she was more uncertain than she had been before the discussion had begun, since the opinions of the practitioners differed so widely. Some thought the cause was a polypus [clot] in one or other chamber of the heart. Some thought the asthma was of hypochondriac origin. Others decided that the suffocation was hysterical. I alone, relying on the certainty of the sign which has been mentioned previously, constantly asserted that the asthma came from an extravasation of serum in the chest. Edematous swelling of the feet subsequently appeared and, to be brief, an autopsy performed in Cracow abundantly confirmed my opinion.

Let my opinion stand firmly, summarized correctly as follows: in one or other patient the danger of suffocation, attacking suddenly, breaks up the first sleep; therefore extravasated serum or lymph is present in the thoracic cavity. On the other hand I would not be responsible for the following opinion: this or that patient, at the time already mentioned, does not develop difficult respiration, therefore he does not have watery matter in his chest. In addition to the example adduced on page 4 of my observations on dropsy of the chest, previously cited, Francesco Contarini, doge of Venice, had in the cavity of his chest about five pounds of serous matter. Yet his respiration was never greatly impaired. This was told by Joannes Pr[a]evotius on pages 9 and 10 of the *Observat*[*ionum*] *Medic*[*inalium*] *Episagm*[*ata Centum*] of the distinguished G. H. Velschius.[9]

But after these digressions let us return to our case. My colleagues did not oppose me and readily acknowledged that the disease was quite severe and underlay a catarrhal fever from which they believed the patient to be suffering and which they had declared to others. And so it was clear to all of us that all our thoughts should be directed to evacuating, as much as possible, the fluid which had accumulated in the lungs and chest and to repairing the damage to the organs, but we could

9. Velschius, G. H.: *Observationum Medicalium Episagmata Centum*, pp. 9-10. In Velschius, G.H.: *Sylloge Curationum*. Augustae Vindel., 1667. An English translation is in preparation.

in no way see by which defences of the art this could be attained in the presence of such debility of powers and fear of lipothymia. We chose a mixture of ammoniacal gum, hyssop, syrup of helenium, etc. We also prescribed an essence of diuretic and alexipharmacic roots with which the essence of amber was mixed. For two days the patient used these drugs to no benefit. Indeed, although she took them faithfully she grew worse and, adding convulsions to her heap of troubles, suddenly died.

After her death the cadaver was sectioned at the request of her distinguished husband. When the chest was opened a serous effusion immediately flowed out and abundantly confirmed what I had predicted concerning the presence of extravasated fluid in the thorax. Apart from this the cavity which is bounded above by the clavicles, anteriorly on either side by the ribs and sternum, and posteriorly by the bones of the back, was so narrow that we could not stop wondering how it was able to contain the heart with the pericardium, the lungs with part of the trachea, and the greater portion of the esophagus. This narrowness apparently was due mostly to disease of the vertebrae, for the dorsal vertebrae were twisted forward as if into a concave contour and presented the configuration of a single solid bone, which filled out the cavity of this hollow, so conspicuous by its protuberance and breadth. On both sides the lobes of the lungs adhered to the pleura and were even united to the mediastinum and sternum. It is most probable that this union was the reason that the thoracic space was so narrow.

More than anything else in this hurried examination of the organs, the gall bladder and uterus held our attention a little longer, for they had assumed the hardness of stone. Since this lady had had her menses regularly, even during the mortal illness, it is clearer than the noonday sun that menstrual flow frequently comes from the vaginal vessels alone.

In the left kidney there was a rather large stone.

* * * *

COMMENT ON HELWICH'S ESSAY

Like some of the more prolix 19th century novelists, Helwich combines his main narrative with a number of subplots.

His principal case is that of an obese kyphoscoliotic woman who had had lifelong external dyspnea which very recently had undergone marked exacerbation. In the latest phase the conspicuous feature was dyspnea that attacked the patient after a few hours of sleep. On this symptom alone, and without anything resembling a physical examination, Helwich declared that the woman had hydrothorax. This reasoning was based on the work of Carolus Piso (1617).

Digressing from his kyphoscoliotic patient, whom we may label Case I, Helwich tells us of a Polish lady, one Moristinia, who also was imperiled by nocturnal suffocation. Practitioners had offered such diagnoses as polypus (i.e., coagulum) in the heart, hypochondria, and hysteria. Helwich "instantly asserted that the asthma came from an extravasation of serum in the chest." Later the feet became swollen. Still later an autopsy confirmed Helwich's diagnosis of extravasation.

At this point Helwich states his opinion almost as a Euclidean proposition: if dyspnea occurs after the first hours of sleep, hydrothorax is present. The converse is not true, i.e., if nocturnal dyspnea is absent it cannot be asserted that hydrothorax is absent; this is shown by the case of the Doge Contarini, reported by Praevotius.

After these digressions Helwich returns to Case I. He and his colleagues wished to rid the patient of her thoracic accumulation but feared to cause lipothymia (syncope). They prescribed diuretics, to no avail. A huge hydrothorax was found. The vertebral column is described. Mention is made of pleural adhesions, and a few details are given about the abdominal and pelvic viscera. *Nothing is said about the heart*, since at this time hydrothorax was not attributed to cardiac failure.

In the diagnosis of hydrothorax Helwich was using an empirical method which, so far as is known nowadays, was introduced by Piso and was applied with fair success by Fonseca, Büchner, the Breslau academicians, and European physicians generally. The method rested on ancient humoralism, virtually uninfluenced by more recent physiological and anatomical advances. Our modern concept of heart failure did not as yet exist.

ON CLINICAL MEDICINE
With Notes from the Diary of a Part-Time Researcher*

Alfred Vogl†

Professor of Clinical Medicine
New York University School of Medicine
New York, N. Y.

I greatly appreciate the honor of having been selected to deliver the Pirquet Lecture this year. I am aware that I owe this privilege partly to the role I played in founding the Pirquet Society of Clinical Medicine and partly to my role in discovering mercurial diuresis half a century ago. Therefore, I want to take my cues for this address from these two roles and discuss two topics which are close to my heart: the future of clinical medicine and the contributions that a part-time clinical investigator can make to advances in medicine.

Clinical Medicine, Past and Future

Clinical medicine has been the leitmotiv of our society since its founding. Its name was chosen to express our intention to follow the tradition of clinical medicine which had flourished so brilliantly during the golden age of the Vienna Medical School.[1]

What do we mean when we speak of "clinical medicine"? By definition it is "bedside medicine" (derived from *kline*, the Greek word for bed). It is a concept of medicine that has as its source the observation of the patient, attention to his complaints, and examination by means of our senses, and it has as its purpose the diagnosis and the cure of his ills.

Clinical medicine has a venerable history. It was created 2,500 years ago by Hippocrates, the Father of Medicine; it flourished in ancient Greece and Rome but apparently lapsed into oblivion in the western world during the age of scholasticism. It was revived by revolutionary thinkers such as Boerhaave, Sydenham, Laënnec, and Skoda, who made it the dominant force in medicine in the 19th and early 20th centuries. But where does it stand today? Does it still have and should it rightly keep the exalted position that it used to command?

*Presented as the Clemens von Pirquet Lecture at a meeting of the Pirquet Society of Clinical Medicine held at The New York Academy of Medicine, May 14, 1969.
†Recipient of the Pirquet Gold Medal for 1969.

Clinical Medicine vs. Laboratory Medicine

Many concerned observers[2, 3] believe that medicine is at a crossroad because time-honored and valued concepts of medicine appear uprooted by the rapid advances of scientific techniques. These changes are regarded with anxiety by all those who see in them signs of an ever-increasing trend toward mechanization and the ultimate dehumanization of the practice of medicine.[4]

Is this threat real? Why could not cooperation of clinical and laboratory medicine work as fruitfully in medical practice as it has done in research? Why could the laboratory not continue to serve as a helpful partner instead of becoming the oracle of medical practice? Is there already a noticeable trend to substitute a battery of laboratory tests for sound and carefully weighed clinical judgment? I am afraid there is. And this trend is hastened by a number of factors which favor "laboratory medicine" over the clinical approach.

One of these factors is the need for saving time as the deluge of demands for medical care taxes the working schedule of every physician; another is the patients' waning respect for what they regard as "horse-and-buggy medicine"; a third factor is the undeniable scarcity of physicians who master the difficult art of clinical medicine.

The attempt by some physicians to save time by using laboratory tests as a shortcut in place of thorough history taking and physical examination is spurious. These methods of examination are indispensable not only for their intrinsic value but also because they establish the personal relation between the sick man and his doctor. This relation has no substitute, and it cannot be established in a hurry. An unhurried office visit in the best traditional style will serve to provide the desired rapport; usually it will also result in a working diagnosis. In this way the patient will be spared the days or weeks of waiting anxiously for the final word.

The restlessness of the patient who would rather have "a quick and foolproof cancer test" than submit to a lengthy interrogation can be overcome by making him feel that this is not a tedious routine but something pertinent to his particular problem. And the resentment against a time-consuming physical examination will vanish as soon as the patient becomes aware that due attention is paid to the apparent site or sites of his complaints. It is self-evident that in psychosomatic maladies, which represent the reason for 40 to 80% of all office visits, careful examination is often more than half the treatment.

The most serious threat to the future of clinical medicine stems from the established fact that the practice of medicine is an *art* as much as a *science*.[3, 5]

There is no doubt that the eagerness of patients as well as of doctors to economize with their time and to turn for help to advances in technology runs counter to good medical practice. But the great trouble with clinical medicine at all times has been the simple fact that it can flourish only in the hands of good clinicians.

Why cannot every good student of medicine who is intent upon being a clinician become one? The scientific qualifications can certainly be acquired successfully, given the necessary intelligence, training, and perseverance. Medicine as an *art*, however, can be mastered only by the student with the talents of the artist, the "born clinician." As such he must possess not only the old master's power of keen observation, his memory, and his patience, but also an artist's intuition and imagination to let him create in his mind a harmonious, persuasive, and meaningful picture out of odd fragments of raw material. Without these abilities there can never be a true clinician.

No wonder, then, that not every medical man strives for the laurels of the artist-clinician, and it seems to me that the ranks of clinicians are depleted not only by the attraction of many gifted men to the glories of pure science, but also by the reluctance of others to embark on the difficult road toward mastery of clinical medicine.

From these remarks you may sense my concern that clinical medicine, and with it the role of the clinician, may be in for hard times, and that their golden age may have passed; but this does not mean that clinical medicine is dead. Just the reverse: with the infusion of new blood from the medical sciences a new clinical medicine is developing which promises a brilliant future under the leadership of the new clinician if he combines the qualities of the legendary "old clinician" with those of the modern human biologist.[5]

Work of the Part-Time Researcher

If we leave this brief analysis of the trends and the future of clinical medicine in general, and turn to a discussion of the role of the clinician in research, especially that of the part-time worker, the question will arise at once whether the work that he can perform in his own realm, in the hospital wards, in the outpatient clinic, and in private practice can be meaningful and productive. In this day and age can significant advances in medicine possibly be expected from any source other than highly trained teams of investigators collaborating in well-organized projects and equipped with the most advanced technical facilities? With your permission I shall try to answer these questions on the basis of personal experience.

My esteemed predecessors as Pirquet Lecturers have all been Nobel Laureates or scientists of similar international renown. Each could unfold to you the proud history of successful work aided by outstanding teams of investigators.[6] I make no attempt to compete with the accomplishments of these eminent scientists, but I thought it might be worthwhile and fitting to relate to you on this occasion the more modest but always enthusiastic and sometimes successful work of a life-long part-time clinical researcher.

Many far-reaching, even revolutionary advances in the sciences have had very humble beginnings.[2, 7, 8] Everyone here is aware of the way in which Roentgen detected the penetrating power of cathode tube rays, or how Semmelweis discovered the contagious character of puerperal sepsis. Serendipity has played an important role in these and other major discoveries, but this fact has too often been deliberately suppressed.[9]

Serendipity

Serendipity, as you probably know, is a term which Horace Walpole coined after he had read the fairy tale of the travels of the three princes of Serendip,[10] who chanced unexpectedly upon novel things which they had not been in quest of but which became the starting point for amazing discoveries because of the inquisitiveness and sagacity of these young men. In short, serendipity is a way of making discoveries without planning them. It is obviously not a recognized method for scientific research and, as Rossman noted when writing on the advance of science and the role of serendipity in it, "scientists tend to cover up any part that serendipity may have played in their own work. They do it in order to create the image of logic and purposeful design in pursuing their scholarly goal, a pursuit in which there cannot be a place for accidents, errors or human foibles." Let us not forget, however, that pure accident is only the first step in serendipity. Much more than this is needed to attain its royal rewards: the intuition to recognize the potentials of the accidental observation, never-ending curiosity, and the patience and courage to embark on an adventure of which the duration is unknown and the end not in sight.

The background of discoveries made through serendipity can be related without embarrassment and without any retouching or retrospective alterations. It should be told factually not only for the sake of historical truth, but, most of all, to encourage members of the profession, young and old, to participate in research with the means at their disposal and to accept a challenge wherever they encounter it. My reports will let you glance behind the stage on which the dramas and the comedies of serendipity are enacted. They may reveal some of the fascination, the joys and the troubles, the rewards and the disappointments encountered during research on a small scale but over a wide range. The chapters which I have selected from my diary deal only with subjects whose investigation had not been planned in advance. No wonder then that all of them must truthfully begin with: "as it happened."

The Discovery of Mercurial Diuresis[11]

May I take you back 50 years to recount the curious events that led to the introduction of the mercurial diuretics: the discovery being commemorated this year.[8] We must remember that no effective diuretic agent existed at that time and that it was the common fate of patients in congestive heart failure, as the saying went, to "drown in their dropsy."

As it happened, an 18-year-old girl with congenital syphilis and protracted diarrhea, bed-ridden, emaciated, and dehydrated (not edematous) was admitted in October 1919 to the Wenckebach Clinic in Vienna where I worked as a third-year medical student and clinical clerk. I was told to order a mercury salicylate solution for the girl as antisyphilitic treatment and to administer one injection every other day. But I made a mistake in the way I wrote the prescription. The pharmacy, therefore, never delivered the solution. After waiting a week for it, I was only too glad to accept a professional sample of a currently advertised organic mercurial from a helpful physician visitor and to substitute it for the missing compound. The trade name of this drug was Novasurol. I duly recorded every injection on the bedside chart

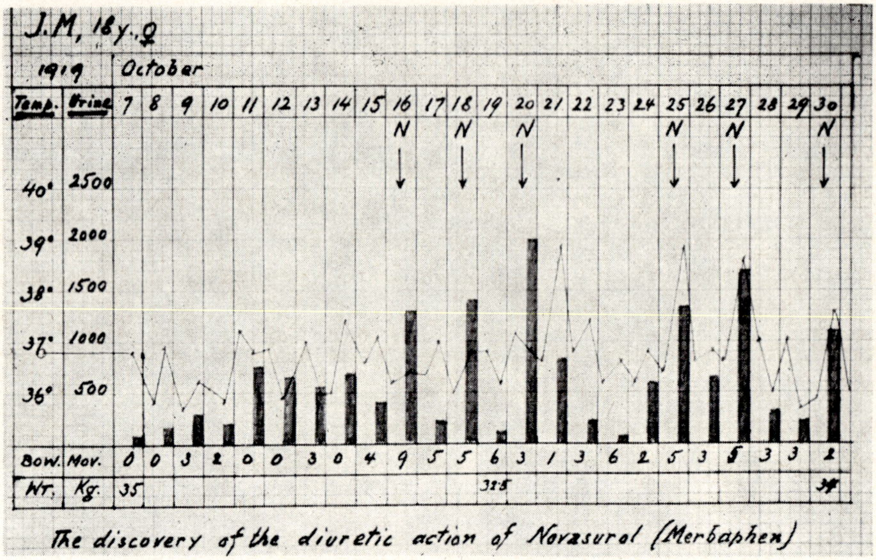

Fig. 1. Bedside chart of the 18-year-old girl on whom the diuretic action of an organic mercurial preparation (Novasurol) was discovered. *N* indicates the day of the Novasurol injections; the dark columns show the daily volume of urine.

on which the nurses also entered pulse, temperature and, in blue columns, the daily urine output (Figure 1). While marking each injection on the chart, I noticed that a tall blue column had appeared on the day of the first injection while previously these columns had been very low. The sudden rise in urinary volume was followed by just as precipitous a drop on the following day. These brief peaks repeated themselves on alternate days, the days of the Novasurol injections.

I reported these startling observations excitedly to my chief. To my disappointment I was informed that it was common knowledge that biological events ran in a wavelike rhythm, a law of nature which could well account for the ups and downs of our girl's urinary volume.

But I remained unconvinced and, being very young and not easily impressed by authority, I challenged this biologic law by simply omitting one ejection during a long weekend. During these days the output or urine remained very scanty again. But when, on Monday, the Novasurol injections were resumed, the flood of urine reappeared in a rhythmic cycle according to the days of injections.

This time I succeeded in getting the chief interested. Question after question was discussed. What had happened? Was it really the mercurial that had produced the urinary floods? How did it do it? Perhaps by a fleeting antisyphilitic action on kidneys or on body tissues? And, if so, would it do the same in other syphilitic patients?

There was one patient in the ward, a middle-aged cab driver with syphilitic heart disease, who was totally water-logged in what was, by the then current criteria, terminal congestive failure. On my chief's order he was to receive the next Novasurol injection. Within 24 hours he voided more than 10 liters and we were sure that we had just witnessed "the greatest man-made diuresis in history." The next day the patient felt "like a new man," and he continued to live and work with the help of repeated injections of Novasurol for more than 10 years. After this first massive diuresis we still assumed that the effect was somehow related to the antisyphilitic action of mercury. But this belief was seriously shaken when other mercurial compounds failed to produce any diuretic effect in our syphilitic patients. So, with much trepidation, Novasurol was tried on a young boy with rheumatic heart disease in advanced congestive failure. To our delight, he, too, had a prompt and massive diuresis.

Now there was no more doubt that we had a new, powerful diuretic in our hands and that we were on the threshold of a new era for the cardiac patient.

All these exciting adventures took place within less than four weeks. We had been blessed with good luck. No severe allergic reactions and no mercurial poisoning occurred until the discovery was reported to the Society of Physicians in Vienna. Soon after this meeting, however, two patients died of acute hemorrhagic colitis. If such catastrophes had happened among our first cases it would, no doubt, have been the end of our experiments with Novasurol.

By the time the diuretic effect of Novasurol was first noted, it had been in use for seven years, and its antisyphilitic effectiveness had been reported in several publications, including a five-year study involving 900 patients who had received a total of 5,000 injections of this drug. It is hard to understand how the diuretic "side effects" could have escaped notice. I kept wondering about this until an older colleague told me why he had given up Novasurol in his treatment of venereal disease. So many of his patients had complained to him of having to urinate all the time and of getting terribly thirsty after their injections, that he had

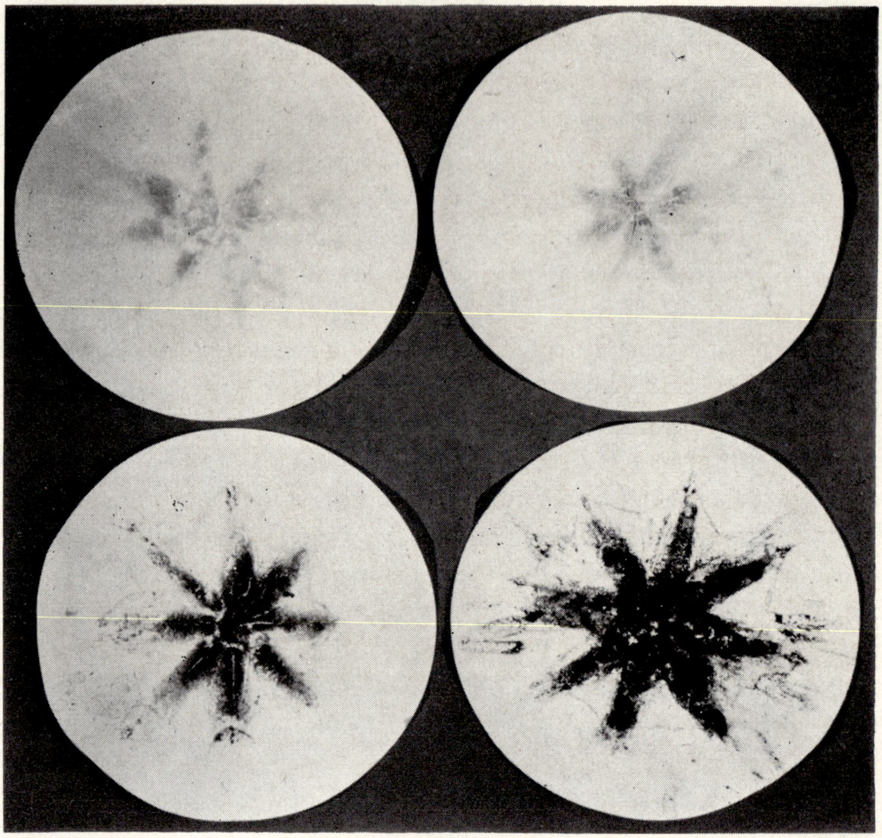

Fig. 2. Four paper filters with the dried plasma precipitated with trichloracetic acid showing the various shades (of green) indicating the bilirubin concentration in patients with different degrees of jaundice.

made up a standard reply to their gripes: "What's all the fuss about? Thank the Lord that you live in Vienna where there is a pub in every block and a comfort station at every street corner." Finally, however, he became tired of all these complaints and simply switched from Novasurol to a bismuth preparation. Thus the observation of the diuretic effect of Novasurol remained unreported for a few more years.

The mechanism of the diuretic action of Novasurol remained obscure for a long time. Many early attempts to elucidate it were all in vain. The time was not yet ripe for successful research in diuresis. Thus the use of mercurial diuretics had become standard therapy all over the

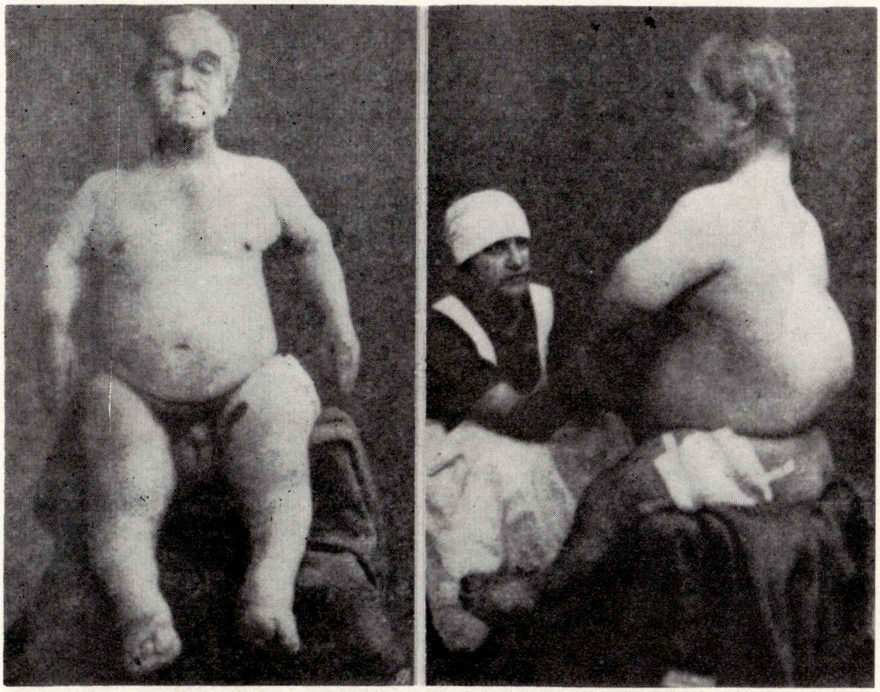

Fig. 3. Achondroplastic dwarf with a dorsolumbar gibbus and paraplegia. Reproduced by permission from: Donath, J. and Vogl, A. Untersuchungen über den chondrodystrophischen Zwergwuchs. *Wien. Arch. Inn. Med. 10*:1, 1925.

world long before advances in renal physiology could provide an understanding of the underlying principles.

The Trichloracetic Acid Test for Hyperbilirubinemia

Another minor but rather useful contribution also had its origin in an accidental observation. As it happened, a series of paper filters, covered with serum protein precipitated by trichloracetic acid, had been left on the work bench in the laboratory and had dried there. I noticed that some of these precipitates had turned various tints of green while most of them remained colorless (Figure 2). The green precipitates were found to have come from blood specimens of patients who had frank jaundice or other disorders of the liver. On the basis of these observations, Berthold Zins and I devised a simple semiquantitative test for bilirubinemia, documenting the course of jaundice by using the filters as a permanent record.[12]

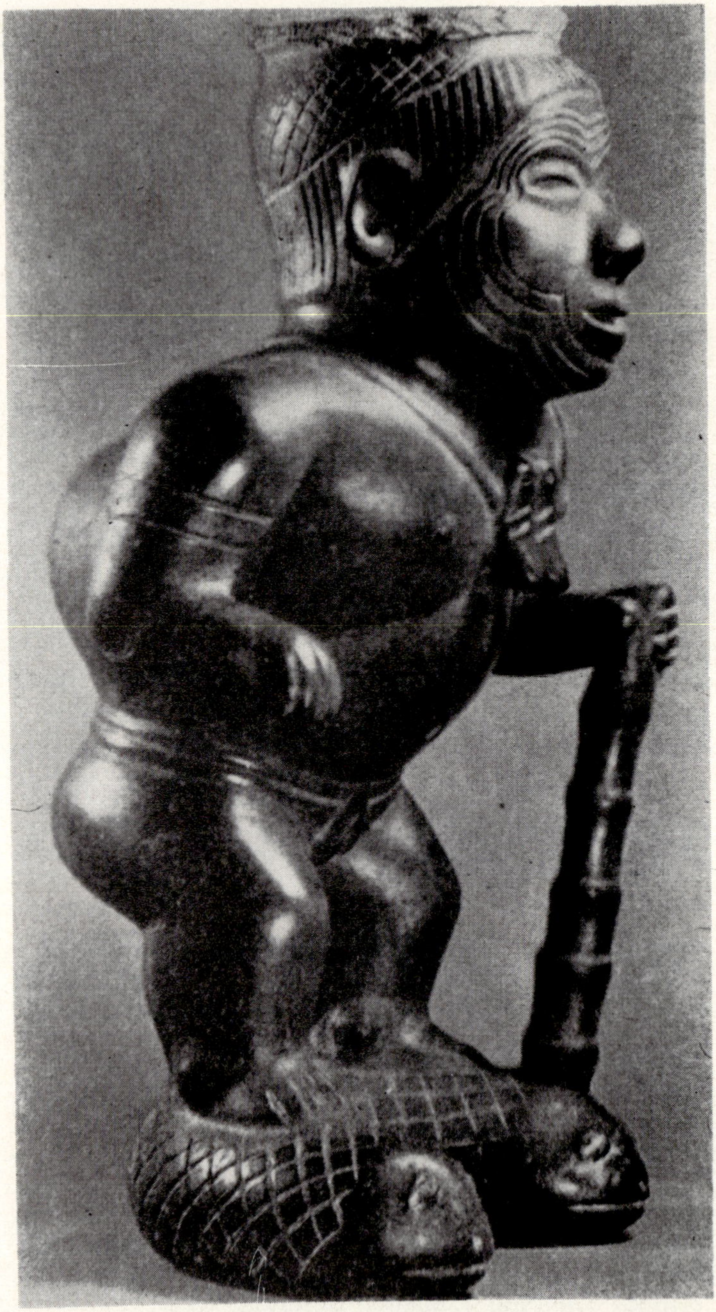

Fig. 4. Pre-Columbian figure of an achondroplastic dwarf with a dorsolumbar gibbus (the heavy cane suggests the possibility of paresis of the lower extremities).

A bit of new basic information also turned up while we were developing the new trichloracetic acid test. At low serum bilirubin levels the test was found positive in some patients but negative in others despite an identical icterus index. These findings suggested the subsequently proved existence of two different types of bilirubin in blood.

The trichloracetic acid test served its purpose well for about a decade when it was superseded by more convenient and exact quantitative methods.

Achondroplasia[13]

Gibbus formation. My next story exemplifies a different road along which the part-time researcher can proceed from a problem encountered in his clinical work.

As it happened, an achondroplastic dwarf was admitted to our ward in 1924. He had a prominent dorsolumbar gibbus and was paralyzed from the waist down (Figure 3). The hunchback had been present since early childhood and was, according to the family, caused by a fall from the crib. The paraplegia, however, was recent.

The unusual kind of gibbus fascinated me and I began to look for achondroplastic dwarfs in the streets, in circuses, among Egyptian and pre-Columbian sculptures (Figures 4 and 5), among Renaissance paintings, and among illustrations in the older medical literature (Figure 6). It became apparent that exactly the same type of gibbus had been depicted in achondroplastic dwarfs often enough to refute the then current notion that the vertebral column was virtually unaffected by the basic disorder of the skeleton, and that a gibbus, when present, was incidental, caused by trauma or Pott's disease. Examination of achondroplastic skeletons in the Rokitansky anatomical museum showed that the spine was not spared and that of four achondroplastic skeletons one had a dorsolumbar gibbus (Figure 7). In achondroplastic babies, however, we could find no angular gibbus but only varying degrees of lumbar kyphosis (Figure 6). We therefore concluded that as soon as the child began to sit the weight of the trunk would increase the kyphosis and tend to convert the curved kyphosis into an angular gibbus (Figure 8). Based on this concept preventive orthopedic measures were devised which have in fact been able to protect achondroplastic children from developing this extreme deformity.

Paraplegia. The investigation of the paraplegia in our patient bore

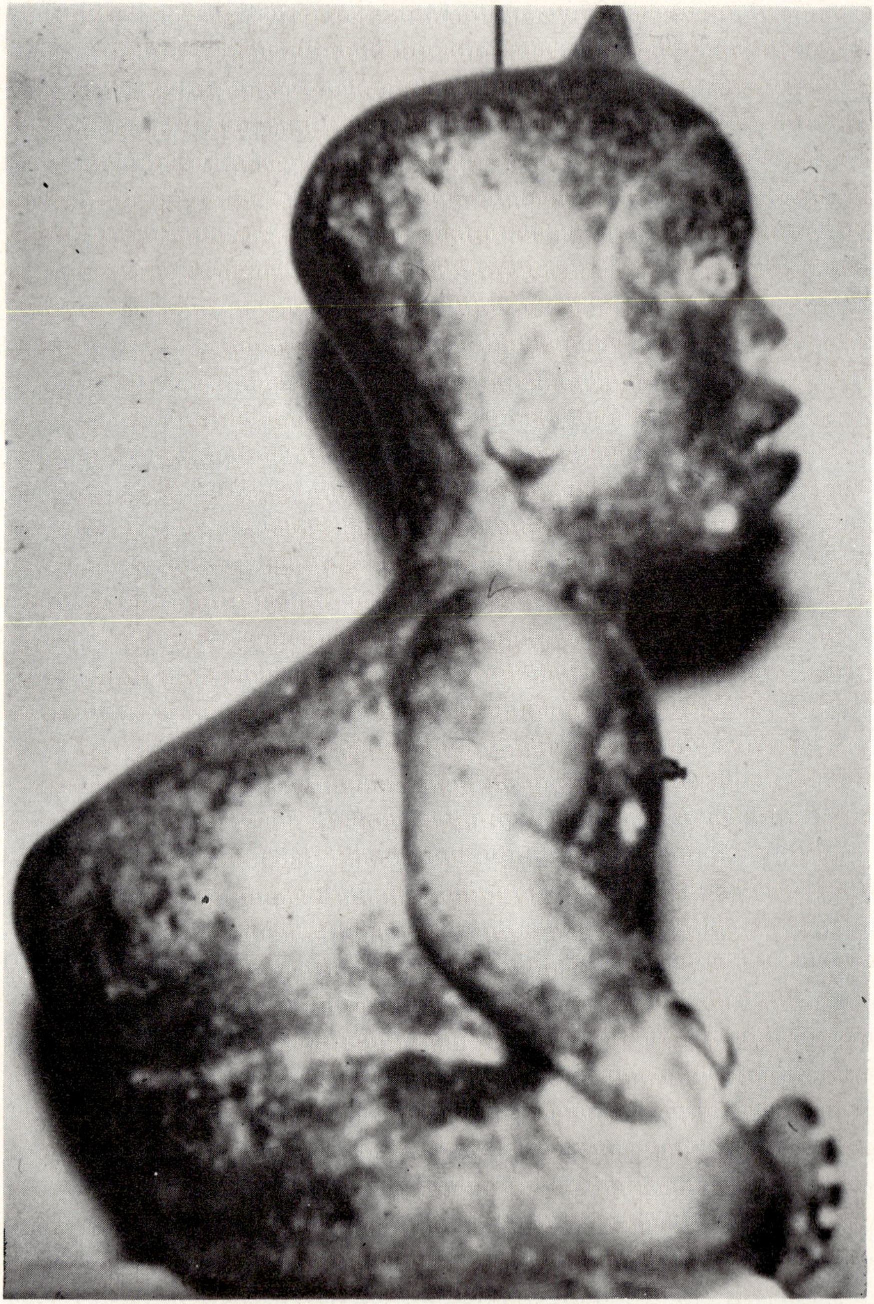

Fig. 5. Pre-Columbian figure of an achondroplastic boy with severe angular dorsolumbar gibbus.

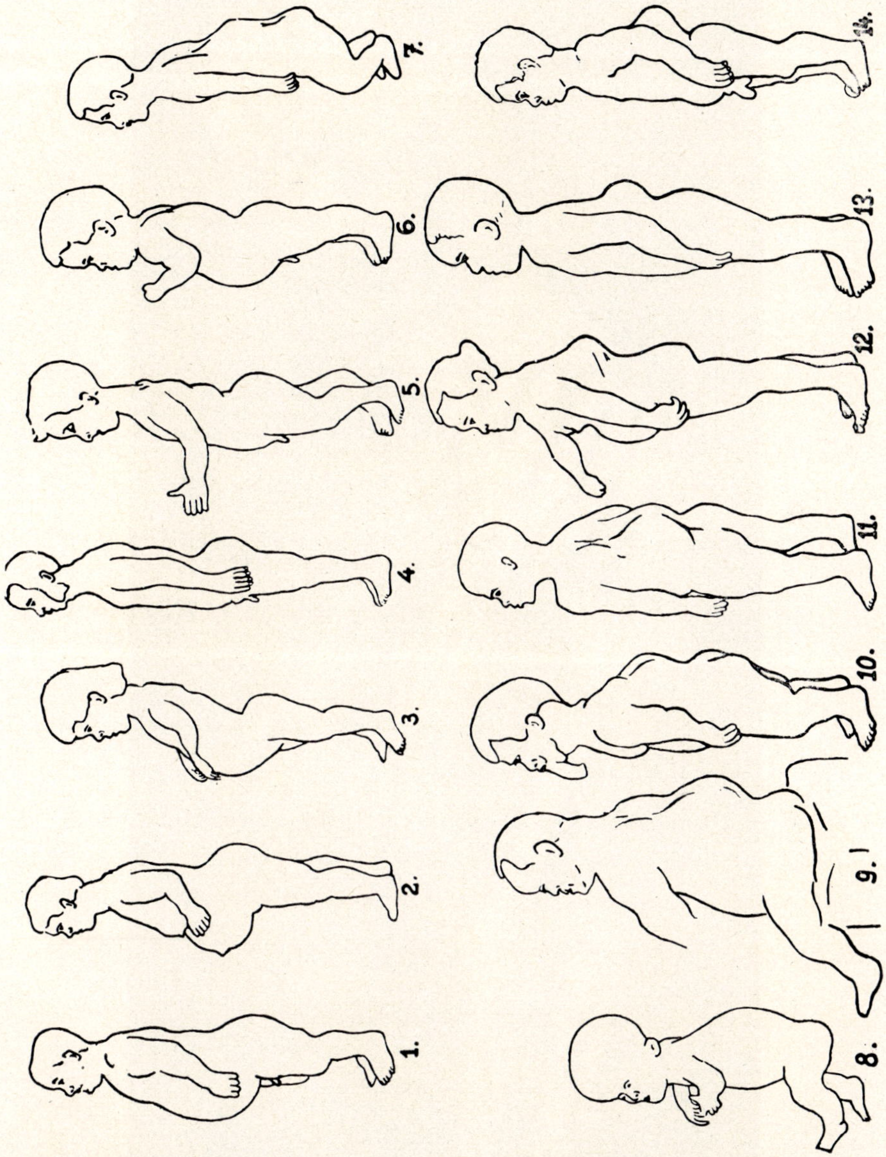

Fig. 6. Profile line drawings of achondroplastic dwarfts showing all degrees of changes of the spine, from the mildest to the most severe degrees of lumbar kyphosis. Note especially the young child (Number 8) with a curved kyphosis when just beginning to sit. Reproduced by permission from: Donath, J. and Vogl, A. Untersuchungen über den chondrodystrophischen Zwergwuchs. *Wien. Arch. Inn. Med. 10*:1, 1925.

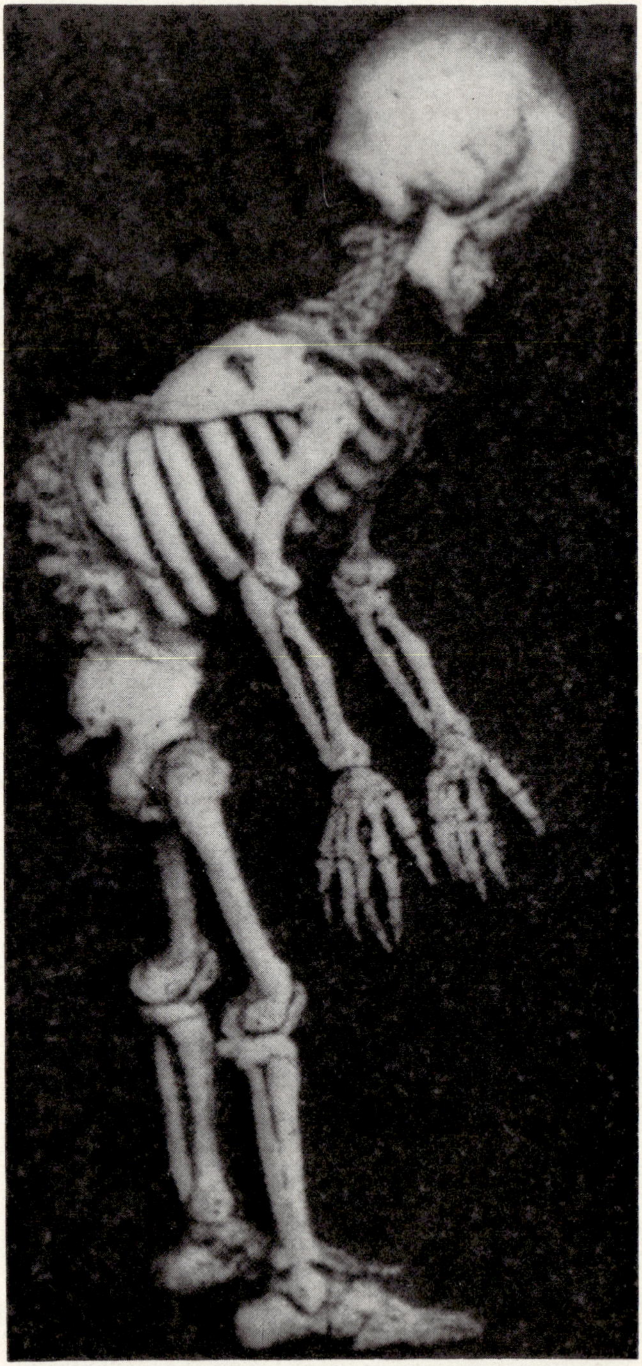

Fig. 7. Skeleton of an achondroplastic dwarf with a dorsolumbar gibbus with a wedge-shaped body of L 1 (forearms and hands of this 18th century specimen do not belong to this skeleton). From the Rokitansky Pathological Museum in Vienna. Reproduced by permission from: Donath, J. and Vogl, A. Untersuchungen über den chondrodystrophischen Zwergwuchs. *Wien. Arch. Inn. Med. 10*:1, 1925.

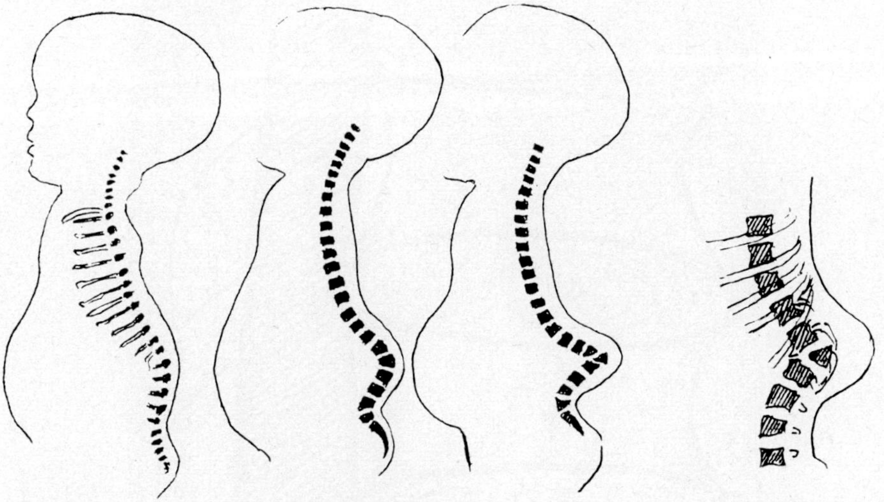

Fig. 8. Sketches indicating the development of an angular gibbus in an achondroplastic child born with a curved kyphosis. After the child begins to sit, the kyphosis increases, the keystone vertebra becomes wedge-shaped and finally dislocated posteriorly. This deformity can be prevented during this period by orthopedic measures.

even richer fruit; it succeeded in bringing about a significant change in the morbidity and mortality of achondroplastic dwarfs. The autopsy of our patient and measurements on the spine of achondroplastic skeletons revealed that the bony canal was just wide enough to fit a normal spinal cord tightly but with no room to spare (Figure 9). Since the spinal cord of an achondroplastic dwarf is normally developed, even minor disc protrusions or osteophytes will produce serious damage to the tightly encased nerve structures. For these reasons most achondroplastic dwarfs sooner or later suffer neurologic complications varying from herniated disc syndromes to complete paraplegia.

Under these circumstances we recommended freeing the cramped intraspinal structures by means of laminectomy. This procedure has now been carried out in many cases with gratifying results.

Through these observations achondroplasia has changed its place in medicine. In the past it had been regarded by the medical profession as the product of a caprice of nature but of no particular interest to any of the medical specialties except obstetrics. But since it has been shown than achondroplasia in itself can be the cause of serious illness and

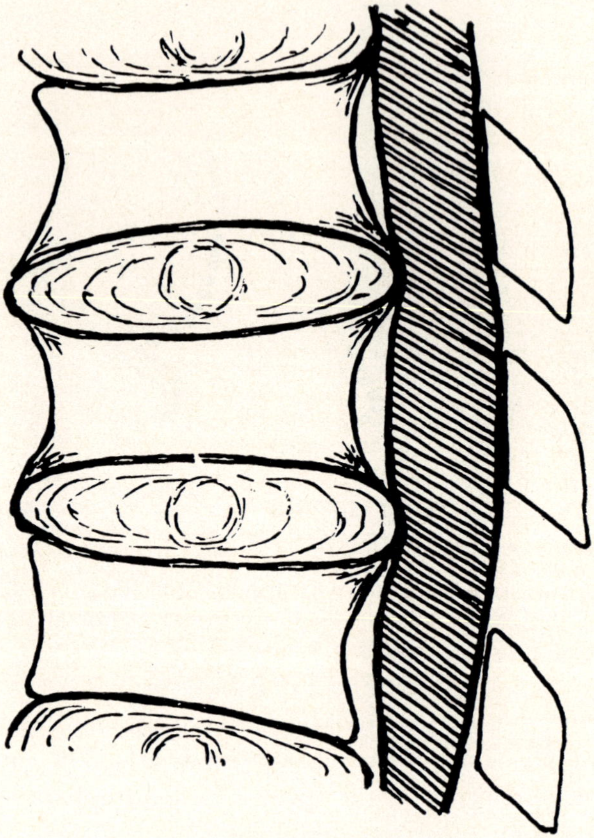

Fig. 9. Diagram indicating the disproportion between the achondroplastic spinal canal and the normally developed spinal cord. Minor osteophyte formations or disc herniations compromise the cord seriously.

death, pediatricians, orthopedists, and neurosurgeons have become aware of the problem and of the therapeutic possibilities. It has given me great satisfaction to have contributed to altering the grim fate of these otherwise healthy and often gifted persons.

Cheyne-Stokes Respiration[14]

Cheyne-Stokes breathing became another target of my interest. Intermittent respiratory standstill has been known since antiquity as an ominous symptom of poisoning and of other serious disorders. No remedies existed. Sedation notoriously made the condition worse.

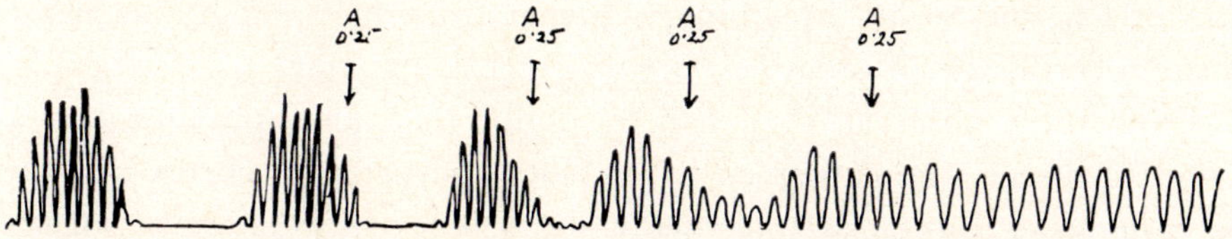

Fig. 10. Diagram indicating the prompt excitatory effect of intravenously administered aminophylline upon the respiratory center, with abolition of the periodic respiration.

As it happened, one day I became a victim of this condition. After an operation in 1926, followed by large doses of morphine, my breathing became distressingly intermittent. Since the start of every period of hyperventilation produced quite some pain in the abdominal incision, I tried to figure out a way by which I could break the self-perpetuating cycle of Cheyne-Stokes breathing and thus avoid the need for the painful hyperventilation. I decided just to go on breathing voluntarily during the periods of respiratory standstill. However, the plan failed. I found myself incapable of using my respiratory muscles intentionally the moment the period of hyperventilation was over.

While recuperating I had time to think about how to abolish the vicious cycle of Cheyne-Stokes breathing, in other words, how to restore the responsiveness of the depressed respiratory center. I remembered then that on several occasions when, for diuretic purposes, I had injected aminophylline too fast by vein, the patient began to hyperventilate forcibly, to the point of dizziness and faintness. This observation indicated that aminophylline above a certain blood concentration may act as a potent respiratory stimulant and possibly be the drug for which I was looking.

Soon afterward I encountered a patient with severe Cheyne-Stokes respiration. He had pulmonary emphysema and had been given an injection of morphine for his air hunger. He was unresponsive and deeply cyanotic, and had periods of apnea. One fourth of an ampoule of aminophylline was injected rapidly by vein before each anticipated phase of respiratory standstill (Figure 10). Even before the entire ampoule was finished, normal respiration was restored and the patient was fully alert. The action was equally rapid and effective in subsequent cases of Cheyne-Stokes breathing, whether caused by congestive heart failure, overdosage of sedatives, uremia, or brain tumor.

From these observations I had no doubt that aminophylline had a powerful direct stimulating effect on both the cerebral cortex and on the respiratory center. It took many years before the pharmacologists accepted the validity of this mechanism of action while the bedside observations had, to my mind, never permitted any other interpretation.

Aminophylline became and has remained the drug of choice for the symptomatic treatment of Cheyne-Stokes. Whenever insomnia is caused by periodic breathing, it is, in fact, the only effective "sleeping drug."

Allergic Thrombocytopenic Purpura[15]

The last chapter selected from my diary for this paper deals with another exercise in serendipity. It goes back to the early 1930's when a veritable epidemic of a mysterious acute hemorrhagic disease swept through Europe. An ever-increasing number of people fell ill with what was considered fulminating Werlhof's disease. Petechiae and bruises appeared rapidly all over the body and bleeding occurred from nose, mouth, rectum, or bladder. This picture, alarming as it was, usually disappeared within a few days, but it was apt to reappear at any time. During these attacks complete or almost complete absence of blood platelets was found.

The public was frightened. The medical profession was puzzled. Treatment was haphazard because every treatment seemed effective for the moment: such as a variety of drugs, irradiation of the spleen and, in case of recurrence, splenectomy. But in at least one case bleeding occurred again after removal of the spleen as soon as the patient had returned home.

As it happened, I had a night emergency call to see an elderly man who had suddenly suffered a shaking chill, soon followed by the appearance of fresh bleeding spots all over the skin, blood-filled blebs on lips and tongue, oozing blood from mouth and nose, and gross hematuria. The absence of blood platelets confirmed the diagnosis of acute thrombocytopenic purpura. The following day the platelet count began to rise, all bleeding stopped and, after 3 days, the patient was well again.

Four weeks later I had to make another night emergency call to the same patient under the same circumstances. Thorough questioning, with the help of the good memory of his housekeeper, revealed that the patient had on both these evenings taken a then popular somnifacient drug called Sedormid. The patient would never have suspected this drug as he had taken it in previous years regularly and with no ill effects.

I felt at that moment that I was on the track of the source of the current epidemic of bleeding. I promptly reached the patient I had seen previously after such episodes of bleeding, and others who, I knew, had suffered such attacks. And, indeed, all of them had taken Sedormid. Among them was the woman who, after being discharged following splenectomy, had suffered another severe attack of bleeding. She told me that, being a poor sleeper she had taken Sedormid frequently before and between her hospitalizations for hemorrhagic purpura. In the hospital, however, she was given some other sleeping pills, and recovered quickly from her hemorrhagic disease; but on returning home after her splenectomy she went back to her favorite Sedormid and promptly started to bleed again.

I was proud of my detective work and was convinced that I had found the key to the rash of bleeding disease and to its instant elimination. I felt that the facts should be made public without delay, preferably by the highest authority. So I hurried with my news to a leading hematologist, but received a cool and skeptical, almost hostile reception and, of course, no cooperation. I was confounded and at a loss to understand this attitude. Only much later I learned that the professor and his associate had just finished a major paper expounding a new theory on the cause of the epidemic and reporting the brilliant results they had obtained in treating the disease with a specially synthesized new drug.

When I just as naively approached the giant pharmaceutical company which produced Sedormid, in order to warn them of the dangers of their drug, I was in for another rude awakening. To my face I was politely admonished not to be hasty and not to let my imagination run away with me and, behind my back, I was accused of being a liar and publicity seeker who had talked patients into making false statements. When I insisted on publication of my findings and conclusions, I was threatened by the company with a suit for damages but at the same time was offered a considerable sum "for additional research" if I were only willing to postpone the publication of my findings for another year.

I realized then that I was on my own and had to face whatever criticism I might encounter in the forthcoming meeting of the Society of Internal Medicine at which I was scheduled to present my observations in a paper titled "Allergic Thrombycytopenic Purpura."

Fortunately I had talked of my observations to another well-known hematologist. He rechecked the cases of purpura that had been admitted to his own service before. He confirmed the use of Sedormid among them and succeeded in opening the discussion on my paper before my adversaries had the opportunity to get up and annihilate me. Soon afterward the company put a warning label on the bottles and not much later withdrew Sedormid from the market.

It was thus established for the first time that in certain individuals a chemical compound would produce an allergic form of thrombocytopenic purpura. The mechanism was still obscure but because of the rapidity and completeness with which the platelets disappeared from the blood stream and then reappeared, I could not visualize depression or destruction of the megakaryocytes in the bone marrow as the cause. I surmised therefore that the circulating platelets must somehow be trapped in the periphery for the duration of the allergic reaction and must be released when it was over.

This hypothesis was essentially confirmed by later investigations that uncovered the complex immunologic mechanism involved.

In telling you these short stories, I followed the Roman dictum: *verba docent, exempla trahunt*. Words can teach but only examples can convince. It was my intention to convince you by these examples that major or minor contributions can be made by the means at everyone's disposal.

The history of my investigations clearly carries the marks of the advantages and the disadvantages that are inherent in part-time research. I have had the advantage of roaming freely in the wide field of medicine, of touching on many fascinating problems, of solving a few and, in other instances, of opening up a tiny window onto new vistas. These far-flung excursions have also broadened my experience as a clinician. The main disadvantage of not being a full-time investigator and a member of a team has been that I have had to leave my studies on completion of the clinical phase and let others work on the unresolved parts of the problems, from diuretics to allergic purpura.

However, I comfort myself with the realization that no research is ever finished, and that even trying to complete the research on all the problems in which I was involved would have taken many busy lifetimes.

May I sum up the message I want to convey to you on this occasion?

Classical clinical medicine reached its culmination at the beginning of the 20th century. It had accomplished the transformation of Western medicine from an empirical and often irrational art of healing into a sound, sober, and well-organized system based on huge autopsy material. Since then the magnificent advances in biomedical sciences have created the miracle of modern medicine. These advances brought with them, by necessity, progressive specialization and fragmentation of medical practice and the tendency to treat diseases instead of human beings. In this manner the holistic approach of traditional medicine toward the sick is replaced by the pragmatic approach of providing expert knowledge and sophisticated techniques for the diagnosis and treatment of each of the patient's problems.

But must these two currents compete in modern medicine? Must the torrent of scientific progress engulf the gentler stream of clinical medicine, in which concern for the sick human being has always been the main motivation? Clinical medicine must dominate medical practice if it is not to become just another field of technology, alienating itself from the patient and losing his confidence. But how can clinical medicine survive the persistent onslaught from its Prometheuslike children, the medical sciences? How can it maintain its traditional role in the care of the patient?

Only by transforming itself into a new clinical medicine which must be a synthesis of benevolent interest and scientific accuracy, and of artistic intuition and scholarly prudence; in short, a synthesis of the ancient heritage of the art of healing and of wise utilization of the advances in medical science. In its forefront we shall find the new clinician, a human biologist with an incisive mind and an enthusiastic physician with imagination and compassion. The tasks of the new clinician will be titanic indeed.

If our medical schools succeed in producing physicians of this type—and the demand for them is overwhelming—then clinical medicine has a future worthy of its past and will be able to retain the role of leadership in medicine that seemed naturally to belong to it. To this end I have ventured, after 50 years in clinical medicine, to reemphasize its merits in the care of the sick, in the making of true physicians of our students, and in providing an inexhaustible source for relevant research in medicine.

REFERENCES

1. Vogl, A. Six hundred years of medicine in Vienna. *Bull. N.Y. Acad. Med. 43:* 282, 1967.
2. Platt, Lord. Medical science: master or servant? *Brit. Med. J. 4*:439, 1967. *J. 4*:439, 1967.
3. Dubos, R. Hippocrates in modern dress. *Perspect. Biol. Med. 9*:275, 1966.
4. Bauer, J. Wie ist es zur Mechanisierung der Medizin gekommen? *Mediz. Welt 20*:1127, 1965.
5. Atchley, D. The evolving art of medicine. *Arch. Int. Med. 112*:455, 1963.
6. Krebs, H. A. The making of a scientist. *Nature 215*:1441, 1967.
7. Cohen, Lord of Birkenhead: The fruits of error and false assumption. *Proc. Roy. Soc. Med. 60*:673, 1967.
8. Palmer, W. L. Tradition and progress in medicine. *Ann. Intern. Med. 47*:383, 1957.
9. Rossman, R. E. The history and significance of serendipity in medical discovery. *Trans. Coll. Phys. Phila. 33*:104, 1965.
10. Remer, T. G. *Serendipity and the Three Princes*. Univ. Oklahoma Press, 1965.
11. Vogl, A. The discovery of the organic mercurial diuretics. *Amer. Heart J. 39:* 881, 1950.
12. Vogl, A. and Zins, B. Eine einfache Methode zum Nachweise pathologischer Bilirubinaemie. *Med. Klinik. 18*:667, 1922.
13. Vogl, A. The fate of the achondroplastic dwarf. *Exper. Med. Surg. 20*:1962.
14. Vogl, A. Ueber den Mechanismus und die Behandlung der zentralen Dyspnoe. *Klin. Wochenschr. 9*:783, 1930.
15. Vogl, A. Die Pathogenese der akuten thrombopenischen Purpura (Ueber Purpura nach Sedormid). *Wien. Arch. Inn. Med. 32*:273, 1938.

STATEMENT

by

THE NEW YORK ACADEMY OF MEDICINE

on

Methadone Management of Heroin Addiction

THE recent *National Conference on Methadone Treatment* held at The Rockefeller University revealed that a significant number of heroin addicts are being managed with methadone by private practitioners on an ambulatory basis. Instances were reported where such office-treated addicts have been dropped from treatment for various reasons. This has caused serious problems for the patients, physicians, and hospitals—as well as for health and enforcement agencies.

The New York Academy of Medicine notes that the methadone technique for managing heroin addicts appears promising. However the Academy believes that indiscriminate management of heroin addicts on an ambulatory basis by individual physicians who are inexperienced in the use of this technique is a dangerous practice and should be discouraged.

While the Academy does not wish to comment at this time on either the short- or long-term merit of the methadone technique, it believes it is necessary to point out that methadone-management programs should be carried out only in association with evaluation procedures of an objective character such as those which are conducted in connection with the work of the group headed by Dr. Vincent Dole in New York City.

The Academy holds the view that the management of heroin addicts by use of methadone is best served when the results are subjected to critical, objective evaluation by an outside, independent agency.

JOHN L. POOL
President

November 19, 1969

ASTERIX THE GAUL

It is not very often that the *Bulletin of The New York Academy of Medicine* or any other medical periodical has occasion to notice the pictorial volumes which we Americans—somewhat to the mystification of Europeans, Asians, and Africans—designate as *comic books*. We are apt to admit, grudgingly and inattentively, that this species of composition reflects, with varying distortion, the appearance, habits, behavior, morality, and fantasies of our times, but we are reluctant to regard it as art or as literature. The comic book is out-of-bounds, substandard, déclassé.

Yet this pariah has noble ancestors. Without laboring the question of genealogy, it is apparent that the comic cartoon, issued singly or serially, is traceable to Hogarth and Rowlandson of the 18th century and to the political and social draughtsmen of the 19th century such as Goya, Gavarni, and Daumier. Much of the more recent development can be credited, or debited, to the United States. Indeed, we have sometimes tended to feel that the comic cartoon is a North American cultural product, exported to Europe and imitated there. This erroneous opinion perhaps owes its origin to the fact that European immigrants are commonly puzzled by the "comic" section of the American newspaper.

It is now evident that in the writing of comic books the Europeans have equaled or outdone us. In 1961 a French draughtsman, Albert Uderzo, joined a writer, René Goscinny, in composing *Astérix le Gaulois*, the first of a series which now includes a dozen volumes, such as *Le Tour de Gaule*, *Astérix aux Jeux Olympiques*, and *Le Bouclier Arverne*.*

The principal scene of action is set in Gaul in 50 B.C. Contrary to the untruthful statements which Julius Caesar made in his *Gallic War*, not all of Gaul has been subjugated by the Romans. A small Gallic village remains unconquered. It is under close observation by the Roman garrisons of Laudanum, Aquarium, Babaorum (baba au rhum), and Petibonum (petit bonhomme). By analogy with Vercingetorix the Gallic heroes of the picture narratives have been given names ending in *ix*, such as: Astérix (Figure 1), the energetic little warrior; his close

*The Astérix books are published in Paris by Dargaud. Volumes issued in the original French and distributed in England contain explanatory four-page leaflets published by the Brockhampton Press of Leicester, England.

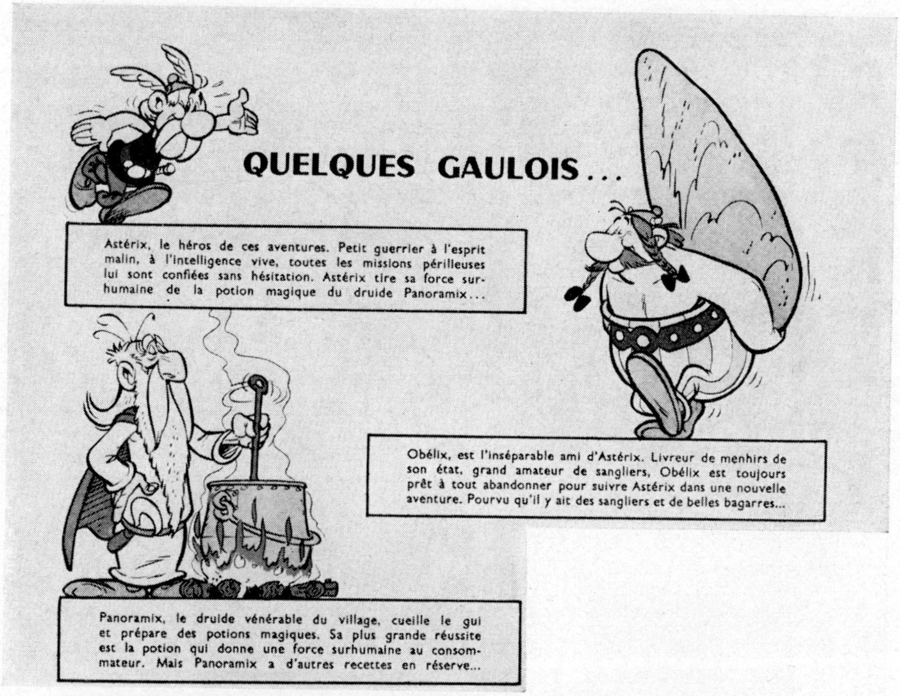

Fig. 1. Principal characters in the Astérix series. Reproduced by permission of the publisher, Dargaud S.A., of Paris.

friend the gigantic Obélix, a maker of menhirs (megaliths); the druid Panoramix, who brews the magic potion that makes his fellow tribesmen invincible; and the intolerably cacophonous bard Assurancetourix (assurance tous risques, all-inclusive automobile insurance).

In *Astérix et Les Normands* we meet a surly long-haired Gallic "hippy," Goudurix (goût du risque, i.e., reckless), who is emotional and cowardly. He dances in an exotic manner and drives a very fast chariot. Also to be mentioned are Pneumatix the courier, named after the Paris postal system, and Idéfix (idée fixe), a tiny dog.

In the course of their colorful adventures our heroes encounter not only Julius Caesar—depicted as thin and hawknosed, unlike the familiar portrait sculptures of the Julian gens—but such imaginary Romans as Claudius Lapsus and Tullius Stratocumulus. In *Le Combat des Chefs* Latin is taught in the Ecole de Langues Vivantes by Professor Berlix.

Egyptians are depicted vividly in *Astérix et Cléopatre* and a Phoeni-

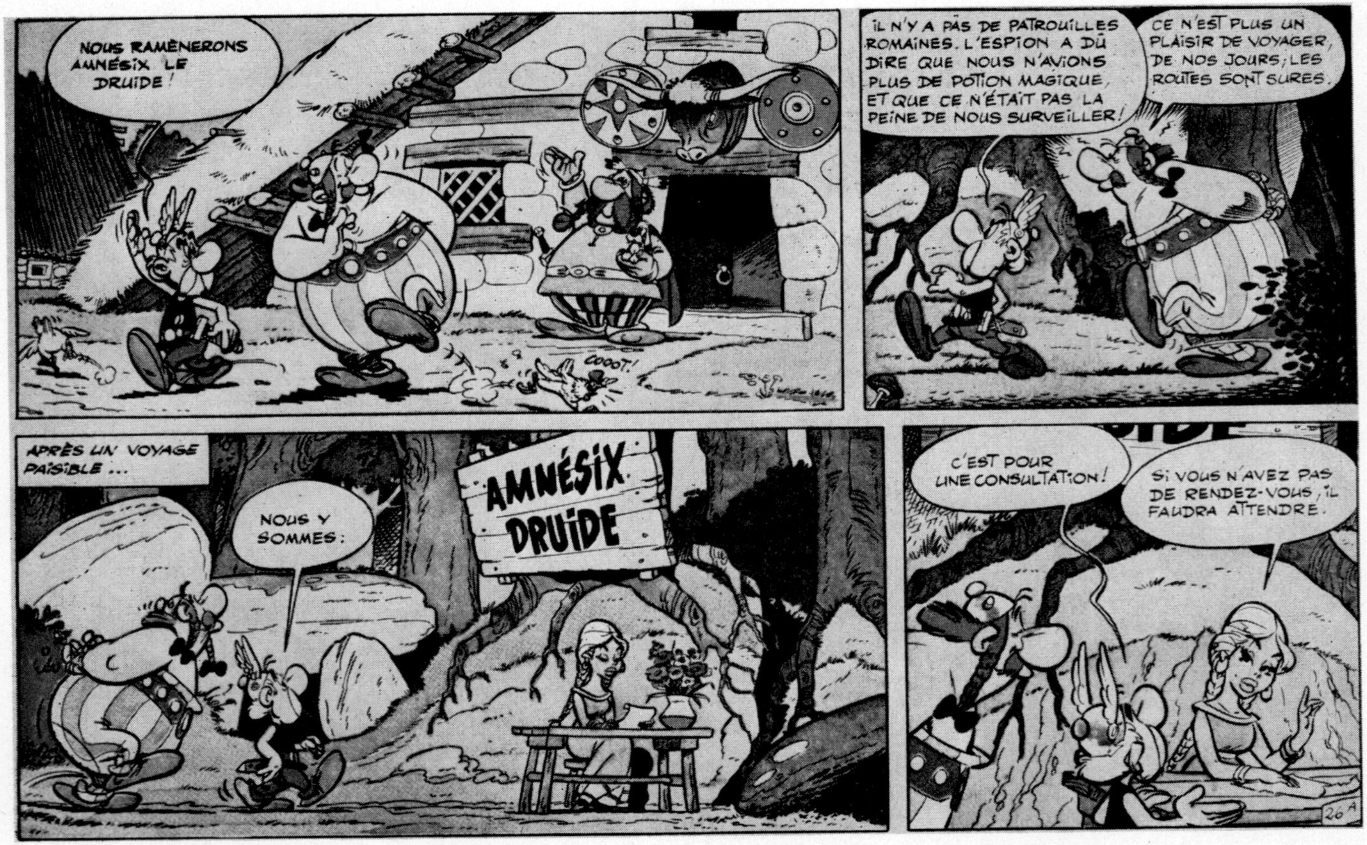

Fig. 2. The office of Amnésix, the Gallic druid-psychiatrist (50 B.C.). From *Le Combat des Chefs.* Reproduced by permission of the publisher, Dargaud S.A., of Paris.

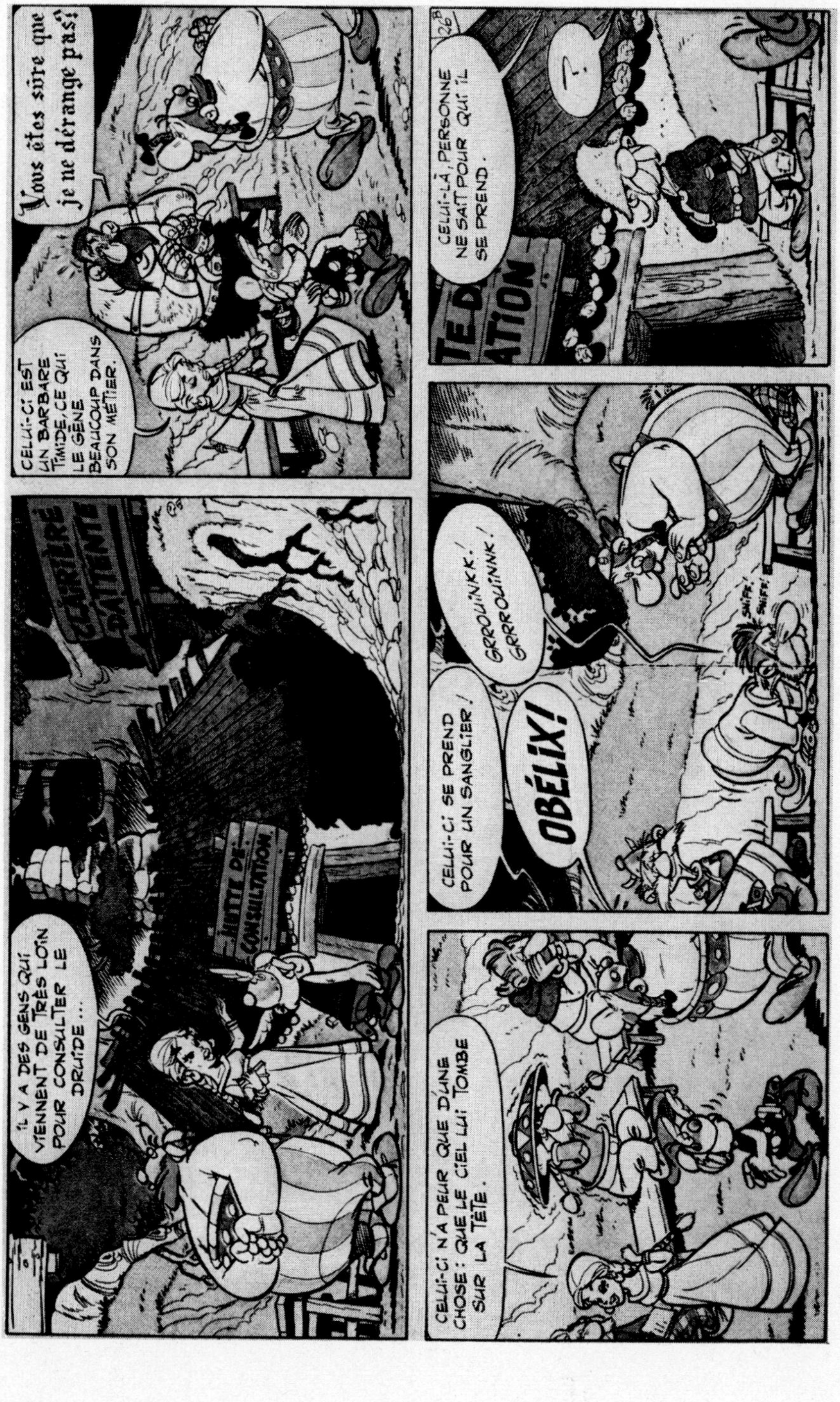

Fig. 2 (continued).

cian merchant captain appears in *Astérix Gladiateur.* Gentlemanly tea-drinking Englishmen are satirized in *Astérix Chez les Bretons.*

The texts are replete with puns, quips, anachronisms, allusions, quotations, and parodies of a thousand kinds. Inevitably science and medicine have attracted the attention of the cartoonist.

In *Astérix Légionnaire* we see the physical examination of recruits in the Roman army. An Egyptian recruit speaks in hieroglyphics, while a Goth and an interpreter express themselves in Gothic type. The examining room is equipped with an eye chart and a mechanical examination table. On the wall are a trephine, two large knives, and a large forceps; these simultaneously suggest the surgical instruments found at Pompeii and the perforated skulls unearthed at various prehistoric sites.

In *Le Combat des Chefs,* Panoramix the druid is struck by a Celtic megalith and loses his memory. For treatment he is taken to Amnésix, a fellow druid who practices psychiatry. The alienist's office is a "hutte de consultation" (consultation hut) in the forest (Figure 2). Beyond the beauteous secretary are patients awaiting their turn: a huge barbarian who suffers from timidity (and whose words are in Gothic letters); a man who imagines himself to be a wild boar and sniffs in the grass of the forest; and a man who struts about in a Napoleonic uniform, his right hand thrust into his coat. "As for this man," says the receptionist, "nobody knows who he thinks he is." The results of the druidic psychotherapy are astounding and will not be disclosed in this review.

It is no wonder that the Astérix books are eagerly read by both adults and children, that they are used in the teaching of French, and that they have been translated into several European languages.

S.J.

UNPUBLISHED PAPERS OF THOMAS HODGKIN

AMONGST the papers of the late Dr. Hodgkin there were found numerous essays and lectures relating to medical and other scientific subjects. These have been placed in my hands with a view to publication if thought worthy of it. Most of them were written about the time of his retirement from Guy's Hospital, which is now nearly forty years ago; of these some have already appeared in print, whilst others are now so antiquated that the opinions they express are obsolete and the statements superseded by those derived from modern research. I find, therefore, I have much less to lay before my readers than I had at first anticipated.

Dr. Hodgkin was born at Tottenham in 1798, took his degree at Edinburgh in 1823, and became a member of the College of Physicians in London in 1825. He belonged to the Society of Friends, as may easily be gathered from the style of his writings. He was possessed of very great literary attainments, being especially complimented on the pure latinity of his thesis on "Absorption" on the occasion of his taking his degree at Edinburgh. He passed a considerable time in France and Italy, where he perfected himself in the Continental languages, and acquired a strong taste for pathological pursuits. This was due, no doubt, to the scientific tendency of his mind, which prompted him to undertake the study of those branches of medicine which possessed a more positive character, as being more congenial to his remarkably simple and truthful nature. On his return to England he engaged himself with others in the foundation of an independent school at Guy's Hospital by becoming curator of the museum and demonstrator of morbid anatomy. The work he did in forming the museum was enormous, both in preparing specimens and framing a catalogue; the result of his labour is seen also in the two volumes of *Lectures on the Morbid Anatomy of the Serous and Mucous Membranes*. That Dr. Hodgkin was actuated by no slight ambition in his work may be gathered from the following lines taken from his opening address:—"I shall conclude by assuring you that it will be my constant aim—whether I may be fortunate enough to reach the mark or not—to co-operate with those who are strenuously endeavouring to render the school of Guy's Hospital the first medical school in the Kingdom." The foundation which he thus laid in the museum and pathological department was one on which many distinguished men have since built by adding their mite to the work he so well began. No one who cares to look upon Guy's as his alma mater but must feel a debt of gratitude to Hodgkin for the important share he took in endeavouring to constitute it a scientific school of medicine. It may be safely asserted that there had been no writer on pathology in this country before his time who had grasped the subject in so philosophic a spirit; for although Baillie, Hooper, and others had already written good descriptions of morbid appearances, Hodgkin was the first to follow in the footsteps of the great Bichat by discussing the diseases and changes in the various tissues of the body. Indeed, few have since copied his example, and the reason may be that the time has not yet come to accomplish what he wished, for probably the descriptive method adopted by Rokitansky and others must necessarily precede the larger one which Hodgkin attempted. The perusal of Hodgkin's manuscripts and notes for lectures has more fully strengthened the high opinion which I have ever entertained of the wide extent of his learning and of that true philosophic spirit by which he made his knowledge of zoology, geology, as well as the history of medicine, all conduce to the perfection of his theme.

The feeling of admiration which arises in one's mind on perusing these documents is not unmingled with the sadness of regret that his career as a pathologist should have been so brief. It was a day ever to be lamented when he turned his back on Guy's, and his philosophic studies came to so premature an end. After having occupied the lecture chair for about ten years, to the special advantage of the school and to the advancement of pathology throughout the world, he retired from the post after his unsuccessful candidature for the assistant physicianship. The lapse of time is too great and the circumstances involved in too much obscurity to make it worth the trouble to dwell upon this episode in his history. Nevertheless it must be said that in him Guy's Hospital lost one of its greatest ornaments, and the profession in England one who was destined to shed a lustre on its ranks. After his severance from Guy's he passed to St. Thomas', where his stay was but short; he continued to practise medicine, but his sources of information on matters of pathology being gone, he turned his mind to more general subjects. He wrote a book "On the Preservation of Health," and some notes for a further work on the subject are now before me. He interested himself in provident dispensaries and in some medico-legal questions. Latterly he almost entirely devoted himself to philanthropic pursuits, and was mainly instrumental in founding the Ethnological Society, in connection with which he devoted himself to the study of philology. Subsequently he travelled in the East with Sir Moses Montefiore for the purpose of rendering aid to the Jews. On their last Journey he was seized with dysentery and died at Jaffa, on the 5th of April, 1866, aged sixty-eight. It may be worthy of note that his successful opponent for the physicianship of Guy's, Dr. Babington, died in London three days afterwards, aged seventy-two. . . .

From Wilks, S. An account of some unpublished papers of the late Dr. Hodgkin. *Guy's Hospital Reports*, 3d series, 23:55-127, 1878. Published by permission.

A FEW COMMENTS BY ARISTOTLE

Some creatures are tame and some are wild: some are at all times tame, as man and the mule. . . .

Some, again, are peculiarly salacious, as the partridge, the barn-door cock and their congeners; others are inclined to chastity, as the whole tribe of crows, for birds of this kind indulge but rarely in sexual intercourse. . . .

The skull has sutures: one, of circular form, in the case of women; in the case of men, as a general rule, three meeting at a point. Instances have been known of a man's skull devoid of sutures altogether. . . .

The part that lies under the skull is called the face: but in the case of man only, for the term is not applied to a fish or an ox. . . . When men have large foreheads, they are slow to move; when they have small ones, they are fickle; when they have broad ones, they are apt to be distraught; when they have foreheads rounded or bulging out, they are quick-tempered. . . .

Furthermore, there is a portion of the head, whereby an animal hears, a part incapable of breathing, the ear. I say "incapable of breathing," for Alcmaeon is mistaken when he says that goats inspire through their ears. . . .

Men that have the inside or sole of the foot clumsy and not arched, that is, that walk resting on the under-surface of their feet, are prone to roguery.

ARISTOTLE, *Historia Animalium.* D'Arcy Wentworth Thompson, transl. Oxford, Clarendon Press, 1910.

ABSCESSES OF THE LIVER; THE DANGER OF MOVING THE PATIENT

NEVERTHELESS, both of these circumstances, which are not to be met with in those histories, has so often occur'd to physicians, and among others, to my preceptor Albertini, that he press'd it very earnestly upon practitioners, not to suffer a patient to be mov'd when there were symptoms of an abscess already form'd in the liver; not because he was ignorant that motion has been prescrib'd, at this time, by authors, who are, in other respects excellent, which I also read has succeeded happily sometimes in our memory; but because he suppos'd, that without using motion, it would, probably, happen, that the pus of an abscess so ruptur'd, without injuring the membrane of the liver, might be carried down to the intestines, through the branches of the biliary duct; and because from a contrary practice, he foresaw how easily the external membrane of the liver might be ruptur'd, so that the pus should be pour'd out into the cavity of the abdomen, and kill the patient instantly, by bringing on a syncopé.

For this he remember'd to have happen'd at Bologna, at the time he was a young man, when an excellent physician, and, at the same time, an eminent surgeon, following the practice of those authors, had prescrib'd motion to a virgin who had a suppuration in the liver; by which means the pus being pour'd out into the abdominal cavity, the patient died soon after, in the arms of the women by whom she was supported. And he had afterwards observ'd the same thing to happen, even without motion, at least with a slight motion, such as we naturally used in bed, or while we are rising from bed, in several persons, but particularly in a noble marquis, who had an abscess in the concave part of the liver. . . .

J. B. MORGAGNI: *The Seats and Causes of Disease*. Translated by Benjamin Alexander. London, Millar, 1769, vol. 2, pp. 185-186. (Letter 36, Article 6.)

NEW FOR EVERYMAN IN MEDICINE FOR 1970 FROM HAFNER PUBLISHING COMPANY, INC.

SHRYOCK, ROBERT H.
The Development of Modern Medicine
An Interpretation of the Social and Scientific Factors Involved.
xv, 457 pages, 10 illus., footnotes, index. (1947) Reprint 1969 **$13.50**

It was said of the 1947 edition:
"... Brilliant and scholarly...." (L.L., *San Francisco Chronicle*)
"... An important contribution to medical history...."
(*New York Herald Tribune Weekly Book Review*)

This reprint is a facsimile of the 1947 edition.

SKINNER, HENRY A.
The Origin of Medical Terms
2nd ed. x, 438 pages, illus., references, a chart of the Greek Alphabet. (1961) Reprinted with corrections 1970 **$15.00**

The English language is based on Anglo-Saxon and has been augmented by various additions from other tongues. This base and augmentation has been influenced by a history of invasions, migrations, inventions, etc. Thus the tracking down of the etymological origin of medical terms as used by English speaking people is a difficult and complex problem. Recently corrected, this volume, written in an informal yet informative style, will find acceptance with anyone interested in medical terminology.

ALL DIRECT ORDERS WILL RECEIVE A 10% DISCOUNT

HAFNER PUBLISHING COMPANY, INC.
P.O. Box 27, Cooper Station, New York, N.Y. 10003

Over 5 million prescriptions already filled at Macy*s

All 13 Macy Prescription Centres *satisfy your patients with efficient professional service*

- You may phone in your patients' prescriptions (except for narcotics, amphetamines, and barbiturates).
- Your patients may charge their prescriptions on their Macy Shopping Accounts or C-T Plans.
- Your patients may have their prescriptions delivered anywhere free of extra charge.
- We serve your patient with a full line of convalescent and diabetic needs.

Macy's Herald Square, OX 5-4400
Macy's Parkchester, TA 8-7000
Macy's Jamaica, OL 7-9000
Macy's Flatbush, UL 6-5000
Macy's Roosevelt Field, PI 6-8200
Macy's Huntington, AR 1-3000
Macy's White Plains, WH 6-5015
Macy's New Haven, Conn. 624-9271
Macy's Bay Shore, MO 5-8400
Macy's Queens, AR 1-9100
Macy's Colonie, 459-1950
Macy's New Rochelle, 633-7700
Macy's Smith Haven, 724-4900

BULLETIN OF
THE NEW YORK ACADEMY
OF MEDICINE

VOL. 46, NO. 2 FEBRUARY 1970

URBAN ECOLOGY, GEOGRAPHY, AND HEALTH PROBLEMS*

GEORGE W. CAREY

Professor of Urban Geography in Planning
Rutgers University
New Brunswick, N. J.

THE urban ecologist is interested in the nature of the city as a life-supporting system for man, while the urban geographer is concerned primarily with the processes of spatial growth and development of the city. Since both of these emphases are closely related to concerns of the health field, it may prove helpful to sketch briefly a theoretical framework for interpreting them before passing to a consideration of our metropolitan ecology in the past, and to make some suggestions for researching its state in the present.

THE SPATIAL STRUCTURE OF AN URBAN ECOLOGICAL SYSTEM

Otis D. Duncan and Leo Schnore,[1] among others, have provided us with a theoretical model of the relation between man and his environment, which may be applied to the study of cities with good effect. As we see from the diagram in Figure 1, the growth of a population and its level of living is closely related to four other interlinked factors. *T* is the

*Presented at a meeting of the Subcommittee on Social Policy for Health Care, Committee on Medicine in Society, The New York Academy of Medicine, May 22, 1969.

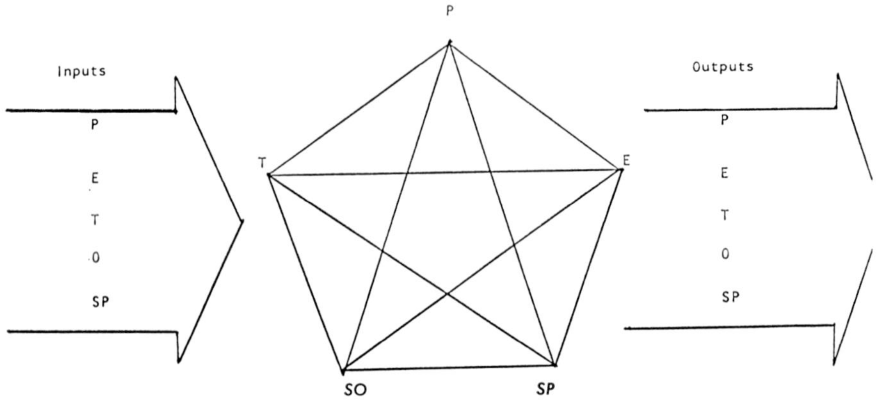

Fig. 1. Metropolitan Systems.

state of technology, *SO* represents the organization of society, *SP* represents the social psychology—the operational world view, so to speak—of the populace, and *E* represents the environment.

The point is that if change is initiated in one or several of these factors, interactions will occur which will induce changes in all. Indeed, several cycles of changes may well occur before a new equilibrium is reached, and the synergistic effects may be such that the aggregate changes may be much larger than anticipated. In a rapidly changing society only transient tendencies toward equilibrium may be noted, while in a relatively static society the ecological system may remain in rough equilibrium for a long time—the city system of the M'zab in Algeria comes to mind as an example often used by geographers.[2]

But the modern metropolis is an open system rather than a closed one. Matter and energy flow into it and leave it, and these flows may be classified in the same fashion as the other dimensions of the system. Thus migration in and out of the city is the dynamic aspect of the *P* factor. Technological flows ranging from goods and skills to manufactured forms of kinetic energy also enter and leave the system. In the area of social organization, managerial decisions made in far-flung capitals, in Federal Reserve Board conference rooms, or in national institutional headquarters may constitute inputs of grave consequence to the metropolis borne into it by the electromagnetic media of modern communication. Social psychological inputs and outputs ranging from pat-

A PARTIAL LISTING OF CLASSIFICATION CATEGORIES: QUICK REFERENCE INDEX—MANHATTAN YELLOW PAGES

Acetate fabrics
Acetate scrap
Acoustical ceilings
Adding and calculating machines
Advertising:
  Radio
  Sound truck
  Subway
  Television
Aerial photographers
Aeronautical engineers
Air conditioners
Airline companies
Air-pollution control
Airports
Automobile dealers

Buses
Business machines
Butane gas

Cadmium plating
Camping trailer
Capacitors
Cathode-ray tubes
Chlorophyll
Chromium plating
Circuits—printed and etched

Data-processing system
Duplicating machines and supplies

Earth-moving equipment
Electrical appliances

Foods-frozen—packers and distributors

Gasoline stations
Germanium
High-fidelity sound equipment

Infrared equipment
Inventories computing service

Lamps—fluorescent
Laundries—self-service
Liquid air
Loud speakers

Magnesium and magnesium products
Missile and rocket-components manufacturers
Mobile homes
Motion picture theaters
Motorcycles

Neon lighting equipment

Oceanographers
Oil burners
Outboard motors

Parking meters
Parking stations and garages
Phonograph records—retail
Plastics—Research and consulting

Radio audience analysis
Radium preparations

Shavers, electric
Silicones
Swimming pools

Television stations
Trucking

Vacuum cleaners

Water heater

X-ray apparatus

terns of prejudice to culture-conditioned preferences and ephemeral fads can also change the landscape and level of life of the region—thereby helping to create ghettos on the one hand and acres of ranch-style or, more recently, split-level suburbs on the other. And we become ever more conscious of environmental flows as they threaten us: air, water, wastes, and pollutants.

As an example of the implications of this framework of reference, consider the accompanying table. Most of these activities, which actually comprise but a small fraction of all which might have been listed, would not have been present in even the largest of cities in 1900, and the rest would have been found in a form which would scarcely reflect the relative sophistication of technology in 1967. "Trucking," for example, in 1900 had quite a different connotation than it has today. Indeed, the very existence of a sufficiently developed telephone network to justify a sizable modern directory depended on switching inventions beginning with the Strowger switch of 1891.[3] Yet every single activity listed in the table has had its effect, great or small, upon metropolitan land-use patterns. In the case of such categories as airports, earth-moving equipment, gasoline stations, motion picture theaters, parking stations, and garages the land-use effects of technological change have clearly been enormous. In the case of other activities, the separate impacts of such activities upon the use of urban land have been small or moderate, but the cumulative effect of clusters of activities has been great. In this category are the electrical and electronic goods-retailing complexes which, together with their supportive services, occupy such a prominent place both in central business districts and in satellite shopping centers throughout metropolitan America. Again, some technological innovations seem to be ubiquitous, and extremely visible wherever urban business enterprise occurs, like neon lighting, air conditioning, and various kinds of central heating. Perhaps the effects of such devices are to be understood more in the social psychological sphere of how we sense the city than in terms of their effects upon urban use of land.

Yet whether the effects of technological change are to be appreciated in terms of our changed perceptions of the city through new visual stimuli and new media of communication, or whether the use of land itself is altered, or whether—as in the case of innovations in data processing and inventory control—the socioeconomic city is reorganized as a flow center, one fact stands out. Virtually all of the technological changes which have so profoundly altered the nature of the city in the 20th century—whether innovations in metallurgical, chemical, manufacturing and process, transportation or health and medical technology—have been inextricably interrelated with major social and demographic changes. And the health-services sector is part and parcel of the changing system. Merely consider the number of problems in safety and health on the one hand, and treatments and supportive services on the other which are related to the list of the table shown. The revolutionary transformation of Manhattan's East River waterfront into an agglomerated subsystem of medical care and research which straddles the midtown central business district on both sides in some of the real estate valued highest in the world testifies to the environmental impact of this metropolitan subsystem.

The urban geographer needs, in addition to an ecological framework, a theoretical structure by means of which he may understand the spatial growth of the metropolis. One very useful approach makes use of the crucial property of the metropolis as a center of flows and communications. It is, as it were, a center of access. Karl W. Deutsch enunciates some of these views in a graphic way:

> Any metropolis can be thought of as a huge engine of communication, a device to enlarge the range and reduce the cost of individual and social choices. In the familiar telephone switchboard, the choices consist of many different lines. Plugging in the wires to connect any two lines is an act of commitment, since it implies foregoing the making of other connections. The concentration of available outlets on the switchboard permits a wider range of alternative choices than would prevail under any more dispersed arrangement. . . . The limits of the potentially useful size of a switchboard are fixed by the capacity of the type of switching and control equipment available.
>
> The facilities of the metropolis for transport and communication are the equivalent of the switchboard.[4]

In this quotation lines of thought ranging from human ecology to systems theory converge in the metaphor of the engine of communication—a system metaphor. But Deutsch extends the range and scope of his analysis by pointing out that the *effectiveness* of a metropolis may be defined as its performance measured in terms of the number of contact choices which it offers to a person in one hour of round-trip commuting time, while its *efficiency* might be measured in terms of the ratio of the effectiveness to some cost unit: how many choices could a given sum make available to a person in the city?

Given the distribution of the population and the pattern of transportation in New York in 1900 the center of access was, no doubt, central Manhattan. The structure of commercial and service activities (including medical services) which arose subsequent to that time probably did reflect the Deutsch criteria of effectiveness and efficiency. Recently intraregional demographic shifts and the revolution in commuter transportation, accompanied by diseconomies of congestion at the core, have considerably diffused the foci of greatest access—a fact reflected in the regional-shopping-center movement.

Peter Haggett has gone into finer detail than Deutsch in specifying the spatial elements which relate to the networks which support the metropolitan flow system. He points out that open-flow systems (such as metropolitan regions) are organized into five general spatial components: 1) *movements* occur along channels which together form a 2) *network;* the network is characterized by intersections of 3) *nodes,* which vary in importance and form a 4) *hierarchy;* the interstitial areas between branches of the network can be interpreted as 5) *surfaces* which may be organized into zones of similar characteristics.[5]

Suppose there is a large lawn behind the main building of a university. Across the lawn other buildings are built. In their passage among these edifices, students in their haste choose not to use the walkway around the lawn, but cut across it without regard to damaging the grass. Eventually, to the despair of the grounds keepers, dirt paths are created. Hoping to restrict the flow, and save at least part of the lawn, asphalt is laid along the paths, which forms a network. At one place, where four paths intersect, an ice-cream vendor positions himself during the warm months and forms a major node, while at minor nodes near the specific buildings students from the schools of journalism, law, medicine, and engineering arrange to meet and gather. Thus a hierarchy of nodes manifests itself, and the lawns around the central node fill up with reclining ice-cream eaters, while those around the minor nodes are less densely occupied by chatting students. If the university accepts as many new students as it graduates, and if the curricular organization is not changed, so that the buildings in the environment do not change, an equilibrium in the pattern may result.

The parable may easily be extended to the case of the growth of a suburb. Consider the pattern of change in the use of land in Staten Island attendant upon the building of the Verrazano-Narrows Bridge and its interlinked highway network. New nodes that manifest an extended range of retailing, service, and other commercial functions and thus occupy a high hierarchical level in the set of all retailing nodes are developing on plazas oriented toward crucial intersections of the new channels. Old nodes eccentric to the new network are relatively—and sometimes absolutely—diminished in hierarchical ranking. Many geographers, by utilizing the mathematics of networks and flows, have done much toward developing quantitative models of the changes in such systems.[6]

In the New York Metropolitan Regional System, the principle node has been the central business district of Manhattan. Figure 2 shows a clay-model conceptualization of the major activity centers in the region

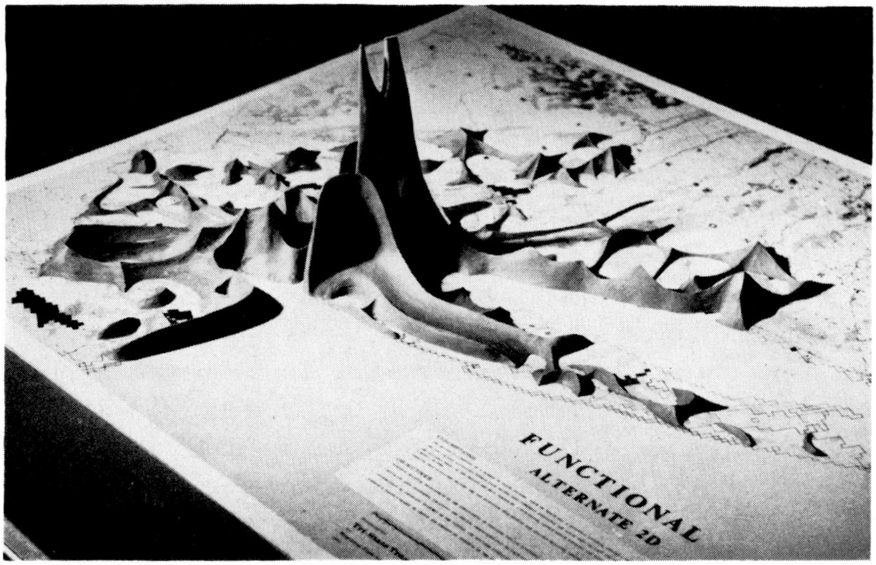

Fig. 2. Commercial activity concentration model: the New York Metropolitan Region. The height of the clay above the map surface is proportional to the commercial activity at the location. Reproduced by permission of Thomas J. Thomas, formerly of the Tri-State Transportation Commission.

developed by T. Thomas. The height of the clay is proportional to the amount of activity at the locus. Variations in the value of land in general follow the patterns of centers of access and activity and, in turn, are of the greatest influence in allocating patterns of the use of land.

In the interstital areas of the model, the "sags" in the clay, we find land surfaces primarily devoted to residential uses. These form the "flesh"—to use the terminology of Berry[7]—which grows around the flow network or commercial "skeleton," which "is determined by broader regional and supra-regional forces."[8]

In the intricate pattern of change and variation of life quality in the "residential flesh," we find concomitant variations in health problems. The pattern of access, land-value determination, and nodal hierarchy established by the skeleton is intimately related to the question of placement of service facilities—including health services. Before considering techniques for studying these let us glance at the ecology of the 19th century city in order to provide us with a benchmark for analyzing the contemporary metropolis.

The Changing Metropolitan Environment

The media assault us on all sides with stories concerning the urban crisis. The themes are familiar. The city of today is becoming uninhabitable because densities are increasing; congestion is increasing; crime and violence, health hazards, and environmental pollution are all increasing.

It is not difficult to show that the core of New York City, at least, has been decreasing in density since 1890. The density of that year, calculated by Weber[9] for Ward 10 (the vicinity southeast of Rivington Street and the Bowery) was in excess of 523 persons per acre—or 335,000 persons per square mile. That census tract of Manhattan with the highest density in 1960 was in Harlem, south of 155th Street, with a density of 247,000 persons per square mile (386 persons per acre), or about 74% of the 1890 figure. This is not an atypical instance in American cities. As the ecosystem responds to transportation advantage, the suburbs extend and the core densities diminish.

When we consider that the 1890 densities in the old Russian-Jewish ghetto were developed on a housing technology of four- or five-story old-law tenement walk-ups, with inadequate sanitation, inefficient garbage removal, and a sewage system which, at best, discharged into the adjacent East River, we may well be appalled at the crowding—in terms of number of persons per room—which the density implies. Modern sites with high-rise apartments can sustain comparable *densities* without crowding owing to the advancement of technology.

As books such as that of Asbury[10] show, crime and vice were rampant in 19th century New York, gaslight nostalgia notwithstanding. Gang warfare and semiorganized street violence can be traced back at least to the cockney gangs which formed after disadvantaged immigrant families came to New York from England following the Napoleonic Wars and the War of 1812.

As to transportation (in 1867) the arrangements were so inconvenient and congested and the pavements so bad that: ". . . a considerable part of the working population . . . spend a sixth part of their working days on the street cars or omnibuses, and the upper part of the city is made almost useless to persons engaged in any daily business of any kind. . . ."[11] Chinitz remarks that already by World War I, pier traffic in New York had slowed to a crawl.[12]

And the inevitable concomitant of congestion in a city relying on animal-powered transportation was an accumulation of urine and manure, not to mention dead animals and offal in the principal streets: a condition that staggers the mind.[13] Mandelbaum tells us that these factors, combined with inadequate sanitary drainage, resulted in a situation in which sewers in the district south of 14th Street clogged and broke, spewing their contents into the streets and turning avenues such as Broadway into sluggish streams of dark brown mud.[14] In the 1850's cellar dwellings (prone to flooding with street effluvium) housed 29,000 persons.[15] Consumption, typhus, typhoid fever, and cholera were frequent pestilences and, before 1823, yellow fever. The death rate per 1,000 in 1865 was 34.2; in 1853, 41.0; in 1849, 60.9,[16] compared to an estimated 1964 rate of 11.0—in an older population. Bearing in mind that these rates were citywide, surely the rates specific to the immigrant wards were much higher. One can conclude that the environment of New York City has improved remarkably in the last 100 years.

This is not to contradict the view that city conditions in many respects—because of neglect—are deteriorating, but rather to put the deterioration in long-term perspective. I find grounds for cautious optimism. Considering how the city as a system for supporting life has improved in the past century in the absence of over-all comprehensive planning from a health standpoint we have every reason to hope that, with diligent application of invested time and money, enough progress may be made not only to reverse the slippage but to score further net advances.

Health institutions which arose in the 19th century, and—to a certain extent—in the early 20th, were oriented toward the control of plague and pestilence in epidemic situations. Since these diseases have been brought under control the emphasis in health problems has shifted to new patterns which have been "unmasked," so to speak, by progress, and which—like urban health problems for hundreds of years—bear more heavily on the poor than the affluent. Many studies correlate the illnesses included in the following diagnostic groups with poverty: heart disease, arthritis and rheumatism, mental and nervous conditions, high blood pressure, visual impairments, orthopedic impairments, mental disorders (including schizophrenia), cancer, and infant mortality. The environment—particularly housing—seems to play an important part in a fivefold classification of complaints developed by Wilner and cited by Schorr:

1) Acute respiratory infections (colds, bronchitis, grippe), related to multiple use of toilet and water facilities, inadequate

heating or ventilation, inadequate and crowded sleeping arrangements.

2) Certain infectious diseases of childhood (measles, chickenpox, and whooping cough) related to similar causal factors.

3) Minor digestive diseases and enteritis (typhoid, dysentery, diarrhea), related to poor facilities for the cold storage of food and to inadequate washing and toilet facilities.

4) Injuries resulting from home accidents, related to crowded or inadequate kitchens, poor electrical connections, and poorly lighted and unstable stairs.

5) Infectious and noninfectious diseases of the skin, related to crowding and facilities for washing.[17]

Schorr also discusses studies which link pneumonia, tuberculosis, and lead poisoning directly to the effects of poor housing, and argues persuasively that stresses arising from crowding and the lack of personal satisfactions in a poverty-stricken environment pose mental and physical health hazards.[18] In animal populations Calhoun and Deevey have called attention to the pathologically self-destructive tendencies of animal populations when exposed to crowding stresses.[19]

But these effects—of crowding, interpersonal tension, stress, environmental hazards, and malnutrition as well—are not independent of each other. As Roemer and Kish point out,

> . . . the aggregate impact of the physical and social environment of the poor, including their housing, nutrition, occupations, and whole style of life, contributed to a burden of disease and death that blights their lives much more than among the well-to-do.
>
> The health handicaps of poverty apply to all places, rural and urban. In the urban slum, however, congested living, air pollution, lack of recreational space, and the general squalor are not mitigated even by sunshine and grass. It is true that access to medical care for rich and poor alike is greater in the cities than in rural areas. The urban poor, however, receive much less medical treatment for their illness than the well-to-do, so that a given sickness is more likely to become advanced, disabling, and even fatal. For the Negro and other ethnic minorities, the problems of poverty and ignorance are compounded by the barriers of prejudice and discrimination.[20]

The foregoing sets the task for the urban geographer interested in health. How is one to sort out—to map, as it were—the variations of these health-associated environmental, demographic, social, and psychological elements of our urban ecology, so that the spatial pattern of the need for health services may be understood? For if that can be done, there is reason to suppose that it may cast light on the problem of deploying medical technology to meet the need.

The mapping and interpretation of complexly related areal data that bear on urban populations is an area of concern to urban and medical geography.[21] The multivariate statistical technique of principal-components analysis is one such tool which I have used in studies of Manhattan and Washington, D.C.[22] It is possible to subdivide an area of study into numerous small subareas (perhaps utilizing the census-tract divisions) and prepare a data matrix of as many as 40 or 60 variables based upon elements of the environment, the population structure, the social structure, and the subcultural outlook of the residents. One may then cluster these individual variables into syndromes of association by the principal-components technique. Each syndrome has the valuable property of statistical independence from the others and can be mapped separately.

The mapped ecological regions might then be used as a guide to the probable incidence of various health problems. This would constitute, as it were, an inquiry into the variation of health needs (in contrast to demands) as they are estimated to vary within the "residential flesh" of the metropolis. There is no real reason, by the way, why mental as well as physical health needs might not be included in the same analysis.

Referring back to the model of Figure 2: these areas of varying need would constitute surfaces on the flanks and in the depressions of the clay model. It is appropriate next, having raised the question of the location of health needs, to ask where health facilities should be located to supply them most effectively.

In studying the nodes, channels, and networks of access which serve the retailing, service, and commercial demands of the metropolis, urban geographers have evolved a body of theory called Central Place Theory, which helps to interpret the spatial arrangement of tertiary activity in general and may be specifically applicable to health planning.

Briefly, every kind of commercial establishment (such as grocery stores, furniture stores, department stores, theaters, etc.) which satisfies the demands of the urban population for goods and services may be characterized in terms of its *range* and *threshold.* The range of a good or service is the distance—often expressed in units of elapsed travel time—which a consumer is willing to travel in order to avail himself of the commodity. Frequently purchased articles and very inexpensive articles tend to have smaller ranges than those which are expensive or infrequently consumed. The small grocery outlet is typical of a small-range establishment, while an opera house has a very large range.

The threshold is defined as the minimum amount of disposable income which suffices to support an establishment selling the good or service in question. Obviously if the circle described by the range of an establishment encloses a market area which possesses an amount of purchasing power less than the threshold, then that establishment cannot survive there.

High-range and high-threshold establishments need to locate at the principal intersections of access in the commercial and transportation "skeleton" of the metropolis by bidding for and securing location at these prized sites in the real estate market. Lower-scale activities seek out less central locations that lead to a differentiation of commercial nodes by a hierarchical level of activity after the manner implied by the model of Haggett. In Figure 2 we discern this effect in the varying heights of the activity peaks and ridges above the plain.

As the central city diminishes in the socioeconomic status of its population the disposable income per acre which provides the thresholds of commercial activities decreases. Low-order, local activities which are not at metropolitan wide-access nodes have their thresholds undercut, and often relocate where the more affluent population has moved.[23] Medical practitioners are typical, in many ways, of small-business entrepreneurs who, as providers of a service, are subject to these stresses. Their movement to the suburbs is akin to the movement of other local tertiary establishments.

Since the density of medical practitioners forms, in turn, the threshold for ancillary and supportive services such as laboratories, pharmacies, and the like, these too will follow; they thereby generate an over-all metropolitan shift toward a geographical pattern resembling an outer ring richer in local medical services that surrounds an inner ring poorer in local services which, in turn, surrounds a core of major medical institutional facilities whose mobility is limited by fixed investment and inertia. How can major treatment facilities be made available to the perimeter? How can local medical services be made available to the inner ring? These questions imply the need for metropolitan area-wide planning.

Kerr White in an excellent paper has elaborated on some of these health-facility supply problems.[24] He criticizes, among other things, the lack of coordination of efforts in the allocation of human medical resources, the inadequate communications which exist between different sources and levels in the hierarchy of personal health services, and the failure of previous attempts to regionalize health services on traditional categorical bases—whether by disease, geography, methods of financing, or traditional functional emphasis. In my view these telling points are reflected in the process sketched above. Berry raises a question which particularly bears on the last point. He finds that the traditional gross categories of tertiary activity often utilized for urban economic study break down when the aim of analysis is to study the fine structure of commercial location, and that "multiple shades of specialization" must be recognized.[25]

We might suggest that—for planning purposes—a major effort be made to catalogue the separate activities—the multiple shades of specialization of activity—that go to make up the body of "health care," and that these activities be studied so as to discover which of them most need to be located together in interdependent clusters. What, then, is the mean range and threshold of each cluster? If this were ascertained then it might be possible to plan the location and spacing of medical facilities in a more rational manner. This kind of study can be done for other types of activities, for instance in planning the location and makeup of regional shopping centers. Recently, in fact, the Regional Planning Association has published a volume in which commercial employment centers are located in connection with transportation development in Manhattan in a manner consonant with many of the views expressed here.[26]

I feel that Kerr White is probably correct *in principle* when he suggests a regionalization of health facilities in a manner resembling that of the United States airlines network, but I prefer to use as a model the network of urban tertiary activity because of its similarities in structure and trend to the health-care network. This also seems to be suggested by the papers of Cherkasky and Pellegrino, which provide interesting insights into the feasibility of the approach suggested here.[27]

In summary, then, it seems to me that urban geography may possibly offer two methodological models applicable to planning for health-care centers. The first would utilize ecological methods to study the distribution of the various differential areas of health needs essential to the estimate of specific-need thresholds. The second might apply some of the approaches of Central Place Theory to the problem of analyzing the supply side of the question. In this regard it might be useful to study the activity structure of the health industry in order to establish activity clusters. These might then be located according to the relations that exist between the surfaces of need and the transportation network in the light of considerations of range and threshold.

REFERENCES

1. Duncan, O. D. Human Ecology and Population Studies. In: Hauser, P. M. and Duncan, O. D. *The Study of Population.* Chicago, Univ. of Chicago Press, 1959. Schnore, L. F. *The Urban Scene.* New York, Free Press, 1965.
2. Carey, G. W. and Schwartzberg, J. *Teaching Population Geography.* New York, Teachers Coll. Press, 1969.
3. Feder, H. S. and Spencer, A. E. Telephone switching. *Scient. Amer. 207:* 133-43, 1962.
4. Deutsch, K. W. On social communication and the metropolis. *Daedalus 90:* 99-110, 1961.
5. Haggett, P. *Locational Analysis in Human Geography.* New York, St. Martin's Press, 1966.
6. Chorley, R. J. and Haggett, P., eds. *Socio-Economic Models in Geography.* New York, Univ. Paperbacks, 1967, p. 34.
7. Berry, B. J. L. Internal structure of the city. *Law Contemp. Problems. 30:* 111-19, 1965.
8. Ibid., p. 119.
9. Weber, A. F. *The Growth of Cities in the Nineteenth Century.* Ithaca, N. Y., Cornell Univ. Press, 1965. Originally published 1899.
10. Asbury, H. *The Gangs of New York.* New York, Knopf, 1928.
11. Mandelbaum, S. J. *Boss Tweed's New York.* New York, Wiley, 1965, p. 15.
12. Chinitz, B., *Freight and the Metropolis.* Cambridge, Mass, Harvard Univ. Press, 1960, pp. 37-40.
13. Mandelbaum, *op. cit.,* p. 65. Duffy, J. *A History of Public Health in New York City, 1625-1866.* New York, Russell Sage Foundation, 1968.
14. Mandelbaum, *op. cit.,* p. 14.
15. Handlin, O. *The Newcomers.* Cambridge, Mass., Harvard Univ. Press, 1959, p. 16.
16. Duffy, *op. cit.,* pp. 575-77.
17. Schorr, A. L. *Slums and Social Insecurity.* Washington, D.C., Govt. Print. Off., 1966, p. 14.
18. Ibid., pp. 14-25.
19. Calhoun, J. B. Population density and social pathology. *Scient. Amer. 206:*139-48, 1962. Deevey, E. S., The hare and the haruspex: A cautionary tale. *Amer. Scient. 50:*339-53, 1962.
20. Roemer, M. I. and Kish, A. I. Health, Poverty and the Medical Mainstream. In: Bloomberg, W., Jr. and Schmandt, H. J. *Power, Poverty and Urban Policy.* Berkeley, Calif., Sage Publications, 1968, pp. 183-84.
21. Armstrong, R. W. Computer graphics in medical geography. *Proceedings IGU 6:*69-74, 1966. Hopps, H. C., et al. *The*

Mapping of Disease Project. Washington, D.C., U.S. Armed Forces Institute of Pathology. Harvard Univ. Institute of Computer Graphics, *SYMAP Program.*

22. Carey, G. W. The regional interpretation of Manhattan population and housing patterns through factor analysis. *Geog. Rev.,* pp. 551-69, 1966. Carey, G. W., Macomber, L. and Greenberg, M. Educational and demographic factors in the urban geography of Washington, D.C. *Geog. Rev.,* pp. 515-37, 1968. Murdie, R. A. *Factorial Ecology of Metropolitan Toronto,* 1951-1961. Univ. of Chicago, Dept. of Geog. Research Paper 116, 1969. Simmons, J. W. *Toronto's Changing Retail Complex.* Univ. of Chicago, Dept. of Geog., Research Paper 104, 1966.
23. Berry, B. J. L. *Commercial Structure and Commercial Blight.* University of Chicago, Department of Geography Research Paper 85, 1963.
24. White, K. L. Personal Health Services: Defects, Dilemmas, and New Directions. In: *Social Policy for Health Care.* New York, New York Acad. Med., 1969.
25. Berry, B. J. L. *Geography of Market Centers and Retail Distribution.* West Englewood Cliffs, N.J., Prentice-Hall, 1967, p. 46.
26. Regional Plan Association. *Urban Design Manhattan.* New York, Viking Press, 1969.
27. Cherkasky, M. Resources Needed to Meet Effectively Expected Demands for Service ,and Pellegrino, E. D. Regionalization: An Integrated Effort of Medical School, Community and Practicing Physician. In: *New Directions in Public Policy for Health Care.* New York, New York Acad. Med., 1966.

THE PROBLEM OF PAIN IN PARAPLEGIA AND TETRAPLEGIA*

L. S. MICHAELIS

Research Fellow
National Spinal Injury Centre
Stoke Mandeville Centre, England

WHEN you invite a foreign speaker you rightly expect him to shed some light on a problem of your work. If he be famous the radiance of his "halo" will do. If he is almost unknown, as I am myself, he will have to bring with him the old two dry sticks and kindling. He will rub the sticks hard to produce a spark, to light the kindling. And if you help me blow, first by your attention and, later, by your discussion, we may see something more clearly than before.

It is odd, is it not, that we should discuss pain in patients whose much more serious problem is that in many cases they cannot and do not feel any pain. This, in fact, is one of the main stumbling blocks for the doctor not experienced in their treatment. The doctor must do without the main indication most patients give as to where he is to look for further guidance in diagnosis. Gross injury may happen in a paralyzed limb, serious disease may go on for years below the level of the complete neurological lesion without either the patient or his doctor suspecting, at least at first, that there is anything wrong.

THREE EXAMPLES OF UNSUSPECTED LESIONS

1) A heavily built man, with severe spasticity from a complete paraplegia, has had extensive pressure sores which have at last been healed during many months in bed. He sits in his wheelchair and tries to put on his shoes. To do this he has to pull up the paralyzed leg, put the ankle across the other knee, and fix the ankle with one hand while he is sliding the shoe on with the other. Just then he has a violent flexor spasm at his hip, as he has had so often before. But this time it occurs while he himself has fixed the ankle. There is a funny noise, he feels a little dazed, and the leg seems much less rigid. If he is in the hospital at the time he may report it or not. The diagonal fracture

*Presented at a combined meeting of the Section on Physical Medicine and Rehabilitation and the New York Society of Physical Medicine and Rehabilitation, October 1, 1969.

through the shaft of the osteoporotic femur may pass unnoticed until days later, when the patient feels weak, looks pale, and finds a dark purple discoloration on the inside of his thigh. Even now an often enormous hematoma from a fracture may not be recognized. An undetected supracondylar fracture of the femur underlying a sudden effusion of the knee joint is not at all uncommon after physiotherapy given for a contracture.

2) A parson injured in the war had become completely paraplegic below the ninth thoracic level. Admitted to our center about two years after his injury, he has made an excellent recovery. His pressure sores are healed. But from time to time he has flare-ups of an established infection of his urinary tract. He reports regularly for controls, is in good general health and works as parson to a residential school. Everyone calls him "the Bishop." Then, about 12 years after his injury, he is admitted with another urinary flare-up, with its rigor, rise of temperature to 104, vomiting, and severe malaise. Appropriate treatment is given, but on the fourth day the temperature is still high and his general condition low. He should have recovered on the fourth day, as so often before. The plain x ray of the abdomen had shown no stones in the urinary tract. An intravenous pyelogram was not done because of his fever and raised blood urea.

The patient is rather stout. There is no tenderness or resistance over either kidney. If his condition is due to urinary infection, which side is responsible? A retrograde pyelogram is the only means to find out. On the right the ureteral catheter does not go beyond the middle third of the ureter and, after injection, a complete block is shown. At operation a right-sided pyonephrosis is found due to a hairpin kink, a stricture, and a minute stone of the ureter. The ureter is split, straightened, and splinted with a T tube. The patient makes an uneventful recovery. Urea and intravenous pyelogram are normal again six weeks after the operation and have remained so until now, almost 15 years later. All this happened without pain which, in the nonparalyzed, would have made the very urgent diagnosis abundantly clear.

3) A young girl, healthy except for meningioma of the spinal cord, had the tumor removed. She remains completely paraplegic below the first thoracic level and very spastic for three years. Then, at home, she develops a sacral pressure sore. She is admitted to the center, the sore is cleaned and, after some weeks, excised and closed. She is nursed in

the prone position. One week after this minor operation she collapses without warning. Pulmonary embolism? Spontaneous collapse of a lung? No proper signs. Reluctantly, because of the recent scar over the sacrum from the operation she is turned on her back. The abdomen is as hard as it often was before, owing to spasms, but now, in collapse, the spasms in the legs are almost gone. Intra-abdominal catastrophe, perforation of an appendix, an ulcer, or acute pancreatitis? A laparotomy is done. A large gastric ulcer of at least three years' standing is found perforated into the lesser sack. A partial gastrectomy results in a very satisfactory recovery. Was it really possible that during those years she had felt nothing? At the end of a long, searching, and entirely negative history-taking she casually mentioned that two years before she had been treated by her doctor for "rheumatism" in her shoulder.

The first two cases are examples of the dangers of the inability to feel pain; the third shows how pain in the shoulder—via the phrenic nerve—can be the only signal, easily mistaken, of an insidious and potentially killing condition below the level of the neurological lesion.

So far we may say that if a paraplegic feels any pain at all, it may quite easily be due to causes other than the common ones. From no pain and misleading pain we now come to pain proper. Here the accompanying tentative diagram may help.

Pain Above the Level of the Lesion

There is, of course, no reason why a para- or tetraplegic should not feel pain above the lesion as would any other person. Toothache and earache are examples. Where injury of the head and spinal cord are combined, as they not rarely are, the recognition and assessment of level and completeness of cervical or lower lesions can be very difficult owing to diminished or absent consciousness, even after full recovery from cerebral concussion or contusion. But headache may be the predominant pain. And headache, hard enough to diagnose properly in the nonparalyzed, acquires quite a new significance in paraplegia and tetraplegia.

The most striking cause, of course, is vasodilatation of the meningeal and cerebral vessels as part of the distension syndrome of the bladder, less so of the bowels, but occurring most severely during childbirth when there are high lesions.

Robbed of normal communication with the brain by the physio-

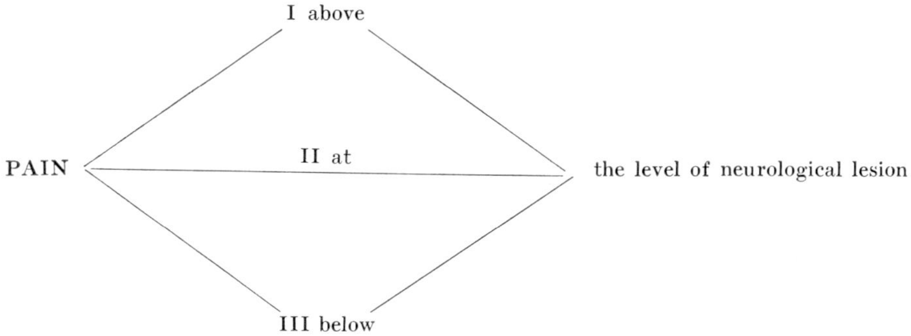

logical interruption of the main cable, the cord, the body has to mobilize all it has in the way of substitutes to get its message past the barrier. The situation corresponds to that in an enemy-occupied country with all communication by telephone, radio, and television interrupted or watched. The "underground" must get messages through on foot, bicycle, rowboat, or cart. Slow, uncertain, but eventually effective, the vegetative nervous system, only temporarily stunned in the first few days or weeks of spinal shock, takes on more and more of these functions. Its signals are not known outside paraplegia or tetraplegia. They are less specific, but they must be watched for and acted upon promptly, so that no serious harm should be done to the patient. The automatism of the bladder, defective for any reason, the blocked catheter, extreme constipation, or pseudo-Hirschsprung dilatation of the colon may all produce the distension-syndrome with its violent pounding headache, the high-red face, stopped-up nose, and profound sweating. In many cases the blood pressure rises considerably, nowhere more than during labor pains in the tetraplegic woman whose systolic blood pressure normally is no more than 90 to 100 mm. We have monitored rises to and beyond 250 mm. exactly coinciding with the uterine contraction and have recognized the danger of cerebral hemorrhage which has been reported elsewhere but not seen by us.

Patients may be having attacks of migraine or trigeminial neuralgia both before and after becoming paraplegic. They will have to be treated as before, except that all paraplegics and, particularly, tetraplegics have an altered reaction to drugs; mostly they need fewer high doses as, e.g., in general anesthesia; all of them are in greater danger of becoming addicts. The warm-hearted but uninstructed physician who prescribes for the "poor cripple" too much of whatever he asks for does him no good and, in the long run, causes serious harm.

Pain at the Level of the Lesion

In the newly injured two facts stand out.

1) Many a patient who receives an open or closed injury of the spinal cord, without losing consciousness or without even being dazed, recalls no pain, but rather a dull violent thud in the neck or the back; another may feel a violent pain from fracture either at once or on being moved or turned.

2) In combined injuries, let us say a fractured humerus and a dorso-lumbar fracture-dislocation with paraplegia, the pain in the arm often is so much greater than the pain in the back that it almost hides the other. In this way a fracture of the spine and paraplegia may be overlooked.

In both instances pain close to the level of the neurological lesion occurs during the first week or two due to the splinting spasm of the most distal normally innervated part of the erector trunci. With reduction, conservative or operative, it quickly subsides. But while it lasts it may require some analgesic aid.

This pain will disappear entirely if immobilization is continued long enough to assure stability of the bony injury. Any pain at this site that occurs during the first or second week after the patient has been allowed to sit up and bear weight must be taken as a warning of as yet incomplete stability or formation of callus. Bedrest and x-ray controls are needed again until this "fracture pain" is gone.

In the meantime, however, a different type of pain may have made its appearance, starting one or two months after the accident, sometimes earlier, sometimes later. It is true root pain, radiating into the arms in cervical lesions, encircling the chest or abdomen in dorsal and lumbar lesions, into the legs in cauda equina lesions or in incomplete lesions at all levels. We believe that such pain is due to irritation of an only partly damaged proximal segment and to its recovery over a few months. One can reassure the patient that, in time, it will disappear, even if it is not just pain and hyperalgesia but that strange and terrible phenomenon: hyperpathia.

As you know, hyperpathia is a form of paraesthesia in which the sensation of pain is radically altered. If you prick a hyperpathic zone with a pin, even if you touch it or permit it to be touched by pajamas or bedclothes, an apparently unbearable form of profound discomfort is produced which makes the most placid patient want to hit the doctor. This feeling of hyperpathic pain stays longer and spreads wider than does an ordinary prick or touch.

It rarely extends over more than one or two dermatomes, bilaterally or on one side only, not always symmetrically. While it lasts everything must be done to protect the patient against its being provoked. All staff members must be instructed, bed cradles must keep off pressure or rubbing, turning must be done without touching the areas. Drugs are rarely much help, but the truthful reassurance that hyperpathia will first diminish and then, in the majority of cases, disappear, will encourage the patient to "grin and bear it" while it lasts. Hyperpathic pain is not the most severe but the most upsetting form of pain in patients with injury or disease of the cord.

Another form of ordinary pain at, above, and below the spinal lesion is purely and simply iatrogenic. Happily we see less of it, since fixation in plaster—either in corset or in bed—have been almost universally abandoned, and passive and active movement by the physiotherapist from day one onward has become standard.

This was diffuse, often intense pain in the back due to adhesions between the superficial fascia of the back and the fasciae of the back muscles several weeks or months after the accident. Such cases are easily recognized from the history and from other signs of neglect (urinary infection, pressure sores, and contractures), and they are distinguished by a particularly low morale, due to despair as much as anemia. Blood-transfusions, gradual withdrawal of analgesics and active mobilization of all joints by every possible form of physiotherapy and occupational exercise and, later, athletics will transform such victims of the "ancien regime" into effective, ambitious, and successful members of society again.

That they have lost months or even years of their lives and cost thousands of their own or someone else's money, that they have not produced anything and have not paid taxes, is the fault of their doctors, not theirs.

Pain Below the Level of the Lesion

In complete para- or tetraplegia normal pain impulses cannot get through. Such impulses, as we have already seen, are translated into the much less well-defined messages sent via sympathetic pathways, particularly those of the blood vessels. These pains may take many forms of varying intensity and location. They may be defined in many individual ways by patients who, according to their pain threshold, self-control and, most of all, morale, will call them "heavy," "dull aches," "fullness to bursting point," "stabbing," "burning or busting," "tight bands," "hot pins." They may extend over one or both lower limbs or be located in patches not conforming to individual dermatomes. They may start on the day the patient sits up in a wheelchair or stands upright for the first time, they may disappear as soon as the legs are lifted or the patient lies down, or they may last through day and night. They may be worst at night. In trying to assess the severity and type of such pain the physician who has treated the patient without interruption or transfer from the day of the accident to later stages of rehabilitation has the very real advantage of already knowing character, temperament, pain threshold, motivation, and resistance to optimum collaboration. He will either succeed or fail to gain and maintain the trust of his patient.

The specialist in rehabilitation who does not see his patient until weeks or months after the onset of involvement of the cord, either traumatic or medical, has to start from scratch. And not rarely primary treatment has been either technically or psychologically faulty, if only because the patient was the only paraplegic in a traumatic, neurosurgical, or neurological service—a "foreign body" in a community of patients with whom he had little in common. The psychological advantages arising from immediate and uninterrupted treatment of a para- or tetraplegic in a special center are far-reaching; and incidence and severity of pain as problems are much less in such facilities than outside them.

No facile distinction between "organic" and "functional" pain is possible. A wide spectrum of psychosomatic influences, varying according to age, sex, education, race, familial and financial circumstances, guilt feelings or their absence, endogenous or exogenous depression, etc., all play a part. The cause for suddenly increased pain may be constipation or receipt of a disappointing letter, jealousy for the interest of the doctor, dislike of a physiotherapist, an outcry of self-pity, or the wish to dominate all around him or, more frequently, all persons around her.

This kind of "pain" turns out to be not pain as we feel it, but an intense discomfort; happily, it tends to diminish and, in most cases, disappear as rehabilitation progresses. One rare location for it is the anus and rectum. Having patiently and persistently trained our patients to acquire strictly timed habits of automatic emptying of the bowels, we may find that this has led to a morbid obsession, of which intense local discomfort is the outward sign. This is by no means restricted to neurotic personalities. My most striking example of such a case was a highly intelligent and educated naval officer with a complete tetraplegia who, on many special neurological examinations, never showed any signs of "sacral sparing" which would have rendered this discomfort more understandable as a kind of hyperpathia.

Very rare are the instances of persistent true root-pain, characterized by their intensity and strict conformity to one or two dermatomes. They are more common after gunshot or stab wounds, myelograms, and operations on the spine than after conservative postural reduction of closed injuries. Such pain can produce a lasting and serious problem of choice of therapy.

Therapy

There are a few basic points to be made on the choice of therapeutic measures.

1) The general physical condition of the patient must be raised. The anemic patient, toxic from infected pressure sores, with a roaring urinary infection and severe constipation, will—rightly—moan and rationalize his feeling of weakness and dependence into pain. He needs blood transfusions, a high-protein diet, proper treatment of sores, bladder, and bowels—not analgesic drugs which do not help and only make him an addict to drugs when he is already an addict to "pain."

2) The emotional state of the patient so treated will respond, sometimes within a week. With such patients we used to receive accompanying letters which explained that the patient was uncooperative and full of complaints. The sad truth is that in such cases the patient is dead right if not yet right dead.

You can set such a patient upon the road to active participation in your program. The need for analgesics can be abolished by vitamins B and C. As you fight the toxicity and infection with appropriate antibiotics, you must mobilize him, find out his hobbies, and keep him occupied all day; pain will then retreat into oblivion.

I am not an expert in applied pharmacology and I am a skeptic as far as the effect of analgesics is concerned. After all, each patient is his own laboratory. In any case, since the pharmaceutical firms persist in giving different names in different countries to identical drugs, and since the higher reaches of chemistry are Chinese to me, I could not recommend any special medication suitable in New York. My advice is: give as little medication as possible, as rarely as possible, and mix tranquilizers with analgesics rather than raise the dosage. Beware of alcohol—at least for the patient—since his kidneys cannot stand it. Many a fracture of a paralyzed limb has occurred when a patient in a wheelchair has lost control after a few glasses of beer and has fallen out of it.

Where there is persistent, severe, strictly localized pain in an otherwise stable patient it may be necessary to try phenol blocks of individual peripheral nerves or of posterior roots.

In complete neurological lesions of older patients intrathecal alcohol blocks for pain may be indicated. But this is rare. Only about 5% of more than 200 alcohol blocks have been done in our center for pain, none in the last 10 years or so.

The intrathecal alcohol block is a sledgehammer method, to be reserved for those in real despair from either pain or spasticity. It is permanently effective in the large majority of cases. However, it has disadvantages. It destroys a well-established automatism of the bladder and bowels. The bladder will have to be expressed or a stay catheter worn, to be changed at least twice weekly. Constipation may be very difficult to overcome. It weakens potency in young men and it transforms any incomplete paraplegia into a complete one. Constipation must therefore be handled with great care and, for at least a week, the patient is in a kind of spinal shock threatening pressure sores unless nursing and turning is perfect.

The need for operations should not arise. Rhizotomy is made superfluous by its chemical equivalent, the alcohol block. Chordotomy is resorted to only in extreme instances, where unfortunately "addiction to pain" not rarely recurs after some weeks or months, and leukotomy goes, perhaps, a little too far, even if the direction may be right.

I must have disappointed many of you who hoped for sophisticated neurophysiological data, for pharmaceutical breakthroughs, or for what the great sardonic Karl Kraus of Vienna called psycholozelachs. All I could invite you to was a walk through my garden of experience to look at the weeds.

MOUNT SINAI'S APPROACH TO THE EAST HARLEM COMMUNITY*

CHARLES H. GOODRICH

Associate Professor of Community Medicine
Director, Division of Health Care

MARGARET OLENDZKI

Assistant Professor of Community Medicine
Coordinator of Research

KURT W. DEUSCHLE

Lavanburg Professor and Chairman

Department of Community Medicine
The Mount Sinai School of Medicine
New York, N. Y.

INTRODUCTION

LIKE most medical schools in the United States today, The Mount Sinai School of Medicine is concerned about the widening gap between the capabilities of medicine and the actual delivery of medical care services at the community level. The gap is especially noticeable in deprived communities such as exist in nearly every major city. Rich resources are available in the medical schools and hospitals in our cities, but a number of barriers exist between them and the health problems in their communities. With few exceptions the hospitals serve only the patients who apply to them for care or whose private physicians are on the staff and have admitting privileges. A local person may fail to be admitted to the inpatient service of a hospital in his area if the hospital does not operate an ambulance service or if he does not have an "interesting" disease. Ambulant patients may be discouraged by clinic quotas, inconvenient hours, long waits even in the emergency room, or fees beyond their means.

As a result of these rigid and dysfunctional policies, the hospital may find its excellent specialty resources devoting more and more of their expertise to less and less of the pressing health problems of society. The task of community medicine, as envisioned at Mount Sinai, is to

*Presented at a meeting of the Subcommittee on Social Policy for Health Care, Committee on Medicine in Society, June 17, 1969.

identify health problems in the community by means of epidemiological techniques, and then unlock resources in the medical center and bring them to bear on the most urgent problems of the community. The Department of Community Medicine should form an important bridge between the specialized services of the medical center and the people outside who need these services.

Mount Sinai, through its various affiliated hospitals and other health institutions, has a number of communities it can try to serve in this way. It is perhaps appropriate to begin with Mount Sinai Hospital's own neighborhood of East Harlem, and to discuss the approach of the medical center to this community as a prototype. This model may be found to have wider applicability to other teaching medical centers and other urban areas.

In this paper we review first the structure of the Department of Community Medicine that has been developed to attempt this linking task. We describe briefly the East Harlem community and the existing health resources. Then we review the hospital-based programs and community-based projects that we have begun to develop in response to the community's expressed desire for help. A discussion follows of the methods being developed to establish baseline data and to monitor the results. In the concluding section we consider the principles upon which this approach to the health-care system of the community is based.

Development of the Department of Community Medicine

The chairman of the Department of Community Medicine has organized practitioners of the traditional public health disciplines, such as epidemiology, biostatistics, and nutrition, and the newer behavioral sciences, such as health economics and medical sociology, into a team which will attempt this new role of identifying and solving health problems in the community. The Division of Health Care is the operational or service arm of the department, responsible for utilizing the talents of these academic disciplines in attaining this goal. We believe that the new health-care system for East Harlem should combine the traditional responsibility of the public-health sector and the clinical medical-care system into a health-care system which unites preventive, curative, and environmental medicine. The medical students will play an important role both in developing the new system and in working within it in the future.

The functions of the Department of Community Medicine can be summarized as follows:

1) to apply the techniques of epidemiological and behavioral science to the identification of health problems in the community;

2) to attempt a solution by unlocking available "numerator" medical resources and putting them in touch with the "denominator" community health problems;

3) to develop an appropriate body of knowledge—the science of community medicine; and

4) to train health professionals in this work.

The objective is eventual improvement of the health-care system.

Dr. George James, formerly commissioner of health of New York City, was the first chairman of the department for the two years following its inception in July 1966. Under his leadership a team representing the various disciplines relevant to community medicine began to assemble. In July 1968 Mount Sinai appointed Dr. Kurt Deuschle, who originally coined the term "community medicine" and in 1960 established the first department of that name at the University of Kentucky Medical School, as chairman of the Mount Sinai Department of Community Medicine.

Between 1966 and 1968 a clinical base within the hospital was established by Dr. Charles Goodrich, the director of ambulatory care. The role of community medicine within the medical center evolved into a coordinating one, with the increasing academic resources of the department being brought to bear on the priority medical problems in the institution, particularly in the area of ambulatory care. Working jointly with the other clinical departments, a family-care unit was established and the emergency-care area was upgraded. Various other programs were instituted to change the character of the hospital's relation to the community: for instance, an ombudsman was placed within the outpatient department to handle the complaints of patients and to guide patients in danger of getting "lost" in the administrative machinery; and a community-relations department was set up to coordinate approaches to the community. At the same time there was widespread and increasing contact with representatives from local groups in East Harlem. A special effort was made not to promise too much too soon. It was made clear that no medical-care programs in the community were going to be forthcoming quickly: the problems of

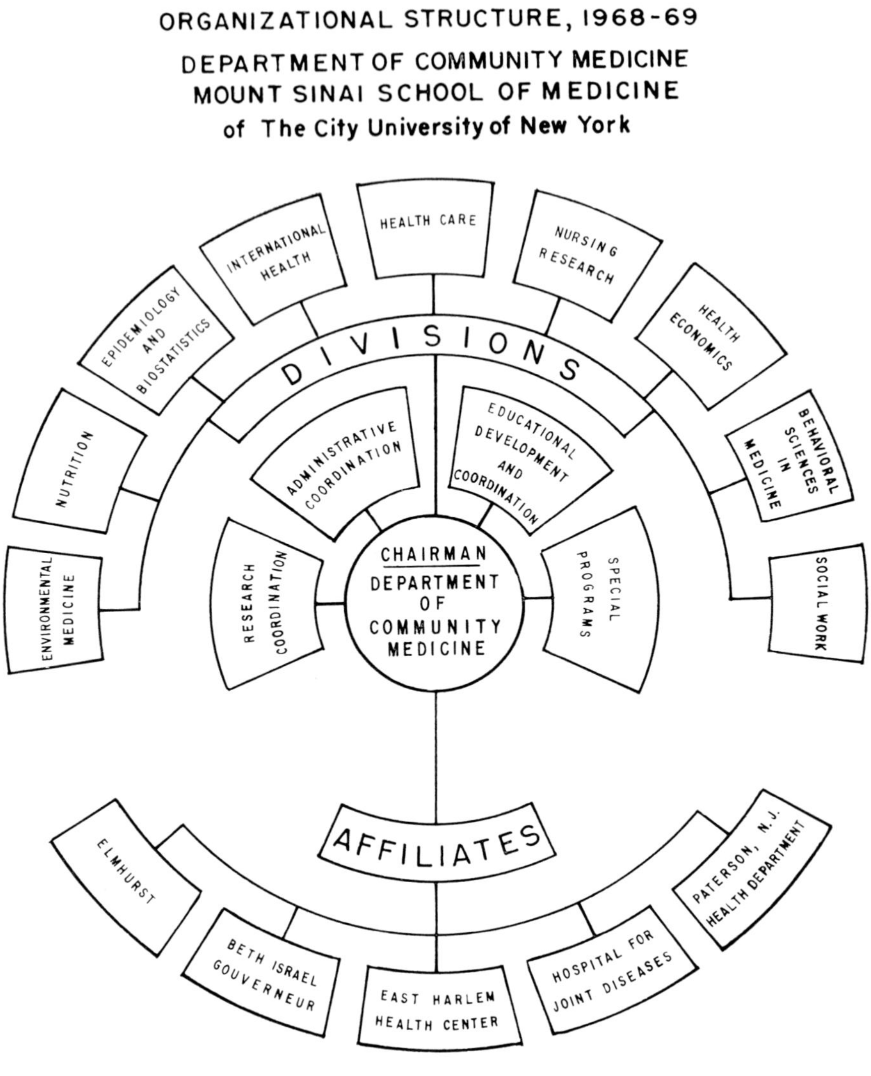

Figure 1

caring for patients within the institution itself, especially in the Outpatient Department (OPD), comprised the first priority.

Dr. James began to attract leaders in health economics (Dr. Victor Fuchs), medical sociology (Dr. Samuel Bloom), and international health (Dr. Rodolphe Coigney). When these had been added to the existing faculty in environmental medicine (Dr. Irving Selikoff) and nutrition (Dr. George Christakis) and the groundwork for the department had

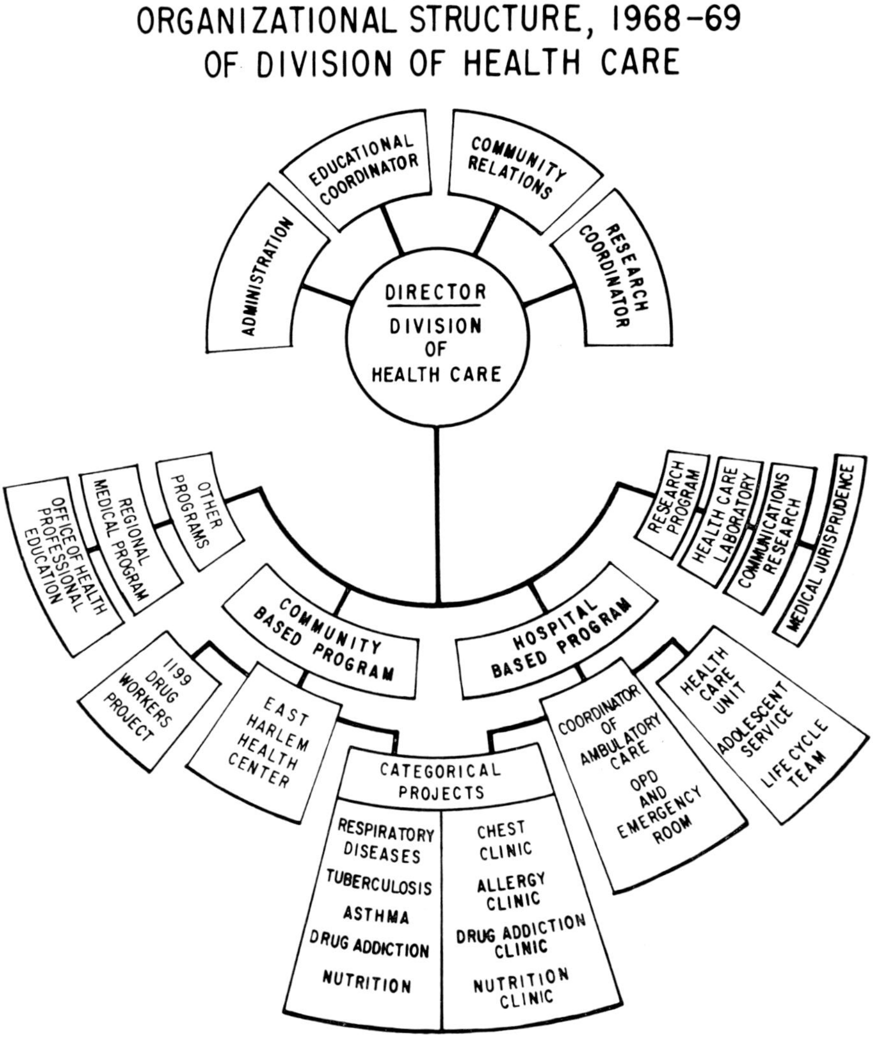

Figure 2

been laid, Dr. Deuschle joined the staff and organized the department into a clinical whole.

New faculty members for the Department of Community Medicine were recruited, and the department was consolidated into nine divisions (Figure 1). The public-health disciplines—environmental medicine, nutrition, epidemiology and biostatistics, and international health—were joined by the appropriate behavioral science disciplines—health economics, behavioral science in medicine—and by social work and

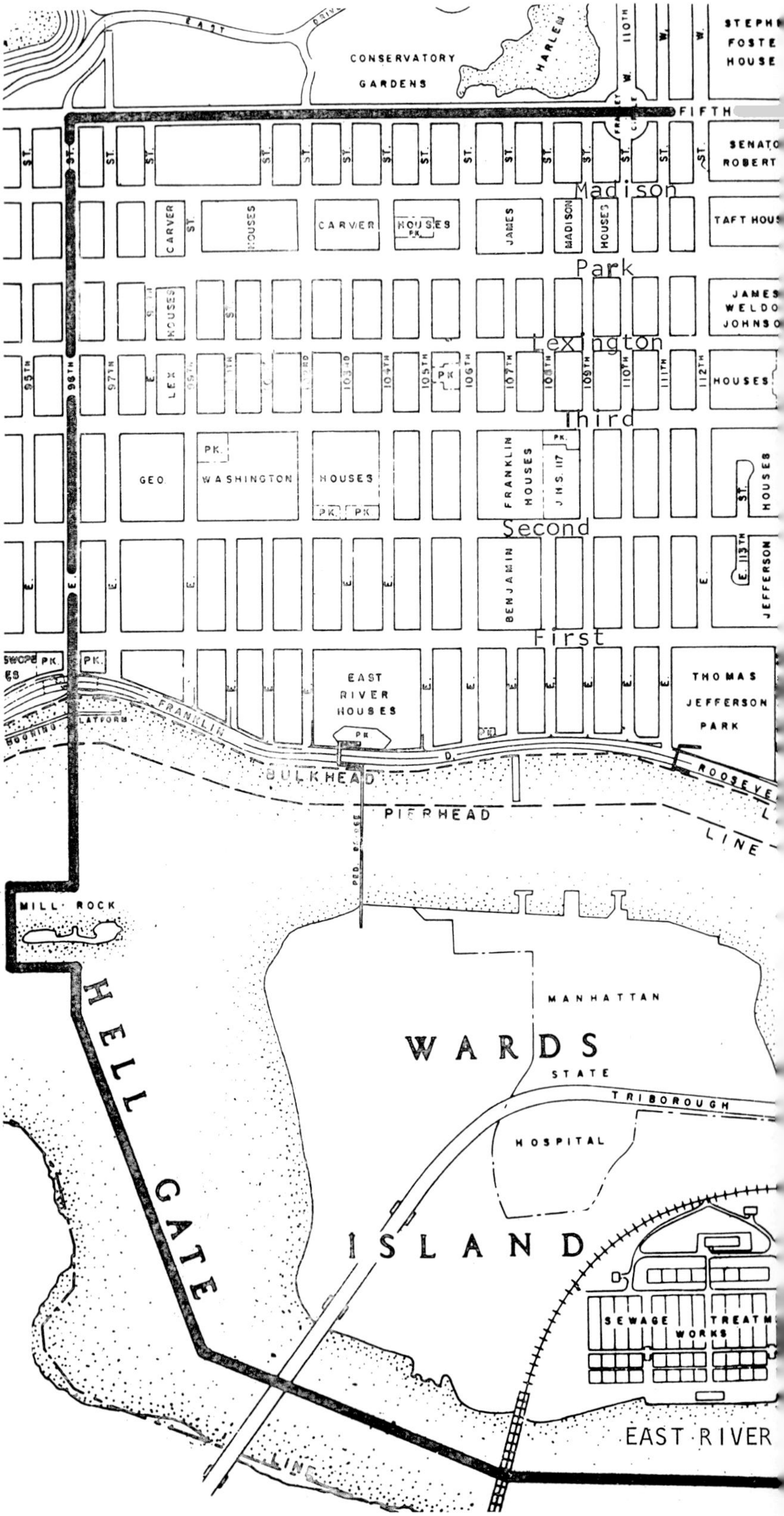

EAST DRIVE
CONSERVATORY
GARDENS
HARLEM
FIFTH
FOSTE
HOUSE
SENATO
ROBERT
Madison
CARVER
HOUSES
CARVER HOUSES
JAMES
MADISON
HOUSES
TAFT HOUS
Park
JAMES
WELDO
JOHNSO
Lexington
95TH
96TH
97TH
LEX
105TH
106TH
107TH
108TH
109TH
110TH
111TH
112TH
HOUSES
Third
GEO.
WASHINGTON
HOUSES
PK.
FRANKLIN
HOUSES
J.H.S. 117
HOUSES
Second
BENJAMIN
E. 113TH
JEFFERSON
First
PK.
EAST
RIVER
HOUSES
THOMAS
JEFFERSON
PARK
FRANKLIN
D.
ROOSEVE
BULKHEAD
PIERHEAD
LINE
MILL ROCK
HELL GATE
MANHATTAN
WARDS
STATE
TRIBOROUGH
HOSPITAL
ISLAND
SEWAGE
WORKS
EAST RIVER

Figure 3

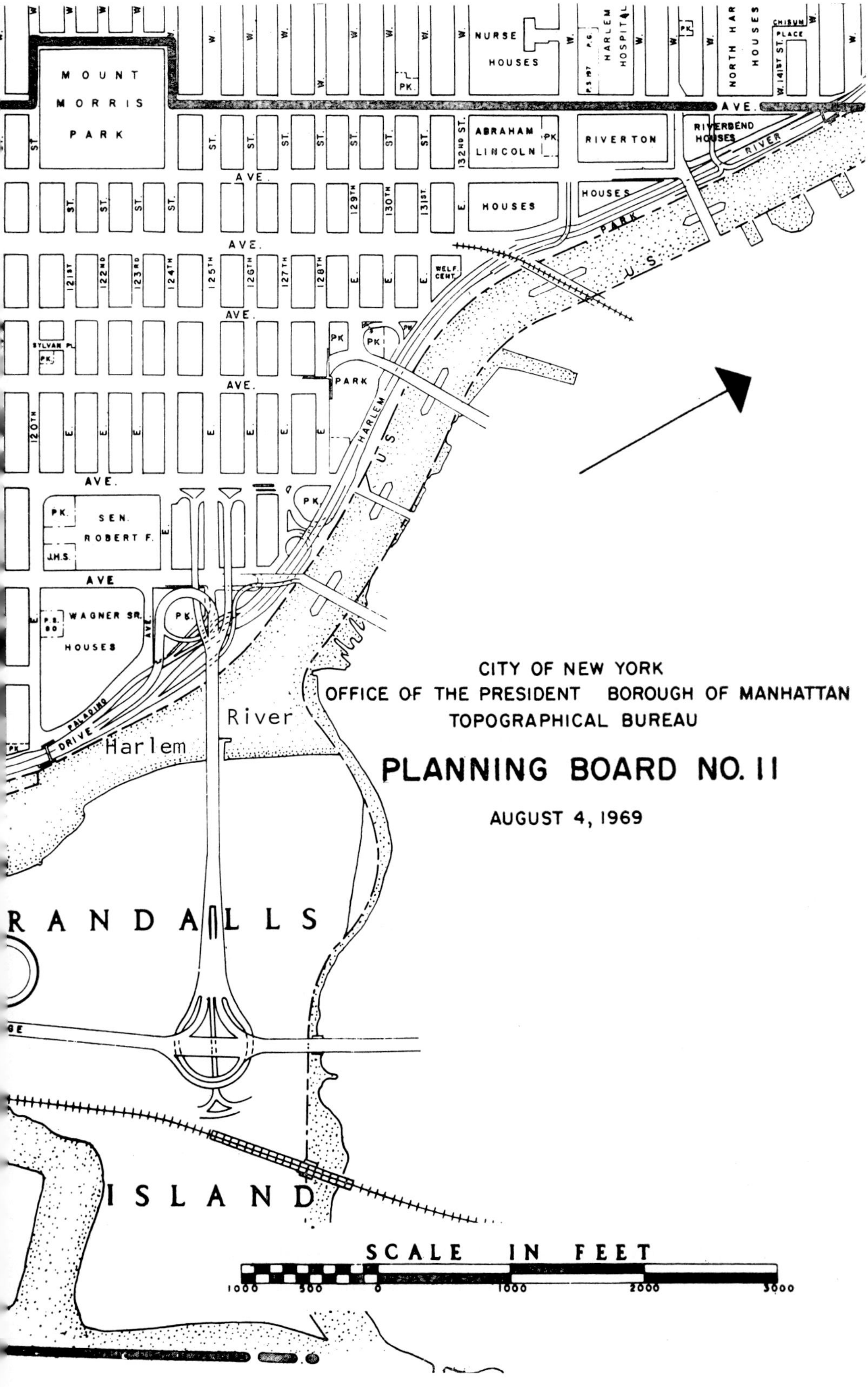

Figure 3 (continued)

nursing research. Thus was created the academic divisional framework for supporting an operational arm in the community, namely, the Division of Health Care.

Outside the divisional structure of the department are the representatives of the affiliated institutions (including Elmhurst Hospital, Beth Israel Hospital, Gouverneur Hospital, the Hospital for Joint Diseases, and the Paterson, N. J., Health Department), and persons in coordinating positions in administration, education, research, and special programs such as the Regional Medical Program.

The Division of Health Care (Figure 2) fuses the traditions of the medical-care system with its base in the hospital ambulatory care service, and the public-health sector with its base in the health center. Within the hospital, the director of the Division of Health Care holds the title of director of ambulatory care. There are separate coordinators for the hospital-based and community-based programs (see below).

The operational division has developed a Health Care Laboratory under a four-year grant from the National Institutes of Health. The threefold purpose of this laboratory is to study the delivery of health care, especially to large groups; to investigate health levels and health needs in the community; and to stimulate interdisciplinary research in community medicine in the department and the medical center. It also serves as a data bank, a source of consultative help in research, and a training ground for medical and other students. Its present activities include long-term follow-up of welfare recipients to measure the impact of Medicare and Medicaid on their use of health services; development of a statistical information unit for Mount Sinai; and a household survey of East Harlem to ascertain present and potential demands for medical care.

The academic instrument designed to bring about change in the local health system has been described at some length. It is time to turn to consideration of the community itself.

East Harlem

East Harlem, for practical purposes, can be considered to cover the area bounded by 96th Street, Fifth Avenue, the East River, and the Harlem River (Figure 3). The census of 1960 reported that about 180,000 people lived in this area. It was estimated in 1965 that about 41% are Puerto Rican and 38% black; the remaining 21% are white, mainly of Italian extraction. There is some evidence that the proportion of blacks is increasing, as the Puerto Ricans continue to move to the Bronx and other boroughs.

East Harlem is one of Manhattan's most conspicuous slums, composed of both badly deteriorated housing and many public low-income housing projects. Its population is not, however, without variety of income and race, since some middle-income housing developments dot the central area, and the western boundary and southern section both contain groups of upper, middle, and high income, composed primarily of white residents. The census of 1960 supplied information rating each census tract according to its citywide quartile standing on income, education, and unemployment; the highest quartile represented the most deprived. This showed that the great majority of census tracts in East Harlem appear in the most deprived quartile standing on all three measures, with some exceptions in the northernmost tract of middle-income housing and in the residual Italian colony on the east side near 116th Street. The complete break in communities at 96th Street was readily apparent by this analysis; the tracts to the south of this street, especially near Central Park, immediately switch to the quartile showing highest income, education, and employment.

Approximately one third of East Harlem's residents live in housing projects. For the other two thirds there are very few modern elevator-equipped buildings; the old "walk-up" tenements predominate. There are a considerable number of small industries scattered through the area. These, incidentally, are of considerable interest to the health officer, since they are mainly too small to have industrial health facilities, yet some may present significant health hazards.

In 1968 there were 207 practicing physicians with their offices within the geographic limits of East Harlem. But when their exact location was mapped, an extraordinary concentration of doctors around the two medical schools was disclosed. Elsewhere there are extremely few practicing physicians. A cluster of doctors along 116th Street consists mainly of elderly Italian general practitioners, who are believed to serve mainly the dwindling Italian community in that area. Very few private practitioners serve the bulk of the East Harlem population. Dentists, formerly scarce, have come into the area in considerable numbers since the advent of Medicaid, but the latest Medicaid cutbacks may make this increase a temporary one.

The bulk of hospital inpatient and outpatient care given in East Harlem—although not necessarily, be it stressed, primarily to East Harlem residents—is provided by two medical schools and their affiliates. New York Medical College operates Flower and Fifth Avenue Hospitals (406 beds; 30,536 ambulant visits in 1968) and is affiliated with Metropolitan Hospital (983 beds; 448,008 visits). The Mount Sinai School of Medicine is located in The Mount Sinai Hospital (1,205 beds; 270,094 visits in 1968) and affiliated with the Hospital for Joint Diseases (330 beds; 78,095 visits). The East Harlem Health Center and its satellite health stations recorded a total of 168,100 visits in 1965.

Strategy for an Improved Health Care System in East Harlem

The departmental structure of community medicine at Mount Sinai has been completed only in recent months, so the programs described are in an early phase of development. Nevertheless some solid beginnings have been made both within the hospital and in the community.

Hospital-based programs. Within the hospital, coordination of the program has been delegated to a physician who has had experience in general practice in Harlem, in hospital ambulatory care, and in the administration of public-health and welfare medical care. As part of his responsibilities this physician staffs the outpatient committee and represents The Mount Sinai Medical Center for the Regional Medical Program.

The immediacy of the community's health problems is felt by a medical center such as Mount Sinai primarily in the emergency room. Studies in the hospital have recently established that although the OPD handles twice as many *visits* as the emergency room, the emergency room in any given year sees twice as many *different* patients as the OPD. Until recently the emergency room functioned in only a small fraction of the space allocated to the OPD.

The first part of the strategy for change was to enlarge the emergency room. The space was doubled and full-time directorships were established for pediatrics, surgery, and medicine. Pediatric acute care was completely integrated with the general pediatric clinic so that children with acute problems are now triaged and cared for promptly. In the next stage, the administration plans to build a set of eight beds for 24-hour admissions, and the Department of Medicine will develop a triage and walk-in service similar to the pediatric acute-care service. A health-surveillance unit with a routine set of general health tests will be attached to the triage and walk-in service; this will assure the episodic-care patient of at least some form of general screening and will initiate the work-up of the patients referred for longer care.

Two examples of several hospital-based programs will be described in some detail to show the principles of linking specialty services to community need. Both these programs originated in the emergency room: one from an individual patient and one from a statistical survey.

A 16-year-old Puerto Rican boy with hepatitis came to the attention of the staff of the Department of Medicine when an attempt to hospitalize him at Mount Sinai revealed that all available beds were full, some with hepatitis cases. The departments of Medicine and Community Medicine with the help of students undertook a pilot epidemiological survey and uncovered an endemic and possibly an epidemic outbreak of hepatitis in East Harlem, particularly among adolescents. These young patients were being denied admission in successive emergency rooms in different hospitals; some were being treated at home but many were not being seen at all. When the chief of the Liver Clinic was alerted to this problem he turned the attention of his special service to it. With the assistance of an epidemiologist and student clerks he is extending the epidemiological survey. He will initiate a general preventive and therapeutic program once this study is completed. His clinic, which until now had a population of patients with rare liver disease, is now beginning to care for patients with a health problem of primary importance in East Harlem.

Another health problem identified initially in the emergency room as of prime importance was bronchial asthma. A one-year study of many facets of the health problems in the emergency room revealed asthma as the most troublesome, persistent, and time-consuming disease for both patients and the staff. A review of the literature showed that although the term "ghetto asthma" had already been coined, there was very little sound epidemiological knowledge about it. One study* in Aberdeen, Scotland, indicates that asthma is more prevalent among lower socioeconomic groups. The chief of the allergy service in the hospital was interested in the problem, and he welcomed the oppor-

*Dawson, B., Gordon, H., Illsley, R. and Mitchell, R. A survey of childhood asthma in Aberdeen. *Lancet 1*:827, 1969.

tunity to collaborate with a specialist trained in public health recruited by Community Medicine to work on this problem. An epidemiological study of asthma is being launched; it starts with the cases in the Mount Sinai emergency room and extends to other primary-care resources in East Harlem. An ad hoc committee of nurses working in the community (Visiting Nurse Service, Public Health Nurses, Little Sisters of the Poor, etc.) has committed itself to a study of the asthma cases it has encountered. The committee developed the pilot phase of a questionnaire survey in consultation with The Mount Sinai Health Care Laboratory. In this way the community-medicine specialist is beginning to connect the scarce resource within the hospital with the true need in the community.

Community-based programs. The East Harlem Health Center is the natural focus of any community-based program in health. In cooperation with the New York City Department of Health the Department of Community Medicine was able to recruit a young public-health physician to apply for the job as health officer of East Harlem. The Health Department has had difficulty with such recruitment in recent years. This addition of academic technological support for the health officer without changing the existing administrative structure of the Health Department holds promise as a model for helping to revive interest in public health by connecting it to the academic mainstream of the medical center through a clinical Department of Community Medicine.

Within the Health Center itself, plans for a model program are being developed by the health officer, based on the community's perception of its health needs. Fortunately, the community has recently developed a Health Council, and this council is now asking all the health institutions in the community to review the entire health program and to make recommendations. The Health Council is beginning to focus on the problem of lead poisoning and is seeking help from the Model Cities program for this project. Other projected programs include the establishment of a "bed bureau" to act as a clearing house of information about available hospital beds in the area, and a project to prevent drug addiction, especially among young adolescent boys.

Three other community-based programs in the early stages of development may be described briefly as follows:

1) The problems of high-infant mortality and poor-child health care

will be approached by a physician who is a board-certified pediatrician and holds a doctorate in international health. Drawing on his experience with a similiar program in Africa, he will develop a nurse-practitioner program with the intention of converting the child-health stations in East Harlem to child-care stations. A pilot phase of the project began in the fall of 1969.

2) The Mount Sinai Hospital Medical Board has asked the Department of Community Medicine to develop a complete health-care program with Local 1199 of the Drug and Hospital Workers Union. The union represents Mount Sinai's nonprofessional workers and is planning a housing project on 107th Street. Nearly 10,000 persons of East Harlem within this project will be under care of the hospital. A young physician with training in epidemiology and public health has been recruited to supervise this program, which started in September 1969. He has already written a general proposal which is supported by the medical center and the union. Twenty thousand square feet have been set aside for a health facility. The details of the program remain to be worked out in collaboration with its future beneficiaries.

3) Recently the administrators of Intermediate School 201 asked the department for help with its school-health program. Through the mediation of the coordinator of the community-based program, a meeting was arranged and the Pediatrics Department agreed to take care of the ocular, auditory, and nutritional defects discovered by a screening program of the 3,500 children in that complex. As this program unfolds it may establish a pattern for connection between hospital resources and the schools in the community.

Finally we return full circle to the categorical projects that were developed from the hospital-based program. Here we see the numerous possibilities of connecting the resources of both community and hospital and of applying them, together, to identify and solve health problems.

Evaluation and monitoring. Evaluating the results of the various hospital- and community-based projects and their impact on the health levels and behavior of the local population will be a long-term preoccupation of the department's research staff. Detailed research plans must await the further development and specification of the programs themselves; but in three areas a beginning has been made in establishing baselines and evolving methods for measuring change.

First, a system for the identification of patients and for obtaining statistics on them has been developed within The Mount Sinai Hospital in the last two years. Before that time Mount Sinai, like so many hospitals, tabulated only transactions and not people: one could tell the number of outpatient visits or inpatient days, but not the number of different individuals served in any one area in a given year. Still less could one tell the extent of overlap of patients between the different areas (inpatient service, outpatient clinic, and emergency room) or how often a given patient visited the hospital. Staff from the Health Care Laboratory of the Department of Community Medicine took advantage of the opportunity offered by the hospital's automation of its billing for outpatients to propose a patient-statistics system that would be the by-product of the billing procedure. Under a contract from the Public Health Service, a system of outpatient statistics has been developed that shows the total number of patients seen in each area, their demographic characteristics, and patterns of utilizing the hospital's resources. Volume of visits per patient, clinics per patient, constellation of clinic use, length of episode of care, and so on can be related to age, sex, pay status, borough of residence, etc. Patients making an inordinate number of visits or attending a large number of different clinics can be flagged for medical review; the system accordingly serves the interests of administration and quality control and provides data of research interest.

One example of the light thrown by the study on the hospital's relation to its East Harlem community is the discovery that most of Mount Sinai's ambulatory patients do indeed come from East Harlem. They are in fact closely clustered between 96th Street and 125th Street. An enlarged map of this area (not shown here) shows that they are fairly evenly distributed throughout East Harlem and not particularly concentrated in the western half, as the presence of Metropolitan Hospital on the southeast corner might suggest. On the other hand, Mount Sinai inpatients come from all over the city, with no particular concentration in East Harlem.

As Mount Sinai's programs begin to go into effect, statistics on the patients will be ready to monitor changes in the characteristics of patients and in utilization patterns within the hospital. For instance, there may be a decrease in the turnover of patients; fewer of them will be making only one visit; and perhaps also fewer patients will make an extremely large number of visits or attend many clinics. The next step is to add diagnosis to the report on visits to the emergency room—this has already been tried on a pilot, nonautomated basis for one year—and a valuable additional epidemiological tool will be available. As the computer gains enough experience to flag unusual events (rise in the number of visits, above-average number of a certain diagnosis, and so on) it is hoped that epidemics such as the outbreak of hepatitis may be detected in advance.

This system of monitoring the acute health problems of East Harlem for which patients seek medical care will be much improved once it can be extended to other sources of primary care, such as the emergency rooms of affiliated hospitals and the offices of private practitioners who will be working closely with Mount Sinai.

Another area being widely studied by many different staff members in the department is that of published and unpublished statistics concerning the East Harlem community. Summer students have assembled census data, statistics of the Health Department, data on housing and voting behavior, medical manpower and health facilities; and they made a series of maps that show this information in graphic form. A series of background papers about East Harlem is being prepared, and these will be constantly revised and updated to see if changes in health and health care are eventually mirrored in some of these statistics. Vital statistics kept by the Health Department will be watched to see if, for instance, the maternal and child-care programs the Department of Community Medicine is planning in conjunction with the East Harlem Health Center have any influence on the present high infant death rates. Members of the research staff are already examining the more detailed analyses by health area which the Health Department collects but summarizes for publication into the larger health-district tabulations. The finer analyses thus made available will enable the programs to concentrate especially on those areas that have the most acute needs.

Finally, a household survey is planned which will measure community demands for health care and seek to find out systematically what kinds of improvements residents think are most urgently needed. The consumer must be a collaborator in this health assessment, which could carry the seeds of many epidemiological studies. The respondent should also be able to see the connection between clarification of demand and service response: he should feel that his opinions truly affect the services offered to him. Then reassessments may be made at a later date to measure the extent to which goals have been met and to ascertain the number of persons satisfied with the changes.

Principles Underlying this Approach

To summarize this approach to the health problems of the community, seven underlying principles may be distinguished:

1) *Breadth of approach*, Community medicine is interested in more than medical care: it is concerned with the total health problems of the community.

2) *Community initiative*. The intention is to respond to community demand and requests for help, rather than to impose our own ideas on the community.

3) *Affiliation*. Our method is to link up the viable parts of the present health-care system rather than bypass or reject them. If the present system is fragmentary, we shall try to bring about affiliations between the various sources of care, rather than attempt to replace it with a whole new system.

4) *Diversity*. We welcome the chance to try as many different models of health-care delivery as opportunity will offer in the expectation that the resulting system will be both flexible and diverse.

5) *Interlocking services*. The service offered should be no more elaborate than the patient needs at that particular time. Ideally, primary care, as close and convenient to the patient as possible, should be provided by small, simple units offering only routine services. If the various resources can be made to interlock, then the patient who needs tests, special care, or complex facilities can be readily referred to the parent or supporting facility.

6) *Cross-fire technique*. By tackling health problems from many different angles the probability that a particular problem will receive appropriate attention is greatly enhanced. A child with a hearing defect, for instance, if missed at the child-care station, may be detected by a school-screening program, or through medical services offered to a neighborhood house, or through a clinic for adolescents.

7) *Economic feasibility*. Above all, an approach to the health needs of a whole area that, it is hoped, will be relevant to other parts of the country as well must be economically feasible. If one keeps in mind the need to distribute scarce health resources over a large area and constantly monitors the effect on the whole population of East Harlem and not the select few in specific programs, it should be possible to see what can be accomplished with realistic staffing and adequate resources.

GROUP PRACTICE DEVELOPMENT: A SERVICE OF THE DEPARTMENT OF HEALTH, NEW YORK CITY*

LOUIS L. FELDMAN

Director
Office of Group Practice Development
New York City Department of Health
New York, N.Y.

I APPRECIATE this opportunity of discussing with you the activities and objectives of the Health Department's newly established Office of Group Practice Development.

Dr. Mary C. McLaughlin, New York City's Health Commissioner, offers the professions, the providers, the community, and officialdom a new resource for the development, organization, and operation of group practices. The objective of this new resource is the effective utilization of available public and private skilled manpower and existing capital facilities to expand the availability and accessibility of acceptable health-care services and to facilitate their delivery.

During the month of May 1969 the commissioner established the Office of Group Practice Development—the first and only health department activity of its kind in the nation. Personnel costs are financed by the Health Services and Mental Health Administration of the United States Department of Health, Education, and Welfare. This new effort represents a combined program of the city of New York and the Health Services and Mental Health Administration to establish an Office of Group Practice within the New York City Health Department. It is financed by a grant of approximately $106,000 for a period of approximately 19 months. The government provides money for staff personnel; the city provides space, equipment, and its total cooperation in achieving the office's goals.

A Health Department service to assist the private sector to develop mechanisms (please note the plural) to coordinate with tax-supported activity—without cost—was unprecedented.

The purposes of the government contract, which are clear and in accordance with the city's objective, are as follows:

*Presented at a meeting of the Committee on Medicine in Society, November 24, 1969.

1) To encourage, initiate, and assist in planning and implementing group-practice health units throughout the five boroughs of New York City.

2) To encourage and organize group-practice medical units that offer comprehensive family health care in the Ambulatory Care Program of the New York City Department of Health and hospital-based units in the affiliated hospitals program of the Department of Hospitals.

Announcement of the contract which appeared in an article by Peter Kihss in the *New York Times* on March 9, 1969, brought requests for assistance from practitioners, hospitals, community organizations, and others as well as evidence not only of interest, but support from other city agencies and their state counterparts.

The program began operation on May 22, 1969. Despite delays in securing funds for staff support, considerable progress has been obtained in developing an interest in group practice and in coordinating the interest of state and city official agencies. One of the outstanding results of the early months of operation was to define more clearly the term "group practice," which means many things to many people. So, prior to discussing the details of the office and its efforts, aims, objectives, and aspirations, let us discuss the words "group practice" as interpreted by practitioners and evolve an approach to a definition for a unit acceptable to the professions and the city.

Prevailing Concepts: Confusion and Impressions

Group practice is interpreted in many ways. Often the meanings held by practitioners have little if any resemblance to each other. The definition of the American Public Health Association (APHA) is the systematic relation between physicians or dentists organized for the conduct of practice.* The United States Public Health Service defines it as three or more physicians (full-time or part-time) formally organized to provide medical services, with income from medical practice distributed acording to some prearranged plan.

To some, group practice as a form of organization means two or more practitioners utilizing a single facility; to others, it means a unit of physicians, dentists, or other health-care practitioners formed to provide care to subscribers to a group-practice prepayment plan such as the

A Guide to Medical Care Administration. Concepts and Principles, vol. 1, p. 78, Donabedian, A., ed. New York, Amer. Public Health Ass., 1969.

Health Insurance Plan of Greater New York or the Permanente Medical Group; to others, it means salaried physicians or others operating a hospital, community, or government ambulatory care unit. The term group practice also defines a storefront in a ghetto area with a sign marked "clinic" or "group" where practitioners with other office facilities provide services to poor people during specified daytime hours on weekdays; it also describes a medical unit comprised of individual practitioners who utilize central administrative services, etc.

Another interpretation, almost a conviction, held by proponents and opponents, considers group practice as health care financed and operated under the auspices of a nonmedically directed organization such as a prepayment plan, a labor union, a community organization, government, etc.

Still another view represents group practice as a device for hospital-based staff to seek payments from insurers or government-funded programs; often such units are used to funnel additional income to hospitals and related institutions.

Another set of impressions about group practice relates to the schedule of Medicaid fees: report requirements, delays in confirming eligibility, further delays in receipt of payments, factoring, and the spectre of audits. The dominant emphasis here is on a registered population—prompt payment of capitation or a fixed amount per registered person; no fee-for-service reports; no medical audit; and protection against public exposure of the individual physician's productivity or, even more worrisome, his income.

Other ideas relate to economic and professional relations administrative and overhead savings, a new way of living, vacations, income during illness, opportunity for and financing of continuing education, accumulation of assets and equity, security, etc.

Thus group practice has no single universal meaning other than a combination of practitioners who occupy a common facility.

The American Dental Association at its November 1969 meeting amended its Principles of Ethics by adopting the following definition:

> Group Practice is that type of dental practice in which dentists, sometimes in association with members of other health professions, agree formally between themselves on certain central arrangements designed to provide efficient dental health service.

There are an ever-increasing number of group practices in New

York City, many of them established since the advent of Medicaid in low-income areas. Lucille Niebur of the Blue Shield professional-relations staff described these emerging and established units, both private and neighborhood, in a presentation before the Committee on Medical Economics of the New York County Medical Society, as follows:

> There does not appear to be any thread of continuity or uniformity in the direction of these groups. None knows what the others are doing. There is no sharing of ideas.

In discussing the stimulus for group practice, Miss Niebur concludes that:

> The community or the consumers, as a group, are becoming more involved with health care and are demanding that medicine find more effective ways of delivering care. Many group administrators believe that traditional medical care will not make an impact on the community. They want to see medicine develop programs which will be continually responsive to changing needs.

In this chaotic hodgepodge of conflicting understandings (and there are many more) it was evident that the prime prerequisite for a health-department development service was the establishment of a concept of a group-practice unit acceptable to government. Such a unit would have to be professionally qualified and financially able to fulfill a contract to provide tax-supported services.

Thus a development activity of the Health Department of New York City must start by defining a group-practice program which meets the needs of the community and of the professional manpower, and has the ability to utilize existing capital resources for maximum effect. The intent of the office is to *help*—to assist practitioners and providers to develop units beneficial to them and to the community. The basic purpose of the office is to bring coordinated medical care and health services into areas where they are nonexistent. Its corollary purpose is to establish a mechanism or mechanisms that provide for practitioners a method of practicing together in an environment which encourages economic and professional satisfaction.

Group practice from the point of view of the department therefore facilitates the coordination of outpatient and inpatient care and assures equal care for all persons without regard to economic status, race, color, or any other factor.

There is no one mechanism. The department would have an active monitoring role in safeguarding the expenditure of public funds and insuring the adequacy and quality of care made available through the facility and its practitioners. Private groups are important. Hospital-related and hospital-associated groups are important. Multidiscipline groups are important. Single-discipline groups used as support for multidiscipline groups are important. The goals are all the same, that is, to establish a mechanism to assure effective utilization of the scarce skilled manpower and fuller employment of increasingly expensive capital facilities. This is a broad order; it requires innovation and often necessitates changes in the thinking of both officials and practitioners. The community is ready. Present-day emphasis in New York City and the nation centers on: 1) universal health insurance, 2) high costs, 3) entire communities without any medical resources, 4) physicians who are aging, and 5) the environment in which younger physicians will practice.

How then do we properly utilize this rare opportunity of combining an official agency's resources with the needs, requirements, and hopes of practitioners to utilize their skills and gain a most effective series of mechanisms? Each variation is to be demonstrated separately, and it is to evolve, from the combination of experience, group-practice forms that enable fuller utilization of scarce manpower and facilities and to provide a mechanism for the expansion of the availability and accessibility of acceptable health-care services.

Establishing a Foundation: Guidelines For Initiating Discussions

Because of a shortage of personnel the efforts of the office have had to be focused on prospects with the potential of developing into an effective program that would serve all components of the community. The objective is the organization of group-practice units that would be self-perpetuating and sufficiently stable (financially and professionally) to enter into binding contracts with the city. To meet the demand guidelines for initiating discussions were developed and cleared within the department. Dr. McLaughlin has directed that peer organizations shall have full opportunity to review and participate in the further development of the professional aspects of these guidelines and in the evolvement of the department's rules and regulations governing ongoing operations of acceptable group practices. The department's responsibility for assuring the adequacy and quality of care mandated by Article

5, Title 11, of the State Social Services' Law extends to all care provided by medical or other groups approved for Medicaid. One requirement must be a uniform standard of high-quality care for all members of the community without respect to economic status or any other factor.

The initiating guidelines are designed to provide for a substantive effort realistically interested in the development of a group practice. The rules establishing priority for assistance from the Office of Group Practice that require a group to "tool up" to provide equal care for all community members are stated in the guideline letter as follows:

> Any combination of licensed practitioners can arrange to provide services from a central location, achieve operating efficiency through sharing of overhead, joint utilization of administrative and technical personnel, and facilitate continuity of care. This type of combined practice provides administrative and other operating benefits as well as the opportunity to establish the fundamental personal and working relationships prerequisite to the organization and effective conduct of a group practice unit.
>
> Due to limited resources, our services for the present will be made available only when a proposed "group" is substantive and can produce evidence that it is prepared to maintain an adequate facility and assure the combination of professional, technical skills and administrative implementation to provide family health care. The core professional composition of such a "group" should meet the following minimum criteria:
>
> 1) Founding members include general practice, internal medicine, pediatrics, obstetrics-gynecology and general surgery.
>
> 2) Retainer, fee-for-service, or other arrangements can be made to assure the availability of medical specialty, sub-specialty care and other health care services.
>
> 3) Hospital care can be provided in one or more institutions in which a majority of the "group" have privileges.
>
> 4) The "group" has the number of practitioners and other personnel (technical, supporting disciplines and administrative) needed to assure coordinated care for 15,000-30,000 persons.

There was a need to find an inducement for practitioners to begin actively to associate with each other to develop a group practice. To provide an incentive and an opportunity to establish a working relation, the interim arrangement providing tangible recognition of the group in process of formation—termed a combined practice—developed with the Department of Social Services, is described as follows:

A combination of practitioners jointly utilizing an adequate facility may apply for a temporary arrangement to provide services to Medicaid eligible persons as a combined practice unit. If approved, this arrangement will provide for a central billing and fee-for-service payments to be made to the "group" for a period not to exceed six months while the "group" is in process of formation. A basis for providing for advance payments is under consideration. When established, such payments will be subject to a final settlement based on the actual services provided to group-served Medicaid eligible persons at the appropriate fees. The objective is the development of a procedure for capitation payments for a wide array of health care services for qualified groups.

Central billing will be made available if the combined practice can meet the Department of Health regulations and demonstrate that:

1) The founders have executed an interim agreement and made a substantial financial and professional commitment to develop a group-practice unit.

2) The professional skills can provide for a wide range of preventive and therapeutic family care.

3) The practice will be conducted at one or more central locations adequately staffed and equipped to assure the provision of initial and continuing patient care.

4) Each practitioner is certified for Medicaid and agrees to designate the combined-practice unit to bill and collect on his behalf for services provided to "group" Medicaid-eligible persons and to execute and file such documents as may be required with the Departments of Health and Social Services.

5) A central family medical record will be maintained for all services provided to "group" patients, without respect to source of payment; these records shall be available for review, upon request, by Department of Health personnel.

6) All monies received from Medicaid will be distributed on a basis established by the "group" and filed with this office. A fiscal audit of all group activities shall be made available to the Departments of Health and Social Services.

At this time only one group, the Mayflower Medical Group, with a facility in Bensonhurst, has this arrangement. Efforts are now in process to provide for a reimbursement basis other than fee-for-service for medical groups that meet health-department requirements. Such an arrangement for Medicaid patients will be available only to groups prepared to serve all members of the community.

Essentially the guidelines seek to establish a group capable of entering into a contract with an official agency. Thus it must be a unit that has the ability to fulfill its obligations. In addition, to enter into a substantive relation, a group must have the professional competence to provide the wide range of services required to meet day-to-day family health-care needs. A prime necessity is the assurance of the availability and accessibility of acceptable care over a 24-hour period, 7 days a week, whether provided through a central facility or provided during working hours at one facility and during off-hours through an arrangement with a nearby hospital or similar facility.

Thus an initial requirement is that the partnership or unincorporated association of physicians with appropriate bylaws requires, at minimum, practitioners in general practice, internal medicine, pediatrics, obstetrics-gynecology, and general surgery. There would have to be more than a physician of each discipline, since one might for reasons beyond his control become unavailable. For the other disciplines, it is required that there be retainer, fee-for-service, or other arrangement to assure the availability of subspecialty care and other related health-care services to persons under group care. It is to be expected that in a group operation ancillary personnel would be utilized to the greatest possible extent. This would include the social worker, the nutritionist, the speech therapist, the physiotherapist, the optometrist, the podiatrist, etc., all of whom would become available to the group although not members of it.

Administrative Implementation

To establish a base whereby it would be possible to evaluate the combined practice units a separate Medicaid participation number is used. Each physician files a statement with the Department of Social Services that designates the group that is to receive his Medicaid fees. A separate bill for each type of service (Form 303G) is submitted to the Department of Social Services and a check is issued in the name of the group. Also in the planning stage is the establishment of a group practice evaluation unit in the department's Bureau of Medical Care.

Preparation for Orderly Development

Tax-supported health-care services are provided through employee benefit and public programs by city, state, and federal agencies. The city's Department of Social Services is responsible for disbursement of Title XIX—popularly termed Medicaid.

The health department provides services through neighborhood family-health units, specialty clinics, and other ambulatory-care activities. The Hospital Department provides directly operated in- and outpatient health care. In addition, there are overlapping community-directed activities funded by government and private services. The coordination of services to assure better use of manpower, facilities, and skills is the assigned task of the comprehensive health-planning unit now in process of organization. The dimensions of the problem are highlighted by the fact that about one third of New York City's 8 million inhabitants have health-care coverage paid for in part or whole by tax-derived funds. Group-practice units, acceptable to government and the community, can be a type of mechanism for establishing a unified community health-care service whether operated by private practitioners, government (directly or through the community), or in combination.

The universal governmental interest in developing new approaches to health care in general is motivated by the desire: 1) to do good and find solutions to meet increasing public demand and, 2) to define more efficient effective methods and to achieve full value for public and private expenditures. Although the interest has common focus there is a wide variation in concepts and understanding of group practice among practitioners.

An inevitable outcome was the decision that the Office of Group Practice Development had multimajor areas of activity. These are: 1) to provide a resource to officialdom to facilitate the acceptance of group practice, both within the Health Department and elsewhere and, 2) to evolve group practices acceptable to the community and an agreed-upon enforceable basis for review, evaluation, and improvement.

Progress had been made in developing liaison with other city agencies which now include on a regular working relation the following:

1) Department of Personnel; 2) Department of Social Services; 3) New York City Housing Authority; 4) City Planning Commission; and 5) Model Cities Program.

Health Department activity is coordinated by a recently established Health Care Council appointed by Dr. McLaughlin. The chairman is Dr. Lowell E. Bellin, first deputy health commissioner, and includes staff members assigned to: 1) ambulatory care activities, 2) group practice, 3) Medicaid. Dr. Bellin's memorandum to the members of the committee summarizes its mission as follows:

> I see the Health Care Council transmuting the City Health Department into a regulatory agency for health care. This obviously means standard setting, quality and fiscal surveillance and enforcement. These in turn mean development and refinement of administrative techniques currently embryonic, if at all existent. I see the Health Care Council as promoting group practice together with ancillary health care personnel.

The present-day status and future activity for the office is summarized in Dr. McLaughlin's letter accompanying a report to the Department of Health, Education, and Welfare on the first five months of the program, as follows:

> An ever-increasing number of practitioners, hospitals and community groups are requesting assistance from this new Health Department activity. The practitioners often are professionals with established practices in depressed areas as well as younger practitioners, seeking to locate in low-income sections of the City. It has been most gratifying to me that many of these interested practitioners represent ethnic groups indigenous to low-income areas.
>
> Hopefully, the funding obstacle will soon be overcome and an intensive effort can be exerted to recruit the much-needed staff support 1) to achieve the objectives of the contract, 2) to develop an adequate budget and program for an ongoing Health Department Office of Group Practice Development.
>
> We now seek an early opportunity to discuss with you the development of a program to accomplish the purposes and meet the needs set forth in the interim report as well as to define and effect the research functions to chronicle and evaluate the office's activities. The purpose of such a meeting would be to explore in detail the program and staffing required to develop, evaluate, and monitor

group practice units, as well as an orderly method for financing operating and research activities.

It is our intention to develop such a program with the long-term objective of establishing this office as a regular activity of this Department.

Comment

The Health Department's new Office of Group Practice Development offers a community service for the organization and operation of combinations of health-care units for the delivery of health services. The office, which was activated on May 22, 1969, is financed in part by a contract with the Health Services and Mental Health Administration of the United States Department of Health, Education, and Welfare. It is the first and, at present, the only such official health department activity in the nation.

The office, in its first six months of operation, has established direct working relations with other city agencies concerned with health-care service in regard to their availability, accessibility, acceptability, and costs. Its current activity is focused on: 1) evolving new bases of reimbursement for tax-supported services; 2) defining the composition and criteria for an acceptable group-practice unit; and 3) developing and implementing a health department program for initial and ongoing evaluation of services provided by group practice and their costs.

The office upon written request will provide peer and provider organizations with the opportunity to participate in establishing:

1) criteria for acceptable group-practice units;

2) rules and regulations for initiating and continuing a contract for the provision of tax-supported health-care services;

3) methods for assuring the necessity, adequacy, and quality of services; and

4) bases for evaluating the effectiveness of group practice as mechanisms:

a) to expand the availability, acceptability, and accessibility of care;

b) to minimize unnecessary, duplicating, and overlapping service and administrative costs;

c) to coordinate ambulatory and inpatient care;

d) to develop definitions of health-care costs and the development of a mutually acceptable basis for cost review and adjustment.

THE INDIA OFFICE RECORDS: A SOURCE FOR HISTORIANS OF PSYCHIATRY

Since human activities are endlessly diverse, it is not surprising that man has left the imprint of his presence in many ways and in all the corners of the world. And wherever man has been and in whatever pursuit he has been engaged he has enjoyed good health or endured bad. Hence the physician is held responsible for a detailed knowledge of human affairs, since a man could hardly be a guide if he did not know the highroads, the crossroads, and the byways.

What is true of general clinical medicine is true *a fortiori* of psychiatry: the psychiatrist attempts to know man both in health and in disease and to understand any conditions that may influence the transition from one to the other.

The disturbed states of body and mind that we wish to elucidate and also the concepts that we employ in our search for understanding have undergone change with time. Hence it is valuable to resort to the records of earlier periods in order to clarify our vision by means of temporal perspective. Such early records are sometimes revealed unexpectedly.

During a meeting of the Friends of the National Libraries held in London on June 19, 1969, the author of this note was presented to Miss Joan C. Lancaster, M.A., F.S.A., and to Mr. S. C. Sutton, C.B.E., who are respectively Deputy Keeper, and Librarian and Keeper, of the India Office Records. Miss Lancaster pointed out that the India Office, now situated at Orbit House in Blackfriars Road, London, contains among its volumes and files, which number more than 160,000, a valuable collection of psychiatric records. How were these obtained?

The early part of the story appears in an essay written by A. J. Farrington,[1] who states:

> Before 1819 servants of the East India Company were detained in various institutions there. On July 30, 1818, however, the Company reached an agreement with Dr. Rees of Pembroke House, Hackney, for the transfer of private patients from India

1. Farrington, A. J.: Ealing Lunatic Asylum. *Local Historian* (Ealing Local History Society), 1965, Part I, pp. 15-17.

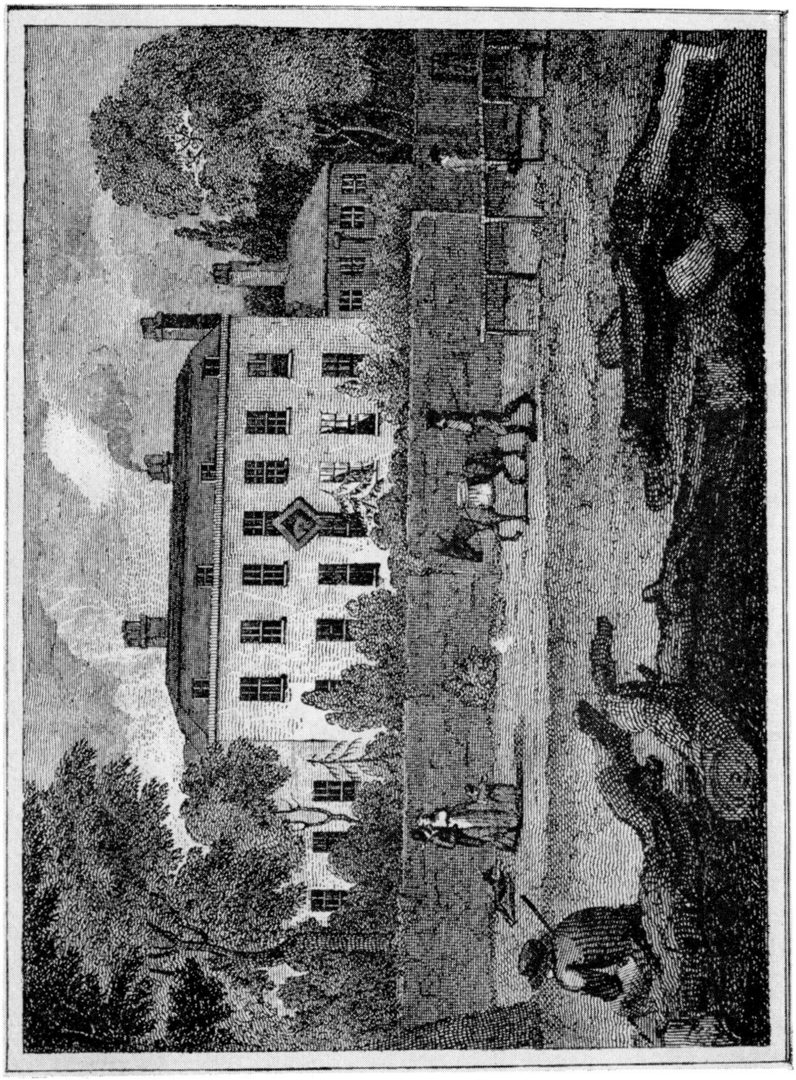

Fig. 1. Elm Grove. From Edith Jackson, *Annals of Ealing*, London, Phillimore and Co., 1898, p. 214. Courtesy of Central Library, Walpole Park, Ealing.

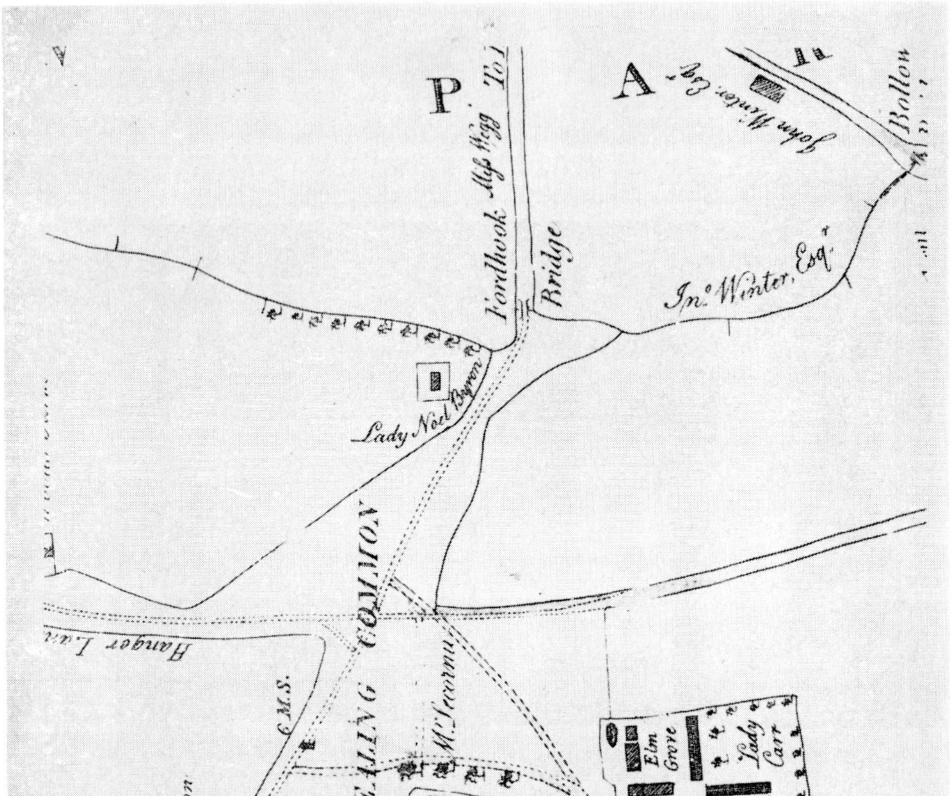

Fig. 2. Elm Grove and Ealing Common. Immediately to the east of Ealing Common is a property then owned by Lady Noel Byron; at this place Henry Fielding, a previous owner, wrote *Tom Jones*. From *An Historical Map of the Parish of Ealing* by William Nichols. Surveyed and drawn by A. Bassett and W. Nichols. Engraved by W. Haydon. Revised 1822, published ca. 1830. The map from which this area has been selected measures 45.6 × 55.2 cm. Reproduced by courtesy of Central Library, Walpole Park, Ealing.

> to his private asylum. Charges were fixed at £100 p.a. for 1st class patients (officers and senior civil servants) and £40 p.a. for 2nd class patients (soldiers, sailors, and minor civil servants). . . .

Farrington goes on to state that in 1870 this arrangement was felt to be unsatisfactory, and on March 25, 1870, the India Company acquired the Elm Grove estate of Mrs. Spencer Perceval (see Figures 1 and 2). The house with its fixtures and 38 acres of land were bought for £24,500. On August 25, 1870, the building was opened as an asylum. On June 24, 1892, after more than two decades of service, Ealing Asylum was closed and the building was demolished. It usually housed 156 patients, classified as follows: 1st class, 23; 2d class, 110; females, 23.

Additional information is found in an essay by Messrs. H. Holt and F. Toufar,[2] who state that the building at Elm Grove was used as an asylum not only by company personnel but also by their wives and children. The superintendent was a Dr. Christie. After his death in 1892 the patients were removed; the males went to the Royal Naval Hospital at Yarmouth, the females to an institution at Stafford. At this time the extant records were transferred to the India Office Military Department.

The records of Pembroke House and of the asylum at Ealing have been mentioned briefly in several published lists,[3] which are being deposited in the Library of The New York Academy of Medicine. Also to be deposited in the Library is a detailed typewritten list furnished in photocopy through the kindness of Mr. H. Holt and Mr. N. E. Binns of the Central Library at Walpole Park, Ealing. This statement mentions medical certificates (1830-1889); registers of admission; case books (1846-1892); medical visitation books; registers of discharges, deaths, and removals; correspondence; and numerous financial accounts.

It is obvious that a careful study of the case records supplemented by examination of financial records and correspondence would provide valuable insight into mental disease which occurred among Englishmen in the Orient during a great part of the 19th century, especially with respect to causative and conditioning circumstances. The diligent inquirer will delve profitably.[4]

S. J.

2. Holt, H. and Toufar, F.: *Elm Grove*. Ealing, Oct. 1962. 5 pp. Mimeographed, 8 × 6 in. Through the kindness of Mr. Holt a copy is being deposited in the library of The New York Academy of Medicine. A copy examined at the Ealing Public Library contains additional notes in manuscript.
3. Foster, William: *A Guide to the India Office Records, 1600-1858*. London, H. M. Stationery Office, 1966 (reprint of edition of 1919), p. 120. Sutton, S. C.: *A Guide to the India Office Library*. London, H. M. Stationery Office, 1967, p. 75. Lancaster, Joan C.: India Office Records. *Archivum* 15:293-302, 1969 (for 1965); see esp. p. 296.
4. The author acknowledges with thanks assistance graciously given by Miss Joan Lancaster, Mr. S. C. Sutton, Mr. H. Holt, Mr. N. E. Binns, Mr. N. Scoales, and Mrs. Richard North.

Over 5 million prescriptions already filled at Macy*s

All 13 M*acy* P*rescription* Centres

satisfy your patients with efficient professional service

℞

- You may phone in your patients' prescriptions (except for narcotics, amphetamines, and barbiturates).
- Your patients may charge their prescriptions on their Macy Shopping Accounts or C-T Plans.
- Your patients may have their prescriptions delivered anywhere free of extra charge.
- We serve your patient with a full line of convalescent and diabetic needs.

Macy's Herald Square, OX 5-4400
Macy's Parkchester, TA 8-7000
Macy's Jamaica, OL 7-9000
Macy's Flatbush, UL 6-5000
Macy's Roosevelt Field, PI 6-8200
Macy's Huntington, AR 1-3000
Macy's White Plains, WH 6-5015
Macy's New Haven, Conn. 624-9271
Macy's Bay Shore, MO 5-8400
Macy's Queens, AR 1-9100
Macy's Colonie, 459-1950
Macy's New Rochelle, 633-7700
Macy's Smith Haven, 724-4900

Include MILK *in your* LOW-SALT DIETS

It's no longer necessary to deny patients fresh, fluid palatable Milk in low-salt diets. Walker-Gordon fresh Lo-Sodium Milk (Certified Milk with 90% of Sodium removed) contains less than 50 mg. Sodium per quart. *Guaranteed free of antibiotic residue.* Paper half-pints for hospitals, quart bottles for home delivery. Write or phone for literature, low-sodium diet sheets, and professional sample.

WALKER-GORDON *Fresh* LO-SODIUM MILK

Walker-Gordon Certified Milk Farm, Plainsboro, N. J. ★ (609) 799-1234

New York: (212) WAlker 5-7464 ★ Phila.: (215) MArket 7-6338

Also Certified Raw, Homogenized Vitamin D and Skimmed Milks; available through leading Milk Dealers or call Walker-Gordon

BULLETIN OF
THE NEW YORK ACADEMY
OF MEDICINE

VOL. 46, NO. 3 MARCH 1970

RADIATION CARCINOGENESIS*

SHIELDS WARREN

Emeritus Professor of Pathology
Harvard Medical School
Cancer Research Institute
New England Deaconess Hospital
Boston, Mass.

ONE hundred twenty-five years ago it required a singularly far-sighted group of medical men to found a society focused on the then new field of pathology. Theodor Schwann had discovered the cell as the basic unit of the animal body five years earlier. The year before the founding of the New York Pathological Society, Virchow graduated from the University of Berlin, and three years after the society was founded the first issue of *Virchow's Archiv* appeared in 1847. The society antedated by two years the discovery of ether as an anesthetic; by more than a quarter of a century both the discovery of bacteria and the dawn of modern surgery; and by more than half a century the discovery of ionizing radiation. In the healthy growth of this society such men as Francis Delafield, James Ewing, Milton Helpern, Eugene L. Opie, Theophil W. Prudden, Fred W. Stewart, Arthur P. Stout, Doug-

*Presented at the 125th Anniversary Meeting of the New York Pathological Society, held in affiliation with the New York Academy of Medicine at The Rockefeller University, New York, N.Y., November 13, 1969.

This investigation was supported by U.S. Atomic Energy Commission Contract AT (30-1)-3777 and U.S. Public Health Service General Research Support Grant FR-05591 from the General Research Support Branch, Division of Research Facilities and Resources, National Institutes of Health, Bethesda, Md.

las Symmers, and Francis Carter Wood have played a significant part. I hope that the group will continue its good work for many centuries more.

Long before that, however, I hope the various causes of cancer will have been clearly understood and preventive measures against the disease brought into effective use. Indeed it may be soon that a viral causation will have been established for some cases of leukemia in man as has been so well demonstrated for leukemia in mice[1] by Dr. Ludwik Gross. In the ultimate solution of the problems of cancer etiology the evidence contributed by radiation carcinogenesis will play a helpful role.

Five years after the discovery of x rays the first skin cancer resulting from exposure to them was reported.[2] Knowledge of the induction of other kinds of cancer by radiation followed slowly. Two intriguing facts about radiation and cancer have helped to spark scientific interest in their relations. Radiation cures cancer and also causes it and, further, does not cause it out of hand but usually after a latent period of years. This latent period might imply that cancer is not produced by a single cellular change but by a series of them.

The exact mode of action of radiation on the cell is not understood but, whatever it is, it must involve damage caused by transfer of energy to controlling mechanisms, either of the cell's metabolic and proliferative activities or of its enzyme systems. The amount of physical energy delivered to the cell by the radiation absorbed is usually far too little to account directly for the effect produced and hence must have been multiplied by some such means as these.

Several hypotheses have been developed to explain the mechanism of radiation carcinogenesis. The production of a somatic mutation leading to uncontrolled cell growth, acceleration of aging with its attendant high incidence of cancer, the activation of oncogenic viruses, altered environment of cells, and abnormal proliferation of cells following repeated attempts at repair of injury have all been proposed. I believe that more than one of these may well be involved, and probably additional hypotheses as yet undeveloped will be required to explain all the accumulated facts.

Thus far morphologic clues, the province of the pathologist, have provided not only the sure criteria for the diagnosis of cancer but also important leads as to the behavior of its many different forms.

The facts relating to the epidemiology of radiation-induced cancer now have impressive impact. I shall present some of them, drawing largely on the data of the many workers in this field, with a few additions from my own experience. The earlier radiologists and radium workers showed excessive incidence of cutaneous cancer and of leukemia. The names of hundreds of scientific martyrs from among these pioneers are inscribed on the base of the monument at St. George's Hospital in Hamburg, Germany. Radium-dial painting provided many victims, among whom were those with osteogenic sarcoma and antral cancer, studied by Martland,[3] Evans,[4] and others. The mysterious pulmonary disease of the miners of Joachimsthal (now Jáchymov), Czechoslovakia, known and feared there since the Middle Ages, had been identified as lung cancer[5] and its causation related to radon and its daughter products present in the air of the mines. More recent examples of radiation carcinogenesis are the increased incidence of pulmonary cancer among some of our own uranium miners,[6] of cancer of the thyroid as demonstrated by Hempelmann and others[7] among those irradiated prophylactically for assumed thymic hyperplasia, and of leukemia among the Hiroshima-Nagasaki survivors studied by the Atomic Bomb Casualty Commission.[8] I propose to examine the incidence and nature of cancer in several of these groups in some detail in the hope of throwing some light on dose-effect relations and of stimulating interest in additional basic and clinical studies in this field.

Radiation dermatitis, sometimes followed years later by skin cancer, was seen all too often among early radiologists, usually on the left hand, which they placed in the x-ray beam for want of an easier way to check the efficiency of their crude devices. Sometimes doses of thousands of rads were accumulated. Atrophy, ulceration, focal hyperplasia, and eventually cancer developed in the epilated, dry, telangiectatic skin.[9] As might be expected from the relative number of epithelial cells contrasted with fibrocytes and also the relative frequency of mitosis between the two, carcinoma is many times more frequent as a manifestation of malignant change than is sarcoma. Sir Stanford Cade,[10] who has had long clinical experience, estimated that only a few of those with heavily irradiated skin developed cancer as a result. Fortunately, these lesions are rarely encountered today. Recently Albert[11] has studied cases here in New York where skin cancer had been induced by x irradiation in the scalps of some of those who had been temporarily epilated as children for the treatment of tinea capitis. Radiation-induced cancer

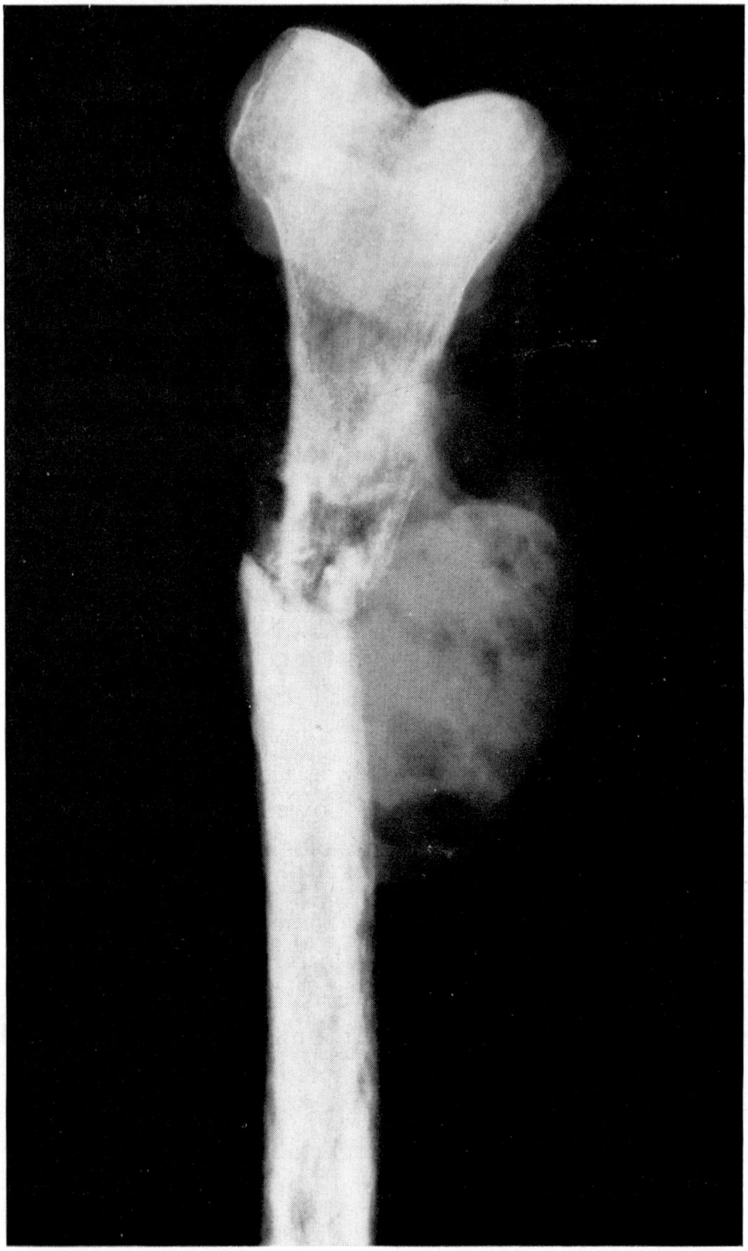

Fig. 1. Roentgenogram of dissected specimen. Radiation osteitis, osteogenic sarcoma, and pathologic fracture occurring in femur of a woman who had ingested radium-containing paint over 40 years previously.

of the skin cannot be differentiated from skin cancers caused by other noxious agents, nor for that matter can any form of cancer on the basis of histopathologic appearance or clinical behavior. Indeed, so far as any radiation-induced tumor is concerned, historical, epidemiologic, and other supporting evidence must be brought to bear. One possible exception is the characteristic and rare anaplastic hemangioendothelial sarcoma that sometimes develops as a sequel to thorium injection.[12] When tissue from the primary site is available, ionizing radiation can be deduced as a factor in causation by the changes suggestive or characteristic of radiation effect present in adjacent non-neoplastic tissue such as hyalinization of collagen, abnormal fibrocytes, and damaged blood vessels.

The dial painters, who pointed the brushes with their lips and so ingested and absorbed radioactive paint in minute amounts, accumulated this radium and in some instances thorium in their bones through selective absorption from the blood stream. The actual exposures to the paint were often brief, the occupation lasting only a year or so, but the difficulty of excretion of the radioactive metals and their deposition in bone produced life-long body burdens. From these deposits the alpha radiation bombarded for years osteocytes, osteoblasts, and osteoclasts. If the damage is less to osteoblasts and osteocytes than to osteoclasts the radiation osteitis that results is manifested chiefly by an increased density of bone to varying degrees, even eburnation. If damage to osteoblasts predominates, continuation of osteoclasis with insufficient bone formation results in rarefied foci. Both types often coexist in adjacent portions of bone, both are associated with pain, both may be present for long periods antecedent to the development of osteogenic sarcoma (Figure 1). As a result of the production of radon from the radium deposited in bones of the skull, high levels of radioactive gas may accumulate in the cavities of the bony sinuses (total local doses to the walls have reached 82,000 or more rads).[4] The resultant radiation damage to the mucous membranes of the walls caused epidermoid carcinoma to develop in some. The careful studies of Evans[4] and others have made dose-effect estimates possible. Evans has introduced the concept of a "practical threshold" below which cancers do not appear. This concept is somewhat unpopular in a period in which the hypothesis of a linear relation between dose and neoplastic effect has gained much support, especially as the application of linearity provides an

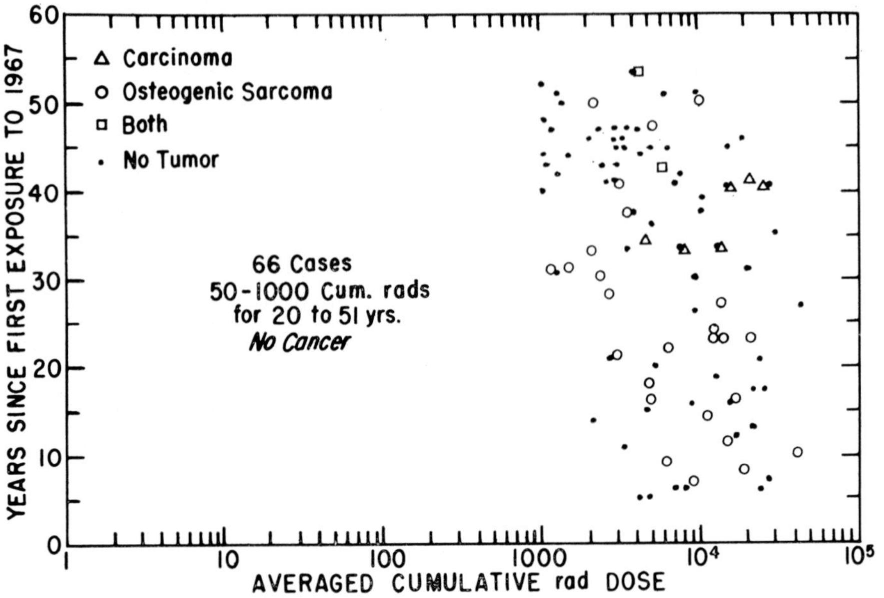

Fig. 2. Diagram showing the occurrence of osteogenic sarcoma and antral cancer in exposed radium watch-dial cases. Modified from Evans' diagram.[4]

added margin of safety in establishing permissible dose levels. Evans' data, based on 496 cases, are presented here in modified form (Figure 2). Until the dose level exceeds 1,000 rads there are no cancers. This, then, might be considered a "practical threshold," as Evans has suggested. At higher dose levels from one third to two thirds of the patients developed cancer, with a probable but ill-defined upward trend with increasing dose. However there is a drop in incidence at the highest dose levels, about 12,000 rads or more, perhaps due to the small size of the sample. This phenomenon of less carcinogenic effect at high dose levels has also been seen in some experiments in animals.

Osteogenic sarcoma, fortunately always a rare neoplasm, is a form of cancer that appears to be decreasing rather than increasing in incidence in the general population as is shown in the accompanying graph (Figure 3) of deaths from the disease in the United States. The rapid and unexplained decrease in mortality, curiously enough, coincides with the time when the level of radioactive fallout, supposed by some to be one of the causes of osteogenic sarcoma, was increasing. The fall-

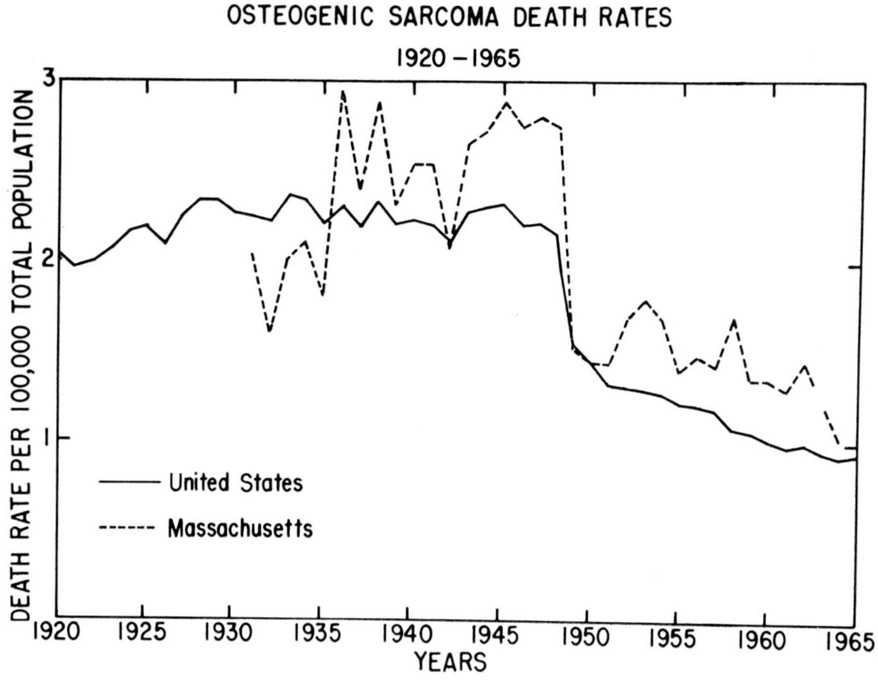

Fig. 3. Osteogenic sarcoma death rates.

out obviously did not reach a level that increased the prevalence of the disease.

The occurrence of another well-known cancer, that of the lung in uranium miners, is less well related to etiology. It is believed that inhaled alpha-emitting daughter products of radon present in the air of the mines and plated out in particulate form are inhaled and retained for long periods in the respiratory tree.[13] The alpha particles from these deposits are poorly penetrating; they reach only the more superficial cells but they have high linear energy transfer and so cause injury or death in those reached. Thus prolonged injury to bronchial epithelium results, which culminates in cancer in some instances. As already mentioned, exposure to the radon-rich air of the mines at Schneeberg, Germany, and Joachimsthal had long been known to increase the prevalence of lung cancer, and the same appears true of our western uranium mines. The risk there is now being lessened by ventilation and other protective measures. Exact dosimetry has been very difficult to establish, and current estimates are subject to revision as additional data become available. These estimates have been made in the form of "working level months" (a combination of radiation level and time of exposure), each of which may indicate a dose to lung tissue of about 7 ± 5 rads.[6] Among 3,414 white underground miners working from 1950 to 1967, 62 lung cancers occurred, six times the expected number. This is much in excess of the rates reported for other United States miners, either hard rock or coal. Miners as a whole tend to show more pulmonary fibrosis and other lung diseases than the population as a whole. Meyer and Liebow[14] have noted that there may be a potentiating effect toward cancer in the combination of widespread pulmonary scarring of the so-called honeycombing type and exposure to cigarette smoke. Sixty of the 62 lung cancers appeared in men who were also cigarette smokers. However only one probable lung cancer has been found among 761 Navajo miners, largely nonsmokers. Other factors, such as chronic infection and inhalation of dust may play a potentiating or cocarcinogenic role. For example, in mice spontaneous cancer of the bronchus is rare. It may be induced, however, by a combination of influenza virus and artificial smog, though neither agent alone will produce the cancer. Bronchogenic cancer is also produced in rodents and other animals by large doses of radiation.

Epidemiologic studies of the uranium miners of the Colorado plateau have shown a rough dose-effect relation between radiation levels in the air of the mines and lung cancers. At higher dose levels (over 840 working level months of about 4,000 to 8,000 cumulative R) there has been consistent increased risk of lung cancer, which rose with exposure. At lower exposure levels there is still increased risk, but it is less and not clearly related to amount of exposure to radiation.

There has been much interest in the fact that many of the bronchial cancers have been of the undifferentiated or oat-cell type, as pointed out by Saccomanno.[15] However, general experience has been that cancers caused by radiation are not distinctive in type. The one example of a Joachimsthal uranium miner's lung cancer that I have, thanks to the late Dr. H. Sikl, happens to be a well-differentiated and heavily keratinized tumor, although a number of them have been undifferentiated. Many lung cancers seen in persons with no radiation exposure vary widely in histologic structure in different parts of the same tumor, so differentiation of cells can be relied upon for classification only if adequate sampling of the total tumor mass has been done.

The evidence is strong that the excess lung cancer among white uranium miners is caused by radiation exposure and that the prevalence of the disease is increased by cigarette smoking, and possibly by other modes of pulmonary injury.

Another example of increased cancer prevalence due to radiation which also illustrates the long latent period involved is afforded by some cancers of the thyroid. These developed in some of those who had been irradiated as infants (90% were less than six months old) to reduce assumed thymic enlargement. Hempelmann and his associates[7] found not only an excess of thyroid cancer, some developing more than 20 years later, but an apparent excess of some other tumors as well, as compared with untreated siblings. Among the other tumors were leukemia and a benign bone lesion, osteochondroma. The range of exposures to x radiation in infancy that produced cancer later ranged from below 120 R to over 600 R. The excess incidence was clear-cut, nearly 100 times the expected incidence. However the incidence of thyroid cancer has not been shown to be clearly related to dose, perhaps because an insufficient number of cases have been available for study. Most of the thyroid cancers were of papillary type. In addition to these cases and series reported by other investigators, there are data from the Atomic Bomb Casualty Commission which indicate that the incidence of thyroid cancer among the Hiroshima-Nagasaki survivors has risen above that in other Japanese.[16] The natives who were exposed in 1954 at Rongelap and Uterik in the Marshall Islands to radiation from fresh fallout rich in radioactive iodine are being studied by Conrad[17] and his colleagues. A number of the exposed children have developed thyroid nodules. They may well provide further information on dose-effect relations.

There is evidence from sheep experimentally exposed to radioactive iodine produced from chemical processing of used reactor fuel in Hanford, Wash., that nodularity of the thyroid gland may be produced and that this nodularity may progress in some instances to the development of cancer.[18] As one would expect, because this nodularity is caused by damage to the thyroid and its attempted repair, there is a much better correlation between dose and the presence of nodules in the thyroid than there is between dose and the development of cancer. Likewise in man the frequency of appearance of nodules in the thyroid is greater

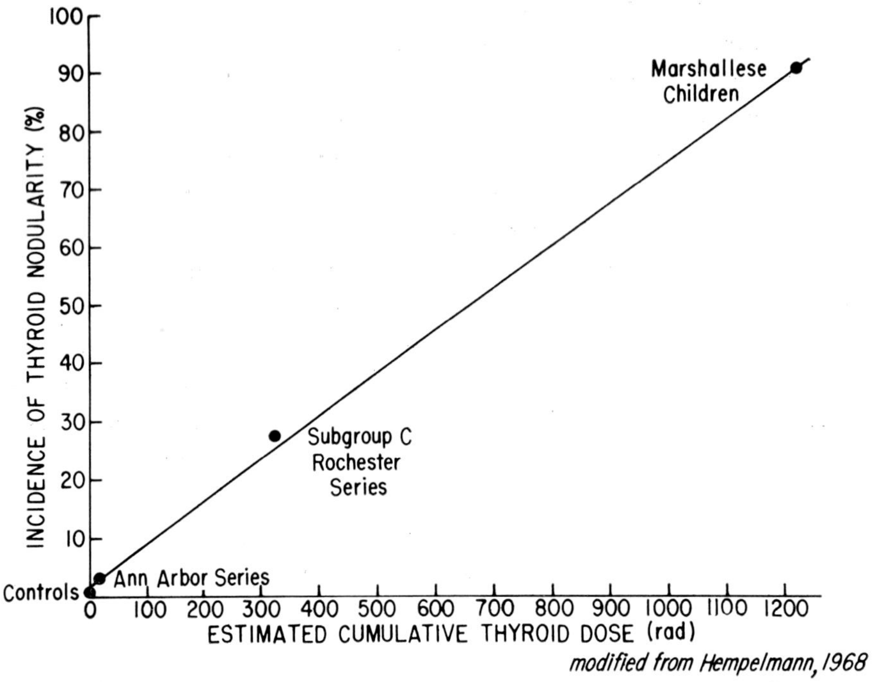

Fig. 4. Incidence of nodules in the thyroid as presented by Hempelmann[19] from his own data and that of others. Note the relative linearity of this type of thyroid damage.

than that of cancer and appears to precede the development of cancer. In the graph (Figure 4) the incidence of thyroid nodules is plotted as they have been encountered in several groups reported by Hempelmann[19] and others. With a low cumulative exposure of the thyroid there is a slight and probably questionable increase as evidenced by the Ann Arbor series.[20] In patients from the Rochester group who received more than 300 R the incidence is about 20%, and in the Rongelap children the incidence at 1,200 rad exposure is better than 90%. Here then, there appears to be a rough linear relation between cause and effect. If one adjusts the dose to allow for the protracted rate at which the radiation was received one finds an even steeper rise of thyroid nodularity with dose.

At present one can say that the incidence of thyroid cancer is increased by radiation, and that those exposed in infancy and childhood appear more susceptible than those exposed in adult life.

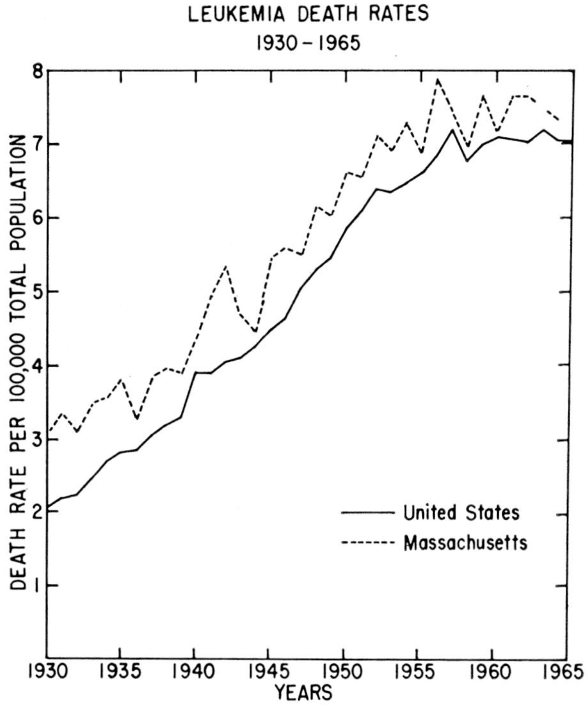

Fig. 5. Death rates from leukemia in the United States and in the Commonwealth of Massachusetts from 1930 to 1965. Note the sharp increase in incidence since 1960 and the tendency for the rate to level off in the late 1950s.

Blood dyscrasias have long been associated with exposure to radiation. Mme. Curie herself died of an unusual type of aplastic anemia. The fluctuations of blood cells following radiation exposure, small or large, have long been studied. In fact, the fluctuations in white blood cell count in survivors as well as mortality figures at Hiroshima and Nagasaki provided more accurate dosimetric information than did the initial calculations of the physicists. The most carefully studied of blood dyscrasias, both experimentally and clinically, is leukemia. A special challenge exists in that the leukemia death rate in the United States rose sharply from 1930 (well before the atomic age) and continued to do so until about 1955 where it seems to have leveled off (Figure 5). Induction of leukemia by radiation is perhaps better documented and correlated with dose than any other form of malignancy. A generation ago radiologists in the United States were found by March,[21] Ulrich,[22]

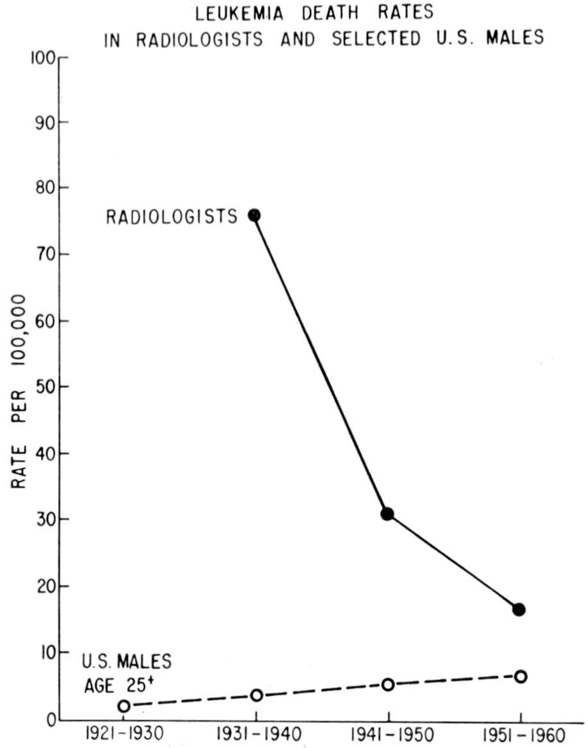

Fig. 6. The incidence of leukemia in radiologists compared with that of the population of the United States. Note the marked decrease in incidence among radiologists as greater precautions against overexposure have been taken.

and others[23, 24] to have a tenfold greater incidence of leukemia than control groups. As they learned to protect themselves better and reduced sharply the occupational exposures received, March's investigation[25] and my recent studies[26] (Figure 6) show the incidence has also been sharply reduced and indeed approaches the level in the general population. Among more than 3,000 Massachusetts dentists whom Miss O. M. Lombard and I[27] have followed for a decade, many of whom had long used x-ray apparatus but with caution, only one case of leukemia has been found.

The population most intensively studied in this regard is the group of Hiroshima-Nagasaki survivors. DeCoursey, Leroy, Liebow, Oughterson, and I,[28, 29] with our Japanese colleagues at the two cities, studied the

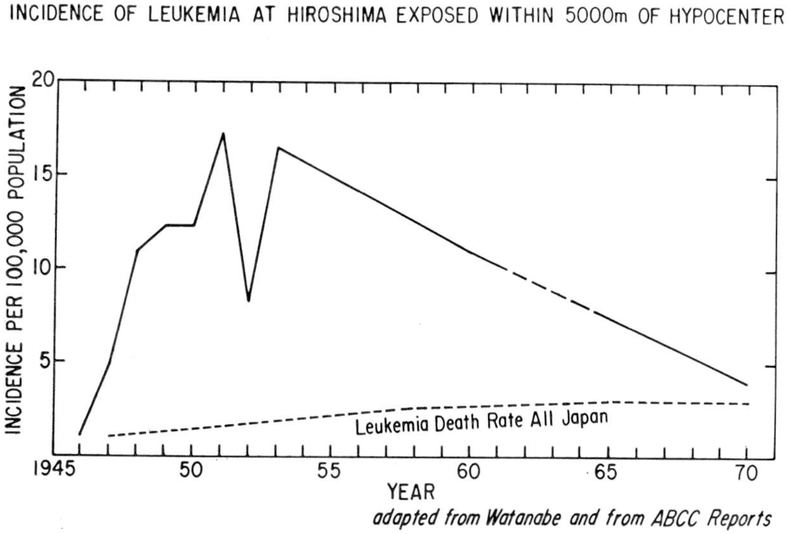

Fig. 7. Incidence of leukemia at Hiroshima among persons exposed within 5,000 meters of the hypocenter. Note the sharp rise in incidence subsequent to the atomic bombing and the decrease in incidence following the mid-1950s. Note also the steady increase in the death rate from leukemia for all Japan and the tendency of the rates in the two populations to approximate each other.

pathology of the bone marrow in those who died within a few months of exposure, noted foci of a typical cellular regeneration in a few and suggested that leukemia might well appear among the survivors. Unfortunately this prediction has been borne out. More than 400 cases have been reported, most of which were of acute myelogenous leukemia.[30] The bulk of the cases thus far reported[31] occurred between 1949 and 1960; the rate, now falling, is now nearing that for all Japan[30] (Figure 7). When the incidence of leukemia is related to distance from the hypocenter of the bomb explosion and thus to estimated dose there is an apparent correlation of increased incidence with dose at levels of 400 rads and above[8] (Figure 8).

These data from Japan, derived from persons who had received a single whole-body exposure, reinforce those reported by the late Dr. Court-Brown[32] as to the dose-effect relation in the development of leukemia among patients whose spinal column had been treated with x rays to relieve the pain of ankylosing spondylitis. In these partial-body, repeated exposures a linear relation could be deduced from the data,

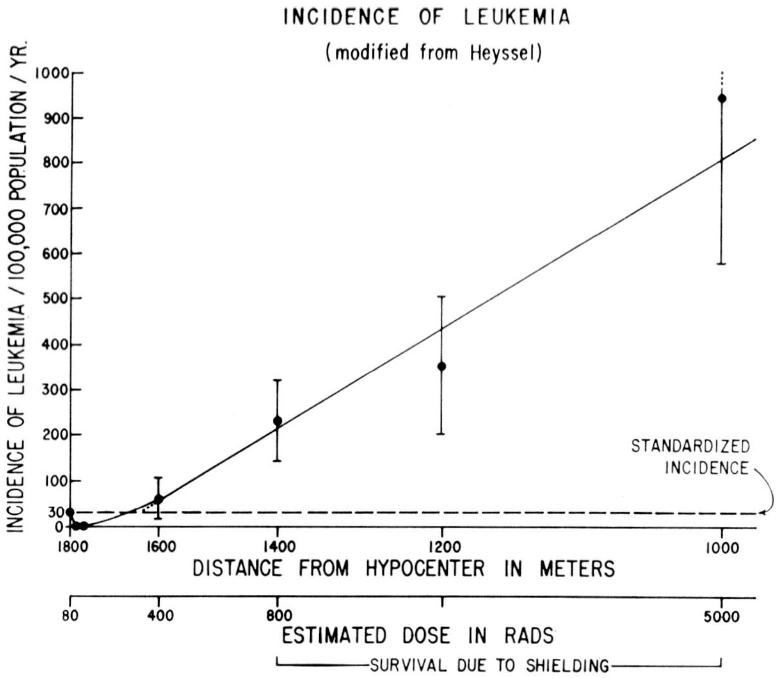

Fig. 8. Incidence of leukemia related to distance from the hypocenter in meters and the estimated dose in rads. Note the approximate linearity of response with increasing dose from 400 rads upward. Survivors in the upper range almost certainly had had partial shielding of their bodies. Reproduced by permission from: Warren, S. *The Pathology of Ionizing Radiation.* Springfield, Ill., Thomas, 1961.

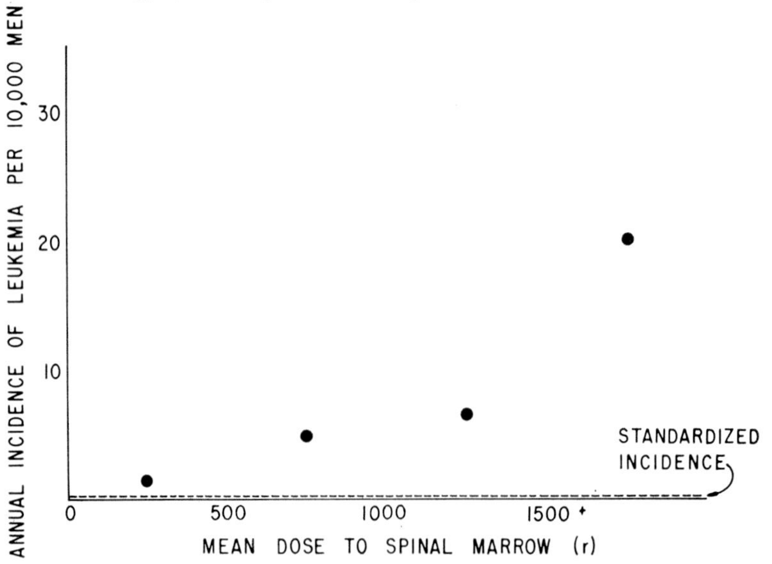

Fig. 9. Annual incidence of leukemia among cases of ankylosing spondylitis[32] with reference to mean dose to the spinal marrow. The data points only are plotted.

PATIENTS WITH CANCER OF THE CERVIX
AGE-ADJUSTED OBSERVED INCIDENCE PER 100,000 PER YEAR*

	Leukemia	*Lymphatic malignancy*	*All hematologic malignancy*
Radium alone	0	0	0
External therapy alone	0	0	0
Radium plus external therapy	8.4	12.7	21.0
No radiation	22.5	0	22.2
All patients	7.3	8.8	16.2
Expected rate	9.0	11.0	20.0

Leukemia and lymphatic malignancy observed in survivors of cervical cancer treated with and without radiation.
*Adapted from Hutchison, G.B.[33]

although the findings were reasonably compatible with a sigmoid type of curve as well (Figure 9).

A puzzling contradiction is found in the international study reported by Hutchison.[33] Here many clinics cooperated to report subsequent development of leukemia in those women treated for cancer of the cervix, many of whom had received radiation to a large portion of their hematopoietic tissue in the course of treatment (see accompanying table). No cases of hematologic malignancy appeared in those cases treated with radium alone and none with external radiation therapy alone. In those receiving a combination of the two the rate was 21/100,000; in those cases that received no radiation and were treated with surgery only the rate was 22/100,000; the expected rate was 20/100,000. In other words, in these patients with thousands of years at risk there was no increase in leukemia. This might be due to the fact that insufficient time has passed; this possibility will be indicated by the continuing character of this study. It might also mean that the considerable unirradiated portion of the marrow had protected the irradiated portion to some degree.

However it is clearly established that leukemia, usually but not always of the myeloid type, is induced in man by exposure to ionizing radiation, although the incidence-dose relation is less clearly established. The percentage of leukemia cases among those exposed is always small, usually under 5%. Apparently an exposure of less than 100 rads is not effective.

To summarize: adequate data have been obtained to establish a variety of types of ionizing radiation as a cause of cancer. This holds for a number of different kinds of malignant tumors derived from different cell types. The dose-effect relations are not clear, but in general a greater dose may be correlated with a higher-incidence rate of cancer. The mechanisms for radiation carcinogenesis are more probably multiple than single.

REFERENCES

1. Gross, L. "Spontaneous" leukemia developing in C3H mice following inoculation in infancy with AK leukemia extracts, or AK embryos. *Proc. Soc. Exp. Biol. Med. 76*:27, 1951.
2. Frieben, A. Cancroid . . . nach langdauernder Einwirkung von Röntgenstrahlen. *Fortschr. Röntgenstr. 6*:106, 1902.
3. Martland, H. S. The occurrence of malignancy in radioactive persons. *Amer. J. Cancer 15*:2435, 1931.
4. Evans, R. D., Keane, A. T., Kolenkow, R. J., Neal, W. R. and Shanahan, M. M. Radiogenic tumors in the radium and mesothorium cases studied at M.I.T. In: Mays, C. W. *et al. Delayed Effects of Bone-Seeking Radionuclides.* Salt Lake City, Univ. of Utah Press, 1969.
5. Sikl, H. Uber den Lungenkrebs der Bergleute in Joachimstahl (Tschechoslowakei). *Z. Krebsforsch. 32*:609, 1930.
6. U.S. Congress Joint Committee on Atomic Energy, Subcommittee on Research, Development, and Radiation. *Radiation Exposure of Uranium Miners.* Washington, D.C., Govt. Print. Off., 1968.
7. Toyooka, E. T., Pifer, J. W., Crump, S. L., Dutton, A. M. and Hempelmann, L. H. Neoplasms in children treated with x-rays for thymic enlargement. II. Tumor incidence as a function of radiation factors. *J. Nat. Cancer Inst. 31*:1357, 1963.
8. Brill, A. B., Tomonaga, M. and Heyssel, R. M. Leukemia in man following exposure to ionizing radiation: Summary of findings in Hiroshima and Nagasaki, and comparison with other human experience. *Ann. Intern. Med. 56*:590, 1962.
9. Wolbach, S. B. The pathological histology of chronic x-ray dermatitis and early x-ray carcinoma. *J. Med. Res. 21*:415, 1909.
10. Cade, Sir Stanford. Radiation-induced cancer in man. *Brit. J. Radiol. 30*:393, 1957.
11. Albert, R. E., Omran, A. R., Bauer, E. W., Dove, D. C., Cohen, N. C., Schmidt H., Baumring, R., Morrill, S., Schulz, R. and Baer, R. L. Follow-up study of patients treated by x-ray for tinea capitis. *Amer. J. Pub. Health 56*:2114, 1966.
12. MacMahon, H. E., Murphy, A. S. and Bates, M. I. Endothelial-cell sarcoma of liver following thorotrast injections. *Amer. J. Path. 28*:585, 1947.
13. Morken, D. A. and Scott, J. K. *The Effects on Mice of Continual Exposure to Radon and its Decay Products on Dust.* Univ. of Rochester, Atomic Energy Commission Project Report No. UR-669, 1966.
14. Meyer, E. C. and Liebow, A. A. Relationship of interstitial pneumonia honeycombing and atypical epithelial proliferation to cancer of the lung. *Cancer 18*:322, 1965.
15. Saccomanno, G., Archer, V. E., Saunders, R. P., James, L. A. and Beckler, P. A. Lung cancer of uranium miners on the Colorado plateau. *Health Phys. 10*:1195, 1964.
16. Socolow, E. L. and Hashizume, A. Thy-

roid carcinoma in man after exposure to ionizing radiation. *New Eng. J. Med.* *268*:406, 1963.

17. Conard, R. A., Rall, J. E. and Sutow, W. W. Thyroid nodules as a late sequela of radioactive fallout: In a Marshall Island population exposed in 1954. *New Eng. J. Med.* *274*:1391, 1966.
18. Bustad, L. K., George, L. A., Jr., Marks, S., Warner, D. E., Barnes, C. M., Herde, K. E. and Kornberg, H. A. Biological effects of I^{131} continuously administered to sheep. *Radiat. Res.* *6*: 380, 1957.
19. Hempelmann, L. H. Risk of thyroid neoplasms after irradiation in childhood. *Science* *160*:159, 1968.
20. Pifer, J. W., Hempelmann, L. H., Dodge, H. and Hodges, F. J. Neoplasms in Ann Arbor series of thymus-irradiated children: A second survey. *Amer. J. Roentgen.* *103*:13, 1968.
21. March, H. C. Leukemia in radiologists. *Radiology* *43*:275, 1944.
22. Ulrich, H. Incidence of leukemia in radiologists. *New Eng. J. Med.* *234*:45, 1946.
23. Henshaw, P. S. and Hawkins, J. W. Incidence of leukemia in physicians. *J.A.M.A.* *4*:339, 1944.
24. Warren, S. Longevity and causes of death from irradiation in physicians. *J.A.M.A.* *162*:464, 1956.
25. March, H. C. Leukemia in radiologists, ten years later: With review of pertinent evidence for radiation leukemia. *Amer. J. Med. Sc.* *242*:137, 1961.
26. Warren, S. and Lombard, O. M. New data on the exposure of the human population to ionizing radiation. Proc. 11th Internat. Congress of Radiology, Excerpta Medica Internat. Congress Series No. 105, pp. 1508-13, 1967.
27. Warren, S. and Lombard, O. M. Mortality and radiation exposures of Massachusetts dentists. *J. Amer. Dent. Assoc.* In press.
28. Liebow, A. A., Warren, S. and DeCoursey, E. Pathology of atomic bomb casualties. *Amer. J. Path.* *25*:853, 1949.
29. Oughterson, A. W. and Warren, S. *Medical Effects of the Atomic Bomb in Japan.* Division VIII—Vol. 8. National Nuclear Energy Series. Manhattan Project Technical Section. New York, McGraw-Hill, 1956.
30. Atomic Bomb Casualty Commission, Fact Book, 1969 ed. Tabular and graphic presentation of ABCC research findings.
31. Bizzozero, O. J., Jr., Johnson, K. G. and Giocco, A. Radiation-related leukemia in Hiroshima and Nagasaki, 1946-1964. I. Distribution, incidence and appearance time. *New Eng. J. Med.* *274*:1095, 1966.
32. Court-Brown, W. M. and Doll, R. *Leukaemia and aplastic anaemia in patients irradiated for ankylosing spondylitis.* Medical Research Council Report 295. London, Her Majesty's Stationery Office, 1957.
33. Hutchison, G. B. Leukemia in patients with cancer of the cervix uteri treated with radiation. A report covering the first 5 years of an international study. *J. Nat. Cancer Inst.* *40*:951, 1968.

AMERICAN MEDICINE: TECHNOLOGY OUTRUNS SOCIAL USEFULNESS*

George A. Silver

Executive Associate
Health Program
The Urban Coalition
Washington, D.C.

American medicine is at a pinnacle of technical advance and success that could not have been dreamed of a generation ago. From the ultramicroscopic nature of life itself to complex transplant surgery, from computer diagnosis to antibiotics, the scientific achievement is incalculably brilliant. Public health activity has eliminated the bulk of epidemic disease. Three million people work in association with health services in the United States in more than 7,000 hospitals and 20,000 other health institutions. And we are not stingy in supporting this medical establishment. This year close to $60 billion, about 6.5% of the Gross National Product, will pay for our health services.

At the same time there is a desperate crisis in health services. Millions of people are without health services or poorly served. A majority of the population expresses dissatisfaction with the arrangements and their cost—they find difficulty in getting the health service they want, when they want it, and in a personally satisfying way. Minor political skirmishes such as the imbroglio over the recent proposed appointment of Dr. John Knowles to the post of assistant secretary of health become bitter controversies over the organization and cost of medical services and the proper role of the medical profession.

A great deal is made of the deficiencies of health services to the poor, and this is surely the case. The poor do suffer disproportionately and unduly from the inequities of the system. But let us not delude ourselves. We are all victims of the disorganization and maldistribution of health-care services. The poor suffer the deficiencies in more exaggerated form.

The inability to find a doctor on Wednesday afternoon or Sundays,

*Presented at a meeting of the Subcommittee on Social Policy for Health Care, Committee on Medicine in Society, October 30, 1969.

frustration in the emergency room, overcrowded clinics, the desperate search for the right doctor for the right condition, the hazardous hospital situation, all of these are ominously developing into worse and worse conditions for the poor, for the middle class, and for the well-to-do as well. There needs to be change, and not just for the poor. In many ways, when we talk of "ghetto health needs" we are like the physicians who used to talk about tropical medicine as if it were a unique type of medicine. Now we know disease in the tropics is compounded by poverty and lack of medical resources.

We have gone beyond the "Negro problem" to recognize the complex of social failure that it epitomizes. We need to go beyond the "ghetto health problem" to see the professional and social problems there. Poor people of whatever color are sicker and need more care; as a matter of fact, some of their poverty may be due to their illness. But there is less health care available to them.

It is fashionable today to talk of crisis: in the cities, in the ghetto, in the schools, in the dollar. There is hardly a place, institution, or idea that is not in crisis. It seems to escape us that crises are not accidents that come upon us without notice, without our fault or contributory guilt. Crises have histories too.

We have already been deep in the crisis in health care much longer than in some of the other crises we talk about. The report of the President's Commission on Health Manpower a few years ago stated flatly that medicine was in crisis. To go back even further, the Committee on the Costs of Medical Care, which was set up in 1928, and reported in 1932, made a similar announcement. The conditions describing the grave nature of the deficiencies in health services and the opportunities for resolving them were clearly spelled out in that report about 37 years ago.

The crisis in health care arises from the nature of our health-care system. The structure is out of date, and the more we tinker with it the more we expose its failure to respond to expressed need.

Why is it more urgent now to do something about it? As one folk singer says, the times they are changing and new winds are blowing. There is an increasing awareness that the demands upon us in every aspect of our social life require that we be more attentive to gross defects in the social fabric. Recognizing this, we must do what can be done to make effective change. John Gardner has said, "History is not going to deal kindly with a rich nation that will not tax itself to cure its misery."

De Tocqueville wrote, "The evils which are endured with patience as long as they are incurable, seem intolerable as soon as hope can be entertained of escaping from them."

The unfortunate fact is that those who see about them the possibilities of change do not want to accept the bitter realities.

In the days of the five-cent beer with free lunch, not too much was expected of medicine or of doctors. In those days doctors were well distributed throughout the country, even in the most isolated places. As a matter of fact there was a better distribution of physicians in rural than in urban America. Hospitals were scarce, but then, most medical practice was outside hospitals—even surgery, and certainly childbirth. We did not have to worry about long-term care, nursing homes, middle medical institutions, convalescent homes, and the like, because the extended family took care of its own. There were always spinster aunts, young cousins, and all sorts of other people to look after the aged, the feeble, the handicapped, the mentally deficient, and those recovering from or failing to recover from chronic illnesses. As a matter of fact, there was very little in the way of chronic illness because people did not live long enough to fall prey to it. Birth rates and infant death rates were high. Life expectancy was no more than 40 or 50 years; degenerative diseases did not begin to have their marked effects on demand for medical services and social institutions until later.

But the character of the physician-advisor, guide to the family, possessor of a few remedies that sometimes worked and many more that did not, his location and easy availability, set in people's minds a certain pattern of what medicine is or ought to be, and they would like to have it again.

In the interval technological advance has changed the capability of the physician enough to make a difference in the outcome, although actually most of the credit should be given to the public-health activities of nonphysicians (usually over the strenuous objections of organized medical bodies): to chlorinate water, eliminate infectious disease and, by preventative measures socially applied, to reduce the major causes of death that carried away our grandfathers and grandmothers in early life.

And the technological changes have had other effects. They brought with the blessings of science the concentration on and worship of the scientific method. As a consequence medicine has been diverted from dealing with people to dealing with "problems." This meant being concerned more about the fascinating variety of illness than about the people who were beset by these illnesses. The students of medicine flocked into scientific training. They stayed on to continue their scientific endeavors and concentrated around the institutions committed to science. They failed to distribute themselves appropriately and clustered around universities rather than in areas where people live. The emphasis on quality and specialism, with the attendant cost of long-drawn-out training appreciably reduced their numbers and broke up the multivalent physician into a multitude of physicians, which made it necessary to see five or six or 20 doctors for appropriate diagnosis and treatment. This multiplied the number of doctors that would be needed at a time when their number was failing to increase.

Parallel with this, of course, was the machinery that accompanied technological advance, which necessitated the employment of hundreds of thousands, and even millions, of technically expert people to deal with the new mechanical, electrical, and other devices that went into the making of modern medicine and multiplied its cost.

And the advances created new problems as they solved old ones. The changing population which resulted added demands on the medical-care system: an aging population; the decline in infant mortality, which gave us more children who needed to be cared for; the associated increase in chronic and degenerative diseases that made increasing demands on the complicated equipment, technical expertise, and specialized qualifications of the diminishing pool of physicians.

Of course we must not forget that, as more could be done, advances in communications spread the word, informing larger and larger numbers of people, giving them hope, and sending them clamoring for the helpful curative services.

There was more recognized need, more demand, and fewer available doctors; there was more technical capability, more patients, more institutions to give care, and more cost.

Frustration began here. No one likes paying more and more for less and less.

Since these facts are all so plain, why have not the intelligent, well-educated, rational human beings who compose the professional personnel and the patients—all of us, in other words—moved in step to make all these things available? When Henry Ford produced his car it did not take too long to get cars to everyone who wanted them and could afford them; now we have more cars than we know what to do with as we pave this country with concrete.

We are not lacking in solutions. There is hardly a person who, having suffered in consequence of the deficiencies in medical-care services, has not come up with a solution. There is the manpower solution: more hands will solve the problem. Organization will solve the medical-care problem. Group practice is the solution. Others prescribe national health insurance, twice as many medical schools, a nationalized health service.

And the result of 30 or 40 years of talk and argument and recommendations is—nothing.

An able British student of these affairs, Professor Thomas McKeown of Birmingham, wrote (20 years ago!): "Both political parties practice a form of political contraception, in which no matter how suggestive the preliminary movements, there are no embarrassing legislative consequences."

It is of no real value to assess blame, because there is more than enough blame to go around. We may recall, in this connection, Pogo's telling us "We have met the enemy and they is us."

Among the responsible elements we must rate ignorance very high. Many people know the problems, but few can cope with the answers because there are so many different threads that must be woven together. Most people prefer simple solutions.

Then there is apathy—"those who ain't hurtin' ain't fightin.'" Too many people are getting just enough out of the system to make them believe it is unnecessary to make major changes.

And there is fear of the unknown by patients who believe that they may be disestablished if they antagonize the professional and lose access to medical care altogether. There is fear on the part of the professional of losing his privileged position. In a sense this stems from the guild character of professional groups, who tend to do whatever is necessary to retain their status, to maintain a scarce labor pool, and to keep salaries high.

There is the vested interest of rich doctors, administrators, and hospital boards who want no change that would put them in secondary roles or make them less likely to earn as much as they do now.

Private insurance, whether nonprofit like Blue Cross, or commercial, has failed us. Knuckling under to the professional interests, such insurance has failed to protect the consumer against exploitation and quality defects and has sold him into bondage for financial considerations.

Some great organized consumer bodies, such as trade unions, have been remiss too. They have not used their united strength to bargain collectively for the 60 million people they represent to obtain more national and satisfactory organized health services.

There is racism; and discussion of this topic cannot be omitted in today's world without a clear recognition that something desperately needed by blacks, Mexican-Americans, and Indians is not necessarily what the rest of us think we ought to pay for out of our taxes.

There is a standard disposition in our public-private partnership to be stingy with the poor and generous with the rich. This is evidenced by the road-building mania and payments to rich farmers while public transportation and food programs for the poor go begging.

There is the obsession left by generations of intimidation about communism and "socialized medicine," so that anything that smacks of effective government action will be immediately labeled as such.

And, of course, there is bureaucracy, that great dragon that lies across all federal, state, and local programs. Of the many sins of which we are guilty no doubt the greatest is bureaucracy.

Still, it is hard to separate out the victims and the villains. Like wars in which there are no victors, only survivors, this battle is also one in which all are vanquished. The federal establishment may bear a heavier share of the blame because of its larger share of responsibilities.

The tangle of federal programs spawned sporadically and capriciously with no design or goal or over-all policy is inexcusable. A dozen agencies have health-care responsibilities: Health Services and Mental Health Administration for comprehensive planning and services; the Children's Bureau for child and maternal health services; the Office of Economic Opportunity, for comprehensive care to the poor; Model Cities programs; the Department of Labor, for training subprofessionals; the Veterans Administration; the Department of Defense. And as if this were not enough, think of all the congressional committees which have to hear testimony and prepare legislation in these various areas, and of the additional committees that have to do likewise for appropriations for programs enacted into law.

And, of course, the programs are run by officials.

Bureaucrats are a special breed. They need not say "no" and risk being fired for insubordination. They can merely do "no" by failing to carry out what was intended because they know better than the people, the Congress, and the policy makers what ought to be done.

State bureaucrats are no better. There is a comprehensive health-planning law, yet from most states there have been no plans. Model Cities programs preoccupy the states and local committees with structural problems, not programs.

Regional Medical Programs offer universities, teaching hospitals, and medical schools a golden opportunity to improve their staff and facilities. The services that did not serve the people before are now more deluxe.

Medicare and Medicaid are payment mechanisms that insure doctors and hospitals against the possibility of loss from indigent patients. They serve only to guarantee providers of care (not poor consumers!) against financial loss.

In the past two years national expenditures for health went up 25%, medical care prices 17%, medical services hardly at all. "Reasonable cost" and "reasonable charges" provide a license for freedom from cost restraints.

There is a cruel insensitivity to social need in this area on the part of the professions. But there is a heavier insensitivity on the part of officials who hesitate to apply the law in a way to make it work for people. And our leaders are no help. There is no coherent long-term policy. We move from problem to problem, never solving one before we jump into another. If we continue to buy fee-for-service medicine for the old, the young, and the poor through Title 19, through Medicare, and through private insurance programs, the cost of the services will go up and up. We might say, "So what, why shouldn't we spend that much money on health?" Well, of course we can, but we will not be getting our money's worth for the money spent. Sweden spends 3½% of its Gross National Product for health services and gets in return better medical service, more satisfactory medical care, lower infant mortality, and longer life expectancy, and fewer people die in the productive years of their lives—all for less money. It is not money that is the problem, it is the policy which is not there that is the problem.

The present efforts to sail the health ship of state without a rudder are doomed to failure. There is no national-health policy. Until we establish one and rearrange our laws, programs, and management to achieve the results desired, more and more confusion and failure await us.

It seems to me that the strategy of the proponents of improved health care in this country in the past has been off-center. This strategy has been largely devoted to national educational programs and efforts to influence national legislation. So long as the vast majority of lay persons and of professionals have the reservations and fears that have been expressed earlier, just so long will national approaches fail. Until there are grass-roots knowledge and pressures it would seem almost hopeless to look for national solutions. The remedy will have to come from large numbers of local efforts for change. The sum of these local efforts will, in my opinion, create the formidable pressures needed for a national effort.

Yes, these national goals must be achieved. But until everyone is aware of the kinds of defects and the kinds of possibilities there will be rhetoric but no action. Right now, in every community in the country, money is being wasted, misused, or unused, because of inappropriate programs and misdirected activities. By working at the local level to improve health services, important lessons can be learned and taught as to how the whole system of health-care services can be improved.

At the very least, more than is now being done can be accomplished by introducing efficiency and economy into the local health-care system. Consumer participation will give each community the opportunity to analyze the needs, propose priorities, and get action.

We have prepared a booklet, *Rx for Action*, to help communities see how they can establish local health-task forces, what such task forces might do, and how health services can be improved locally. It is more like a menu than a cookbook. It describes what can be done, rather than how to do it. But for those communities which elect to move in this direction the Urban Coalition will provide technical assistance and consultation. Among the action programs suggested—which will vary from community to community, naturally—are such things as the improvement of hospital service through overhauling the outpatient clinic, improvement of emergency services; manpower-training programs to add the health workers needed to eliminate sanitation and environmental hazards; cooperative actions with medical societies for supplying added medical services where needed; developing new programs in the fields of mental health and mental retardation. The basic emphasis is on better use of existing resources rather than further multiplication of programs. The emphasis is on efficiency and economy, underlining the added services that can result from better use of existing monies and better services for the same dollars. For a more complete review I recommend *Rx for Action* to you.

Here is where we come to the joining of forces with the strong drive in this country to improve the condition of the poor and of minority groups. Until now the effort has been concentrated on the creation of improved health services for the poor.

In reviewing the variety of solutions that have been proposed in the past there is good reason to question efforts that focus on improving medical care for the poor alone. In a sense this must be a dual system, a poor system, in both senses of the word. In some cases, of course, the effort has resulted in a striking improvement of health services available, and it would be unfair to describe it as "poor" medicine. On the other hand, in the long run the creation of a dual system must have the same effect as the creation of two currencies. In addition, of course, it will tend to drain off manpower and multiply the needs and expense unnecessarily. A unified single system would undoubtedly be preferable.

Medical care for the poor in sufficient quantity and satisfactory quality will be achieved only when we have a system that guarantees equal access to all—rich and poor, black, Chicano and white, urban and rural—all over this country.

To achieve this a number of things must be done. To talk about simply increasing manpower, for example, is useless if all we are going to do is create more people like the ones we have. We need not only physicians who are oriented differently toward their profession and technicians who will do more than simply produce a mechanical response: we must have new and differently trained people to meet this society's needs for health services. Manpower will not be the answer unless it is coupled with changes in organization and structure of medical practice, and also changes in the way health care is financed.

A thoughtful administrator, Irving Lewis of the Health Services and Mental Health Administration, has written, "The great social dilemma is that liberals, conservatives, and reactionaries have all fallen victims to the myth that the only barrier standing between a person and good medical care is his inability to pay for it. The concept that the problem of distribution can be handled by mere availability of money has proved unworkable."

As far as using the money made available in any scheme, how the providers will be reimbursed also presents problems.

The prevalent mechanism for paying physicians in this country is through fee-for-service. Under these conditions, no plan of trying to distribute medical services more equitably and of providing them in poorly served areas can be successful. Fee-for-service has a built-in inflationary character, as Title 19—the Medicaid Act—has shown. In examining mechanisms of reimbursing physicians in various countries in the world, it has been found that the method of reimbursement to which physicians are most fiercely attached in any country is the direct product of the system that provides the largest income to physicians. One must take the "ethical" stance of physicians with regard to fee-for-service with a grain of salt. It happens to be the method that assures the physician the highest possible income in this country.

When we talk of "national health insurance" or "national financing" the idea of a universal compulsory federal system springs to mind immediately. This need not be the case. The United States is uniquely blessed with a pluralistic tradition. This can be taken advantage of in designing a system that covers private and public insurance efforts, federal-tax revenues, voluntary participation, and involuntary contribution. The Scandinavian countries have a mixed insurance and health-service financing mechanism. There is no reason why we cannot adopt similar measures.

Let us lay at rest the bugaboos of "compulsory health insurance" and "socialized medicine." Let us think and talk in terms of universal national financing and how to accomplish this.

A National Commission should be directed to recommend to the federal government *how to*, not whether to, introduce a national, universal arrangement for financing health care.

We need national financing of health care on an equitable basis, and reimbursement of physicians on a basis that overcomes the inflationary effect of fee-for-service payment.

The current system of organization of practice depends to a large extent upon solo practitioners, and this system cannot possibly provide the needed complicated services people must have in the places where they must have them. Certainly solo practitioners are not going to practice in rural areas and ghettos: they have been fleeing these places for years. Urban physicians have fled to the suburbs along with all the other middle-class white people who can pay for their services.

Therefore those who recommend group practice are right. Solo practice will have to be modified to become group practice. But none of these arrangements can be imposed upon physicians and patients by fiat. Patients must have an experience with something other than solo practice to convince them that group practice will be advantageous. Physicians, too, will have to have the same experience. So far in this country there are few such examples; only 10% of the population may have had such experience and have been quite satisfied with it.

In addition, of course, the introduction of new types of health practitioners to create a level of service between that of the highly qualified specialists in group practice and general practitioners will have to be developed. So far very few of these experiments have been demonstrated and, as a consequence, very few persons in the United States are prepared to give up their nostalgic longing for the family doctor who lives a few steps away, who is available 24 hours a day, and who will provide kind and compassionate, albeit rational and scientific, quick cures for their complaints and illnesses at very little cost.

A program of action to improve the system of delivering health services is also necessary. We need a Health Policy Council, a high-level group of knowledgeable people to lay out the general outlines of what we ought to do and where we ought to be going. A further significant step would be the rationalization of our disorganized approach to the funding of health services—at least a coordinated federal attack through amalgamation of the various agencies responsible plus the amalgamation of the Congressional committees responsible.

You have heard all this before. We need better organization, national financing, more and different kinds of health workers, a straightforward national health policy.

First will have to come more consumer input. Major policy decisions in health must have the participation of citizens as well as of professionals. Every committee, every board, every advisory and operating group must have such participation, especially from among groups now specifically ignored or deprived. The voice of the people must be heard.

More participation by consumers is merely a restoration of American democratic principles. Harold Laski said we must keep the experts "on tap, not on top." We need to keep our technical expertise in the health field on tap rather than on top.

If these things can be done, many of the other things will be carried out more easily: universal national financing of health services organization along modern lines, more and newer kinds of health workers, team practice. But without the input of people on national policy I doubt if anything can be done.

In a real sense, of course, this merely reiterates what has been said of other segments of society and their responsibility. Are we not our brothers' keepers? Should a drug company sell a drug it knows to be useless or dangerous only because it is in line with "business ethics"? Should institutions starve and mistreat their occupants because the profit margin is narrow? Are patients or doctors the hospital's clients?

Of course this is true of all the rest of our environment—air and water pollution, decayed and execrable housing, inadequate transportation, and the use of police instead of doctors for drug addicts.

Let us not delude ourselves, either, that we can restrict our concern to personal health-care needs. The environment is causative of a good part of the disease we have to spend so much money to treat. We must clean up the environment, eliminate air and water pollution, provide decent housing and neighborhoods, and make our living space clean. We must get rid of situations that lead kindergarten children to identify a picture of a teddy bear as a rat!

At the moment the best hope seems to be through local action in providing the educational matrix, the demonstrated experience, and some of the logical and rational ways in which these things can be done. The Urban Coalition is moving in this direction through stimulating the formation of local health task forces that will examine their own local situations and, by discussing with local people how improvements can be made on a local level, show the country at large what changes can be made nationally in these same directions.

Professionals can play a critical role in this effort. Health services for all Americans depends on concerted, intelligent action by all the people. The education of Americans in health-care needs and in solutions to health-care problems will flow from effective local organizations for the improvement of health services. If physicians will put aside narrow guild interests, address themselves in a statesmanlike way to social problems and social needs, and participate in health task force deliberations and efforts success will be assured.

DISCUSSION OF PAPER BY DR. GEORGE A. SILVER: "AMERICAN MEDICINE: TECHNOLOGY OUTRUNS SOCIAL USEFULNESS"

Mack Lipkin

Clinical Associate Professor of Medicine
Cornell University Medical College
New York, N. Y.

I have heard Dr. George A. Silver present his paper, but unfortunately I have had no opportunity to read it. However, I was able to read the pamphlet just published by his group, the Health Task Force of the Urban Coalition.† In my judgment there is no planning document anywhere in the medical literature which contains a more comprehensive statement of the problems, greater wisdom, or more pertinent suggestions.

Having said this, may I offer a few comments. Medical care is an intensely personal matter, delivered very commonly in a setting of apprehension and confusion on the part of its recipients. If changes are to be made there is great need for them to be made at such a pace and in such a manner that they can be acceptable to persons in search of care and caring. For example, Medicare by and large has been successful in achieving much of its purpose, that is, making more medical care freely available for most older people. It changed medical care *only* by supplying more funds. To be sure it has not created more doctors, more nurses, more hospitals, or more nursing homes, and all of these are in short supply. Its costs have been too great, but these will eventually be controlled. In contrast Medicaid has created a sea of confusion for which, as usual, medical practitioners have been blamed—in my judgment with virtually no justification.

If we are to have planning for medical care on a national scale it seems clear that we really need a separate secretary of health to coordinate health efforts. We shall probably need a national Council of

*Presented at a meeting of the Subcommittee on Social Policy for Health Care, Committee on Medicine in Society, October 30, 1969.

†*Rx for Action.* Report of the Health Task Force of the Urban Coalition. Washington, D.C., Urban Coalition, 1969.

Health Advisers. But above all we need careful planning, careful setting of priorities, and great care not to arouse false hopes which can result only in more disappointment, more hasty corrections, and further confusion.

The public at all levels now seems ready for some kind of national health-care insurance, perhaps some type of national Medicare. The unions, the Nixon administration, and the American Health Administration are all ready for a national plan: the time for one is ripe. This now seems to be the only possible way to wipe out the inequities of our present patterns of insurance. Currently the kind of medical care available depends partly on where people happen to be living—in which state, in which county, in which city. Partly it depends on membership in which union, partly on private funds. This is not to ignore the fact that there is a dearth of facilities of every kind.

One facet of Medicare is the payment of hospital bills, a sort of national Blue Cross. It would be feasible to establish a complete national Blue Cross at the same time that national medical care insurance begins. Of course there will be many difficulties.

After the confusion of these first steps has ended—a matter, I should think, of two or three years—it would be time for the next step: namely, a governmental takeover of all except proprietary hospitals. This is the usual pattern in Europe. It also seems the only reasonable way of clearing this hodgepodge of control of our hospitals. At present some of them are federal, some of them are state, county, municipal, church, voluntary, or privately controlled. At the beginning, costs would be huge, but medical and hospital fees can be controlled. Perhaps if we had some national system it might be possible to arrange for the use of management consultants and perhaps for studies like those made by the Rand Institute. Anybody who has worked in large hospitals knows how grossly inefficient they can become. And perhaps we might have an end to the monstrous temples of administrative empire building, the ever-larger medical centers.

As far as payment for medical care as distinct from hospital care is concerned, perhaps the next step might be that all operations be done in the hospitals, and that all surgeons be on salary rather than on fee-for-service arrangements. First, this would wipe out most of the objections to whatever fee-for-service arrangements remain. The greatest advantage of capitation is the reduction in surgical procedures (a great boon quite apart from the reduction in cost), since it removes all incentive toward unnecessary surgery. Second, it would reduce the number of surgeons being trained. At the present time this seems to be the only field of medicine which is generously supplied with personnel.

Once surgeons have been put on salary, a similar arrangement could be extended easily and quickly to those in the departments of medicine whose work is largely confined to the hospital: for example, those in charge of coronary-care units, intensive pulmonary-care units, radiologists, etc. All of these changes could be effected in the first few years after a national Medicare is established. What happens then is problematic.

I should like to turn now to another question. The lack of manpower and facilities represents perhaps the greatest risk in establishing national health insurance. Since there are simply not enough doctors, nurses, hospitals, and nursing homes to go around, there will inevitably be dissatisfaction and a major outcry. One of the first steps must be a vast increase in our output of doctors.

I agree with the authors of the pamphlet of the Urban Coalition that our medical schools are in need of drastic overhaul. There must be a vast and immediate increase in admissions. There is a need for somebody with the power to cut this gordian knot. I asked two deans of medical schools what would happen if the federal government made further funding of schools conditional on a 10 to 15 to 20% increase in the student population annually for the next five years. What if the medical schools were told by the authorities to have five, then six, then seven, then eight students where they now have four students in a group? What would happen if schools were told that two students would have to use each seat? Each of the deans replied that if just one ingredient were added, money to build more teaching facilities, including perhaps dormitories, it could certainly be done, and done quickly. Each specified that money would have to be earmarked not for research, not for the care of patients, but for teaching. Think of the difference in cost, in time and money, between building a new medical school which costs at least $100,000,000 and five to ten years of planning, as compared with just building facilities.

I then asked both of these very thoughtful, concerned men what would happen if they were told to revert to wartime conditions and to graduate men in three years with the understanding that students would be attending school 11 months a year. Both commented that some of the preclinical people might leave for graduate schools. Both, on second thought, said perhaps not. Perhaps if salaries were raised this would be overcome. And then there was final agreement that this not only could be done but should be done. And that at Dartmouth and perhaps other places, this will be done.

Another notion is the possibility of subsidizing all or most medical students, that is, offering free tuition and perhaps all or most living expenses. After all, we presently pay for the education of virtually all our Ph.D. candidates in the sciences. The cost of doing this for all our medical students might amount to several hundred million dollars a year. In return could we then not ask for two or three years of service at an appropriate salary in the areas of greatest need?

The next spot for careful scrutiny, it seems to me, is the kind of teaching our medical schools are now providing. At present, as far as the interests of the majority of the full-time faculty of most medical schools are concerned, research and publication are accorded the highest priorities, education receives a lower priority, and the care of patients receives the very lowest. As one recently appointed head of a department said to me a few years ago when he was on his way up: "I really don't like to teach. You don't get anywhere teaching. You get no credit for it and besides teaching is infantilizing. To teach successfully you have to bring yourself down to the level of the medical student and that is infantilizing." Is any further comment necessary? And somebody remarked: "I have never met a medical student who was much interested in his teacher's number of publications. In contrast, I have never met a dean or department head who was primarily interested in anything else." But there is a change coming. At Stony Brook, N.Y., and at Hershey, Pa., the emphasis will apparently be on training people for medical care.

Medical schools represent, in their governance, one of the really oligarchic institutions in our society. Every nonmedical top-level academic official I have ever talked with has commented on the unbelievably backward management of medical schools. At a time when so many colleges have elected chairmen, these are almost unheard of in medical schools. There is a great need for a greater voice for the clinical faculties, for the students, and perhaps even for the knowledgeable members of the community in determining the policies of the medical school. Perhaps in this way we might profit from the comment of a European sociologist who happened to require care in an American hospital and used the opportunity to talk at length with interns and attending physicians. This man said: "You American doctors have made of your hospitals your private—how do you call it?—playground. You care mostly for your learning and for your research, and if you have a little time left over, you take care of your patients." Obviously this viewpoint stems from the current overemphasis on research, an emphasis fostered by the flow of money for research and the publicity and prestige which go with research.

May I turn briefly to some of Dr. Silver's other points. Every discussion I have heard by community representatives and especially those union leaders concerned with medical care has emphasized the need of the patient for a personal physician. It is perfectly true that any well-run group can furnish personal physicians. But often enough they simply do not. It can be more easily done in the pattern that Dr. George Baehr suggested a few years ago. Dr. Baehr suggested that we have two- or three- or four-man groups scattered near community hospitals. The members of these small groups would be recruited from the staff of the local hospital. This means no construction of great health centers; it means offices in housing projects and street corners. It solves the transportation problem for mothers of children and others. The trip of 20, 30, or 40 blocks to a medical center, to a community health center, is a problem for poor persons which can be met by busing and other ways, it is true. But this plan means that the person in this area can have a personal physician whom we can hold responsible for his medical care. That physician can refer him to all the consultants he needs at the local hospital, a hospital which would be familiar with and to the physician. In a small unit a physician soon learns what his aides can do and what they cannot be trusted to do. He uses personnel more efficiently and appropriately than any large institution can manage. As a matter of fact, in every large group in which I have ever worked, assistants change all the time and one never knows the personnel very well.

As to fee-for-service: I too should like to see it ended. But let me point out what you already know. At one end of the scale there will be dedicated people who do the best they can no matter how you pay them; at the other end there are men who never do well no matter how you pay them. But in between, in our society, the majority of persons—doctors being among them—will work harder and better if they get immediate rewards. I do not like this system but I think if society is going to get the best out of the medical profession, it will have to have some kind of reward for additional effort. Capitation and salaries tend to reward the lazy and penalize the concerned and the industrious. Fee-for-service, to be sure, encourages unnecessary medical care and, as I have already indicated, there are ways of solving this problem.

RICHARD WISEMAN: HIS CONTRIBUTIONS TO ENGLISH SURGERY*

ALAN DEFOREST SMITH

Emeritus Professor of Orthopedic Surgery
Columbia University College of Physicians and Surgeons
New York, N. Y.

RICHARD WISEMAN was an eminent 17th century surgeon, whose position has been likened to that of Thomas Sydenham in medicine in the same period. He was sergeant-surgeon to King Charles II. Wiseman is best remembered for his book called *Severall Chirurgicall Treatises*,[1] which was the most important text on the subject for many years and was reprinted in several editions (Figures 1 and 2).

This was a momentous period in English history. After the civil war Charles I was beheaded in 1649 and Cromwell ruled as the Protector until his death in 1658. The monarchy was restored in 1660 with the return of Charles II.

London was devastated by the plague in 1665. It is said that 1,000 persons died each week and that a total of 100,000 perished. The epidemic was ended by the great fire which ravaged the city in September 1666.

Among the notable persons of the era in the field of science were William Harvey, who published his treatise on the circulation of the blood in 1628; Isaac Newton; and Robert Boyle, the physicist and author of Boyle's law. In literature were John Milton, Izaak Walton, whose *Compleat Angler* appeared in 1653; and Sir Thomas Browne, noted for his *Religio Medici* and *Urne-Buriall;* Browne was a physician and Osler's favorite author. John Locke, the philosopher who wrote the famous *Essay Concerning Human Understanding*, practiced medicine at one time.

The greatest physician of the time was Thomas Sydenham, although he was not so recognized then. The prominent architects were Sir Christopher Wren and Inigo Jones. We have a very complete picture

*Presented at a meeting of the Section on Historical Medicine, October 22, 1969.

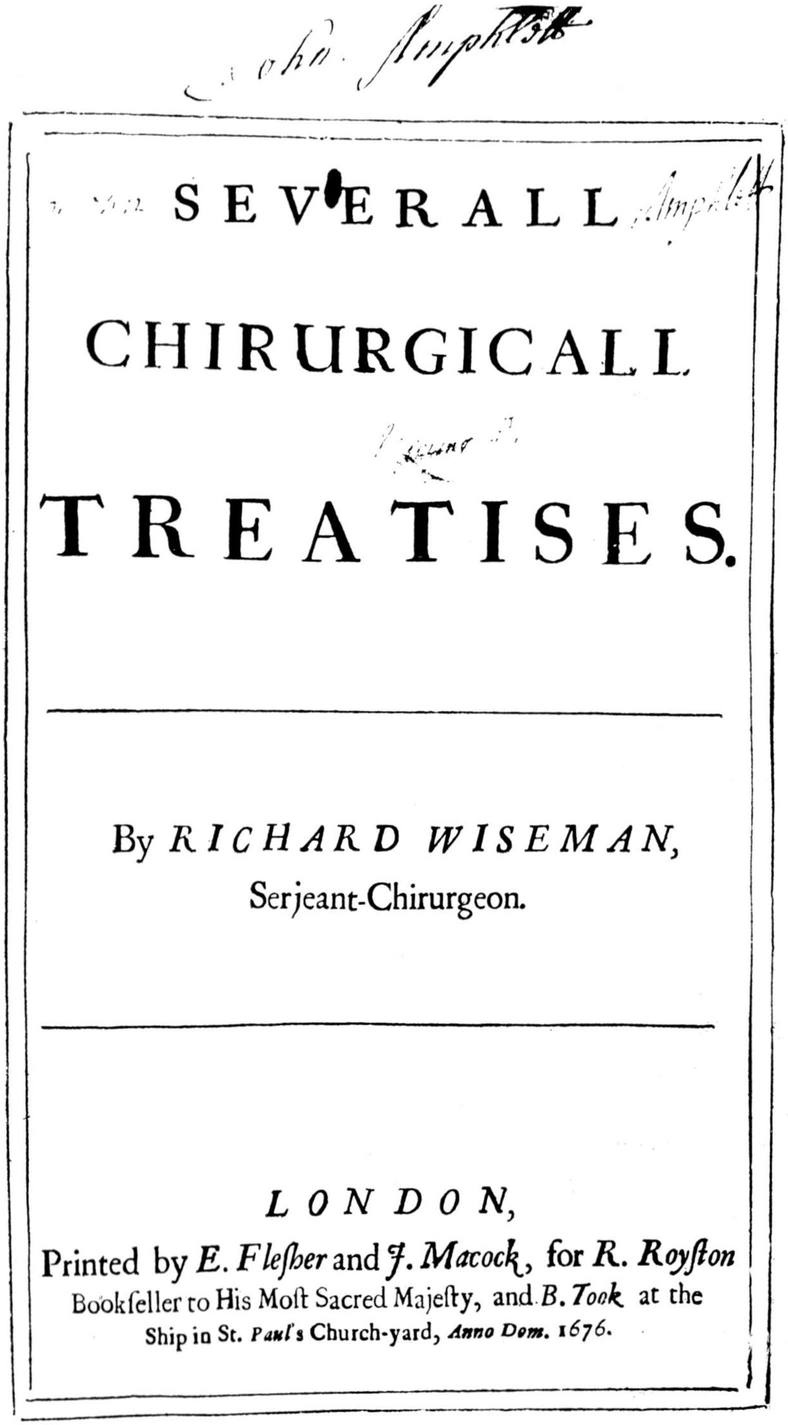
SEVERALL

CHIRURGICALL

TREATISES.

By *RICHARD WISEMAN*,
Serjeant-Chirurgeon.

LONDON,
Printed by *E. Flesher* and *J. Macock*, for *R. Royston*
Bookseller to His Most Sacred Majesty, and *B. Took* at the
Ship in St. *Paul's* Church-yard, *Anno Dom.* 1676.

Fig. 1. Title page of Richard Wiseman's *Severall Chirurgicall Treatises* (1676). Library of the New York Academy of Medicine.

of the life and character of the period in the diaries of Samuel Pepys and John Evelyn.

Wiseman's parentage and the date of his birth are obscure. Circumstantial evidence places the time of his birth between 1621 and 1623; this appears to be quite accurate. His parents are not known. The name Wiseman was quite common in England at the time and there were three baronets of that name. There is speculation that he may have been the illegitimate son of Sir Richard Wiseman, who died in 1641, but there is no proof of this. At his request he was acknowledged by Sir Robert Wiseman as a kinsman, but he did not specify the relation, and the statement was not accepted officially. Wiseman had an apprentice named Jacques Wiseman, to whom he referred as a kinsman. Jacques was the son of a merchant in London, and it is probable that Richard's father also was an obscure tradesman. The greater part of the hall of the Barber Surgeons was consumed in the great fire and with it the records which may have contained more information about Wiseman.

It is known that Richard Wiseman was apprenticed to a surgeon named Richard Smith in 1637. His history between then and 1645 is not clear but it is certain that he served for part of that time in the Dutch Navy, and it may have been that Richard Smith also was in that service. Many surgeons at that time had their training in military service, as did John Hunter in the following century. It also was quite customary for Englishmen to enlist in the Dutch army or navy, since Holland was then an ally of England.

Wiseman next appears as a surgeon in the Royalist army. He was in the battle of Weymouth and narrowly escaped capture by the parliamentarians under Colonel Sydenham. He was in southwest England in the forces under the prince of Wales as surgeon to the guards of the prince. He escaped with the prince to Scilly in March 1646 and accompanied him to Jersey, France, and Holland. He was with the prince, later Charles II, and the duke of York when they went to Jersey in 1649 and to Scotland in June 1650. He was a surgeon in the king's army which went south into England.

Wiseman was taken prisoner in the battle of Worcester, which was the final blow to the Royalist cause. From Worcester he was taken to Chester and there detained until near the end of 1651, when he received a pass to London. When he arrived there in February 1652 he was placed under arrest but was released on bail. He then obtained his freedom of the Company of Barber Surgeons, which gave him the rights and privileges of a citizen of London. This was about 15 years after he was bound as an apprentice, but he had had no previous opportunity to become a member of the Company.

Wiseman then became assistant to Edward Molins but he soon went into practice for himself and took a house in the Old Bailey. Apparently he prospered. Colonel Barkstead, lieutenant of the Tower of London, said of him several years later that "he had been living in the Old Bailey at the Signe of the Kings-head in great practice."

In March 1654 Wiseman was arrested on a charge of having connived in the attempt of a Royalist prisoner named Read to escape from the Tower. Wiseman was taken to the Tower and from there transferred to Lambeth House, which had been expropriated from the church and was used as a prison. Although confined to Lambeth, he was given a good deal of liberty and was permitted to see his patients there. It would appear that there was much doubt as to his guilt. Wiseman said in a petition for his freedom that Read had sent for him to treat an ulcer, which he did reluctantly. A jailer in the Tower appears to have tried to implicate Wiseman but the evidence was very unconvincing, and he later was released. Had there been any certainty about his guilt he would have been punished severely.

Wiseman continued to practice but life was difficult for a Royalist. In 1657 he took service in the Spanish Navy, where he remained until early in 1660 when he returned to London, doubtless in the assurance that the monarchy was about to be restored. Wiseman moved to better quarters in Covent Garden where many of the more successful medical men lived; this area was the equivalent of today's Harley Street.

Charles II returned to London on May 29, 1660. Wiseman was appointed "Surgeon in Ordinary to the Person" in June. This was confirmed by royal warrant in the following year. With this went a salary of 40 pounds per annum and a pension of 150 pounds. When later he was made sergeant-surgeon the stipend was increased to 256 pounds. There were three sergeant-surgeons at the time, all of whom had held that office under Charles I and thus outranked Wiseman. It was not until 1672, on the death of Humphrey Painter, that he was made sergeant-surgeon and principal surgeon to the king.

The sergeant-surgeons at that time acted in the capacity of the sur-

TO THE

MOST SACRED MAJESTY

OF

CHARLES II.

KING

OF

GREAT BRITAIN,

FRANCE and IRELAND, &c.

ARE

HUMBLY DEDICATED

THESE

Chirurgicall Labours

OF

His MAJESTIES

most faithfull Servant,

and loyall Subject,

Ri. Wiseman.

Fig. 2. Dedication to Charles II in Wiseman's *Severall Chirurgicall Treatises* (1676).

geons general of the armed forces today. Wiseman, however, was prevented by poor health from assuming these duties; he became ill in 1660 with what evidently was pulmonary tuberculosis. From then on he had repeated hemoptyses. He described how on one occasion he was trepanning a depressed fracture of the skull when "going presently out of his close Room (where I was crowded up with great Lights burning near me) into the fresh Air, I presently burst out with a violent Coughing of bloud: yet the next day I drest the Patient again . . . ."[2]

On another occasion: "In the year of the great Sicknesse, whilst I was in the North-country, a Gentleman sent his Servant to me, who had some half a year before luxated his right shoulder. He had been with a Bone-setter, who took some pains in stretching it, and made him believe that he had set it: but upon sight of it, I concluded it luxated, and felt the head of the Humerus lying in his Arm-pit. I being then lame of my fractured Leg, and indisposed with coughing bloud, advised the man to return to his Bone-setter, and tell him what I had said. . . ."[3] Wiseman later reduced the dislocation by means of a pulley and coulstaffe.

In the preface to his book he says:

> In doing this, Reader, I have made a vertue of necessity and imployed those hours for the publick service, which a frequently-repeated Sickness for this twenty years last past deny'd me the use of in my private occasions. It hath pleased God by casting me into such a condition to give me opportunity of reading and thinking, as practising. Both which are necessary to the accomplishment not onely of an Authour, but indeed of a Chirurgeon. I cannot be so uncharitable to my Brethern, as to wish them the like Sickness to oblige them to the like Retirements for contemplation and study. But I do heartily wish, that what was necessity in me may be the choice in them, viz. that they would set apart some time for reflection upon their Labours, and for comparing the Empiricall part of the Profession with the Rationall.[4]

Wiseman was married twice, the second time one year after his first wife's death and only a short time before his own. He died in Bath, where he had gone in search of better health, and was buried in St. Paul's Church, Covent Garden, on August 29, 1676.

In a dissolute age Wiseman was an unusually temperate man. He described himself as a water drinker, but advised alcoholic drinks for patients who were accustomed to them. He indulged in few amusements or diversions, devoting his whole time and efforts to his profession. Many of his patients were poor persons from whom he could expect little or no remuneration, but his efforts to help them were unstinting.

He wrote well with a good style and had the faculty of giving a clear account of a case with a graphic picture of the patient and the circumstances, all in a few words. He was well-versed in Latin, which was the universal language of science and medicine, and a knowledge of which was required of apprentices in surgery. A number of letters written to him by physicians about their patients were in Latin. Although his book was written in English, it was frequently interspersed with Latin phrases or sentences.

In the preface of his first book he said: "I do pretend to have spent my time in Armies, Navies and Cities, not in Universities nor to have been much conversant in Books, through my constant Employment in and the little leisure I had, from my Profession."[5] After this, however, he must have read a good deal. Although acquainted with the authorities such as Hippocrates, Galen, and Celsus, he stated that his work was based on his own judgment and observations. He wrote:

> For my part, I have . . . thought it no disgrace to let the world see where I failed of success, that those that come after me may learn what to avoid: there being more instructiveness in an unfortunate case than in a fortunate one. . . . Thou wilt also learn one necessary piece of Humility, viz. not to trust too much on thy own judgement, especially in difficult cases; but to think fit to seek the advice of other Physicians or Chirurgeons, whose long experience hath enabled them to assist thee in preventing the Accidents, and encourage thee to go on in the work, or forewarn thee of the danger. After thou hast thus defended thyself from the censure of Rashness, proceed boldly, and let thy sincerity in thy acting be the warrant to hope for God's Blessing on thy endeavors: and if these Papers prove any advantage to thee in them, remember with kindness the Labours of Thy Friend and Servant, Richard Wiseman.[6]

Wiseman's first book appeared in 1672. It was intended primarily for naval surgeons who, he said, seldom troubled their cabins with books. It dealt largely with gunshot wounds, fractures, and venereal diseases. Its reception encouraged him to publish an enlarged and more comprehensive edition in 1676. This he called *Severall Chirurgicall Treatises*. It was very successful and became the authoritative work on surgery for many years. New editions were printed in 1686, 1696, 1705, 1719, and 1734. A fraudulent edition was sold in 1692, which really consisted of copies of earlier versions in which a new title page and date had been pasted. As a matter of fact the editions subsequent to 1676 were simply reprints with no change in the text. Wiseman died a few months after the publication of the book in that year, and it was not altered after that.

The 1676 or, as it usually is considered, the second edition, bore the name "Richard Wiseman, Serjeant-Chirurgeon." It was dedicated to His Most Sacred Majesty, Charles II, King of Great Britain, France, and Ireland, and was printed by E. Flesher and J. Macock for R. Royston, "Bookseller to his Most Sacred Majesty and B. Took at the Ship in St. Paul's Church-yard, A.D. 1676." The book consists of eight treatises on tumors, ulcers, diseases of the anus, the king's evil, wounds, gunshot wounds, fractures and luxations, and lues venerea. Each treatise is subdivided into chapters. The discussion of each topic includes definition, cause, signs, prognostics, and cure. These are followed by case reports, of which there are 634. They are the most interesting part of the book. It is evident that Wiseman kept notes of his cases, since otherwise he would scarcely have remembered them in such detail years afterward.

It was generally believed that the king had the power by his touch to heal those conditions which were included under the name of the king's evil. From time to time Charles held public audiences to which the afflicted came. They cost the king great sums of money, for with each touch he bestowed upon the unfortunate a gold piece which was believed to play some part in the magic. Wiseman says in his treatise on the subject: "He will find reason of acknowledging the goodness of God; who hath dealt so bountifully with this Nation, in giving the Kings of it, at least from Edward the Confessor downwards, (if not for a longer time) an extraordinary power in the miraculous Cure thereof."[7] Whether or not Wiseman actually believed this, he was in duty bound to say so, for to deny it would have been an act of serious disloyalty.

To explain why in these circumstances the services of a surgeon were necessary he said: "But since the infidelity of many of this fanaticall Age, and want of opportunity of others, doth deprive them of this easy and short remedy. . . I think it will not be amiss, if I do here give an account of what Nature and Art have supplied towards the relief of Mankind. . . ."[8] He said that the Latins called the disease struma or scrofula, but he defined it as a tumor arising from a peculiar acidity of the serum of the blood. In any event it was meant to be what we know as tuberculosis. Diagnosis then was inexact and doubtless other infections were included. Wiseman mentions diet and air in the cure. He preferred extirpation of the lesion when feasible, but used caustics when this was not possible. His chief contribution to the understanding of the disease was the differentiation of tuberculous joints from other infections. He described the former as tumor albus or white swelling.

In the treatment of wounds he mentions the suture of arteries. He had little patience with the bungling efforts of some surgeons as in the following case:

> A fat Gentleman came from Rochester, wounded in the Thigh with a Tuck. It was much inflamed, by reason of the Tent in it, which was very long; his young Chirurgeon supposing the Wound could not be cured unless the Tent reached to the bottom of it. I threw out the Tent, and dressed the wound with a Pledgit of unguent. basilic. embrocated it with ol[eum] ros[ae] and applied empl E' bolo, then let him bloud. He being feverish, I also prescribed a Clyster, and sent him an Anodyne draught to dispose him to rest that night. The next day I found him in good temper, and his Wound inclined to heal. . . . About two days after I visited him again, and taking off the Dressings, saw his Wound perfectly cured: so it continued, and he walked abroad the next day.[9]

In abdominal wounds he emphasized the necessity of suturing the peritoneum to avoid hernia. If the large intestine was wounded "it may be reasonable to lay open the Wound and stitch the Gut[10] and reducing it back, stitch up the externall Wound of the Belly. . . ." He operated on incarcerated or strangulated hernias.

> A man was brought to Lambeth wounded transverse the Belly a little below the Navel on the left side; the Omentum and Intestines were thrust out, and kept close to the wound with a Handkerchief in his hand. The Omentum was much out; but not being

> altered by the Air, I caused warm Cloaths presently to be held upon them very close, and the Patient to be placed low with his Head, and his Hips raised up: then by the help of his Friend raising them yet higher, and shaking his Body, I reduced them . . . and passed my Needle first through the Peritonaeum, and then to the opposite side. . . .[11]

Wiseman used a trepan in operating on depressed fractures of the skull.

> . . . the Battel of Worcester, a Soldier came to us where we were dressing, with his Sword in his hand, the Blade broken off near the Hilt, with many Wounds on his Head. I seeing the Hairy scalp of one side of his Head hanging down his Neck, went to him and, calling my Friend, Will. Clarke to me with a Sponge to cleanse the Wound, we saw six pieces of the Scull sticking on it: some of them were of the first Table, others of both Tables. Besides which there were various Fissures, Sedes, and some Fractures, with Depression, made by Sword, Musket-stock, &c. We freed the Scalp of those Bones, and returned it upward so far as we judged it necessary; then cutting off what was superfluous, tacked it to the sound parts by severall Stitches distant from one another, leaving a space to dress the Depression and greater Fractures. Then we dressed up the Wounds with Digestives ex terebinth, &c. . . . The Alarm growing hot of the Enemies entring the Citie, I left Will. Clarke to bind it up, and made my way out of the Town. But this young Chirurgeon, being taken busied in dressing the wounded Souldiers, had liberty, after the heat of the Fight was over, to employ his Charity in dressing some of them; and writ me since this Souldier's particular Case: viz. The third day he found him pretty hearty, and his Wounds mattering so very much, that he was necessitated to cut loose two of the Stitches, to give vent to it: then he dressed the penetrating Wounds with mel ros. and the Cranium with Lint pressed out of spir[itus] vini; and proceeding accordingly in the Cure, saw the depressed and mangled Bones cast off, incarn, and cicatrize with the rest. The Souldier thus being cured by him, made a Voiage to the Indies, and since that served a Souldier in the Tower of London.[12]

The treatise on gunshot wounds is one of the best.[13] Wiseman insisted on removing all foreign bodies at the first dressing, enlarging the wound if necessary in order to do it.

The Part is at first dressing to be cleaned with what diligence you can of all such foreign Bodies as have made violent intrusion into it; when the Patient is warm with the heat of Battel and the Wound fresh, and very little altered by Air or Accidents; upon which consideration less Pain must necessarily follow upon Extraction.

In the Armado Navall of Dunkerk, where we Chirurgeons were oft imployed in this kind of work, we after every Fight, went together visiting one anothers wounded men. It was thought amongst us a great shame, if any thing of this work of Extraction were then to be done: for after the first and second day the Wound proveth tumefied, also the neighbouring Parts are inflamed, and so changed in their temper, that they conceal from your sight both the Bullet and his companions, so that the place they are coucht in can hardly be known; or, being discovered, you cannot without hazzard of your Patient, or great trouble of the Part, make Extraction of them. . . .

. . . while any of the Rags remain in the Wound, it will never cure: but the extraneous bodies drawn out, there is little difficulty in the healing these Simple Wounds if drest rationally.[14]

Wiseman performed primary amputation in gunshot wounds of joints:

In heat of Fight, whether it be at Sea or Land, the Chirurgeon ought to consider at the first Dressing, what possibility there is of preserving the wounded Member; and accordingly, if there be no hopes of saving it, to make his Amputation at that instant whilst the Patient is free of Fever, &c.[15]

In fact, except that he adhered to the common practice of the day of bleeding his patients frequently, and that he used many salves, ointments, embrocations etc., Wiseman's treatment of gunshot wounds differed little from that used in our own Civil War. Surgery could make no real advances until the advent of anesthesia and the discoveries of Pasteur and Lister.

Wiseman reduced fractures by traction and manipulation and immobilized them with splints of various materials after an elaborate system of bandaging. He emphasized the importance of early reduction before the onset of swelling. His ingenuity is illustrated in the following cases.

> A Commander at Sea, valiantly fighting in the midst of the Enemie's Fleet, had his Leg fractured by the fall of his Mizzentop-mast it breaking his Leg transverse near the Ancle, the edge of the Bone thrusting out through the Skin. He not suffering the Bone then presently to be set while it was warm, afterwards, when it was swelled and stiff, it did not yield to Extension, but became painful and inflamed.[16]

A deformity resulted which caused weakness and disability. Wiseman saw him later in London and "caused a bar of Steel to be fixed to his Shoe with joints, and by a Bracer of Cloath to be laced on, or tied with Ribbons on the outside of his Leg; by which it was marvellously strengthened."[17]

In another instance:

> Some years before the Fire, I was sent for to a poor Widow inhabiting near Bridewell, whose little Son, of about eight years of age, playing about the Wharf, was struck by one of those great Cart-horses full in the Face, beating the Ethmoides quite in from the Os cribriforme, without any great Wound. The Boy lay for dead a while, and dozed longer. It appeared a strange sight at first to me, his Face being beaten in, and the lower Jaw sticking out: nor did I presently know how to help him, or by what Art to make my Extension. But after a while, he a little recovering his Senses, was perswaded to open his Mouth. And there I saw the Os palati and Uvula beaten so close backwards, that it was not possible for me to get my finger behind, as I designed; and other way of Extension there was none. Upon which I presently formed an Instrument bended up at one end, by which I got up behind the Uvula; then raising it a little upward, pulled it forward with the bone into its former place very easily. But I no sooner let go my Extender then the fractured body returned back again. I then contented myself with dressing up the Face with a restrictive Cerate, to prevent the influx of Humours, and let him bloud, and within a few hours after caused an Instrument to be made, whereby the fractured body was more easily brought into its naturall place, and also kept there by the hand of the Child, his Mother and my servants helping him some while: other way there was none. Thus by their and our care, the Tone of the Part was preserved, and a Callus thrust forth, which as it hardened, the Part grew stronger and the

Face was restored to a good shape, better then could have been hoped for from such a Distortion in that place. The Patient is yet alive and well.[18]

The fortitude of the patient and the courage of the surgeon in undertaking some of these operations is illustrated by the following case. Wiseman was consulted by letter, written in Latin, about a young gentleman with a tumor on his maxilla which was thought to be due to the king's evil. Wiseman saw him half a year later with a large exostosis on the outer side of his jaw. He hesitated to operate but three or four months later the patient returned with his uncle earnestly desiring him to cut off the exostosis. Wrote Wiseman:

In order to the Operation, the Patient having seated himself in a clear light, I passed my Knife between the outside of his jaw and his Cheek close to the basis of the Exostosis the length of it, and at that instant attempted the cutting of it: but it was too hard. I declared so and asked them whether I should pull out the Knife. They all unanimously, with the Patient and his Uncle, declared that I should proceed with the Saw; of which there were two provided of equall size with the Knife. I pulled out the Knife, and passing in the Saw to the very basis, made a track: then put the handle of the Saw into one of the Physician's hands, desiring them they would severally help in the sawing off the Bone; so should they be more satisfied in the work, and ease me, who was too much indisposed in my health for such a business. They did severally take their turns, and had at that time sawed off the Bone, if we had not been interrupted by the weariness of the Patient, and the bleeding of a small Capillary Artery. . . .

The operation was completed later by Jacques Wiseman, Richard not having the strength to do it. On the third day following, the patient died in convulsions. A postmortem examination was made at which "the Bone was found sawed off without the least impairing of the Jaw, but it was very much eaten into by the Caries and was spongie."[19]

Wiseman performed an autopsy whenever it was possible and described the findings in a number of other cases.

If the surgery of that day seems crude it should be compared with the practice of internal medicine, which is exemplified by the treatment of Charles II during his final illness. This is related by Sir Charles

Scarburgh in a manuscript which was preserved in the history of the Society of Antiquaries, London, and which is quoted by Haggard.

Scarburgh himself had an interesting career. He was born in 1616. He took his A.B. degree at Caius College, Cambridge, in 1637 and his M.A. in 1640. Because of his Royalist sympathies he was forced to leave Cambridge and enter Merton College, Oxford, where he became a friend of Harvey. He took his M.D. at Oxford in 1646 and was awarded an M.D. at Cambridge in 1660 with the restoration of the monarchy. In addition to his principal vocation as a physician, he had a great interest in mathematics and lectured on that subject. He also was an anatomist and studied the action of muscles. Christopher Wren came under Scarburgh's influence at Oxford and became his assistant in anatomy; Wren followed his dissections and prepared pasteboard models of the muscles.

Scarburgh became anatomical reader to the Company of Barber Surgeons in 1649 and continued in that capacity for 17 years. There, and also as physician to the king he became acquainted with Wiseman, who was his counterpart as the king's surgeon. They frequently consulted and treated patients together.

Scarburgh was elected a fellow of the College of Physicians in 1650 and succeeded Harvey as Lumleian lecturer in 1656. He attended Harvey in his last illness and was one of the pallbearers at his funeral in 1657. Harvey bequeathed his cloak to him. Scarburgh was one of the delegation sent to the Hague to bring Charles back to England. He was a member of parliament for several years and was knighted in 1669.

Although of equal prominence in surgery, Wiseman was not knighted. Surgeons were then considered inferior to physicians both socially and professionally and it was not until the early 19th century that the honor was conferred upon them.

Scarburgh accompanied the duke of York with the fleet to Scotland in 1682. His ship struck and sank in the Humber and Scarburgh was picked up by the ship carrying Samuel Pepys, who was his friend. Scarburgh died February 26, 1694: "By no violent distemper but by a gentle and easy decay he departed this life."

According to Scarburgh's description, on the morning of February 2, 1685, while Charles was being shaved he fell back with a cry and had a convulsion. Scarburgh was the chief physician but he called in 12 or more others to share the responsibility. Sydenham was not among them. He had been a captain of horse in Cromwell's army, and besides that he was unpopular with his colleagues because of his unconcealed contempt for their practices.

A phlebotomy was done in the right arm and a pint of blood was removed. An incision was made in the king's shoulder and with cups another eight ounces of blood was extracted. Following this an emetic and purgative were given, and then a second purgative. After that came an enema containing antimony, sacred bitters, rock salt, mallow leaves, violets, beet roots, camomile flowers, fennel seed, linseed, cinnamon, cardomon seed, saffron, cochineal, and aloes. This was repeated in two hours and another purgative was given. Next the head was shaved and a blister raised. A sneezing powder of hellebore root was administered and also a powder of cowslip flowers in order to strengthen the brain. Cathartics were repeated frequently and at the same time a soothing drink composed of barley water, licorice, and sweet almonds. In addition to this white wine, absinth, and anise were given, together with extracts of thistle leaves, mint, rue, and angelica. A plaster of burgundy pitch and pigeon dung was applied to the feet. In addition to more bleeding and purging further medications included melon seeds, manna, slippery elm, black-cherry water, extract of flowers of lime, lily of the valley, peony, lavender, and dissolved pearls. After this, gentian root, nutmeg, quinine, and cloves were given. The king's condition becoming worse, 40 drops of extract of human skull were prescribed to allay convulsions. There followed a dose of Raleigh's antidote containing large amounts of herbs and animal extracts. Bezoar stone was given. Scarburgh then wrote:

> Alas after an ill-fated night his Serene Majesty's strength seemed exhausted to such a degree that the whole assembly of physicians lost hope and became despondent; so as not to appear to fail in doing their duty in any detail, they brought into play the most active cordial.

Fortunately the king was unconscious during most of these ministrations.

CITED REFERENCES

1. Wiseman, R. *Severall Chirurgicall Treatises.* London, E. Flesher and J. Macock, 1676. The eighth and last treatise is paginated separately. All references in this essay are to the first pagination.
2. Bk. V, chap. 9, p. 394.
3. Bk. VII, chap. 5, p. 490.
4. Epistle to the Reader (unpaginated), second page.

5. Epistle to the Reader, fifth and sixth pages.
6. Epistle to the Reader, final paragraph.
7. Bk. IV, chap. 1, p. 245.
8. Bk. IV, chap. 1, p. 247.
9. Bk. V, chap. 6, pp. 364-65.
10. Bk. V, chap. 8, p. 372.
11. Ibid.
12. Bk. V, chap. 9, pp. 399-400.
13. Bk. VI, pp. 407-38; appendix, pp. 439-59.
14. Bk. VI, chap. 2, pp. 410-11.
15. Bk. VI, appendix, chap. 2, p. 451.
16. Bk. VII, chap. 1, p. 475.
17. Ibid.
18. Bk. VII, chap. 1, pp. 472-73.
19. Bk. IV, chap. 4, pp. 290-91.

GENERAL REFERENCES

Longmore, T. *Richard Wiseman, Sergeant-Surgeon to Charles II: A Biographical Study.* London, Longmans, Green, 1891.

Power, D'A. Richard Wiseman. *Brit. J. Surg. 16:* No. 63, 1929.

Garrison, F. H. *History of Medicine,* 4th ed. Phila., Saunders, 1929, pp. 276, 288, 293.

Keevil, J. J. Sir Charles Scarburgh. *Ann. Sci. 8:*113-21, 1952.

Charles Scarburgh. In: *Dictionary of National Biography,* vol. 17, pp. 886-87. London, Oxford Univ. Press, since 1917.

Haggard, H. *Devils, Drugs and Doctors.* New York, Harper, 1929, pp. 334-35.

THE USE OF AN AUTHORITY FOR HOSPITALS*

Harvey Sherman

Director
Organization and Procedures Department
The Port of New York Authority
New York, N. Y.

Let me make clear, first, that I know nothing about hospital administration except what I have learned from being a patient in one. The lesson was clear: hospital administration can be improved.

One of the questions that is crucial in solving the problem of the governance of hospitals is whether hospitals can be self-supporting. Proprietary hospitals apparently are. The question, then, is: are proprietary hospitals self-supporting because they cater primarily to a certain wealthy group, or could they be self-supporting with a cross-section of patients, given Medicare, Medicaid, and other available federal aid, and given efficient operation? The answer does make a difference in solving the problem of whether it would be desirable to operate hospitals with some kind of "authority" device.

Before The Port of New York Authority assumed operation of the airports in this region few if any airports in this country were self-supporting. We demonstrated that self-maintenance could be achieved, and our airports are now self-supporting. So what has happened in the past need not happen inevitably in the future.

Obviously, with my background I am sympathetic to the idea of establishing an authority for public hospitals. Indeed, partly because of my work for the Task Force on Education of the New York City Urban Coalition, where I have had an intense exposure to some of the problems of the New York City school system, I recognize the great desire and probably the great need to try to escape from bureaucracy and from partisan political controls and influence.

Nevertheless I do think that some very fundamental questions are involved in making such a major change in direction. The first question is really a question of basic political science: should hospitals be financed

*Presented at a meeting of the Subcommittee on Social Policy for Health Care, Committee on Medicine in Society, March 27, 1969.

by their users—whether the users pay for themselves directly or through insurance or through federal or state aid—or should hospitals be financed by the general taxpayer, or by some combination of both? In other words, who should pay for what? Certainly I think one can argue that the general taxpayer receives a benefit from hospitals even if he is never a patient in one: from the training of doctors and from the research and general development of medical science that take place there. So one might well argue that just as the general taxpayer pays for our schools, he should also pay for the cost of maintaining hospitals. The answer depends on one's basic political values.

A second basic problem is: If you proceed in the direction of an authority or district, how do you achieve the proper balance between freedom from central administrative controls and from partisan politics on the one hand, and the attainment of necessary controls on the other? Or, to put it in terms of public responsiveness: where do you draw the line? One wants freedom from red tape and from partisan politics; but certain kinds of public-policy controls are necessary. For example, how does one relate hospital expenditures to all governmental expenditures? What proportions should be allotted? Someone with a broader perspective than a hospital administrator alone has to decide.

To be even more specific, how are hospital expenditures to be related to other health expenditures, and who is to make these decisions? And should civilian control over the hospitals be exercised as lay control is maintained over educators? How are public demands and needs to be determined and met? In other words, the question of community control is as relevant to hospitals as to education. Each community may have different desires and different needs—but how are these needs to be met and to what extent should they be met?

At this point let me tell you a little bit about The Port of New York Authority. I raise this question about control because the Port Authority is sometimes criticized as being arrogant, uncontrolled, and unresponsive to the public. Since it is governed by an appointed board of commissioners, not an elected board, how is control over it to be maintained?

Here are some of the answers that have been found to work for us. One is, of course, the power of the two governors (of New York and of New Jersey) to appoint and remove Port Authority commissioners. Each governor appoints six commissioners to six-year, overlapping terms, and can remove them under certain circumstances. A second control is that either governor has the right to veto the actions of the commissioners from his state. In effect, this establishes a veto by either governor of any action taken by the board of commissioners.

A third major control is that no important new activity is undertaken without the passage of identical legislation in both states, which insures legislative control. A fourth control is that the Port Authority is subject to audit by the state auditor of either state. A fifth is that the Port Authority can be sued in court.

Also, the Port Authority does its capital financing by selling bonds, and the public will not buy bonds unless it feels that the management of the agency is competent, that its revenues are adequate, and so on. This is an additional effective control. We must satisfy the bond holders or we cannot exist.

Another effective control is that we must submit an annual report to the governors and the legislatures of both states. Still another is that a number of our facilities, such as the major airports, are operated under leases with New York City and the city of Newark, and there are many controls under the leases by which we must be governed.

There are also many federal government controls: for example, the Interstate Commerce Commission has close control over our interstate railroad (PATH), and the Federal Aviation Agency has close control over many aspects of our airport operations. Surprisingly, for many years the army engineers had the right, now belonging to the Department of Transportation, to approve the tolls that we set on our bridges.

There are, accordingly, many formal controls over the policies and operations of the Port Authority. In addition to all the formalized controls cited, there is also the more informal but very important control of meeting the needs of our patrons, of the public, of the press, and of the civic groups that watch over us continuously. Thus a variety of controls are available to insure that an authority remains responsive to the public and to its representatives, even though it is free from certain outside administrative controls and from partisan political interference.

In setting up an authority, then, a major question to be resolved is the proper balance between freedom and responsiveness to the public. An additional question arises: if it is desirable for the hospitals to be set up as an authority or as a district in order to escape bureaucracy, partisan politics, and so on, then why should not other agencies of the government be established on the same basis?

You might argue that hospitals are, in a sense, revenue-producing units, which many other government agencies are not, and this might be a deciding factor. A second argument might be the critical nature of the hospital problem. It might also be argued that one authority is good but that many authorities are bad. While certain advantages are obtained from setting up an authority, a penalty is paid as a result of the increased difficulty of integrating the total government program. That penalty may be small when only one authority is established. When 2, 3, 4, or 20 authorities are set up it becomes more and more difficult to integrate them into a unified, coherent administration.

If the purpose of setting up an authority is to obtain greater efficiency and economy and less political interference, one might well ask why this goal cannot be achieved for the more traditional government agency. In theory, of course, it can. But in practice it may be a long and difficult process—if the goal is achievable at all.

Another decision that must be made is whether to adopt the authority device or the district-government device. What is the difference between them? Generally, the district has taxing powers with an elected governing board, while the authority is self-supporting with an appointive board. What are the implications of these differences? Let me discuss them briefly.

One advantage of choosing the district would presumably be the availability of more money; if the district cannot be self-supporting, it can obtain needed funds through taxes. If one believes that the general taxpayer does benefit from government (public) hospitals and should therefore help pay for them then this is the thing to do. Another advantage (or disadvantage, depending on the point of view) is that the district tends to have more independence from the state or the city. Another important advantage of the district is that jurisdictional lines can be crossed more easily.

But there are also disadvantages. When a jurisdiction has taxing power it is not faced with the necessity of being self-supporting. Now self-support is very important: it is a tangible measure that requires an organization to operate efficiently, to obtain able employees, and to get rid of incompetent ones. If a deficit cannot be met through taxes some other way must be found. Conceivably this could be done by cutting public service. In the case of hospitals, the quality of service clearly comes first and cost second. Therefore I think that under the self-support concept, there would be great pressure to find more efficient ways of doing business to meet any potential deficit.

Moreover, the power to tax and to hold elections—through the district method—puts one right into politics. Elections are always political. Taxation, especially because of the current revolt of the public against high taxes, increases the political factor again. And if politics is what one is trying to get away from, then adoption of the district approach is not the appropriate action to take.

Further, adding another tax further complicates the tax structure as seen by the citizen. There are many citizens in this country who must meet 5, 6, or as many as 13 tax bills. If a hospital district is created, the citizen is faced with one more tax bill. And, of course, a certain percentage of the returns must be used to pay for the collection of the tax.

There are many other questions to be answered that I do not have time to discuss. For example: Who should appoint the governing body? Should such a body include elected officials? Should it include ex-officio officials? Should such officials be appointed for fixed terms, or should they be removable at will? What costs should be self-supporting and what costs should be subsidized? Who should decide whether there is to be a subsidy of some kind? Who should determine how much it will be? Who should decide what kind of controls the provider of the subsidy will maintain over its expenditures? What freedom should the authority or the district have to set charges? What should the relation of the authority or district be with the universities, including financial relations? All these questions, it seems to me, ultimately will have to be answered.

And now to summarize. As far as I am concerned, the creation of an authority, which I know more about than a district, is certainly not a panacea. It is a specific approach designed to solve certain specific problems. I quote to you on this point from one who is an authority, Austin Tobin, executive director of The New York Port Authority, who said in a recent speech:

"I certainly do not believe that the public authority is the answer to all governmental problems. It is a specific, not a cure-all. It should not be used to displace the permanent and regular governmental agencies. But it can be used to break off certain appropriate pieces of the total governmental function and handle them effectively. It is particularly well suited to the financing, construction and operation of public enterprises. As guidelines for using the public authority, I would suggest that it is most effective where the program to be carried out cuts across political and geographical boundaries; where the decisions to be made are primarily of a commercial or business character and the program is to be self-supporting, or the revenues principally based on user charges; where continuity of policy, planning, financing, and operation is crucial to the success of the program; and where the undertaking is neither attractive to private industry nor so deficit-ridden as to be impossible of self-support. Freedom from partisan political influence is also important, but it is not so much a reason for creating an authority as a necessary condition for its effective performance."

THE CHELSEA PHYSIC GARDEN

According to a recent and unauthoritative estimate, more than 2 million visitors came to England in 1969. How many of these were Americans our demographers and customs officials have not yet revealed, but it is certain that the charm of Britain and the civility of its inhabitants combine to strengthen the bonds of history and to draw our compatriots across the ocean in their thousands and their tens of thousands. Most of these travelers go to London and some go to London only. The metropolis has attractions for all.

After one's first or second visit to the classic shrines, after the layman has been to Trafalgar Square, the Bank of England, or Soho, and the physician has been to Guy's Hospital, the charm of planned travel is gradually replaced by the charm of planless wandering.

If you wander in the district of Chelsea and are accompanied by your wife, it is best to bear southward toward the Thames, since a walk along Brompton Road may lead you to Harrod's, a department store irresistible alike to man and woman. Of Harrod's we need remark only that it is equipped with futuristic computerlike devices: you press a button and out come typewritten directions for the route to any department you may choose to visit, e.g. "BOOKS—Face the machine & turn left into the Linen Hall, then turn right—the Book Department now faces you." One of the direction machines is trilingual and on demand will print out "Bücher: Blickrichtung zur Maschine, dann Links . . . ." or "Livres: Faites face à la machine et tournez à gauche. . . ."

Going southward from Harrod's you traverse Chelsea and reach the Thames. Turn right, walk along the Chelsea Embankment, and presently you are passing a walled enclosure, whose pylons read "The Botanic Garden of the Society of Apothecaries of London, A. D. 1673" and "Granted to the Society in Perpetuity by Sir Hans Sloane, Bart. A.D. 1723."

It is advantageous to visit this site—now called the Chelsea Physic Garden—under the guidance of its hospitable curator, Mr. W. G. MacKenzie, a medalist of the Royal Horticultural Society. An area slightly larger than three and a half acres now supports a hundred natural families of plants in the open and an additional collection in greenhouses. Early medicinal plants and contemporary pharmaceutical plants are

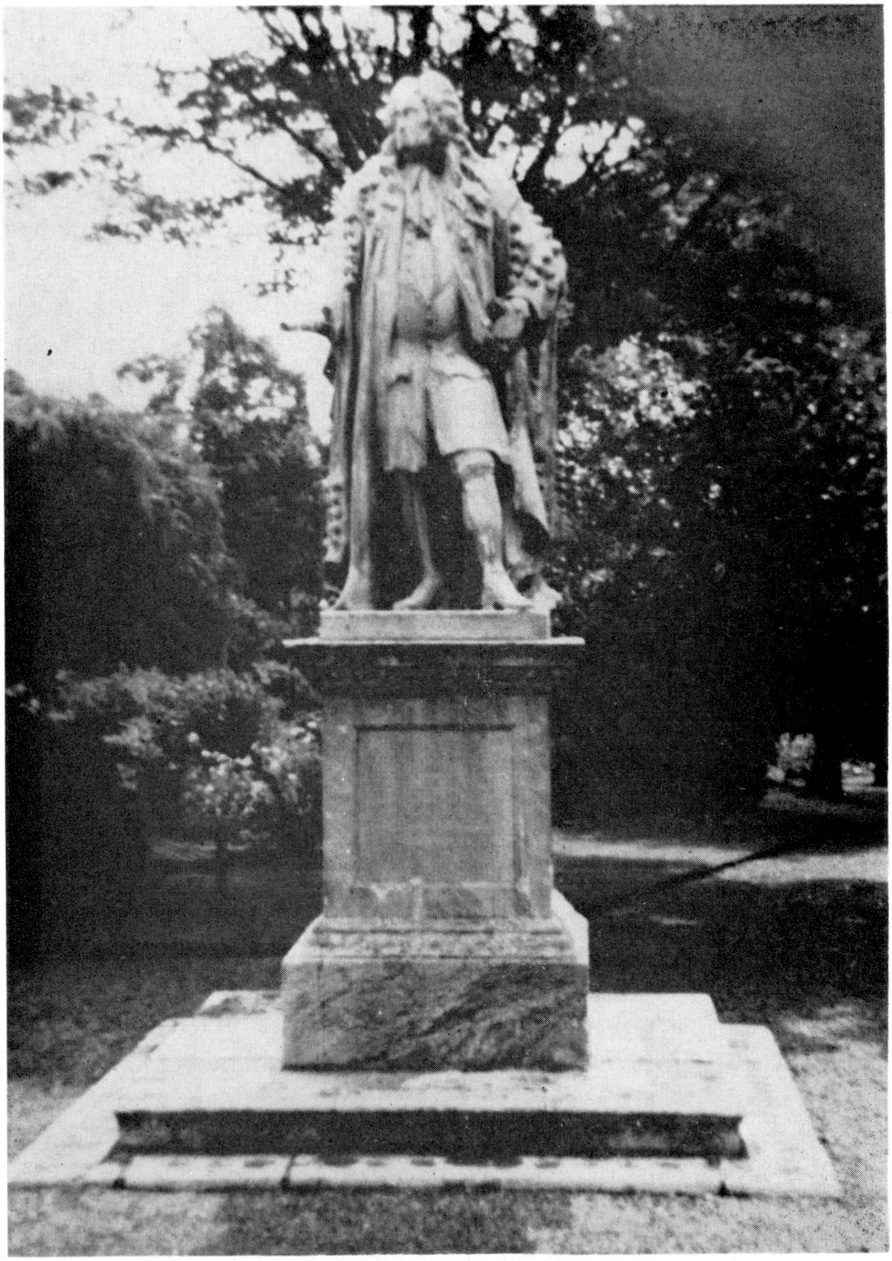

Fig. 1. Sir Hans Sloane (1660-1753). Statue by Rysbrack in Chelsea Physic Garden, London.

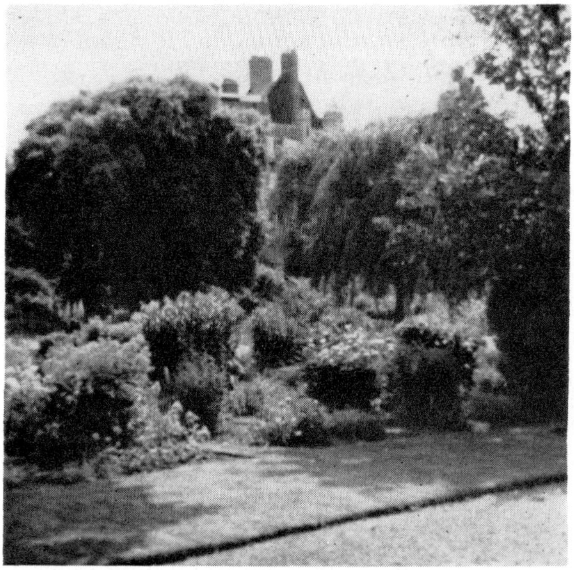

Fig. 2. The Chelsea Physic Garden.

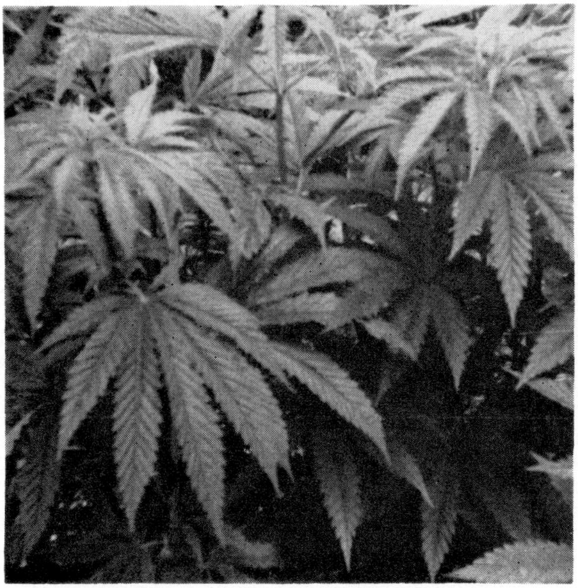

Fig. 3. *Cannabis indica*, Chelsea Physic Garden.

included, as are numerous ornamental, exotic, esculent, and incidental forms (see Figures 2 and 3). The indoor collection is used chiefly for teaching. At the end of the 19th century botany replaced pharmacy and pharmacognosy as the subject of principal emphasis. At present the garden supplies about 30,000 specimens a year to universities and other educational institutions. Research is carried on actively and this includes advanced genetic investigation and the use of radioactive isotopes.

The Garden still possesses its original library. Here one can see Gerarde's *Herball* in the desirable second edition (1633); Sir Hans Sloane's *Voyage to Jamaica* (1707); Sloane's copy of the *De historia stirpium* by Leonhart Fuchs (Basel, 1542); and a student prize awarded to James Paget at St. Bart's—the *Plantae Aequinoctiales* of Humboldt and Bonpland (1808).

The library and the Garden bear the imprint of three centuries. In 1673 the Worshipful Society of Apothecaries of London obtained the land by lease. Before long the functioning garden was used for the instruction of medical students, including the young Hans Sloane. In 1712 Sloane, now a distinguished and wealthy physician, purchased the manor of Chelsea and thus became ground-owner of the Garden. A decade later he deeded it to the Society of Apothecaries. His services commemorated by a statue (Figure 1) which stands in the Garden.

During the course of three centuries the Garden has established a notable place in botanical history. Here Linnaeus visited and collected specimens. Here Sir Joseph Banks sent plants acquired during his famous voyages. Here William Forsyth worked, for whom the forsythia is named. And from this garden seeds of the cotton plant were sent across the Atlantic to the impecunious North American colony of Georgia—of which Sir Hans Sloane was a promoter—as an innovation that might prove economically beneficial.

Like the old-fashioned anatomical theater, the pharmaceutical garden is an educational device that served an important purpose during earlier phases of medical education. It has yielded its primacy but it is not forgotten. Times have changed and we have changed with them.

S. J.

NOTES

I thank Mr. W. G. MacKenzie, curator, and Doctors Noel Poynter and W.S.C. Copeman, who helped me make arrangements for a visit to the Garden. The photographs were taken by Thomas Jarcho.

The following works will be helpful to those who seek additional information:

E. A. Underwood, editor: *A History of the Worshipful Society of Apothecaries of London*, vol. 1, 1617-1815, by C. Wall and H. C. Cameron. Publications of the Wellcome Historical Medical Museum, new series, no. 8. London, Oxford University Press, 1963.

W. S. C. Copeman: *The Worshipful Society of Apothecaries of London; A History, 1617-1967*. Oxford, Pergamon Press, 1967.

C. R. B. Barrett: *The History of the Society of Apothecaries of London.* London, Stock, 1905.

W. H. Godfrey: *The Parish of Chelsea (Part I)*. London, London County Council, 1909-1927.

J. Strype: *A Survey of the Cities of London and Westminster . . . written at first in the year MDXCVIII by John Stow*, vol. 2, p. 233. London, Churchill, et al., 1720.

T. Faulkner: *An Historical and Topographical Description of Chelsea*, 2 vols. in 1. Chelsea, Faulkner, 1829.

THE ANTHROPOLOGICAL WRITINGS OF THEOPHIL MITCHELL PRUDDEN (1849-1924)

The roster of the New York Academy of Medicine[1] lists many eminent physicians who are alumni of the Columbia University College of Physicians and Surgeons and whose memories reach back to the grim edifice on West 59th Street where serious students were grounded in a difficult art. The oldest living alumni remember having studied pathology under Dr. T. Mitchell Prudden, a highly esteemed teacher and the collaborator of Dr. Francis Delafield in the authorship of a leading textbook on pathology.

It is not regularly granted to students to have more than a vague appreciation of the scientific eminence attained by their teachers. In the early decades of this century, when the distance between student and professor was great, few students can have known that Dr. Prudden had earned distinction both in pathology and in anthropology.

Dr. Prudden was graduated with honors from the Sheffield Scientific School at Yale in 1872. During the next two years he was instructor there and at the same time was a student at the medical school. In 1873, while still a medical undergraduate, he joined Othniel C. Marsh, the world-famous paleontologist, in an expedition to Nebraska, where they collected fossils. Even at an early stage of his scientific development Prudden was simultaneously pursuing two divergent courses.

He was graduated from the medical school of Yale University in 1875 and then spent a year in German centers with Rudolf Virchow and others. While Virchow was capable of stimulating and expanding Prudden's interest in anthropology, there appears to be no evidence that he actually did so.

On returning to New York Prudden commenced to teach pathology and microscopic anatomy at the College of Physicians and Surgeons. As his biographer Francis Carter Wood points out,[2] Prudden's scientific training (somewhat of a rarity in the United States in those days) enabled him to appreciate the importance of the research done by Koch, von Behring, and Roux on tuberculosis and on dipththeria, and Prudden, following their lead, was the first to make diphtheria antitoxin in the United States. Prudden later became an adviser to Herman M.

Biggs. He returned to Europe for a short time and studied with Koch (1885).

His contributions to pathology and bacteriology need not be recounted here. It is sufficient for present purposes to mention that he was a member of the Board of Scientific Directors of the Rockefeller

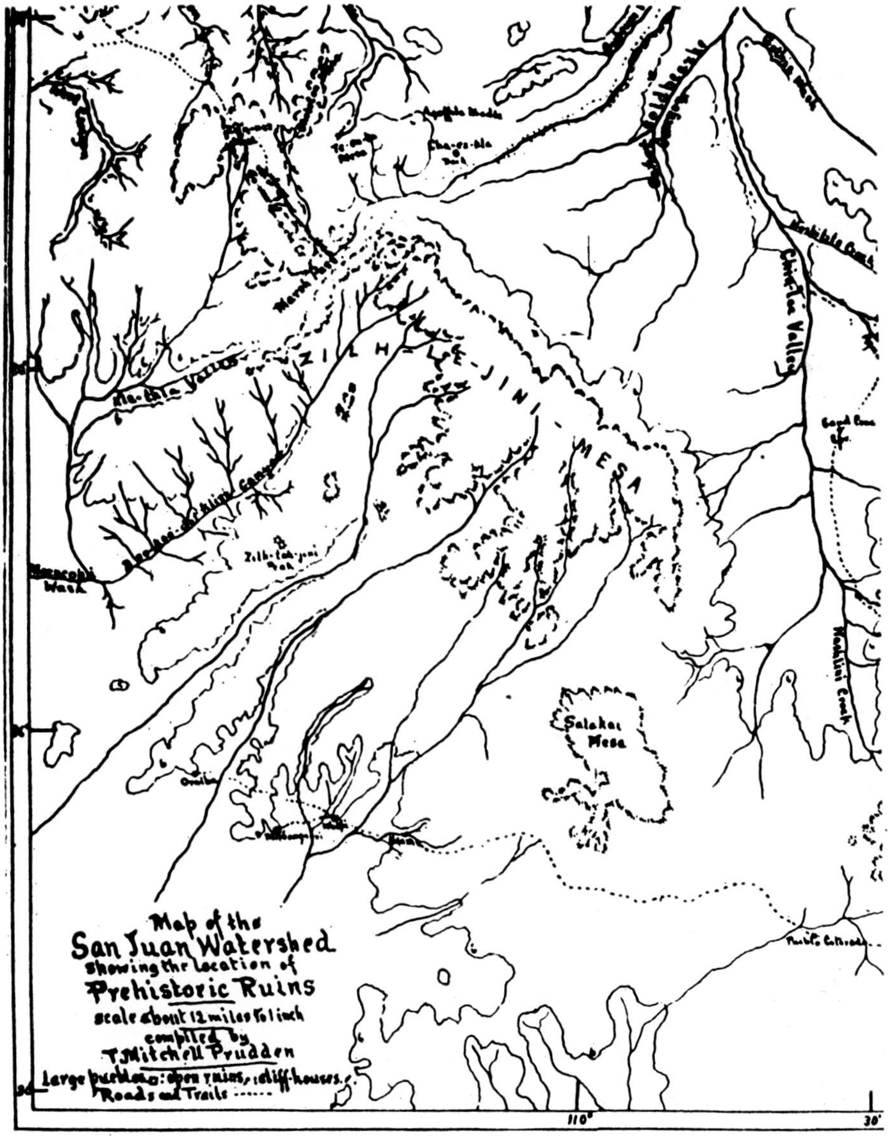

Part of map drawn by Prudden. From his essay "The Prehistoric Ruins of the San Juan Watershed."[5] Reproduced by permission of the American Anthropological Association from the *American Anthropologist, 5*:224-88, 1903.

Institute, a member of the International Health Board of the Rockefeller Foundation, and a member of the National Academy of Sciences.

Toward the end of the century he started to spend his summer vacations regularly in exploring the desert regions of the American Southwest. According to another of his biographers, Ludwig Hektoen,[3] a disinclination to mingle with people generally has been mentioned as one reason for this practice. For no less than eight summers he traveled with pack train to prehistoric ruins in Arizona, New Mexico, Colorado, and Utah. The thoroughness of his explorations was not then exceeded, and he prepared maps (see illustration), sketches, scale models, and photographs of what he saw. His work was facilitated and fortified by a considerable knowledge of geology.

In the realm of anthropology his chief interest was in problems of cultural development as revealed by houses and other artefacts. According to A. V. Kidder[4] his description of early Basketmaker culture in *Harper's Magazine* (1897) was the first to appear in print, and his study of prehistoric ruins in the San Juan watershed[5] was "a model report of reconnoisance, accompanied by a most invaluable map, but especially important in that it . . . laid the foundation for all subsequent research on the developmental side of Southwestern civilization."

In view of Dr. Prudden's incontestable eminence in morbid anatomy and in view of the fact that his explorations were done in the Southwest, an area rich in well-preserved human remains, one would expect to find in his writings some observations on human paleopathology. Somewhat surprisingly such is not the case, and I have examined his major contributions without being able to come upon anything of the kind. It would seem that he kept anthropology and archeology as a relief or refuge or distraction from his winter work in morbid anatomy.

S. J.

REFERENCES

1. Dr. Prudden was elected to fellowship on December 2, 1886 and served as vice president in 1905 and 1906.
2. Wood, F. C.: Theophil Mitchell Prudden. *Dictionary of American Biography,* vol. 8, part 1. New York, Scriber, 1935. pp. 252-253.
3. Hektoen, L.: Biographical memoir of Theophil Mitchell Prudden. *Nat. Acad. Sci. Biog. Memoirs 12:* 71-98, 1928.
4. Kidder, A.V.: Theophil Mitchell Prudden. *Amer. Anthropol. 27:* 149-50, 1925.
5. Prudden, T.P.: The prehistoric ruins of the San Juan Watershed in Utah, Arizona, Colorado, and New Mexico. *Amer. Anthropol. 5:* 224-88, 1903.

THE EFFECTS OF ALBUMINURIA UPON VISION

It is well known that impairment of sight is one of the occasional phenomena of albuminuria. In the first paper by Dr. [Richard] Bright, published in *Guy's Hospital Reports* for 1832, in which, out of one hundred reported cases, he gives a detailed statement of the symptoms of ten, five of these latter had deterioration or loss of vision. Before Dr. Bright brought to light the kidney disease, cases of dropsy were recorded seventy years ago in which attention was called to the remarkable loss of vision of the patients. The origin of this symptom was ascribed to the brain, or left unaccounted for by covering up entire ignorance of the matter under the name of amaurosis. So little attention did this important damage of function excite, that at post-mortem examinations the eyeballs were not examined; and as late as 1852, in *Guy's Hospital Reports,* will be found one hundred cases of Bright's disease tabulated by Dr. Wilks, in which among the columns of symptoms no mention is made of eye lesions. In France the visual disturbance first awakened investigation. The first paper upon it was published by M. Landouzy in the *Annales d'Oculistique* for 1851. This was the year in which Prof. Helmholz of Heidelberg, studying why, when the media of the eye are transparent, the pupillary aperture through which the light enters should not permit light to come out again, but should always appear dark, in solving this problem fell upon the invention of the ophthalmoscope. Aided by this simple yet wonderful instrument, the pathology of the deep textures of the eye may, when our limited knowledge of former days is remembered, be said to have advanced to the precision and value of an exact science. We now know that the amaurosis of albuminuria is due to a lesion of the retina, and not of the brain, in the vast majority of cases. Still further, so accurate is the knowledge afforded by the ophthalmoscope, and so great the possible diagnostic skill, that whereas the eye trouble was once regarded as simply an interesting phenomenon in the progress of Bright's disease, it has now become an index of unsuspected renal disease, and a means of diagnosis. It has happened to not a few oculists of the present day to have pointed out the lurking malady of the kidney by the ophthalmoscope. This fact gives the occurrence of visual disorder a peculiar significance, and is reason why it should have been assigned special consideration in this discussion before the Academy.

We now are made aware that the eye trouble does not belong to the later stages of the disease exclusively, when anasarca and other symptoms, threatening life, command attention; but it occurs often at a very early period before any such grave danger has been thought of and no alarm taken. . . .

NOYES, H. D.: The effects of albuminuria upon vision. *Bull. N. Y. Acad. Med. 2*:14-20, 1862.

SMALLPOX IN NEW YORK CITY, 1868-1870

As there had been a period of exemption for several years, when the disease appeared it created alarm, for it was not known to what extent the public was protected. Private practitioners have always endeavored to support the Jennerian theory in their families, and thus those who have the services of regular medical attendants were, to a considerable extent, secure from the disease. The poorer classes, however, who depend upon charitable institutions and midwives, were not all so fortunate. It is true, those who reside in the neighborhood of dispensaries, and those children attending the public schools, were generally vaccinated; but those living more remote from dispensaries, and children attending the various mission and ragged schools, were not so generally protected, making about eight per cent of the children of New York unvaccinated. The extent to which the very poor classes were exposed, was illustrated in one of the schools under the care of the Managers of the Home for the Friendless, and located among the shanties between the Sixth and Seventh avenues south of the Central Park. In the latter part of January, 1869, smallpox broke out in this school, and the Sanitary Inspectors upon examination found of the 151 children in attendance, only 50 that presented any evidence of having been previously vaccinated, and that in many of these the marks were of a very imperfect character. All of the children in this school were vaccinated, and the progress of the disease checked in this immediate locality; but it soon became more general, breaking out in different parts of the city. Small-pox has previously appeared in many of the western cities, and had been attended with a high rate of mortality, notwithstanding repeated efforts at protection by vaccination, until the profession as well as the public began to lose confidence in vaccination. It was at length found that the stock of virus had so degenerated as to be wholly unreliable. This was particularly the case in San Francisco, and not until a fresh stock of virus was obtained from the East did the practice of vaccination prove effectual in arresting the progress of the disease. In New York we had plenty of virus, but a large unvaccinated population; and, although we can probably never ascertain the exact number of cases, yet the number of deaths during its greatest prevalence we know to have been about 18 per cent of all the cases, which, however, if we deduct those brought here in ships, would probably be reduced to about 15 per cent, the disease attacking a large number of adults who had been vaccinated in infancy, but had either not been seen by the inspectors during the house-to-house visitation, or had refused the offer of revaccination. At this time the disease prevailed mostly in the East Houston Street district and became so serious a matter, that it was found expedient to dissuade from holding public assemblages within the infected districts by persons from other portions of the city, with the exception of the public schools, where vaccination had been so thoroughly performed that the disease did not reappear, except among a few of the children that were not in attendance at the time the work of vaccination was being done.

That small-pox is readily controlled when connected with conditions under control, is readily proved by the events of the past season. The disease appeared early in the spring, and had made considerable progress, when a plan was organized for visiting, block by block, and vaccinating all who were unprotected, or who would submit to the operation. This duty was discharged as well as faithful officers could do it, and it was noticed that the virus used produced a good effect, as the number of cases began to diminish at once, and continued to diminish until October, when there was again a gradual increase.

During this fresh outbreak about 380 died. At this time the disease attacked, to an unusual degree, a certain class that apparently had been well vaccinated in infancy, as, for instance, Bohemians and others from the northern part of Germany. Though a large number of the Irish population were not well vaccinated, they did not suffer so much as the German class. Our native population suffered somewhat, but the Germans suffered about five times as much as Americans. This was probably due in a great measure to the change of climate experienced by that particular class of immigrants. . . .

From Discussion on the teachings of Jenner and the lessons of experience concerning vaccination, by E. Harris et al. *Bull. N.Y. Acad. Med.* *4*:137-42, 1872.

BULLETIN OF
THE NEW YORK ACADEMY
OF MEDICINE

Vol. 46, No. 4 April 1970

MADNESS AND POETRY: A NOTE ON COLLINS, COWPER, AND SMART

William B. Ober*

Director of Laboratories
Knickerbocker Hospital

Associate Professor of Pathology
New York Medical College

New York, N. Y.

Precision in textual criticism is no guarantee of profundity in poetic analysis. In his Leslie Stephen lecture of 1933, *The Name and Nature of Poetry*, A. E. Housman wrote that

> Meaning is of the intellect, poetry is not. If it were, the eighteenth century would have been able to write it better. As matters actually stand, who are the English poets of that age in whom pre-eminently one can hear and recognize the true poetic accent emerging clearly from the contemporary dialect? These four: Collins, Christopher Smart, Cowper and Blake. And what other characteristic had these four in common? They were mad. Remember Plato: "He who without the Muses" madness in his soul comes knocking at the door of poesy and thinks that art will make him anything fit to be called a poet, finds that the

*Now Attending Pathologist, Beth Israel Hospital, and Clinical Professor of Pathology, New York Medical College, New York, N. Y.

> poetry which he indites in his sober senses is beaten hollow by the poetry of madmen!

Not every reader would concur in the dogma of the first sentence, and the judgment of the second sentence is rhadamanthine; the anathema seems to be personal rather than professorial. But Housman's selection of William Collins, Christopher Smart, and William Cowper with respect to their poetic language is the shrewd comment of a professional philologist and requires examination. For the purpose of this essay I shall exclude William Blake, partly because of chronology, partly because his may be a special case.

The passage from Plato is taken from the *Phaedrus*, and the text as rendered seems to be Housman's own paraphrase. The key word is "madness," and shortly after the Stephens lecture was published Ezra Pound took issue with Housman in a polemic titled *Mr. Housman at Little Bethel:**

> If the Greek word there translated means "madness" in the sense of Smart's and Collins' and Willie Blake's being occasionally sent off to do a week-end in an asylum; if it means anything more than a certain tenseness of emotion, a mental excess, no more insane than the kind of physical excess . . . that enables the sabre ant to cup a spider . . . Mr. Housman can pack that sentimental drool in his squiffer, and turn his skill to throwing the dart in the pub next adjacent.

Pound's tone is so ill-mannered and inappropriate that one does not hesitate to recall that a few years later his come-uppance was somewhat longer than a mere weekend in the "happy house." But his point about the word "madness" is well taken, albeit not made with the usual precision of *il miglior fabbro.*

Plato's word for the muses' madness is μανική (mania) which he contrasts in the passage preceding Housman's excerpt with μαντική the "madness" of prophecy (cf. the suffix "–mancy" as in necromancy). Plato distinguished clearly between prophetic insights and intuitive insights into the nature of reality. He distrusted the latter as being nonrational, but his use of the term "mania" does not necessarily imply irrationality or psychosis. Even today, in English usage, mania encompasses a wide range of attitudes and behavior, from folly through uncontrollable impulses to overt psychosis; it is not a restrictive term.

**Criterion,* January 1934.

Housman, who should have known better, chose to disregard the continuum of rational-nonrational-irrational in favor of the oversimplified dichotomy between madness and sanity. (Later in the Stephens lecture Housman describes his sympathomimetic correlative for his own poetic inspirations. His muse, it appears, would draw nigh when he was shaving and induce a dermatopathic response, his arrector pili muscles contracting to produce something akin to gooseflesh.) It is bad enough to be hoist by one's own autonomic nervous system, but for the professor of classics at Cambridge to be taxed with misconstruing a simple Greek word out of a familiar context implies that there is more to the relation between madness and poetry than "allusions to profound emotions rigidly controlled." Mania in the classical sense can imply that the mind has been taken over by a god or by the muses.

Pound, too, oversimplifies; there is more to the muses' madness than a certain tenseness of emotion and a mental excess. The sterilized vocabulary of latter-day psychology uses such phrases as "rapid restructuration of the cognitive field" to describe the intuitive perceptions which Plato held suspect. Shakespeare assigns the image (but not the seat) of poetic inspiration to the poet's eye "in a fine frenzy rolling," and we are fortunate that in his day the anatomy of the inner ear had not yet been unraveled, else we might have had "the poet's ear, its cochlea in a fine frenzy spiralling." There seems to be no dearth of psychopathology among poets past *(praetereo* poets present), and we cannot doubt that poetic frenzy does involve some disturbance of the sensorium.

But no reader is so naive as to imagine that Collins, Cowper, or Smart wrote poetry because they were mad or that they went mad because they wrote poetry. Rather, we are concerned with the idea that they wrote the kind of poetry they did and used the language of poetry in a particular fashion because their mental condition enabled them to perceive reality in a fashion different from the ordinary run of men (alternatively, *dis*abled them from perceiving reality as most men do). To apply rational analysis to a nonrational (not *ir*rational, but beside or beyond reason) perception of the world is fraught with danger. Our concern is with the *use of language* to describe such perceptions and what such usage tells us about the poetic process; at a further remove we may be able to discover what the practice of poetry tells us about mental disease.

Certain precautions have to be taken: "... instruments / To take the measure of all queer events...." It is reasonable to interpret the life and works of poets in the light of what has happened to poetry since their time and even with the illumination of modern psychology. But it is not proper to credit them with prescience; the term "preromantic" is dangerous. Neither Collins, Cowper, and Smart, nor Thomas Gray, Mark Akenside, and others knew in the 1740's and 1750's that William Wordsworth would publish *Lyrical Ballads* in 1798 and that the romantic movement in English poetry would dawn with a thunderclap. Nor can one safely attribute to them a deliberate disavowal of Plato's distrust of mania. One of the central themes of romanticism is its acceptance of the irrational, its interest in the unnatural as contrasted with the natural, be it in attitude, vision, or behavior. None of the poets who flourished between the death of Alexander Pope in 1744 and the revolution of 1798 tried to solve his personal and poetic problems by adopting a romantic stance: "Unluckily they were their situation." That Collins, Cowper, and Smart went mad was not the result of their choosing an incorrect solution; madness does not stem from failing a multiple-choice examination.

Another precaution is to delimit the field. Poets who were not mad need not apply. Richard Savage (1697-1743) occupies a problematic position in the poetic demimonde. Samuel Johnson liked him and gave credence to his story of being the rejected illegitimate son of the unchaste countess of Macclesfield by Earl Rivers; Johnson's *Life of Savage* is disproportionately long by comparison with Savage's poetic gifts and our sympathies are earnestly solicited. In retrospect, there are three possible solutions: 1) Savage's account of his birth and rejection is true, and his bizarre conduct is explained by his quest to establish his correct identity. 2) Savage's account is false and he knew it. If so, we must account him a scheming rogue. A rogue may be a good poet, and a good poet may be a rogue, but Savage was not a good poet. 3) Savage's account is false but he was convinced of its truth. If so, it was a well-systematized paranoid delusion but, as is often the case in true paranoia (monomania), his intellectual powers were not impaired. Documentary evidence fails to establish any of these three possibilities beyond doubt. The record of Savage's life—his murder of James Sinclair in a tavern brawl, presumably in self-defense, his vituperative quarrel with Lord Tyrconnel, his irregular habits, viz., roaming the streets at night and consorting with low company, his continuous alienation of his would-be friends by petulant letters—all these point to what we should now classify as a personality that was psychopathic but not psychotic. Savage's personality may have been "assumed," but there is no evidence of disturbed reason or perception in his pedestrian poetry nor his language.

Professor Tracy[1] construes Savage's notion of the poet as bard in *The Wanderer:*

> He takes his gifted Quill from Hands divine,
> Around his Temples Rays refulgent shine!

to indicate the stereotype of the mad poet receiving revelations from heaven and being transformed at his death into a seraph complete with flowing vestments and halo, a concept of the poet "we have grown accustomed to call romantic."[1] The point is open to rebuttal: that poets were divinely inspired and elevated to demigod status *post mortem* is well within the canon of orphic verse; only the nimbus is an accretion of the Christian era, and a purely decorative one at that. This study is confined to three poets who had overt psychoses and who had to be institutionalized. To be sure, many poets are queer and have been known to behave in extraordinary ways, but we are on safer ground if we stick to those who, in the judgment of their peers, were certifiably insane.

A final precaution is to maintain a position of clinical detachment and not to inflict subjective or doctrinaire interpretations upon a 20th century readership. To gauge at a remove of two centuries the intent and meaning of the words chosen by "a mind unhing'd" invites speculation. Exuberance of a poet's metaphor is to be expected; exuberance of a reader's interpretation all too often defeats its own aim. One must avoid the pitfall of the archer whose accuracy was achieved by shooting his arrows, then drawing a circle around the place they hit. I have taken one liberty with chronology: because of the nature of their psychiatric problems the sequence of Collins, Cowper, and Smart provides a more coherent pattern than the sequence by birth dates of Collins, Smart, and Cowper.

William Collins (1721-1758)

Biographical materials about Collins are scanty and are likely to remain so; his sister Anne Sempill burned his papers after his death.

What we know of Collins comes to us from a few public records, recollections by friends, memoirs by literary annotators, a few passing comments in miscellaneous writings of the period, two manuscript letters of little importance, and a few *Drafts and Fragments*[2] of verse preserved by chance among the Warton papers at Trinity College, Oxford. There is, however, enough information for us to trace the outline of his life and arrive at reasonable inferences about his mental status.

Collins' father was a successful hatter who had risen twice to become mayor of Chichester before Collins was born in 1721. His only siblings were two sisters, 17 and 16 years older. We have no data on the obstetrical history of Collins *mère* to explain the 16-year interval between her second and third children; one may conjecture a series of miscarriages, a period of infertility, the successful practice of contraception followed by a "menopause baby"—but it remains a matter of conjecture. The only established fact is that Collins' two sisters were almost grown women when he was an infant and he grew up in a household of adults. Whether his having "three mothers" played any role in the subsequent development of his mental disease is pure speculation. We do know that Collins gave early promise of intellectual talent; precocity is not uncommon in children living almost exclusively among adults. After preliminary education at Chichester he was sent in 1733 to public school at Winchester. Among his fellow Wykehamists was Joseph Warton* and the close friendship between them was a decisive element in Collins' development. It is not difficult to imagine the hatter's son being impressed by the greater intellectual sophistication of the ex-professor's son. Together they shared an interest in poetry; Collins appears to have had the greater poetic gift, but Warton, one infers, was superior in critical analysis and dialectic. Presumably the two boys debated the aims and methods of poetry, and Warton's ability to articulate his ideas in a coherent, logical argument helped shape Collins' poetic aspirations. Collins' first published poem dates from 1739; he, Warton, and a schoolfellow named Tomkins each sent a poem to the *Gentleman's Magazine* in a single packet. Collins' contribution was the charming lyric *When Phoebe Form'd a Wanton*

*Joseph Warton (1722-1800) was the elder son of Thomas Warton (1688-1745), professor of poetry at Oxford from 1718-1728, and older brother of Thomas Warton (1728-1790), professor of poetry at Oxford from 1757-1767, author of *The History of English Poetry,* created poet laureate in 1785. Joseph Warton returned to Winchester in 1755 as master, became headmaster in 1766, and served in that post to 1798. He is best known for his *Essay on the Writings and Genius of Pope* (2 vols., 1756, 1782).

Smile, published over the signature "Delicatulus." The conceit of Venus rising from a lover's teardrops is pleasant and fully realized. Confirmation of Collins' intellectual promise was seen when he stood first on the list of successful candidates for New College in 1740; Warton was second to him. There was no vacancy at New College, and Collins had to settle for admission to Queen's College as a commoner. This, Samuel Johnson tells us, was "the original misfortune of his life." Joseph Warton entered Oriel, but the friendship between the two budding poets continued unabated. The following year Collins was elected to a demyship at Magdalen.

At Oxford, Collins' first footsteps conformed to Johnson's description of the young scholar:

> When first the college rolls receive his name,
> The young enthusiast quits his ease for fame;
> Through all his veins the fever of renown
> Burns from the strong contagion of the gown.

Collins applied himself industriously to poetry; in 1742 he published anonymously his *Persian Eclogues* (republished as *Oriental Eclogues* in 1757). The following year saw the publication of his *Verses Humbly Address'd to Sir Thomas Hanmer on his Edition of Shakespear's Works* by "a Gentleman of Oxford." He revised the poem for its second edition in 1744 and subjoined to it the agreeable *Song from Cymbeline.* Despite these successes, Collins was unhappy at Oxford. Whether this can be attributed to his disappointment over failing to be placed at New College or the unfulfilled vague hope for patronage from Hanmer, who had retired from his political career, is uncertain, even doubtful. In any case he was dissatisfied with the undergraduate curriculum of those days and, despite his brilliance, soon acquired the reputation for indolence. This may be the first hint of his later mental depression. According to a few contemporary hints he indulged in occasional dissipations. Graduating as B.A. near the end of 1743, Collins went to London to embark on a literary career and enjoy the pleasures which the metropolis had to offer. He rejected the Aristotelian rigidities of the academic life

> Where Science, prank'd in tissued Vest
> By Reason, Pride, and Fancy drest,

Comes like a Bride so trim array'd,
To wed with Doubt in Plato's shade!

in favor of

. . . that ampler Range,
Where Life's wide Prospects round thee change.

and

To learn, where Science sure is found,
From Nature as she lives around. . . .

Collins' attitude is not unlike that of the undergraduates in the 1930's who were "fed up and going down."

Collins managed to follow Nature's example and "live around" in London. We catch glimpses of him leading the life of a young man about town, enjoying the pleasures of Ranelagh and Vauxhall, listening to music, indulging in a few casual love affairs. His father had died in 1734; his mother died in 1744 and left him a modest legacy. His gay life in London soon disposed of his financial resources. In the meantime he had not neglected his literary ambitions entirely. He had made the acquaintance of many of the figures on the literary scene; these included James Thomson and Samuel Johnson, and in 1746 he proposed a plan to bring out a volume of odes in conjunction with Joseph Warton. The joint project seems to have foundered when Collins, who was in financial straits, asked for 10 guineas as his solatium. The two volumes of odes appeared separately, under different publishers' imprints, in December 1746. Warton's 17 *Odes on Various Subjects* received favorable notice and reached a second edition. Collins' 12 *Odes on Several Descriptive and Allegoric Subjects* went unnoticed. Bitterly disappointed, he had to account them a failure. This failure marks a decisive point in Collins' career. Though he subsequently projected several other literary schemes, none of them ever came to fruition. In fact, he completed only two major poems thereafter: the touching *Ode on the Death of Mr. Thomson* and the somewhat overrated *Ode on the Popular Superstitions of the Highlands of Scotland*, both dating from 1749. Collins had never been a *vielschreiber*, but the sharp decline in his output after 1746 coincides with the disaster of the *Odes*, and from this date we can trace the decline in his mental powers and energies which culminated in his psychosis.

Information about Collins' life and movements between 1747 and 1750 is fragmentary and sometimes contradictory. Collins was able to solve his financial problems, but whether it was from the estate of his uncle Colonel Edmund Martin who died in 1749 or that of his uncle Charles Collins who had died in 1745 remains debatable. A legend has developed that when he came into his inheritance he purchased the unsold copies of his *Odes* from A. Millar, the publisher, and burnt them. The onset of his mental disorder seems to have been gradual, and at first his associates were probably unaware of the serious nature of his illness. Johnson tells us that after his melancholia began he "snatched that temporary relief with which the table and the bottle flatter and seduce." No stranger himself to melancholy, Johnson recognized the inadequacy of such psychotherapy. He also reports that Collins tried to dispel his unhappiness by a trip to France, the well-known "change of scene" which affords little benefit to patients who carry their mental disease within themselves. It seems likely that after 1749 Collins retired to Chichester and lived under the care of his sister Anne, now married to Captain Hugh Sempill. There is evidence that he collected a considerable library there, and one infers from the *Drafts and Fragments*[2] that he tried to write poetry on occasions when he felt well enough but gradually sank into a depressive psychosis from which he never emerged.

Writing in his *Lives of the Poets* some three decades later, Johnson describes his symptoms as

> . . . not alienation of mind, but general laxity and feebleness, a deficiency rather of his vital than his intellectual powers. What he spoke wanted neither judgment nor spirit; but a few minutes exhausted him, so that he was forced to rest upon the couch, till a short cessation restored his powers, and he was again able to talk with his former vigour.

Johnson was probably drawing upon his memory of Collins in the early stages of an uncomplicated depressive psychosis; he was not aware of the occasional manic episodes. In 1754 Collins visited Oxford to be near his friends, Joseph and Thomas Warton. He is described as lacking the energy to drag himself from his lodging in St. Aldate's to Warton's rooms in Trinity, but a few days later Gilbert White of Selborne writes of seeing him

> . . . in a very affecting situation, struggling and conveyed by force, in the arms of two or three men, toward the parish of St. Clement's, where there was a house which took in such unhappy objects.

This was Collins' last public appearance away from the seclusion of Chichester where he spent his last few clouded years, visited occasionally by the Wartons and by a few other friends. A letter to Thomas Warton from the vicar of St. Andrews at Chichester, who buried Collins in 1758, tells us that in the last stages agitated depression had supervened:

> Walking in my vicarial garden one Sunday evening, during Collins' last illness, I heard a female (the servant, I suppose) reading the Bible in his Chamber. Mr. Collins had been accustomed to rave much, and make great moanings; but while she was reading, or rather attempting to read, he was not only silent but attentive likewise, correcting her mistakes, which indeed were very frequent, through the whole of the twenty-seventh chapter of Genesis.

Our own skeptical age will readily accept the vicar's evidence of raving and moaning, but there is a suggestion of self-serving religiosity which makes suspect the vicar's image of Collins on his deathbed correcting the servant's mistakes in the Holy Writ.

Edmund Blunden's *Study of William Collins*, which introduces the handsomely printed 1929 edition of Collins' poems, preserves one important anecdote from Collins' last year. About 1756 William Smith, treasurer of the ordnance, who had shared chambers with Collins at Winchester, came to visit him at Chichester. Collins was asleep when Smith arrived, and the visitor's entrance aroused the poet

> . . . whose first remark was, "Smith, do you remember my dream?" Smith remembered it well. His schoolfellow had been seen one morning "particularly depressed and melancholy. Being pressed to disclose the cause, he at last said it was in consequence of a dream: for this he was laughed at, but desired to tell what it was; he said, he dreamed that he was walking in the fields where there was a lofty tree; that he climbed it, and when he had nearly reached the top, a great branch, upon which he had

got, failed with him, and let him fall to the ground. This account caused more ridicule; and he was asked how he could possibly be affected by this common consequence of a schoolboy adventure, when he did not pretend, even in imagination and sleep, to have received any hurt; he replied that the Tree was the Tree of Poetry."

We must eschew the easy interpretation that climbing a tree is a dream-equivalent for the sexual act and that to fall out of it before reaching the top signifies premature ejaculation, a common source of worry among schoolboys. We have no information about Collins' psychosexual development nor his sexual activities when mature; in the absence of any objective events to which this dream can be related, such an interpretation cannot be affirmed. We are on safer, though less imaginative ground, to interpret the dream as reflecting Collins' youthful anxieties about whether his abilities would match his aspirations. In point of fact, they did not; and in this sense the dream is prophetic.

The antistrophe of the *Ode on the Poetical Character* reinforces Collins' image of himself as failing to attain the poetic height to which he aspired. After alluding to Milton as an oak and paying honor to Waller's myrtle shades, Collins closes with

My trembling Feet his guiding steps pursue
  In Vain—Such Bliss to One Alone,
  Of all the Sons of God was known. . . .

that is, to Milton, whom Collins admired more than any poet other than Shakespeare. To the extent that poetic expression of such autobiographical emotion lies beyond the classic Augustan canon, Collins is taking a small step in the direction which romanticism was later to explore at length and in some depth.

Given the known facts, it seems reasonable to assign Collins' feelings of inadequacy as a major cause of his depression. Whether this emotional state was superimposed on some unknown (at this date unknowable) constitutional predisposition or organic factor is a matter of idle speculation. If Collins was haunted by a sense of inadequacy as a schoolboy, it is quite plausible that when confronted by real failure as an adult—the lack of favorable notice toward the *Odes* of 1746—a reactive depression should develop. Failure to bring any subsequent major literary projects to completion can be seen as both the result of the initial depression and the mechanism whereby the depression was intensified and persisted. To have produced only two odes between 1747 and 1749 must have been a certain sign to Collins that his powers as a poet were not great and that the top of the tree would continue to elude him.

An undated fragment of a poem by Collins recovered among Warton's papers includes the line: "No more, sweet Maid, th' enfeebling dreams prolong!" It is tempting to assign this fragment to the period of his melancholia, implying as it does an invocation to the muse to relieve him of the cause of his depression, but actually it is more likely part of a rejected stanza in an ode of 1746 *To Simplicity*. We may ask ourselves if Collins' schoolboy dream was recurrent, but there is no evidence that this was the case.

What evidence of poetic mania can we find in Collins' poems? In what respect is his "true poetic accent" related to his mental state? The *Persian Eclogues* cast no light on these questions. They were written before any mental disturbance was evident. Pleasant though they are, their substance is little more than that of a gifted undergraduate experimenting in an established form. The *Odes* of 1746 furnish a few modest clues to Collins' mental state, but before examining these clues it may be helpful to consider Joseph Warton's *Odes on Various Subjects* which were coeval with Collins'. Collins sent his *Odes* naked into the world, but Warton prefaced his with an essay setting forth their raison d'être, a preface which might well have served for the odes of both of them had the original plan of a joint publication been carried out. Like other young men of their generation Warton and Collins chafed at the restraints of the neoclassic heritage of Dryden and Pope. Feeling that the moral and didactic poetry of their predecessors had exhausted that vein, they wished to enlarge their experience and free their language. Imagination was in the air; two years previously Akenside's *The Pleasures of Imagination* had stirred the literary world, and the emphasis of the rising generation was on "fancy." The year before, Akenside had revived the Pindaric ode in a somewhat different form from Cowley in order to have a vehicle in which to express more personal emotions. Warton warned his readers against identifying the true subject matter of poetry with the moral and didactic themes to which writers at the time had confined their efforts.

Historically, there is a convention of revolt in English poetry. Each new generation tries to replace the values of the generation just past with material based on its own values and interests. Sometimes the revolution is real, vide *Lyrical Ballads* in 1798, but more often it is merely a shift in tone, a slight change in the direction of the poetic compass. Rupert Brooke did not revolt effectively against the tradition of Byron; Wilfred Owen did. Neither Collins nor Warton had sufficient intellectual strength or poetic energy to mount a full scale revolution. There is some justice in Professor Garrod's comment[3] that "There was . . . a change of taste, not a change of heart." Joseph Warton was very explicit about his aims, and there is no reason to believe that Collins was not in substantial agreement. "The Advertisement" to Warton's *Odes on Various Subjects* states his position bluntly:

> The Public has been so much accustomed of late to didactic Poetry alone, and Essays on moral Subjects, that any work where the imagination is much indulged, will perhaps not be relished or regarded. The author therefore of these pieces is in some pain lest certain austere critics should think them too fanciful and descriptive. But as he is convinced that the fashion of moralizing in verse has been carried too far, and as he looks upon Invention and Imagination to be the chief faculties of a Poet, so he will be happy if the following Odes may be look'd upon as an attempt to bring back Poetry into its right channel.

But the language of the *Odes* of 1746, whether one reads Collins' or Warton's, is much the same. Thomas Gray thought he could distinguish between the two. In a letter dated December 27, 1746 he wrote:

> Each is half of a considerable man, and one the counterpart of the other. The first [i.e., Warton] has but little invention, very poetical choice of expression, and a good ear. The second [i.e., Collins] a fine fancy, modelled upon the antique, a bad ear, great variety of words, and images with no choice at all.

Posterity has reversed Gray's judgment, but the rhetoric of personification, prosopopoiea, and language of generality is common to both Collins and Warton, and one might add Akenside and Gray himself to the list. However, Collins went mad and Warton did not. Given random passages in a "blindfold test," one would be hard put to decide whether Collins or Warton was the author of a given passage.

The personified lyric was a form characteristic of the 18th century, and personification was the figure of speech used to give structural unity to the poem, as in Collins' *Ode to Peace*. The device can be traced back, if necessary, to Greek and Latin lyrics, but the immediate source for the use of personification in English poetry was Milton, who found it irresistible and whom Collins much admired. Collins, Warton, and Gray tended to use personification in an allegorical sense; other poets tended to use it more metaphorically. But no diagnostic inference can be made from Collins' frequent use of personification; it was common coin among all poets of the age, didactic or nondidactic as they might choose their odes to be. Poets with so varied neurotic syndromes as Pope, Johnson, and Gray—not to mention a host of lesser talents—all used personification. In this respect Collins' use of language is the product of chronology; it represents no advance, nor the "true poetic accent emerging," nor a result of his disordered mind, nor even a liberation of his thought and feeling.

Yet even before the *Odes* of 1746 Collins had indicated his espousal of the cause of "poetic imagination." Speaking of Shakespeare's works in the *Verses to Hanmer* (1743) he had written

> Where'er we turn, by Fancy charm'd, we find
> Some sweet Illusion of the cheated Mind.

Much as Collins admired Shakespeare's inventive genius and imagination, when he came to use his own, he found it deficient, stored with furniture from the lumber room of a "classical" education, filled with abstractions which led him to write odes *To Pity*, *To Fear*, etc. His imagination, even *en rêve*, could lead him only so far up the tree of poetry.

An occasional line in the odes can be taken to indicate that Collins had some insight into his deficiency of affect. Alluding again to Shakespeare at the end of the ode *To Fear*, he exclaims

> Teach me but once like Him to feel . . .

and near the close of *The Manners*, he apostrophizes Nature

> If but from Thee I hope to feel,
> On all my heart imprint thy Seal!

But Collins' hope for rich personal emotions was never to be realized. His emotional experiences did not expand; they contracted as his melancholia progressed. It is, possibly, noteworthy that in *The Passions* he never once refers to love, and in his *Ode on the Poetical Character* he devotes most of his language to the magic girdle whose possessor becomes endowed with the gift of poetic speech. The lack of references to love in these poems may bear some obscure relation to the idea that the cestus (magic girdle) which endows its wearer with fancy in the *Ode on the Poetical Character* is the girdle which, as Collins states at the poem's opening, was the test of chastity in the *Faerie Queene*. One might speculate whether in Collins' mind Fancy depended upon chastity, a virtue he had lost, hence a possible cause for feelings of guilt and unworthiness. Collins may have experienced deep emotional upheavals, but he was either unable or unwilling to express them in his poetry. To that extent he was a poet manqué.

The modified Pindaric elements in his odes enabled Collins to liberate his feelings and his language to a limited extent. A hint of the depressive psychosis which was to develop three years later can be found in *The Passions:*

> With Eyes up-rais'd as one inspir'd
> Pale *Melancholy* sate retir'd,
> And from her wild sequester'd Seat,
> In Notes by Distance made more sweet,
> Pour'd thro' the mellow *Horn* her pensive Soul:
> And dashing soft from Rocks around,
> Bubbling Runnels join'd the Sound;
> Thro' Glades and Glooms the mingled Measure stole,
> Or o'er some haunted Stream with fond Delay,
> Round an holy Calm diffusing,
> Love of Peace, and lonely Musing,
> In hollow Murmurs died away.

The variable number of feet in the lines is quite suitable for verses to be set to music, as indeed the poem was, but the landscape is pedestrian Gothic with Pale Melancholy appearing as an abstract personification. The same limitation applies to the anxieties, so common in the content of the psychopathology of depression, described in the ode *To Fear:*

> Ah *Fear!* Ah frantic Fear!
> I see, I see Thee near,
> I know thy hurried Step, thy haggard Eye!

Like Thee I start, like Thee disorder'd fly.
For lo! what *Monsters* in thy Train appear!
Danger! whose limbs of Giant Mold
What mortal Eye can fix'd behold?
Who stalks his Round, and hideous form
Howling amidst the Midnight Storm,
Or throws him on the ridgy Steep
Of some loose hanging Rock to sleep:
And with him thousand Phantoms join'd,
Who prompt to Deeds accurs'd the Mind:
And those, the Fiends, who near allied,
O'er Nature's wounds, and Wrecks preside;
While *Vengeance*, in the lurid Air,
Lifts her red Arm, expos'd and bare:
On whom the rav'ning Brood of Fate,
Who lap the Blood of Sorrow, wait;
Who, *Fear*, this ghastly Train can see
And look not madly wild, like Thee?

This is as close as Collins came to expressing "the grandeur of wildness and the novelty of extravagance," and the lines coincide with his personal experiences. The final line of *To Fear* indicates Collins' recognition that his fears and anxieties would abide with him, but it is doubtful that he could foresee a psychotic breakdown:

And, I, O *Fear*, will dwell with *Thee!*

In the next century poets who avowed their romanticism were to place a high value on the validity of such subjective experiences. These are "the terrible dreams that shake us nightly," and Collins was somewhat in advance of the poetic content and diction of his day when he wrote them. It was as far as he could bring himself to express his mania in poetry. We read the lines, sense his disturbance, but are stopped from closer inspection of its content by Collins' lack of specific, denotative imagery.

But there is no evidence in such passages to indicate that Collins' perception of reality was disordered nor that the images he created were nonrational or irrational. The Monster and his ghastly train are not Goyaesque hallucinations; they are spirits summoned from the vasty deep for rhetorical effect. Their personifications are abstract and the emotion they denote is generalized rather than personal. That the arm of Vengeance should be red is wholly reasonable, even pedestrian, and the Blood of Sorrow is its natural result. Collins' prosopopeia might safely be illuminated by the linear outlines of neoclassic figures in the mode of John Flaxman. The midnight storm with the Monster's victim lying on a ridge of loose-hanging rocks is a stage set waiting for thunder; the blood follows the thunder a few lines later. In an epoch during which one of the prime functions of poetry was supposed to be to elicit visual responses from its readers (cf. Lord Kames's axiom, "the eye is the best avenue to the heart")—Collins' visual imagery was conventional. If, in fact, he was seeking for visual novelty, his efforts fell wide of the mark. Collins may have had visions or been a visionary poet, but he was not a visual one. Whatever mania he had was not manifest in unusual perceptions which he could communicate; if anything, his perceptual range was limited and inhibited.

The two odes of 1749 furnish no further evidence of the content of Collins' anxieties and fears. The *Ode on the Death of Mr. Thomson* compares the late poet to a druid, but Collins injects none of his own personality. Collins' failure to express a more personal involvement in the grief at James Thomson's death may be ascribed to a sense of classic reticence, but it may equally be symptomatic of a blunting of his own affect and power to be affected by the death of a friend. The *Superstitions Ode*, though incomplete, is Collins' last poem, and it contains the ominous line in which the poet, referring to a "luckless swain," asks:

What now remains but tears and hopeless sighs?

A number of biographers have suggested that Collins may have been thwarted in love by a young lady who did not reciprocate his feelings. Documentary evidence of this is lacking, and the argument is based on one or two of the lyric poems and this passage in the *Superstitions Ode*. Was the posture of being disappointed in love based on real events or was it a stance within the poetic convention? Did Collins identify himself with the "luckless swain"? But the verse quoted seems to describe, if not predict, the last nine years of Collins' life.

The *Superstitions Ode* is likewise one of the clearest examples of Collins' use of an adjectival vocabulary in which participial forms are strikingly frequent. Patricia Spacks[4] has commented that although Collins used individual adjectives with sensitivity and precision, there are simply too many of them, particularly at the expense of verb forms in the active voice. And the verbs which Collins does use tend to describe appearances rather than suggest action. This type of diction is consistent with, though not necessarily diagnostic of, an attitude of passivity and withdrawal. To predict that any poet who uses adjectives to excess and active verbs too little is destined to develop a depressive psychosis would be an exaggerated claim. Gerard Manley Hopkins comes immediately to mind as an adjectival poet who was withdrawn from this world but not psychotic. Diction alone does not establish the diagnosis of a pre-psychotic personality. The tabulations by Miles[5] demonstrate that Collins' proportionate use of adjectives, nouns, and verbs was average for his decade; both Joseph and Thomas Warton as well as James Thomson used a higher proportion of adjective-noun combinations and fewer verbs, yet none of them went mad. Miles' further tabulation of majority and minority vocabulary as well as individual word usage does show that Collins used such words as "joy," "life," and "love" less frequently than most poets of his time, but again he shares this characteristic with nonpsychotic poets. His excessively frequent use of the word "*maid*" might be consistent with a preoccupation with frustrated love, but this solitary idiosyncracy is susceptible to a variety of interpretations.

Possibly more significant than vocabulary or diction is Collins' "repeated unconcern for syntactical logic or consistency."[4] A striking example is the entire strophe of the *Ode on the Poetical Character*, a single 22-line sentence which has been described as grammatically impenetrable. Another syntactical flaw is Collins' knack for separating a relative pronoun an unconscionable distance from its antecedent. If we add to a passive, withdrawn diction the disjunctive, incoherent syntax and both of these to a poetic content expressing fear and anxiety as well as an inadequacy of affect, it is possible to outline a constellation of effects which, taken together, suggest depressive psychosis as that form of mental disturbance most likely to develop. To this extent Collins' mania was expressed and can be detected post hoc in his poems. Whether this constitutes a poetic accent which is "true" in Housman's sense is a question best decided by readers who can conceive of a poetic accent in true-false terms. But such interpretations are subject to the caution that many poets wrote on melancholy, on thwarted love, on their fears and anxieties, and only a few developed clinical psychosis. It would be unwise to apply the argument in reverse, that one can predict from the diction, syntax, and content of a group of poems that the poet is doomed to madness. Nor do the life and work of Collins lend credence that poetry written by a man "in his sober senses is beaten hollow by the poetry of madmen," that is, provided the man of sober sense is a poet of equal gift.

William Cowper (1731-1800)

How many examination papers have put the question "Compare and contrast Cowper with Collins"? A fair question, and the alliteration makes it a pretty one: every man his own Plutarch. Unlike Collins, William Cowper has been the subject of extensive biographical study. Without difficulty one can find over 20 full length biographies; Lord David Cecil's *The Stricken Deer*[6] is the most readable, and Professor Ryskamp's *William Cowper of the Inner Temple, Esq.*[7] provides as much information about his formative years as we are likely to have. Cowper's letters occupied four volumes when edited by Thomas Wright in 1904; by 1925 Wright had collected enough additional letters for a fifth volume, and there are papers yet unsifted. We do not lack for information about Cowper, nor do we lack for opinion; the scholarly literature contains more than 300 articles and special studies. Collins' literary career lasted for only a decade (1739-1749), *aet. sua* 18 to 28, and his literary remains comprise four eclogues, a verse essay, 16 odes, and a handful of short lyrics. Cowper's first extant poem dates from 1748, when he was a lad of 17, and he continued writing for more than half a century; the Oxford Standard Authors' edition runs to 600-odd pages with two appendices. Such riches embarrass the short essayist; he can barely touch the peaks.

Most schoolboys first encounter Cowper through his ever-popular recitation piece, *John Gilpin's Ride*, and it is difficult to reconcile its good humor with the later knowledge that Cowper described himself as the "stricken deer that left the herd . . . to seek a tranquil death in distant shades." But for all his productivity and outward geniality, Cowper was a psychotic who suffered from mental depression with suicidal tendencies. His madness was colored strongly by religious delusions centering about his own damnation. To his friends and physicians Cowper was a man of sorrow and acquainted with grief. Yet when placed in the shelter of a well-structured environment, when protected from the stress of making decisions, Cowper's psyche and its disorders were kept in a reasonable state of compensation. In such a milieu he was able to write a considerable body of poetry which is effective and durable.

It is not difficult to sketch the biographical background against which Cowper's madness developed, but despite the wealth of factual data, many important questions remain open for lack of evidence, evidence which is no longer retrievable. Cowper's family was of some consequence. His father, John Cowper, the rector of Berkhamsted, was a son of Spencer Cowper the judge, and a nephew of William, first Earl Cowper, twice lord chancellor. His mother was Ann Donne, a collateral descendant of John Donne, a member of a family which proudly traced its ancestry back to Henry III and was distantly related to the great families of Boleyn, Mowbray, Carey, and Howard. The poet's father became rector of Berkhamsted in 1722, married Anne Donne in 1728, and proceeded to get his wife with child six times in the nine years of their marriage. Their home was no stranger to the high infant mortality of the age. The birth of William Cowper, who survived, had been preceded by the neonatal deaths of a firstborn son in 1729 and twins in 1730. Following William's birth a daughter was born in 1733 who died at the age of two, then a son in 1734 who lived for only two weeks and, finally, in 1737, the birth of William's younger brother John, who survived to become a Fellow of Corpus Christi College, Cambridge. Ann Cowper died six days after the birth of this last child; William lacked but two days of his sixth birthday. Knowledge of death and grief must have surrounded him almost from the cradle.

More than 50 years later, when his cousin, Ann Boham, sent him a copy of his mother's picture, Cowper wrote:

> Oh that those lips had language! Life has passed
> With me but roughly since I heard thee last . . .
> Voice only fails, else, how distinct they say
> "Grieve not, my child, chase all thy fears away!" . . .
> And, while that face renews my filial grief,
> Fancy shall weave a charm for my relief—

Cowper's fancy enabled him to recollect his nursery, his being escorted to school by the gardener, his mother's tenderness:

Thy nightly visits to my chamber made,
That thou might's know me safe and warmly laid;
Thy morning bounties ere I left my home,
The biscuit, or confectionary plum; . . .
All this, and more endearing still than all
Thy constant flow of love, that knew no fall . . .

His visual memory in 1790, aided by fancy, was so keen that he even remembered his mother's funeral:

I heard the bell toll'd on thy burial day,
I saw the hearse that bore thee slow away,
And, turning from my nurs'ry window, drew
A long, long sigh, and wept a last adieu!

Surely Cowper missed the constant flow of mother love and quite possibly these were real memories; the lines have often been quoted by others to indicate the sharpness and persistence of Cowper's grief. Without minimizing the trauma of losing a mother at the age of six, one can question whether Cowper actually remembered the scenes and incidents he described or whether he seized the occasion to discharge an emotion by using conventional poetic imagery and speech. The Cowper household was an upper-middle-class menage with several servants, and his mother had her share of social obligations attendant upon her being the rector's wife as well as being pregnant three times during William's infancy. At that time parent-child relations were more formal than today; it is reasonable to think that most of the boy's waking hours were superintended by servants and that he saw his mother and father at appointed hours. Without impeaching the credibility of the nightly good-night kiss, one notes that Cowper, by 1790 more deeply religious than either parent, fails to mention whether his mother heard his nightly prayers. Though there is sufficient evidence from Cowper's later relations with women that part of his psychological problems involved a quest for a lost mother or a mother-substitute, one must leave unanswered the question why he went mad while his infant brother John, who never knew a mother, did not.

A few weeks after his mother died Cowper was sent to the Reverend William Pittman's* boarding school at a village some seven miles away; the nearby school at Berkhamsted had fallen on evil days. This marked

*Pittman or Pitman? Authorities differ.

the last time he lived continuously under his father's roof. The remainder of his childhood and youth was largely spent away at school or visiting relatives. One cannot tax Cowper's father with being indifferent to his son's welfare, nor is there any but inferential evidence that young Cowper interpreted his being sent away to school so soon after his mother's death as a form of rejection. But the Reverend John Cowper seems to have been a dutiful rather than an affectionate father. Certainly he was occupied with running the affairs of his parish, and possibly he was preoccupied with his own grief. Nonetheless, he provided for his older son's material needs and saw to it that he had a proper education. The 18th century was not a period notable for its attention to the emotional needs and sensitivities of young children. John Cowper's relation with his son was consistent with the standards of his class in his day. Cowper never reproached his father; he dutifully respected him. But it seems to have been a formal relation without warmth.

Had Cowper been happy in the Reverend Pittman's school, his separation from the parental home might not have proved so disastrous. But Cowper soon became the victim of a school bully. His autobiographical *Memoir*[8] written in 1766, three years after his first major depression, recalls that

> . . . my chief affliction consisted in my being singled out from all the other boys by a lad about fifteen years of age as a proper object upon whom he might let loose the cruelty of his temper. I choose to forbear a particular recital of the many acts of barbarity with which he made it his business continually to persecute me; it will be sufficient to say that he had by his savage treatment of me impressed such a dread of his figure upon my mind that I well remember being afraid to lift up my eyes upon him higher than his knees, and that I knew him by his shoebuckles better than any other part of his dress.

It is a clear enough statement of juvenile sadism with Cowper as victim, but we shall never know whether there was a sexual element in the bullying which Cowper's modesty and the literary standards of his age made it impossible for him to commit to writing. Concomitantly, he had his first brush with using religion and religious texts as a way of solving his personal problems. The *Memoir* continues:

> One day as I was sitting alone on a bench in the school, melancholy and almost ready to weep at the recollection of what I had already suffered . . . these words of the Psalmist came into my mind, "I will not be afraid of what man can do unto me." I applied this to my own case with a degree of trust and confidence in God that would have been no disgrace to a more experienced Christian.

Again, much like the poem on his mother's picture, one questions whether the event occurred as stated or whether Cowper was creating the literary expression of a religious emotion suitable for the occasion. But the oppression by the adolescent bully was real, all too real.

At this moment it may be profitable to consider another open, unanswered question about Cowper. Since 1834 there has been an undercurrent of rumor in literary circles that Cowper suffered from some form of genital malformation. The rumor is based on letters from the Reverend John Newton, Cowper's friend, to John Thornton, an Evangelical philanthropist. These letters were transmitted 34 years after Cowper's death to Robert Southey, who was then writing a biography of Cowper. Southey suppressed this particular anatomic detail, and the datum was first published in Charles Greville's memoirs in 1874, which hinted at "some defect" in Cowper's "physical conformation." To a pathologic anatomist this may mean any number of things, but according to Ryskamp,[7] the most recent and authoritative edition of the text (1938)[9] reads: "He was an Hermaphrodite; somebody knew his secret, and probably threatened its exposure." That Cowper was an hermaphrodite as we now define the term is most unlikely; that he had a hypospadias is possible; that the genital deformity was a delusion founded a sense of sexual guilt overlaid by a depressive's preoccupation with his own anatomy and physiology is just as possible. The presence of an anatomic abnormality might account for Cowper's being considered an unsuitable suitor for his cousin Theodora's hand, for the peculiar relation he later had with Mary Unwin, and for the generally asexual nature of his life and poetry. But the answer to the question lies beyond proof. There is no extant report of an examination performed. Like Byron's club foot, Cowper's penis remains an object for idle speculation.

We are on surer ground if we stick to the chronologic record. Cowper's experience at the Reverend Pittman's school was damaging.

The bully was found out and expelled; Cowper was withdrawn. But two traumatic years had passed, and Cowper at the age of eight developed what may well have been his first psychosomatic ailment; he complained of what is reported as "specks of the eyes." Cowper underwent no surgical correction nor in later life did he wear eyeglasses. According to unimpeachable biographic sources he passed the next two years in the home of a Mrs. Disney, described as "an eminent oculist." We may take as fact that young Cowper did have an ocular or visual disturbance, but it does not seem to have been an error in refraction, a cataract, or a tumor. Iritis or uveitis would not produce such a symptom. It might have been due to a chronic conjunctivitis which resolved slowly, but more likely his symptom was *muscae volitantes.* That the symptom disappeared and did not recur permits us to raise the question whether it might not have been a reaction to the emotional strains of the two years preceding its onset. Again, this is speculation.

In 1742 Cowper, then 10½ years old, was entered at Westminster, where his father, grandfather, and other Cowpers had gone before him. It was a training and proving ground for future leaders of the Whig establishment, and Cowper's father had hopes that his intelligent but timid son might enter a career in law and politics, as many other members of the family had. In retrospect we can see that this was not Cowper's *métier*. In later years he satirized such parental ambitions in *Tirocinium, or a Review of Schools (1784):*

They dream of little Charles or William grac'd
With wig prolix, down-flowing to his waist;
They see th' attentive crowds his talents draw,
They hear him speak—the oracle of law!
The father, who designs his babe a priest,
Dreams him episcopally such at least. . . .

Tirocinium, lines 360-65

Despite his later reservations Cowper was happy and well adjusted at Westminster. He made friends easily, enjoyed living in London and visiting the homes of his many relations there. At Westminster he acquired his taste for literature and his skill at translation; here he began to compose verses, juvenilia which have not survived.

It was only after his mental breakdown and religious conversion that he assailed the quality of instruction in public schools:

There shall he learn, ere sixteen winters old,
That authors are most useful pawn'd or sold;
That pedantry is all that schools impart,
But taverns teach the knowledge of the heart. . . .

Ibid. lines 210-13

and that the curriculum contained

No nourishment to feed his growing mind,
But conjugated verbs and nouns declined,
Nor such is all the mental food purvey'd
By public hacknies in the schooling trade. . . .

Ibid. lines 618-21

to say nothing of the droll comment:

The management of tiros of eighteen
Is difficult, their punishment obscene.

Ibid. lines 220-21

One can only speculate whether he had his father's image in mind when he, having become intensely religious, indicted the conventional non-Evangelical clergyman trained at England's public schools:

Let rev'rend churls his ignorance rebuke,
Who starve upon a dog's-ear'd Pentateuch,
The parson knows enough who knows a duke. . . .

Ibid. lines 401-03

and, at a somewhat greater eminence:

Behold your bishop! well he plays his part—
Christian in name, and infidel in heart,
Ghostly in office, earthly in his plan,
A slave at court, elsewhere a lady's man!
Dumb as a senator, and, as a priest,
A piece of mere church-furniture at best. . . .

Ibid. lines 420-25

Regardless of how his view shifted, it was at Westminster that Cowper became acquainted with the poetry which served as a model for his own—"Butler's wit, Pope's numbers, Prior's ease."* Successful though his poems may have been, Cowper was gifted with great originality in devising poetic forms. He was content to express his ideas in the stanzas and meters of the century of English poetry which had

*Table Talk, line 764.

preceded him: "He lisped the numbers he'd been taught at school." Converts to religious enthusiasm rarely acknowledge their indebtedness to the previous intellectual training which has equipped them to marshal their arguments, debate, exhort, and proselytize.

From Westminster Cowper readily acceded to his family's design for a career in law and public life. Articled to Mr. Chapman, a solicitor, from 1749 to 1752, he then entered the Middle Temple and was called to the bar in 1754. He finally bought chambers in the Inner Temple in 1759 and about this time was appointed a commissioner in bankruptcy. His interest in the law was superficial and he soon fell in with the convivial bonhomie of a group of old Wykehamists of good family, the so-called Nonsense Club, comprising such poetasters and bon vivants as Charles Churchill, Bonnell Thornton, George Colman, Robert Lloyd, and others. Cowper's father died in 1756, but no elegiac verses from his son's pen are preserved. A few premonitions of impending mental disaster can be traced in extant verses of this period. The lines written to Lloyd in 1754 tell us that he composed light verse as a means of escaping from depressing thoughts:

> . . . to divert a fierce banditti
> (Sworn foes to anything that's witty),
> That, with a black infernal train,
> Make cruel inroads in my brain,
> And daily threaten to drive thence
> My little garrison of sense:
> The fierce banditti which I mean
> Are gloomy thoughts led on by spleen.

Cowper suffered a recurrent attack of spleen about three years later, but this can be traced to adequate external causes: his father's death, the loss by drowning of William Russell, his "favourite friend," and his uncle Ashley's permanent interdiction of his courtship of Theodora. Now in 1757 he wrote:

> Doom'd as I am in solitude to waste
> The present moments and regret the past;
> Depriv'd of ev'ry joy I valued most,
> My friend torn from me, and my mistress lost:
> Call not this gloom I wear, this anxious mien,
> The dull effect of humor, or of spleen!

Fits of melancholy were not unknown to 18th century English psychiatry, and much has been made of the influence of George Cheyne's *The English Malady* (1733), but his views of mental depression had been largely anticipated by Nicholas Robinson in *A New System of the Spleen, Vapours, and Hypochondriack Melancholy . . . to which is subjoin'd, a Discourse upon the Nature, Cause, and Cure of Melancholy* (1729) as well as by Sir Richard Blackmore, F.R.C.P., a poet himself, in his *Treatise of the Spleen and Vapours: or Hypochondriacal and Hysterical Affections* (1725). Blackmore was among the first to distinguish severe (or psychotic) depression from mild (or neurotic) ones, as some do today; he also wrote the first reasoned account for and against the prolonged use of "pacifick Medecines." Robinson's text was one of the most advanced of its century; he stressed the unity of mind and body; for him psychological processes were expressions of physical events in nerves, a view which was not to find laboratory validation for over a century. Cheyne's *The Englsh Malady* served to popularize interest in melancholia among the reading public, then a select few, and his catchy title gave the dubious blessing of chauvinism to a malady which is universal.

Nonetheless, as Quinlan[8] points out, "the mental depression of Johnson, Boswell, and Cowper was largely the result of religious doubts, scruples, and conflicts. Many, it would appear, suffered from a fear of ultimate damnation. While this prospect has harassed Christians at all times, it may have been stronger in an age when Calvinism, though no longer the positive force it had once been, still cast a lingering shadow of doubt and despair over the minds and hearts of men." To such names as Johnson, Boswell, and Cowper, Quinlan might well have added numberless inarticulate souls of various denominations and national origins who took literally the doctrine of eternal damnation and whose lives were permanently discolored by this form of theological masochism, lacking the compensatory satisfaction of the flagellant's orgasm. For the time being, Cowper's versifying had helped him "to keep the silence at bay and cage / His pacing manias in a worldly smile."

He managed to find an antidote for his low spirits by translating parts of Voltaire's *Henriade*, a joint project with his brother John, and he turned for further comfort to the poems of George Herbert. Without dispraise for Herbert's religious verses, their sadomasochistic images, viz.:

Ah! how they scourge me! yet my tenderness
Doubles each lash: and yet their bitterness
Windes up my grief to a mysteriousness:
  Was ever grief like mine?

or,

Love is that liquor sweet and most divine
Which my God feels as blood; but I, as wine.

To say nothing of the lines

That when sinne spies so many foes,
Thy whips, thy nails, thy wounds, thy woes
All come to lodge there, sinne may say
No roome for me, and flie away.

These are scarcely likely to restore balance to a mind already disturbed by religious guilt. Shortly after dissuading him from perusing Herbert's poems, Cowper's friends took him to Southampton for a change of scene. It was there, circa 1758, that he developed the not uncommon delusion that he had committed the unpardonable sin.

The precise nature of the unpardonable or unforgivable sin seems to vary somewhat with the psyche of the person who claims to have committed it. Clearly, it cannot be defined as a simple physical act; the variety of possible misfeasances is too various and too idiosyncratic to permit a simplistic description. Rather, the unpardonable sin must consist of a voluntary mental act, perhaps that state of mind which denies that a sin, real or imagined, can be forgiven. For to deny forgiveness of sin is to deny the omnipotence of God or the all-merciful gift and sacrifice of our Savior. Such denial serves to place the minuscule mortal sinner *praeter salvationem*. If a rational man believes he has committed an unpardonable sin, he is guilty of hubris; if an irrational man believes this, it is merely a symptom of his loss of reason, and God will forgive him, though literary critics may not.

Cowper's fragile psyche could not long endure the strain of maintaining the façade of the well-adjusted inner templar. The crisis struck in 1763 when Cowper, whose finances were dwindling, was offered patronage by his cousin, Major Cowper, as either "reading clerk and clerk of the committees" or to the less valuable post of "clerk of the journals of the House of Lords." Political opposition to his proposed appointment to either of these sinecures developed, and Cowper was informed that he would have to stand examination for his qualifications. He manfully attempted to familiarize himself with the duties of these offices, but the thought unnerved him. His *Memoir*[8] offers the clearest picture of his mental state:

> I now began to look upon madness as the only chance remaining. I had a strong kind of foreboding that it would one day fare with me, and I had wished for it earnestly and looked forward to it with impatient expectation. My chief fear was that my senses would not fail me in time enough to excuse my appearance at the bar of the House of Lords.

In October 1763 he made three maladroit suicidal gestures, first by drinking laudanum, then an attempted drowning in the Thames, and finally by suspending himself by his scarlet garters, which broke. Were these gestures not cries for help from a sorely troubled soul they might have their comic value; at least his competence as a suicidal actor is called into question. But Cowper was too far gone in psychosis; the content of his disordered mind hinged on fantasies of religious persecution, his own guilt and unworthiness. After failing to take his own life he tried to say the Creed, but had mysteriously forgotten the words:

> I laid myself down, howling with horror, while my knees smote against the other. In this condition my brother found me, and the first words I spoke to him were, "Oh, Brother, I am damned!"[8]

His brother, according to the pious custom, sent for Martin Madan, who attempted to impress on Cowper his utter sinfulness for attempting suicide. Not surprisingly, he awoke the next morning with a sense of terror and depression even stronger than before. His brother and Madan arranged for his care in the private asylum of Dr. Nathaniel Cotton at St. Albans. "One should not give a poisoner medicine . . . nor a rifle to a melancholic bore."

Cowper remained in Dr. Cotton's Collegium Insanorum from December 1763 through June 1765. At first his improvement was slow and "Satan still plied (me) closely with horrible visions and more horrible voices." But Dr. Cotton was a man of sympathetic understanding with minor poetic gifts himself; his works may be found in Anderson's and Chalmer's collections. He proved a wise choice as a psychotherapist for Cowper. Leigh[10] comments that "to the eighteenth century physician the role of emotion in disease was all too evident. He moved in the same small social group as his patients, dined with them, heard their confidences, dealt with their excesses, their jealousies, their ambitions, and their weaknesses. No laboratory stood in the way of this human, personal relationship; no recondite theory of a personal or collective unconscious as yet obscured his clear and simple vision." Cowper paid eloquent tribute to Nathaniel Cotton as a physician:

> I was not only treated with kindness by him when I was ill, and attended with the utmost diligence; but when my reason was restored to me, and I had so much need of a religious friend to converse with, to whom I could open my mind upon the subject without reserve, I could hardly have found a fitter person for the purpose. The doctor was as ready to administer relief to me in this article likewise, and as well qualified to do it, as in that which was more immediately in his province.

Cowper dates his restoration of reason to a sudden revelation from a text in the New Testament: "Whom God hath set forth to be a propitiation through faith in his blood to declare his righteousness for the remission of sins that are past through the forbearance of God" (Romans 3: 25). To this revealed truth he prefixed the comment: "Thus may the terror of the Lord make a Pharisee, but only the sweet voice of mercy in the gospel can make a Christian."

His spirit now exalted, possibly hypomanic, Cowper felt "unspeakable delight in the discovery and was impatient to communicate a pleasure to others that I found so superior to everything that bears the name. This eagerness of spirit . . . made me inprudent, and, I doubt not, troublesome to many. . . ." His relations arranged for a brief visit to Cambridge, then saw to it that he was comfortably installed at Huntingdon in the home of the Reverend Morley Unwin and his pious wife, Mary. When Morley Unwin was killed by a fall from his horse in July 1767, Cowper continued to live with Mary Unwin, whose relation to him was that of a mother. By this time he was a passionate advocate of the Evangelical Movement, and in September 1767 Cowper and Mary Unwin moved to Olney, an unattractive town on the Ouse where lacemaking was the principal industry.

At Olney Cowper came under the influence of the Reverend John Newton, a zealous convert to Evangelicism, who had passed his earlier days as captain of a slave ship. Cowper served Newton as a lay assistant; he visited the sick, conducted prayer meetings, and even organized parish affairs. Whether Newton's driving religious zeal—"he could preach men mad"—or Cowper's engagement to marry Mary Unwin was the responsible factor, by 1773 he was again suffering from religious hallucinations, was convinced he was irrevocably damned, and attempted to hang himself. Again, he was a suicide manqué. The net effect of this attempt at suicide was to convince Cowper that he had forfeited God's grace and mercy and was forever damned. He never again attended public worship; when grace was said at the table, he would remain seated, his knife and fork in hand, to show that grace was denied to him alone.

However, it was at Olney, chiefly between 1771 and 1773, that Cowper made his first significant attempt at poetry. His juvenilia and later *vers d'occasion* would scarcely entitle him to a footnote, but the *Olney Hymns* published in 1779 by Cowper—282 by John Newton—are one of the great glories of English hymnology. It may be true that some of Cowper's contributions are more of a personal devotion than a public choral chant, but this detracts neither from their fervor nor their grace. Taking for an example the famous hymn, *Oh! For a Closer Walk with God*, Norman Nicholson[11] comments that it is "a private devotional poem rather than a congregational hymn" and that "the second and third stanzas refer to Cowper's own life and have a delicacy of sentiment which could hardly be shared by the ordinary hot-gospelling convert of the time." But Nicholson justly adds the observation that "the lines are astonishingly good for congregational singing, for the imagery is so simple, so clear and glowing, that everyone can recognize its truth. An intensely personal experience has become the expression of a universal longing." Such other familiar hymns as *God moves in a mysterious way—His wonders to perform*, and *The Contrite Heart* succeed in breathing personal life and conviction into a form which was all too often stereotyped, devoid of substance, and stamped with the mediocrity of the *routinier*.

Considerable attention has been directed toward Cowper's *Olney Hymns* with respect to their prosody, their theologic content, their relation to the credo of Evangelicism, and there is little need to recapitulate the pieties and impieties of past commentators. It will not be considered out of place, however, if a morbid anatomist takes notice of their conspicuously sanguinary imagery. Cowper's hymns have a hemoglobin level somewhat in excess of normal values. Added to this rich measure of blood is a strong affinity for Old Testament sadomasochism; biblical Judaism was not an unbloodthirsty culture. The point is readily clarified by a few citations:

Hymn II* reminds us that "This Abraham found, he rais'd the knife. . . ." and Hymn V tells us that Jesus's blood "so freely streamed to satisfy the law's demand," a thought which leads us directly into Hymn VIII in which "Comfortable thoughts arise / From the bleeding sacrifice." Such comfort was ambivalent and found its expression in *The Contrite Heart* (Hymn IX) in an image not devoid of its metaphysical wit:

> I hear, but seem to hear in vain,
> Insensible as steel;
> If aught is felt, 'tis only pain,
> To find I cannot feel.

Finding himself a failed masochist, unable to take pleasure in his spiritual pain, Cowper turns to God in the final stanza and asks him to arbitrate upon what can only be a subjective judgment based on afferent neural pathways:

> Oh make this heart rejoice, or ache;
> Decide this doubt for me;
> And if it be not broken, break,
> And heal it, if it be.

Fortunately, despite his religious trauma, Cowper had had the saving grace of a public school education in the classics and some experience with the conventional modes of the Church of England. In Hymn XI he recognizes his standing in the form at Westminister; likening God to a headmaster and himself to a boy receiving instruction prior to confirmation, he writes:

> My God, how perfect are thy ways!
> But mine polluted are;
> Sin twines itself about my praise,
> And slides into my pray'r

*The numbering of the hymns follows that used in Cowper's *Poetical Works,* Milford, H. S., ed. English Standard Authors series, 4th ed. New York, Oxford Univ. Press, 1934.

When I would speak what thou hast done
To save me from my sin,
I cannot make thy mercies known
But self-applause creeps in.

Like Eton in the mid-19th century, Wesminister in the late 17th and early 18th centuries had a singular reputation for its floggings. In Thomas Shadwell's *The Virtuoso* (1676) the hypocritical Snarl solicits flagellation from his mistress, Mrs. Figgup, saying "I was so us'd to't at Westminster School I could never leave it off since. . . . Do not spare thy pains. I love castigation mightily." (*III*, ii, 67-71.). Schoolboy masochism recurs in the image of the first line of the following Hymn XII:

My God! till I receiv'd thy stroke,
How like a beast was I!

But the whippings of clever schoolboys with a gift for versification leads inevitably to fantasies of blood (cf. Swinburne et al.), and in Hymn XIV Cowper speaks of Jerusalem, informing us that

Jehovah founded it in blood,
The blood of his incarnate Son.

There is considerable biblical as well as archeological evidence to the contrary, and the blood shed in and near Jerusalem seems to be fairly evenly distributed among Christians, Jews, Moslems, and even disbelievers. One may pardon Cowper's evangelical fervor, but images so palpably lacking in historicity indicate that their writer's grasp of reality might have profited from further psychotherapy. It may be the victor's prerogative to rewrite history to favor the justice of his own cause, but such a position is untenable for a hymnodist committed to Truth.

The *locus classicus* for Cowper's morbid affection for blood in his hymns is found in the familiar Hymn XV, "There is a fountain fill'd with blood / Drawn from Emmanuel's veins." The image is extended to sinners who, "plung'd beneath that flood" are redeemed and made virtuous, to the penitent thief as he lay gasping his last on the cross, and to other situations in which the hemoglobin-rich fluid is endowed with special virtues exceeding the claims of the most optimistic latter-day hematologists. Remembering from laboratory experience that blood becomes sticky before it coagulates, we learn that Cowper has washed all his sins away in blood, that the Lamb's blood never loses its redemptive (curative) powers, and that Cowper has purchased his celestial harp with an offering of blood. Nicholson[11] has commented that "the combination of sacramental and anatomic imagery . . . is of immense interest both to the anthropologist and the psychologist, for in it we are aware of rituals even older than the Old Testament: of the dying gods of the fertility cults and of primitive symbols that probe deeply into the subconscious mind." That fertility cults loomed large on Cowper's impuissant horizon is doubtful; he was both insular and pre-Frazerian. His morbid interest in blood seems more of a schoolboy's attraction to Count Dracula and Bela Lugosi with overtones of the 18th century classroom as in Hymn XIX where

> In vain by reason and by rule,
> We try to bend the will;
> For none but in the Saviour's school,
> Can learn thy heav'nly skill . . .
> How light thy troubles here, if weigh'd
> With everlasting pain!

Pain and bloodshed seem to have been the key elements in Cowper's psychopathology. But if we seek a visual correlative for Cowper's agony of blood, we do not see the tortured souls of Bosch's purgatory nor Michelangelo's *Last Judgement.* Rather we see the style of painting depicted in a crucifixion at Pommersfelden in Franconia. An angel collects the bleeding drops from Christ's wounds after the blood has run through an elaborate system of gutters and drain pipes which discharge it through a large gilt spout several feet below where the Savior stands.

In Hymn XX Cowper deals in a sanguinary fashion with the Old Testament legend commenting on the paschal sacrifice and the blood-besprinkled door, the Lamb and the Dove whose blood of matchless worth serves as the soul's defense, and the idea of salvation *per sanguinem:* "Dipt in his fellow's blood, / The living bird went free." All this bloody imagery was written before the public execution by guillotine in the French Revolution became commonplace, though England had not been without its share of public decapitations.

Hymn XXIX is titled *Prayer for Children* and alludes with happy relish to the Lord's angel who

Slew with an avenging hand,
All the first-born of the land,
Then thy people's doors he pass'd
Where the bloody sign was plac'd;
Hear us now upon our knees
Plead the blood of Christ for these!

In a country where primogeniture was a pillar of the social structure this hymn could not have failed to be a stirring example of Christian virtue applied to an Old Testament legend.

In Hymn XXVIII we learn that Jesus himself was excited by the prospect of bloodshed, in this case, his own; Cowper tells us that as He entered Jerusalem

He longs to be baptiz'd with blood,
He pants to reach the cross.

The received legend is, of course, that Jesus was baptized not in blood but in running water by John the Baptist who later was decapitated by Herod at the behest of Salome. Perusal of the Gospels by Matthew, Mark, Luke, and John fails to reveal authority for Christ's desire to be rebaptized by his own blood.

Masochism without overt bloodshed returns in Hymn XXXVII:

Long unafflicted, undismay'd,
In pleasure's path secure I stray'd;
Thou mad'st me feel thy chast'ning rod,
And strait I turn'd unto my God.
What though it pierc'd my fainting heart,
I bless thine hand that caus'd the smart;
It taught my tears awhile to flow
But sav'd me from eternal woe.

The image most readily conjured to one's mind is the flogging block at Eton, but doubtless a similar apparatus was in use at Westminster in Cowper's youth. Many a lad was whipped for straying into pleasure's path and being late for chapel. E. e. cummings has told us that "punished bottoms interrupt philosophy," but the different tradition of the English public school is best exemplified, not so much in the pathologic verses of Swinburne, circa 1869-1888, but in the more contemporary lines addressed by Lytton Strachey to Roger Senhouse in 1929:

How odd the fate of pretty boys!
Who, if they dare to taste the joys
That so enchanted Classic minds,
Get whipped upon their neat behinds;
Yet should they fail to construe well
The lines that of those raptures tell
—It's very odd, you must confess—
Their neat behinds get whipped no less.

But it is possible that the element of sadomasochism shown in the preceding examples can be overemphasized. Cowper may have intended little more than the literary conventions common to the poetry of Christianity tinged with Evangelical passion. Christ's sacrifice is central to all Christian sects. As in many other religions there is a strong, almost mystical, use of blood, either symbolic or transubstantiated in Christian rituals. Even in the application of Christian principles to politics, so gentle a man as Thomas Jefferson wrote that "The tree of liberty must be refreshed from time to time with the blood of patriots and tyrants. It is its natural manure." To say nothing of the constant allusions to the blood of martyrs and the blood of the lamb. That Jesus' blood "so freely streamed" in Hymn V may merely echo Faustus' last speech in Marlowe's *Doctor Faustus:* "See, see where Christ's blood streams in the firmament." And the image of the aching heart broken by God finds its correlative in "Batter my heart. . . ." in Holy Sonnet XIV by John Donne, Cowper's collateral maternal ancestor. Cowper's Jerusalem in Hymn XIV is "not historical but typological: Jehovah's Old Jerusalem will be reincarnate as the New Jerusalem through Christ's sacrifice." But it is evident, regardless of the conventions of Christian poetics, that Cowper had a heightened sensibility toward blood and that his general posture was that of a sufferer on this earth. Both his attitude toward the evangelical creed and the hymns which it inspired satisfied whatever masochistic elements were represented in his psychopathology.

Like most boys educated in the upper-middle-class tradition, Cowper was not unmindful of his duty to the poor. In Hymn LIII, titled *For the Poor*, he reminds us that

When Hagar found the bottle spent . . .
A message from the Lord was sent
To guide her to a well.

One is a bit surprised that she did not send Ishmael round to the corner grocer for a liter of blood, but gin was the drink of the lower classes in the 1770's, and Cowper was too conscious of his own class and that of his readers to invoke an image which would lower the tone of his hymn.

But, best of all, Cowper found incredible therapeutic powers in blood of religious origin. Hymn LXV informs us that

> Of all the gifts thine hand bestows,
>   Thou giver of all good!
> Not heav'n itself a richer knows
>   Than my Redeemer's blood.
> Faith too, the blood-receiving grace,
>   From the same hand we gain . . .
> Yet fly that hand, from which alone
>   We could expect a cure.

It is not difficult to conjecture that Cowper's propensity for images of masochism, punishment by the rod, and the shedding of blood as a means of redemption from guilt all stem from his juvenile exposure to the unnamed bully at Dr. Pittman's school. Leslie Stephen's remark that "Cowper is an instance of a thinker too far apart from the great world to apply the lash effectually" is a clue to our understanding that even in his satires such as *Tirocinium* he fell short of the corrective aim of satire because he was the victim of a lash, specifically his own sense of guilt and failure in the public world. Biographic details about other disciplinary practices are lacking but were in all probability no different from those prevailing in other English schools of the time. That the emotion engendered by these experiences was intensified during his period of preclinical depression circa 1754 to 1763, and that his final release from the bonds of overt psychosis through Romans 3: 25 with its emphasis on remission of sin *per fidem in sanquine Dei* were the decisive landmarks. Many of the interstices cannot be filled in for lack of documentation, but excessive proliferation of anamnestic data might serve only to muddy the outline.

Spacks[4] speaks of Cowper's lack of control of his images, citing examples from the *Olney Hymns*. But his occasional imperfect control of language is not due to mania but rather maladresse. Cowper was far more concerned with the substance of his poems than with technique. After mildly disparaging stylistic refinement,

> Manner is all in all, whate'er is writ,
> The substitute for genius, sense, and wit.
>
> *Table Talk,* lines 542-43

Cowper goes on to demonstrate that his chief interest lies in the poet's message:

> To dally much with subjects mean and low
> Proves the mind is weak, or makes it so . . .
> Else, summoning the muse to such a theme,
> The fruit of all her labour is whipt-cream.
>
> Ibid., lines 544-45, 550-51

This attitude is not uncommon among poets with a religious or social message, but it is not a symptom of mania. It would not be unfair to compare Cowper's poems written under the impulse of 18th century Evangelicism with Herbert's written under the influence of 17th century Anglicanism. Cowper, like other poets of his time, viewed in the historical perspective as falling between Augustan self-confidence and romantic energy, looked backward and forward at the same time, adrift on a current of slow change which neither he nor they could govern nor understand.

Following Newton's departure for the pulpit of St. Mary Woolnoth in London, Cowper's overt, public involvement in the Evangelical movement became less intense. His later poems, inspired or instigated by Mary Unwin, Lady Hesketh (formerly Harriet Cowper, Theodora's sister), and Lady Austen dealt with more secular moral subjects and conspicuously avoided the self-revelation of the *Olney Hymns* and other poems of the 1770's. Much of his newer poetry was rurally pictorial, and he combined the two strains in the oft-quoted aphorism: "God made the country, and man made the town." Less intensely Evangelical, his poetry was more in harmony with the popular ethos of his day.

His moral essays and agreeable social verses interspersed with an occasional mock-heroic made him the most widely read and influential poet in England of his day. *Table Talk* (1782), *The Task* (1785), and *Tirocinium* (1785) served to established his preeminence. The popular success of *John Gilpin's Ride,* published anonymously in 1782 and under Cowper's own name in 1785, put his name on everyone's tongue; its only rival in that light-hearted genre is *The Colubriad*, written in 1782 but not published until 1806. Cowper also contributed many topical poems to magazines of the day. Apart from a recurrent episode of depression and attempted suicide in 1784 he remained in his customary spirits and functioned efficiently. Except for the personal revelations in the *Olney Hymns*, Cowper at this time seems to have deliberately avoided poetry in which either form, content, or use of language might expose the carefully constructed defences in his persona. Norman Nicholson[12] has summarized this aspect of his career with insight:

> He was at times a madman, and he was always one whose mental powers were unstable, yet his poetry is essentially the poetry of the sane. . . . The good common sense of the average intelligent man. . . . Living a life of extreme oddity, (he) became by far the most popular poet of his time . . . the spokesman for the conscience of the middle classes. . . . Though he lived in an out-of-the-way village, though he met scarcely anyone but a few selected friends, he was able to exercise a tremendous influence over a large section of society . . . his verse had more direct effect on politics than that of almost any other poet in English literature. Dryden, Pope, and Wordsworth no doubt made a deeper impact on their readers, but these belonged in each case to a small group: Cowper, on the other hand, influenced an enormous public, many of whom gave little attention to any other literature but the Bible and, maybe, The *Pilgrim's Progress* . . . because, through the Evangelical Revival, he was able to join in a great movement of popular thought.

In addition to the *Olney Hymns* three of Cowper's poetical projects have psychobiographic interest, one for its design and purpose, the others for their content. In 1784 Cowper, then 53 years old, began to translate Homer at the instigation of Lady Austen. Despite an interruption by a serious recurrence of melancholia in 1787, Cowper continued this laborious task for more than seven years until it was completed and published. Eschewing Pope's example of heroic couplets, Cowper translated the *Iliad* and the *Odyssey* into blank verse. Richard Bentley, the great classical scholar, had said of Pope's translation, "It is a very pretty poem, but you must not call it Homer." Cowper's translation has the virtue of accuracy, and Bentley might have praised it on that score, but it lacks the Homeric vigor; it fails to recreate the atmosphere of primitive myth. Though many passages may be singled out for their beauty, on the whole it fails to catch the fire of the original. Nonetheless an accurate translation of Homer by a man aged 53 to 61 whose history is marked by depressive psychosis can be taken as evidence that dementia was not present.

Somewhat more revealing are the five stanzas entitled *Lines Written During a Period of Insanity*. If they were written circa 1774 (cf. H.S. Milford, ed., *Cowper: Poetical Works*, 4th ed. Oxford Standard Authors, 1934), they refer to his episode of depression and attempted suicide in 1773 but if, as Ryskamp[7] claims, they were written in 1763, they refer to his first major breakdown. The regular stanza form and use of language is too controlled for the lines to have been written during Cowper's acute madness, but he may well have jotted down notes and polished his verses later. The reader is scarcely surprised to find that they again relate to Cowper's conviction of his own damnation—"Hatred and vengeance, my eternal portion, / Scarce can endure delay of execution. . . ." After proclaiming that God has disowned him and that he is encompassed with a thousand terrors, Cowper finally develops an image in the last stanza which combines his masochism with the ideas of a unique funerary monument:

> *Him* the vindictive rod of angry justice
> Sent quick and howling to the centre headlong;
> *I*, fed with judgment, in a fleshly tomb, am
> Buried above ground.

By contrasting himself with Abiram (Numbers 16), who had placed his holiness on a level with Moses and was punished by being swallowed alive with his kith, kin, and substance into a bottomless pit, Cowper presented the image of his life on earth as a living tomb. In Nicholson's terms[12] "The earth, in fact, was a knife-edge on which Cowper walked between the heaven he thought he had lost and the hell he feared would gain him." It is not a position which lends itself to equipoise, but Cowper was able to state his dilemma, both spiritual and intellectual, in a language which did not betray mania, but rather explained it with lucidity.

Several reasons combined to keep Cowper's poetry within the usual bounds of sanity. To some extent he used the act of composition as a form of occupational therapy, and in *The Progress of Error* (1780-1781), written after Newton had left for London, he was able to give voice to the relation between the mind-body problem;

> Faults in the life breed errors in the brain;
> And these, reciprocally, those again
> The mind and conduct mutually imprint
> And stamp their image in each other's mint."
>
> Lines 564-67

At the same time the public intensity of his Evangelical fervor subsided; Newton was no longer at Olney to serve as a goad, Cowper did not obtain his beliefs; he merely kept them private, for himself and a small circle of friends. This limitation is the point of the closing lines of *The Progress of Error:*

> I am no preacher, let this hint suffice—
> The cross, once seen, is death to ev'ry vice:
> Else he that hung there suffer'd all his pain,
> Bled, groan'd, and agoniz'd, and died, in vain."
>
> Ibid., lines 621-24

In such lines Cowper recognized the individual, subjective nature of neurotic ecstasy, a feeling which may combine both suffering and despair. Kenneth MacLean[13] presents one aspect of this view when he says that "in time Cowper discovered that the poetic creation of language was very helpful in drowning out inner voices of despair:

> There is a pleasure in poetic pains
> Which only poets know. . . .

as he wrote to save his own soul, he developed . . . an aesthetic which had something to do with saving the soul of poetry in his day. . . . The sense of terror . . . is most skillfully transferred into the symbols of those excellent poems frequently enclosed in a [private] letter. In some of these Cowper has drawn upon his beloved sea imagery as in *The Castaway*, his last poem and an ultimate image in lonely terror."

The last few years of Cowper's life were those of slow decline. In 1791, the year his translation of Homer was published, Mary Unwin suffered the first of a succession of paralytic strokes which progressively crippled her body and mind until she died in 1796. By 1793-1794 Cowper himself had entered his last phase of melancholy; at this remove it is difficult to decide whether it was a recurrence of his former depressive psychoses, the slow onset of senility, or a combination of both. One last poem, *The Castaway*, written in March 1799, barely more than a year before his death, is Cowper's most self-revealing poem since the *Olney Hymns* and *Tirocinium*. It is, as MacLean[13] labels it, "an ultimate image in lonely terror," but it is more than that. It is based on an incident described in Richard Walter's *A Voyage Round the World . . .* by George Anson (1748) and deals with the death of a sailor fallen overboard whose shipmates are unable to rescue him. Cowper compares his own fate with that of the gallant sailor on life's voyage. "No poet wept him. . . ." but Cowper describes the brave man's death agony and the helplessness of his friends, concluding with a comparison to his own unhappy lot:

> I therefore purpose not, or dream,
> Descanting on his fate,
> To give the melancholy theme
> A more enduring date:
> But misery still delights to trace
> Its 'semblance in another's case.
>
> No voice divine the storm allay'd,
> No light propitious shone;
> When, snatch'd from all effectual aid,
> We perished, each alone:
> But I beneath a rougher sea,
> And whelm'd in deeper gulphs than he.

The image of the soul lost in a tempest at sea is not unique to *The Castaway* of 1799. Cowper had used it before in verses *To Mr. Newton on his Return from Ramsgate:*

> I, tempest-toss'd and wrecked at last,
> Come home to port no more. . . .

and also in the lines *On the Receipt of My Mother's Picture:*

> Always from port withheld, always distress'd—
> Me howling winds drive devious, tempest-toss'd. . . .

For Cowper this must have been a very personal image, suggesting perhaps the need for a mother or father figure to guide him through what he interpreted as life's perils. It is without doubt a subjective image of an emotion deeply felt, but the actual language in which the image is expressed is metaphorically coherent. The mere fact that Cowper used metaphor rather than personification does not indicate poetic mania, but merely a shift in the poetic practices of the latter half of the century. Surely Housman could not have intended us to believe that the use of one form of figure of speech in preference to another was the "true poetic accent emerging from contemporary dialect."

Cowper shared an interest in natural science with other poets of his day, and many of his observations on the natural—especially botanical—aspects of the English countryside exceed the powers of observations granted to his contemporaries. But when he witnessed the growing atheism of his contemporary scientists, he rebelled with traces of his old evangelical passion. It is in this sense that his use of language reveals the paradox of his conflict. Reared in a classic or Augustan school in which metaphor was a condensed simile or had a common-sense basis in likeness, he slowly turned his metaphor inward. In this sense Northrop Frye[14] has focused attention on the central problem of the transition in poetic language: ". . . where metaphor is conceived as part of an oracular and half-ecstatic process, there is a direct identification in which the poet himself is involved. . . . In the age of sensibility some of the identifications involving the poet seem manic, like Blake's with druidic bards, (cf. also Collins' druids in the ode on Thomson's death), or Smart's with Hebrew prophets, or *depressive, like Cowper's with a scapegoat figure, a stricken deer or castaway. . . .*" It was in this last poem, *The Castaway*, that Cowper most surely used the old language to express the new personal metaphor. His "deeper gulph" was not merely the physical and spiritual fact that each man dies alone, but a gulf of language which in his last utterance he successfully bridged.

Christopher Smart (1722-1771)

Literary stereotypes die hard, and we are all familiar with Dr. Johnson's famous dictum that Smart ought never to have been confined:

> His infirmities were not noxious to society. He insisted on people praying with him, and I'd as lief pray with Kit Smart as with anyone else. Another charge was that he did not love clean linen; and I have no passion for it.[15]

Less familiar and less charitable is Thomas Gray's comment in a letter to Thomas Warton, written in 1747 when Smart was getting into difficulties at Pembroke College:

> As to Smart he must necessarily be *abimé* in a short time. His debts daily increase. . . . Addison, I know, wrote smartly to him last week; . . . [as] for his Vanity and Faculty of Lying, they are come to their full maturity. All this, you see, must come to a Jayl, or Bedlam, and that without any help, almost without pity.[16]

Both statements reveal as much about their authors as they do about Smart. Johnson was a man of broad sympathy and human understanding; Gray was too preoccupied with his own neuroses to develop insight into the problems of a fellow member of his college. Yet there are more important ways of leaving one's mark on history, and neither Johnson nor Gray tells us more than a fragment of Smart's story and nothing of his poems. Professor Sherbo's recent biography[17] makes it unnecessary to recite in detail the facts of Smart's unhappy life, wasted gifts, madness and confinement and, finally, death in a debtor's prison. But a few salient features must be outlined if only to frame the picture in historical perspective.

Smart's father, who died when the boy was only 11, was the steward for the large estates of the Vane family in Kent. We are told that Christopher, his first child and only son, was a sickly boy, and there are many comments about his small stature. We are also told that he developed an adolescent "crush" on Anne Vane, even carrying it to the extent of a juvenile "elopement"! After his father's death in 1733, his impecunious mother was enabled to educate Christopher, whose intellect gave promise, through the kind assistance of the Vane family, and the lad was sent to Durham School, many miles northwest of his native Kent. Any one of these particular items might have contributed to his later mental instability, and they have all been duly noted by his psychobiographers. But for the 15 years after his father's death he led a straightforward, successful life, well adapted to his gifts as a student and scholar.

In 1739 he was admitted as sizar to Pembroke College, Cambridge, was graduated A.B. in 1742, and elected Fellow in 1745. He had shown a happy facility for writing verse and was adept at translating from English into Latin. An omnivorous reader, he was truly a "scholar of the university," and many considered him "the pride of Cambridge and the chief poetical ornament of the university."[18] He was elected praelector in philosophy, then in rhetoric, and received his M.A. degree in

1747. But the signs of disaster were at hand, as Gray noted. Popular with both fellows and students, Smart could not resist living beyond his means, standing his share for rounds of drinks in local taverns, dressing expensively, and leading "the good life" in mid-18th century Cambridge.

Smart's chief motive for leaving Cambridge circa 1748-1749 was to establish a financially successful career in London literary circles. He had some acquaintance with literary figures of the day, including a letter of praise from Alexander Pope of recent memory, and he was known to several publishers. At one time he developed an attachment for Anna Maria Carnan, the daughter of a printer and publisher. He married her in 1752, which made it necessary for him to give up his Fellowship at Pembroke which the college authorities had kindly let him maintain in absentia. Devlin[19] has developed a case that Smart's bride was a practicing Roman Catholic, that his guilt about the education of his two daughters in that faith may have played a precipitating role in his madness, and that Smart was actually committed at the instigation of his wife's father and brother, lest his religious mania lead to an official investigation of her religious practices and subject her to civil penalties. The question remains open, but the significant events in Smart's life between 1749 and 1755 were not his hack work in Grub Street but his labors on the Seatonian Prize poems.

The Seaton Prize was awarded annually with its stipend of £30 for a poem written on "the attributes of the Supreme Being." Smart won it for four consecutive years, 1750-1753, did not enter in 1754, and won it again in 1755. One reason advanced for his being kept on the rolls of Pembroke even though he was in some disfavor was his success in the Seatonian competition, and he was even allowed to enter and win after his Fellowship had been revoked. More important than the external circumstances and even the welcome stipend was that the Seatonian poems were the only meaningful contact Smart had with his former academic life during his lean years in Grub Street. His victories were his badge of belonging to the intellectual community, albeit indirectly and at a distance. His earlier poems had dealt with more mundane and conventional topics. *The Hop-Garden* (1750) was a successful Georgic which recalled the landscape of his native Kent, and he had a felicitous turn of phrase in some occasional verses, *viz.*, in the lines *To my Worthy Friend, Mr. T.B.* (1752):

Where Light and Shade in varied Scenes display
A Contrast sweet, like friendly *yea* and *nay*.
My Hand, the Secretary of my Mind,
Left thee these lines upon the poplar's Rind.

But on occasion he descended to passages worthy of *The Stuffed Owl*, as in the epilogue spoken by Desdemona in a 1751 revival of *Othello:*

True Woman to the last—my *peroration*
I come to speak in spite of Suffocation. . . .

Like other poets of the post-*Dunciad* era, Smart tried his hand at literary satire in the Martinus Scriblerus tradition. In 1753 he wrote *The Hilliard*, poking fun at one Dr. John Hill, a notorious but versatile scientist and writer. It is accompanied by *Notes Variorum* which attempt to explain obscure points in the text but which add nothing but academic mirth. *The Hilliad* contains such gems as:

Sweet boy, who seem'st for glorious deeds design'd
O come and leave that clyster pipe behind.

It would be idle to pretend that Smart's odes, addresses, epigrams, and occasional pieces, even *The Hop-Garden* and *The Hilliad,* had any great poetic merit or substance. They are the pleasing effusions of a well-educated man who made his living by his pen. There is no hint of madness or incipient mania. The substance and language are well within the conventional canon of the time.

The first clue we find to Smart's later problems in reconciling mid-18th century science with religion is in one of his earliest preserved poems, the *Secular Ode on the Jubilee at Pembroke College, Cambridge, in 1743*. For a recent A.B. to have been chosen to write such an important poem in a high academic festivity was indeed an honor, and Smart began with an invocation appropriate to the occasion, but it contains the germ of the Seatonian Odes, from which one can trace the origins of his religious mania.

God of science, light divine,
O'er all the world of learning shine;
Shine fav'ring from th' etherial way:
But here with tenfold influence dwell,
Here all thy various rays compell
To dignify this joyful day.

There is nothing, however, in the poem which foreshadows his anti-Newtonianism[20] so evident in *Jubilate Agno,* the poem of his "madness."

Unlike some religious-obsessives Smart has not left a day-by-day record of his spiritual grapplings with faith and reason, but we can trace his growing concern with religious questions in the Seatonian Odes of 1750 to 1755. They represent a way station in his spiritual growth and reveal some of his conflicts. The first of the group, *On the Eternity of the Supreme Being* (1750), deals with the problem of creation and the last judgment. Smart asks the question which has baffled geologists and paleologists for the past three centuries:

> Thou art—all glorious, all beneficent
> All Wisdom and Omnipotence thou art,
>   But is the Era of Creation fix'd
> At when these Worlds began?

He does nothing more than pose the question, almost as an aside, but he makes it plain that mid-18th century natural science had taught him to look for scientific answers, or at least to ask questions which could be answered in the language of science. There is no need to revive the old controversies about fossils, e.g., Arbuthnot vs. Woodward, but Smart was of a generation of university men who could not accept explanations of nature on the basis of revealed truth alone, at least not in 1750. The remainder of the ode is given over to conventional rhetoric about the "flaming sword's intolerable blaze" and "forms Seraphic with their silver trump," culminating in a climax to the effect that

> . . . for Thou art holy,
> For thou art One, th' Eternal, who alone
> Exerts all goodness, and transcends all praise.

Apart from the single question whether the time of creation is "fix'd," Smart presents no unconventional ideas about the eternity of God, and the poem's language is decorous enough to merit the prize it won.

The second Seatonian Ode, *On the Immensity of the Supreme Being* (1751), employs the same iambic pentameter form, but Jones[21] points out that a decisive element is Smart's notion that "The mind loses its way in searching out the immensity of God, whether in the sky where the planets go harmoniously around the sun . . . or in the sea with its coral gardens and whales, or inside the earth with its rich jewels and hidden streams, or on [the surface of] the earth with its varied beauty that defies human art." Here we find Smart's first admission that the human mind, specifically his own, can be overwhelmed by the Newtonian concept of a mechanical universe. Until this time, the scientific essay or scientific poem, of which Pope's *Essay on Man* is the best known example, had usually illustrated and amplified the idea that God's wisdom, goodness, and power were the saving grace. True, in 1746 Collins and Joseph Warton had begun an abortive revolt against the moral poem, but they had met with little success. For Smart to admit that the mind was not equal to the strain was a novel idea. It surely opened a chink in his intellectual armor.

The third of the series, *On the Omniscience of the Supreme Being* (1752), threw down the gauntlet to science. Smart glorifies both man's powers of reason and the animal's instincts, but then takes to task that "proud reasoner, philosophic man" for failing to perceive through his reason that which the animals know by instinct. He casts doubt on the value of some types of scientific investigation:

> The venerable sage, that nightly trims
> The learned lamp, t' investigate the pow'rs
> Of Plants medicinal, the earth, the air,
> And the dark regions of the fossil world
> Grows old in following what he ne'er shall find;
> Studious in vain! till haply, at the last
> He spires a mist, then shapes it into mountains,
> And baseless fabric from conjecture brings.

One does not nowadays consider the work of Robert Boyle, Robert Hooke, James Tyson, Newton, or even Harvey's successors in medical physiology, to have constructed a "baseless fabric," but for Smart, who could not foresee the purpose and direction of natural science, the appeal to God's omniscience was a more satisfying alternative. Greene[20] summarizes the anti-intellectual attitude: "Newton was very clever, but we must not forget that God is even cleverer." By 1752 Smart's position was close to Berkeley's anti-Newtonianism, and from this unsafe ground he never retreated.

The fourth poem, *On the Power of the Supreme Being* (1753), shows no change in Smart's moral or intellectual position. Smart deals chiefly with God's power to perform miracles and with some of the more terrifying aspects of nature: earthquakes, hurricanes, and electrical storms—and he implies that these are supernatural phenomena which will not yield their mystery to rational analysis. Magnetism and electricity come in for their share of disparagement on theological grounds:

> Survey the magnet's sympathetic love,
> That woos the yielding needle; contemplate
> Th' attractive amber's power, invisible
> Ev'n to the mental eye' or when the blow
> Sent from th' electric sphere assaults thy frame,
> Shew me the hand that dealt it!—baffled here
> By his omnipotence, Philosophy
> Slowly her thoughts inadequate revolves,
> And stands, with all His circling wonders round her,
> Like heavy Saturn in th' etherial space
> Begirt with an inexplicable ring.

It is supererogatory to point out that the next century provided explanations for what Smart felt was inexplicable. The point in his mind was that science had failed to furnish the explanations he sought, and he preferred to place his trust in God's powers and a supernatural interpretation of the cosmos.

The fifth and last Seatonian Ode, *On the Goodness of the Supreme Being* (1755), eschews the conflict between faith and reason. It is a paean praising God's goodness for the plenitude of Nature, exhibiting "in an imperceptible point, as well as in an unbounded sphere, the perfections and attributes of an infinite God."[21] The net effect of the Seatonian poems was to deepen the channel of Smart's thought and cause him to be more preoccupied than ever with the relation of the human soul to God. They prepare the way for Smart's three most revealing religious poems, the *Hymn to the Supreme Being* (1756), *Jubilate Agno* (1759-63), and *A Song to David* (1763). By 1755 Smart's mind, not exactly at peace, somewhat beset by external problems, had committed itself to a religious outlook on life, and the last 15 years of his life were devoted to the literary expression of that faith, even at the expense of mania.

The precise date of onset of mental illness is always a biographical problem, and after two centuries the details of psychopathology tend to become blurred. Sherbo[17] cites constant financial pressures as a precipitating factor and minimizes the role of Smart's drinking. It seems reasonable to believe that he drank to excess only when troubled, and that it was a symptom of ill-directed self-therapy rather than a cause. Devlin[19] emphasizes Smart's concern about his wife's Roman Catholicism and his doubts about his daughters' religious education as a major event in the development of his mental disease. Some writers have taken an allusion in the *Hymn to the Supreme Being* (1756) as denoting Smart's recovery from his first bout of madness. Support for this theory has been found in the comparison with Saul, king of the Israelites, in the opening stanzas and in the later lines:

> When reason left me in the time of need,
> And sense was lost in terror or in trance,
> My sick'ning soul was with my blood inflam'd,
> And the celestial image sunk, defac'd, and maim'd.

Smart records his recovery from this illness by writing

> The lamp of life renew'd with vigour burns,
> And exil'd reason takes her seat again.

Sherbo argues with some force that Smart's illness in 1756 was not a mental breakdown but more probably an acute infectious disease, now undiagnosable, but accompanied by high fever and toxic delirium. That the delirium was colored by hallucinations reflecting Smart's predilective religious bent satisfies both possibilities, organic and functional. There seems to be no cause to doubt from the sense of the poem that Smart's contact with reality during his illness was abnormal and that on recovery he recognized it as such. It is clear that his friends and associates did not consider him *non compos mentis* at the time, for between this illness and his confinement publishers were willing to enter into contractual relations with him, advancing monies with reasonable expectation that marketable literary wares would be delivered.

The "official" onset of Smart's overt madness is revealed in a letter written many years later by his eldest daughter. The pathetic text informs us*[17] that

> Previous to my father's showing any symptom of insanity, my sister, a child of three years old, awoke one night screaming and saying that her *papa had lost his head*. This singular presentiment

*Pp. 111-12

> ... was soon after verified, and it was found necessary to confine him. He was committed ... to the care of a Mr. Potter who kept a private house at Bethnal Green. There I remember to have been taken to see him by my mother, and I retain a faint recollection of a small neat parlour in which we were received. He grew better . . . He never recovered the clearness of his intellect, though he continued to write and publish.

This letter was written in 1831, and it is possible that Smart's daughter was confusing his second confinement with his first. The records at St. Luke's Hospital in its *Curable Patients' Book* show that Smart was confined there from May 6, 1757 through May 11, 1758. He did not become a patient at Mr. Potter's until an unspecified date in 1759 and he left there in 1763. Smart was discharged from St. Luke's as incurable, and the interval between May 1758 and his admission at Bethnal Green was largely occupied by petitions from his friends to have him admitted to the Incurable Ward at St. Luke's.

Parenthetically, there is no record of Smart's having been a patient at Bethlem. The literary anecdotes about friends visiting him there and finding his health improved by gardening are to be taken with caution. Sherbo*[17] informs us that his treatment at Mr. Potter's was humane and enlightened: "Provided with pen and ink and paper, allowed visitors, digging in the garden, playing with and talking to his cat, reading books and periodicals, possibly even allowed a few hours, accompanied freedom ... Smart spent almost exactly four years in the private madhouse at Bethnal Green. Part of each day . . . was ritually devoted to the composition of one, two, or three pairs of lines that were then written down neatly in the document he entitled *Jubilate Agno*." This effectively disposes of the romantic myth of Smart laboriously scratching his verses on the wall of his cell with a pin. No doubt some of his time at Bethnal Green was spent writing *A Song to David*, which appeared in print on April 8, 1763, nine weeks after Smart's discharge. He must also have written some of his *Translations of the Psalms of David*, for on the last pages of the *Song* he solicited subscriptions for them, stating that copy was already in the hands of the printer, but the Psalms were not published until 1765.

Two contemporary comments, each by a redoubtable raconteur,

*P. 130

give us a clue to the nature of Smart's aberrant behavior. First, Dr. Johnson writes[22]

> Madness frequently discovers itself merely by unnecessary deviation from the usual modes of the world. My poor friend Smart showed the disturbance of his mind, by falling on his knees, and saying his prayers in the street, or in any other unusual place. Now although, rationally speaking, it is greater madness not to pray at all, than to pray as Smart did, I am afraid there are so many who do not pray, that their understanding is not called in question.

This is the authentic voice of the Great Cham making a general proposition and supporting it with the ideals of a staunch and regular communicant of the established church. It provides little insight regarding the cause and nature of Smart's madness and merely attempts to rationalize his conduct. A more penetrating comment comes from Hester Thrale Piozzi:[23]

> The famous Christopher Smart . . . would never have had a commission of Lunacy taken out against him, had he managed with equal ingenuity (that is, kept his eccentricities private)—for Smart's melancholy showed itself only in a preternatural excitement to prayer . . . taking *au pied de la lettre* our blessed Saviour's injunction *to pray without ceasing*. So that beginning by regular addresses at stated times to the Almighty, he went on to call his friends from their dinners, or beds, or places of recreation, whenever the impulse towards prayer pressed upon his mind. In every other transaction of life no man's wits could be more regular than those of Smart's for this prevalence of one idea pertinaciously keeping the first place in his head, had in no sense except what immediately related to itself perverted his judgment at all. . . . Now had this eminently unhappy patient been equally seized by the precept of *praying in secret*, as no one would have been disturbed by his irregularities, it would have been to no one's interest . . . and the absurdity would possibly have consumed itself in private . . . for mean observers suppose all *Madness* to be *Phrenzy*, and think a person *Insane* in proportion as he is wild, and disposed to throw things about—whereas experience shows that such temporary suspensions of the mental faculties are oftener connected with delirium than with *mania*, and, if not en-

couraged and stimulated by drunkenness, are seldom of long duration.

Mrs. Piozzi is garrulous to a fault, but her social and clinical acumen are sound and to the point. Had Smart been content with private devotions, however elaborate, he would have come to little harm. But when his public praying disturbed more than the small community of literary London, it became necessary to confine him for the convenience of others. Smart may have suffered from hallucinations and his public conduct was often aggravated by inebriety, but in essence his disease was religious monomania. Unfortunately, it became a community scandal.

From *Jubilate Agno* we know that he created public disturbances by praying in St. James's Park and in Pall Mall.

> Let Shobi rejoice with the Kastrel blessed be the name of JESUS in falconry and in the MALL.
>
> For I blessed God in St. James's Park till I routed all the company . . .
>
> For the officers of peace are at variance with me and the watchman smites me with his staff.

He prayed on the rooftops, the flat leads of the neatly porticoed, commonsense, 18th century houses:

> For a man should put no obstacle between his head and the blessing of Almighty God . . .
>
> For the ceiling of the house is an obstacle and therefore we pray on the house-top.

There was very little need for such a muezzin in Georgian London, but Smart also committed the solecism of praying naked in the rain which gave him a sense of added purity:

> For to worship naked in the Rain is the bravest thing for refreshing and purifying the body.

Creating a public disturbance and praying "in the Emperor's clothes" are likely to come to judicial notice, and magistrates often commit persons to psychiatric institutions despite their protestations of sanity simply because their behavior is at variance with accepted norms.

But Smart never considered himself insane, regardless of the opinion of his family, friends, neighbors, and of the fact of his confinement. In this sense his estimate is not wholly false; society confines many persons because their beliefs and the manner in which they exercise them constitute "disorderly conduct." There is no evidence that Smart developed intellectual deterioration or dementia; he was not a depressive like Collins, nor did his religious mania lead to guilt feelings and attempts at suicide as in the case of Cowper. Smart's religion was one of exaltation and ecstasy. Curiously, he derived his religious notions not from the use of drugs nor from an exotic, Oriental cult but from such mundane sources as the King James Bible and the *Book of Common Prayer*. He was a Tory and an Anglican; he believed in the Apostles' Creed and the Thirty-nine Articles. His offense was that he enjoyed them. He even took them seriously. In the age of reason this was sufficient cause to be put away.

The test of Smart's mental status in relation to his poetry rests chiefly on *Jubilate Agno*, written during his confinement at Mr. Potter's between 1759 and 1763, and *A Song to David*, surely conceived, probably drafted, and possibly corrected in 1763 toward the end of his confinement. The literary history of *Jubilate Agno* is well known and requires only brief mention. The manuscript came into the possession of the Cawardine-Probert family which generously permitted Stead[24] to publish it in 1939. It was not known to Housman when he delivered the Leslie Stephen lecture in 1933, and Housman's estimate of Smart's madness can be based only on *A Song to David*. In evaluating *Jubilate Agno* we must always remember that the manuscript represents a mutilated original of the poem with a subtitle of Stead's own devising, "A Song from Bedlam," indicating he felt it was the product of a deranged mind. Stead described it as a "strange composition . . . the fundamental brainwork was broken down, the walls, as it were, are cracked . . . frequent intrusions of the meaningless and grotesque." His introduction and notes show that he did not credit Smart as having anything more preserved in his mental faculties than a good memory.

Smart's reputation was more fortunate in his next editor. In 1954 Bond[25] revised Stead's order and fundamental plan of the fragments. He described *Jubilate Agno* as a "discarded experiment . . . an attempt to adapt to English verse some of the principles of Hebrew verse as expounded by Bishop Robert Lowth in his pioneering study, *De Sacra Poesi Hebraeorum*, first published in 1753 . . . Smart was on familiar terms with Lowth himself." Bond emphasizes the antiphonal nature of the "Let" and "For" sections and their origin in both Hebrew and early Christian liturgy. He advances the claim that Smart's experience in the asylum permitted him to "contemplate his past life and present condition, [in which] he worked out a poetic theory and a personal philosophy, and he experimented with form and style in a manner wholly original and unconventional. He was forced to give up the world, and in so doing he found himself." This may be idiosyncrasy, but it is not madness, at least in any medical sense of the term. That Smart was able to conceive a complex aesthetic theory and compose a highly organized poem, albeit incomplete, is substantive evidence of the soundness of his ratiocination. His use of language and personal allusions are other questions whose consideration for the moment can be deferred.

More recently Hope[26] has developed the idea that *Jubilate Agno* is an apocalyptic vision, a poem cast as a *Magnificat,* written to glorify and praise a systematic cosmology, a theory of the universe based on Smart's extensive scholarly reading—"a single fairly coherent theory of the universe which must have been elaborated before his confinement and which he probably continued to hold after his cure—or, should one say, his release? Citing in detail Smart's reading lists when he was praelector in philosophy at Pembroke, a literary experience which ranged from Sir Isaac Newton's theological speculations to Patrick Delaney's *An Historical Account of the Life and Reign of David, King of Israel, in Four Books . . . by the Author of Revelations examined with Candour* (1740-42) and included Thomas Burnet's *Sacred Theory of the Earth,* William Whiston's *The Accomplishment of Scripture Prophecies,* and Richard Burthogge's *Of the Soul of the World and of Particular Souls.* Hope points out that "such theories, however wild they may look today, were held by learned and rational men." In Smart's era this was a legitimate effort to replace a materialistic cosmology with a spiritual and animistic one, an attempt to reconcile imagination with reason. Smart viewed himself as the bearer of the Lord's cross, the heir to the tradition of the Old Testament psalmists, writing under divine inspiration in praise of that view of God's creation and creatures which he had excogitated.

One reason advanced for Smart's abandonment of *Jubilate Agno* is that he was able to rephrase and crystallize his personal philosophy in *A Song to David* toward the end of his confinement. Hope[26] tells us:

> To the later eighteenth century [it] seemed an insane poem, demonstrating that though the author had been discharged from

> the asylum, he was as mad as ever. To the nineteenth century it seemed a glorious extravaganza displaying a wild and unusual imagination, but not insane. Only in the last forty or fifty years has it become apparent that it is . . . a highly organized poem, extremely complex in its design and as intellectual as it is ecstatic. Admittedly, it conceals a system of ideas which no one has quite succeeded in making explicit and a mysterious symbolism of numbers and correspondences which still eludes complete explication. But it is neither an insane poem in itself nor does it suggest an insane mind.

It is not difficult to recognize that the Seatonian *Odes* were the precursors for *Jubilate Agno* and *A Song to David*. This accounts for the point of view, prevalent until recent years, that *A Song to David* was a unique poem, an outpouring of deeply felt personal religious emotion quite startling in a man like Smart whose only other known poems were conventional, even dull. It was even thought that the poem was "a lucid interval" in the life of a madman. It remained for Havens[27] to demonstrate that *A Song to David* with its 86 six-line stanzas follows a careful plan, the stanzas being arranged in groups of three or seven, or multiples of these mystical numbers. In one sense *A Song to David* is the finished product from the blueprint of *Jubilate Agno;* it was the one poem of Smart's to achieve any reputation for a century and a half after his death. Not long before the manuscript of *Jubilate Agno* came to light, Laurence Binyon[28] achieved a remarkable insight:

> Obsession with a fixed idea is a common form of insanity. But such obsessions are a mental imprisonment; whereas the *Song to David* is unmistakably the expression of a great release. I speak as a mere layman in these matters, but it seems to me that, while there is nothing in the poem to betray an insane mind—no confusion of the real with the unreal—the mental disturbance must have indirectly affected Smart by shaking him out of his normal self, so that *for the time he was freed from the inhibitions which had dominated till then his creative impulses.* [Italics supplied.]

If this is true of *A Song to David*, it is equally true of *Jubilate Agno.*

But even in his obsession Smart was orthodox. Unlike Blake, who was a visionary and a rebel from his youth, Smart's education and mental outlook were conventional. Binyon[28] asks the same question as Housman: "Does poetry need a kind of madness for its liberation?"

His reply was that Smart was exploiting his unconscious but, to his advantage, was unaware of it. "No effort of intellect will ever produce . . . the propitious state. One cannot tap the unconscious at will." But Binyon and Housman, writing before *Jubilate Agno* was published, estimated the liberating effects of Smart's religious monomania on *A Song to David*, and Binyon asked whether, if we knew nothing, should we say that this poem was the work of a madman. The net effect of Smart's mental disturbance was, according to Binyon, "an estrangement of his mind from his century, a liberation of the vein of true and impassioned poetry that was in him but so long disguised and hidden." In that sense *A Song to David* is a Dionysiac poem, a religious poem of an intensity rarely found in England, except for such poets as Thomas Traherne and in occasional passages in Richard Crashaw and George Herbert. Smart's "estrangement"—or alienation, to use a term now in fashion—merely took him back a century in terms of religious feeling, and in *Jubilate Agno* to a Hebraic rather than an English rhetoric.

That the language of *Jubilate Agno* is idiosyncratic, even eccentric, no one can deny. But the text contains accurate references to classical and contemporary literature, the new science, philosophy, religious and theologic controversies then current, as well as to astrology, occultism, and numerology. As Stead[24] demonstrated, Smart retained unimpaired the wide range of knowledge he had acquired while a scholar at Pembroke and from his reading assignments necessary to fulfill his work as a Grub Street hack. The many scattered strokes of imagination, arresting images, gnomic utterances, flashes of wit and insight enable us to put in perspective the occasional passages of self-justification, *e.g.:*

> For I have abstained from the blood of the grape, and that even
> at the Lord's table—

a bit at variance with the known fact of Smart's intermittent trips to the local tavern from which he had to be carried back. Contrasted with trivia of that sort are lines rich in magical incantation:

> For in my nature I quested for beauty, but God,
> God hath sent me to sea for pearls—

an image so autobiographical that it echoes forever. Nor can one even mention Smart's freedom of vision without recalling the famous passage about his cat Jeoffry:

> For at the first glance of the glory of God in the East he worships in his way.

> For this is done by wreathing his body seven times round with elegant quickness. . . .

The famous comments about Sir Isaac Newton—

> For Newton nevertheless is more of error than of the truth, but I am the Word of God.

and with specific reference to Newtonian optics

> For Newton's notion of colours is ἀλόγος unphilosophical, for colours are spiritual.

are to be taken in the sense of an attempt to refute the mechanistic theory of the universe which developed from Newton's theories; they are not an attempt to refute him at the level of experiments in physical science.

Spacks[4] traces Smart's verbal freedom to Lowth's lectures *De Sacri Poesi Hebraeorum*, where the claim is made that

> The origin and first use of poetical language are undoubtedly to be traced in the vehement affections of the mind. For what is meant by that singular frenzy of poets, which the Greeks, ascribing to divine inspiration, distinguished by the appellation of *enthusiasm*, a style and expression directly prompted by nature itself, and exhibiting the true and express image of a mind violently agitated.

This is not far removed from Laurence Binyon's "shaking him out of his normal self." The idea of enthusiasm was scarcely new to poetics, either in classical theory and practice or in English poetry, but Smart was *par excellence* the poet moved to enthusiasm by religious ideas. Because of the circumstances of his life, especially conduct which led to his confinement in an asylum, his enthusiasm was confused with mania.

In *Jubilate Agno* the experiment with enthusiasm and the Hebraic antiphonal mode was uncontrolled, and it is not to Smart's discredit that he abandoned the experiment. We, of a later generation, can only admire its fragmentary successes. Conversely, *A Song to David* was a controlled expression of his enthusiasm. Its recent exegesis by Blaydes[29] has served, in her own words, to "justify Smart's sanity, his adherence to the codes of his age, and his particular genius which transformed many dicta into brilliant poetry."

The physiognomy of the poem is not disturbing. The six-line rhyming stanza in *aabccb* pattern with *aa* and *cc* in iambic *tetrameter* and the *bb* lines in iambic trimeter was not unusual for the century. It recalls many of the strophic odes set by Handel, William Boyce, William Felton, and lesser composers, and the musical analogy is surely apposite for the century's psalmist. The vocabulary is well within the canon of 18th century usage. Take, for example, stanza XVIII in which Smart describes David as a psalmist praising God:

> He sung of God–the mighty source
> Of all things–the stupendous force
> On which all strength depends;
> From whose right arm, beneath whose eyes,
> All period, pow'r, and enterprise
> Commences, reigns, and ends.

There is nothing in these lines which could cause even the most conservative Anglican divine to raise an eyebrow, nor is the general thrust of the poem with its emphasis on adoration and glorification of God outside the tradition of religious poetry at any time, except perhaps in its fervor and the vigor of its expression.

A Song to David is notable for the richness and variety of its images, the number of objects Smart conjures up to fit into his hierarchial scheme of the universe for which he lauds God. This is surely enthusiasm rather than mania, and Callan[30] describes Smart as "a poet with the eye of a painter developed to an unusually high degree. He has the stereoscopic vision which makes the object leap to the eye, the painter's sense of physical texture, and his skill in 'composing' a picture." Similar comments can be made about Blake, who actually was a painter and illustrator, but with respect to Smart one can select such examples of painterly vision as:

> The pheasant shows his pompous neck;
> And ermine, jealous of a speck,
> With fear eludes offence:
> The sable, with his glossy pride,
> For ADORATION is described,
> Where frosts the wave condense.

It is a striking fusion of natural imagery set down with almost scientific accuracy to illuminate the adoration by the animal kingdom. For this sort of writing Smart was rejected by his own age and almost sanctified by the Victorians. Is it too much to expect that the 20th century, which prides itself on enlightened insight into psychopathology, should achieve a more balanced view? One test of the value of a religious poem, not necessarily the best, is whether the poem will have enduring interest, even excitement, in a nonreligious age, and this much we can claim for Smart and his language.

Smart lived for eight years after his release from the asylum. He did not return to his wife and children but took lodgings, first near St. James's Park, later in Chelsea. Not wishing to be returned to custody, he was careful to avoid associations or involvements which might lead to a public profession of his enthusiasm. There is no reason to believe that he modified his idea of a hierarchical universe; his personal cosmology remained unaltered. It is erroneous to believe, as some critics have, that his writings reverted to the conventional level of his early work; once begun, the transformation continued. But the critical response was discouraging. *A Song to David*, published in 1763, elicited a lukewarm response: "his friends were too ready to be saddened, and his enemies too eager to be pleased, by discovering signs of madness in everything he did."[25] Admittedly, his two oratorio texts, *Hannah* (1764) and *Abimelech* (1768), set to music by John Worgan and Samuel Arnold respectively, are not memorable achievements, but his four-volume verse translation of Horace (1767) is a vigorous and felicitous rendition, redeeming his hackwork, prose translation that dated from his Grub Street days.

Smart's most important works during his last few years were his metrical translation of the *Psalms of David*, published in 1765, including with it a cycle of hymns for the Christian year, followed by the versification of the *Parables of Our Lord and Saviour Jesus Christ* (1768), and finally the *Hymns for the Amusement of Children* (1770). These works were consonant with his image of himself as the man chosen to carry on the psalmist tradition. Unconscious of any incongruity, he infused Christian imagery and ideas into his translation of the *Psalms*. Though he translated each verse, the rendering was "free," to say the least. Two examples will suffice to exhibit the limitations:

The passage in Psalm 98:3, which in the King James version reads: "He hath remembered his mercy and his truth toward the house of Israel; all the ends of the earth have seen the salvation of our God. . . ." in Smart's hands becomes

Christ Jesus has declar'd
That sinners shall be spar'd.
And that through him salvation came;
The world could not convince
Of sin the righteous prince,
So manifest his spotless fame.

And Psalm 95:6—"O come, let us worship and bow down: let us kneel before the Lord our maker" is transformed into

Come, O come with Christian union
Let us these our frames abase.
And approach to his communion
Kneeling, falling on our face.

Disregarding their intrinsic lack of poetic merit, they are not so much translations as propaganda at the level of a religious tract, far beneath the attainments one might expect from a one-time praelector in philosophy at Pembroke. They indicate not madness but Anglican insularity. But Smart's later religious poems lie beyond the scope of this essay.

His last years were not easy. His daily life was one of continual financial harassment. He could not make a living from his writing and he had no other trade. In 1770 he was arrested for debt, confined to the King's Bench Prison, where he died in 1771, ending as Thomas Gray unkindly predicted "in Jayl . . . almost without Pity."

Epicrisis

When we apply medical psychology to the cases of Collins, Cowper, and Smart, we fail to find any unifying principle, any common denominator in their clinical states. Collins was a case of simple depression or melancholia. As his emotional status deteriorated, his poetic output declined. If there is any effect of his depression to be seen in his poetry, it lies in the absence of any strong emotional expression. Whatever syntactical incoherence is present is more likely the result of technical maladresse than disordered cerebration. The account of his dream of falling from a tree before he reached the topmost branches has its psychodynamic and symbolic implications, but there is too little factual data about his life and personal relations to permit further exploration. Insofar as Collins' own poetical intentions are concerned, we learn them not from him but from his friend Warton's "Advertisement," a modest desire to expand the ode form into the area of invention and imagination, replacing thereby the "moralizing in verse" which till then had been in fashion. Only a handful of poems followed the *Odes* of 1746. By 1749 he was sufficiently depressed to have to retire to Chichester, and his career as a poet was finished.

Cowper's psychopathology was more complex, and clues to its pathogenesis was better documented. The major episodes are best described as agitated depression with attempts at suicide. The traumas of his childhood, loss of his mother at six, and sadistic treatment at school may have sensitized his impressionable mind. Whether a congenital organic defect, specifically a penile malformation, was a contributing factor must remain an open question in the absence of clear anatomic evidence. But the precipitating factors in Cowper's episodes of agitated depression can be traced to a set of religious beliefs: guilt-ridden, he believed himself eternally damned. He deliberately adopted the writing of poetry as a form of occupational therapy, and only occasionally can the reader gain a glimpse into his conflicts. Most notable are the blood motif in the Olney hymns and passages in *Tirocinium* which reflect a latent sadomasochistic component, and his last poem, *The Castaway*, which brings into the open his fear of loneliness and his sense of alienation. It would be difficult to make a case for Cowper as an imaginative poet, but it is the subject matter of selected poems rather than the language in which he clothes the subject that reveals his mental state. Theory would outrun data were one to claim that his psychological state freed his language in advance of the idiom of his day.

Collins and Cowper were both overtly psychotic; whether Smart was psychotic is debatable. In retrospect, the most suitable diagnosis is religious monomania without intellectual deterioration. Both Cowper and Smart shared the element of intense religious feeling at the centers of their mental disturbances, but the operation of religious sentiment was completely different in each. In Cowper it led to a sense of guilt, depression, and attempted suicide. In Smart it led to a sense of exaltation and enthusiasm; his conviction of his sense of divine mission, rather than mental deterioration, led to the conduct which precipitated his confinement. Yet the two poems to which "madness" has been imputed were written when he was in the asylum, and even critics who defend his sanity agree that his psychological experience was a "release" or that it freed him from inhibitions. Even though one judges an incomplete manuscript, *Jubilate Agno* is different from and possibly more freely expressive than any poem theretofore written in English. Whatever the form may owe to an imitation of Hebrew antiphonal verse, the language is not that commonly used by English poets to that time. Tightly as *A Song to David* may be constructed, impeccable as its private logic may be, the work is unusual among English devotional or adorational poems and a departure from those written before it; both its form and language may be more controlled than *Jubilate Agno*, but apart from Blake and Gerard Manley Hopkins, who came later, it achieved an intensity of language which was new.

Returning to the opening theme, the only evidence of Plato's divine mania in these three "mad" poets can be found in Smart's *Jubilate Agno*, which does transcend the rational, physical world into a spirit of nonrationality, but not to the point of irrationality. Whether his insights are prophetic rather than intuitive lies beyond the purview of a 20th century antinomian and skeptical reader. But the use of poetic language by Collins and Cowper is generally that of men in their "sober senses," and whatever insights they achieved were more anamnestic in light of their personal intrapsychic problems than prophetic. In none of the three cases can we claim that an "assumed personality" freed their language. The poems of Collins and Cowper all stemmed from the previous tradition of English verse and were a logical outgrowth from it. The same stricture applies to most of Smart's poems; only in *Jubilate Agno* did he seek a different tradition of poetical rhetoric, and indeed he was not able to complete that poem.

REFERENCES

1. Tracy, C., ed.: *The Poetical Works of Richard Savage.* Cambridge, Cambridge Univ. Press, 1962.
2. Cunningham, J. S., ed.: *William Collins: Drafts and Fragments of Verse.* Oxford, Clarendon, 1956.
3. Garrod, H. W.: *The Poetry of Collins.* Warton Lecture on English Poetry, from Proc. Brit. Acad., vol. 14. London, Humphrey Milford, 1928.
4. Spacks, P. M.: *The Poetry of Vision.* Cambridge, Harvard Univ. Press, 1967.
5. Miles, J.: The primary language of poetry in the 1740's and 1840's. *Univ. Calif. Publ. in Eng. 19*:161-382, 1950.
6. Cecil, D.: *The Stricken Deer.* London, Constable, 1929.
7. Ryskamp, C.: *William Cowper of the Inner Temple, Esq.* Cambridge, Cambridge Univ. Pres, 1959.
8. Quinlan, M. J.: Memoir of William Cowper, an autobiography edited with an introduction. *Proc. Amer. Phil. Soc. 97*:359-82, 1953.
9. Strachey, L. and Fulford, R. J., eds.: *The Greville Memoirs,* 8 vols. London, Macmillan, 1937-1938.
10. Leigh, D.: The form complete. *Proc. Roy. Soc. Med. 61*:375-84, 1968.
11. Nicholson, N.: *William Cowper.* Published for the British Council and the National Book League. London, Longmans, Green, 1960.
12. Nicholson, N.: *William Cowper.* London,

Lehmann, 1951. esp. pp. 7-8.

13. MacLean, K.: William Cowper. In: *The Age of Johnson.* Essays presented to Chauncey Brewster Tinker, pp. 257-67. Hilles, F. W., ed. New Haven, Yale Univ. Press, 1949.
14. Frye, N.: Toward defining an age of sensibility. In: *Fables of Identity,* pp. 130-37. New York, Harcourt, Brace, 1963.
15. Boswell, J.: *The Life of Samuel Johnson, LL.D.,* vol. 1, p. 397. Hill, G. D., ed. Revised and enlarged by Powell, L. F. Oxford, Clarendon Press, 1934-1950.
16. Toynbee, P. and Whibley, L., eds.: *The Correspondence of Thomas Gray,* vol. 1, pp. 273-75. Oxford, Clarendon Press, 1935.
17. Sherbo, A.: *Christopher Smart, Scholar of the University.* Ann Arbor, Michigan Univ. Press, 1967.
18. Anderson, R.: *The Works of the British Poets,* vol. 11, p. 117. London, Arch, 1795. *XI.*
19. Devlin, K.: *Poor Kit Smart.* London, Hart-Davis, 1961.
20. Greene, D. J.: Smart, Berkeley, the scientists and the poets, a note on eighteenth-century anti-Newtonianism. *J. Hist. Ideas 14*:327-52, 1953.
21. Jones, W. P.: *The Rhetoric of Science.* Berkeley, Univ. Calif. Press, 1966.
22. *Boswell's Life of Johnson,* Oxford Standard ed., vol. 1, p. 265. New York, Oxford Univ. Press, 1933.
23. Piozzi, H. T.: *Thraliana,* p. 728. Balderston, K. C., ed., 2d ed. Oxford, Clarendon Press, 1951.
24. Smart, C.: *Rejoice in the Lamb, a Song from Bedlam.* Stead, W. F., ed. New York, Holt, 1939.
25. Smart, C.: *Jubilate Agno.* Bond, W. H., ed. London, Hart-Davis, 1954.
26. Hope, A. D.: The apocalypse of Christopher Smart. In: *Studies in the Eighteenth Century.* Brissenden, R. F., ed. Toronto, Univ. Toronto Press, 1968.
27. Havens, R. D.: The structure of Smart's *Song to David. Rev. Eng. Studies 14:* 178-82, 1938.
28. Binyon, L.: *The Case of Christopher Smart.* English Association Pamphlet No. 90. London, 1934.
29. Blaydes, S. B.: *Christopher Smart as a Poet of his Time, a Reappraisal.* The Hague & Paris, Mouton, 1966.
30. Callan, N., ed.: *The Collected Poems of Christopher Smart,* 2 vols. p. xxxi. Cambridge, Harvard Univ. Press, 1967.

MOZART: HIS TRAGIC LIFE AND CONTROVERSIAL DEATH

Louis Carp*

At eight o'clock on Sunday evening, January 27, 1756, Wolfgang Amadeus Mozart, one of seven children, first opened his eyes in the Austrian city of Salzburg. The child was baptized Johannes Chrysostomos Wolfgangus Theophilus. This last name was derived from the Greek θεός (*theos*), meaning God and φιλέω (*phileo*), meaning to love; accordingly it became Amadeus, from the Latin *amo*, to love, and *deus*, meaning God. Leopold Mozart, the child's father, also showed love in his diminutive for Wolfgang: "Wörfel." The boy was destined to become the most sensational infant prodigy and one of the greatest musical geniuses of all time. Mozart has not had an equal for swift composition and great spellbinding music that has an unmistakable personal musical style full of variety and beauty. His manuscripts have very few corrections. During the last 17 years of his life-span of 36 years there flowed from his pen on the average a major work every fortnight. In spite of recurrent prostrating illness, economic woes, frustrations, and humiliations, Mozart nevertheless nourished the astonishing talents that produced, according to the official thematic catalogue of Ludwig von Köchel, a priceless and stupendous output of 626 works. These works include, among others, 22 operas, 50 symphonies, 28 piano concertos, violin concertos, sonatas, chamber music to include 27 string quartets, 17 masses, vocal and choral works, and dance music. Mozart's music brought him great critical acclaim (sometimes unpleasant reviews), royal welcomes, and hero worship from his infancy to his death.

Even at the age of three he could pick out chords on the clavier and memorize passages he heard when his musician father gave lessons to his sister Nannerl, who was five years older. At the age of five he composed minuets and violin sonatas which were transcribed by his father. Endowed with a highly sensitive musical ear, he could detect the

*Dr. Carp is a consultant surgeon to the Goldwater Memorial Hospital, New York, N. Y., and to the Nyack Hospital, Nyack, N. Y. He lectures as a guest of the Program of Continuation Education, Columbia University School of Public Health Administration, New York, N. Y. He is a member of the Board of Directors of the City Center of Music and Drama, Inc., New York, N. Y., and is on the Advisory Council of the Hospitalized Veterans Music Service and of the Musicians Emergency Fund.

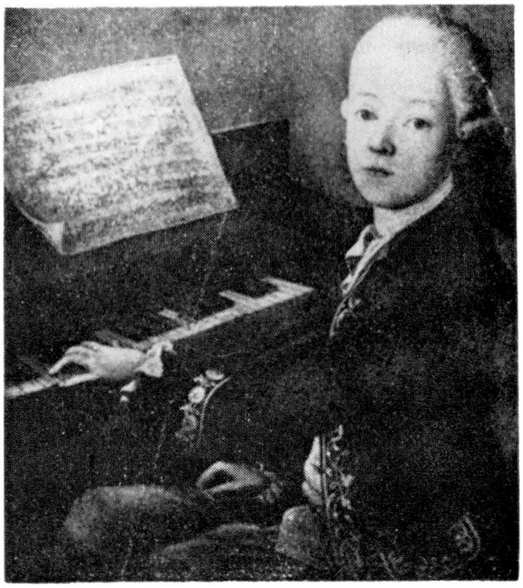

Mozart as a boy. From a portrait by Thadäus Helbing. Reproduced by permission of the Mozart Museum, Salzburg, Germany.

slightest error in pitch. He played the violin without any formal teaching. Once when his father assembled a few musicians for chamber music, Wolfgang, then five, sporting his powdered wig and sword, walked in uninvited and, to the astonishment of all, played second violin and then, amidst laughter, first violin. His father said that if the youngster had practiced enough he would have been "one of the first violinists of Europe." Emperor Joseph II of Austria, during a command performance, referred to him as the *kleiner Hexenmeister* (little magician). Leopold liked to show how the child, whose tiny fingers could scarcely reach a sixth on the harpsichord, could strike the proper notes on a keyboard covered with a piece of cloth. Wolfgang at five was already conversant with the principles of composition. His arithmetical mind helped, for he was scribbling the solution of problems on the walls of his house. At this period of his life his path toward recognition was strewn with petals.

As an adult Mozart demonstrated a remarkable memory; he could compose a new opera in his mind for subsequent transposition into a score. With extraordinary facility he injected into his music what came through to listeners as pathos, humor, drama, malice, sweetness, sunshine. He was prolific in new melodic ideas, especially for the voice. It may be said to his credit that he worked very hard from early morning until 10 at night, when he ate his only meal of the day. He wrote in a letter, "Believe me, I love work and not idleness." On request, he improvised and played an aria or song—for example, *Affetto*, a love song, and *Perfido*, a song of temper and rage. He sight-read symphonies and transposed at sight into any key.

Mozart's physical stature was against him. He was unimpressive, short, and thin, with small, plump hands, blue, near-sighted eyes, and a disproportionately large head and long aquiline nose. His head and nose were frequently caricatured. His ears were deformed, but the narrow, slitlike entrance to the auditory canal had no untoward effect on the acuteness of his hearing. His hair, a source of vanity, was thick and fair. During the years 1784 and 1785, when he was at the height of his earning capacity, he squandered a good part of his income on clothes, which were handmade, embroidered, and colorful, with red predominating. Jewelry was another fetish of his. Wolfgang's letters, usually signed Wolfgang Amade, were witty, frank, incisive, chatty, sophisticated, and full of earthiness. They contained some of the most striking pornography in the German language, especially as it related to physiological functions. Casual to a fault, indecisive, careless, and extravagant, he did not seem to face reality, and he lacked adroitness in business and financial matters. It was difficult for him to withstand the jealousies and intrigues of competitors. Strangely enough, he did not care much for literature or the static arts. A gay blade with pretty women, he is alleged to have been oversexed. Was he overcompensating for what society viewed as physical defects? He once wrote, "If I had to marry every girl I've jested with, I'd have at least two hundred wives by now." Dancing and billiards were his entertainment. Wolfgang liked wine but he was never a drunkard. His house pets were a canary and a dog. Although his sharp and tactless tongue frequently got him into trouble, he was basically a gentleman—cheerful, affectionate, honest, cooperative, and proudly independent. A personality of quicksilver!

Mozart came of a nice, middle-class family of business people and mechanics in the Swabian city of Augsburg. His father, whose name in full was Johann Georg Leopold Mozart, was born in 1719, the son of a bookbinder. He married pretty Anna Maria Pertl of St. Gilgen, near Salzburg. Leopold began the study of law at the age of 18, but dropped law and took up music as a vocation. At that time it was customary for musicians to be in the employ of a noble or rich family and to function additionally as house servants, such as valets or footmen. Leopold's slim livelihood was augumented by a public post as organist and later as a fourth violinist. When he was appointed vice kappelmeister in Salzburg, he attained his height of professional recognition. An accomplished and versatile musician, he taught violin and clavier, including keyboard instruments such as the harpsichord and pianoforte but not the organ.

Leopold, industrious, handsome, austere, irascible, and a strict disciplinarian, had a profound influence on his son. He has been criticized for the alleged exploitation of Wolfgang from the age of six. There began irregular hours of arduous, slow, dangerous, and uncomfortable tours in jolting coaches through Austria, Germany, Italy, and England; on these tours Nannerl was a musical participant. Roads were bad, mechanical breakdowns unavoidable, wayside inns intolerable. The adverse effects on Mozart's health seem obvious. His third tour began at the age of seven and lasted three years. The itinerary included many cities in Germany and Austria and the cities of Brussels, Paris, and London. It was in London, at the age of eight, that Wolfgang met Johann Christian Bach and was cordially received by George III and Queen Charlotte, both of whom were musical. Wolfgang sight-read difficult pieces and played accompaniments for the queen, who showered favors on him at court. Suspicions were aroused that he was not a mere boy. This illusion came to an abrupt end when, during one of his concerts, a cat walked onto the scene. Wolfgang deserted the keyboard to play with the cat. At times he would prance around the room with a stick between his legs, playing horse. A horse race introduced him to one of the favorite sports of the time. He stayed in England 15 months and during this time he wrote his first symphonies, K 16 and K 19. The *Public Advertiser* for July 11, 1765, described him as "The greatest prodigy that Europe or even Human Nature has to boast of."

The criticism of Leopold's exploitation of his young son is open to argument. It is true that Wolfgang was dragged through many countries in Europe and exhibited as a wunderkind. But he himself was on his father's side much later when he wrote Archbishop Hieronymus Colloredo in Salzburg requesting leave of absence as kappelmeister. "Parents endeavour to place their children in a position to earn their own bread. . . . The greater the talents which children have received from God, the more they are bound to use them for the improvement of their own and their parents' circumstances." To be sure, Mozart missed two of the assets of boyhood—playmates and exercise—at a time when the child prodigy was escalating into a musical genius. Was not the father justified in exposing his little boy not only for the entertainment he gave and the contacts he made, but also to add to the meager family income, even though the financial rewards were not in keeping with Wolfgang's genius? The boy's first three tours netted a profit of 7,000 gulden* in addition to gifts of numerous watches, rings, jewelled snuffboxes, and other trinkets. Some of these are on exhibit in the Mozarteum in the Getreidegasse in Salzburg, including a ring from Empress Maria Theresa and another from the prince archbishop in Augsburg.

At the age of 13 Wolfgang wrote his little German operetta, *Bastien and Bastienne*, which was performed in the private theater of Dr. Anton Mesmer, the physician hypnotist. Already conversant with Italian (in addition to his native German) Mozart also knew French and Latin. The opera *La Finte Semplice* was produced next in the same year in the palace in Salzburg. The young composer toured Italy three times, the last time when he was 16 years old, when his opera *Lucio Silla* was partly successful. This was his last commission in Italy. Pope Clement XIV bestowed on him the order of the Golden Spur and the title *signor cavalier*. At Bologna, Mozart was elected a member of the Academia Philharmonica. His ninth tour lasted until he was 23 years old. No longer a boy prodigy, he went through a difficult age transition and was received politely as an adult. In our own time Yehudi Menuhin, Ruggiero Ricci, and others have gone through a similar transition.

Idomeneo, produced in 1781, helped to establish him as a recognized composer in Germany. Wolfgang had some upleasant problems when he was engaged as kappelmeister in the home of Archibishop von Colloredo in Salzburg. He was unhappy because he disliked sitting at the same table with cooks and other servants. The archbishop called him a knave, a scamp, and a dissolute young man. Enraged, Mozart sent in his resignation. When he returned a month later, the detested, grim martinet von Colloredo dismissed him with the help of Count Arco, his high steward and toady, who unceremoniously kicked him out the door. Young Mozart was articulate about a reciprocal plant of a well-aimed shoe on Arco's posterior. The humiliating experience was a pronounced

*It is difficult to evaluate the currencies of 18th century Austria as they related to other countries because of the different economies. Marcia Davenport in her book *Mozart* wrestled with the problem. She figured one gulden or one florin (silver) to be worth about $0.45 and one ducat (gold) about $2.25 in the currency of the United States in 1792.

setback for Mozart, but he determined to make a success of his career independently.

Even when Mozart was a youngster love affairs crept into his life. He was alert to petticoats and to the kissing games and bawdy jokes that were then current. At the age of six, after one of his concerts in the palace in Vienna, the Empress Maria Theresa was fondling him in her lap when he slipped down and fell on the polished floor. The Archduchess Marie Antoinette, only two months older than Wolfgang, helped him to his feet. The story goes that her reward was a marriage proposal. At the age of 21 he stayed for a while in Mannheim with a family whose bread-winner was Fridolin Weber, a prompter and singer at the opera. The calculating matriarch, Frau Caecilia Weber, drew a net around him for one of her four daughters, Aloysia, a young opera singer. Mozart's father objected to the affair in a strong letter, "Off with you to Paris, and that immediately! . . ." Wolfgang was accompanied on the trip to Paris by his mother, who died there in convulsions and of an unknown illness. Subsequently Aloysia became a prima donna in Munich and despite Wolfgang's insistent advances she rejected him for Lange, a painter, sculptor, and actor. About two years later Mozart carried on an intense love affair with a girl cousin, Maria Anna Thekla, "the Basle," who was three years his junior. His ardent love letters to her, in which pornographic four-letter words were incorporated, finally won her over. "I knew you wouldn't be able to resist me much longer. Why, of course, I'm sure of success." He was known to pass a sly, slithering hand over her thigh under a dinner table. She eventually gave him an illegitimate child, Marianne Victoria.

Mozart, determined to maintain his contact with the Weber family, at the age of 26 married Aloysia's sister Constanze, a serious musician. In nine years of married life, Constanze had six pregnancies, but only three babies came to term. Two of them survived. Karl (September 17, 1784 to December 30, 1858) became a career government official and Franz Xaver Wolfgang (July 26, 1791 to July 29, 1844) a frustrated musician. Both remained unmarried.

After his marriage, Mozart made the romantic music-struck city of Vienna his home for the rest of his life; he lived in a shabby, narrow, and smelly street. There he wrote some of his best and popular operas: *The Abduction from the Seraglio*, *The Marriage of Figaro*, and *Don Giovanni*, for the last of which he accepted a compensation of 100

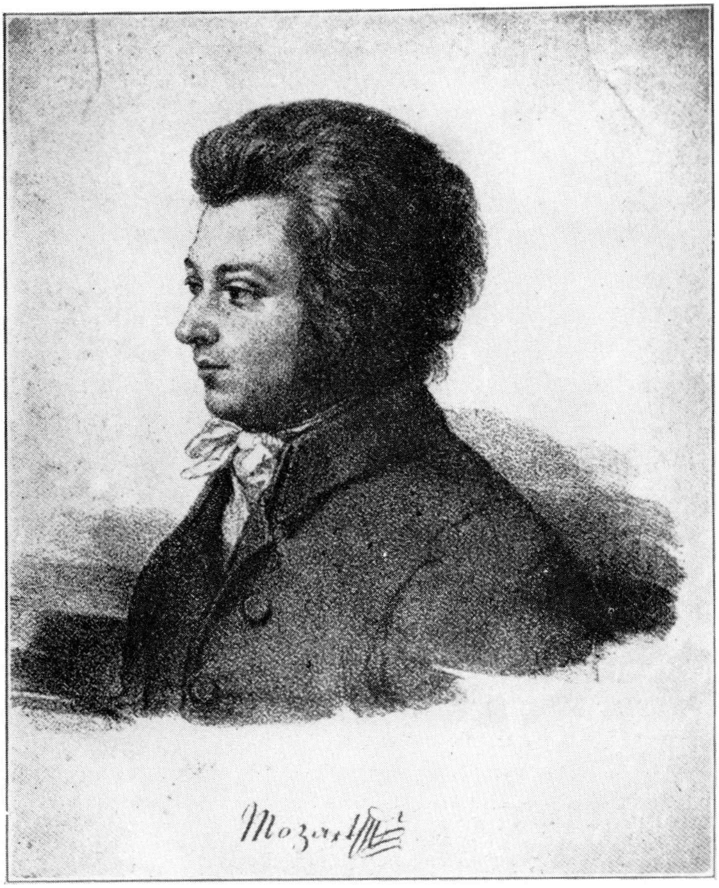

Mozart in his manhood. From a portrait by Joseph Lange. Reproduced by permission of the Mozart Museum, Salzburg, Germany.

ducats. Winthrop Sargeant, distinguished music critic, has described *Don Giovanni* as "the greatest opera ever written" with "supremely beautiful music . . . breathless suspense . . . unsurpassed delineated character."

In great demand in musical and social circles, Mozart continued to pour out concertos and chamber music. Franz Josef Haydn, the most celebrated composer in Europe and a great friend of Mozart, told his father in 1785, "I tell you before God as an honest man that your son is the greatest composer known to me either in person or by reputation. He has taste, and what is more, the most profound knowledge of composition." Two years later the domineering father was dead at the age of 68, crippled with arthritis. It was a severe blow to Wörfel, who idolized him to such an extent that he would frequently say, "Next to God comes papa." During the next year, 1788, Mozart composed three great symphonies in six weeks: the E flat, the G minor, and the C major (Jupiter)—the last full of the most complicated counterpoint. Meantime, his wife Constanze became ill with phlebitis and frequently went to Baden for the cure.

At the age of 33 Mozart was back in Vienna, where he began to suffer from the tribulations of outrageous fortune and declining income, even though he was a most popular and fruitful composer. Failing health, bad marketing of his extraordinary talent and virtuosity, jealousies, and intrigue did not help. Financial distress compelled him to sell or pawn his valuables, some of his clothes, furniture, and plate. A viola on which he played quartets with Haydn went for two dollars. Rent was in arrears. Pupils were in short supply and creditors were hounding him and pounding at the door. Karl, five years old, had to be cared for by strangers.

Although Mozart was a pious Catholic, he also sought refuge and comfort in freemasonry and became an active member of the order in 1785. There were pitiful and degrading requests to brother masons for loans. In 1788 a letter to one of them, Michael Puchberg, a wealthy merchant in Vienna, emphasizes the plight to which Mozart had descended. "Your true friendship and brotherly love embolden me to ask a great favor of you. I still owe you eight ducats. Apart from the fact that at the moment I am not in a position to pay you back this sum, my confidence in you is so boundless that I dare to implore you to help me out with a hundred gulden until next week, when my concerts in the Casino are to begin. . . ." And again, ". . . In short, being unable to find a friend to help me, I have been obliged to resort to the money-lenders; . . . I am at the moment so utterly penniless that I have to beg you, dearest friend, by all that is sacred, to help me with whatever you can spare! . . . If you only knew how this worries and troubles me!" Mozart also appealed to Franz Hofdemel to ". . . lend me 100 florins till the 20th of next month." He was victimized by loan sharks and became a target for cheats and leeches. To make a little money he wrote *Cosi fan Tutte*, which was produced in January 1790. In the face of all his adversity and progressively bad health, necessity spurred him on to write and, between May and July 1791, he composed *Die Zauberflöte* (*The Magic Flute*). Emanuel Schikaneder, a mercenary and uncouth producer, paid 100 ducats for the score. To celebrate the coronation of Leopold II as king of Bohema, Mozart wrote the opera *La Clemenza di Tito*. It failed. The strain of meeting deadlines and his failing health had shown their effects. Mozart left Prague for Vienna in sunken spirits.

His strenuous life, anxieties, failures, precarious financial situation, and many illnesses began to take their toll. He became neurotic, moody, and unsociable. A fragmented personality! Then a mysterious, tall, and cadaverous visitor, clad in gray, appeared and gave him an advance fee of 50 ducats to commission a *Requiem*. It turned out that the visitor, Leitgeb, was the steward and go-between for a Count Franz van Walsegg, an amateur musician who was scheming to have it performed as his own. Mozart worked hard on it, although he had an obsession that it would be a sign of his own approaching death, and that he was writing it for himself. "I know I will not last very long," he tearfully told his wife. Sickness prevented the completion of the *Requiem* and it became his last musical testament. "My music making is drawing to an end. I feel a cold which I cannot explain—winter is coming." Violent headaches, blackouts, nausea, and tell-tale swelling of the extremities and face plagued him. "I am at the point of death. I have finished before I could enjoy my talent. Yet life is so beautiful, my career opened so auspiciously—but fate is not to be changed. . . ." Mozart was so exhausted that the thought of death was sweet as compared with the fear of life.

Constanze returned home from Baden and gave birth to a son in July 1791. Sick as he was, Mozart conducted the first two performances of *The Magic Flute*, which ran for 100 consecutive nights in Vienna. His health continued in a serious decline. Run down, nervous, and feeble, he was highly susceptible to infection. His eyes had lost their lustre and they stared into space. Dr. Sigmund Barisani, an intelligent and conscientious family physician, had treated him for rheumatic fever when he was 28. After this doctor's death, Dr. Nickolaus Closset assumed charge. Much later, Dr. Closset called in consultation Dr. Mathias von Sallaba, chief of the Allgemeine Krankenhaus in Vienna. They agreed on the hopeless outlook. Mozart struggled on, impoverished, sick in body and spirit, and continued as best he could to work on the

Requiem. Although the composition was unfinished, friends* gathered at his bedside to sing it on Sunday, December 4th. Only seven bars of the "Lacrimosa" were finished. Mozart started to sing the alto part and even puffed out his cheeks in an attempt to imitate the trumpets (maybe respiration was difficult), but he broke into a bad weeping spell. "Here is my death song. I must not leave it incomplete." He asked his good friend and former pupil Franz Xaver Süssmayr to finish it. He begged his sister-in-law, Sophie Haibel, to stay at his bedside. "You must see me die. . . . I already have the taste of death on my tongue." Constanze was hysterical. Dr. Closset was called from a theater. Cold compresses were ordered for the feverish brow of the delirious and comatose Mozart. A priest delivered the last sacrament. On attempting to rise, Mozart fell back dead, 55 minutes after midnight, December 5, 1791. Thirty-six years later, his *Requiem* was performed at the solemn high mass during the funeral of Ludwig van Beethoven.

On December 6, in a third-class funeral that cost $5.50, the plain coffin was carried through the streets in such inclement weather that it prompted the accompanying mourners, who numbered nine and included Süssmayer and Salieri but not Constanze, to return home. The hearse arrived at the St. Mark cemetery in a suburb of Vienna and without a note of music, a sad and tragic irony and an inconsequential event. The coffin was deposited in the mortuary chapel. The following day it was lowered into a pauper's grave that has never been positively identified. The city of Vienna later erected a handsome monument by Hans Gasser, on what was dubiously considered to be Mozart's grave; the monument was unveiled on December 5, 1859, 68 years after Mozart's death. There is no certainty that the skull exhibited in the Mozarteum and alleged to be that of Mozart is actually his.

"Even his funeral was a failure," wrote George Bernard Shaw. "Depend on it, they no sooner put up their umbrellas and bolted for the nearest shelter than he got up, shook off his bones into the common grave of people and soared off into immortality." Rubenstein characterized the master's genius as "Eternal sunshine in music, thy name is Mozart." Great composers acknowledged their debt to him: Beethoven, Rossini, Donizetti, Schubert, Wagner, Gounod, Massenet, Debussy.

There is some lively and simmering controversial literature in

*Schack, soprano; Hofer, tenor; Gerle, bass: members of the cast of the first performance of *Die Zauberflöte* at the theater on the Wieden, the so-called Freihaus Theater, on September 30, 1791.

German, French, Russian, and English which embraces Mozart's illnesses, with wide speculation on the cause of his death. Was his death natural or was he poisoned? It has been difficult to separate fact from fiction. In Mozart's day diagnoses were clinical and philosophical without the help of laboratory tests such as are available today. Perhaps one of the most comprehensive and painstaking research treatises on the subject, *Gewiss, man hat mir Gift gegeben* (Surely, I have been given poison), was written by Gunther Duda, a German physician, and published in 1958. The bibliography is extensive. After a lapse of almost 200 years, Duda, Dr. Dieter Kerner, and a Russian physician, Igor Belsas, have become the chief proponents of the theory that Mozart died as a result of a slow poisoning by a mercury salt. One version has it that the Venetian Antonio Salieri, director of the Vienna Opera and an arch rival and jealous composer-conductor, admitted the crime in a confessional (how could such a secret get out?); according to another version, he stoutly denied the crime on his death bed on May 7, 1825. Can it be that the poison theory was triggered by Mozart's tearful exclamation to his wife ". . . I will not last longer. I have been given poison. I cannot get this out of my head"? Indeed, it has not been shown anywhere that this claim was factual. Toward the end of his life Mozart was very sick, and his claim, a pathological obsession, was a pure figment of his delirious and paranoid moments, the result of fear of imagined or actual enemies.

According to Duda, the first poisoning occurred in the summer of 1791, by means of a small dose of mercury. This was followed by a large dose on November 20th. This would be hazardous pinpointing. But one month earlier Mozart was apparently well enough to conduct *The Magic Flute* and to write a clarinet concerto. In that same month Constanze went to Baden where she received long letters from her husband. On October 14 he brought her back to Vienna. There were, then, two months during which he had no outstanding complaints. Duda and others have drawn conclusions from detective stories, and use unproved dates and non sequiturs. The poison legend became so fixed that Pushkin seized upon it and wrote the tragedy *Mozart and Salieri.*

Over the years the myth became a source of idle or malicious gossip. Even during a performance of Beethoven's Ninth Symphony as late as May 23, 1824, circulars were passed around which stated that Salieri had put containers of poison at Mozart's bedside. How much credence can this be given?

Mozart's physicians did not suspect foul play. Their diagnoses of the cause of death were recorded as malignant typhus (*ein hitziges Frieselfieber*) or meningitis. In the light of our present knowledge, after analysis of the clinical picture, these diagnoses were incorrect.

What, then, are the facts? Perhaps it is possible to be more realistic and conservative after analysis of the historical records which seem to indicate why Mozart died so young and what pathological processes in his various infections took the life of this burning and creative genius. To begin with, Mozart was one of seven children; it was fortunate that he and his older sister, Nannerl, survived infancy and childhood. His father and mother thought that the proper feeding for babies was water. It is probable that the infant suffered from malnutrition. The family lived in dampness and poor sanitation in an otherwise fine house. A high fever and scarlet rash, diagnosed scarlet fever by the physician to the Countess von Ginseldorf, struck Wolfgang at the age of six. He was sick for four weeks. This infection was the inception of kidney damage which undermined his health for the rest of his life. The administration of *Schwarzpulver* (black powder), a cathartic, and *Markgrafenpulver*, an antiperspirant, had little if any remedial effect. Concerts were canceled for eight days and there was a financial loss of 50 ducats. The next year painful knees and fever (rheumatic fever?) were so severe that Mozart could not stand up. At the age of nine, he had what probably was a septic sore throat, which disabled him for a month and left him emaciated. Smallpox attacked him at the age of 11, made him desperately ill, and closed his eyelids for nine days. More sore throats followed. Cramps and vomiting with high fever attacked him several times and disabled him when he was 28. Many bad toothaches with swollen jaws and many bad colds added to his ailments. It must be emphasized that five years before his death, at the age of 31, he was so sick that he wrote, "I never lay myself down in bed without reflecting that perhaps I, as young as I am, shall never see another day." Because of his bad health, he delayed writing the overtures to *Don Giovanni* and *The Magic Flute* until just before their dress rehearsals.

Late in 1790 he was critically ill, but his iron will, residual stamina, and rallying power enabled him to give concerts in Frankfurt during the coronation of Leopold II. Challenge and financial necessity pushed him far beyond human tolerance.

From then on, the massive insult to his kidneys from repeated bacterial maladies became evident by the superimposition of acute on chronic nephritis,* a recognized clinical entity. He had uremia from kidney failure and infection, with significant and symptomatic black-outs, abdominal pain, splitting headaches, vomiting, fever, and extensive and more pronounced edema of the upper and lower extremities and face. In fact his lower extremities were so swollen that he could not turn in bed. His kidneys could not properly eliminate chemical waste products, urine was scanty, his breath was foul, his muscles twitched and were weakened, and his face took on a waxy pallor. There were terminal episodes of delirium and coma. Hypertension was a natural complication. The battle against degenerative disease was lost. With modern technologies and therapy, the story might have been different.

Mired in poverty, Mozart was dogged to the very end by desperate financial problems. He left six florins and a destitute wife, except that she received from the emperor a paltry pension of 22 gulden a month. Happily, in 1809, she married a Danish diplomat, G. N. Nissen. She died in 1842.

Mozart, bedeviled with tragedy, was a man who received intermittent recognition of his greatness. He went from ecstacy, financial and social success to pauperism, mendicancy, rejection, despair, and depression. Covered with glory in his best years, he nevertheless had an inglorious finale. He failed in success. With comparatively good health and longer life, it is probable that he would have surpassed his extraordinary productivity in even higher standards of music as an added legacy for the civilized world.

One may appropriately paraphrase Callimachus, the Greek architect and poet:

> Somewhere, lapped in hallowed slumber Mozart lies,
> Asleep, not dead: a great man never dies.

*Vide Duda. J. Barraud, Casseroller, H. Holz, A. Marx, and J. Willms concur in the diagnosis of nephritis and they do not substantiate that of mercury poisoning. After a perspective of many years, the *Neustadter Tageblatt* of October 10, 1957, concludes that Mozart died of severe chronic nephritis.

REFERENCES

Brockway, W. and Weinstock, H.: *Men of Music: Their Lives, Times and Achievements.* New York, Simon and Schuster, 1939.

Sanborn, P.: *International Cyclopedia of Music and Musicians,* pp. 1391-1406. Thompson, O., Ed. New York, Dodd, Mead, 1964.

Groves Dictionary of Music and Musicians, vol. 5, pp. 923-83. Blom, E., ed. New York, St. Martin's Press, 1959.

Newman, E.: *Stories of the Great Operas,*

vol. 1. New York, Garden City Pub., 1930.

Abeshouse, B.: *A Medical History of W. A. Mozart.* Norwich, N. Y., Eaton Laboratories, 1966.

Cyclopedia of the Arts. Read, H., consulting ed. New York, Meredith Press, 1966.

Girdleston, C. M.: *Mozart and his Piano Concertos.* Norman, Okla., Univ. of Oklahoma Press, 1962.

Roseberry, E.: *W. A. Mozart, The Story of his Life and Work.* New York, Boosey and Hawkes, 1960.

Davenport, M.: *Mozart.* New York, Scribner's, 1932.

Anderson, E.: *The Letters of Mozart and his Family,* vol. 1. Prepared by King, A. H. and Carolan, M. New York, St. Martin's Press, 1966.

Mozart Letters, Readings and Musical Illustrations. Goldovsky, B., annotator. Philharmonic Hall, Lincoln Center for the Performing Arts, New York, August 20, 1968.

Duda, G.: *Gewiss, man hat mir Gift gegeben.* Pähl, Obb., Germany, Hohe Warte, 1958.

Shapiro, S. L.: Medical history of Wolfgang Amadeus Mozart. *Eye, Ear, Nose, Throat Monthly 47*:17-20, 1968.

Weiss, D.: *Sacred and Profane.* A novel based on the life of Mozart. New York, Morrow, 1968.

Sergeant, W. Manuscript Events. It's the Tops. *The New Yorker,* Dec. 28, 1968, pp. 60-61.

Eagle, N.: Variations on a theme (travel) by Mozart. *New York Times,* Section 10, November 23, 1969.

THE PRESENT STATUS OF ABORTION LAWS*

A STATEMENT BY
THE NEW YORK ACADEMY OF MEDICINE
PREPARED BY THE COMMITTEE ON PUBLIC HEALTH

"A small and temporary improvement may really be the worst enemy of great and permanent improvement, unless the first is made on the lines and in the direction of the second." –Morley, J. *On Compromise,* vol. 3., p. 129. London, MacMillan, 1921.

THE New York Academy of Medicine has issued three opinions on therapeutic abortion since 1943. In that year, after a grand jury investigation of so-called "abortion specialists," the Committee on Public Health of the Academy recommended that the state penal law should be amended to legalize therapeutic abortions in order to preserve the health of a pregnant woman. By way of implementing its recommendation, the Committee drafted the proposed amendment in appropriate phraseology:

> Definition of abortion and therapeutic abortion and punishment of one who performs a non-therapeutic abortion.
>
> 1) an abortion is an interruption of an intrauterine pregnancy before the period of viability (up to 28 weeks gestation) is reached.
>
> 2) a therapeutic abortion is the artificial interruption of an intrauterine pregnancy before the period of viability (up to 28 weeks of gestation) is reached where the continuance of such pregnancy would jeopardize the life of the woman or so aggravate the physical or mental disease from which she suffers as seriously to impair her health or threaten her life.
>
> 3) may be performed only by a physician duly licensed in the State of New York, and only in a hospital recognized by the Department of Social Welfare of New York State, or the

*Approved by the Committee on Public Health of the New York Academy of Medicine, December 1, 1969.
Approved by the Council of the New York Academy of Medicine, December 17, 1969.

> Department of Health of New York State, or approved by the American College of Surgeons and/or the American Medical Association. After written opinions of its necessity have been obtained from competent qualified and recognized consultants in the respective specialties involved, which said written opinions shall be incorporated in the records of the hospital.

In 1953 the Committee on Public Health recommended that its previously proposed amendment be broadened to include the likelihood of impaired health or disability of a child as an indication for therapeutic abortion.

In 1959 the American Law Institute suggested a Model Penal Code governing abortion. This code would authorize therapeutic abortion when a licensed physician believes there is substantial risk that continuance of the pregnancy would gravely impair the physical or mental health of the mother, or that the child would be born with grave physical or mental defects, or that the pregnancy resulted from rape by force or incest. Two physicians must certify in writing their belief in the justifying circumstance.

In a statement issued in 1965 the New York Academy of Medicine reaffirmed its previously expressed opinions that changes in the abortion law were necessary. This statement contained the following recommendation:

> The New York Academy of Medicine therefore strongly recommends that the Penal Law of the State of New York be amended to legalize therapeutic abortion where there is substantial risk that the continuance of pregnancy would gravely impair the physical or mental health of the mother, or that the child would be born with grave physical or mental defects. Safeguards should also be included in the legalization of the procedure on these grounds: therapeutic abortion should be permitted only in officially recognized or accredited hospitals after review and approval in each instance by a competent committee established by the hospital; and the operation should be performed only by a physician licensed in the State of New York.

In the intervening years many resolutions from diverse authoritative bodies and changes of statutes here and abroad have called attention to the appalling inadequacy of the New York law.

TABLE. INDICATIONS FOR THERAPEUTIC ABORTION
Statutes Enacted 1967-1969

	Life	*Health*	*Mental health*	*Fetal defects*	*Rape*	*Incest*	*Limit weeks*
Arkansas	X	X		X	X	X	12
California		X	X		X	X	20
Colorado	X	X	X	X	X	X	16*
Delaware	X	X	X	X	X	X	20†
Georgia	X	X		X	X		
Kansas	X	X	X	X	X	X	
Maryland	X	X	X	X	X		26†
Mississippi	X				X		
New Mexico	X	X	X	X	X	X	
North Carolina	X	X		X	X	X	
Oregon	X	X	X	X	X	X	21‡

*Applies only to cases of rape or incest.
†Exceptions in the case of serious threat to the mother's life or in cases of fetal death.
‡Time limit does not apply in cases of danger to life.

In 1967 the House of Delegates of the American Medical Association went on record as supporting reform of the abortion laws to conform with the general guidelines set forth in the Model Penal Code. The American College of Obstetricians and Gynecologists recommended, in addition to the provisions of the Model Penal Code, that social and total economic environment—actual or reasonably foreseeable—be considered as having a bearing on the health of the mother.

For more than two years the Medical Society of the State of New York has formally approved reform of the present "inadequate" abortion law.

The American Public Health Association at its 1968 annual meeting took the final step; it formally advocated repeal of the existing statutes regulating therapeutic abortion.

Between 1967 and 1969 eleven states have amended their abortion laws by extending the indications for therapeutic termination of pregnancy as indicated in the accompanying table.

The new abortion act in Great Britain (1967) is potentially the most permissive of all recently enacted statutes. It contains two significant clauses in respect to the ascertainment of health of the mother.

a) Account be taken of the pregnant woman's actual or reasonably foreseeable environment.

b) Account be taken not only of the effect of pregnancy on the mother but on any existing children of her family.

If liberally construed, the current British abortion law could amount to virtual unrestricted abortion.

The report of Governor Nelson A. Rockefeller's special commission to review the New York State abortion law was published in March 1968. The recommendations follow the Model Penal Code, but add two additional indications for abortion as follows:

a) The pregnancy commenced while the female was unmarried and under 16 years of age, and is still unmarried.

b) When the female already has four living children.

The principal arguments in favor of a more permissive abortion statute have been summarized by the governor's special commission as follows:

1) The deaths, sterility and harmed physical and mental health, resulting from the large number of illegal abortions each year, could largely be prevented if such abortions were performed by competent physicians in proper hospital surroundings, within the framework of reasonable legislation.

2) The wide disparity between the statutory law and actual practice encourages disrespect for the law and places upon the conscientious physician an intolerable conflict between his medical duty to his patients and his duty as a citizen to uphold the law.

3) The present law places an unfair discrimination on the poor. Persons with money may obtain safe abortions either by travelling to other jurisdictions, by going to high-priced, competent though illegal abortionists, or by obtaining legal abortion here based on "sophisticated" psychiatric indications.

The divergence between the literal interpretation of the law and current medical practice has led today's physician into an area of grave legal risk. There are indications that the courts may take action when reputable medical practice in accredited hospitals does not conform to strict interpretation of rigid abortion laws.

In 1969 there were two court decisions of major importance in this field. On September 5 the California Supreme Court in the case of People v. Belous declared the pre-1967 California abortion law unconstitutional on the following grounds:

1) The phrase "necessary to preserve life" is vague;

2) "The fundamental right of the woman to chose whether to bear children" is a right of privacy which the statute abridges;

3) The statute violates the Fourteenth Amendment because of the "delegation of decision making power to a directly involved individual," (i.e., the doctor might be penalized for approving a request for abortion but not for denying a request).

In November a decision in the United States District Court for the District of Columbia declared unconstitutional that part of the statute that outlawed abortions other than those done "for the preservation of the mother's life or health." The reasoning was similar to and in part relied upon that in the Belous decision.

At present the New York law is being challenged in the Federal Court for the Southern District of New York. The complaint in the case alleges that the abortion law is unconstitutional on grounds approximately similar to those cited in the California case.

In view of these circumstances, the New York Academy of Medicine recommends repeal of those sections of the criminal code referable to the performance of abortion by qualified physicians and further supports the legal changes that would place abortion under the general provisions of the medical-practices act of the various states.

REFERENCES

1. American Law Institute. Model Penal Code, Sec. 230, 3, 1962.
2. Committee on Human Reproduction, American Medical Association. A.M.A. policy on therapeutic abortion. *J.A.M.A.* *201*:544, 1967.
3. American Public Health Association resolution on therapeutic abortion. Editorial. *Amer. J. Public Health 59*:155, 1969.
4. British Abortion Act, 1967. Elizabeth II, chap. 87. London, Her Majesty's Stat. Off., 1967.
5. *Pioneering in Public Health for Fifty Years.* Committee on Public Health, the New York Academy of Medicine, pp. 108-10, 1961.
6. Report of the Governor's Commission to Review New York State Abortion Law. Hon. Charles Froessel, chairman, 1968.
7. Resolution 69-96. Criteria for revision of abortion laws introduced by the Medical Society of the County of New York. *N. Y. J. Med. 69*:1660, 1969.
8. State laws:
Arkansas, 1969; HB 189. An Act to Define Abortion.
California, 1967; Calif. Laws C 327, chap. 2.
Colorado, 1967; Col. Laws, C 190, Art. 2, chap. 40, Colorado Revised Statute 1963, as amended 1967.
Delaware, 1969; chap. 17 of Title 24. Delaware Code Relating to Licensure to Practice Medicine and Surgery, the Termination of Pregnancy, etc.
Georgia, 1963; Penal Code, chap. 26-11.

Foeticide and Infanticide.
Kansas, 1969; Penal Code 31-3407. Criminal Abortion.
Maryland, 1968; Sec. 145, Art. 43. Annotated Code, 1967 Suppl.
Mississippi; Sec. 2223, Miss. Code of 1942, as amended 1966.
New Mexico; 1953; Sec. 40A-5-1 through 40-A-5-3, NMSA. An Act Relating to Abortion, etc.
North Carolina; N.C. Laws, Art. 2, chap. 14. General Statistics Relating to Abortion and Kindred Offenses.
Oregon; ORS465-110; 677.18 and 677.190. An Act Relating to Abortion, etc.

9. *Therapeutic Abortion.* Statement by the New York Academy of Medicine; prepared by the Committee on Public Health, April 1965.

LEPERS, PARIAHS, AND CHURCHES

Those who visit Norway are well advised to take the three-day tour from Oslo to Bergen. Of the wondrous scenery of mountains, ravines, valleys, and fjords, and the less conspicuous wonders of universal urban and rural electrification, no mention need be made in this brief note. Instead, attention is invited to an unusual antique product of human culture.

In mountainous central Norway on the road between Fagernes and Laerdal stands the "stave church" of Borgund[1] (see figure). As the name suggests, the structure is supported by wooden pillars; indeed, the entire structure is wooden, including the floors, the windowless walls, and the steep gabled roofs which rise tier upon tier to a spindlelike steeple. These tiered gables and their shingles combine to make a singularly distinctive impression, which gains additional force from the weird wooden dragon heads that stretch forward from the higher gable ends.

One of the side doors of the church was reserved for lepers. This portal leads to a small and partly secluded indoor area where lepers were obliged to remain if they wished to attend services.

The Borgund edifice is dated at approximately 1150 A.D. Of the 1,300 churches estimated to have been in existence in Norway as late as 1300 A.D.,[2] about two thirds were stave churches. Approximately 25 are still extant, in most instances with the help of restoration.

The presence of a leper's portal in Borgund church reminds us that leprosy attained high incidence and wide dissemination in Europe during the Middle Ages. While it is safe to assume that other diseases such as psoriasis were sometimes mistaken for leprosy, the high incidence of true leprosy in the Middle Ages is well established and recently has gained additional support from archaeological and paleopathological investigations in Scandinavia.[3]

The decline and virtual disappearance of the disease in Europe has been attributed partly to an improvement in general hygiene and nutrition and partly to the special restrictions that were imposed on lepers.[4] Often lepers were isolated in special institutions, which traditionally were placed under the patronage of Saint George (in Scandinavia, St. Jørgen). When permitted to be at large they were obliged to wear

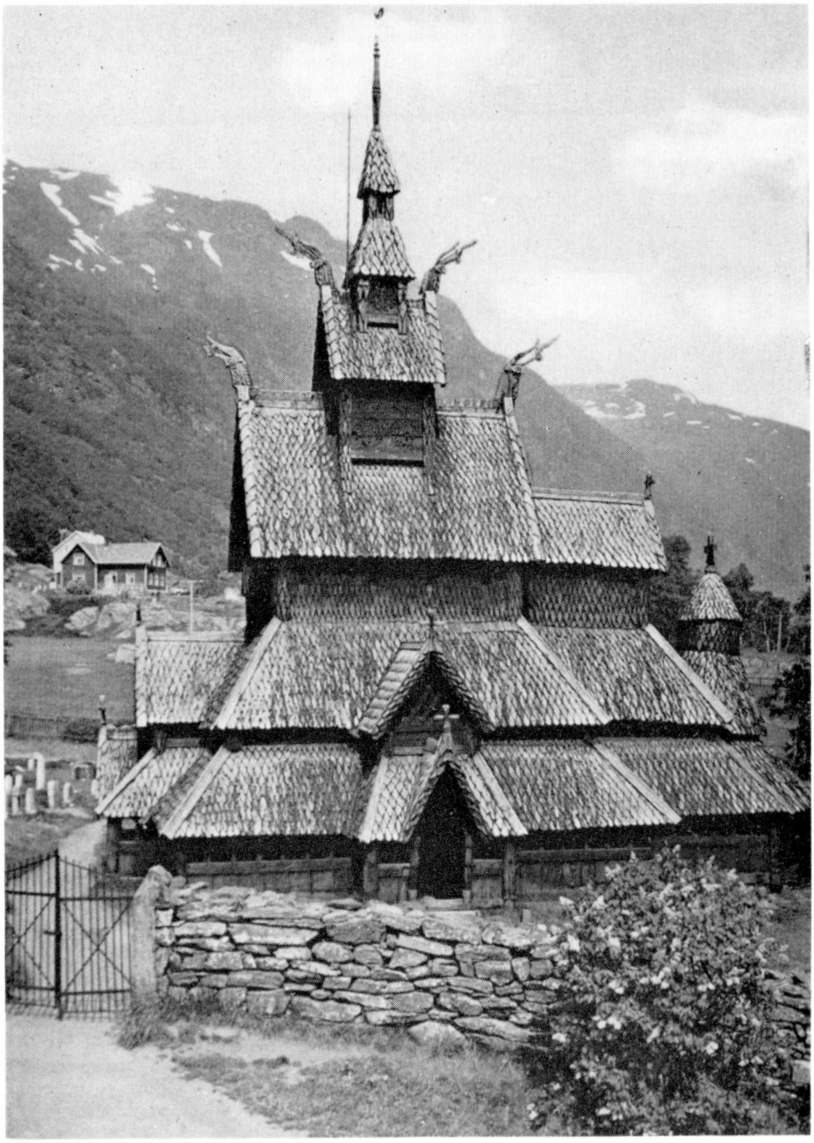

The stave church at Borgund, Norway. The doorway at center of foreground was reserved for lepers. Photograph by courtesy of Normanns Kunstforlag A/S, Oslo, Norway.

distinctive clothing, to carry bells or clappers,[5] and to avoid contact with other persons, especially children.

Where they were permitted to come to churches, they were obliged —as at Borgund—to use special entrances, and to remain within specially designated parts of the edifice. In some places they might view the services through special holes known as *leper squints* or *leper holes.* In some districts, especially in parts of France, they were regarded as officially dead; the service for the dead was read over them and earth was thrown at their feet.

Restrictions of this type were not limited to lepers. Until recent times there existed in France, especially in the southwestern part of the country, a class of pariahs known as *cagots*, or *cacous*, or *gahets.*[6] These persons are variously regarded as having been sufferers from attenuated leprosy or as descendants of lepers. Another possibility, which I have not found adequately discussed in the literature, is that they were bearers of anomalous genetic traits which produced conspicuous malformations of the face and limbs.[7]

Whatever the nature and origin of their abnormality, the *cagots* were subjected to a wide range of restrictions. They were obliged to live in isolated areas; they wore distinctive clothing; they were limited to a small number of occupations, chiefly carpentry; they were often mocked and insulted, and were sometimes accused of sorcery.

Like lepers, they had special doorways reserved for their use in churches. If they entered the church they were compelled to stay within an area specially designated for them. Often they had their own holy-water fonts, which were attached outside the churches.[8]

The leper's doorway and the outdoor font of the *cagot* may be regarded as architectural evidences of man's attempts to limit the spread of disease. The cruelty that accompanied these preventive measures expresses a human trait more resistant and more persistent than leprosy.

S. J.

NOTES AND REFERENCES

1. Borgund is situated approximately at 61° N, 8° E.
2. United Nations Educational and Cultural Organization (UNESCO): *Norway; Paintings from the Stave Churches.* With preface by R. Hauglid and introd. by L. Grodecki. New York, New York Graphic Society, 1955, p. 5. Photographs and plans of the Borgund church are in A. Bugge, *Norwegian Stave Churches.* Transl. by Ragnar Christophersen. Oslo, Dreyer, 1953.
3. Møller-Christensen, V.: New knowledge of leprosy through paleopathology. *Int. J. Leprosy 33*:603-10, 1965.
4. For details see Danielssen, D. C. and Boeck, W.: *Traité de la Spédalskhed.* Paris, Baillière, 1848, pp. 120 ff.
5. A leper's clapper is included among the collections of the Library of the New York Academy of Medicine.
6. Fay, H. M.: *Histoire de la Lèpre en France; Lépreux et Cagots du Sud-Ouest.* Paris, Champion, 1910. See also review of this book by W. Dubreuilh in *Lepra 9*:160-62, 1910. See also P. Delaunay: Le Cagots du Sud-Ouest, *La France Médicale 57*:161-63, 1910.
7. Here is an excellent subject for paleopathologic investigation.
8. Photographs will be found in Fay, *op. cit.*, pp. 576-77.

LORD BRYCE ON INTELLECTUAL PRODUCTIVITY

THOSE who have discussed the conditions of intellectual productivity have often remarked that epochs of stir and excitement are favorable, because they stimulate men's minds, setting new ideas afloat and awakening new ambitions. It is also true that vigorous, unremitting labor is, speaking generally, needed for the production of good work, and that one is therefore less entitled to expect it in an indolent time and from members of the luxurious classes. But it is not less true, though less frequently observed, that tranquillity and repose are necessary to men of the kind we are considering, and often helpful even to the highest geniuses, for the evolving of new thoughts and the creation of forms of finished and harmonious beauty. He who is to do such work must have time to meditate, and pause, and meditate again. He must be able to set his creation aside, and return to it after days or weeks to look at it with fresh eyes. He must be neither distracted from his main purpose, nor hurried in effecting it. He must be able to concentrate the whole force of his reason or imagination on one subject, to abstract himself when needful from the flitting sights and many-voiced clamor of the outer world. Juvenal said this long ago about the poet; it also applies, though possibly in a lower degree, both to the artist and to the serious thinker or delicate workman in any field of literature, to the metaphysician, the theologian, the philosophic historian, the economist, the philologist, even the novelist and the statesman. I have heard men who had gone from a quiet life into politics complain that they found their thinking powers wither, and that while they became far more expert in getting up subjects and speaking forcibly and plausibly, they found it harder and harder to form sound general views and penetrate beneath the superficialities of the newspaper and the platform. Interrupted thought, trains of reflection or imaginative conceptions constantly broken by a variety of petty, transient calls of business, claims of society, matters passing in the world to note and think of, not only tire the mind, but destroy its chances of attaining just and deep views of life and nature, as a wind-ruffled pool ceases to reflect the rocks and woods around it. Mohammed falling into trances on the mountain above Mecca, Dante in the sylvan solitudes of Fonte Avellana, Cervantes and Bunyan in the enforced seclusion of a prison, Hegel so rapt and lost in his speculations that, taking his manuscript to the publisher in Jena on the day of the great battle, he was surprised to see French soldiers in the streets: these are types of the men and conditions which give birth to thoughts that occupy succeeding generations; and what is true of these greatest men is perhaps even more true of men of the next rank. Doubtless many great works have been produced among inauspicious surroundings, and even under severe pressure of time; but it will, I think, be almost invariably found that the producer had formed his ideas or conceived his creations in hours of comparative tranquillity, and had turned on them the full stream of his powers, to the exclusion of whatever could break or divert its force.

In Europe men call this a century of unrest. But the United States is more unrestful than Europe, more unrestful than any country we know of has yet been. Nearly every one is busy; those few who have not to earn their living, and do not feel called to serve their countrymen, find themselves out of place, and have been wont either to make amusement into a business, or to transfer themselves to the ease of France or Italy. The earning of one's living is not, indeed, incompatible with intellectually creative work, for many of those who have done such work best have done it in addition to their gainful occupation, or have earned their living by it. But in America it is unusually hard for any one to withdraw his mind from the endless variety of external impressions and interests which daily life presents, and which impinge upon the mind, I will not say to vex it, but to keep it constantly vibrating to their touch. Life is that of the squirrel in his revolving cage, never still even when it does not seem to change. It becomes every day more and more so in England, and English literature and art show increasing marks of haste. In the United States the ceaseless stir and movement, the constant presence of newspapers, the eagerness which looks through every pair of eyes, even that active intelligence and sense of public duty, strongest in the best minds, which make a citizen feel that he ought to know what is passing in the wider world as well as in his own,—all these render life more exciting to the average man than it is in Europe, but chase away from it the opportunities for repose and meditation which art and philosophy need, as growing plants need the coolness and darkness of night no less than the blaze of day. The type of mind which American conditions have evolved is quick, vigorous, practical, versatile; but it is unfavorable to the natural germination and slow ripening of large and luminous ideas, it wants the patience that will spend weeks or months in bringing details to an exquisite perfection. . . .

Bryce, J.: *Social Institutions of the United States.* New York, Chatauqua Press, 1891, pp. 176-79.

THE CONDITION OF AGRICULTURAL LABORERS IN ENGLAND

I HAVE no disposition to obtrude my opinion, in any form, so as to give offence. Indeed, it has always seemed to me unreasonable in any case, or on any subject, that the honest opinions of any man should be the occasion of offence, as though we had the same control of our opinions as we have of our limbs; as though we should have any other object, in any matter, but the attainment of truth; and as if there were any way of attaining truth but the utmost freedom of discussion; and, above all, as though men should, under any circumstances, feel at liberty to exercise the same tyranny over the mind which physical force and political stratagem give them over the person.

One cannot help seeing that wealth and prosperity are not always coincident; that wealth is not therefore the infallible index of prosperity. In many cases,—and perhaps it may only be rendered more striking from contrast,—the extraordinary accumulations of wealth on one side are followed by a corresponding depression on the other; while the rich are made richer, in the same proportion the poor are made poorer. As wealth increases, avarice is more powerfully stimulated, and labor more severely taxed. In the richest communities, the price of labor is always the most depressed; and with the increase of luxury the desire of indulgence is quickened with all classes: what might properly be termed luxuries and superfluities become absolute necessaries of life, and the expenses of living are proportionally increased to all. We may deplore such results, and deem it easy to suggest a remedy; but what remedy is of general or of practical application? The more artificial the state of society becomes, the more difficult it becomes to provide the means of living; and yet who would return to the state of nature, or abate one tittle in the actual refinements of life? Communities are growing up among us upon the principles of perfect equality of rank, the equal combination of labor, and an entire community of goods; and there are examples, where such communities, bound together by a strong religious tie, and subject to a most despotic government within themselves, have been maintained, and are still flourishing. But without this religious tie, or some strong personal and pecuniary interest, and without an absolute head, does any sober man dream that such communities can be sustained, excepting within the narrowest limits? or that such principles can be applied, to any great extent, to society at large, without an entire change in the whole structure of society, and, I may almost add, an entire renovation of human nature itself? Far be it from me, however, to suggest that the evils of society are without a remedy, or at least beyond alleviation. Our own country, under a free constitution of government, and with an almost unlimited extent of the most fertile territory, accessible upon the easiest terms, presents, perhaps, the most favorable condition, which has been known, for a security of the rights of labor, and the just fruition of its products; but it would be a great injustice to infer that there are not to be found in England many generous and just persons, devoted to the maintenance of the rights, and the welfare and improvement, of the humble and laborious classes. There cannot be a doubt, that, in a noiseless and unobtrusive way, much is, and infinitely more can be, done for these objects; and the aim of every good man, as far as he has any power, should be to diffuse, to the greatest extent possible, the means of subsistence and comfort to all, and to remove every impediment to the most equal distribution of the products of labor among those whose labor in their production gives them certainly a fair claim upon these products. Now, whether it be by large farms or by small allotments, by plough or by spade husbandry, that mode of husbandry by which the largest amount of product, and at the least expense, can be drawn from the soil, and with the least injury to its productive powers, is to be preferred. This great point is not yet ascertained; and its determination must necessarily be different in different places and conditions. But it is with England a question of tremendous importance, what is to become of the vast accumulations of people, which are continually increasing here at the rate of from seven hundred to a thousand per day. It is impossible to become accurately, though it may be slightly, acquainted with the condition of things in England, the actual suffering for a want of the means of subsistence, which prevails among large portions of the population, especially in some of the agricultural districts, and not to feel that there are powerful elements of disease at work in the social body, whose disastrous effects must presently be felt in all their violence. Men with families dependent upon their labor, earning not more than 7 s., and in some instances even less, per week, and often times with only occasional employment at that rate, present objects of deep interest to a philanthropic mind. Men living themselves upon a single meal per day, and that potatoes only, for the sake of keeping a wife and children from absolute starvation,—and there is ample evidence that such cases exist,—present a sad spectacle. What are the remedies for such a condition of things, if remedies there are to be found, it is not within my province, in this case, to discuss. It is a hard lot, where the most severe and unremitted labor will not avail to procure a subsistence for one's self and family, and where, with immense tracts of uncultivated land, the opportunity even of exerting this labor, however cheerfully it might be rendered, is, for any cause whatever, refused or prevented.

The subject, it appears to me,—and perhaps wholly from my being unaccustomed to a condition of things in any degree resembling it,—is daily assuming a fearful aspect; I do not mean of danger to the government,—for the government of the country seems never to have been stronger,—but fearful in its bearings upon the public peace, the public morals, the security of property, and the state of crime. . . .

Colman, H.: *European Agriculture and Rural Economy, from Personal Observation*, vol. 1, part 2, pp. 133-35. Boston, Phelps, 1844-1847.

Over 5 million prescriptions already filled at Macy*s

All 13 M*acy* P*rescription* C*entres*
satisfy your patients with efficient professional service

- You may phone in your patients' prescriptions (except for narcotics, amphetamines, and barbiturates).
- Your patients may charge their prescriptions on their Macy Shopping Accounts or C-T Plans.
- Your patients may have their prescriptions delivered anywhere free of extra charge.
- We serve your patient with a full line of convalescent and diabetic needs.

Macy's Herald Square, OX 5-4400
Macy's Parkchester, TA 8-7000
Macy's Jamaica, OL 7-9000
Macy's Flatbush, UL 6-5000
Macy's Roosevelt Field, PI 6-8200
Macy's Huntington, AR 1-3000
Macy's White Plains, WH 6-5015
Macy's New Haven, Conn. 624-9271
Macy's Bay Shore, MO 5-8400
Macy's Queens, AR 1-9100
Macy's Colonie, 459-1950
Macy's New Rochelle, 633-7700
Macy's Smith Haven, 724-4900

Not Just "Milk" But . . .

WALKER-GORDON CERTIFIED MILKS

There are many reasons why thousands of discriminating families have been raised from infancy on Walker-Gordon Certified Milks. Among the reasons:

- *Super-Sanitary Production Methods.* From cow to bottle, milk is never exposed to air or human touch.
- *Cleanest.* Lowest bacteria count. Laboratory on the farm.
- *Freshest.* Bottled immediately after milking, usually delivered the following day. Keeps for weeks under normal refrigeration.
- *Uniform.* No variance in flavor or nutritional value, 365 days a year.

Guaranteed Free of Antibiotic Residue

Certified Milks available through Leading Milk Dealers: Raw, Homogenized-Vitamin D, Skimmed, Fresh Lo-Sodium. *Write for complete information.*

WALKER-GORDON CERTIFIED MILK FARM

Plainsboro, N.J. ***(Code 609) 799-1234***

NEW YORK: 212 WAlker 5-7464 ★ PHILA.: 215 MArket 7-6338

BULLETIN OF
THE NEW YORK ACADEMY
OF MEDICINE

VOL. 46, NO. 5 MAY 1970

SYMPOSIUM ON MEDICINE AND DIPLOMACY IN THE TROPICS

Opening Statement*

THE HONORABLE ANGIE BROOKS

President, The General Assembly of The United Nations

I am delighted to open officially this *Symposium on Medicine and Diplomacy in the Tropics,* for I have always felt that medicine, like music, is a universal language. The healing arts permit and promote international understanding—and international understanding is the way to international peace and security.

Medicine as a universal language knows no boundaries of race, religion, or sex but operates in the interest of all humanity. Dr. Kevin M. Cahill, who knows so well our needs in Africa, has called attention to medicine as an untapped resource in diplomacy. We in the tropics, the developing nations, have great need for medical assistance and we ask your help. Those with respect and love for the human family will not want the benefits of health restricted to a particular geographical area, and efforts such as yours today should assure a better future for all mankind.

On behalf of the United Nations I wish you all success.

---

*Presented as part of a *Symposium on Medicine and Diplomacy in the Tropics* sponsored by The Tropical Disease Center, St. Clare's Hospital, New York, N. Y., and The Merck Company Foundation, Rahway, N. J., held at the Center, December 13, 1969.

SYMPOSIUM ON MEDICINE AND DIPLOMACY IN THE TROPICS

Introduction*

KEVIN M. CAHILL

Director
The Tropical Disease Center
St. Clare's Hospital

Associate Professor of Clinical Medicine
New York Medical College

New York, N. Y.

MEDICINE is one of the last, and certainly the finest, untapped resources of international diplomacy.

This conference began more than five years ago when the concept that the developed nations could profitably incorporate medicine to a greater extent in their endeavor to communicate with the developing world was propounded.† This sentiment has strengthened to a conviction, and from my own continued experience with the newly independent nations of Africa I feel that such a course is inevitable in the 1970's.

In the United States our leaders must obviously seek alternative methods of providing assistance to and promoting areas of cooperation and communication with the developing world. As the financial resources for overseas aid programs are diminished annually by Congress, expensive and often unsuccessful projects such as providing airports and major dock facilities or underwriting the cost of entire armies will become as unfeasible as they have been unsuccessful. Few areas of overseas aid are immune to the sensitivities and misinterpretations of recipient nations. Few forms of aid can be offered with the assurance that both donor and recipient countries will experience the dramatic impact of immediate benefit, as well as the long-term effect of hard-won mutual respect. Few aid projects can be completed with the assurance that later political changes will not confuse or diminish the good that is done. Medicine is such a field, especially in the developing

*Presented as part of a *Symposium on Medicine and Diplomacy in the Tropics* sponsored by The Tropical Disease Center, St. Clare's Hospital, New York, N. Y., and The Merck Company Foundation, Rahway, N. J., held at the Center, December 13, 1969.

†Cahill, K. M.: Medicine and diplomacy in the tropics. *N.Y.J.Med. 67*:2229, 1967.

nations where infectious diseases and epidemics remain the great scourges

Medicine, in a relatively inexpensive manner, can alter or even save the future of a newly independent nation on the verge of chaos and collapse. Further, physicians and medical workers have the unique opportunity and privilege of entering far more rapidly than in any other profession into the closed and often suspicious inner political circles and power structures of developing lands. Needless to say, this privilege brings responsibility. If a program of medical aid is to be incorporated into a diplomatic effort it must be entrusted to extremely sensitive physicians who know not only the realms of their own profession but are attuned to the limitations of diplomatic intercourse and who have courage to bridge the transient differences that separate nations. There will be difficulties in the marriage of medicine and diplomacy, but I see no alternative if we, as one representative of the developed world, still care about the needy in many other parts of the globe. Medicine must inevitably be recognized as a necessary bridge, not merely to serve the health needs of the developing world, but to link those of widely divergent political and philosophic views to one another.

Some of the problems in joining medicine and diplomacy are pointed out by Dr. John Badeau, former ambassador of the United States to the United Arab Republic and currently director of the Middle East Institute at Columbia University. During more than a quarter of a century in the turbulent world of the Middle East, Dr. Badeau as a foundation worker, university president, and finally ambassador, has sought and thought deeply about possible links between nations and how these could be forged into a viable chain. The use of medicine as a link is not new but its significance has been poorly appreciated and inadequately supported in recent years. Dr. Badeau's thorough review of the philosophic basis for incorporating medicine with diplomacy is completed by a suggestion that we consider the establishment of a completely new administrative channel to permit overseas medical activity to function untainted by politics.

Ambassador Abdulrahim Abby Farah of Somalia, a nation on the eastern tip of Africa, whose medical needs are poignantly detailed in his address, represents the developing world at this conference. In his capacity as chairman of the Special Political Committee of the United

Nations' 20th Session, he had the opportunity of traveling extensively throughout the tropics. His descriptions of medical problems and goals can be applied to many other areas outside Somalia. For the past 25 years, the Most Reverend Edward Swanstrom has been director of the largest American voluntary agency that provides overseas aid. The change from merely distributing surplus food to the incorporation of nutritional supplements with self-help programs and with preschool health projects provides one example of medical-diplomatic efforts at a nongovernmental level. Such is the basis of the diplomacy of persuasion.

Congressman Hugh L. Carey has served for more than 10 years on the Subcommittee on Health, Education, and Welfare of the Appropriations Committee of the House of Representatives and, as chairman of the Subcommittee on Micronesia, has had ample opportunity to consider carefully the health problems in one tropical area. His presentation is a clarion call to our government to consider alternative methods for overseas aid, and he provides specific recommendations as to how this might be done.

Dr. Gustav Dammin's involvement in the tropics goes back to World War II. He is very well qualified to discuss America's research commitment overseas. As president of the Armed Forces Epidemiological Board and as a member of the Board of Directors of the Gorgas Memorial Laboratory, he is intimately acquainted with most of the military, governmental, and private university research activities overseas. His review of the extent of America's international research commitment, with its relatively minuscule proportion of our total research budget, and the decrease in even this amount since the days of the early Kennedy Administration, is a definitive, though somewhat depressing review.

Finally, Dr. George Lythcott's reflections, based on seven years in West Africa both as associate director of the National Institutes of Health program in Ghana and as field director of the highly successful Smallpox Eradication Program, abound with the common sense born of experience, and the call, "if we care," in his peroration, born of hope.

It is our hope that the views expressed in this conference will provide the basis for planning an alternative approach in foreign aid for the 1970's, and will serve to link nations together through medicine.

DIPLOMACY AND MEDICINE*

JOHN S. BADEAU

Director
The Middle East Institute
Columbia University
New York, N. Y.

To place medicine and diplomacy in the same equation is neither new nor novel. The diplomatic records of ancient Egypt tell us that about 29 centuries ago the famous physician-priests of the Nile Valley sometimes accompanied Egyptian missions to neighboring countries and sometimes acted as ambassadors. We find that millennia later during the Crusades Arab doctors played a part in the contacts between Saladin and his Frankish opponents. On more than one occasion the Christian leaders appealed to their Arab foe for Muslim physicians, whose skill was superior to anything Europe then knew. Contemporary accounts from this period do not record a high level of medical skill on the part of the Frankish practitioners. One Arab doctor tells of being called to treat the ulcerous leg of a Christian knight—which he did with unguents and poultices. The Christian doctor who watched the process was then invited to give his prescription. This consisted of having the camp executioner chop off the affected limb since, said the doctor, "Cases like this are hopeless and I don't know how to cure him."

This ancient although incidental connection between medicine and diplomacy reflects the fact that health (even more than wealth) is a common and prized goal. Political allies sought not only financial and military assistance from their neighbors but also the services of healing when these were available. Moreover, medicine has often been one of the first professions to emerge in a society; hence doctors were an early part of the intellectual elite. It was natural that some of them should be called upon to serve their governments in capacities other than that of their profession. I was interested to note that during my term at the American embassy in Cairo the diplomatic corps had a number of

*Presented as part of a *Symposium on Medicine and Diplomacy in the Tropics* sponsored by The Tropical Disease Center, St. Clare's Hospital, New York, N. Y., and The Merck Company Foundation, Rahway, N. J., held at the Center, December 13, 1969.

doctors in it—including, notably, some from African and South American countries.

It is not this ancient and simple connection between the doctor and the diplomat which concerns this conference. The question is more complex: do current international relations offer a special challenge to medical and health services? We are really asking whether there is a new diplomacy which creates a new role for the medical profession—or whether there may be a new profession of health care which has a unique contribution to make to current diplomacy.

In what sense is there a new diplomacy today? If we go back to the classical age of foreign affairs (roughly from the Congress of Vienna to the end of World War I) we find that diplomacy was a limited operation carried on under generally accepted rules by recognized professionals. It was said that foreign policy was like an orchestra—a harmony produced by the interchange of notes among highly skilled professional artists. This meant that the conduct of foreign affairs was in the hands of a restricted group that staffed the foreign offices of the world. It was among this corps of professional diplomats that most of the discussions of international politics went on, usually behind the hushed doors of foreign offices. Thus at the Congress of Vienna the professional diplomats of Europe met for an extended discussion on the problems created by the collapse of Napoleon's empire, to emerge finally from their seclusion with a series of agreements which set the pattern of international relations in Europe for the next 50 years.

This state of affairs began to change shortly after World War I. A number of elements entered the world scene which made it inevitable that diplomacy should take on new characteristics. One of these was the rapid expansion of public communication through the cable, press and, later, radio and television. The rapid and wide dissemination of news about national and international affairs made it increasingly difficult for the professional diplomats to treat foreign affairs as their special preserve with the masses excluded from it. Increasingly the public became aware of, and thus interested in, national policies both domestic and foreign. Incidents between nations which in the past would have been quietly and quickly worked out between diplomats before they became public knowledge now became the immediate possession of all who could read or tune in the airwaves. One

British administrator in Africa told me how this had complicated the task of diplomacy. "Before the war," he said, "when there was a border incident I would get in touch with my opposite number in the neighboring territory and we quickly worked out a solution. Only after the matter was settled did it become public knowledge. Today the most insignificant border incident is on the radio almost before it happens. By the time I get in touch with the other chap it has become a matter of national honor and patriotic dignity, from which it is difficult to find any retreat."

To the impact of widely disseminated information has been added the effects of nationalism and popular education. Decades of struggle for national independence in colonial areas taught the masses that they had a role to play in their nation's life. During the protracted campaigns for independence, crowds were organized for street demonstrations, students for protest and rioting, and every citizen was urged to support "national liberation." A voiceless and politically inert class, seldom before called upon to play a role in national affairs, suddenly discovered that it had a place in them. Having been awakened to this fact during the struggle for independence this class was unwilling to lapse into passivity once independence had been gained.

This popularization of political concern was aided by the spread of education. Traditionally the educated elite in colonial and undeveloped areas was only a minute fraction of the population. The common man had neither the opportunity nor the expectation of going to school. But with the founding of national systems of education and the resulting rapid proliferation of schools, many more people are being educated than ever before. Figures vary from country to country but, as an example, about 80% of the children of primary school age now attend school in the United Arab Republic; 20 years ago less than one third of them did so. The increase is not only absolute in terms of the number of pupils, it is also relative to the classes of society who are being educated. A different kind of person is going to school today in many emerging countries—the peasant, the laborer, the urban poor, some tribesmen—all of them typical of that elusive but ubiquitous "common man" who is the foundation of all society. Whatever the education given in school, its invariable effect is to broaden the horizons of the students and their families; this breaks down their isolation from national affairs and makes them feel they have entered the class of educated people who traditionally have guided the affairs of the nation.

As a result of these factors, diplomacy and the foreign policy with which it deals has been given a new constituency which it addresses and to which it must listen. The day when a small intellectual elite could settle the foreign policy of a country and negotiate diplomatic relations through a professional corps without reference to popular opinion is gone. In every country there is now a public opinion which must be taken into account by the diplomat. This is as true in emerging countries under authoritarian rule as in more democratic societies. Foreign affairs can no longer be the preserve of the professional; it now includes the dimension of popular interest and opinion.

This is illustrated clearly by the impact of the war in Vietnam on the conduct of American foreign policy. The United States has participated in other wars to which objections could be raised; the most recent was the Korean war, which began in 1950. Why is there so much more outcry over Vietnam? I believe it is largely because of the constant flow of radio news bulletins, the television reporting which brings the sights and sounds of war into the living room every night and to a generation of students who have been awakened to international affairs. It may be true, as Senator Hugh Scott said, that foreign policy cannot be made by the crowds in the streets and the byways, but obviously it is impossible for any administration to frame a policy for Vietnam without taking into account what is being said in the streets and byways.

Another new factor affecting the conduct of diplomacy arises from the same ease of communication which generates popular participation in national affairs. It is now possible for a chief of state to speak about foreign affairs not only to his own citizens but also to the citizens of other countries. President Richard M. Nixon on television or President Gamal Abdel Nasser in Liberation Square in Cairo are going over the heads of their own foreign officers and diplomatic corps to present policies to popular audiences and to appeal for their support. This not only increases the consciousness of the citizenry of their political role, it also may affect popular opinion in another country with which a diplomatic problem exists. There can be no doubt that part of North Vietnam's diplomacy has been to seek direct appeals to the American public for the purpose of arousing opinion in the United States against the policies of the American government. Similarly statements made by American leaders, some broadcast throughout the nation over television and some relayed abroad by satellite, are aimed at influencing public attitudes outside as well as within American borders. Diplomacy is thus no longer a matter of diplomats talking to diplomats; it often involves governments talking over the heads of their diplomats to the citizens of other countries in the hope of affecting their attitudes.

Since World War II the conduct of diplomacy has been profoundly affected by an unprecedented number of new, if small, nations. The future historian may well conclude that the most significant feature of these past decades has not been the emergence of atomic power, but the emergence into political freedom of a large segment of the world's population. Since the ending of World War II more than one billion people in about 30 countries have passed from foreign control to their own independence and sovereignty. Diplomacy today does not operate in a world composed of a few great powers around whom cluster colonies, protectorates, mandates, and spheres of interest. It must function amidst a multicentric system of political power where the majority of nations is composed of smaller states—many of them new—and where all claim the full prerogatives of their sovereignty.

Out of this situation has grown a new dimension of diplomatic activity that concerns the economic and social development of emerging states. In the past, people struggling for independence often appealed to world powers on the grounds that political freedom is an inherent human right and that the great powers had a responsibility for ensuring that this right was given to all who sought it. Thus during the Algerian struggle in the 1950's the Algerian independence movement despatched emissaries to foreign governments, including the United States, to urge that the world community owed them political freedom. This view is still widely held, but most newly independent nations have now added to it a further demand: the right to economic and social growth. Emerging nations discovered that political independence did not, as expected, solve all their problems. It was not enough to be free, it was also necessary to be progressive and prosperous. As the world owed them a debt of political freedom, so, these nations maintained, it owed a debt of economic and technical assistance.

Thus the diplomacy of the postwar period has had to respond to new demands. Even though a particular economic situation might not vitally affect the immediate interest of a great power, it was often impossible to pursue political ends without meeting some of the economic demands of the recipient country.

But it was not merely pressure from developing countries which added this dimension to postwar diplomacy. Stability, economic growth, and progress in developing areas were quickly recognized by some great powers as favorable to their own interests. Poverty, backwardness, and unfulfilled expectations could easily create both political and economic instability and set off clashes which might well imperil the peace of the world. Thus one of the two major global objectives of the United States after World War II was to support in vital areas the forces which made for political and social stability, so that the danger of "brush-fire" wars would be reduced and external radical forces would not be tempted to exacerbate domestic conflicts.

One final factor in postwar diplomacy must be noted. Although the war resulted in the emergence of two superpowers, the United States and the Soviet Union, neither of these has retained the capacity to have its way absolutely in world affairs. It might be thought that the vast armaments and political prestige of either country would make possible the enforcement of almost any foreign policy desired if important enough. Yet this has not proved to be the case. The proliferation of independent states with the status in world affairs given them by membership in the United Nations has circumscribed the direct influence of the great powers. It was not difficult for a major power to control and direct the policies of its colonies, protectorates, spheres of influence, and clients in the old imperial days: but today these same areas, now fiercely independent and proudly sovereign, do not easily come to heel. The very extent of military force available to either superpower has militated against its use for diplomatic ends. The continued balance of terror between the Western and the Communist blocs is such that neither side can use its weapons to maintain diplomatic pressure on other nations. Both the East European clients of the U. S. S. R. and America's partners in Europe and Asia have been able to pursue freer foreign policies because of this situation.

This means that diplomacy today must more often use a diplomacy of persuasion rather than a diplomacy of pressure. Both American and Soviet attempts to order their alleged clients around have not proved very successful, as the continued stalemate between Israel and some of the Arab states clearly shows. Unless a diplomatic problem affects its most vital national interests, a great power must depend upon its ability to persuade another power to accept a mutually satisfactory course of action. This means that common interests and shared objectives become central to diplomatic practice.

From this brief description emerges the picture of a new diplomacy closely related to the popular mind in emerging countries, based upon shared interests and expressing itself in economic and technical as well as in political terms. Foreign aid and technical assistance have become a large part of foreign policy in the postwar years. Subsidies, grants, loans, and limited technical services have long played a role in the relations between nations, but never before have there been such comprehensive, massive, and sustained programs of aid as during the past two decades. Beginning with the Marshall Plan, Western and Communist nations have made foreign aid a substantial and vital part of their policies. In some relations between countries these programs have been the major instrument of diplomacy; they may account for the largest expenditure of funds, the most numerous personnel, and the most frequent contacts with the host governments.

It is at once obvious that it is in this field of diplomacy—i.e., technical and developmental aid—that the services of health and healing have an opportunity to play a significant role. Every emerging country is challenged by its own independence to provide better health for its citizens. One of the first steps of modernization is usually the establishment of government-directed health services, in the fields of preventive and curative medicine both. The demand for such services comes not only from the government but equally from the common people. Go into even the most remote villages of the Middle East and ask: "What do you want?" and the answer usually will be: "A doctor and a school."

This being true, health programs would seem to meet some of the needs of the new diplomacy in almost ideal fashion. Since health is desired and readily understood by the common man, any foreign contribution to public health would immediately be recognized as valuable by the recipient. Long-range technical programs of development may be essential for building the economic strength of a new country, but often they take years to mature and are not quickly recognized by those they are designed to serve.

Moreover, health is one of the basic, universal human interests—the kind of "shared concern" for which the diplomat is often searching. The utility of and the need for health does not require argument either in a giving or a receiving country, and contributions of assistance in the health field are immediately apprehended and eagerly sought. One sign of this is the fact that in the United Arab Republic the Naval Medical Research Unit (NAMRU) was quickly reestablished after the Six Day War and is operating today—even though political and diplomatic relations between Egypt and the United States remain broken.

But the contribution of medicine and health is not simply one of charity and compassion, represented at its best by the missionary hospital and doctor who have contributed so much to the emerging world. New governments and emerging countries want to establish their own health services, and the problem is how to render assistance in this field with the primary object of developing the capability of the receiving government to operate its own health program. It is comparatively simple for a foreign doctor to go into another country, open a clinic or hospital, and personally attack the problems of ill-health and disease. It is much more difficult and complicated to refrain from doing this in the interest of helping national doctors, hospitals, and clinics to perform the work. Yet this should be the goal of true technical and medical assistance.

It might be concluded from all this that every embassy ought to have a medical staff attached to it and that every American aid program should include a technical-assistance team working in the field of public health. Yet this is highly questionable. Although the contribution of health obviously is important and useful, it is a particularly difficult one to make within the limitations of a diplomatic mission.

There are several reasons for this. One is that programs of assistance closely tied to diplomacy cannot escape the pressures of political objectives. Congress does not make appropriations for programs of aid out of the goodness of its heart—or as one Congressman put it—"United States aid programs are not meant to play Santa Claus." While there is a genuine interest in economic and social development, appropriations are scrutinized increasingly by legislators with a view to winning host governments to the acceptance of American policy.

The use of aid for political ends is always resented by those who receive it, but it is particularly resented when that aid deals with such basic human needs as food and health. Our experience with the Food for Peace program in the United Arab Republic was that any alteration in that program which appeared to be dictated by political ends brought an immediate outcry from Egyptians: "You are using the threat of starvation to coerce us." This is equally true in the field of health. Given current attitudes in Congress and the virtual certainty that aid programs will expand or contract in proportion to their success in securing support for the United States, to tie the services of health closely to the diplomatic mission might be disastrous.

Undersecretary of State Nicholas deB. Katzenbach recognized this when he said: "Aid can be a liability as well as an asset to bilateral relations. These countries strongly resent the use of aid for purposes they consider extraneous to the aid relationship; namely, as a lever to compel conformity to our foreign policy."

How then can health services be used in the relations between two countries, yet remain insulated from the impact of political diplomacy? In some cases, where we are working with allies with whom we have few political problems it is possible to place health programs under the general direction of aid operations. Yet often such programs are in areas which need these services least and where their usefulness as an international bond is greatest. I suggest that what is needed is a more complete separation between that assistance which deals with basic human needs—health, education, and food—and other types of economic and technical assistance. This could be accomplished best by a private professional organization responsible for furthering health programs abroad yet financed in large measure by grants from the United States government.

An example of this type of administration (rare in the United States) is the British Council, which for long has played an important role in bringing British culture to emerging nations. The British Council is financed by grants by Parliament, but is itself a nongovernmental agency conducted by professional specialists who are responsible for defining and conducting its program. While the council represents British influence and serves the general cause of Anglo-foreign understanding it has been remarkably free from the accusation of serving immediate political or diplomatic ends.

I suggest that the contributions of medicine to the needs of developing countries could best be made under some such form as the British Council. The initial leadership would have to come from the ranks of the medical and health professions rather than from the United States government, but a sustained concern and the formation of a private organization seeking government support might succeed. Some private American universities abroad have received government funds, especially from counterpart monies, and it is not impossible that health programs cast in a similar relation could win support. Certainly we should not allow either the current temper of Congress or the difficulties in depoliticizing aid programs to deter us from pressing for a larger role for medicine in the relations of the United States with other countries.

In the last analysis, the success of the affluent Western world in dealing with the emerging areas will not be determined by military might or diplomatic pressure. It will come from the success of the developed countries in identifying themselves with the urgent problems of new nations by contributing to their solutions. This is true of the Soviet-American rivalry in the Middle East as well as elsewhere. Surely we must press for a new and imaginative approach to the use of health services as we seek this long-range goal.

HEALTH PROBLEMS AND GOALS OF A RECIPIENT NATION*

ABDULRAHIM ABBY FARAH

Permanent Representative of Somalia to the United Nations
New York, N. Y.

MANY African states today are in the midst of a process of transformation as traditional ways of living meet the challenges involved in contact with technologically advanced societies. If it were desirable to ignore this challenge, the radio, jet plane, and television have made it impossible to do so. The emergence of African states to political independence itself demands, as they take their places in the family of nations, that they embark on a course of modernization aimed at reducing, as rapidly as possible, the economic inequality of their societies vis-a-vis those societies where technological and scientific knowledge have ensured a higher standard of living.

It is right that people in Africa, as elsewhere, should want to achieve material progress, but tremendous problems have been created by increasing demands from expanding populations for better services, more educational facilities, and more opportunities for jobs. Since many of the developing countries are poor—either because their resources have not yet been fully developed or because they have few natural resources—governments have to make agonizing decisions when they try to assign priorities for the long list of developmental needs. It is against this general background that the health problems and goals of a recipient nation such as my own—the Somali Democratic Republic—must be viewed.

Somalia's basic health needs are similar to those of the majority of the developing countries of Africa. First, we have most of the diseases that beset other countries as well as some which apply particularly to Africa: we need, for example, campaigns both for tuberculosis control and for the eradication of smallpox; second, we suffer from an acute shortage of doctors, nurses, and other medical personnel;

*Presented as part of a *Symposium on Medicine and Diplomacy in the Tropics* sponsored by The Tropical Disease Center, St. Clare's Hospital, New York, N. Y., and The Merck Company Foundation, Rahway, N. J., held at the Center, December 13, 1969.

third, we need assistance in the form of financial, material, or technical aid, in order to carry out the services which are necessary for maintaining good standards of health including additional hospitals and laboratories; fourth, we need to plan very carefully to ensure that the best use is made of our financial resources and that health programs will be suited to the needs of a predominantly nomadic population which adheres strongly to its cultural traditions.

A look at some of the health programs which are being carried out in Somalia by WHO and UNICEF will pinpoint our most obvious problems of disease.

A WHO malaria preeradication campaign aims, in the words of that organization, "to build up the technical, administrative and operational facilities for a full-scale malaria eradication program and, at the same time, to develop the rural health services, so that they may provide efficient collaboration in the eradication program."[1] An example of the kind of information that such preliminary surveys elicit is the discovery that the use of medicated salt—successful among the Iranian nomads—is not feasible in Somalia since the nomad herdsmen consume almost no salt.[2] Mass drug distribution has not been found to be a satisfactory approach to the eradication of malaria either, as Somali nomads scatter during the malaria transmission season. Spraying operations were carried out successfully in urban areas, but particular problems were encountered when these were applied to the nomads. In the northern region of the country an attempt to spray caravans moving to and returning from "wet" grazing areas met with little success because of the impossible task of keeping track of thousands of caravans moving over widely scattered areas and because of insufficient propagation of the scheme and the consequent lack of cooperation from the people.

The United Nations International Childrens Emergency Fund (UNICEF) is carrying out a tuberculosis-control program to test, in certain areas, a simple, practical, and effective method of preventing and treating tuberculosis, including vaccination and the examination of sputum.[3] WHO is working on a program for the eradication of smallpox and a survey of yellow fever.[4] Dr. Kevin Cahill, our distinguished chairman, has done extremely valuable work—as you are no doubt aware—in tracing the incidence of various types of diarrheal diseases in Somalia.[5] The importance of this research is underlined by the fact that such diseases account for more deaths in the "under-four" age group than any other single cause.[6]

As far as our goal to increase the supply of doctors and other medical assistants is concerned there are two important needs that have to be considered in planning for the training of medical personnel for a country like Somalia. The experience of other African countries has shown the need for a special curriculum for our students who study medicine abroad. African students are usually trained in the European tradition and it is often difficult for some of them to adjust to the fact that medicine in Africa cannot be practiced in the consulting room or operating theatre alone, but must be related to the social and community aspects of disease.

The other consideration is that recognition must be given to the special role played by local medical assistants in the total picture of medical services. In Somalia, these workers—usually males—have risen from the ranks through the level of the dresser and, because of particular economic and social conditions, have played and should continue to play a very important part in our health programs. Most of them are skilled and highly intelligent persons; they lack all but the academic background necessary for professional training and are able to perform a great part of the more routine work of doctors. Since doctors are in short supply it is extremely useful to have a cadre of assistants whose work ensures that the best use will be made of the professional talents of fully trained doctors. Our government, in consultation with WHO and UNICEF, has given priority to the training of such people, and a Health Training Institute has been set up which will instruct various categories of auxiliary personnel.

With regard to the third factor on my list of basic health needs: namely, assistance in the form of financial, material, and technical aid, successive Somali governments have welcomed and continue to welcome aid from many different countries. As a nonaligned nation we accept such offers on their merits and quite apart from any political considerations. May I add here the assurance that a change of government such as has recently taken place in our country does not signify any change in the health needs and goals of the nation which, after all, remain the same, whatever government is in power.

The question of the financial and other resources available for health programs is closely bound up with our fourth basic need: careful planning to ensure the best use of these resources. Planning for health must take several factors into account. First, priorities must be established between health and other developmental programs aimed at educating the population and raising the standard of living. Then, priorities for different types of health programs must be ranked. Next the implications of health programs which are to be introduced must be studied carefully.

The difficulty of assigning priorities between different developmental schemes becomes immediately apparent if one agrees that a sound medical program can be established only on the basis of progress in the field of education and, more fundamentally, on the basis of general economic progress. Raising the standard of education in general is a necessary step toward achieving goals for health, but attempts to educate the people will be of no avail if the standard of living is not improved. Dr. H. B. L. Russell, WHO Liaison Officer with the Economic Commission for Africa, posed the problem in this way: "No amount of talking and lecturing will persuade people on a very low economic level to adopt measures for which their social situation does not make the need clear: as the standard of living rises, so does the call for better sanitation and housing and improvements in the environment."[7]

What then is the prospect for improving the standard of living in Somalia so that benefits such as a general improvement of the health of the population may occur? The economy of the country is fundamentally a subsistence economy. Of the estimated 246,000 square miles which comprise the territory approximately 20% can be used for agricultural purposes and about 60% for grazing; the remainder is barren. More than 70% of the population are nomadic herdsmen whose lives are spent with their flocks of sheep, camels, or goats in an unrelenting search for grazing and water.

The life of the nomad is supported by his animals, which provide him with milk, meat, and transport. The sale of sheep and goat skins to local traders provide him with the simple necessities of life, and the export of the skins as the raw material for fine kid leather provides a long-established export trade. This trade has declined somewhat of late because of the introduction of synthetic leather. However, there is also a lively export trade in camels, sheep, and goats on the hoof, particularly to the Middle Eastern countries.

Agriculture, carried on in the south between the two permanent rivers—the Juba and the Webi Shabele—provides the country's most profitable export: bananas. Attempts are being made to diversify agriculture and to make a country which formerly imported all its food except meat and milk self-sufficient in staples such as grain, sugar, and rice.

Prospecting for oil has been carried on for several years without result but an exciting development has been the discovery of uranium after a United Nations survey of mineral resources. Concessions have been given to United States, Italian, and West German companies, and these firms are attempting to ascertain if mining the deposits is economically worthwhile.

One of the great drawbacks to economic, social, and health programs in Somalia is the shortage of water in our largely semiarid country. Every few years we have to proclaim certain areas as famine areas because of drought. There are two permanent rivers in the southernmost region of the country but elsewhere the people depend on boreholes, wells, and water pans for their water supply. Many of the wells and water pans become exhausted during the dry season and the consequent lack of water presents a real threat to life. When the seasonal rains fail, as they do periodically in many areas, the perennial problem takes on the proportion of a disaster. In 1969, for example, an emergency situation necessitating international relief was declared in substantial areas of the northeastern part of Somalia, where over 200,000 nomads were affected.

Scarcity is not the only problem connected with water supplies in Somalia. In the region where the two rivers lie there is the question of being able to utilize the river waters for developmental purposes. The particular hazard to be faced is the spread of parasitic diseases, in particular bilharziasis. A Food and Agriculture Organization (FAO) project to design irrigation schemes in the Shabele River Valley has been provided by the World Health Organization (WHO) with a team composed of an epidemiologist and a sanitary engineer whose task is to assess the health hazards of the project.

Again there is the problem presented by the absence of environmental sanitation and the ignorance of precautionary health measures; this means that often the water available is not safe to drink—certainly not by normally accepted hygienic standards.

This is a very brief outline of our resources but it should be sufficient to show that only with a great deal of external assistance—both financial and technical—can the necessary infrastructure for economic development be established and sustained. Assistance is presently being received from the European Economic Community (EEC), of which we are an associate member, and from a number of countries, but the needs and the problems are monumental. Take the question of developing our agricultural resources. Even if the technical personnel and capital were available for irrigation schemes (extremely costly ventures in a country which is mainly semiarid) there would still be the difficulty of persuading the proud nomad, who looks with disdain on the agriculturalist, to settle down and practice farming.

It is clear that for the foreseeable future the main pattern of life for a large proportion of the population will be that of the nomadic pastoralist and high priority must be given to development plans aimed at making his lot easier. These plans are mainly centered around the provision of more water for the nomad and his animals through the drilling of boreholes and providing treatment for animal diseases. Such treatment will make his livestock more useful to him and more suitable for export—on the hoof and in the form of skins; also, the animals will be more suitable for use in the small but growing meat-canning industry.

High priority must also be given to the difficult task of educating the nation. In Somalia this task is complicated by the fact that few settled communities exist outside the main towns. It has been estimated that 2,000,000 Somalis are on the move over this part of Africa at any one time. Providing education and other services for a largely illiterate and predominantly nomadic population is a tremendous task which calls not only for large-scale financing but also for new approaches to deal with our particular educational problems. An approach now underway is that of giving short intensive courses to the traditional holy men or *widads* who have always traveled with nomadic communities in order to teach the Koran to the young boys of the tribe. The *widads* now teach the children to read, write, and calculate, and give them some knowledge of the outside world and Somalia's relation to it. They also give talks to adults and children on land conservation, first aid, and hygiene.

But unless a boy has relatives with whom he can stay in a town where there is a school, his formal education ends with the *widads'* limited store of knowledge. With the help of United Nations Educational, Scientific, and Cultural Organization (UNESCO) surveys have been made and plans formulated for providing more educational facilities in settled communities, and for boarding schools in interior areas where nomads congregate seasonally. But a few statistics will show how far we have to go before we can arrive at an educational standard comparable to that of more advanced countries. For an estimated population of approximately 3.5 million, the enrollment of children in elementary schools is approximately 30,000; in intermediate schools, 12,000, and about 3,000 in secondary schools. Just over 1,000 Somalis are pursuing degree courses overseas.[8]

The problem of education in general—and of education in health also—is compounded by the language difficulty. The Somali Democratic Republic is composed of the former British Somaliland and the former Trusteeship Territory of Somalia administered by Italy. When it acquired independence, the country had three official languages: Arabic, English, and Italian. The common tongue—Somali—has never been written, since the question of whether it should be written in Arabic, or Latin, or in a locally devised script known as Osmania has long been a subject of contention between philologists and politicians. So children begin to learn Arabic at the elementary level; then English or Italian is added at the intermediate level.

Also, the fact that Somali is not written means that it is extremely difficult for government authorities to give even simple instructions—for example on hygiene, on agricultural methods—to the majority of the population. Our new government has promised that it will address itself promptly to the task of creating a written script for the Somali language and it is to be hoped that this great need will soon be filled.

A very useful method of communicating is by radio. In recent years Somalia has made increased use of its broadcasting services to reach the nomads. The ubiquitous transistor radio set is an ideal receiver for this purpose and has found its way into some of the nomadic hamlets. Unfortunately it is beyond the means of the majority of the people. If it were economically possible to make transistor radios available to a larger proportion of the nomadic population, this would be an important contribution to the problem of adult education.

I have dealt at some length with Somalia's economic and educational problems because obviously our health needs and goals can best be seen in relation to those problems. I have already said that in establishing priorities one must rank health needs with economic and social requirements and that one must also consider the needs for various health programs. It must be decided, for example, whether increased provision of medical treatment is more important than an intensive program of preventive and health education. Obviously there should be provision for both, but if funds are limited, it must be decided if the greater proportion of the resources available should be put into one area, or whether modest advances should be made in a number of directions.

Over-all planning for Somalia's health services is being done with the advice and technical assistance of WHO. Modest programs have been initiated with the aim of providing the most basic health requirements of each area rather than emphasizing any one area. I have already mentioned the Health Training Institute for auxiliary personnel. In addition, the nursing services are being strengthened by an improvement in the program for education in nursing. Improved services in surgery and anesthesiology are being provided and a public-health laboratory is being established. An important project planned for the area of public health is the setting up of a rural demonstration and training program that will provide practical training and experience in the development of an integrated public-health service in a rural area.

The difficulty of deciding on medical priorities in Somalia can be illustrated by the fact that there were 67 doctors—mostly attached to hospitals—serving the entire population of between three to four million people in 1967.[9] These figures point to a need for more doctors and more facilities for medical care. But there is perhaps an even greater need for extensive programs of preventive medicine and health education in a country where ignorance, suspicion of the methods and ideas of the outside world, and the strong prejudices of a proud and individualistic people militate against progress.[10]

I have already mentioned that the nomad looks with scorn on agricultural pursuits. There are many other things which he views with contempt: fishermen and fish, for example. A Somali family might prefer to go without sufficient food and suffer the consequences of malnutrition rather than take advantage of the vast, mainly untapped source of protein that lies in the waters of the longest national coastline in Africa. In a land where malnutrition, especially among children, is common during the frequent periods of drought it is ironic that eating habits exclude many nutritionally valuable foods.

That a variety of factors must often be taken into consideration when plans are being made to launch a campaign for health was vividly illustrated in 1943 when the colonial medical authorities attempted to introduce a campaign for vaccination in what was then the Somaliland Protectorate. Political unrest, together with the normal suspicion of foreign motives and methods, led to the spreading of a rumor that the vaccinations were meant to make Somali women sterile. In one of the main townships there were serious riots in opposition to the campaign and many people were seriously injured.

Once the process of modernization has been set in motion there are inevitable clashes with the forces of tradition. The main hospital in Hargeisa once had to be closed down temporarily because the European medical superintendent—an otherwise well-qualified man but sadly deficient in his knowledge of Somali customs—ordered the local hospital staff to give bedpans to patients. He was unaware that social custom had apportioned jobs of that nature to a particular clan and that it was infra dig for other clans to undertake such tasks. This happened 20 years ago and, fortunately, incidents of that kind are less likely to occur now that Somalis have replaced foreigners in positions of authority. But, generally speaking, social customs and local prejudices must be taken into account in the formulation of development plans.

Somalis possess a considerable body of native medical practice, and while certain practices and principles are not without value, many of them hinder the acceptance of modern medicine. It is interesting to note that Sir Richard Burton reported in a footnote to his account of his travels in East Africa in the 1850's that the Somalis believe that malaria is transmitted by mosquitoes. He added that they held this "superstition" because mosquitoes and malarial fevers both appeared at sundown.[11] The principle, at least, behind modern malaria eradication comes as no surprise to Somalis. They have also long been aware of the gravity of tuberculosis and of its contagious nature. Persons suffering from this disease have always been housed separately and, before the advent of modern methods of treatment, they were always given the salutation "God have mercy on you" instead of the more customary "may God restore your health"—a reflection of the realization that nothing could be done for the victim.

Many Somalis, too, are expert bonesetters and surgeons and can perform tonsillectomies and trepanning operations.

By and large, however, Somali medicine is reminiscent of medieval medicine. Blood-letting is considered valuable for many ailments; it is carried out in such painful ways as cutting the veins under the tongue and under the eyelids or by drawing off blood in affected areas of the body through small incisions. While the Somali belief that fire and disease cannot exist together is compatible with modern knowledge of bacteriology, the practice of branding areas of the body in certain traditional patterns in order to cure a variety of illnesses ranging from tetanus to appendicitis is one that certainly requires reassessment.

It is clearly important for psychological and practical reasons to take into account local beliefs and practices. In medicine, as in other fields, traditions that are valuable can best be preserved by incorporating them into the mainstream of scientific and technological progress. Certainly education for health must aim at replacing widespread reliance on questionable or outmoded practices with respect for modern medical procedures.

It is pertinent to emphasize here the need for foreign governments and international organizations that offer assistance to developing African nations to pay particular attention to the special conditions prevailing in each recipient country, and to orient their approaches accordingly. There is great diversity in Africa, and it would be imprudent to expect that a medical program applied successfully in one country would automatically succeed in another, even though the countries concerned might be neighbors.

It might seem that taking the traditional culture of a people into account when planning health projects for developing countries would make the process complicated enough, but there are other social, economic, and health implications which are perhaps more practicable but need careful study. For example, it has been found in some countries that a successful program for eradicating malaria has resulted in the survival of a large number of infants and children who formerly would have died from malaria or allied causes. This is not to say that such programs should not be carried out for this reason. But it does mean that additional facilities in services such as education—and later in job opportunities—have to be provided, and planning should take account of this.

I think I have said enough to show that the Somali Democratic Republic is faced with a complex pattern of interlinked problems. But progress, however small, is being made in every area. Our new government is particularly aware of the deficiencies of the program for health and is determined to end the stagnation caused in the past by inefficient organization and the maladministration of resources.

Specialized agencies of the United Nations—WHO, UNICEF, and FAO—are giving invaluable technical and material assistance. In addition, the republic has benefitted from the services of medical teams, medical equipment, and medicine provided by many governments, including those of the Soviet Union, Italy, China, the United Arab Republic, West Germany, and the United States. If our problems are large, so is the good will which continues to be shown toward our country and the energies of our government and people that are being used toward their solution.

REFERENCES

1. UN document EM/RC 19/2, p. 170.
2. Simon, J. *Men and Medicine in the Middle East.* WHO Regional Office for the Eastern Mediterranean, 1967.
3. UN document EM/RC 19/2, p. 171.
4. Ibid., pp. 172-75.
5. Cahill, K., Davies, I. and Johnson, R. Report of an epidemic due to *Shigella dysenteriae. Amer. J. Trop. Med. Hyg. 15*:52, 1966.
6. Simon J. Ibid., p. 154.
7. Ciba Foundation Symposium. *Man in Africa.* Wolstenholme, G. and O'Connor, M., eds. Boston, Little, Brown, 1965.
8. *Somalia: Survey of Technical Education.* UNESCO serial No. 1254. New York, UNESCO, 1969.
9. Simon, J. Ibid.
10. Cahill, K. *Health on the Horn of Africa.* London, Spottiswoode, 1969, 69 pp.
11. Burton, R. F. *First Footsteps in East Africa.* 1856.

THE EVOLUTION AND DELIVERY OF MEDICAL PROGRAMS IN DEVELOPING LANDS*

EDWARD E. SWANSTROM

Director
Catholic Relief Services
New York, N. Y.

I CONFESS to an understandable diffidence–even reluctance– in joining medical experts and diplomats in a symposium dealing with medicine and diplomacy in the tropics. The organizers of the symposium deliberately included a person who is alert to the multiple problems of the developing world but is not a medical professional. As the executive director of a large American voluntary agency, and as one member of a council of 24 voluntary agencies, I decided to offer what I might call "Notes from the Medical Underground."

My vantage point of observation is the dark underside of life, the isolated rural areas, urban centers newly swollen with rural migrants, and refugee communities located in 30 countries between the tropics of Cancer and Capricorn. Because of the absolute urgency of scientific direction, our agency has added medical personnel to our staff in Africa and Central America; I shall draw on their reports and on the reports and critiques of field personnel in what I offer you today.

In the past quarter of a century, since I first began visiting our projects in India, the Philippines, Africa, and Latin America, there has been a tremendous surge in medical aid from private, governmental, and intergovernmental sources. In the days after World War II the health centers we visited were mostly scattered and heroic outposts conducted by various religious groups.

I gratefully note recent signs of interdenominational cooperation and planning. Much more is needed.

Many of the missionary medical centers dealt with the old scourges that had afflicted these areas from time immemorial. Leprosy is a prime example. Denominational bodies have been dunned for generations for

*Presented as part of a *Symposium on Medicine and Diplomacy in the Tropics* sponsored by The Tropical Disease Center, St. Clare's Hospital, New York, N. Y., and The Merck Company Foundation, Rahway, N. J., held at the Center, December 13, 1969.

the support of hospitals for the segregation and care of lepers. Perhaps because leprosy is a biblical disease it has elevated the international Christian community to a worldwide preeminence in the care of a disorder that made outcasts of those afflicted with it.

Progress in this one field has been dramatic. Instead of collecting the enormous funds necessary for the construction of a leprosarium and the administrative planning necessitated by a staff of lay or religious missionaries, the approach today is simpler and, I feel, more effective. Take the well-known case of Calcutta, for example, where all the health problems of Asia meet in one choking and glutted city. Little nests of lepers cluster with their families in many of the *bustees* or slum sections. The lepers sally out to beg at certain times and in certain areas, outside churches, temples, and mosques. The well members of the family often hold jobs as food-handlers and servants, so that leprosy has appeared in some of the wealthiest families of the city.

A new group, headed by a woman of Albanian origin known as Mother Teresa, asked for a mobile clinic so that she could visit the groups of leprosy patients she had met in her *bustee* schools and training centers. Rather than expect the afflicted people to come to a center, the clinic went to them. The Institute for Tropical Diseases of Calcutta supplied doctors, and American sources supplied a key factor: food. When a significant amount of food was given to each patient and his family, the number of patients increased enormously. Oxford Famine Relief joined the project to supply the latest antileprosy medicaments in quantity.

Will this development resolve the leprosy problem of this refugee-swollen city? Of course not, but the improved nutrition and regular treatment will accomplish two very desirable goals: a certain number of leprosy patients will be rendered noninfectious, and a large number of what are referred to as "untainted children" will be saved from the affliction through the educational adjuncts of the program. After a few years of cooperation between Mother Teresa, the Institute of Tropical Medicine, and two voluntary agencies, the Calcutta community became interested and is now concerned with housing and work for the hitherto invisible lepers.

In Korea, a country outside the latitudes mentioned earlier, the rate of leprosy is very high. Persons do not come forward for treatment because they fear being branded for the rest of their lives. A counterpart voluntary group with the aid of the American Catholic Medical Mission Board operates five mobile clinics, called by their clients "skin clinics." Through this service skin diseases are cared for and the first signs of leprosy are detected. The developments cited indicate not only the evolution of medical programs but the delivery of medical care to those who would not otherwise receive it and who would almost inevitably infect family and community. They are also evidence of a particular service of the voluntary agency: namely, the "finger-pointing exercise."

Although it lacks larger resources available to governments and intergovernmental organizations, the voluntary agency is often strong on personnel who are close to the realities of a given area. Such personnel, sometimes a sister-doctor, a few trained nurses, or a midwife, will often dare to start a pilot project that is no more than a finger pointing at a huge unmet need. The incessant finger-pointing inherent in a manifestly inadequate but zealous health unit often stimulates communities and official organizations into taking more adequate action.

Certainly the new mobility of peoples, often forced, as in massive exiles and expulsions, often voluntary, as in the movement of families and parts of families to the cities of Latin America, Africa, and Asia has demanded a mobility in medical programs. A vastly increased mobility is needed. How else can even emergency medical care be brought to the poor who inhabit new agglomerations of shanties and huts around such Latin-American cities as Buenos Aires, Bogota, and Caracas? Increased mobility will enable international voluntary agencies to serve better the more than 17,000,000 refugees who straddle the world as a virtual "refugee nation"; this may help develop a new "medicine for the poor."

The middle-class doctor who waits passively for his adequately housed middle-class patients to come to his consultation room has little or no relevance for the developing world. And yet the doctor who is trained in the United States all too often goes back to the main metropolitan areas of his own country and attempts to develop this type of lucrative and tragically selective medical practice. Such incidents put in doubt the transferability of medical training from developed to lesser developed areas, not only in the case of doctors but of nursing and administrative personnel.

Thus far I have been referring to the curative aspect of medicine, and this, of course, is where medicine began. In the developing world, unless medicine can move dramatically from its heavy emphasis on the simply curative, it will isolate itself from the realities of living. Even the witch doctor stresses preventive medicine in his propitiatory rites to the spirits.

Let me attempt to clarify what I mean. Our field staff has stressed to me that the medical profession must think, in the developing world, in terms of educative and preventive programs over and above the practice of cure. Further, much of this education must be in the fields of nutrition and public health. Dr. René Dubos has expressed "a deeply felt conviction that the extent of health improvement that ensues from building ultramodern hospitals with up-to-date equipment is probably trivial in comparison with the results that can be achieved at much lower cost by providing all infants and children with well-balanced food, sanitary conditions, and a stimulating environment."* We add to this the need for educative medicine.

Our medical adviser in Africa, Dr. Carlo Capone, has written a monograph entitled *Child Health and Food Aid in Developing Countries* in which he gives evidence that the child under five bears the chief brunt of the social, economic, and nutritional problems of deficit areas. On the other hand, the child of this age lags far behind in benefits accruing from the economic development of a country. The only chance he has of receiving benefits is for the country to plan a *direct* and *specific* program on his behalf. Current programs demonstrate that national health care is first focused on the productive segment of the population. Tracy May says "Tropical medicine is the 'midwife of economic progress' in the underdeveloped areas of the world. Where mass diseases are brought under control, productivity tends to increase . . . through augmenting strength and ambition to work. . . ."

Senegal, whose national budget can afford no more than 30 cents per inhabitant per year for medical aid and vaccines, cannot afford a health project designed specifically for the "under fives" in the population. Fortunately, governments such as our own are recognizing malnutrition for what it really is: the cause not only of a large percentage of disease problems but also of irreversible damage to physical and even mental development. The onslaught on hunger and malnutrition both

*Dubos, R. *Man and His Environment,* Washington, D.C., Pan American Health Org., 1966.

here and abroad is a most important step in preventive medicine.

Our own agency under the leadership of Dr. Carlo Capone has created a Child Health Scheme for children under five in Senegal and in almost all the countries of sub-Saharan Africa. At least 600 clinics are presently engaged in providing extra nutrition to mothers of preschool children. The foods come from the stocks of the U.S. Food for Peace. The contact with the mothers in their fertility period offers an unexampled opportunity for training in child and family nutrition. In addition to its supply of high-protein foods each clinic or health center uses scales and charts (known as Health Indicators) to plot the weight changes of the child in such a way that even an illiterate mother can see graphic indications of her child's health.

To women of child-bearing age the opportunity is given to learn basic hygiene as well as the prerequisites to having and rearing a healthy child. Dr. Capone, who points out that the child is the chief victim of underdevelopment, maintains that unless practical steps are taken for infants and children here and now *it is the child who will defeat all other development programs.* This is a sobering thought as we enter the second development decade of the United Nations in 1970.

It may be helpful to consider the implications of this warning and to take action. First, the prime need of developing countries is for supplemental supplies from outside them. These countries cannot provide the extra foods needed to combat the vast malnutrition. The extra foods exist in such rich and developed nations as Canada, the United States, and parts of Europe and Australia. If there is a focus on the needs of the children under five, plans can be made for the transfer of the needed and available foods, including powdered milk and high-protein cereals, from the rich countries to the poor. Health Indicators are already being printed for nations in Asia as well as Africa.

The latest extension of this type of program in nutritional education is being prepared for six Central American countries with the cooperation of the U.S. Agency for International Development. The general supervision is in the hands of Dr. Frances Rothert, our medical and public health adviser for Central America. Food will again be the real "hinge" of the program.

The availability of food ensures the presence of mothers with children under five. We cannot expect illiterate mothers to come to the village school or church hall for a lecture. The food is also a spur to community leaders; it can thus spark a many-pronged effort not only for nutritional improvement but for community action in general.

The educational program will eventually reach tens of thousands of the most deprived families. These are the families whose access to curative medicine is minimal. For them the preventive aspect of the nutritional education program is crucial. What is especially significant about the organization of the growing network of under-five health schemes is that a single doctor can put it in motion. That same doctor, tied to a stationary clinic and a line of patients would play a far less valuable role in promoting health in any tropical country.

Another medical channel in the developing world is the radio. The omnipresence of the transistor radio has been put to marvelous use. Village mothers in the most remote sections of Colombia, for instance, have learned child care and elementary sanitation in lectures transmitted through the transistor. Arrangements were made for village women to listen in groups and to take a test at the end of a given course. When clothing was offered as prizes, thousands more participated.

Dr. Capone is not alone in pointing out that "Foods are the principal item the developing nations are short of and will be short of for many years to come. . . . It is also the commodity that the developed world can produce, and must produce, above commercial requirements."

Those of us who see our United States overseas aid budget shrink each year (while our arms budget has grown until it swallows well over half of our federal budget) will become more and more vocal about the needs for a radical change in priorities. Maximum utilization of the food resources of developed countries calls for larger foreign-aid outlays from the United States as well as the provision of skilled personnel who will be available to places such as Latin America, Africa, and Asia and to their public-health officials.

In this connection I must also mention another facet of the utilization of foods from developed lands. There is need to prepare the foods in such a way that they may be immediately usable by the recipient. When, in the late 1940's and early 1950's, the United States had enormous surpluses of wheat, the voluntary agencies could obtain large supplies of flour for their aid programs in the hungry areas of the world. But flour presumes baking, and millions of the poorest people—Asians, for example—had nothing resembling an oven. Voluntary agency leaders, from their close acquaintance with the living habits of the needy, explained that wheat would have to be supplied in a form that could be cooked by boiling. It was suggested that the wheat be supplied in the form of bulgur wheat, a cracked wheat used in tropical areas since biblical times. Bulgur wheat has become the basis for many development programs in India and elsewhere in the past decade and a half.

Many new forms of food, especially such high-protein concentrates as CSM (Corn-Soya-Milk), and various fish flours are among the contributions that science has made to nutrition. Science has shown that in many deficient areas of the earth local resources that were never believed to have nutritional value can be processed for human consumption. These untapped sources can be tapped only through committed research.

Even more fruitful results can be achieved in the future if funds are channeled more liberally into research for projects of human welfare and nutrition. Here is where the medical men today must raise their voices if we are to have a better tomorrow, or even any tomorrow. Who can estimate the billions of dollars that went into research to produce hydrogen bombs that can cremate alive the populations of the world's greatest cities? The inhabitants of the developing world are very sure that such weapons can be delivered. They have every reason to doubt that in the next developing decade there will be much improvement in the delivery of even the most basic of health services.

Lest I sound apocalyptic, let me sound a note of hope. At the Child Welfare Conference held in Stockholm this year, the only essentially cheerful note concerned progress in the health field in developing countries. Mortality rates and infant mortality specifically have decreased in the last several decades. The decrease is attributable to the fight against endemo-epidemic and infectious diseases, and the efforts made in the field of environmental sanitation, health, and *nutritional education.*

The medical profession must, then, be constantly looking toward the future, using every available means to prod society away from its ignorant, lazy, and even lethal tendencies and toward those aspects of knowledge and practice that strengthen and conserve life. This is not easy. It would be much easier for a medical man to cure one by one the cases of worms that debilitate his patients than to mount a tiring and difficult *campaign* against intestinal worms in a province of India or in the rural part of Taiwan. Vigorous campaigns are needed to promote the medicine of the poor and the medicine of the illiterate.

Someone commenting on an East African scene described a condition which kills 14% of all babies before the 10th day of life, namely, tetanus of the umbilical cord. Curative medicine using all forms of modern treatment *might* save four out of ten cases, whereas antitetanus injections will immunize the fortunate mothers. This is preventive medicine. Teaching natives not to use dirty bamboo knives in severing umbilical cords could save thousands of mothers and infants. This is educative medicine.

Every doctor in a developing area must be in great measure a public and environmental expert if he is to avoid the stigma of being a sort of commercial agent who sells his medical product to the highest bidders. As a man with scientific credentials he should play the role of a guru for society in all health matters: in the necessity for latrines, for example. No aspect of the environment should be beyond his ken – and he must become a multidisciplinary man if he is to talk to the community as a guru.

Thus far I have been discussing preventive medicine as it relates to education and to education in such basic matters as nutrition. I should like to stress a necessity of life as basic as food. Dr. Dubos tells us "There are indications that general dietary improvement, better practices of infant feeding and handling, and *simply an abundant supply of water*, would be a far more effective and less costly approach to the control of intestinal disorders, than are prophylaxis and treatment with drugs and vaccines."

The phrase "an abundant supply of water" is hardly more than a dream in the *favelas, barriadas,* or *callampas* that have mushroomed around Latin America's cities where the poorest of the poor often have to buy their drinking water from vendors. Abundant water is hardly more than a dream in great parts of India where, according to a recent conference at Wardha, only 120,000 of India's 570,000 villages have a good and adequate supply of drinking water. Of the remaining 450,000 villages, it is estimated that one third have inadequate sources of drinking water and another third have unhygienic sources. The last third have no sources at all, meaning that the villagers have to fetch all water from a distance of a mile or more.

A doctor serving in such an area might well make himself an expert on wells and water levels. Our director for India worked with Indian officials and representatives of other voluntary agencies and decided on a health project to mark this Gandhi centennial year of 1969. Again, food became the "hinge" on which the whole program turned. The wells were to be dug in such parched areas as Bihar by voluntary effort, but the workers needed supplementary food. Here again, Food for Peace mobilized people to participation. Squads of workers recruited by Indian voluntary agencies in the Gandhian tradition constructed 2,000 wells in Bihar alone. Close to 4,000 wells have been constructed in other areas of India. Of course a cash outlay was necessary to purchase the cement and other supplies needed to complete the wells. Here is a challenge to a medical team: to motivate and stimulate support for construction of wells for the villages of India without wells and for those villages whose water supply is unhygienic. What a massive work of preventive medicine that represents.

But that leads us to the question of motivation, and that is where all such schemes for the betterment of man either flounder or sail into port. Motivation comes out of our commitment, out of the deepest recesses of our consciences. I hope that many more professional medical people will be motivated to join people-to-people programs of the long-standing service groups that have a mission to raise people by their educative and preventive medical programs around the world, and that they will offer aid through a permanent corps of medical professionals to assure constant attention to the medical problems of the developing world. I make this point to emphasize the need for *longer terms* of volunteer or semivolunteer services so that the personnel can absorb the language or the special mores of an area. Our young people now are motivated by a desire for service rather than profit; they desire peace rather than conflict. Even the medical profession should open its doors for young people to serve the needs of the poorer nations in paramedical assistance as a form of field work. I also hope there will be a unification of the efforts of all religious groups in the planning and execution of their medical programs so that they can present a united appeal to governments, foundations, and specialized agencies of the United Nations.

Nikolai A. Berdyaev, the Russian philosopher, has said that the question of bread for one's neighbor is not a material question but a spiritual one. I accept that in its widest application, for I believe that the question of healing our neighbor in this global village is a spiritual matter. The spiritual eye must see the whole human family as actually one; it must pierce us with pain at another's suffering. Otherwise how can we be moved to the healing acts that our sick society and our sick world so tragically need?

A WAR WE CAN WIN*

Health as a Vector of Foreign Policy

Hugh L. Carey

United States Congressman
15th District
Brooklyn, N.Y.

It is time our country won a war. In my lifetime I have fought in one war and helped to finance four others, and I have not felt like a winner yet. In the past 50 years more than a million American casualties and the expenditure of trillions of dollars have not secured peace on earth.

In the 1970's, for a change, I should like to see us enter a war we can win. Let me suggest a winning strategy for the war of the 1970's: first, we should pick an old opponent already on the downgrade: man's most ancient enemy—disease and its allies, hunger and ignorance. Next, I should enlist the largest possible army—all mankind—in a common and united front to wage an all-out assault on an aggressor who respects no borders: premature death. For leadership I should seek the ministers of the healing arts, such as those whose efforts are like those of Albert Schweitzer, of Thomas A. Dooley, and of Father Damien. A foreign-policy effort that would utilize medicine and health care has proved its soundness in the past. I believe it would justify a new initiative in the 1970's.

The Historical Basis

Every time we have supported medical leadership in international health we have won battle after battle and inflicted all the casualties among the insects and microscopic organisms which prey upon man and the other animals.

Medical leadership and foreign policy are not new companions. We are indebted to Dr. Kevin M. Cahill, the organizer of this symposium, for an excellent review of the role of medicine in international diplo-

*Presented as part of a *Symposium on Medicine and Diplomacy in the Tropics* sponsored by The Tropical Disease Center, St. Clare's Hospital, New York, N.Y., and The Merck Company Foundation, Rahway, N.J., held at the Center, December 13, 1969.

macy. In his report "Medicine and Diplomacy in the Tropics,"[1] Dr. Cahill traces the history of the humanitarian alliance of health and statecraft. He tells us that six of the signers of the Declaration of Independence were physicians and that the last president of the Republic of Texas was a doctor. He identifies leaders in other lands as physicians: Georges Clemenceau in France; Isidro Ayora in Ecuador; Juscalino Kubitschek in Brazil; and H. Kamuza Banda in Malawi. Representative Thomas E. Morgan of Pennsylvania, chairman of the Committee on Foreign Affairs in the House of Representatives, is a practicing physician. It would be an error to depict the doctor in diplomacy as a practitioner in rhetoric or a surgeon in striped pants: in reality he is a pioneer.

Historically, American medical help has been used to open new frontiers in our hemisphere and around the world. Significantly, our major efforts to employ overseas health care as a measure of our national interest have in many cases followed the end of military operations. In 1798, in postrevolutionary America, President John Adams signed the law to establish the Marine Hospital which became our U.S. Public Health Service. One hundred years later, in 1899, after the Spanish-American War, Walter Reed led the U.S. Army Yellow Fever Commission in the assault on yellow fever in the Caribbean and, by 1901, the disease had been completely eradicated in Havana. The construction of the Panama Canal was made possible through the program led by Dr. William Crawford Gorgas. Sixty years later in Havana, American medicine came to the rescue of our foreign policy after the abortive mishap of the Bay of Pigs, Cuba: 1,700 prisoners were released from Cuba in exchange for $25 million worth of drugs supplied by American firms through the Pharmaceutical Manufacturers' Association as a result of adroit negotiations conducted by Attorney General Robert F. Kennedy and James B. Donovan.

In wartime I witnessed how Europeans esteemed Dwight D. Eisenhower, our commanding general, and President Franklin D. Roosevelt for their leadership in liberation. But Herbert Hoover was revered as well for his mission after World War I that had supplied food, medicine, and other necessities to millions of victims of that war.

However, it was Harry S. Truman, our postwar president in 1949, who set forth with historic determination the humanitarian commitment as it is, or should be, today.

The Foreign Policy Pathmark

In his Inaugural Address, 1949, President Truman stated:

> For the first time in history, humanity possesses the knowledge and the skill to relieve the suffering of these people.
>
> The United States is pre-eminent among nations in the development of industrial and scientific techniques. The material resources which we can afford to use for the assistance of other peoples are limited. But our imponderable resources in technical knowledge are constantly growing and are inexhaustible.
>
> I believe that we should make available to peace-loving peoples the benefits of our store of technical knowledge in order to help them realize their aspirations for a better life.[2]

This policy became the Marshall Plan, which has had no equal as an effective instrument in furthering American foreign policy. Most of its success was due to the fact that it incorporated extensive public-health programs that were made available to needy nations. Out of such efforts emerged the World Health Organization (WHO), which has served to portray vividly the needs of the health-poor peoples of the earth.

Because disease respects no boundaries, President John F. Kennedy pointed up in his foreign policy, through the Agency for International Development, the principle of interdependency of nations in health planning and operations.

Caught up in a tragic war, President Lyndon B. Johnson saw that violence in and among nations results when suffering people lose confidence in their governments. This is particularly true in small nations but it is becoming painfully evident now in great powers also. Speaking as the leader of the world's greatest power in 1966 he called for action in international health and education in his message to Congress:

> We have committed ourselves for many years to relieving human suffering. Today our effort must keep pace with a growing world and with growing problems. Therefore, I propose a program to create an international career service in health; help meet health manpower needs in developing nations; combat malnutrition control and eradicate disease; co-operate in world-wide efforts to deal with population problems.[3]

The president had reason to feel that his words fell on sympathetic ears. Congress has been saying for years in the language of the Foreign

Assistance Act: "Ignorance, want and despair breed extremism and violence which lead to aggression and violence."

It is sad to relate today that the International Health Education Act, calling for an expenditure of only $10 million, died in the Rules Committee in 1966 and has yet to be resurrected. This happened despite the fact that John Gardner, then Secretary of Health, Education, and Welfare, had said before the Congressional Committee which considered this bill:

> One of the necessities of our time is to create the kind of relationships with other countries which will enable all of us to live in peace. More than ever before, all of us recognize that the hazard of war is greater than any other.
>
> There may be many ways to reduce this hazard, but there are few which are better than establishing constructive working relationships in those fields of human endeavor in which all men share the same aims, the same hopes, the same goals. Health is such a field. There are no better grounds on which we can meet other nations and demonstrate our own concern for peace and the betterment of mankind than in a common battle against disease.
>
> To this field, we can bring special competence, we can address ourselves to the alleviation of serious but soluble problems. We can relate ourselves constructively to others in improving international understanding and co-operation.
>
> Furthermore, when we engage in such shared work with the health professions in other lands, particularly in the developing nations, we are relating ourselves to key groups and individuals, destined to play vitally important roles in shaping the future of their countries.
>
> It is important to note that any aid to improve the health of people in other countries—especially in the developing nations—will be a substantial contribution not only to their health status and their freedom from disease, but also to their educational status, their food production, their economic strength, their social stability, and the attainment of that level of social and economic development which will permit them to be self-sufficient and self-supporting.
>
> We could bring these benefits to many nations simply by exporting our know-how, at relatively little cost to ourselves.[4]

Exporting Our Know-How: A Boon and a Bargain

"Exporting our know-how, at relatively little cost to ourselves"—this would seem to be the kind of boon at bargain price which should appeal to even the most cost-conscious Congress. The 89th Congress, however, was not convinced even though the Committee, in favorably reporting the bill, stated that this would mobilize slightly less than 1% of America's total health-manpower pool.

With unusual Congressional chagrin the Committee further stated:

> It will be noted that this number (of trainees) is considerably less than the number of M.D.'s licensed in the U.S. which is draining scarce medical manpower from other nations in the world for our domestic health problems.[5]

On this same point, in an address titled "Medicine: The Global Diplomat," former Secretary of State Dean Rusk pointed out how we are "sopping up" medical talent from developing countries. Mr. Rusk stated:

> Now, if there is a country which can produce its own resources for its own medical care, surely it must be the United States. For if we cannot do it, who can? And if we get in a position of absorbing from countries who are in desperate need of their talents and their manpower, then we have some very major problems in front of us.[6]

The unfortunate history of this legislation serves to illustrate that Congress is not moving to win this war that we can win against disease and premature death. What is even more tragic is that in this hour, in the most affluent period in the history of this or any other nation, we propose to do even less in the year ahead. Our arsenal of aid in the war we can win in health is provided basically in the Foreign Assistance Act. Under this we provide for our cooperation in the World Health Organization, our aid to developing nations for the needs in health and sanitation, and our programs to cope with the crisis in population.

The record of recent months shows a unilateral withdrawal—a retreat from man's most ancient and newly vulnerable enemy: disease. Since 1948 and the Marshall Plan, Congress has appropriated about $47 billion for foreign assistance. As a percentage of our gross national product this equaled 2% in 1949; declined to two thirds of 1% in 1954; and one half of 1% in 1962. The $1.6 billion proposed by Congress in the pending appropriation for FY1970 is less than one fourth of 1% of our 800 billion of the total production of the United States. In our effort as compared with that of other industrial nations who provide assistance in development to our weaker neighbors the United States has fallen from first to eighth place.

I recently asked a representative of the Agency for International Development (AID): "At what point does this program become marginally effective in terms of being funded at levels too low to have significant impact?" Sadly he answered, "I believe we may have passed that point two years ago."

Recognizing the status of Congressional antipathy to universal technical-assistance programs and the failure of the present administration to exercise leadership as yet in this field, is it realistic to talk of a new initiative in world health on the part of the United States?

Is a New Initiative Feasible?

My answer is that it will take some hard selling, but I consider it possible to convince Congress that health care is an effective instrument of foreign policy in at least four ways:

First, I submit that health care is our lowest cost form of international security and protection against war and violence. In a recent eight-year period 87% of the very poor nations, 69% of the poor nations, 48% of the middle-income nations and just 4% of the rich nations suffered serious violence.[7] The recent overthrow of governments in developing and less-developed countries proves that the smaller nations are a long way from stability and that disorders in their countries tend to bring the great powers into conflict on one side or the other. Recently in Dahomey and in recent months, Peru, Ecuador, and Panama have erupted, to say nothing of Nigeria, Biafra, and Libya.

Corpsman to Mankind, Not Policeman of the World

As we watch these seemingly superficial eruptions on the various continents we might well remember that the great wars of this century started in backyard quarrels. Conflict among remote neighbors in the Balkans, in the Rhur and Saar valleys, and in Vietnam eventually involved the United States. It is true that we became involved under the notion that we had a function as policeman of the world. It is apparent from the statements of the Nixon administration and of many Congressional leaders that we no longer regard ourselves as such even though we carry the "biggest stick" in history, referred to by the administration as our "nuclear umbrella." The difficulty, of course, is that there are also sticks of similar if not equal weight in other hands so that we cannot afford the least instability in smaller nations lest that instability trigger the "last world war."

If our country is not to act as a policeman of the world and wield the bomb as a club, then perhaps in our own interest and in the interest of humanity we might consider ourselves as corpsman to mankind, bearing the balm of healing and helping. Exporting our know-how in health care at relatively little cost to ourselves should be an attractive alternative to some high-cost, low-yield programs of foreign aid that we now support under the name of mutual security.

For decades we have scattered our hardware among weakling autocracies, old colonial powers, and juntas passing through the palaces of developing nations as though they were swinging doors. From Sherman tanks to surplus ships we have dispensed so-called defensive weapons to nations we have described as our eligible friends.

All too often, unfortunately, these weapons have been used to sustain governments which must perpetuate themselves in power through the force of "borrowed" arms. Such governments must use arms to promote stability through force because they have failed to win the loyalty and support of their people. I believe it would be worth our effort to see if the ill and starving people of the weak nations would prefer a ton of food or a kilo of vaccine to a ton of ammunition.

An American Corpsman Health Program could aid any government interested in the preservation of life in its own country; this could also be done on a regional basis.

It is not an abstraction that health programs can promote stability and protect against chronic anarchy.

Health as an Instrument of Stability

Herbert Singer, chairman of the board of The World Health Foundation, has discussed "Health as an Instrument of Foreign Policy." He pointed out: "Health and health programs have a unique capacity to touch the lives of individuals and families and to do so more dramatically than perhaps any other service of government."

Mr. Singer cites the following examples, which I believe are persuasive:

In Colombia where guerilla warfare has had, for years, fertile territory within which to function, health has recently taken on a new and significant role. A successful program is now in operation by the Colombian Navy who, in addition to their prime mission of policing the Magdalena River have added a medical and dental service for an area previously deemed isolated and unfriendly to the military. This health program, built around the gun boat and rendering service to people living within range of the river, has changed the image of Navy personnel in that territory from that of enemy to that of friend. It has produced vital intelligence of the hinterland of the river never before known or understood. In bringing the people of the area into league with the Navy, it has generated an extraordinary loyalty to the government in a vast area previously deemed, at the very least, unfriendly. The program has been so successful that a new vessel is now being completed to bring the program to the head waters of the Amazon River on the other side of the Andes.

It is not accidental that the Feldsher System of medicine was incorporated in the Soviet health system in the very early days of their revolution and has been built upon vigorously ever since. To provide a broad and immediate base of medicine for the people of the Soviet Union, the Feldsher System provides medical coverage to a community, not through graduate doctors, but through specially trained personnel to deal, on a personal level, with a limited scope of medical needs. The system may not produce the highest quality of medicine, but it has permitted the Soviet government to give to the masses of its people, broad, immediate, and effective health coverage. It is said that the Soviet people consider their medical system one of the fundamentally important dividends from their government.

It is interesting to note that, at a recent conference of the Pan American Health Organization in Trinidad, the Cuban Delegation wished to dramatize its health program (which follows the Soviet system) and requested a comparative examination of health programs in Latin America. This request was for the obvious purpose of demonstrating Cuba's superior coverage of its peoples' health needs as against the relatively low health coverage of the "imperialistic" oriented governments of Latin America. Castro, very early in his regime, endeavored to dramatize to his people his concern for their health: and it is not at all surprising that Castro insisted on drugs and medical supplies as the consideration for his release of prisoners captured in the Bay of Pigs incident. It is particularly interesting to note that Castro is presently using the Cuban health structure and personnel as a means of communicating with his people on a political as well as health level.

Negatively, we have seen the strong reaction of people when a government health service is withdrawn or curtailed, as took place in England and in other countries in recent years.[8]

The horror of our experience in Vietnam should teach Congress something about the present instability of small governments. The Thieu regime there is the latest administration in a series which sought to win the loyalty of its citizens by both democratic and undemocratic means.

In Vietnam experience shows that one of our most successful efforts in pacification has been in the field of health services. There is another lesson for us. We have spent as much on Vietnam—$120 billion—as we have on the entire Foreign Assistance Program since it began 21 years ago!

The second way in which Congress may be sold on health is to point out that a new priority program which has found favor with the White House and Congress—population control—may be ineffective without companion programs in public health. This will be particularly true in the poorest nations with the highest birthrates unless we also provide or help to promote a system for the delivery of health services that include maternity and child health and nutrition as integral to family planning.

This we have not done. Instead, in order to underwrite a new national and international emphasis in family planning, Congress has earmarked a rising level of funds for family planning while decreasing the level of technical assistance, which includes health services. As a result little assistance is now available for the improvement of the basic structures of developing countries for providing health services at the local level.

In Africa, in fiscal year 1968, 80% of all the AID funds available for health, population, and nutrition were allocated to just two projects: the Regional Measles Control-Smallpox Eradication Project that serves 19 countries and the Ibadan Water Supply Project in Nigeria.

No amount of money for family planning will have the desired effect on fertility rates, disease, or nutrition until we achieve some simple way of handling all three.

Notestein, Kirk, and Segal in 1963 observed: "No efforts of socio-economic development can be successful in a disease-ridden population, nor will a desire for small families be likely to emerge. Better health and improved chances for survival of the individual child lie at the root of the motivational change we are seeking."[9]

Dr. Walsh McDermott agrees with Barbara Ward,[10] the economist, that the population question has "suffered badly from misleading simplifications. The very broad generalization is true, however, that as long as there continues a high infant and early childhood mortality it is very hard to make sustained high fertility seem disadvantageous. Thus the high early mortality blocks creation of the preconditions necessary for reduction in fertility that is, in itself, necessary for reduction of early mortality.[11]

Population control as an element of our foreign policy in health, then, if it is to succeed, turns on the readiness of Congress and the president to support the development of a new system of health-care delivery adaptable to the traditional societies in the underdeveloped countries.

To be adaptable such a system need not and should not be the kind of sophisticated system common to western civilization. Our highly developed health system is outstripping our means so fast that it is obviously too costly to export all over the world.

Further, it is of little use in the treatment of illiterate patients who know neither when they were born nor how old they are in terms of our years or who must observe local taboos by sticking pins in a doll to describe their symptoms or must communicate their aches and pains in West Nigeria through the *dokita* (native doctor), *babalawos* (Ifa priests), or the *onisegurns* (herbalists).

Since our American system of health care is too advanced in practice and in cost to be feasible for use in the developing countries how are we to export our know-how in health care? The answer is neither to ignore the challenge nor the opportunity to serve mankind but to adapt ourselves to the varieties of need.

When President John F. Kennedy saw the need for a new instrument for technical assistance to the developing nations he did not conscript the graduate schools at the Massachusetts Institute of Technology, at the California Institute of Technology, or at the Georgetown School of Foreign Service. Rather he founded the Peace Corps as a broadly based agency for voluntary service tailored to interface the needs of the host country with the talents of American volunteers.

Anyone who has priced our Peace Corps effort in cost-benefit terms will reach the conclusion that the return to our nation, to the host countries, and to the individuals involved has been profitable beyond measure.

On the basis of this record I suggest that a third way to persuade Congress and the administration to support a new initiative in this war we can win is that we should begin with an economical low-cost developmental project which would entail neither a vast financial nor skilled manpower commitment.

I urge, therefore, that the United States undertake the foundation of an International Health Corpsman Program. Such a program would be multilateral; it would involve both the personnel and resources of other willing nations in cooperation with but not under WHO.

I suggest the latter because of the presently limited resources of WHO (approximately $100 million worldwide) as well as the political structures which bind WHO as an agency of the United Nations.

The program would be one of training and placement at the invitation of host countries in need of mobile medical and paramedical, technical and subtechnical personnel, specifically trained for the needs of the area to be served.

Miss Julia Walsh, a senior at New York University School of Medicine who recently attended the World Health Assembly as student representative, describes such a plan in her excellent article "Medical Education and World Health."[12] Miss Walsh suggests the need for measurements of productivity of health personnel and she says that "with the increasing use of labor-saving devices a health worker is able to serve more people or larger areas in a shorter time but first he must be skilled to use these devices." She further points out that the particular combination of medical and paramedical personnel to meet best the needs of the specific country and to use most efficiently its resources can be determined; this of course will differ in each instance. The educational system for the development of the health personnel requires variations suited to the particular country. The training plan, according to Miss Walsh, should take into account the nature of services to be provided and tailored to fulfill the needs defined.

A nation which has learned to train technicians such as we have for space, for military purposes, for agriculture, etc., should have little difficulty in developing a versatile system of training medical and health personnel in such an effort. The advances we have made in programmed instruction, the available trained medical-corps personnel discharged from the armed forces, and the ability we have to train others by example are factors in our favor.

In fact it is precisely because we have the competence that I feel we have a moral as well as humanitarian imperative to undertake such a program. We have the know-how to prevent, to cure, to immunize, and we have done so on an isolated basis in the tropics, in the ghettos, in Appalachia, and in the war-ravaged areas of the world.

Not only have we the know-how but we have mastered the technique of mobility necessary for on-the-spot delivery of services as well as the needed support and communications vital to such a program. The world would benefit from our helicopters, field radios, massive airlift capacity, and all-round logistical competence gained in military activity.

It is no small coincidence that our system of national security and our leadership in international security will equip us to move from a post of policeman of the world to corpsman to humanity in need.

There are few legislators now in Congress who are as knowledgeable on health matters as our present Secretary of Defense and former Congressman Melvin Laird. Over many years in the House, as a member of the Subcommittee on Health, Education, and Welfare of the Appropriations Committee of the House of Representatives, he provided vital leadership, particularly in the support of research and international cooperation in health. How fitting it would be for us to now apply some of the savings we forecast in defense to a modest initiation in winning the war against disease. Defense of medical manpower resources could be of significant help in another way. We have scarce medical personnel "locked" into our Selective Service, a commissioned-medical-officer system to a greater degree than seems justifiable at this time. As of June 1969 in the Department of the Army, the branch with the highest rate of hospital patients, there were 32,000 inpatients. There were 7,132 Medical Corps officers on duty or approximately one doctor for every five patients. Armywide, among 1,500,000 personnel in uniform, the doctor-patient ratio is 4.72 per 1,000—or three times better than that among civilians.

Couple this with the fact that most doctors in the armed services are under a six-year obligation for two years of active duty during which their professional skills are usually devoted to a limited range of practice. The figures cited for the army alone, extended by the similar situations in the air force and navy, should provide some basis for a possible alternative as we move toward voluntary service in the armed forces. Such an alternative might well be for doctors to serve for a limited period in training and preparing the mobile medical and auxiliary units which would be the heart of this program. It need not be emphasized that the staffing of such units would provide an opportunity for young Americans who are seeking an alternative to serving in combat. Young people today are in search of unconventional careers. What I am suggesting is a radically different and unconventional approach to the practice of medicine. The medicine we know involves a doctor-patient ratio of 1:1,000. The ratio among foreign persons would be 1:20,000. Medical tasks which are fairly simple and occur frequently would devolve onto auxiliaries. Simple health centers, mobile units, and guided self-care could bring millions of lives into productive activity and turn the tide against death at infancy, death at adolescence, death from privation at any age.

As an original site for a training unit and staging area for movement into Asia and Africa, regions of need, we might consider Saipan, in the Mariana Islands, or other tropical sectors in the Trust Territory of the Pacific Islands under control of the United States. Our strategic trust agreement with the United Nations would permit this kind of activity and would in fact be of benefit to Micronesia.

We now have in Micronesia a health-training facility that turns out vocational-school-age male and female health assistants in nursing and allied health programs, almost all of whom will return to their native districts. In addition, in American Samoa we have the new Lyndon Johnson Tropical Disease Center, which could provide technical aid and research to such a facility. A similar undertaking in Puerto Rico or the Virgin Islands could be organized to serve Latin and South America.

It is apparent that we have the basic elements needed to originate this program without any vast new budgetary expenditure. More effective support for present limited efforts to prevent disease would be one dividend from a better organized system.

Present Programs Could Be Improved

Such a system would serve as a multiplier of medical skills at low cost and would implement our present programs more effectively in all phases of health care from fertility control to treatment of infectious disease. With a clinical program such as this we could both accelerate and intensify not only the campaign against yellow fever and smallpox but also against measles, scarlet fever, diphtheria, and all the other killing and crippling diseases we have eliminated in this country. For example, on November 30 we announced that in Bourbon, Niger, a medical aide vaccinated the 100 millionth African in a campaign that has freed 120 million people from smallpox in 19 countries of West and Central Africa.

This is progress, but we know that more than half of all the children born in Africa die before the age of five, not just from yellow fever. I asked an official of our AID program why we did not give multiple vaccinations at the same time for tetanus, diphtheria, typhoid, typhus, measles, scarlet fever, etc., as we do in this country. I was told there was not enough money for the cost of the serum, even though these vaccines are the lowest-cost pharmaceuticals that money can buy. I have learned since that many American pharmaceutical houses such as Merck, Pfizer, SKF, etc., have donated much of these drugs. More could be used if we had a system of clinical inoculation. An additional fact that should appeal to Congress would be that American tourist taxpayers and traveling Congressmen now spend more than $20 million a year in getting immunization shots for overseas travel which we should not need if we could expedite our immunization and control programs.

We Can Succeed

The fourth and last reason why a new and greater effort should be made to win the war against disease is that we can anticipate the kind of success factor that Congress and the administration seek in new programs.

We can expect success because of the example set for our government by private agencies which have proved their effectiveness under most trying conditions all over the world. Eighty-two American organizations under private auspices are working overseas alone or in cooperation with the Public Health Service, AID, the Peace Corps, or branches of our Armed Forces Medical System. Care-Medico, the Dooley Foundation, Project Hope, the major religious groups—Catholic, Protestant, Jewish, and others—are the best emissaries of the United States we have in the world.

Here again, by more imaginative and innovative utilization of overseas diplomatic agencies, we could augment and assist the work of these organizations and individuals. Instead there are instances, as in Paraguay, where our policies actually hinder and hamper the efforts of voluntary missions working at the local level in the war against hunger and disease.

I advocate that the president use diplomatic efforts in aid of a war that we can win against disease in several other specific ways.

1) As we now do in the International Postal Agreement and the early-warning service of hurricanes and other meteorological phenomena, we can organize a network for world health in cooperation with all willing nations.

Such a communications system is now tied in to a limited degree with the Communicable Disease Center in Atlanta, Ga., which we use to alert us in our successful programs in Foreign Disaster Emergency Relief under AID. We know we can defeat and eliminate kwashiorkor or yaws or snail disease or tropical infections wherever they appear.

2) By international negotiation similar to the Geneva Convention in Warfare, we can take the lead in freeing doctors and other health professionals from all restrictions to travel on professional and health missions. It simply does not make sense to deny our health and medical skills to nations from whom we have withdrawn diplomatic recognition. The best way to get diplomacy going again would be to have our health scientists in constant communication with their colleagues throughout the world.

3) To broaden this understanding of health needs and opportunities I urge the federal government to assist educational institutions in studies in this field. The new institutes on campus for African, Asian, and Hispanic studies, for instance, could well help win the war against disease in the developing countries.

In conclusion I am convinced that no cause can prevail today unless it has earned the confidence and gained the support of young people. I believe the cause of international health and winning the war against disease is that kind of cause.

I am inspired, therefore, to see that the *New Physician*, the journal of the Student American Medical Association, in its issue of October 1969, devotes its entire issue to international health. That issue reveals the desire of young doctors and students who are working in remote and primitive corners of the world to better their skills and extend them to those most in need.

The editorial in this issue is eloquent:

> It is the two central aspects of medicine which have given it universal appeal as a humanitarian discipline. The first is its basic act, which is that of one human being helping another in need. The second is its basic method, which is science. The human crises of illness and death are universal, knowing no political, economic, or social boundaries, and science, in an age where advocacy silences dialogue and caps the ear of reason, is a last redoubt of a healthful cultural relativism, which sees mostly wonder in a fellow human's different way of life without a dimming veil of xenophobic arrogance.[13]

Our student doctors give us hope that in this century we can win our greatest conquest. In the 19th century Sir Ronald Ross prayed for help in his research to find the "unseen, small million murderous killer"; we now pray for victory also, mindful of his words:

This day relenting God
  Hath placed within my hand
A wondrous thing. And God
  Be praised, at his command
Seeking his secret deeds,
  With tears and toiling breath,
I find thy cunning seeds,
  O million-murdering death,
I know this little thing
  A myriad men will save,
O death, where is thy sting?
  Thy victory, O grave?

We can win the war against the unseen "million murdering killer." We have the means. Let us call forth the will.

FOOTNOTES AND REFERENCES

1. Cahill, K. M. Medicine and diplomacy in the tropics. *N.Y. J. Med. 67*:2229-38, 1967.
2. Truman, H. S. Inaugural address. Congressional Record, January 20, 1949, pp. 447-78. Washington, D.C., Govt. Print. Office, 1949.
3. Johnson, President Lyndon B.: Message to Congress on International Education and Health Acts. Congressional Record, February 2, 1966, pp. 1738-41. Washington, D.C., Govt. Print. Office, 1966.
4. Hearing before the Committee on Interstate and Foreign Commerce, House of Representatives, 89th Congress, on H.R. 12453, International Health Act of 1966, pp. 6-7. Washington, D.C., Govt. Print. Office, 1966.
5. House Report No. 1317, House of Representatives, 89th Congress, to accompany H.R. 12453, International Health Act of 1966, p. 8. Washington, D.C. Govt. Print. Office, 1966.
6. Rusk, D.: Medicine: The Global Diplomat. Fourth Conference on International Health (American Medical Association). Chicago, Ill., May 17-18, 1969. Unpublished.
7. McNamara, R. S. Address before the American Society of Newspaper Editors. Montreal, Canada, May 18, 1966. Unpublished.
8. Singer, H. M. Health as an Instrument of Foreign Policy. Congressional Record, February 19, 1968, p. E-870. Washington, D.C., Govt. Print. Office, 1968.
9. Notestein, F. W., Kirk, D. and Segal, S. The Problem of Population Control. In: *The Population Dilemma.* Hauser P. M., ed. pp. 125-42. Englewood Cliffs, N.J., Prentice-Hall, 1963.
10. Ward, B. Development: The irreversible revolution. *J. Med. Educ.,* Sept. 1966, p. 5.
11. McDermott, W. Environmental factors bearing on medical education in the developing countries. *J. Med. Educ.* (Part 2) *41*:137, 1966.
12. Walsh, J. Medical education and world health. *New Phys. 18*:819-22, 1969.
13. Douville, A. Medical education and world health (editorial). *New Phys. 18*:803-04, 1969.

MEDICAL RESEARCH ACTIVITIES OVERSEAS*

GUSTAVE J. DAMMIN

Pathologist-in-Chief
Peter Bent Brigham Hospital

Elsie T. Friedman Professor of Pathology
Harvard Medical School

Boston, Mass.

THE time for an analysis of medicine and diplomacy in the tropics is now. I congratulate Dr. Kevin M. Cahill for having planned this symposium and I thank him for including me among the participants. As workers in the health and medical fields, we are more needed in the tropical countries today than ever before. For those of us who were planning our international health programs a decade ago, today must be a sad day, for there has been a great reduction in funds for health and medical research programs in general and for work in the tropical countries in particular. Because of the reduced financial support for overseas programs, I believe that we have been forced into a two-phase effort: today's, for the development of our plans, and tomorrow's, for their implementation. We must pursue our planning in the hope that the day when overseas work can be resumed and new momentum generated by it will be in the foreseeable future. We must see progress soon because there is an urgency about reviving programs now in limbo and initiating new ones, in part because of the broad drive among today's youth to work with the unfortunates of the developing countries in the tropics. This urge to serve is very evident among today's medical and health-science students, and it is a relatively new phenomenon. We should respond to it so that when today's younger students of medicine and the other health sciences are ready to apply themselves in their professional capacities we shall be prepared with plans, programs, and funds.

The extension of medical and health aid by this country to the developing countries of the tropics has been viewed by those countries

*Presented as part of a *Symposium on Medicine and Diplomacy in the Tropics* sponsored by The Tropical Disease Center, St. Clare's Hospital, New York, N.Y., and The Merck Company Foundation, Rahway, N.J., held at the Center, December 13, 1969.

in various lights. However, almost irrespective of its origin—whether the assistance has been offered by governmental, industrial, philanthropic, religious, or other agency—such aid in general has been welcomed and accepted in the light in which it has been offered. Until a few years ago our allocations of funds for overseas medical research were still expanding. We are now at the end of a decade which began with a breadth of national purposes that included the extension of our medical knowledge and wherewithal to the many developing countries so badly in need of them. It was in 1959 that the National Academy of Sciences-National Research Council (NAS-NRC) undertook, as Dr. Keith Cannan summarized it, "a study of the needs and resources for research in the broad field of tropical health."[1] When the study was published in 1962, Dr. Albert Sabin recorded in its preface the collective opinion of his group, the NAS-NRC Advisory Committee on Tropical Medicine:

> It is an inescapable fact that history, having brought the United States to a position of leadership in the world, has imposed on it a responsibility to support the efforts of other peoples to improve their health and welfare.[2]

The Committee also noted:

> Specifically there is need to establish authority to support research on problems that are important as problems of the tropics and not because their solutions may contribute indirectly to the health of the people residing in the United States.[3]

It was during the deliberations of the committee on the problems of tropical health that the International Health Research Act of 1960 was passed; this stimulated a substantial increase in research activities in this field. Unfortunately the last years of this decade have seen a serious reduction in such support, and to a level from which recovery will be slow, difficult, and costly.

Planning for tomorrow requires that we know about past efforts, especially those of the recent past, since we must plan for a world which is in many ways new. The United Nations, which now represents 126 countries, tells us in one way how new today's world is. As we look for guidance on the development of overseas medical research programs we find that medical research itself is a relatively new development in this country.[4, 5] In writing about the beginnings of organized medical research in the United States, Sigerist[6] set the date as

1893, the year in which the Johns Hopkins Medical School was opened. Shryock,[7] a fellow medical historian, chose 1895 as the year in which American medical research entered its independent stage; previous efforts in American medical research had been dominated in succession by Great Britain, France, and Germany. There can be little dispute with this choice of dates if one refers to the beginnings of independent and organized medical research in this country. However, there had been occasional American medical research efforts that were truly pioneering, neither prompted nor guided from abroad. In this category belongs the work of William Beaumont, the first and the leading American clinical investigator for many years. Beaumont's studies of gastric function more than 100 years ago led Sir William Osler to describe him as "The pioneer physiologist of the United States and the first to make a contribution of enduring value, his work remains a model of patient, persevering research."[8]

A search for the beginnings of American medical research overseas shows that they coincided with the first military effort that took large numbers of American troops overseas, namely, the Spanish-American War. It was the scientific developments of the latter decades of the 19th century that provided the stimulus to examine the infectious diseases that assumed such great importance in the tropics. The bacteriological discoveries in France and Germany were cheered and welcomed in this country, and by no one with more enthusiasm than George Miller Sternberg, Surgeon General of the Army from 1893 to 1902. General Sternberg exploited these discoveries to benefit American medicine and launched the "bacteriological era" in this country. He founded the Army Medical School soon after his appointment as Surgeon General and appointed the Reed-Vaughn-Shakespeare Typhoid Board in 1898 and the Walter Reed Yellow Fever Commission in 1900. He was responsible also for research programs in the tropical diseases of the Philippines and of Panama.[9] Thus, armed with the newer methods for the investigation of the infectious diseases of the tropics, the army took the lead in epidemiological and laboratory research on the major bacterial, viral, mycotic, and parasitic diseases of the tropics.[10]

That was certainly another time and another day. The leaders in military medicine—Sternberg, along with Walter Reed, John Shaw Billings, and William Gorgas among others—ranked in eminence with the outstanding figures in medicine of that day: Osler, Pepper, Welch, Councilman, Delafield, and Fitz.[11] Their associations through common interests were such that whatever distinctions may have existed between military medicine and medicine in that day are not perceptible today.

It should be noted that the then newly organized Association of American Physicians held its first annual meeting, in 1886, in Washington, D.C., in the reading room of the Army Medical Museum. It was at this meeting that Councilman presented a paper on certain elements found in the blood in malarial fever. Councilman suspected that by staining he had demonstrated the plasmodia of malaria. Osler, in his discussion of Councilman's paper, drew on the blackboard the structures he had seen in fresh preparations of the peripheral blood which he thought to be vacuoles rather than organisms in the erythrocytes. Sternberg entered the discussion and sided with Councilman against Osler; he stated that by staining the red cells parasites and not vacuoles could be visualized.[12] Sternberg mixed not only with this elite group, but ultimately rose to the presidency of both the American Medical Association and the American Public Health Association.

Although work on the diseases of the tropics continued in this country and abroad during the early decades of the present century, efforts to continue overseas research stations did not thrive, and few survived. Not until 1939, when a limited national emergency was proclaimed by President Franklin D. Roosevelt, were plans developed for a resumption of overseas work. Early in 1941 the Surgeon General of the Army announced the establishment of a system of corps area and department laboratories.[13] These were to be essentially public health laboratories for field and laboratory research. The former were to serve the corps areas in the continental United States and the latter were to be located in the Canal Zone, Puerto Rico, Hawaii, and the Philippines. In the Canal Zone the Gorgas Hospital and the adjacent Board of Health Laboratory together served the Panama Canal Department as a Department Laboratory. For the Puerto Rican Department a laboratory building was constructed in San Juan. This was begun in mid-1941 and opened for service in February 1942. In Hawaii and the Philippines existing laboratory facilities were designated as Department Laboratories. However, the Hawaiian Department became part of a larger command and was served first by a Medical Field Laboratory and then a Medical General Laboratory. Because of enemy action, the

Philippine Department was never served by a Department Laboratory although the services of such a laboratory would have been provided by the Sternberg General Hospital in Manila. With World War II under way, a wide variety of medical laboratories served in tropical areas. The army had Medical General Laboratories in Hawaii and the southwest Pacific, and half of its Medical Field Laboratories were stationed in tropical areas. The navy established its famous Naval Medical Research Unit No. 2 (NAMRU-2) on Guam, and one of the army's medical field laboratories, the well-known 406th Medical Laboratory, was stationed first in the Tokyo-Yokohama area and then transferred to Zama, west of this area. The build-up of overseas installations continued after the end of World War II, and NAMRU-3 was established near Cairo. NAMRU-2 was reactivated and located in Taipei. The army, in coordination with the Southeast Asia Treaty Organization, set up a research laboratory in Bangkok, Thailand; and in Malaysia a medical-research institute was activated near Kuala Lumpur. The air force inaugurated its epidemiological flight-laboratory system with so-called "epi flights" at Clark Air Force Base in the Philippines and in Izmir, in western Turkey.

This brings us almost to the beginning of the present decade when a unit of the Southeast Asia Treaty Organization (SEATO) laboratory in Bangkok was moved to Dacca, East Pakistan, under the auspices of the State Department and of the National Institutes of Health (NIH), with support from the governments of Pakistan and the United Kingdom. Founded in 1960 as the Pakistan-SEATO Cholera Research Laboratory, the unit has a record of remarkable achievement in the development of newer diagnostic and management procedures and in its studies of the pathogenesis, epidemiology, and control of cholera. This was also the time of the launching of the International Centers for Medical Research and Training (ICMRT) in Calcutta, India; Lahore, West Pakistan; Cali, Colombia; Kuala Lumpur, Malaysia; and San José, Costa Rica. These centers were organized and staffed by American medical schools and funded by the National Institutes of Health. At this time also, funds were increased for the congressionally funded Gorgas Memorial Laboratory in the Republic of Panama, and the Middle America Research Unit was organized by the army and the NIH and installed in the Canal Zone. The Institute for Nutrition in Central America and Panama (INCAP) was founded earlier with assistance from the Pan American Health Organization but then, for a period, also received funds from the National Institutes of Health and the U. S. Army Medical Research and Development Command.

It is clear from a survey of present efforts of governmental agencies that the peak of our commitment and activity in overseas medical research has passed, and that the decline is continuing at a worrisome rate. We should heed the urging of the National Academy of Sciences-National Research Council Advisory Committee on Tropical Medicine, mentioned earlier, to establish an authority which could organize our efforts both here and abroad; we could thereby restore the position of this country in international health research and recapture much of the esteem and goodwill of the rest of the world.

In this summary of overseas medical research I have concentrated on the work of our governmental agencies only because their programs have been so much more familiar to me. More detailed accounts of some of their notable achievements are contained in Dr. Williams' history of the Public Health Service,[14] Dr. Corner's account of NAMRU-2 in his *History of The Rockefeller Institute*,[15] and in a historical review of the army's medical laboratories.[16]

The substantial contributions of agencies not supported by governmental funds are widely known. The outstanding programs of the Rockefeller Foundation in international health research were cited in the National Academy of Sciences-National Research Council's report, *Tropical Health.* The high cost of this important report was shared by the foundation, the National Institutes of Health, and the U. S. Army Medical Research and Development Command; these organizations in concert served as sponsors of the report. Other contributors to the study were the Pan American Health Organization of the World Health Organization (WHO), the Pharmaceutical Manufacturers Association, and the Louisiana State University School of Medicine. The director of the staff that conducted the study was Dr. Willard H. Wright. In referring to sources of information on the several major categories of tropical diseases, Dr. Wright cited the great value of the epidemiological reports of WHO and the epizootiological data published by the Food and Agricultural Organization (FAO). Since the preparation of its report, *Tropical Health*, WHO has shown increasing leadership in the fields covered by the report and has planned larger financial outlays for the coming years.[17]

Over-all funding of tropical-health research about 10 years ago was not large, but was rising. The average annual expenditure of funds from federal sources for the five-year period ending in 1958 was about $6 million, of which almost three fourths was for intramural research. This annual expenditure represented less than 3% of the total allotted from federal sources for biomedical research. In the medical schools tropical health research comprised an even smaller percentage of total biomedical research, somewhat over 1%. The country's drug companies were expending over $5 million per year for tropical health research, and the country's largest private institution, the Rockefeller Foundation, allotted over $1 million for such research.

The recent reduction of funds from federal sources has been accompanied, fortunately, by a rising interest and support from the country's larger foundations and corporations. This encouraging movement is exemplified by the number of private sources which are identified with financing the construction of a health-sciences laboratory building for the Harvard School of Public Health and the funding of some of this school's overseas programs. Helping in the former venture are the Colonial Research Institute, the Rockefeller Foundation, the Kresge Foundation, the John A. Hartford Foundation, and the Wellcome Trust. Among the contributing corporations are the country's leading industrial, banking, and drug companies. In the accompanying table are listed governmental and other contributors to the tropical-health programs sponsored by the Harvard School of Public Health. This tabulation is presented only as a sample of the activities of one educational institution interested in tropical health problems, and this school is selected primarily because of my familiarity with its programs.

There still exist today many of the overseas installations that had their beginnings almost a decade ago. The programs of most have been curtailed and some have been inactivated. Each of these research installations represents an enormous investment in persons and in their careers in the health sciences, in programs, and in goodwill—an investment which should be protected. Support for these installations should be increased so that they can pursue their missions and obligations in the respective geographic areas they serve. However to assure their continued operation, these installations would have to be part of an over-all plan for funding overseas medical research so that a resetting of priorities within any one organization would not jeopardize the op-

HARVARD SCHOOL OF PUBLIC HEALTH — INTERNATIONAL ACTIVITIES

Country	*Program*	*Consultant and/or participant institutions*	*Financial sponsor*
North and Central America			
Canada	Mental health in rural communities	Digby-Annapolis Mental Health Centre, Nova Scotia	NIMH
Bahamas	Tropical public health; family planning clinic; mosquito control studies	Colonial Research Institute	CRI, GRSG
Puerto Rico	Maternal and child health	University of Puerto Rico, Department of Preventive Medicine and Public Health	USPHS, WHO, Children's Bureau and other sources
Haiti	Tropical public health; population studies and family planning clinic	Hôpital Albert Schweitzer	HSPH
Mexico	Rickettsial infections	Instituto de Salubridad y Enfermedades Tropicales	Commission on Rickettsial Diseases, AFEB
South America			
Chile	Epidemiology of abortion; evaluation of fertility control program	University of Chile Medical School, Department of Preventive Medicine	The Rockefeller Foundation
Brazil	Training program for medical students in tropical medicine	University of Bahia Medical School, Bahia	NIAID, USPHS
Colombia	Training program for medical students in tropical nutrition	University of Antioquia (Medellin); National Institute of Nutrition (Bogota)	NIH, AMA
Yugoslavia	Rickettsial infections	Faculty of Medicine, Sarajevo	Commission on Rickettsial Diseases, AFEB
The Middle East and North Africa			
Israel	Nutrition	Hadassah Medical School, Department of Nutrition, Hebrew University	Julian Mack Fund
	Epidemiology of heart disease in siblings	Hadassah Medical School, Department of Medical Ecology, Hebrew University; Israel Institute of Applied Social Research	GRSG, NHI
Lebanon	Trachoma	American University of Beirut, Department of Ophthalmology and Epidemiology	NIAID
Tunisia	Relation between economic development and public health	University of Tunis; Ministries of Health, Education and Foreign Affairs	AID
Saudi Arabia	Trachoma	Arabian American Oil Company, Medical Department	ARAMCO
Asia			
Ceylon	Health care of mothers and children in a rural demonstration area	Department of Preventive Medicine, University of Ceylon	Social and Rehabilitation Service, Children's Bureau
India	Population pressure and health	All-India Institute of Medical Sciences	Ford Foundation, HSPH
	Population analysis in Ganges-Bramaputra Basin	Officials of Governments of India and Pakistan	HSPH

eration of an overseas unit and thereby the over-all plan. At the present time and in the recent past there have been government-supported tropical-health research activities in Japan, East and West Pakistan, India, Panama, Colombia, Costa Rica, Malaysia, Thailand, the Philippines, Taiwan, Turkey, and Egypt. The funding of their programs is determined largely by the mission of the governmental agency responsible for each. Unfortunately, as emphasis on certain components of the mission may change, so will financial support for an activity be altered. It would seem wise therefore, for the future of this government's position in international health research, to have one agency, preferably a nongovernmental one, take the leadership in organizing our assets and capabilities, to assure an optimal breadth of operations in our overseas installations, and to seek to establish others where needed. The Advisory Committee on Tropical Medicine of the National Academy of Sciences-National Research Council saw the need for such an organization and recommended that the academy itself, with its Council, establish a "national program for National research in tropical health." Such a move by the Academy would give a program its most appropriate support and would be in essential accord with the proposal made earlier in this symposium by Dr. John S. Badeau, director of the Middle East Institute.

In closing this review of our country's medical research activities overseas, I must place considerable emphasis on the importance of a matter which, a decade ago, was only beginning to receive attention: namely, control of population. In the developing countries this matter deserves as much attention as the control of infectious diseases and the drive for better nutrition. We must recognize what has been accomplished by the containment of some of the mass-killing diseases and how much of a hazard to world stability and peace the continued increase in the world's population would be if it were concentrated in the economically most depressed areas. The emphasis on family planning and control of population must be even greater today. A grim forecast of the consequences of a lack of planning were well expressed by Dr. Sabin in his report when he stated:

> . . . there are many who believe that the continued acquisition and application of knowledge designed to prolong life and to eliminate the miseries and handicaps of disease, without comparable concurrent activities directed at fertility control, will in

effect, before long, result in the even greater miseries of hunger, poverty and war, and thereby create the greatest potential threat to human survival in all parts of the world.[18]

REFERENCES

1. *Tropical Health: A Report on a Study of Need and Resources.* Division of Medical Sciences. Publication 996, National Academy of Science—National Research Council. Washington, D.C., 1962, page v.
2. Ibid., p. ix.
3. Ibid.
4. *Patterns of Incidence of Certain Diseases Throughout the World. Opportunities for Research Through Epidemiology.* Prepared for the Committee on Government Operations, U.S. Senate, and its Subcommittee on Reorganization and International Organizations; 86th Congress, first session. Washington, D.C., Committee Print, November 9, 1959 (45675).
5. *International Medical Research.* A compilation of background materials. Subcommittee on Reorganization and International Organization pursuant to S. Res. 347, 85th Congress and S. Res. 42, 86th Congress. Senate Report No. 160, April 10, 1969 (38996).
6. Sigerist, H. E.: *American Medicine.* New York, Norton, 1934.
7. Shryock, H.: *American Medical Research.* New York, Commonwealth Fund, 1947.
8. Myer, J. S.: *Life and Letters of Dr. William Beaumont with an Introduction by Sir William Osler.* St. Louis, Mosby, 1912.
9. Bayne-Jones, S.: *The Evolution of Preventive Medicine in the United States Army, 1607-1939,* pp. 118-121. Office of the Surgeon General, Department of the Army. Washington, D.C., Govt. Print. Off., 1968.
10. Ibid., part VII, pp. 123-46.
11. Means, J. H.: *The Association of American Physicians—Its First Seventy-five Years,* chap. 1. New York, McGraw-Hill, 1961.
12. Ibid., pp. 12-13.
13. Letter from the Surgeon General, signed by Col. Larry B. McAfee, M.D., Executive Officer: *Corps Area and Department Laboratories.* January 15, 1941.
14. Williams, R. C.: *The United States Public Health Service, 1798-1950,* pp. 612-768. Washington, D.C., Washington Commissioned Officers Association of the U.S. Public Health Service, 1951.
15. Corner, G. W.: *A History of the Rockefeller Institute, 1901-1953, Origins and Growth,* chap. 20, pp. 523, 571. New York, Rockefeller Inst. Press, 1964.
16. Dammin, G. J. and Robinson, E.: *The History of Preventive Medicine in World War II,* vol. 9. Special Fields, Chap. 7 — The Medical Laboratories. Office of the Surgeon General, Department of the Army. Washington, D.C., Govt. Print. Off., 1970.
17. *WHO Chron. 23*:453, 1969.
18. Sabin, A. B.: *Tropical Health: A Report on a Study of Needs and Resources.* Division of Medical Sciences. Publication 996, National Academy of Sciences — National Research Council, Washington, D.C., 1962, p. x.

OBSERVATIONS ON AMERICA'S INTERNATIONAL MEDICAL PROGRAMS*

GEORGE I. LYTHCOTT

Associate Dean
Office of Urban and Community Health Affairs
Associate Professor of Pediatrics
and Preventive Medicine
Columbia University College of Physicians
and Surgeons
New York, N. Y.

THE subject of American programs of medical assistance for developing countries is one of considerable importance and one in which I have a deep and abiding interest. In my view such programs can have, on the one hand, vast positive implications and rewards and can become a real source of pride for both donor and recipient; on the other hand, without thorough cognizance of the delicate nature of international affairs, without proper thought in its planning and attention to detail in its implementation, official American involvement in international medical programs can indeed become a fiasco.

My experience in the tropics extended over the seven-year period between June 1962 and June 1969; during that time I was stationed in Accra, Ghana, and later in Lagos, Nigeria. I still have continuing involvement in West Africa, which takes me back to the area from time to time, though on a different basis. My responsibilities involved all of West and Central Africa (except for Portuguese Guinea) with limited experience in East and South-Central Africa as well. West and Central Africa is the vast territory bounded on the north by the Sahara Desert, on the west by the Atlantic Ocean, on the south by the Gulf of Guinea and the Bight of Benin, and on the east by the Congo River. This area is inhabited by an estimated 120 million people who speak more than 500 major tribal dialects; the official language of this area, however, is English, French, or Spanish. By 1962 all these countries except Equatorial Guinea had recently become independent of their colonial governments, although the influence of the parent country was

*Presented as part of a *Symposium on Medicine and Diplomacy in the Tropics* sponsored by The Tropical Disease Center, St. Clare's Hospital, New York, N.Y., and The Merck Company Foundation, Rahway, N.J., held at the Center, December 13, 1969.

still manifest to a greater or lesser degree within most of them. By 1962, however, at least three of these newly independent nations had for all practical purposes repudiated their parent countries. The ecology of this 19-country area varies from sandy desert land, with nomadic tribesmen roving willy-nilly across country borders in search of water or commerce, to tropical rain-forest country, inundated with up to 400 inches of rain annually and inhabitated by a virtually stationary population. Customs, culture, and the rhythm of day-to-day living are represented by patterns almost as numerous as the dialects. This cultural heritage, unchanged for centuries, is a source of great pride for each tribe and tribesman. There are several fairly large port and capital cities with quite a cosmopolitan air, and the language, customs, and culture of the ages have inevitably become so dissipated in these urban melting pots that a casual visitor to this area could easily be completely unaware of the very different perspectives, values, and attitudes that make Africa the exciting continent that it is. Common to all these countries, however, are economic instability, poverty, and disease.

My experiences were based on two American international medical programs: the first, a research laboratory created through bilateral agreement between an agency of the U.S. Public Health Service and one of the independent governments in West Africa; the second, a regional program for all 19 West and Central African countries, under the general auspices of the Agency for International Development but under the technical direction of a Bureau of the United States Public Health Service.

The 19-country regional program for the eradication of smallpox has been eminently successful; it is reputed by some to be not only the best medical program mounted by the government of the United States in the developing countries, but also one of the most dramatic and successful American foreign-assistance programs ever—a testimony to the enthusiasm, dedication, knowledge, and meticulous attention to detail of those responsible for it. On November 30, 1969, in the little market village of Burbon, Niger, the 100 millionth vaccination was given, less than three years after the program had begun and more than one year ahead of the timetable the project had set for itself.

The research laboratory, by contrast, was considerably less successful for both the donor and the recipient, culminating for all practical purposes in a premature withdrawal of American personnel. This program, unfortunately, was doomed from its inception by an unusual set of circumstances that included some naïvete, ignorance, and questionable judgment on the parts of many, including myself. Further, the original agreement was drawn up and the American team recruited and dispatched at a time when diplomatic relations between the governments concerned were extremely tenuous. In addition, the scientist responsible for this program in the host country was himself a political refugee from his native country, and his political ideologies were completely antagonistic to those of the West—especially the United States. With more forethought and planning, and especially at a different time in political history, this could have been a most successful venture. Its dedicated senior scientists deserved a better fate.

Despite the second program's lack of success, however, *both* programs offer valuable experiences—some positive, some negative—for medical-assistance programs. Additional insights were provided during this period by my constant exposure to other official and private-sector medical programs in West Africa, including the Peace Corps and the whole spectrum of missionary effort. My observations, therefore, issue from all these experiences and reflect the pertinent practical issues that have crystallized during the last several years.

I use the terms "official American programs" or "official programs" in this discussion to refer to programs federally supported through active government agencies such as the Agency for International Development (AID), the Peace Corps, and the military—as distinct from medical programs sponsored by private groups, including missionary activity. Before approaching some of the practical aspects of the official American medical experience in emerging countries, I should like to examine the relation between this experience and the broad issues of politics and diplomacy. For these are the issues that significantly influence international medical programs, and discussion of them is essential in creating a frame of reference for my subsequent observations.

By technical definition, politics and diplomacy are not synonymous. "Politics" carries the unfavorable connotations of deviousness, of capriciousness, of expediency, and of partisan scheming. "Diplomacy," on the other hand, is reserved for the epitome of sophisticated social intercourse and it somehow seems very grand, even exemplary, and most palatable indeed. In practical parlance and in colloquial use, however, the onus of politics frequently attaches itself to diplomacy. It is important in this discussion, then, to recognize that to many people these terms are kissing cousins. This will help us appreciate the problems inherent in a discussion of medicine and diplomacy in the tropics. One could not hope to find two more incongruous bedfellows than medicine and politics—with medicine enunciating the brotherhood of man under the Hippocratic oath and politics enunciating its philosophies of expediency and factionalism. Yet in my experience I found them inseparable.

Dr. Kevin M. Cahill, writing in the *New York State Journal of Medicine* in 1967 on the subject of this symposium,* stated, "Anyone visiting or working in a foreign country becomes involved—willingly or unwillingly, wittingly or unwittingly—in the political intercourse of his native and the host nation." A tourist, an itinerant working student, a sailor calling in port are all similarly affected. When that person visiting or working in a foreign country is an American, representing the richest and one of the two most powerful nations in the world, it is difficult for him to escape the onus of being a political animal —no matter how apolitical he might be or may feel in this situation. Further, when an American is an official government representative visiting or working in an emerging country, the responsibility of coping with the politics of the United States and the host nation becomes impossible to escape. An official American in medicine overseas is no more and no less fortunate in this respect than his counterparts in agriculture, technology, education, or business enterprise. Medicine delivered in this context has no special license that would elevate it beyond this realm.

This phenomenon—which sometimes attracts suspicion, sometimes antagonism—may on the other hand force the official American into the role of a savior, a harbinger of all solutions—and he may well fall heir to the ensuing disappointment when "all" things fail to materialize. The thrust of the American position on issues must never be underestimated, even when our judgment is being made solely in the context of American affairs and when no real attempt is being made to influence the position of other nations. The U.N. Food and Agriculture Organization, for example, is becoming deeply concerned by the reaction in many emerging countries to the American position on DDT. Because the United States decided to ban the use of DDT by

*Cahill, K. M. Medicine and diplomacy in the tropics. *N.Y.J. Med. 67*:2229, 1967.

1971 for reasons we all know, the developing countries are suggesting that they must take the same position—thus discounting the necessity of DDT and dieldrin for their proved beneficial effects on health, agriculture, and economics in these countries.

Most physicians feel that medicine is a pure discipline which, ideally, should be extracted from the suspicion and vagaries that surround other forms of foreign assistance and that medical aid should be offered solely according to the needs of the recipient, rather than according to the political strategies of the donor nation. Moreover, we know well the great need for medical assistance to the emerging countries. And while one can hardly separate the priorities for assistance in health, education, technology, or agriculture, it is evident that health is the common denominator for the effective implementation of all these. We know that infectious diseases and malnutrition, singly and especially in combination, impose the greatest threat to life. Further, accumulating evidence indicates the direct relation between malnutrition and mental retardation—that malnutrition is capable of producing irreversible damage to the learning apparatus of children. Thus when we consider the ecology of human societies, physical well-being must be considered one of the most important limiting factors in this dynamic equilibrium.

We know that half the deaths in the developing countries occur among children under six years of age. In many African countries a mother must bear five children to assure that even one reaches the age of 15. We know that in Northeast Brazil, 48% do not survive the first year of life; by the age of four, 63% have succumbed. In parts of Southeast Asia 40% of the children die of disease in their first four years. This proportion of deaths is not reached in the United States until the age of 60.

Thus the potential for spectacular improvement in the health of the populations of emerging countries stems from two factors: 1) the health problems are so great to begin with, and 2) the present facilities and technology for dealing with them are generally so limited. Medical assistance, then, should be provided because the need is there—a lesson learned long ago by the missionary groups in their broad and redounding experience in the emerging countries. When the missionary groups first ventured into the underexplored areas of the world, medical personnel generally accompanied the missionaries abroad for the sheer survival of the clergy. Survival in those days was of paramount importance—in Accra, Ghana, there is a cemetery which was used only for the Europeans who arrived during the early 19th century. The gravestones are marked with the date of arrival in Accra and the date of death; all but three of some 250 persons succumbed during the first year in the tropics. Indeed, the coast of West Africa earned the name "The White Man's Grave."

As the years passed and medical knowledge increased, the physicians in the missionary groups, due to their growing familiarity with the communities they had come to love, began responding on an ad hoc basis to the desperate health needs of the indigenes. More recently church boards have changed their emphasis from proselytizing, with medical assistance as a secondary goal, to providing medical assistance as a separate objective with no strings attached, in concert with the primary goal of proselytizing. This medical assistance now often includes preventive as well as curative medicine. That some identity has been lost in this change in focus has disturbed the international Christian community not at all.

Today's official agencies would do well to heed this imperative: to heal the sick *because they are sick.* It took the Peace Corps several years to embrace this point of view. Like the missionaries, the Peace Corps originally recruited physicians solely for the medical care of Peace Corps volunteers. The Peace Corps too has been through the intermediate ad hoc phase, but it now expects to mount structured medical programs in public health for its host communities, with the same sort of emphasis and care given to its successful projects in education, agriculture, and so on.

Nonetheless, even if government agencies do gradually respond directly to the pressing health needs of the host communities, medical-assistance programs delivered in this setting will still carry political overtones. If we are to operate official medical programs, we must be prepared to accept this political element as a fact of daily life; otherwise we must go outside the government enclave altogether and create new vehicles for the delivery of medical assistance. I realize that creating mechanisms outside the political environment by no means guarantees freedom from politics. It would, however, reduce the political onus to a level with which most people here and abroad could live.

Yet operation of medical-aid programs within the official government setting seems to be the working reality for the time being. And if we are to operate successful programs in this setting we must recognize the unfortunate image our official setting evokes abroad and accept the political responsibilities that come with the program. It then becomes incumbent upon us to create programs with so much relevance, quality, and appeal that their success is assured even in this political milieu. It also behooves us to take the same great pains in their planning and administration that we do in the more obvious arenas of political and diplomatic intercourse. It is naïve indeed to acknowledge in principle that medical programs are perceived through a politico-diplomatic prism, but to plan, develop, and implement them as if they constituted a pure, uncomplicated scientific venture—and then expect them to be successful. As with programs of the highest political and diplomatic priority, a successful medical-assistance project must be based on research in depth that not only provides a theoretical knowledge of the proposed program but that also assures its practical relevance and adaptability to the foreign clime. The details of implementing the program must also reflect these political and diplomatic considerations.

The overriding principle in medical assistance to emerging nations is to create, develop, and administer programs that satisfy a priority *need* of the recipient, bringing to bear the particular skills which the donor possesses. The determination of that priority need must rest ultimately with the recipient, for only he knows what his priorities are at a given time and only he can assess the full gamut of factors that must influence his judgment.

On the other hand, of course, the donor and other international authorities can *assist* the recipient in arriving at its priorities. The donor might make available modern technological approaches to research and fact-finding, or he might lend personnel to work in concert with indigenous experts to help them put the issues into better focus. For example, according to all significant parameters, medical assistance to emerging countries should take the form of preventive rather than curative medical programs, although this concept still presents problems both at home and abroad. A donor who is asked to advise on an issue can only negotiate: if he fails in negotiation, he fails, and that's part of the game, for the ultimate judgment on needs and priorities must rest with the emerging country.

I am reminded of an incident that occured in India about two years ago. India, a huge area of endemic smallpox, was in the upswing of its epidemic curve for this disease when the program director was informed that the stock of smallpox vaccine was rapidly becoming depleted. India accordingly made a request to the World Health Organization for 10 million doses of multiple pressure vaccine to be administered by the traditional method of scarification. WHO passed the request on to the United States government, and from there it went to the National Communicable Disease Center in Atlanta, Ga. All of us in the smallpox program, both at headquarters in Atlanta and in the field, were delighted with the request. Here at last was a chance to help India solve its smallpox problem with the mass vaccination techniques which had proved so effective in West Africa: by use of the jet-injector, an instrument capable of vaccinating 1,000 people an hour. The response to the request for 10 million doses of multiple pressure vaccine was answered, then, with 10 million doses of *jet-injector* vaccine (and the promise of more to come), 50 jet-injectors, and two epidemiologists to advise on mass programs and train personnel in use of the jet-injector.

The epidemiologists arrived with all their gear, began training people, and mounted pilot projects to demonstrate the efficacy of the injector and their techniques. Finally they were ready for the mass campaign to begin. But nothing happened. Meeting after endless meeting, one fruitless conference after another occurred until it became patently clear that the Ministry of Health had no intention of mounting the type of campaign envisaged by the visitors. Confused and frustrated, the epidemiologists were moved to ask at a meeting what the problem was. An official of the ministry replied with a rhetorical question that demonstrated how completely the needs and desires of the recipient nation had been neglected in the enthusiasm of the donor. He responded most politely, "Gentlemen, if someone gave you an elephant as a sign of friendship, what would you say?"

The skills offered by the donor must not only be oriented toward the recipient's concept of its needs but must also reflect the specific characteristics of the country involved–its cultural attitudes, logistics, geography, climate, systems of administrations, and its economic and human resources. These differences among countries and peoples often make it impossible to mount a program in country *Y*, even when it has worked effectively in country *X*. If medical-assistance programs are to be planned carefully, well-developed, and efficiently administered, they must be formulated not only on the basis of the solid theoretical knowledge available on the subject but also on appropriate prior homework for each program site.

A true story is told about a physician who became alarmed over his inability to keep a generator-driven freezer at optimal levels to preserve the heat-labile vaccine he was administering. The man cabled his headquarter base for advice and the answer came by return cable: he was advised to park his truck under a tree, where the temperature would be a few degrees cooler—not an unreasonable answer if he were working in a park, but distinctly inappropriate for a physician working in a sub-Saharan country on the fringes of the desert in an ambient temperature of 120 degrees. This example underscores the value of doing the proper homework, and that, before the fact.

It is also important both in negotiating programs and in implementing them to take into consideration the growing nationalism in the newly independent countries. Implicit here is an awareness of the sensitivities one can expect to encounter at all levels of activity. These nations are just now developing their technology, to be sure, but they have a culture which has been fully developed for centuries and of which they are justifiably proud. It is often difficult for some who have been indoctrinated into thinking of these areas as the "underdeveloped" world to recognize that they have *anything* of value to offer or to be taken into account when programs are being developed there.

It is certainly in the interest of the donor country to see that its medical assistance has a unique appeal for the host country and is perceived in as favorable a light as possible. And it is in the interest of the recipient country for assistance to be delivered as efficiently as possible. These are not incompatible interests!

With competent leadership it is easy to make a basically good program successful. On the other hand, even with genius at the helm, it is impossible to sustain one badly conceived.

The success of the 19-country program for the eradication of smallpox illustrates the effectiveness of giving full consideration to the factors we have discussed. First, the program was designed to respond to a long-standing medical priority in many of these West African countries, and this need had been enunciated for a long time by the

World Health Organization as well as by the involved countries. Smallpox had been a scourge to many communities, killing and maiming countless thousands for generations. In 1965 the World Health Organization reaffirmed an earlier unsuccessful position it had taken on global eradication, but this time the assembly requested that its more affluent member states provide bilateral assistance to those countries in which smallpox was endemic. In immediate response to this request, the government of the United States committed itself to work with other interested countries in eradicating the disease and agreed to take the original 19 contiguous sub-Saharan countries of West Africa as its responsibility. The Agency for International Development delegated the responsibility for vaccinating 120 million people in an area larger than the United States itself to the National Communicable Disease Center in Atlanta. The center then set out to plan and develop this program.

I recall that active planning for this program began more than a year before the first American advisor departed for his assigned country. I recall that American experts were in the field visiting each of the 19 countries a year before the American teams arrived in order to familiarize themselves with all the practical data necessary for complete and efficient planning. I also recall that 10 months before the American teams arrived in Africa, the National Communicable Disease Center convened an expert committee on the subject "Smallpox Eradication in a Developing Country"—a group made up of professionals from all over the world who assisted in planning the technical aspects of the program. I recall our scouring the nation to find Americans with firsthand knowledge of modern Africa to recruit some of the finest young men and young women in our land who would serve either as physician-epidemiologists or as public-health administrators and who would be the program's envoys and resident advisors in each country. These men and women were carefully selected not only for their expertise in epidemiology, disease control, and public-health practices but also with specific regard to their motivations and general suitability for the envisioned African experience. Further, the health workers were given a 10-week course before departure that covered not only the technical aspects of the program but also every recognizable discipline that might prove advantageous to their advisory function: culture, geography, politics, and economy plus extended training in the official language of the country to which they were to be assigned.

Unfortunately, however, the principles underlying this program represent the exception, not the rule. Too many medical programs theoretically designed to assist emerging countries are in fact developed around the needs or priorities of the donor country or, to put it in truly colonial terms, are based on what the donor country *believes* the needs of the recipient country are or should be. Even when overriding evidence indicates that the needs identified by the donor nation are valid, it is in my view a crass error—and, indeed, an inappropriate assumption of prerogatives—for a donor nation to attempt to force acceptance of medical programs on emerging countries. If we foist a medical principle upon an emerging country by threatening to withhold all other assistance unless the country complies we must stand guilty of the worst kind of political intrigue; and under these circumstances we can forget whatever remains of the humane principles underlying the medical assistance offered.

Because of the growing crescendo of utterances on population control, I am constrained to present this as a pressing example. There is a suggestion that the federal government may well withhold all types of assistance from countries which fail to subscribe to modern concepts of population control and which do not set out to implement them. Equally deplorable is the suggestion attributed to a spokesman for the World Bank that all future development loans to emerging countries may be contingent upon the adoption of population-control programs. In addition, there are the unconscionable expressions of some experts who would have our government put sterility drugs in reservoirs and in food shipped to foreign countries in order to limit human multiplication.*

Many ongoing health programs that are saving lives daily in emerging countries are already in jeopardy of being curtailed or eliminated because of the cutbacks in foreign aid and foreign spending by the United States and other countries, and also because of the presently inadequate funding of the World Health Organization.† To limit these

*Dr. Paul Ehrlich, at the U.S. National Commission for UNESCO 1969 Biennial Conference on *Man and His Environment* held at San Francisco, Calif., November 23 to 25, 1969. Quoted in the *New York Times,* November 28, 1969.

†See, for example, R. W. Apple, Jr. Vital foreign aid drying up in black Africa. The *New York Times,* November 24, 1969.

programs even further by attaching a population-control prerequisite is completely unjustifiable in humanitarian or ethical terms.

How do the potential recipients of population-control assistance view this issue? Specifically, in most of sub-Saharan Africa, promotion of population-control measures is perceived by many native health authorities and statesmen as a subtle but hostile attempt to limit the power of these countries. These officials firmly believe they need *more* people, not less, in order to become viable nations. This position is more understandable when one recalls that in 1967 a South African "expert" recommended compulsory birth control for black Rhodesians and birth promotion with incentives for whites!

And in fact this problem of interpretation is by no means limited to the African continent. In travels around the country attending meetings and seminars on urban and community health—in San Francisco, in New York, in Los Angeles, in Boston—one hears loud outcries from ghetto residents expressing their distaste and suspicion of family-planning programs as separate activities, when there are so many inequities and gaps existing in the more conventional health services. It behooves us, then, not only to listen, but to heed!

And, indeed, in West Africa several objective factors lend support to the opposition of inhabitants to population-control measures. First, in terms of population distribution, West Africa is relatively underpopulated. Second, as we have already noted, the mortality rate for children in the emerging countries is exceptionally high. Everyone has a basic right to "immortality," and in affluent societies the probability of achieving it exists through many mechanisms. For the desperately poor farmer in Ghana or Mali, however, his only hope for such immortality lies with his descendants, and I am concerned that we weigh this consideration so lightly.

Third, since West Africa lacks formal governmental systems for welfare and old-age assistance, children represent the only form of social security that aging parents have. The extended-family system common throughout West Africa represents more than a familial sharing of benefits and misfortunes: it means that whatever belongs to one member of the family becomes the property of the whole family, so that old age accompanied by the growth and production of many children and grandchildren is eagerly anticipated, not dreaded, as contrasted with our more impersonal social system. There are myriad factors governing human multiplication, and all these factors must be taken into consideration.

So, I submit, we must show parents in these emerging countries that their children can survive to adulthood, show them the fullness of life through health, education, and economic development, and they will limit their own families. The educated and affluent African knows what family planning is all about. But he represents only about 2% of the population, and this proportion must be increased enormously before the posture of the population-control experts can become comprehensible—or even tenable.

In summarizing this particular issue, let me add that there are strong, logical arguments which clearly indicate the wisdom of population control, and with these I have no contention. This issue, however, is so provocative and so emotionally charged that under no circumstance should acceptance of family-planning measures be stipulated as a prerequisite for anything — certainly not for desperately needed programs of foreign assistance! Such an approach is not only likely to be rejected itself but would also reduce receptivity to other more rational approaches—and half a loaf is better than none.

Instead of single-thrust or forced population-control measures, foreign assistance in medicine should be offered through a comprehensive, integrated program focusing on the total family. It should provide ongoing assistance in preventive public-health measures, health education, home economics, and sanitation, along with complete family-planning programs which should address themselves to the problems of subfertility as well. When these public-health programs are available in concert with traditional foreign assistance in education, agricultural development, and industrial development—all within a comprehensive foreign-aid philosophy—the ethics of birth control will become academic for many, and acceptance or rejection as a principle will lie where it belongs: with the individual, according to his own personal values.

Beyond satisfying a priority need in a recipient country, the basic justification for foreign medical assistance, it seems to me, is the building and development of institutions and the training of personnel, both planned so they can be expanded or modified to accommodate the delivery of other health programs at a future time. Programs planned and developed without heed to this underlying goal, no matter how well meant, how prestigious, or how glamorous, represent a luxury that developing countries can ill afford and beg the question of total national development in an emerging country.

In the West African program for the eradication of smallpox, fewer than 50 American trainer-advisors participated in the development of more than 4,000 indigenous Africans who learned to function in all program disciplines and at every level of supervision, based on their specific talents and experience. The African personnel actually carried out the smallpox program—a system that provided at least three rewards:

1) It developed a multidisciplined cadre of health workers specifically trained in the skills necessary to carry out their own duties; moreover, these workers were exposed to a complex program that allowed them to appreciate the relation of their contribution to the many other disciplines involved in the total effort.

2) These health workers developed the pride in accomplishment that is so necessary to continued involvement, morale, and fulfillment.

3) The institutions developed and the skills learned by the personnel can be modified to meet the delivery of other health services for the nation. For example, all these countries now have a built-in mechanism for responding to epidemics in the future or, more routinely, they can deliver other immunizations, as for polio, tetanus, and yellow fever. And with appropriate retraining these teams could effectively tackle the delivery of altogether different health services.

One final consideration seems essential in discussing how to make programs for foreign medical assistance more attractive and useful to the emerging countries. The developing countries in which I have had experience have created or are creating "development plans" for five-year periods. Some countries have already consummated their five-year plans and now have 10-year development plans in operation. These development plans, unique for each country, are created within a system that establishes priorities, coordinates related activities and programs, and reconciles the envisioned programs with available manpower and budgetary determinations. These plans are predicated to some extent, of course, on certain expectations of foreign assistance from given sources.

These long-term guidelines and priorities in the emerging countries would seem to offer an excellent opportunity for coordinated multiple-donor-nation activity. If each nation would coordinate its contribution with those of other donors, measurable portions of the five- and ten-year plans could be expedited from year to year in an orderly fashion. Unfortunately, since donor nations regard their assistance programs to emerging countries as private preserves, as tools of political strategy, each seeks to develop so complete a package that the recipient cannot possibly resist. This would be the best of all possible worlds if the recipient nation could actually accept all the packages offered. Paradoxically, however, one important factor prevents this: the recipient country's own lack of resources, both human and financial.

I am reminded of a provocative suggestion made by the Director General of Health in the Gambia, that tiny slip of a country along the shores of the Gambia River with a population of about 285,000. When asked at an early stage why the Gambia was progressing so slowly in the organization and planning of its smallpox program, he replied, "Why don't you donor countries and agencies get together and coordinate your offers of assistance in health programs instead of coming to us individually with something new and attractive? Our needs are so great that we can use almost any sort of assistance in health programs, but our personnel and financial resources are so limited that developing a new program frequently means removing personnel from other programs." The pièce de résistance was his statement that "We don't dare turn you down for fear that you'll become provoked, and then you may not make us another offer for several years."

A look at one small coastal West African country of 2.3 million inhabitants amply illustrates this point. No fewer than nine Western nations supply assistance to this country for health programs, agricultural and industrial development, and education. The support is channeled through 12 independent projects which are totally uncoordinated —even within the health field itself. This lack of coordination among the donors has forced the recipient government to shift national priorities, rotate civil servants from project to project, and juggle the budget of the realm to meet its commitments to each foreign donor.

As a result of this uncoordinated donor activity, the ministries of health in emerging countries find themselves embroiled in foreign-assistance programs which are begun and abandoned or are staggering along with no hope of successful conclusion, programs which represent scattered thrusts in terms of meeting the total needs, and programs which at best overlap and frequently duplicate effort. Clearly this situation is a luxury that none can afford.

I have tried to present some of the influences and observations that have surfaced during my active participation in official American medical programs and from my exposure to others in developing countries. I should like to summarize these as follows:

We have examined at some length the gap between the ideal and the real relation between medicine and diplomacy. While I share the view of many that, ideally, these disciplines should provide a unique and effective resource for the delivery of health assistance to emerging countries, the fact is that they do not. We have suggested, then, some influences that must be taken into account if we are to overcome this unfortunate situation.

We have pointed out that infectious diseases and malnutrition in childhood pose the greatest threat to life in the developing countries, and we have given evidence to support the overwhelming mortality rate among children in these countries as contrasted with our own. The desperate *need* for assistance, then, is there.

We have emphasized the importance of the donor's satisfying a priority need of the recipient and have stressed that the determination of that need must, in the final analysis, rest with the recipient.

A related tenet is that in responding with the required skills to recipient-set priorities, the donor country must do its homework *before* developing programs—taking full account of all the vagaries that may exist in a given program site.

We have deplored the blackmail implicit in making foreign medical assistance contingent upon *anything* and have made a special issue of population control, which looms as the most forbidding example in this context. We have suggested a reasonable alternative to this all-or-nothing approach.

We have suggested that the pervading philosophy in the development of medical programs in emerging countries must be the building of institutions and the training of skilled personnel—both capable of adaptation to the delivery of other health efforts in the future.

We have emphasized that the increasing reliance of the emerging nations on five- and ten-year development plans affords an excellent opportunity for donor nations to coordinate their programs of medical assistance. Such a coordination of health assistance would avoid duplication and wasted efforts and, most important, would allow the recipient nations to deploy their limited personnel and financial resources far more efficiently than at present.

Finally, if we really cared, we could and should rethink and restructure our entire administrative mechanism for delivering programs of medical assistance to developing countries. If we really cared, we should be willing to forego a bit of national prestige and, if necessary, to dilute our official identity in order to provide medical assistance where it best meets the need. Are there not areas other than the delivery of health services in which we could sustain our prestige and identity if we really cared? And could we not let the virtue of providing medical assistance to those who need it be its own reward, if we really cared?

EMPYEMA OR HYDROTHORAX IN THE NINETY-FIFTH DOGE OF VENICE*

SAUL JARCHO

BEFORE the concept of heart failure reached its present stage of clarity and acceptance, the subject was enmeshed in almost hopeless confusion. This can be demonstrated readily if we take as a test object a single important gross alteration, namely hydrothorax. Until comparatively recent times hydrothorax caused by disease of the heart could not be differentiated from hydrothorax caused by inflammation (including tuberculosis) or by neoplastic disease. Moreover, until thoracic percussion and auscultation gained general application—at least a decade *after* Laennec—the diagnosis of hydrothorax depended chiefly on the clinical history, and historical data often did not allow the physician to ascertain whether an effusion was unilateral or bilateral.

The difficulties of the clinician can best be understood by the selection, examination, and analysis of old clinical reports.[1] While this usually involves the tedious labor of translation and must often be complicated by a protracted search of supplementary sources, the process yields rewards. It clarifies the problems which the physician confronted and the conceptions that underlay his incomplete knowledge. And often it brings in a harvest of incidental detail, usually in the form of social or political information.

In the present case the background is exceptional and impressive. The patient was Francesco Contarini (1556-1624), 95th Doge of the Venetian Republic. He belonged to a family which had been regarded as patrician as early as the 11th century and which had given the republic eight doges and many other eminent citizens.

Francesco Contarini[2] was both a cultivated and an experienced man. He had written a history of the wars of the Turks. He had held 10 ambassadorial posts and had filled important positions in the central administration of the republic. He had been sent to England in 1609

*Based on research assisted by the National Institutes of Health (HE-10948).

as a special envoy to James I.[3] He had been given the rank of *chevalier* by Henry IV of France.

His physician, Johannes Praevotius (Jean Prevost, 1585-1631),[4] was likewise a man of distinction. After early studies in theology he turned to medicine and was graduated at Padua in 1607. He later held professorships of medicine and botany at that university. His writings dealt chiefly with materia medica and therapeutics. The most famous, the *Medicina Pauperum*, was first published in Frankfurt in 1641 and was reprinted repeatedly. A collected edition of Praevotius' writings appeared in 1656 under the editorship of J. Stephanus.[5]

The present case report was published by Georgius Hieronymus Velschius (1624-1677) as Section 7 (pp. 7-10) of his *Observationum medicinalium episagmata centum*, which forms the seventh and penultimate part of his *Sylloge curationum et observationum medicinalium*, published by G. Goebelius at Augsburg in 1667.[6] As the reader will observe, Velschius states that he records the case "in the words of that most distinguished man Johannes Prevotius." Although this signifies direct quotation, I have been unable to find a corresponding original in the writings of Praevotius.

Velschius (Georg Hieronymus Welsch)[7] was *Stadtarzt* at Augsburg. His published works consist largely of casebooks, of which the *Sylloge* is a typical example. He also wrote an *exercitatio* or essay on the dracunculus or guinea worm, published at Augsburg in 1674.

Fever from Abscess and Dropsy of the Lungs

Very rare is the disease which was fatal to a great prince and which I record in the words of that most distinguished man Johannes Prevotius.

His Most Serene Highness Francesco Contarini, the doge of Venice, died on December 6, 1625 at the twenty-third hour. I had been summoned to Venice on three occasions because of his illness and had debated it under various designations with other physicians who disagreed with me.

On the very day of the summer solstice the patient had fallen into very sharp colicky pains, to which he was subject. On the following day he had hardly been relieved by means of hot remedies when he developed a fever which had the character of a double tertian and returned, sometimes ahead of schedule for a few days and sometimes delayed for an equal length of time or even longer. Insomnia and thirst were annoying until the seventh day. At that time after mild medication a bilious diarrhoea started; it continued until the fortieth day. From the eleventh day the urine always appeared to be of moderate consistence. It was usually reddish and abundant, now with a white and thin sediment, now with a suspension that was of good color, thin, and sufficiently coherent. The patient also had a mild little cough, by which he brought up a small amount of thick phlegm. His breathing was quite free. However it was hard for him to lie on either side. He always responded well to whatever was done for him. His pulses were large and stronger than was appropriate to his age. At the fortieth day the fever seemed to remit and no exacerbation was present. The stools began to have consistence and proper color. The pulses continued to be vigorous but still had a certain unnatural rapidity. The patient never recovered his appetite.

The fever would return manifestly at intervals of 8 to 10 days and ended in two or three attacks after a gentle evacuation of the bowel, either spontaneous or produced by an enema or by very mild medication.

The patient continued to have a slight cough and to experience difficulty when he lay down. Toward the equinox his usual cough and catarrh increased; in other respects he remained as before until the beginning of October, greatly emaciated. At that time the fever came back twice on alternate days, but was accompanied by such great difficulty in breathing and such anxiety at the beginning of the attack that he could hardly overcome these two recurrences. However, after much bile had been evacuated by the help of a clyster, the fever manifestly stopped. Then he passed almost a whole month quietly and, if you except the slight cough, the difficulty in lying on either side, and the lack of appetite—these never subsided—His Highness appeared to have reached convalescence. He would sleep; he would eat without nausea; he sometimes arose from bed, even alone and without support; he walked about for a short while and his pulse was constant and strong, just as it had been at the beginning of the illness.

About the beginning of December he had sudden difficulty in breathing, with anxiety and a lower fever that was indistinct in its approach on alternate days, with anxiety, laborious panting, and remarkable inequality and smallness of the pulse. He had to sleep almost upright and could not rest on either side. Loud abdominal noises were heard and because of flatulence it was often difficult for him to swallow food and drink. With difficulty he spat up thick ashen and yellowish matter that resembled something rotten. The urine was thick and had an abundant thick sediment. On December 6 at the beginning of an attack he died of the vehemence of the aforementioned symptoms,[9] although from the condition of pulse, examined a short time previously, it was believed that he could live until the next day.

The Venetian physicians constantly attributed his sickness to intense heat of the liver and to dryness of the lung, which they believed to be consumed and dessicated. Therefore they never wanted to use honeyed and sugared substances and other aperient and cleansing substances and drugs that to a moderate extent remove catarrh and also strengthen the stomach and the lungs.

On the seventh [of December] the body was opened while I was present as an observer. All the intestines, small and large, were distended with flatus. The liver was swollen and resembled a sponge full of a white matter which had removed all the redness of the organ so that the parenchyma, cut in different directions, appeared white all over. The cavity of the chest contained about five pounds of watery matter. The flaccid right part of the lung appeared to be full of thick mucous fluid. The left had turned entirely into a whitish gore, which was contained in the pulmonary tunic[10] as if in a sac. When this was cut apart, about 16 ounces of matter flowed out into the thoracic cavity. No trace of lung remained on the left side except the mark of the membrane which adhered to the ribs. The heart was very large but was not contaminated by matter either internally or externally.

Despite these conditions the respiration had never been conspicuously hindered until almost the time of death. The cough was never continuous; sometimes the patient did not cough for hours, even a short while before his death. Certain physicians inferred from this that there was no disease in his chest, especially in the deep parts of the lungs. They concluded instead that a mild irritation of the throat from some deposit of catarrh caused the slight cough. The latter on rare occasions was laborious and was caused by dryness of the lungs. This prevented the free contraction necessary for the expulsion of remains of catarrh that slipped down through the trachea.

Comment on the Case of The Doge Francesco Contarini

The patient was a distinguished man, 68 years of age. His habitus is not described and nothing is said about his manner of living. From other sources we know that he was unmarried. From his biographers we know also that he was wealthy and had traveled widely. If he was the author of the book that is ascribed to him, he was probably studious. He had been subject to attacks of "colic," the location and duration of which are not stated.

On June 23, 1624, five and a half months before his death, he had a severe return of colic, followed by protracted fever. About July 1 he began to have diarrhea, which lasted until August 1. The urines (use of the plural implies that more than one specimen was examined) were of moderate consistence, reddish and copious, with light pale sediment. A mild cough was present. Respiration was free but the patient could not lie on either side. The pulse was strong and somewhat fast.

Toward the autumnal equinox the cough increased. Early in October the fever continued to recur and was now accompanied by respiratory difficulty and anxiety. Later a degree of improvement set in, but the cough, anorexia, and pain during recumbency continued persistently.

Early in December there was distinct respiratory difficulty, with anxiety and fever. The pulse was small and irregular. Orthopnea became prominent. The sputa were produced with difficulty and appeared to be "corrupt." On December 6 the eminent patient died.

He had had fever for about five and half months, a light cough, and emaciation. He could not lie on either side. Toward the end he had orthopnea, foul sputum, and arrhythmia. Nothing is said about edema.

Venetian physicians had attributed the symptoms to excessive heat in the liver and to dryness of the lungs. Praevotius, the professional consultant from Padua, allows the reader to smile at this diagnosis but does not offer an opinion of his own.

At autopsy about five pounds of watery material was found in the chest. The right lung contained a thick mucoid fluid; the left had turned into a whitish gore, which was contained within the pulmonary tunic (abscess or empyema?) and which replaced the lung almost entirely. The heart is said to have been very large but is not otherwise described. The liver was the site of a puzzling alteration. It was swollen and spongy and was filled with a whitish material; this may have been amyloid or perhaps tumor in a passively engorged organ.

Despite the hazards of retrospective diagnosis undertaken three and a half centuries *post mortem*, we may venture to say that the Doge Contarini suffered from cardiac hypertrophy and in addition had *both* hydrothorax due to heart failure *and* either empyema thoracis or a lung abscess. In addition he may well have had amyloidosis of the liver, a concomitant of protracted suppuration.

Although, as has been stated above, Praevotius refrained from offering a diagnosis *ante mortem*, he ventured a few *post-mortem* comments in the last few sentences of his report and these are relevant to the problem of diagnosis. He says that "despite these conditions," i.e., fluid and purulent material in the thoracic cavity, respiration had never been markedly impaired until almost the very end of the patient's life. This probably means that the inability of the patient to lie on either side was not regarded as a respiratory symptom.

Moreover, since cough was not present continually, certain physicians inferred that there was nothing wrong in the chest, especially in the deeper parts of the lungs. Hence the discontinuous and inconspicuous cough was attributed to minor irritation of the throat. By a further elaboration of hypotheses it was imagined that the occasional laborious quality of the cough was caused by dryness of the lungs which impeded the expulsion of catarrhal material. The latter, in accordance with old doctrine, was thought to have originated in the upper respiratory tract and to have descended by way of the trachea. It is implied, but not explicitly stated, that the presence and character of the effusions in the chest and the extensive loss of pulmonary tissue were surprising to the attendant physicians. No relation is stated or implied between the hydrothorax and the condition of the heart.

The Significance of Velschius' Report

Velschius has been forgotten, Praevotius has been forgotten, and the Doge Francesco Contarini is scarcely remembered even by historians of Venice. What, then, is the significance of the present case report, if any?

The significance becomes apparent if we consult a case report published by Christianus Helwich in 1722.[11, 12] Helwich had been attempting to ascertain the relation between hydrothorax and dyspnea. In one case he had offered the diagnosis of hydrothorax *intra vitam* because the patient had been awakened at night by dyspnea. The autopsy corroborated the diagnosis. Helwich felt that if nocturnal dyspnea is present, hydrothorax is present. However if dyspnea is *absent*, no conclusion could be drawn as to the presence or absence of hydrothorax; this, he says, *is shown by the case of the Doge Contarini*, who had had little impairment of respiration despite the fact that his chest contained five pounds of fluid.

Therefore the case of Contarini is important because it was one of a small number of exceptional cases which showed the limitations of dyspnea as an indicator of hydrothorax. The entire tenor of the problem points to what may be called the dawn of modern clinical medicine, when individual clinical phenomena were being assessed and their limitations were being discovered.

It should also be noticed that the clinical and anatomical observations in the case of the Doge Contarini were made in 1624 and presumably were recorded at about the same time. The report was published by Velschius in 1667. Fifty-five years later, in 1722, it was still considered to be the record of a crucial case in the development of semeiology.

NOTES AND REFERENCES

1. Jarcho, S.: An eighteenth century treatise on dropsy of the chest (Büchner, 1742). *Bull. N.Y. Acad. Med. 45*:799-806, 1969 (esp. footnotes 1-7).
2. Nani, B.: *Degl' Istorici delle Cose Veneziane,* Venice, Lovisa, 1720, vol. 8, p. 276.
   Gambier, H.: *Histoire de la République de Venise.* Venice, Ongania, 1955, p. 192.
   Da Mosto, A.: *I Dogi di Venezia.* Venice, Ongania, 1939, pp. 224-27.
   Romanin, S.: *Storia Documentata di Venezia.* Venezia, Fuga, 1914, vol. 7, pp. 274-75.
   L***: *Histoire de la République de Venise.* Paris, Duchesne, 1767, vol. 11, p. 163 ff.
3. Smith, Logan Pearsall: *The Life and Letters of Sir Henry Wotton.* Oxford, Clarendon Press, 1907, vol. 1, p. 106. See also vol. 1, pp. 192, 399, and n.l, 474, 489; vol. 2, pp. 277-80, 492.
4. Pagel, J. In: Hirsch, A.: *Biographisches Lexikon,* 3d ed. Berlin, Urban and Schwarzenberg, 1962, vol. 4, pp. 672-73.
5. Stephanus, J., ed.: *J. Praevotii Opera Medica Posthuma.* Frankfurt, Beijerus, 1656.
6. I am indebted to the National Library of Medicine for furnishing a microfilm of the *Episagmata,* which has been deposited in the library of the New York Academy of Medicine.
7. Seitz. In: Hirsch, A.: *Biographisches Lexikon* (see footnote 4, above), vol. 5, p. 895.
8. Almost all biographers give the date as December 6, *1624.* Allen B. Hinds *(Calendar of State Papers and Manuscripts, Relating to English Affairs Existing in the Archives and Collections of Venice,* London, 1921, vol. 18, p. 532, n.)

gives the date as Saturday, December 7, 1624.

9. Da Mosto (op. cit., p. 227) says he died "suffocated by catarrh."
10. The visceral pleura.
11. Helwich, C.: Observata quaedam ex anatome matronae difficiliori respiratione per totum vitae spatium laborantis. *Academiae Caesareae-Leopold. Carol. Nat. Curiosorum Ephemerides,* Centuria 10, observ. 32, pp. 307-10. Augsburg, Kühtz, 1722.
12. Jarcho, S.: Christianus Helwich on difficulty of respiration. *Bull. N.Y. Acad. Med. 46*:34-38, 1970.

THE *JACKDAW* SERIES ON THE HISTORY OF MEDICINE AND SCIENCE

During the last few decades increasing dissatisfaction with classical pedagogic methods has led to a search for new educational materials and novel pedagogic techniques. In the teaching of history this movement has revealed itself especially in the efflorescence of well-planned and well-produced supplementary materials, which have developed from older source books that resembled the chrestomathies used in the teaching of exotic languages. The newer source books, which are numerous, range from simple collections of documents and excerpts to collections of documents accompanied by commentaries, to collections of documents selected in order to present different aspects of a single issue.[1] Another sequence consists of rare source materials reproduced in facsimile.[2]

In 1963 a new and unusual series, the Jackdaw Publications, was inaugurated by Messrs. Jonathan Cape of Bedford Square, London. In this series[3] there are now 53 so-called History Jackdaws, which range from *King John and Magna Carta* to *Assassination at Sarajevo*. Science Jackdaws thus far issued deal with Newton and gravitation; the discovery of the galaxies; Pasteur and the germ theory; Darwin; Faraday; and Harvey and the circulation of the blood.

We may use the last-named as an example. The material on Harvey, compiled by Jonathan Miller and edited by Gerald Leach, is presented in a stout and brightly-colored envelope measuring approximately 13½ by 9 inches. It contains 11 numbered items, such as: a portrait of Harvey; four facsimiles of manuscript pages from John Aubrey's *Brief Lives* (with transcription); the opening pages of the First Folio *Coriolanus*, containing the physiological parable of the belly and the members; the arterial system as depicted in the *De Humani Corporis Fabrica* of

1 Kriegel, L., ed. *Essential Works of the Founding Fathers.* New York, Bantam Books, 1964.
Baritz, L., ed. *Sources of the American Mind,* 2 vols. New York, John Wiley, 1966.
Friede, F. and Pollack, N., eds. *American Issues in the Twentieth Century.* Chicago, Rand McNally, 1966.
Hofstadter, R., ed. *Great Issues in American History,* 2 vols. New York, Vintage Books, 1958.
Boorstin, D. J., ed. *An American Primer.* Chicago, Univ. Chicago Press, 1966.

2 The *March of American Collection* (directed by H. H. Peckman, Louis B. Wright, and P. A. Knachel). Ann Arbor, Univ. Microfilms, 1966- .

3 In the United States the Jackdaw series is issued by Grossman Publishers of New York, N. Y.

Vesalius; part of Harvey's diploma from Padua, with translation; and pages from the writings of Harvey. These objects are supplemented by modern materials such as an x-ray film of the chest and part of an electrocardiogram. The final component consists of five illustrated broadsheets (7½ x 16 inches), which explain the history of our ideas of the circulation from antiquity to the days of the open-heart operation. The historical exposition is sound.

It is evident that on the Harveian theme the publishers have provided an impressive quantity of material and have set it forth in an impressive way. The device of detached presentation in loose pages allows the reader to make selection according to his capacity or his fancy. It is evident further that, while most of the material is within the scope of an intelligent high school student, nothing has been included which would draw disdain from a medical student or a physician. Indeed the materials are such as most physicians could hardly assemble without skilled help and large resources.

The Science Jackdaw on Pasteur is analogous to the envelope on Harvey but contains in addition an ingenious cut-out chart which makes vivid the gradual destruction of the hypothesis of spontaneous generation.

Here at last we have a series of nonbooks, issued by an eminent publisher and capable of conveying serious instruction in a superior manner. The unconventional use of broadsheets and packets is refreshing and, to the youngest students, will appear less didactic and hence less odious and onerous than the traditional bound book.

S. J.

now for your non-hospitalized patients

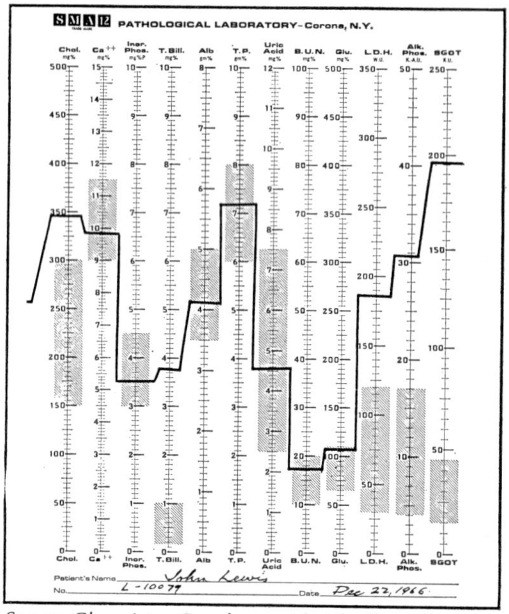

Serum Chemistry Graph provided is 8" x 11"

blood chemistry profiles

run on

TECHNICON®

Sequential Multiple Analyzer

only $15⁰⁰

FOR A ~~12~~-TEST BLOOD CHEMISTRY PROFILE

COMPUTER AUGMENTED TO 14 TESTS

Heretofore available only to patients in a few large hospitals, PATHOLOGICAL LABORATORY *now provides* this *rapid* automated analytical service for the non-hospitalized patient.

A Serum Chemistry Graph of each analysis summarizes in graphic form the results of *all 12 tests together,* superimposed over a background of normal values.

Patients may be directed to the laboratory; or blood samples can be mailed in post-paid containers provided by our laboratory. The Serum Chemistry Graph and a report in the usual numerical format will be mailed the same day samples are received. Free messenger pick-up is available in select areas.

PATHOLOGICAL LABORATORY

40-03 NATIONAL ST., CORONA, N.Y. 11368 TELEPHONE 212-639-5403

send for post-paid blood sample mailing containers

PATHOLOGICAL LABORATORY • 40-03 National St., Corona, N.Y. 11368

Gentlemen:

☐ *Please send additional literature*

☐ *Please send post-paid containers for blood samples*

Dr. ....

Street ....

City .... *State* .... *Zip* ....

BULLETIN OF
THE NEW YORK ACADEMY
OF MEDICINE

Vol. 46, No. 6 June 1970

METHADONE MANAGEMENT OF HEROIN ADDICTION*

A Report by
The Committee on Public Health
of
The New York Academy of Medicine

In 1955 the Committee on Public Health of the New York Academy of Medicine issued the first of a series of reports on the problem of narcotics addiction. In that first report the Committee reviewed the existing situation from the viewpoint of prevailing law and its administration, the prevalence of addiction, the problem of illicit narcotics traffic, the interrelation of addiction, financial gain and crime, as well as the federally mandated approach to treatment and rehabilitation. At that time the Committee noted: "Today a number of cities are raising a hue and cry of apprehension and alarm over drug addiction. Charges and claims about it appear in the headlines, coupled with demands for action of the usual kind: crackdown by the enforcement officials." That comment is still applicable.

Viewing the addict primarily as a sick individual rather than as a criminal, and reflecting that prevention of addiction was of the essence, the Committee formulated a comprehensive program whose purpose was to eliminate the supply of narcotic drugs and to punish the im-

*Approved by the Committee on Public Health, February 2, 1970.
Approved by the Council of the New York Academy of Medicine, February 18, 1970.

porters and suppliers. It also proposed to take the profit out of illicit drug traffic and, by emphasizing the medical rather than the criminal aspects of narcotics addiction, to provide an adequate program of therapy.

In a later report in 1963 the Academy, through the Committee on Public Health, reaffirmed its opinion that addiction is an illness and recommended the formulation of a national policy emphasizing the medical and social aspects of the problem. In addition, it suggested a more realistic and less rigid governmental approach to its solution.

Again, in 1965, the Committee reviewed the addiction situation and recommended that a procedure be instituted that would "bring all addicts under medical supervision" since they are sick people. The report also noted that "because of the psychological element in addiction and the high frequency of recurrence, the addict should not be removed from narcotics until another and salutary crutch is provided"; that "treatment varies with the individual patient . . . and should be tailored to the addict"; that "maintenance therapy on a narcotic . . . should be restricted to highly selected subjects"; and that "the Academy does not favor indiscriminate dispensing of narcotics to addicts but . . . would not object to a demonstration project."

In January 1969–in response to a request from Dr. Bernard Bucove, Health Services Administrator of New York City, the Committee on Public Health undertook a review of the New York City methadone maintenance programs for opiate addicts. This approach to the management of the addiction problem was initiated by Drs. Vincent P. Dole and Marie Nyswander in 1964.

Methadone maintenance therapy of addicts is based on the premise that, although it is itself an analgesic narcotic similar to morphine, methadone is effective in blocking both the euphoria and craving for heroin in individuals addicted to the latter. It is also potentially addicting–although less so than either heroin or morphine. It is effective when taken orally and is relatively long acting–from 12 to 48 hours. Appreciation of this long duration of action is particularly important in the management of overdosage.

Usually a single daily oral dose of methadone is effective in the prevention of euphoria in heroin addicts. It is specific for narcotic drugs of the opiate type and has no beneficial effects in the management of alcoholic patients, or of those dependent on barbiturates or amphetamines. When properly administered methadone permits the addict to function normally in society—no sedative effect or euphoria ensues (even if challenged with heroin) and there is little or no impairment in somatic or psychological reactions, or intellectual capacity.

Drs. Dole and Nyswander at The Rockefeller University have treated more than 2,000 heroin addicts since 1964. They have pointed out that all of their patients were able to resist the necessity for heroin as long as they continued on methadone and that over 80% of their group have been returned to a useful role in society: in school, at work, or in the home. On the other hand, of the 17% of patients who withdrew from the program, almost all have returned to the use of heroin. Dole and Nyswander conclude that the use of methadone maintenance, supported by a proper rehabilitation program, is an effective method of managing heroin addicts on an ambulatory basis.

The experience of The Rockefeller University group has been confirmed by other treatment centers in New York City and elsewhere. The results presented at the Second National Conference on Methadone Treatment in October 1969 reinforced the value of this approach. In all the successful programs the medical management has had an associated program of social and psychological rehabilitation.

The Committee, having studied the available literature, having met with experts in the management of opiate addiction (including methadone maintenance), and having considered and discussed the matter at length believes that methadone maintenance therapy, properly administered and supervised, offers a substantial hope for the rehabilitation of selected heroin addicts.

Motivation on the part of the patient appears to be the most important element for a successful result. This regimen has proved to be effective in the management of narcotic addicts who have volunteered for the methadone treatment after other approaches have failed.

Methadone maintenance, properly managed, induces a high tolerance to narcotics and the patient is thereby protected to a degree against overdosage from methadone or other narcotic drugs. However, this tolerance must be built up gradually since too rapid an increase in dosage may produce confusion and sedation. The usual daily maintenance dose of an addict is dangerous to a person who has not built up such tolerance. The management of methadone overdosage differs markedly from that of heroin or morphine in that the duration of action of the former is long—as long as 48 hours. Accordingly treatment of overdosage of methadone with narcotics antagonists, such as nalorphine, requires careful observation of the patient as well as frequent and prolonged treatment with the antidote.

Although methadone has proved to be an effective treatment in selected heroin addicts the legal status of maintenance programs remains unclear. As noted in the 1955 Committee report, "The present federal regulations control the practice of medicine in relation to drug addiction to such an extent, and so look upon the physician as a potential criminal, that he prefers not to include the treatment of drug addiction in his practice." This lack of clarity inhibits the practitioner in the management of addicts by any method including the use of methadone. However, the delay that exists before a motivated addict can be admitted to an organized methadone maintenance program places a tremendous responsibility on physicians, hospitals, and governmental agencies.

In a recent statement the Academy pointed out the difficulties that might be encountered in having heroin addicts managed with methadone by physicians unfamiliar with the method. In our view such treatment, including that of ambulatory patients, should be carried out by practicing physicians in association with organized programs in an institutional or team setting.

Currently a crisis exists in New York City. The number of treatment programs is insufficient at present for proper handling of the problem. The number of physicians experienced in the technique is also inadequate. As a result many candidates for methadone management have no place to turn. Interested physicians without the necessary support provided by an organized unit cannot properly handle the individual addict. Provision must be made promptly for expanding the number of programs so that these individuals can be properly treated. In addition, operative treatment centers should institute educational programs so that interested practicing physicians could participate with subsequent involvement in a program on a continuing basis. Present law should be revised to eliminate any legal obstacles to such an arrangement. Thus addicts could be managed effectively while awaiting entrance into organized programs with benefit to themselves as well as to society.

The Committee recognizes the fact that treatment of heroin addiction with methadone substitutes one addiction for another. Evidence suggests that such treatment may be a life-long affair. However, the Committee feels that no other regimen currently available offers as much to the chronic addict. At the present time the Committee does not recommend this method of treatment for the occasional user or for individuals whose dependence has been newly acquired. More conventional methods, including social and psychiatric approaches, should be utilized for the latter group.

Neither does the Committee feel that methadone management is the final solution to the management of the addict. As new approaches become available they must be carefully evaluated in a supervised and controlled manner.

After reviewing the available information on methadone maintenance, the Committee feels that the following comments are justified:

1) The drug-addiction problem is real and serious. Resolution will require a comprehensive and coordinated approach involving enlightened legislation as well as active involvement of the medical and lay communities.

2) No totally satisfactory method of prevention or treatment of narcotics addiction is currently available. Research into the causes and prevention of addiction should, of course, continue.

3) Methadone maintenance is an effective method of treating selected chronic addicts, but it should be used only in conjunction with a program of social and psychiatric rehabilitation. At present this approach should not be used for the occasional user or for individuals whose drug dependence has been newly acquired.

4) Properly organized and evaluated methadone maintenance programs should be expanded promptly.

5) Physicians should keep abreast of new developments in the field of addiction. Interested practitioners should be encouraged to accept the responsibility for managing addicts in association with organized programs, and organized centers should involve such citizens in their ongoing programs. However, indiscriminate use of methadone management by physicians unfamiliar with the method should be discouraged.

6) Federal, state, and local laws should be reviewed and revised, where necessary, to separate the criminal from the medical aspects of the drug problem. Barriers preventing the qualified practicing physician from managing the addict in association with an organized treatment program should be removed.

HEMOLYTIC ANEMIA

*A Symposium**

LEON N. SUSSMAN, *Chairman*

Hereditary Hemolytic Disorders

Ernst R. Jaffé 397

Disease-Associated Autoimmune Hemolytic Anemia

Arthur Sawitsky and Panfilo B. Ozaeta, Jr. . . . 411

Drug-Associated Hemolytic Anemia

Ralph Zalusky 427

*Held at a meeting of the Section on Medicine, February 17, 1970.

HEREDITARY HEMOLYTIC DISORDERS*

ERNST R. JAFFÉ

Professor of Medicine
Albert Einstein College of Medicine
Bronx Municipal Hospital Center
New York, N. Y.

A DECREASE in the average life-span of the human erythrocyte to less than 120 days is the hallmark of hemolysis. This decrease is manifested by evidence of increased destruction of erythrocytes (unconjugated hyperbilirubinemia, increased urinary and fecal urobilinogen, decreased free serum haptoglobin), and increased production of erythrocytes (reticulocytosis, erythroid hyperplasia of the bone marrow). Hemolytic *anemia* develops only when the rate of destruction exceeds the capacity of the bone marrow to manufacture erythrocytes. Compensated hemolysis without significant anemia probably is more prevalent than frank anemia. Compensated hemolysis, however, may still bring the patient to the physician because of unexplained jaundice, splenomegaly, or the development of cholelithiasis at an early age.

Knowledge about the disease processes which cause increased destruction of circulating erythrocytes has developed at a rapid rate during the past 20 years. Despite this "information explosion," the reasons for the premature death of the erythrocytes are still poorly understood. Diagnostic criteria have been developed to permit a reasonable classification of most of these disorders. A fundamental but not invariable division can be based upon whether the destruction of erythrocytes is due to something in the environment of the cell (extrinsic or extracorpuscular) or is due to something abnormal in the cell (intrinsic or intracorpuscular).

This discussion will be concerned with those disorders which are associated with a decreased life-span of the circulating erythrocytes and which have been attributed to inherited abnormalties. To date all of the hereditary hemolytic disorders appear to be associated with intracorpuscular abnormalities.

*Presented at a *Symposium on Hemolytic Anemia* sponsored by the Section on Medicine, February 17, 1970.

The investigations in the author's laboratory are supported by Public Health Service Research Grant AM-13698 from the National Institute of Arthritis and Metabolic Diseases, Bethesda, Md.
The author is a Career Scientist of the Health Research Council of the City of New York (1-169).

Classification of the Hereditary Hemolytic Disorders

A) Abnormalities of the erythrocyte membrane(?)

1) Hereditary spherocytosis
2) Hereditary elliptocytosis
3) Hereditary stomatocytosis
4) Hereditary cation-leaking erythrocytes
5) Hereditary alterations in lipid composition

B) Abnormalities of the hemoglobin or its synthesis

1) Sickle cell anemia
2) Hemoglobin C, D, and E diseases
3) Unstable hemoglobins
4) Thalassemia syndromes
5) Erythropoietic porphyria(?)

C) Abnormalities of the enzymes

1) Well-established deficiencies with hemolysis
   a) Hexokinase
   b) Phosphohexose isomerase
   c) Triosephosphate isomerase
   d) Phosphoglycerate kinase
   e) Pyruvate kinase
   f) Glucose-6-phosphate dehydrogenase

2) Deficiencies reported with hemolysis
   a) Phosphofructokinase
   b) Aldolase(??)
   c) 2,3-Diphosphoglycerate mutase
   d) 6-Phosphogluconate dehydrogenase
   e) GSSG reductase
   f) GSH peroxidase
   g) GSH synthetase(?)
   h) ATPase

A classification of the inherited hemolytic disorders can be formulated by beginning with the membrane and proceeding to the interior of the cell (see accompanying table). The simplicity of this classification may be unwarranted. The three fundamental sites where abnormalities can occur may be affected to different degrees in all illnesses associated with hemolysis. Primary membrane lesions are often accompanied by increased but perhaps ineffective metabolic activity, while effects on the hemoglobin have not yet been demonstrated. Abnormal hemoglobins may influence both the metabolism and the membrane of the erythrocyte. Defects in the glycolytic pathways available to the cell may harm the membrane and may lead to alterations in a normal or abnormal hemoglobin. Finally, the spleen, although not necessarily the only site for destruction of erythrocytes, may influence the circulating cell and may affect its life-span.

Abnormalities of the Erythrocyte Membrane

Until recently the membrane of the erythrocyte has received the least investigative attention.[1, 2] The difficulty in obtaining membranes in pure form and the hazards inherent in interpreting both morphologic and biochemical observations have contributed to this neglect. Hereditary spherocytosis, the first familial hemolytic jaundice recognized, probably belongs in the group of membrane abnormalities. Although the fundamental defect has defied definition, the morphologic characteristics, the increased lysis *in vitro* occurring either spontaneously or upon exposure to hypotonic solutions of sodium chloride, and the favorable response to splenectomy have been thoroughly documented. Disagreement persists between the advocates of the thesis that the disorder is the consequence of loss of pieces of the erythrocyte membrane[3] and those who believe that excessive leakage of sodium into the cell with concomitant increased but ineffective metabolic activity is responsible.[4] Recently it has even been postulated that there may be a relative deficiency of aldolase, a glycolytic enzyme, in this disorder.[5] Hereditary elliptocytosis may also belong in this group. The actual shape of the cells appears to be of little importance since patients with this abnormality may have no evidence, or minimal or marked evidence, of increased destruction of erythrocytes.[6] Patients with hereditary elliptocytosis and significant hemolysis may benefit from splenectomy. The clinical picture of hereditary stomatocytosis is similar to that of hereditary spherocytosis or elliptocytosis, but the response to splenectomy is less satisfactory.[7] Recently patients have been described in whom the cation content of the erythrocytes is markedly abnormal with increased intracellular sodium and decreased intracellular potassium concentrations.[8, 9] Although these syndromes resemble hereditary spherocytosis in that the osmotic fragility of the erythrocytes is increased, bowl-shaped stomatocytes and not spherocytes are seen in wet preparations of peripheral blood. The alterations in the concentrations of cations are distinct from those seen in hereditary spherocytosis where the sodium and potassium contents are normal. Stomatocytes, however, do not indicate a specific abnormality because they are seen in other hemolytic disorders without abnormalities in erythrocyte cation content. We have described a hemolytic disorder in a large family from the Dominican Republic in which the erythrocytes of the affected members have an alteration in their phospholipid composition, an increase in the content of lecithin.[10] None of these patients has had a splenectomy. The patients' erythrocytes are more resistant to osmotic stress than normal. While the mechanism for the accelerated destruction of the erythrocytes is unknown, there is evidence to suggest that there may be a deficiency in the pathway for the degradation of lecithin.[11]

In all studies in which sufficient data are available the presumed membrane defects appear to have been inherited as dominant characteristics. The mechanism of hemolysis remains a mystery. Neither hemoglobin nor enzyme defects have been demonstrable. Membrane alterations, regardless of changes of shape, may make the erythrocytes unusually susceptible to stagnation in the splenic sinusoids where they are destroyed by the reticuloendothelial system. Splenectomy, therefore, may be of value in patients with these disorders.

Abnormalities of the Hemoglobin or Its Synthesis

Hemolysis due to an abnormality in the structure or synthesis of hemoglobin is well known.[12, 13] Nearly 100 abnormal human hemoglobins have been described. Only a very few, however, are associated with accelerated destruction of erythrocytes. Hemoglobins S, C, D, and E, as the predominant hemoglobin in the homozygote, or in various combinations, or in association with thalassemia, can give rise to hemolysis. Hemoglobin S can lead to severe anemia, while hemoglobin C causes mild anemia. The mechanism for the minimal hemolysis associated with hemoglobin D or E is unknown. In sickle-cell anemia, the propensity for the hemoglobin S to become a semisolid gel upon deoxygenation, decrease in *p*H, or increase in salt concentration, leads to the formation of the characteristically deformed cell. If the sickled state is prolonged, irreversible changes occur, perhaps as the result of interaction between the abnormal hemoglobin and the red-cell membrane. As a consequence of the decreased deformability of the erythrocytes and increased viscosity of the blood, destruction of the erythrocytes and obstruction of the microvasculature occur. Thus the major clinical manifestations are the result of recurrent vascular obstruction. In hemoglobin C disease it has been suggested that the formation of intracellular crystals or a "precrystalline" state of the abnormal hemoglobin results in the loss of plasticity of the cell with increased rigidity and decreased survival of the cell.[14]

Recently considerable interest has been evoked by the "unstable hemoglobins" which are characterized by the presence of a hemoglobin which is unusually susceptible to precipitation upon heating *in vitro*.[15] In many but not all of these unstable hemoglobins, the structural abnormality involves an alteration at or near the site in the polypeptide chain where the heme moiety is attached or the absence of one or more amino acids. These peculiar hemoglobins have been detected only in heterozygotes, probably because the homozygous state would be incompatible with life. The degree of hemolysis *in vivo* and, therefore, the severity of the anemia are extremely variable, even among different families with the same abnormality. Some of the patients who have these abnormal hemoglobins experience exacerbations of their hemolytic process upon the administration of certain drugs. Dr. Ralph Zalusky considers them in greater detail elsewhere in the present symposium.

The abnormal hemoglobins are inherited as autosomal codominant characteristics. All of the normal hemoglobin component is replaced by the abnormal hemoglobin in the homozygous subject, while somewhat less than half of the affected hemoglobin fraction is abnormal in the heterozygote. The abnormalities are attributable to the replacement or loss of one or more amino acids from one of the polypeptide chains of hemoglobin. These substitutions or deletions can be explained by alterations in the genetic code provided by the deoxynucleic acid (DNA) of the progenitor of the erythrocytes.

In the thalassemia syndromes an inherited defect in the net rate of synthesis of one or more types of globin polypeptide chains is presumably responsible.[12] In beta-thalassemia (thalassemia major, Cooley's anemia), decreased production of the normal beta chains is associated with ineffective erythropoiesis and with accumulation of free alpha chains, which are thought to precipitate within the cells. Conversely, various forms of alpha-thalassemia with impaired formation of alpha chains are associated with accumulation of gamma chains (hemoglobin Bart's) or of beta chains (hemoglobin H). Interaction between the normal globin chains which accumulate in excess in the absence of their normal counterparts and the red-cell membrane has been postulated to cause the accelerated destruction of these erythrocytes, especially in the spleen. The genetic mechanisms resulting in the various types of thalassemia are extremely complex. A heterogeneous group of beta-thalassemia genes and two structural genes for alpha chains have been proposed to explain the variability in the expression of these disorders.

No therapy capable of producing a cure has been found for these inherited disorders. When they are severe, as in sickle-cell anemia, transfusions may be required. Splenectomy occasionally seems to decrease the transfusion requirement in beta-thalassemia and, perhaps, in other types of thalassemia.

For the sake of completeness, the extremely rare disorder, congenital erythropoietic porphyria, with its variable degree of hemolysis, is included in this category. The hemolytic anemia, if present, may respond to splenectomy, and the cutaneous manifestations may improve. Apparently inherited as an autosomal recessive characteristic, the disease is expressed only in the homozygous subject. The mechanisms by which increased porphyrins are produced and lead to hemolysis are unknown.[16] This porphyria reflects an abnormality in the synthesis of the porphyrin precursors of the heme moiety and does not imply a defect in the synthesis of hemoglobin itself.

Abnormalities of the Enzymes

Biochemists, geneticists, and anthropologists, as well as internists and pediatricians, have become extremely interested in the hereditary hemolytic disorders that are associated with deficiencies in the activities of the enzymes of the erythrocytes. Fourteen enzyme deficiencies have now been reported to be associated with hemolytic disorders.[17] Six enzyme deficiencies have been well defined; eight less definitely.

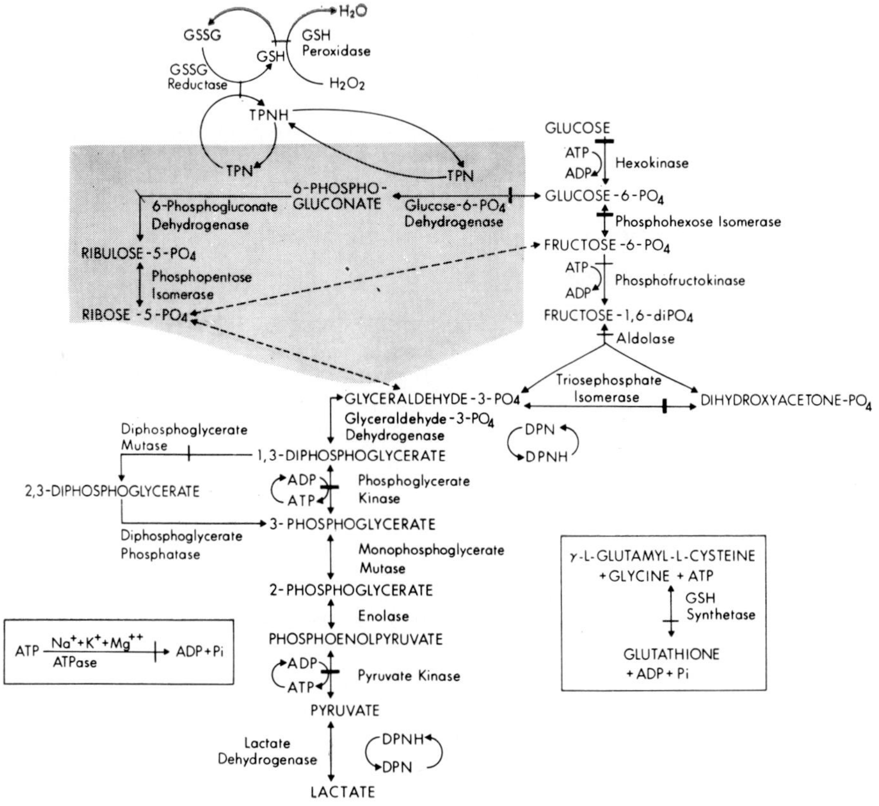

Pathways by which glucose is metabolized in human erythrocytes. Reactions enclosed in the shaded area comprise the hexosemonophosphate (HMP) shunt pathway. Interrupted lines indicate omission of several reactions. Bold bars indicate enzymatic deficiencies whose association with hereditary hemolytic disorders is well established, lighter bars indicate enzymatic deficiencies which have been reported to be associated with hemolytic disorders. Reproduced by permission from: Jaffé, E. R. Hereditary hemolytic disorders and enzymatic deficiencies of human erythrocytes. *Blood: 35,* 116, 1970.

In order to appreciate these enzyme-deficiency hemolytic disorders it is necessary to consider the relation between metabolic activity and the functions of the erythrocyte. Man is endowed with erythrocytes to contain the hemoglobin essential for the transportation of oxygen from the lungs to the tissues. This vital task depends upon the ability of the hemoglobin to bind oxygen reversibly. This binding can be influenced by organic phosphate esters, especially 2,3-diphosphoglycerate (2,3-DPG), which are generated by the cell's metabolic machinery. The binding of 2,3-DPG to deoxyhemoglobin changes the configuration of the molecule and decreases its affinity for oxygen. Increased concentrations of 2,3-DPG may therefore make oxygen more readily available for release to tissues at low oxygen tensions.[18]

The mature human erythrocyte is limited to glycolysis as the only significant source of the energy required for its functions (see figure on page 403). For an expenditure of two molecules of adenosine triphosphate (ATP) per molecule of glucose used, the erythrocyte can generate four, a potential net gain of two. This ATP can be used to maintain the high intracellular potassium and low sodium content characteristic of human erythrocytes against concentration gradients and passive leaks by means of an ATPase system. ATP can also be utilized for the resynthesis of purine nucleotides and the synthesis of pyridine nucleotides, both essential cofactors for glycolysis. Maintenance of the lipids of the erythrocyte also appears to require metabolic activity and ATP. Metabolic activity is involved in maintaining hemoglobin in a state suitable for the reversible binding of oxygen, a process which requires that the iron of the heme moiety be in the ferrous state. Reduced diphosphopyridine nucleotide (DPNH) is required for the reduction of any methemoglobin (ferrihemoglobin) which is formed to (ferro) hemoglobin. The Rapoport-Luebering or 2,3-DPG cycle permits a bypass of an ATP-generating step, may serve to conserve DPNH, and may play a role as a regulator of glycolytic activity.

In addition to the direct pathway from glucose to lactate, the erythrocyte possesses an active hexosemonophosphate (HMP) shunt through which normally 5 to 10% of the glucose utilized passes before reentering the mainstream of glycolysis. This shunt is the only source for the generation of reduced triphosphopyridine nucleotide (TPNH), the preferred cofactor for the reduction of oxidized glutathione (GSSG) to reduced glutathione (GSH). Although the precise function of the latter is still unknown, the human erythrocyte contains about half as many molecules of GSH as of hemoglobin. HMP shunt activity is required to maintain the intracellular concentration of this sulfhydryl-containing tripeptide which may be involved in protecting hemoglobin against irreversible oxidative denaturation, guarding membrane lipids against peroxidation, and shielding essential enzymes against inactivation.

In contrast to the mature erythrocyte, the immature cell or reticulocyte is capable of much more metabolic activity.[19] Reticulocytes contain ribonucleic acids, synthesize proteins, lipids, heme and purine nucleotides, can perform oxidative phosphorylation with an intact cytochrome system and tricarboxylic acid cycle, and may be able to utilize amino acids and fatty acids as sources of energy. The concentrations of ATP and, probably, other organic phosphate esters such as 2,3-DPG are higher, and the activities of several but not all enzymes are considerably greater in these young cells.

With a relatively limited metabolic apparatus the normal mature human erythrocyte can support all of its essential functions for about 120 days. This limited capacity, however, makes it not too surprising that the survival of erythrocytes deficient in the activity of any one of the enzymes involved is jeopardized. The greater metabolic potential of the reticulocytes probably makes it possible for the young cells to survive at least long enough to prevent the death of the patient.

Of the six well-defined enzyme deficiencies associated with hemolysis, five are in the direct glycolytic pathway from glucose to lactate (Embden-Meyerhof pathway); one is in the HMP shunt. Two of the enzyme deficiencies in the Embden-Meyerhof pathway are of particular interest because of their association with syndromes other than hemolysis alone.

Deficiency in the activity of triosephosphate isomerase (TPI) results in a severe, incapacitating, progressive neuromuscular disorder.[20] At least nine patients with this affliction are now known, and all but one died before the age of six. All patients appear to develop normally except for evidence of severe hemolysis during the first six to seven months of life and then suffer progressive neuromuscular impairment with initial generalized spasticity and subsequent weakness. These patients are subject to frequent infections, and their sudden deaths have been attributed to cardiac involvement. Deficient TPI activity has been documented in the erythrocytes, leukocytes, skeletal muscle, serum, and spinal fluid of affected subjects. The generalized nature of this deficiency has led to speculation about the deleterious effect of the metabolic abnormality on the functions of all tissues. While supporting data are not yet available, it is known that both brain and muscle are quite dependent upon anaerobic glycolysis via the Embden-Meyerhof pathway for their energy requirements. This disorder, first described in children of French Louisiana and Negro origins, has subsequently been observed in individuals of Anglo-Saxon extraction. The mode of inheritance is autosomal recessive with intermediate levels of TPI activity demonstrable in the erythrocytes and leukocytes of the clinically normal parents of affected children. We have recently had an opportunity to study a 21-year-old woman of Irish-English ancestry with severe TPI deficiency.[21] Although her early clinical course had been similar to that of the eight other cases, her transfusion requirement has subsided, her intelligence is above normal, and there has been no clear evidence of progression of her disease for several years.

A moderately severe hemolytic disorder associated with a deficiency in the activity of phosphoglycerate kinase (PGK) in both erythrocytes and leukocytes has been demonstrated in a large Chinese kindred.[22] Two young males are most affected and, in addition to hemolysis, they have a neurologic disorder with abnormal behavior, emotional lability, and impaired speech. Five male relatives in the maternal portion of the family tree have died in early childhood and may have had the same disorder. The metabolic block is in the first of the two ATP-generating steps in the Embden-Meyerhof pathway. Despite deficient PGK activity in the leukocytes, recurrent infections have not been a significant problem. The family history and the results of biochemical investigations have been interpreted as indicating that mosaicism for PGK activity may be present in the erythrocytes of affected women with mild or no hemolysis and that the affected males are hemizygotes. Thus PGK deficiency may be a sex-linked disorder.

The remaining three enzyme deficiencies in the Embden-Meyerhof pathway may be summarized briefly. Pyruvate kinase deficiency probably is the most common of the enzyme deficiencies associated with spontaneous nonspherocytic hemolytic anemia. Considerable heterogeneity in the clinical severity and in the biochemical abnormality has been described. Although this disease is most common in persons of northern European origin, it has been found in Italians and Japanese, a Mexican child, an American Negro, and a Syrian girl. Hereditary hemolytic anemia has been observed in a few patients whose erythrocytes are deficient in hexokinase activity or have a hexokinase with aberrant properties. Four patients from two unrelated families have been found to have erythrocytes, leukocytes, and plasma with extremely low levels of phosphohexose isomerase activity. Despite the low leukocyte and plasma activities these children do not have increased susceptibility to infection, and neurologic or developmental abnormalities have not occurred. These three enzyme deficiencies are inherited as autosomal recessive characteristics.

Deficiency in the activity of glucose-6-phosphate dehydrogenase (G-6-PD), the most frequently recognized human erythrocyte enzyme deficiency, has been the subject of extensive investigations.[23] More than 50 different variants of G-6-PD have been defined. Many are associated with no clinical effect and no significant decrease in activity, while others are associated with mild to moderately severe nonspherocytic hemolytic anemia even in the absence of any known precipitating agent. The data from all investigations so far reported are consistent with the thesis that G-6-PD deficiency is sex-linked. The precise mechanism by which G-6-PD deficiency causes hemolysis is still unknown, although it appears to be related to the need for this enzyme in the maintenance of GSH within the erythrocyte. Because of its importance in some of the drug-associated hemolytic anemias, this problem is also considered by Dr. Zalusky.

The eight other enzyme deficiencies listed in the table have not been examined extensively enough to permit definitive conclusions about their roles in hemolysis. The hemolytic disorder associated with extremely low concentrations of GSH in the erythocytes is included in this list because there is only indirect evidence for deficiency in GSH synthetase activity. The well-compensated hemolytic process in GSH-deficient subjects is in marked contrast to the more severe hemolysis in some Caucasian patients with G-6-PD deficiency and nearly normal concentrations of GSH in their erythrocytes. What, therefore, is the role of GSH in the erythrocyte and in the hemolysis associated with deficiency in G-6-PD activity?

Since environmental modifications can have profound effects on the metabolism of erythrocytes these factors must also be considered in studies of enzyme deficiencies. For example, the decreased GSSG-reductase activity noted in many patients' erythrocytes can be increased markedly by the administration of riboflavin *in vivo* or the addition of the enzyme's coenzyme, flavin adenine dinucleotide, to the hemolysate *in vitro*.[24] Therapy with riboflavin has had no effect upon the degree of hemolysis in a patient homozygous for hemoglobin C with approximately 50% of normal GSSG-reductase activity in the erythrocytes prior to treatment; GSSG-reductase activity proved to be normal after treatment.

Diagnosis and Treatment of Hemolytic Disorders With Enzyme Deficiencies

These hemolytic disorders are characterized by their nonspecific but nonspherocytic nature. Large numbers of spherocytes are not detected in the peripheral blood, either on the stained smear or upon determination of the osmotic fragility of the erythrocytes before and after incubation of whole blood for 24 hours. Spontaneous or autohemolysis of erythrocytes *in vitro* is often increased and may or may not be decreased by the addition of glucose or ATP. Unfortunately, the autohemolysis test is not very helpful in the differential diagnosis. The hemolytic process is often apparent from birth, but not infrequently the illness is detected only in adult life. In keeping with the autosomal recessive mode of inheritance of most of these enzyme deficiencies, parent-to-child transmission has been rare and has usually been explicable on the basis of a mating between heterozygous and homozygous subjects. G-6-PD deficiency and, probably, PGK deficiency are inherited as sex-linked characteristics and, therefore, are most manifest in males.

Much of the diagnostic evaluation involves the exclusion of other causes of hemolysis, such as the autoimmune disorders, drug-associated hemolysis, and the disease-associated hemolytic anemias which are considered by Dr. Arthur Sawitsky. The problem of identifying known deficiencies of enzymes in erythrocytes has been eased by the development of several simple screening tests which recently have been evaluated carefully.[25] A definitive diagnosis, however, requires the demonstration of a significant enzyme deficiency by *direct* assay. Enzymes are usually present in great excess over the minimum required for normal metabolic activity, and the activities are rarely if ever totally absent in deficient cells. Attention has therefore been directed to the determination of the concentrations of intermediates of glycolysis to provide clues as to the site of the metabolic block. The definition of an enzymatic deficiency should include: 1) significantly decreased activity of the enzyme in the hemolysate, especially in relation to the activity in a hemolysate of erythrocytes of comparable age; 2) increased concentrations of substrates preceding the metabolic block; 3) decreased concentrations of compounds dependent upon the enzymatic activity; and, ideally, 4) similar but less pronounced abnormalities in erythrocytes of blood relatives with minimal or no evidence of hemolysis.

Treatment of patients with inherited enzymatic deficiencies has not been very effective. While not as curative of the anemia as in hereditary spherocytosis, splenectomy appears to have ameliorated the anemia in many patients, especially those with pyruvate kinase deficiency and, perhaps, in those with hexokinase, phosphohexose isomerase, and phosphoglycerate kinase deficiency. It is sometimes difficult to be certain if this improvement has resulted from the splenectomy or if it is coincident with the subsidence of the rapid growth phase of early childhood. Evidence for a beneficial effect of splenectomy in patients with G-6-PD deficiency and spontaneous hemolysis is equivocal.

Future studies may not only reveal additional enzyme deficiencies in association with hemolytic disorders but may also permit the development of therapeutic procedures that can modify or ameliorate the deleterious effects of some of these inherited abnormalities.

REFERENCES

1. Jamieson, G. A. and Greenwalt, T. J.: *Red Cell Membrane: Structure & Function.* Philadelphia, Lippincott, 1969.
2. Disorders of the red cell membrane. *Semin. Hemat. 7:* July, 1970.
3. Weed, R. I.: The Cell Membrane in Hemolytic Disorders. In: *Plenary Session Papers, 12th Congress International Society of Hematology.* Jaffé, E. R., ed. New York, 1968, p. 81.
4. Jandl, J. H.: Hereditary Spherocytosis. In: *Hereditary Disorders of Erythrocyte Metabolism.* Beutler, E., ed. New York and London, Grune and Stratton, 1968, p. 209.
5. Chapman, R. G.: Red cell aldolase deficiency in hereditary spherocytosis. *Brit. J. Haemat. 16:*145, 1969.
6. Cutting, H. O., McHugh, W. J., Conrad, F. G. and Marlow, A. A.: Autosomal dominant hemolytic anemia characterized by ovalocytosis. *Amer. J. Med. 39:*21, 1965.
7. Lock, S. P., Smith, R. S. and Hardisty, R. M.: Stomatocytosis: A hereditary red cell anomaly associated with haemolytic anaemia. *Brit. J. Haemat. 7:*303, 1961.
8. Zarkowsky, H. S., Oski, F. A., Sha'afi, R., Shohet, S. B. and Nathan, D. G.: Congenital hemolytic anemia with high sodium, low potassium red cells. I. Studies of membrane permeability. *New Eng. J. Med. 278:*573, 1968.
9. Oski, F. A., Naiman, J. L., Blum, S. F., Zarkowsky, H. S., Whaun, J., Shohet, S. B., Green, A. and Nathan, D. G.: Congenital hemolytic anemia with high-sodium, low-potassium red cells. *New Eng. J. Med. 280:*909, 1969.
10. Jaffé, E. R. and Gottfried, E. L.: Hereditary nonspherocytic hemolytic disease associated with an altered phospholipid composition of the erythrocytes. *J. Clin. Invest. 47:*1375, 1968.
11. Shohet, S. B., Livermore, B. M. and Jaffé, E. R.: The mechanism of phosphatidyl choline (PC) accumulation in the red blood cells of patients with familial hemolytic anemia and altered erythrocyte lipids. *Blood 34:*859, 1969.
12. Abel, H. A., Bradley, T. B., Jr. and Ranney, H. M.: Pathophysiology of the hemoglobinopathies. *Clin. Obstet. Gynec. 12:*15, 1969.
13. Lehmann, H. and Carrell, R. W.: Varia-

tions in the structure of human haemoglobin. *Brit. Med. Bull.* *25*:14, 1969.
14. Charache, S., Conley, C. L., Waugh, D. F., Ugoretz, R. J. and Spurrell, J. R.: Pathogenesis of hemolytic anemia in homozygous hemoglobin C disease. *J. Clin. Invest.* *46*:1795, 1967.
15. Carrell, R. W. and Lehmann, H.: The unstable haemoglobin haemolytic anaemias. *Seminars. Hemat.* *6*:116, 1969.
16. Taddeini, L. and Watson, C. J.: The clinical porphyrias. *Semin. Hemat.* *5*: 335, 1968.
17. Jaffé, E. R.: Hereditary hemolytic disorders and enzymatic deficiencies of human erythrocytes. *Blood* *35*:116, 1970.
18. Benesch, R. and Benesch, R. E.: Intracellular organic phosphates as regulators of oxygen release by haemoglobin. *Nature* *221*:618, 1969.
19. London, I. M.: The Metabolism of the Erythrocyte. In: *Harvey Lectures 56*. New York, Academic Press, 1961, p. 151.
20. Schneider, A. S., Valentine, W. N., Baughan, M. A., Paglia, D. E., Shore, N. A. and Heins, H. L., Jr.: Triosephosphate Isomerase Deficiency. A Multi-system Inherited Enzyme Disorder: Clinical and Genetic Aspects. In: *Hereditary Disorders of Erythrocyte Metabolism.* Beutler, E., ed. New York and London, Grune and Stratton, 1968, p. 265.
21. Harris, S. R., Paglia, D. E., Jaffé, E. R., Valentine, W. N. and Klein, R. L.: Triosephosphate isomerase deficiency in an adult. *Clin. Research* *18*:529, 1970.
22. Valentine, W. N., Hsieh, H. S., Paglia, D. E., Anderson, H. M., Baughan, M. A., Jaffé, E. R. and Garosn, O. M.: Hereditary hemolytic anemia associated with phosphoglycerate kinase deficiency in erythrocytes and leukocytes. A probable x-chromosome-linked syndrome. *New Eng. J. Med.* *280*:528, 1969.
23. Beutler, E.: Glucose 6-Phosphate Dehydrogenase Deficiency. In: *The Metabolic Basis of Inherited Disease,* 2nd ed. Stanbury, J. B., Wyngaarden, J. B. and Fredrickson, D. S., eds. New York, McGraw-Hill, 1966, p. 1060.
24. Beutler, E.: The effect of flavin compounds on glutathione reductase activity: in vivo and in vitro studies. *J. Clin. Invest.* *48*:1957, 1969.
25. Fairbanks, V. F. and Fernandez, M. N.: The identification of metabolic errors associated with hemolytic anemia. *J.A.M.A.* *208*:316, 1969.

DISEASE-ASSOCIATED AUTOIMMUNE HEMOLYTIC ANEMIA*

ARTHUR SAWITSKY AND PANFILO B. OZAETA, JR.

Division of Hematology
Long Island Jewish Medical Center
New Hyde Park, N. Y.

"BLOOD-INDUCED ICTERUS" produced by the release of massive amounts of a coloring material from blood cells followed by the formation of bile was recognized and described by Vanlair and Masius[1] in 1871. About 20 years later Hayem[2] distinguished between congenital hemolytic anemia and an acquired type of infectious icterus associated with chronic splenomegaly. In 1904 Donath and Landsteiner[3] suggested that a serum factor was responsible for hemolysis in paroxysmal cold hemoglobinuria. French investigators[4] led by Chauffard stressed the importance of red-cell autoagglutination in patients with acquired hemolytic anemia. In 1930 Lederer[5] and Brill[6] described cases af acute hemolysis with rapid onset of anemia and rapid recovery after transfusion therapy. These hemolytic episodes were thought to be due to infectious agents. A clear distinction between congenital and acquired hemolytic anemia was not drawn, however, until Dameshek and Schwartz[7, 8] in 1938 and in 1940 demonstrated the presence of abnormal hemolysins in the sera of patients with acquired hemolytic anemia and postulated an immune mechanism.

During the past three decades studies[9] defining red-cell blood groups and serum antibodies have produced diagnostic methods that have laid the basis for immunologic concepts relevant to many of the acquired hemolytic states. Of these developments, the antiglobulin test described by Coombs, Mourant, and Race[10] in 1945 has proved to be one of the more importantly useful tools now available for the detection of immune hemolytic states. This technique demonstrated that a rabbit antibody against human globulin would induce agglutination of human red cells "coated with an incomplete variety of rhesus antibody." C. Moreschi[11] had used the same method in 1908 in a goat antirabbit-red-cell system. The test was historically premature and was forgotten. In

*Presented at a *Symposium on Hemolytic Anemia* sponsored by the Section on Medicine, February 17, 1970.

1946 Boorman, Dodd, and Loutit[12] applied the direct antiglobulin test to a variety of hemolytic anemias and laid the foundation for the clear distinction of autoimmune from congenital hemolytic anemia.

A hemolytic state exists whenever the red-cell survival time is shortened from the normal average of 120 days. Hemolytic anemia is the hemolytic state in which anemia is present, and bone-marrow function is inferentially unable to compensate for the shortened life-span of the red cell. Immune hemolytic states are those hemolytic states, both anemic and nonanemic, which involve immune mechanisms consisting of antigen-antibody reactions. These reactions may result from unrelated antigen-antibody complexes that fix to an innocent-bystander erythrocyte, or from related antigen-antibody combinations in which the host red cell or some part of its structure is or has become antigenic. The latter type of antigen-antibody reaction may be termed "autoimmune," and hemolytic anemias so produced are autoimmune hemolytic anemias. A group of patients having such disorders forms the basis of this report.

In our view the following criteria must be satisfied if the diagnosis of autoimmune hemolytic anemia is to be made: 1) there must be a direct positive antiglobulin test; 2) there must be suggestive evidence that the globulin which coats the red cell is an antibody produced by the host; 3) coating antibody must be presumed to be responsible for damage and consequent shortened survival of the red cell.

General clinical observations have emphasized that the autoimmune hemolysis is not a disease but rather a syndrome—the top of an iceberg produced by a series of immune reactions. These reactions in turn may be the expression of an acquired abnormal lymphoid system evoked by antigen and nurtured and given final expression by the lymphoid organ of the host. These immune reactions may therefore stem from diverse underlying or associated diseases.[4, 9] Figure 1 offers a representation of an immune mechanism in which the presence of antigen provokes either a humoral or cellular response. Usually and "normally" the antigen concerned is "nonself," and the antibody produced is directed against "nonself" antigen. Under certain conditions in which there is either alteration of antigen or alteration of host immunocyte, humoral and cellular immune processes may be brought to bear against "self." Let us reserve further discussion of this mechanism.

The presence of direct-positive antiglobulin tests in a hospital

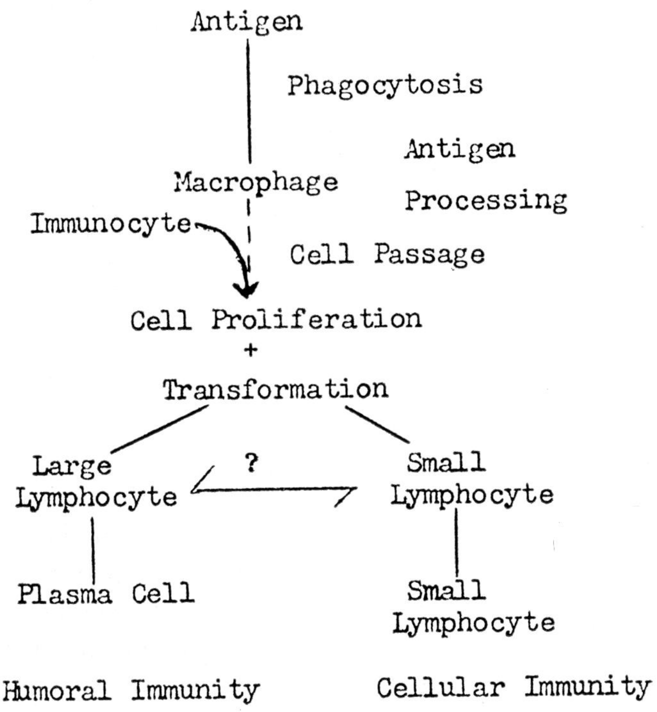

Figure 1

TABLE I. INCIDENCE OF AUTOIMMUNE HEMOLYTIC ANEMIA

	1967	*1968*	*1969*	*Total*	*Percentage*
Direct antiglobulin test done	1,424	1,355	1,478	4,257	100.0
Positive direct antiglobulin test	94	133	149	376	8.8
Hemolytic disease of newborn	34	44	36	114	2.6
Hemolytic state (?)	60	89	113	262	6.2
Hemolytic anemia— Adequate data available	—	—	—	90	—

population will depend upon the enthusiasm and effort with which it is sought.

Table I gives the incidence of positive-direct antiglobulin tests obtained at the Long Island Jewish Medical Center for the years 1967 through 1969. Four thousand, two hundred and fifty-seven bloods were

TABLE II. COMPARATIVE INCIDENCE OF PRIMARY AND SECONDARY FORMS OF AUTOIMMUNE HEMOLYTIC ANEMIA*

Investigator	*Number of patients*	*Incidence per cent primary*	*Incidence per cent secondary*
Dameshek and Komninos[14] (1956)	43	50.0	50.0
Evans and Weiser[15] (1957)	41	54.0	46.0
Lal & Speiser[18] (1957)	97	50.0	50.0
Von Loghem et al.[16] (1956)	122	45.0	55.0
Dausset and Colombani[13] (1959)	128	73.0	27.0
Dacie[9] (1962)	129	70.0	30.0
Yunis and Bridges[17] (1966)	40	42.5	57.5
Pirofsky[4] (1968)	234	18.8	81.2
Sawitsky and Ozaeta (1969)	90	10.0	90.0

*Adapted from Pirofsky.[4]

tested, of which 376 or 8.8% were positive. Of the positive group approximately 30% were in newborn infants with acquired passively transferred hemolytic disease. Seventy per cent were patients with a presumed hemolytic state but there was sufficient data in only a third of the remaining patients to permit their inclusion into the group we have designated autoimmune hemolytic anemia. Autoimmune hemolytic anemia may be primary or idiopathic and, therefore, of indeterminate etiology; alternatively it may be secondary to other disease states. Most commonly the secondary or symptomatic varieties involve the lymphoreticular system (i.e., chronic lymphocytic leukemia and the lymphomas), other malignancies, or systemic lupus erythematosus and other hypersensitivity diseases, or infectious disease of bacterial, viral, or fungal origin. Finally, there is a miscellaneous group which includes mechanical trauma to erythrocytes as well as drug-related syndromes which may provide the stimulus to the production of hemolytic disease.

The comparative reported incidence of the primary and secondary forms of autoimmune hemolytic anemia is listed in Table II. The overall incidence of primary and secondary autoimmune hemolytic anemia as reported during 1950 and to 1956 is almost the same. Data provided by Dausset[13] (1959) and Dacie[9] (1962) show a preponderance of the primary or idiopathic type of hemolytic anemia. Since 1966, however, the symptomatic or secondary type appears to predominate, and Pirofsky[4] in 1968 found that 80% of patients with autoimmune hemolytic anemia were of the secondary or symptomatic type.

TABLE III. SYSTEMIC DISEASES ASSOCIATED WITH DIRECT ANTIGLOBULIN TEST IN 90 PATIENTS

Diseases	*No.*	*Per cent*
I) Idiopathic (primary) A.I.H.A.	9	10.0
II) Secondary (symptomatic) A.I.H.A.		
A) Red blood cell dyscrasia		
Aplastic anemia	1	1.1
Myeloid metaplasia	3	3.3
Pure red-cell anemia	2	2.2
B) Platelet dyscrasia		
Idiopathic thrombocytopenia purpura	8	8.8
C) Lymphoreticular disorders		
Acute leukemias	6	6.6
Chronic lymphatic leukemia	13	14.4
Hodgkin's disease	6	6.6
Lymphosarcoma	4	4.4
Hemangiosarcoma	1	1.1
Multiple myeloma	3	3.3
D) Malignancies—carcinomata	3	3.3
E) Connective tissue disorders and hypersensitivity states	15	16.7
F) Miscellaneous disorders	16	17.6

Our data agree with his findings, and Table III details the incidence of associated diseases found in our patients with autoimmune hemolytic anemia. The differences in incidence noted by the various authors undoubtedly are due in part to differences in the patients examined, laboratory procedures, and reagents used. Our patients have a high incidence of leukemia, lymphoma, and allied disorders. In addition, our blood-bank laboratory does antiglobulin testing on most of the bloods received, and employs a routine serum-enzyme screening for atypical antibodies. Direct antiglobulin tests are then performed on any bloods suspected of atypical reactions. The newer antiglobulin reagents are also more potent than those available 10 years ago. Finally, the proficiency with which the blood bank detects positivity of the antiglobulin reaction influences the incidence of positive findings. It should be emphasized at this point that there is frequently a lack of correlation between the finding of a positive-direct antiglobulin test and clinical hemolysis or a clinically apparent hemolytic state.

In the group of patients we studied, hemolytic syndrome was found in all ages from one through 80 years. Adults predominate, and the largest number of patients were found to be in the 50- to 70-year group. The disease was found to occur in both males and females but in agreement with other reports[4, 9, 13] the female predominated almost two to

TABLE IV. THE DISTRIBUTION OF BLOOD GROUPS IN AUTOIMMUNE HEMOLYTIC ANEMIA IN 47 PATIENTS

ABO (H) Phenotype	*No.*	*Per cent*	*Expected incidence-per cent*
A	21	44.7	44.6
B	7	15.6	8.5
AB	1	2.1	3.5
O	18	38.3	43.6
Rh-hr Genotype			
R_1R_1 or $R_1r + R_1R_2$	30	63.8	62.98
R_2R_2 or $R_2r + R_1R_2$	11	23.4	27.23
R_1R_2	3	6.6	13.95
rr	9	19.1	14.60

one. Although it has been claimed that there is an excess of blood-group O patients with an autoimmune hemolytic anemia[19] our findings do not support this contention.

Table IV indicates no bias, although there is a slight excess of type B patients. This may be due to the small number of patients in whom blood-grouping data were available. Similarly, the Rh-hr phenotype or genotype does not show any significant trend although again a slightly higher proportion of Rh-negative individuals appeared in our hemolytic-anemia series. Our data are too meager for analysis as to race or genetic background. The possibility that genetic predisposition plays a role is strong since familial predisposition for the initiation of various autoimmune disorders has been postulated, i.e., systemic lupus erythematosus,[20] rheumatoid arthritis,[21] pernicious anemia,[22] and thyroiditis.[23] Pirofsky[4] in his excellent text on autoimmune hemolytic anemias cites the reports from the literature involving eight families that showed a familial occurrence of this disorder. He adds a ninth family in which two sisters and a brother developed autoimmune hemolytic anemia. In our own series no familial occurrence was noted. An animal model developed by Bielschowsky, Helyer, and Howie[24] in 1959 lends credence to the concept that genetic factors predispose to the production of autoimmune hemolytic anemia. In this animal model clinical features of autoimmune hemolytic anemia are clear.[25] The homozygous NZB mice develop their anemia at 6 to 12 months of age. A moderate but aggressive icterus and progressive anemia occurs, followed by ataxia and intercurrent infection resulting in the death of the animal. In approxi-

TABLE V. AUTOIMMUNE HEMOLYTIC ANEMIA

Pt. *Dx.*	*N.S.♂54* *lymphosarcoma*	*M.B.♀65* *C.L.L.*	*G.P.♀17* *I.M.*	*G.F.♀13* *IAIHA*
Time to Dx	8 years	---	1 wk.	(?)
Antiglobulin test	+++	+++	++++	+++
Gamma	+++	+++	?	+++
Nongamma	++	+	?	++
Eluate (specificity)	hr″ (?)	Weak (nonspecific)	?	Pan.
Serum antibodies	Pan.	Cold	Neg.	Pan.
Serology	+	+	+	Neg.
Serum Immuno-diffusion	IgM ↑ IgA ↓ IgG ←→	IgM ↑ IgA ←→ IgG ←→	IgM ? IgA ? IgG ?	IgM ←→ IgA ←→ IgG ←→

mately 5% of the homozygous group a positive lupus preparation is obtained; all these mice have a positive direct antiglobulin test. In the heterozygous state, 10% of the animals show intermittently positive direct antiglobulin tests but 35% of the mice have a positive L.E. preparation. It is of interest that in this group females predominate over males almost three to one.

The onset of disease in our patients was referable either to signs or symptoms associated with a progressive anemia, to the onset of icterus, or to the presence of fever. Physical examination usually showed splenomegaly, hepatomegaly, lymphadenopathy, and icterus. The spleen and liver were not much enlarged and were rarely palpable beyond 6 cm. below the costal margin. The liver and spleen were smaller in patients with the idiopathic type whereas the larger spleens and livers were both associated with the secondary or symptomatic type.

Table V lists the characteristics found in four patients who had secondary or symptomatic autoimmune hemolytic anemia.

The first patient is a 54-year-old white male in whom a diagnosis of idiopathic autoimmune hemolytic anemia was made eight years ago. His brother had died previously of multiple myeloma and his mother of breast cancer. During this period he was treated with cytotoxic agents and prednisone. Splenectomy was seriously considered but was continually deferred. The direct antiglobulin test was strongly positive; this was found to be due largely to a gamma-globulin coating of the red cell. The eluate appeared to have "hr" activity, and study of this patient's serum showed the presence of a panagglutinin. The serology was positive and serum immunodiffusion studies showed an increase in IgM, a decrease in IgA, and normal IgG. Within the past two months lymphadenopathy became prominent and a lymph node biopsy was diagnostic for lymphosarcoma. The second patient is a 65-year-old white female with known lymphocytic leukemia of three years' duration who developed hemolytic anemia and a positive-direct antiglobulin test mainly of the gamma type. The eluate showed a weak and nonspecific antibody which had more activity in the cold than in the warm. The serum showed a low-titred cold agglutinin. The serology was positive. There is an increase in serum IgM. The third patient is a 17-year-old black female in whom a diagnosis of infectious mononucleosis followed the onset of acute hemolytic anemia. This patient's serum showed no antibody. Her serology was biologically positive. No immunodiffusion studies were done in this patient. No specific treatment was given this patient, and she recovered from infectious mononucleosis. The positive direct antiglobulin test reverted to negative after 11 weeks. The fourth patient is a 13-year-old white female whose condition was diagnosed idiopathic or primary autoimmune hemolytic anemia. The disease presented itself with severe anemia and icterus. A positive direct antiglobulin test with a strong panagglutinin eluted from the cell and a panagglutinin was easily demonstrated in her serum. Serum immunodiffusion studies were normal. Steroid alone and with azothioprine was unsuccessful. The patient has recently been splenectomized and the hemolysis is controlled.

Survival data in our group of patients indicate that a mortality of 40 to 45% can be anticipated for patients whose diagnoses are idiopathic or primary autoimmune hemolytic anemia. If death occurs it usually happens within two years of diagnosis.[4, 9] Twenty per cent can be expected to be "cured." An indeterminate percentage of the remaining 35% can be expected to develop or manifest underlying lymphomatous or hypersensitivity-state disease. In 29 children under 13 months of age a mortality of 28% was documented by Dacie.[9] With longer and more efficient follow-up the multisystemic nature of abnormalities of immunologic origin becomes more and more apparent.

This tends to eliminate "idiopathic" disease. This, in effect, is what has occurred in many of our patients. Patients who have symptomatic or secondary autoimmune hemolytic anemia have a mortality rate based upon the underlying primary disease. Autoimmune hemolytic anemia secondary to bacterial or viral infection rarely results in death. Pirofsky found that if death occurs in secondary autoimmune hemolytic anemias 26.9% of the patients die within three months and 60.0% within one year.[4] Only 7.8% live five years. Because of the age group involved, associated diseases are common. Arteriosclerotic heart disease is a common concomitant in these patients. Steroid treatment frequently potentiates diabetes, which may in turn have an autoimmune origin. Treatment requires general supportive care with insulin or diuretics where necessary. Total care of the patient cannot be ignored and, with proper management, successful results can be obtained.

As evidence accumulates that autoimmune hemolytic anemia is an immunologically mediated disease, initial treatment is being directed toward immunosuppression. Corticosteroid therapy may produce immunosuppression by lympholysis or by interference with antigen-antibody union and stabilization of lysosomes. In addition, corticosteroids may stimulate erythropoiesis and delivery of red cells to the peripheral blood. The benefit derived from the use of cytotoxic drugs such as azothioprine and six-mercaptopurine[27] or of alkylating agents such as cyclophosphamide is thought to be due to similar immunosuppressive activity against the immune-component lymphocyte, immunocyte, or antibody-producing plasma cell. Local splenic irradiation may act similarly against a large localized mass of antibody-producing tissue, and thereby may be beneficial.[4] The treatment of autoimmune hemolytic anemia advocated by most authorities today is based on the corticosteroids, usually prednisone with or without the addition of a cytotoxic agent, usually azothioprine or cytoxan. If results of this regimen are poor or inadequate, splenectomy is recommended.

The value of splenectomy is debatable, [9, 13, 14] but if prednisone and cytotoxic therapy are ineffective, radioisotope splenic sequestration studies may be carried out and, if strongly positive, may indicate that splenectomy will be beneficial.[26] Unfortunately, we have had patients with a positive splenic-sequestration study followed by splenectomy and minimal benefit. We have other patients with negative sequestration studies in whom splenectomy has provided significant benefits. Further

TABLE VI. PATIENTS WITH AUTOIMMUNE HEMOLYTIC ANEMIA TESTED WITH SPECIFIC COOMBS' SERA[56]

Gamma	*Nongamma*	*No. patients*	*Per cent*
+	—	12	21.4
+	+	34	60.6
—	+	10	17.9

TABLE VII. AUTOIMMUNE HEMOLYTIC ANEMIA

Eluate Study

	Direct antiglobulin reaction		*Test cells*						
	gamma	*non-gamma*	R_1R_2	R_1R_1	R_1r	R_2r	*rr*	*null*	*Pooled cells*
N.S.	+++	++	+/++	0	0	0	0	+	+
M.B.	+++	++	0	0	0	0	0	0	0
C.W.	+++	++	0	0	0	+/++	+/++	+++	+/++
A.S.	++++	++	+++	+++	+++	+++	+++	0	++
G.F.	+++	+++	++++	++++	++++	++++	++++	++++	++++

studies of red cells found to be positive to a broad-spectrum antiglobulin serum indicate that the presence of a positive Coombs' antiglobulin test is not necessarily due to gamma antibody.[9, 30]

Table VI is an analysis of 56 such studies in which approximately 18% of patients showed only the presence of a nongamma globulin attached to the red cell. Presumably the nongamma globulin was complement or complement component. Elution studies of red cells with strong direct antiglobulin tests have indicated that the antibody concerned with the hemolytic state may be related to the Rh-hr system.[4, 28, 29]

Table VII shows the results of one such study. Antibody was eluted from the red cell by heat treatment at 56°C. The eluates were then tested against the panel of cells; the results are indicated in the table. The first patient shows a reaction to R_1R_2 cells and to Rh-null red cells. This pattern of reaction is somewhat difficult to explain. The second patient shows an eluate from a strongly gamma Coombs'-positive cell which did not react with any of the cells tested and was found to be a cold antibody. The reaction of the eluate from the third patient was

TABLE VIII. AUTOIMMUNE HEMOLYTIC ANEMIA SERUM STUDY

	Test cells					
	R_1R_2	R_1R_1	R_1r	R_2r	rr	*null*
N.S.	+	0	+	+	+	–
M.B.	0	+	+	++	+	±
C.W.	0	0	0	0	0	±
A.S.	0	±	0	++	+	0
G.F.	++++	++++	++++	++++	++++	++++

TABLE IX. AUTOIMMUNE HEMOLYTIC ANEMIA ELUATE ABSORPTION STUDIES

Absorb eluate	*with A null cells*		*with R_1R_2 cells*	
Then react with	R_1R_2	*Null*	R_1R_2	*Null*
N.S.	0			
M.B.	0			
C.W.	0			
A.S.	+++	0	+/++	+
G.F.	++++	+++	+++	+++

strongest to the Rh-null cell and against the Rh-negative cell. This antibody is a warm antibody but the exact significance of the finding is not apparent. The fourth patient shows the typical reaction of warm antibody against all red cells with an expressed Rh-hr component but not to Rh-null cells. The antibody of the fifth patient reacts strongly with all cells and does not appear to have any specific affinity for the Rh-hr antigen.

Table VIII shows the reaction of serum against the same panel of cells; this time it would appear that although no specific pattern is noted, the reaction to Rh-null cells is uniformly weak except that of patient G.F.

Eluate-absorption studies shown in Table IX indicate that the eluate of patient A.S. reacts in typical fashion and absorption with Rh-positive cells reduces the strength of antibody in the eluate. Absorption with the Rh-null cell does not change the antibody reaction. G.F. manifests no such pattern.

Lalezari[31] has studied the temperature-gradient dissociation curve

TABLE X. OTHER SERUM ANTIBODIES ASSOCIATED WITH AUTOIMMUNE HEMOLYTIC SYNDROMES

Positive serology	4/16
Latex (RA) floc	3/5
Antinuclear (ANA)	1/10*
Leukagglutinins	4/5
Platelet agglutinins	3/9

*Excluding documented L.E.

TABLE XI. POSITIVE ANTIGLOBULIN TEST ASSOCIATED WITH VARIATIONS IN PERIPHERAL BLOOD COUNTS

Cell type	*Abnormally low*	*Abnormally high*
Platelets	17	4
Leucocytes	5	14
Lymphocytes	23	13*

*All CLL cases

of red cells and serum from patients with acute hemolytic anemia. The curves produced by cells obtained from patients with the idiopathic type reflected resistance by the antigen-antibody complex for dissociation by heat as compared to that produced by cells from a patient with secondary or symptomatic disease.

Table X shows the incidence of other serum antibodies in patients with autoimmune hemolytic syndromes. In 4 of 16 patients positive serology was observed. In three of five, positive Latex (RA) flocculation was present. Excluding patients with known disseminated lupus erythematosus, one additional patient showed the presence of a positive antinuclear antibody test. Leukagglutinins were present in four of five patients so tested and platelet agglutinins in three of nine.

The incidence of antibodies against blood-cell elements other than red cells is high. This finding suggests either that there is widespread alteration of the immune response to different tissue antigens or that there are antigens shared between red cells and at least leukocytes and platelets. It seems probable that these or similar autoantibodies are being directed against other cell types or elements.

Table XI shows the concentration of platelets, white cells, and

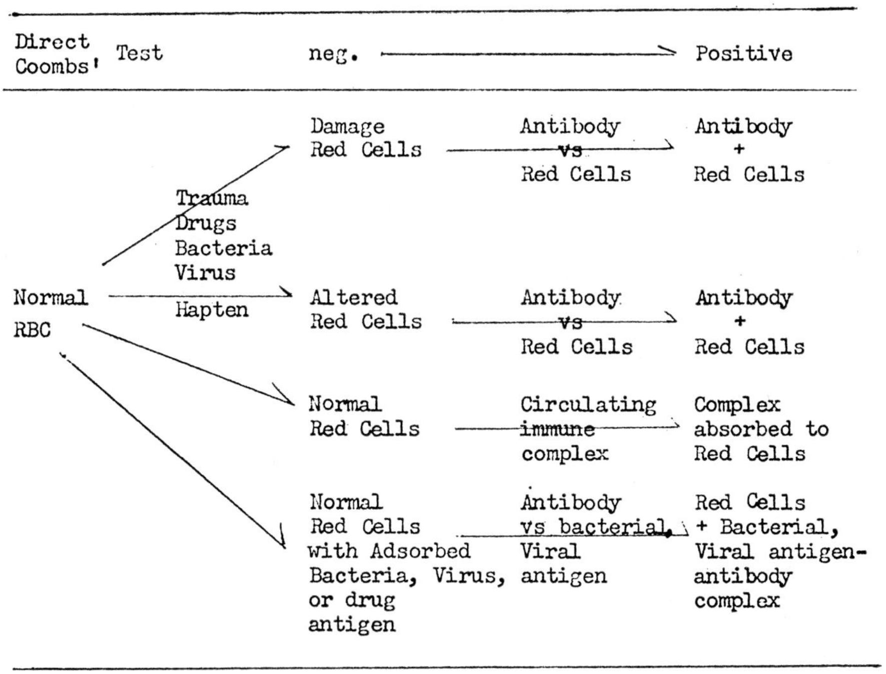

Fig. 2. Pathogenesis—direct-positive antiglobulin test

lymphocytes in the peripheral blood of patients found to have autoimmune hemolytic disease when they first presented for diagnosis. This table includes both primary and secondary autoimmune hemolytic anemia. Simultaneous occurrence of thrombocytopenia and autoimmune hemolytic anemia is now well recognized and is frequently referred to as Evans' syndrome.[32] The larger proportion of patients with changes in platelet count occurred in the secondary thrombocytopenic group. The high proportion of patients with lymphopenia is worthy of some note and suggests abnormality in the lymphoid organ.

Figure 2 suggests a concept for the pathogenesis of the direct positive antiglobulin test. This pattern of reaction suggests that normal red cells may be altered because of physical trauma, drugs, bacteria, or virus, with subsequent damage to the membrane or alteration of surface antigen. Alternatively surface antigen may be uncovered by the event, and antibody against these altered cells may be formed by the host. Ultimate antibody and red-cell reactivity and a positive-direct antiglobulin test would produce alteration in the plasticity of the cell, followed by sequestration and hemolysis. Alternatively hapten may react with the red cell to produce a change in the cell surface or cell antigen, followed by production of antibody by the host. Autoreaction with the host red cells would ensue. On the other hand, normal circulating red cells might absorb to their surface a circulating antigen-antibody-immune complex which, having become absorbed to the red cell surface, would react positively to the antiglobulin test with or without the production of a hemolytic state. Finally, normal red cells could absorb bacteria, virus, or drug antigen and, acting as "innocent bystanders," react to antibody produced against the bacterial, viral, or drug antigen and so develop a positive direct antiglobulin test. Alteration in cell-surface plasticity, sequestration, and hemolysis are then a probable sequence.

Summary

The autoimmune hemolytic anemias are characterized by premature destruction of erythrocytes with antibody bound to the cell surface. The presence of the antibody is demonstrated by a positive direct antiglobulin test. However, the presence of a positive test is not invariably associated with hemolytic disease. Pathophysiologic mechanisms leading to this state may be nonimmunologic, immune but not antoimmune, or autoimmune. Approximately 80 to 90% of these patients have reached this altered state of immunity because of underlying systemic disease or exogenous stimulus. These patients are said to have secondary or symptomatic autoimmune hemolytic disease. In the remaining 10 to 20% no underlying systemic cause can be found. The most common diseases associated with autoimmune states are the lymphoreticular diseases, such as lymphocytic leukemia, lymphoma, and Hodgkin's disease, or the connective-tissue disorders and the hypersensitivity states such as lupus erythematosus. In these patients survival is largely dictated by the prognosis of the systemic disease. In the primary or idiopathic type a mortality of 40% can be anticipated. Treatment is directed toward immunosuppression with the use of corticosteroids and chemotherapeutic agents. Splenectomy is reserved for the unresponsive patient; its value still remains difficult to assess. The antibody related to production of the hemolytic anemia is usually of the incomplete warm type and is in some way related to red cell Rh-hr antigen. The multisystemic aspects of the disorder are demonstrated by the increased frequency in the presence of serum antibodies directed against white cells, platelets, thyroid, and desoxyribosenucleic acid. Abnormalities in the serum-protein pattern are frequent but no characteristic pattern is noted. When viewed in the broadest sense our data indicate that autoimmune hemolytic anemia is only a manifestation of generalized altered immune response.

REFERENCES

1. Vanlair, C. F. and Masius, J. R.: De la microcythémia. *Bull. Acad. Roy. Med. Belg. 5*:515, 1871. Quoted by Pirofsky, B.[4]
2. Hayem, G.: Sur une variété particulière dictère chronique. Ictère infectieux chronique splénomégalique. *Presse Med. 6*:121, 1898. Quoted by Pirofsky, B.[4]
3. Donath, J. and Landsteiner, K.: Ueber paroxysmale Hämoglobinurie. *Munchen Med. Wschr. 51*:1590, 1904.
4. Pirofsky, B.: *Autoimmunization and the Autoimmune Hemolytic Anemias.* Baltimore, Williams and Wilkins, 1969, pp. 1-8.
5. Lederer, M.: Three additional cases of acute hemolytic (infectious) anemia. *Amer. J. Med. Sci. 179*:228, 1930.
6. Brill, I. C.: Acute febrile anemia—a new disease? *Arch. Intern. Med. 37*:244, 1926.
7. Dameshek, W. and Schwartz, S. O.: The presence of hemolysins in acute hemolytic anemia; preliminary note. *New Eng. J. Med. 218*:75, 1938.
8. Dameshek, W. and Schwartz, S. O.: Acute hemolytic anemia (acquired hemolytic icterus, acute type). *Medicine 19*:231, 1940.
9. Dacie, J. V.: *The Haemolytic Anaemias,* part 2, 2d ed. New York, Grune & Stratton, 1962.
10. Coombs, R. R. A., Mourant, A. E. and Race, R. R.: A new test for the detection of weak and "incomplete" Rh agglutinins. *Brit. J. Exp. Path. 26*:255, 1945.
11. Moreschi, C.: Beschleunigung und Verstärkung der Bakterienagglutination durch antieiweis-sera. *Zbl. Bakt. 46*:456, 1908.
12. Boorman, K. E., Dodd, B. E. and Loutit, J. F.; Haemolytic icterus (acholuric jaundice) congenital and acquired. *Lancet 1*:812, 1946.
13. Dausset, J. and Colombani, J.; The serology and the prognosis of 128 cases of autoimmune hemolytic anemia. *Blood 14*:1280, 1959.
14. Dameshek, W. and Komninos, Z. D.: The present status of treatment of autoimmune hemolytic anemia with ACTH and cortisone. *Blood 11*:648, 1956.
15. Evans, R. S. and Weiser, R. S.: The serology of autoimmune hemolytic disease: Observations on forty-one patients. *Arch. Intern. Med. 100*:371, 1957.
16. Van Loghem, J. J., van der Hart, M. and Dorfmeier, H.: Serologic Studies in Acquired Hemolytic Anemia. *Proc. 6th Internat. Cong. Int. Soc. Hemat.* New York, Grune & Stratton, 1956.
17. Yunis, E. J. and Bridges, R. A.: Blood transfusion problems in autoimmune hemolytic anemias. *Minn. Med. 49*:759, 1966.
18. Lal, V. B. and Speiser, P.: Quoted by Pirofsky, B.,[4] p. 35.
19. Hunt, M. C. and Lucia, S. P.: The occurrence of acquired hemolytic anemia in subjects of blood group O. *Science 118*:183, 1953.
20. Leonhardt, T.: Familial studies in systemic lupus erythematosus. *Acta Med. Scand.* (Suppl.) *176*:416, 1964.
21. Fudenberg, H., German, J. L. and Kunkel, H.: The occurrence of rheumatoid factor and other abnormalities in families of patients with agammaglobulinemia. *Arthritis Rheum. 5*:565, 1962.
22. McIntyre, P. A., Hahn, R., Conley, C. L. and Glass, B.: Genetic factors in pre-

disposition to pernicious anemia. *Bull. J. Hopkins Hosp. 104*:309, 1959.
23. Hall, R., Owen, S. G. and Smart, G. A.: Evidence for genetic predisposition to formation of thyroid autoantibodies. *Lancet 2*:187, 1960.
24. Howie, J. P. and Helyer, B. J.: Autoimmune disease in mice. *Ann. N.Y. Acad. Sci. 124*:167, 1965.
25. Holmes, M. C. and Burnet, F. M.: The natural history of autoimmune disease in NZB mice. *Ann. Intern. Med. 59*: 265, 1963.
26. McCurdy, P. R. and Rath, C. E.: Splenectomy in hemolytic anemia. Results predicted by body scanning after injection of $Cr.^{51}$ tagged red cells. *New Eng. J. Med. 259*:459, 1958.
27. Schwartz, R. and Dameshek, W.: The treatment of autoimmune hemolytic anemia with 6-mercaptopurine and thioguanine. *Blood 19*:483, 1962.
28. Wiener, A. S. and Gordon, E. B.: Quantitative test for antibody-globulin coating human blood cells and its practical applications. *Amer. J. Clin. Path. 23*: 429, 1953.
29. Wiener, A. S., Gordon, E. B. and Gallop, C.: Studies on autoantibodies in human sera. *J. Immun. 71*:58, 1953.
30. Vaughan, J. H.: Immunologic features of erythrocyte sensitization. I. Acquired hemolytic disease. *Blood 11*:1085, 1956.
31. Lalezari, P.: A New Approach to the Study of Red Cell Antigen-antibody reactions. Its Application to Autoimmune Diseases. *Twelfth Congress Int. Soc. Blood Transf.* Moscow, U.S.S.R., 1969.
32. Evans, R. S. and Duane, R. T.: Acquired hemolytic anemia. II. The significance of thrombocytopenia and leukopenia. *Blood 4*:1196, 1949.

DRUG-ASSOCIATED HEMOLYTIC ANEMIA*

RALPH ZALUSKY

Associate Professor of Medicine
Mount Sinai School of Medicine
New York, N. Y.

INTRODUCTION

ALTHOUGH the human red cell contains protective mechanisms for the maintenance of membrane and hemoglobin integrity a variety of drugs and chemicals can alter these components and cause early destruction. Drug-induced hemolytic anemias may occur in one of the following ways: 1) *immunologic*—the drug induces serologically identifiable changes in the susceptible individual that may or may not require the continuing presence of the drug for appropriate diagnosis; 2) *metabolic*—genetically determined abnormalities in red cell metabolism may predispose the cell to irreversible injury by "oxidant" drugs; and 3) *hemoglobin instability*—certain amino-acid substitutions in the α or β chain or abnormal tetrameric species are associated with chronic hemolytic anemia which may be greatly exaggerated in the presence of drugs.

DRUG-INDUCED IMMUNE HEMOLYTIC ANEMIA

Fifteen years ago Harris[1] reported a case of acute intravascular hemolysis that developed in a patient undergoing treatment with the drug stibophen. He demonstrated that the direct antiglobulin test was positive and that the patient's serum contained an antibody that in the presence of stibophen caused agglutination of normal cells and sensitized them to antiglobulin serum. Deleting the drug from the system resulted in no sensitization of normal cells. Since this initial report, 40 similar cases of drug-induced immune hemolytic anemia have been described.[2] Table I lists the drugs that have been implicated.

Except for penicillin and alpha-methyldopa, which require special consideration, these drugs cause a hemolytic anemia with the following characteristics: 1) hemolysis is usually acute and intravascular with

*Presented at a *Symposium on Hemolytic Anemia* sponsored by the Section on Medicine, February 17, 1970.
This study was supported in part by the Albert A. List, Frederick Machlin, and Anna Ruth Lowenburg Funds, New York, N. Y.

TABLE I. DRUGS IMPLICATED IN CAUSING HEMOLYTIC ANEMIA*

Underlying mechanism			
Immunologic	*Erythrocyte metabolic abnormalities (primarily G-6-PD deficiency)*		*Unstable hemoglobin*
Acetophenetidin	Acetanilid	Pamaquine	Causyth
Alpha-methyldopa	Acetophenetidin	Pentaquine	Primaquine
Antistine	Acetylsalicylic acid	Phenylhydrazine	Sulfamethoxypyridazine
Chlorpromazine	Chloroquine	Primaquine	Sulfaproxiline† sulfamerazine
Dipyrone	Diaphenylsulfone	Quinine	Sulfisomidine
Insecticides	Fava beans	Quinocide	Sulfisoxazole
Isonicotinic acid hydrazide	Furazolidone	Sulfacetamide	
Mefenamic acid†	Furmethonol	Sulfanilamide	
Para-aminosalicylic acid	*N*-Acetylsulfanilamide	Sulfapyridine	
Penicillin	Napthalene	Sulfamethoxypyridazine	
Pyramidon	Neoarsphenamine	Sulfisoxazole	
Stibophen	Nitrofurazone	Vitamin K	
Sulfonamides	Nitrofurantoin		
Quinidine			
Quinine			

*See Worlledge, S. M.,[2] Beutler, E.,[12] Marks, P. A.[13]
†Hemolytic mechanism similar to alpha-methyldopa.

hemoglobinemia and hemoglobinuria; 2) dosage of the offending drug is low and there is usually a history of prior ingestion; 3) the direct antiglobulin test (γ-Coombs') is frequently negative, while components of complement (complement Coombs') can generally be detected on the red cells; and 4) the sera of affected patients will not react with normal cells unless the drug is present also. This combination may show lytic activity *in vitro*.

Approximately one half of the reported cases of drug-antibody hemolytic anemia have been associated with penicillin therapy. The course of one such patient[3] is shown in Figure 1. Characteristically, these patients have been treated with very large doses of the drug, in the region of 20 million units daily, and hemolytic anemia develops gradually rather than abruptly. Hemolysis occurs by extravascular mechanisms; the trapping of autologous Cr^{51}-labeled cells in the spleen has been demonstrated in one patient. Serological studies invariably show a positive antiglobulin test due to IgG on the red cell. Specificity of this antibody for penicillin-treated cells has been demonstrated by elution methods.

Mechanisms involved in the formation of antibodies and the ensuing hemolysis in these drug-induced immune hemolytic anemias remain to

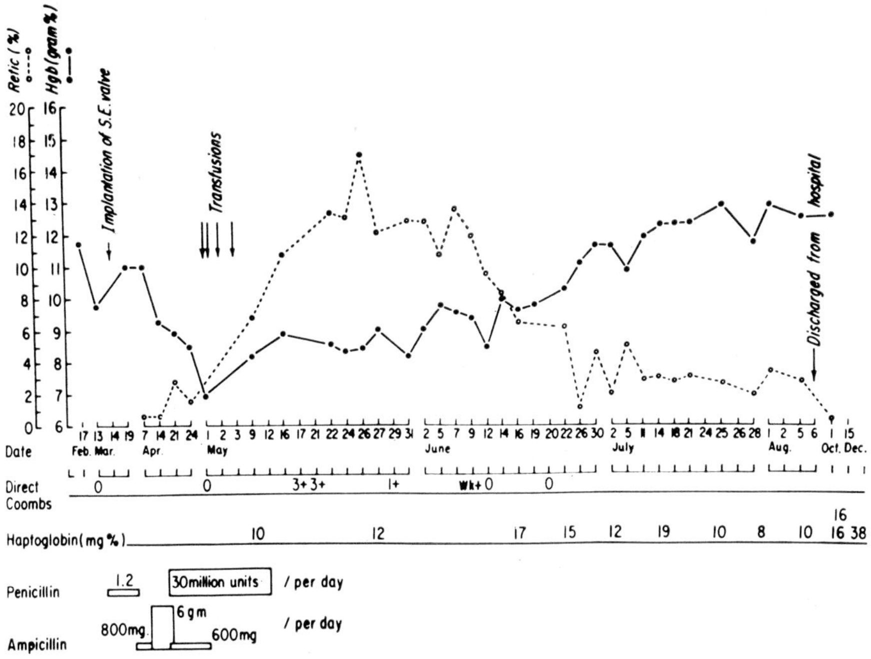

Fig. 1. Course of a penicillin-induced hemolytic anemia after replacement of the mitral valve.[3] Reproduced with permission of the publisher.

be clarified. Two major hypotheses have been offered. Miescher[4] and Shulman[5] have proposed that the initiation of antibody production results from the drug becoming antigenic by combining with a soluble macromolecule. On subsequent reexposure to the drug, drug-antidrug complexes passively adsorb to the red cell, which is merely an "innocent bystander."[6] Either this complex or the initiation of the complement-fixation sequence causes damage to the cell. Alternatively, antibodies may be induced as stated above, but readministration of the drug results in its attachment to the surface of the red cell. Antidrug antibody then combines with this drug antigen on the cell.

Ackroyd and Rook[7] have proposed a second hypothesis: that the red cell behaves as a carrier for the drug or drug-metabolite hapten in the initiation of the formation of antibody. Thus readministration of the drug would lead to a specific interaction between antibody and the drug-carrier (red cell) antigen. The red cell has lost its innocence and is a direct participant.

TABLE II. CHARACTERISTICS OF DRUG-INDUCED IMMUNE HEMOLYSIS

	Drug type		
	General	*Penicillin*	*Alpha-methyldopa*
Type of hemolysis	Intravascular	Extravascular	Extravascular
Drug dose	Low	High	High
Prior ingestion necessary	Yes	No	No
Serology	Complement	IgG	IgG
Drug present in system	Yes	Yes	No

DRUG-INDUCED AUTOIMMUNE HEMOLYTIC ANEMIA

In 1966 investigators in England[8, 9] reported a high incidence of positive direct antiglobulin tests in patients who were administered the antihypertensive drug, alpha-methyldopa (Aldomet). Of 572 patients on this medication, 20% showed a positive test but only two had overt hemolytic anemia. Since these initial reports Worlledge has estimated an over-all incidence of 15% positive direct antiglobulin tests in approximately 1,400 patients studied.[2] Of these, 0.8% developed hemolytic anemia.

Serologic findings in these patients are indistinguishable from those in idiopathic "autoimmune" hemolytic anemia. Red cells are agglutinated by antisera directed against IgG, and free IgG antibody is usually present in the patients' sera. Specificity for Rh antigens has been demonstrated. Presence of the drug is not necessary for this reaction.

Characteristically, the positive direct antiglobulin test develops after three to six months of therapy and becomes negative within one month to two years after discontinuation of the drug.[10] Reinstitution of alpha-methyldopa therapy at a later time does not appear to influence the time necessary to develop a positive reaction. Discontinuance of the drug in patients who have active hemolysis usually results in clinical improvement. Although little is known of the mechanisms that underlie this fascinating phenomenon further studies should be fruitful in unraveling some of the mysteries of "autoimmune" disorders in general.

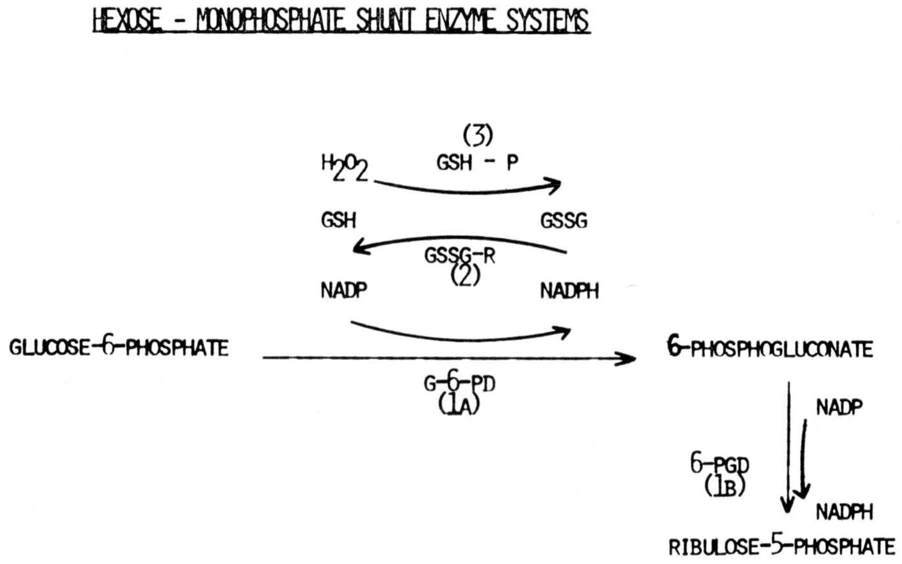

Fig. 2. Hexose-monophosphate shunt pathway of the red cell. See text for details.

Table II summarizes the major distinguishing characteristics of these drug-induced immune hemolytic anemias.

Drug-Induced Hemolytic Anemias Associated with Red Cell Metabolic Abnormalities

Susceptibility to drug-induced hemolysis is found in association with biochemical lesions affecting the hexose-monophosphate shunt pathway in the red cell (Figure 2). Normally, approximately 10% of glucose-6-phosphate is metabolized through this pathway, which serves the important function of maintaining glutathione in the reduced form (GSH). The role of GSH has not been defined completely, but it would appear that it is of major importance in maintaining sulfhydryl-containing enzymes in active form and detoxifying small quantities of hydrogen peroxide. As shown in Figure 2, there are three enzyme systems that must be intact if the red cell is to withstand excessive oxidative stress: 1*a*, 1*b*) the glucose-6-phosphate dehydrogenase (G-6-PD), 6-phosphogluconic dehydrogenase (6-PGD) system which catalyzes the reduction of NADP to NADPH; 2) the glutathione reductase (GSSG-R) system that converts oxidized glutathione (GSSG) with NADPH back to GSH; and 3) glutathione peroxidase (GSH-P) which catalyzes the oxidation of GSH for the reduction of hydrogen peroxide.

G-6-PD deficiency. In his excellent reviews[11, 12] Beutler has described the historical background in the development of our knowledge concerning the metabolic basis of drug-induced hemolytic anemia in persons who harbor a deficiency of G-6-PD. It is now well established that this sex-linked genetic disorder is by far the commonest cause of drug-induced hemolysis. It has been estimated that more than 100 million persons are affected; there is an ethnic incidence as high as 58% in Kurdish Jewish males.[13] Approximately 10% of black American males harbor the defect.

Table I lists many of the agents that have been implicated in causing hemolysis in susceptible individuals. Using Cr^{51}-labeled red cells, Dern et al.[14] performed some classical studies on the hemolytic syndrome associated with the ingestion of primaquine in these subjects. They showed that in the Negro type of G-6-PD deficiency a predictable sequence of events occurred: 1) after two days of primaquine ingestion, during which Heinz bodies could be found in fresh blood, the hematocrit declines abruptly; 2) over the ensuing four to five days the hematocrit reaches its nadir at approximately 50% of its initial value and, with a brisk reticulocytosis, begins to rise toward normal; and 3) despite continuation of the drug, the hematocrit ultimately returns to normal. From these studies Dern and his associates concluded that in these patients the older red cells are most susceptible to the hemolytic effect of the drug. As younger red cells emerged from the bone marrow, refractoriness to lysis induced by primaquine was found.

In 1956 Carson et al.[15] attributed the metabolic abnormality to a deficiency of glucose-6-phosphate dehydrogenase in the red cells. Since that time approximately 45 variants of this enzyme have been identified,[12] but only a few of these are associated with drug-induced hemolysis. The Negro variant (A-) is found in the majority of cases seen in this country with red-cell enzyme activity only 8 to 20% of normal. This probably accounts for the differences seen clinically in comparison with a second common variant, Mediterranean (B-), where enzyme activity is 0 to 7% of normal. In the latter instance, exposure to one of the "oxidant" drugs or Fava beans often results in a fulminating hemolytic anemia with hemoglobinemia and hemoglobinuria. Because even the young red cells have little enzyme activity, hemolysis may continue

TABLE III. GLUCOSE-6-PHOSPHATE DEHYDROGENASE ACTIVITY IN YOUNG AND OLD RED CELLS FOLLOWING TRANSFUSION IN A PATIENT WITH THE MEDITERRANEAN VARIANT OF G-6-PD DEFICIENCY

	Whole blood	*Top layer*	*Bottom layer*
G-6-PD def.			
Reticulocytes (%)	3.6	14.1	0.4
G-6-PD (units)*	619	275	811
Control†			
Reticulocytes (%)	24.9	49.2	12.8
G-6-PD (units)*	2300	3965	2348

*Assayed by the Motulsky modification of the method of Zinkham et al.[25] Normal range is 1200-1800 units/gram hemoglobin.
†Patient with autoimmune hemolytic anemia.

unabated in the presence of the incitant and may lead to death if blood transfusion is not given early. Table III shows the G-6-PD activity in young and old red cells separated by differential centrifugation; the cells were from a patient with the Mediterranean variant one week after a hemolytic episode following the ingestion of acetophenetidin. This patient was given two units of packed red cells upon admission to the hospital, and it is apparent that G-6-PD activity in the reticulocyte-rich layer is abnormally low in comparison to the reticulocyte-poor layer of older transfused normal cells. Control blood from a patient with Coombs' positive hemolytic anemia shows the expected increased enzyme activity in normal reticulocyte-rich blood.

It should be pointed out that in addition to drugs, other factors may lead to active hemolysis in G-6-PD-deficient individuals. Infections, both bacterial and viral, even in the absence of drug therapy, have been incriminated, as has diabetic acidosis. Also a physiological aggravation of the deficiency caused by the relative immaturity of enzymes in the newborn may predispose affected infants to even mild oxidant stimuli such as vitamin K.

Mechanisms of hemolysis in G-6-PD deficiency. Formation of Heinz bodies[16] and loss of GSH[17] are readily observed *in vitro* when enzyme-deficient red cells are incubated with an oxidant drug such as acetylphenylhydrazine. Presence of precipitated denatured hemoglobin adherent to the membrane of the red cell may well diminish the deformability of the cell and may predispose it to early destruction by the reticuloendothelial system. It has been suggested that "oxidant" drugs react with hemoglobin to produce low levels of hydrogen peroxide within the cell.[18] The normal cell is capable of removing this low level of hydrogen peroxide via the glutathione-peroxidase system. The oxidized glutathione formed is then reduced by the enzyme glutathione reductase, and by continuing generation of the cofactor NADPH. When the capacity of the cell to form NADPH is severely restricted, as occurs in G-6-PD deficiency, this mechanism for removal of peroxide is markedly impaired, and peroxidative damage to sulfhydryl-containing enzymes, hemoglobin, and membrane constituents occurs. Although this sequence of events appears plausible, other changes accompanying the presence of drug metabolites that might directly affect red-cell enzymes or hemoglobin cannot be ruled out. Furthermore, since many of the agents responsible for the hemolytic reaction can also induce the formation of methemoglobin, current evidence suggests that methemoglobin may not be necessary for the oxidative damage of hemoglobin.

Other abnormalities of erythrocyte metabolism associated with drug-induced hemolytic anemia. From study of the constituents of the hexose monophosphate shunt pathway it is evident that any abnormality might predispose the red cell to oxidative injury. This is indeed the case, and a few patients with deficiency of glutathione reductase, glutathione, and phosphogluconic dehydrogenase have been reported[12] to show drug-associated hemolysis.

Drug-Induced Hemolytic Anemia Associated with the Unstable Hemoglobins

In 1960 Hitzig et al.[19] described a severe hemolytic anemia in an infant girl and her father following the use of sulfonamides. The red cells contained Heinz bodies during the active hemolytic phase, and hemoglobin electrophoresis showed an abnormal band migrating in a position similar to hemoglobin S. Subsequently this hemoglobin abnormality was characterized as a replacement of arginine for histidine at position 63 of the β chain. Many of the earlier cases of congenital Heinz-body anemia have now been shown to be caused by globin-chain abnormalities and, in addition to Hemoglobin Zürich described above, 20 such abnormalities have been identified.[20]

Clinical features of these unstable hemoglobin-hemolytic anemias tend to show a clearly identifiable pattern. Only heterozygotes have been described; the homozygous state has never been reported and is probably incompatible with life. Hemolytic anemia, often of the compensated variety, is present from infancy. Red cell inclusions, or Heinz bodies, are usually found in patients who have been splenectomized, but can also be demonstrated readily *in vitro* by incubation with redox dyes such as brilliant cresyl blue. Splenomegaly is a common accompaniment of this hemolytic state. Dipyrroluria, caused by a dark pigment of the mesobilifuscin group, has been found frequently. Although methemoglobinemia is not seen clinically, its formation *in vitro* is more rapid than that of normal blood.

Table I lists some of the drugs that have been implicated in increasing the hemolytic disorder in patients with Hemoglobin Zürich. Little information is available concerning the role of drugs in aggravating hemolysis of the other unstable hemoglobins. Mechanisms underlying hemolysis have been suggested by several investigators. The normal hemoglobin tetramer consists of two α and two β chains with their individual heme groups inserted in a hydrophobic pocket of the polypeptide chain. Substitutions in most of the known unstable hemoglobins tend to be found in the globin chain near points of heme contact. Since heme-free globin is quite unstable, it has been suggested that any tendency toward detachment of heme would hasten the precipitation of globin into insoluble residues or Heinz bodies. Methemoglobin, with its greater ease of heme dissociation,[22] may facilitate the precipitation of globin in some of these disorders. Oxidative drugs might thus act by increasing the rate of methemoglobin formation, with consequent increase in the detachment of heme and the precipitation of globin. Alternatively, the substitution may expose a critical portion of the globin chain (such as the β93 cysteine in Hemoglobin Köln), formation of mixed disulfides with GSH or membrane thiols,[21] molecular distortion and Heinz-body formation. However, it is not possible to explain the hemolytic process in all the unstable hemoglobins by this mechanism. In studies performed on Hemoglobin Riverdale-Bronx,[23] we were unable to find any alteration of the heme-to-globin ratio in the course of heat precipitation, and it is apparent that other mechanisms, such as conformational changes or instability due to substitutions at points of subunit contact may be responsible for ease of Heinz-body formation. It is of interest that patients with Hemoglobin H, an unstable tetramer of β chains, show increased hemolysis when given sulfonamides.[24] In any event, since oxidant agents such as acetylphenylhydrazine induce rapid formation of Heinz bodies *in vitro*, the small number of patients who have unstable hemoglobins should not be exposed to these drugs.

Conclusions

Drugs or their metabolites may attack the red cell by immunologic mechanisms or may accelerate breakdown of hemoglobin to Heinz bodies in persons who have inherited enzymatic or hemoglobin defects. Withdrawal of the inciting agent is the first order of treatment but transfusions may be necessary when intense acute hemolysis is present.

REFERENCES

1. Harris, J. W.: Studies on the mechanism of a drug-induced hemolytic anemia. *J. Lab. Clin. Med. 44*:809, 1954.
2. Worlledge, S. M.: Immune drug-induced haemolytic anemias. *Semin. Hemat. 6*: 181, 1969.
3. Lyon, L. J.: Coombs' positive hemolytic anemia due to penicillin. *J. Mt. Sinai Hosp., N.Y. 35*:258, 1968.
4. Miescher, P. and Straessle, R.: Experimentelle studien über den Mechanismus der thrombocyten-schadigung durch Antigen-antikorperreaktion. *Vox Sang. 1*:83, 1956.
5. Shulman, N. R.: A mechanism of cell destruction in individuals sensitised to foreign antigens and its implications in autoimmunity. *Ann. Intern. Med. 60*: 506, 1964.
6. Dameshek, W.: Autoimmunity: Theoretical aspects. *Ann. N.Y. Acad. Sci. 124*: 6, 1965.
7. Ackroyd, J. F. and Rook, A. J.: Allergic Drug Reactions. In: *Clinical Aspects of Immunology*, 2d ed. Gell, P. G. H. and Coombs, R. R. A., eds. Oxford and Edinburgh, Blackwells Scient. Publ. 1968, p. 693.
8. Carstairs, K. C., Breckenridge, A., Dollery, C. T. and Worlledge, S. M.: Incidence of a positive direct Coombs test in patients on α-methyldopa. *Lancet 2*:133, 1966.
9. Worlledge, S. M., Carstairs, K. C. and Dacie, J. V.: Auto-immune haemolytic anemia associated with α-methyldopa therapy. *Lancet 2*:135, 1966.
10. Worlledge, S. M.: Annotation: Autoantibody formation association with methyldopa (Aldomet) therapy. *Brit. J. Haemat. 16*:5, 1969.
11. Beutler, E.: The hemolytic effect of primaquine and related compounds: A review. *Blood 14*:103, 1959.
12. Beutler, E.: Drug-induced hemolytic anemia. *Pharmacol. Rev. 21*:73, 1969.
13. Marks, P. A.: Glucose-6-Phosphate Dehydrogenase: Its Properties and Role in Mature Erythrocytes. In: *The Red Blood Cell*. Bishop, C. and Surgenor, D. M., eds. New York and London, Acad. Press, 1964, p. 211.
14. Dern, R. J., Beutler, E. and Alving, A. S.: The hemolytic effect of primaquine. II. The natural course of the hemolytic anemia and the mechanism of its self-limited character. *J. Lab. Clin. Med. 44*:171, 1954.
15. Carson, P. E., Flanagan, C. L., Ickes, C. E. and Alving, A. S.: Enzymatic deficiency in primaquine-sensitive erythrocytes. *Science 124*:484, 1956.
16. Beutler, E., Dern, R. J., and Alving, A. S.: The hemolytic effect of primaquine: VI. An *in vitro* test for sensitivity of erythrocytes to primaquine. *J. Lab. Clin. Med. 45*:40, 1955.
17. Beutler, E., Dern, R. J. and Alving, A. S.: The hemolytic effect of primaquine: VII. Biochemical studies of drug-sensitive erythrocytes. *J. Lab. Clin. Med., 45*:286, 1955.
18. Cohen, G. and Hochstein, P.: Generation of hydrogen peroxide in erythro-

cytes by hemolytic agents. *Biochem. 3:* 895, 1964.

19. Hitzig, W. H., Frick, P. G., Betke, K. and Huisman, T. H. J.: Hämoglobin Zürich Eine Neue Hämoglobinanomalie mit sulfonamidinduzierter Innenkörperanämie. *Helv. Paediat. Acta. 15*:499, 1960.
20. Carrell, R. W. and Lehmann, H.: The unstable haemoglobin haemolytic anemias. *Semin. Haemat. 6*:116, 1969.
21. Jacob, H. S., Brain, M. C., Dacie, J. V., Carrell, R. W. and Lehman, H.: Abnormal haem binding and globin SH group blockade in unstable haemoglobins. *Nature 218*:1214, 1968.
22. Bunn, H. F. and Jandl, J. H.: Exchange of heme among hemoglobin molecules. *Proc. Nat. Acad. Sci. 56:* 974, 1966.
23. Zalusky, R., Figur, A. M. and Ross, J.: Hemoglobin Riverdale-Bronx (Hb RB): Another example of hemoglobin instability. *Clin. Res. 17*:348, 1969.
24. Rigas, D. A. and Koler, R. D.: Decreased erythrocyte survival in Hemoglobin H disease as a result of the abnormal properties of hemoglobin H: The benefit of splenectomy. *Blood 18*:1, 1961.
25. Motulsky, A. G. and Yoshida, A.: Methods for the Study of Red Cell Glucose-6-Phosphate Dehydrogenase. In: *Biochemical Methods in Red Cell Genetics.* Yunis, J. J., ed. New York and London, Acad. Press, 1969, p. 52.

TEEN-AGE OUT-OF-WEDLOCK PREGNANCY

A Phenomenon of Many Dimensions

W. Godfrey Cobliner

Assistant Professor of Gynecology and Obstetrics
Albert Einstein College of Medicine
New York, N.Y.

The topic of teen-age out-of-wedlock pregnancy has for some time occupied a position of prominence in the professional literature of many disciplines. Most contributions describe the nature and success of service programs that nowadays operate all over the country. Their primary aim is the rehabilitation of teen-age primigravidae and their integration into the community. According to these accounts few of the girls cared for have subsequent out-of-wedlock pregnancies.[9, 14, 17, 18, 20, 21, 22, 26, 27, 30]

This massive remedial effort has evidently not affected the rate of teen-age out-of-wedlock pregnancies. Its index has remained stationary for some years at an alarmingly high level.[23, 25]

One therefore wonders why the insight into the synchronic and diachronic roots of the phenomenon which has been gained from close, long-term contact with thousands of pregnant teenagers has so far not been translated into the implementation of preventive measures of suitable dimensions directed to teen-agers who have never been pregnant. One could cite a number of circumstances for this situation: the multifarious roots of these out-of-wedlock pregnancies, the conflict of values occasioned by preventive action, the generation gap, inaccessibility of subjects, fiscal priorities, etc. All these are frequently discussed. But it is quite possible that another element, rarely mentioned, is a more important obstacle.

Most authors refer to teen-age out-of-wedlock pregnancy as an undifferentiated entity. No distinction is made between the pregnancy of a 13-year-old and that of an 18-year-old, between that of a child grown up in a broken home, or one coming from a stable family. *One label, "teen-age out-of-wedlock pregnancy," is affixed to all cases regardless of the origin, the age, and background of the mother, and the circumstances of her impregnation.*

Most current papers lack a clear-cut distinction between teen-age out-of-wedlock pregnancy and sexual activity. Accordingly motives, opportunities, and risks are merged for two phenomena that have only a sequential and causal link, one which is not valid in the psychological sphere. In fact, for a great many sexually active teenagers the advent of a pregnancy is an unanticipated unwelcome occurrence.

It is clear that a conceptual reexamination of teen-age out-of-wedlock pregnancies on the basis of current data will serve, as it were, for the differential diagnosis of the phenomenon.

Traditionally teen-age out-of-wedlock pregnancy and sexual activity in unmarried teen-agers have been associated with the terms juvenile delinquency and acting out.[6, 8, 10, 11, 12, 16, 19] The first is a sociological category as well as a legal term, the second a psychodynamic term; both connote maladjustment of the individual. The former is linked to a normative disturbance on the social level—deviance; the other is connective with malfunction on the personality level—a psychiatric disturbance.

Two decades ago Lucien Bovet, an eminent Swiss psychiatrist and public official, called attention to the fact that not all delinquents are "maladjusted."[5]

On the basis of his worldwide survey of delinquency, which he illustrated with figures taken from court records in many countries, including those of the United States, he concluded that "as a general rule when times are quiet, community life peaceful . . . the delinquent population contains proportionally few 'normals' but when community life is unsettled . . . when social unrest is allied with poor economic conditions (as in some big American cities where immigration constantly changes the population, giving a special character to the poverty peculiar to large cities) then the number of 'normals' who are the victims of these disturbed times increase considerably." And he suggests that "a social factor" . . . sets "in motion a number of psychological processes" leading to acts of delinquency.[5]

A similar position was taken at the June 1969 Stockholm conference on *Mental Health of Adolescents and Young Persons* in which it was suggested that the fundamental needs of many adolescents were not being met by the environment and that therefore it was not *they who were maladjusted but it was rather society that was not adapted.*[31]

Many psychiatrists hold the view that disturbed social conditions that give rise to stresses and strains impinge on the individual in such a way that the conflict becomes "internalized" and is then manifested as a mental-health problem of a given individual. Adolescents so affected, for example, can "act it out" in the sexual sphere. This process was not noted in a group of 78 pregnant lower-class girls (11 to 16 years of age) seen by a team of professional workers in Chicago. In their conclusion the authors write "we found it impossible to apply psychiatric diagnosis to our patients' difficulties and could not even say that they were emotionally disturbed."[2]

The Chicago findings challenge our current concept of teen-age out-of-wedlock pregnancy and invite a closer look at the stresses in the social fabric which bring them about. For teen-age out-of-wedlock pregnancy is not merely a product of disruption and maladjustment; it is also an agent generating further societal disturbance.

The past few decades have witnessed a series of significant biological, psychological, social, and cultural changes affecting adolescents which, no doubt, have had an impact on the pattern and number of teen-age out-of-wedlock pregnancies. First, the onset of puberty has advanced considerably; boys and girls nowadays mature earlier.[29] Second, boys and girls mix much earlier and are free socially with one another. Third, the family and the school have relaxed their control over the activities of adolescents. Fourth, in the past available free time, recreation, or leisure activities of adolescents were more structured; this provided orientation for them that is now missing. Fifth, the values governing intimacy among adolescents have been liberalized tacitly. In fact in many instances parents pressure adolescents into dating activities.[1] Sixth, the age of economic independence has gradually increased, forcing many otherwise mature adolescents to defer vital decisions regarding life plans and marriage.[6, 7]

In the wake of these changes contemporary youth, particularly in urban areas, now face fundamental contradictions which have sprung up from impersonal social roots and for which they are inadequately prepared. Their biological drives press for an outlet so much earlier than in former days; this happens at a time when their psychological (inner) development has not provided them with the capacity to control and direct these needs toward satisfactory and constructive gratification.[6, 7] Neither parents nor elders, external obstacles, or clear-cut rules give them support or guidance in their struggle to contain the drives that propel them toward immediate gratification regardless of consequences. One therefore encounters many *categories* of teen-agers who nowadays engage in heterosexual experimentation and activities and who in previout times would have pursued and even preferred other activities. One thinks here of the timid, the lonely, the conscience-stricken, the overprotected, the ignorant, and even those who do not enjoy it (and only do it because of peer-group pressure), etc. All these types have greatly increased the numbers of sexually active teen-agers and have thereby widened the range of problems disrupting heterosexual relations, often with permanent consequences for the individual who started early, before his full sexual awakening.

As the opportunities for sexual activities increase and obstacles disappear, risks of destructive consequences (out-of-wedlock pregnancies, venereal diseases, emotional damage) rise proportionately unless something is substituted for the former barriers.[15]

The characteristics of these barriers were immobility and strictness, and they worked as long as society was relatively stable. Suddenly a formidable technological advance set in that did away with many occupations while creating entirely new ones in a matter of years. This process was combined with unprecedented geographical mobility of the population. These two phenomena shook the very fundaments of society and started a transformation of many institutions that is still running its course.

Given the actual social constellation with its emphasis on fun and the exposure to sexual stimulation through the mass media, it would be futile to try to influence the sexual activity of teen-agers through persuasion or any kind of restrictive measure. One cannot reverse the wheels of history.

These facts highlight a prevailing situation: our current values no longer protect our youth from individual or collective damage and society from social disruption, while the adult generation sees in those values the sole barrier to social and moral disintegration.

We shall have to "shift gears," as it were, to keep up with the rate of change that has overtaken our communal life and our human relations. To shift gears with regard to out-of-wedlock pregnancy calls for a closer and open-minded look at the phenomenon.

Up to now the bulk of systematic data on sexual activities of adolescents has been gathered by psychiatrists who, as stated before, link these activities to psychic maladjustment and juvenile delinquency, in accordance with their professional experience, which evidently derives from contact with selected groups of teen-agers.[3] However, psychiatrists do recognize the multiple determinants and subdivisions in the reported behavior. Thus P. Blos recently suggested that the sexual activities of youngsters who came to his attention are rooted in psychic, social, biological, and epidemiological factors. Generally speaking, he says, none of these seems preponderant although for a given case or group of cases one or the other factor may be dominant. In the same paper Blos describes three distinct constellations typical in female delinquency that include promiscuity (and consequently the attendant risk of out-of-wedlock pregnancy). He recommends that for each constellation a specific therapeutic approach corresponding to its origin and dynamics is indicated.[4]

Dr. Helene Deutsch, as adviser on ordinary life problems to single, apparently healthy college girls in the Boston area, was struck by the presence among quite a few of them of an urgent need to become pregnant. Since her observations draw on her recent extensive contacts with normal teen-age girls they add another important category to the phenomenon of teen-age out-of-wedlock pregnancy that stresses the absence of gross mental or social pathology.[6, 7] By contrast, Dr. J. M. Perman, another psychiatrist, reports the same tendency among a group of lower-class adolescents in the New York metropolitan area among whom manifestations of psychiatric disturbance were evident.[24]

Since only a fraction of sexually active youngsters who are in conflict or who need help come to the attention of psychiatrists, one is justified in assuming, pending the collection of systematic data, that many additional constellations exist. Independently from Blos, J. P. Semmens and W. M. Lamers divided the very phenomenon of teen-age pregnancy into three major categories: the accidental cases, the intentional cases, and those arising out of ignorance.[28] Blos is concerned with distinguishing clusters of psychological tendencies occurring in sexual activities of teenagers and their dynamics. Semmens and Lamers also deal with patterns of volitional control of conception.

A recent pilot study I carried out consisted of group discussions and individual interviews with 30 sexually active girls and boys between 12 and 18 years of age who resided in the borough of the Bronx, New

York City. The following preliminary findings, which seem to refer to this particular group as well as to many of their peers, were obtained.

1) Teen-agers in the lower socioeconomic strata residing in the Bronx and also those who come from families that have upward social mobility lack facilities and opportunities to spend their free time together in constructive and self-fulfilling ways. Most of the time they are bored. The girls face unusual difficulties in obtaining gainful employment.

2) During their free time they congregate in territorial groups. Admittance to these groups is on a personal basis, and each group is made up of subunits comprising a few teen-agers of the same sex.

3) Fierce competition is generated among the girls "to have and to hold" desirable boys.

4) In this setting and atmosphere there is little room for spontaneity, for self-growth, or the pursuit of favored pastimes or interests. In fact the concept of leisure time is foreign to these teen-agers.

5) There seems to be widespread sexual experimentation among teen-agers, from necking to intercourse. Some of this exploration definitely derives from external influence. For example, even the more cautious members of the group and the ones not quite ready for such intimacy follow the practice because of group pressure and other circumstances.

6) The sexual exploration and experience are matched by an alarming ignorance of the modes of conception, of venereal infection, symptoms, and prophylaxis. In fact there is not even any indication of the existence of a rudimentary grapevine diffusing any semblance of accurate information. By contrast it would seem that misinformation is in part responsible for the occurrence of out-of-wedlock pregnancy and venereal disease.

7) Some of the sexual experimentation takes place during parties or "gigs" in the basement of the home of one or another youngster. The parties are held with the knowledge of the parents but in their ignorance (deliberate or otherwise) of the specific activities that occur there.

All our informants had satisfactory standing at their respective schools and were members of a peer group. We were impressed by the fact that they did not suffer from any obvious serious personality disturbance that interfered either with their scholastic performance or their social relations within the peer group. All of them reside in a sec-

FACTORS GOVERNING ADOLESCENTS' HETEROSEXUAL ACTIVITY AND ITS SEQUELAE

Motives for or circumstances of sexual exposure.	Curiosity, loneliness, need for affection, extreme passivity (girls), preservation or enhancement of (sexual) self-image, rebellion, spirit of adventure, impulsivity, "disproving" homosexual tendencies, boredom, sexual needs, peer-group pressure, conscious or unconscious desire for a child.
Awareness of associated risks.	Misinformation, ignorance, incomplete information, diffusion of information (correct or incorrect) in peer group.
Intention for protection.	Relation to partner, level of maturity, feeling of responsibility, reality-orientation.
Access to protection.	Available community resources, community attitudes.
Usage of protection.	Personal experience, available practical instruction.

tion of the borough which contains a large segment of the lower class who presently are mobile upward; many of our informants belong to this group.

The work of Blos, of Semmens and Lamers, and of others, as well as our own data, disclose the existence of a few major variables that seem to govern the advent of a teen-age out-of-wedlock pregnancy or venereal disease: 1) motives for or circumstances of sexual exposure; 2) the teen-ager's awareness of associated risks; 3) his intention for guarding against these risks; 4) his access to means of protection; 5) his actual usage of protection. Some of the concrete manifestations exemplifying these variables are shown in the accompanying table.

Theoretically any combination of these variables can give rise to a type or category of teen-age out-of-wedlock pregnancy but few will turn out to be discrete or exclusive.

It would appear from this table as well as from the previously cited data that the incidence of teen-age out-of-wedlock pregnancy as well as that of venereal disease can perhaps be reduced sharply without any major transformation of our social institutions or economic reform. This can be accomplished by strategic intervention at any stage of the sequences listed in the above table.

The following steps seem most promising and practical in this connection: 1) To encourage teen-agers to work out suitable, timely outlets for their energy and needs by providing them with the proper facilities. Among these would be youth centers, recreational arrangements, opportunities to implement their desire for being active for the community in ways that are different from those of adults. 2) To substitute goal-oriented and rational knowledge in the sphere of emotions and sexual behavior for tradition-bound, dated values calling for blind adherence. This should be attained by involving adolescents themselves in the elaboration of new codes of social behavior instead of imposing codes from outside.

This goal is practical. It can be attained by convincing adolescents that one is genuinely concerned with their problems, by conveying vital knowledge to them in a true educational process. True education is radically different from the mere mechanical dispensing of information; it includes the subjective sphere, the human element—the key principal factor governing volitional action.

It is precisely the failure to provide this kind of education to adolescents which contributes greatly to the growing rate of venereal disease and out-of-wedlock pregnancy. What is more, the youngster who has had unsatisfactory sexual experiences lacking in excitement and gratification of basic needs for affection will turn elsewhere; and he may become an easy convert to drug exploration with its attendant risks. This has been observed in several groups of adolescents whom I have followed for a number of months in my pilot study.

Blaming poverty, urban conditions, or psychiatric disturbances in the victims for the occurrence of the two phenomena under discussion will perpetuate the fragmented counteraction which marks our current programs concerned with teen-age problems.[13]

The 1969 Stockholm Conference on Mental Health of Adolescents and Young Persons had this to say on the subject of adolescents: "We must be willing to record our observations within a scientific framework in order to influence the social development of youth and to free ourselves from some of the mythology about youth and society that deludes us into laying the blame on some factor which may be unchangeable, whilst overlooking factors in which change is actually possible."[31]

Systematic collection of data about the thinking of teen-agers, their perception of the world, their values, their conduct and activities—particularly of those among them that do not ever come to the attention of adults who specialize in extending help to them—holds out the promise for discarding our mythology about them. It is the prerequisite for working out a useful typology of teen-age out-of-wedlock pregnancies, useful in the sense that it is an indispensable instrument for opening our eyes to problems that we have overlooked, useful also in the design of preventive policies on the individual, collective, and community levels.

ACKNOWLEDGMENT

Thanks are due to Dr. John Mayer, Dr. Angelo Danesino, Mrs. Marjorie Milton, M.S.W., and Mrs. Vivian Smith, R.N., for their suggestions made during the preparation of this paper.

REFERENCES

1. Anthony, E. J.: The Reactions of Adults and Their Behavior. In: *Psychiatric Approaches to Adolescence.* Caplan, G. and Labovici, S., eds. Sixth International Congress of the International Association for Child Psychiatry. *Int. Cong. Series Excerpta Med.* Amsterdam *108*:46-59, 1966.
2. Barglos, P. et al.: Some psychiatric aspects of illegitimate pregnancy in early adolescence. *Amer. J. Orthopsychiat.* *38*:672-87, 1968.
3. Blos, P.: *On Adolescence.* New York, Free Press Glencoe, 1962.
4. Blos, P.: Three Typical Constellations in Female Delinquency. In: *Family Dynamics and Female Sexual Delinquency.* Pollak, O. and Friedman, A. S., eds. Palo Alto, Calif., Science and Behavior, 1969.
5. Bovet, L.: *Psychiatric Aspects of Juvenile Delinquency.* Monograph Series No. 1. Geneva, WHO, 1951.
6. Deutsch, H.: *Selected Problems of Adolescence.* Psa. Study Child, Monograph No. 3. New York, Int. Univ. Press, 1967.
7. Deutsch, H.: The contemporary adolescent girl. *Seminars Psychiat. 1*:99-112, 1969.
8. Friedman, A. S.: Delinquency and the Family System. In: *Family Dynamics and Female Sexual Delinquency.* Pollak, O. and Friedman, A. S., eds. Palo Alto, Calif., Science and Behavior, 1969.
9. Gordis, L. et al.: Adolescent pregnancy. Hospital-based program for primary prevention. *Amer. J. Public Health 58:* 849-58, 1969.
10. Group for the Advancement of Psychiatry, Committee on Adolescence. *Normal Adolescence: Its Dynamics and Impact.* Report No. 68. New York. Scribner's, 1968.
11. Group for the Advancement of Psychiatry, Committee on the College Student. Sex and the College Student. In: *Report of the Group for the Advancement of Psychiatry,* vol. 6, report No. 60. New York, Group Advance. Psychiat., 1965.
12. Gruenberg, E.: The social breakdown syndrome: Some origins. *Amer. J. Psychiat. 123*:1481-89, 1967.
13. Herzog, E.: Families Out-of-Wedlock. In: *Family Dynamics and Female Sexual Delinquency.* Pollak, O. and Friedman, A. S., eds. Palo Alto, Calif., Science and Behavior, 1969.
14. Howard, M.: Comprehensive service programs for school-age pregnant girls. *Children 15*:193-97, 1968.
15. Leasure, J. W.: Some economic benefits of birth prevention. *Milbank Mem. Fund Quart. 4*:417-25, 1967.

16. Lerner, B., Raskin, R. and Davis, E.: On the need to be pregnant. *Int. J. Psychoanal.* (Part 2) *48*:289-97, 1967.
17. Liben, F.: Minority group clinic patients pregnant out-of-wedlock. *Amer. J. Public Health 59*:1868-81, 1969.
18. Lyons, D. J.: Developing a program for pregnant teenagers through the cooperation of school, health department and federal agencies. *Amer. J. Public Health 58*:2225-29, 1968.
19. Martin, J. M., Fitzpatrick, J. P. et al.: *The Analysis of Delinquent Behavior: A Structural Approach.* New York, Random House, 1969.
20. McMurray, G. L.: Project teen aid: A community action approach to services for pregnant unmarried teenagers. *Amer. J. Public Health 58*:1848-53, 1968.
21. Murdock, C. G.: The unmarried mother and the school system. *Amer. J. Public Health 58*:2217-24, 1968.
22. Osofsky, H. J.: On attempting to reach the "unreachable" individual: A progress report of a program for pregnant schoolgirls. *Obstet. Gynec. 32*:869-81, 1968.
23. Pakter, J.: Out-of-wedlock births in New York City. *Amer. J. Public Health 51*:683-96, 1961.
24. Perman, J. M.: Multi-pregnancies in multi-problem families: The chronic postpartum reactions. In press.
25. Podell, L.: *Families on Welfare in New York City.* New York, Baruch College, 1968.
26. Rashbaum, W. et al.: Pregnancy in unmarried women: Medical and social characteristics. *J. Mount Sinai Hosp. N.Y. 30*:30-46, 1963.
27. Sarrel, P. M.: The university hospital and the teenage unwed mother. *Amer. J. Public Health 57*:1308-13, 1967.
28. Semmens, J. P. and Lamers, W. M.: *Teenage Pregnancy.* Springfield, Ill., Thomas, 1968.
29. Tanner, J. M.: *Growth at Adolescence.* London, Oxford, 1955.
30. Visotsky, H. M.: A Community Project for Unwed Adolescents. In: *Family Dynamics and Female Sexual Delinquency.* Pollak, O. and Friedman, A. S., eds. Palo Alto, Calif., Science and Behavior, 1969.
31. WHO. Conference on Mental Health of Adolescents and Young Persons. Summary and Conclusions. Stockholm, June 1969. Mimeographed.

MEDICAL NUMISMATICS: A DENARIUS COMMEMORATING ROME'S FIRST DOCTOR, ARCAGATHUS (219 B.C.)*

ADRIAN W. ZORGNIOTTI

Clinical Associate Professor of Medicine
Principal Lecturer, History of Medicine
New York University School of Medicine, New York, N. Y.

PLINY, in his *Natural History*,[4] quotes Cassius Hemina as saying that the first doctor (*medicus*) to come to Rome was Arcagathus, who arrived from the Greek Peloponnese in 219 B.C. and was treated with extraordinary kindness. Arcagathus was accorded the rights of citizenship (*ius Quiritium*). With public monies a medical shop (*taberna*) was purchased for his use at the Acilia Cross Roads. Prior to this, Rome had no physicians and home remedies were used.

Because he was an expert wound surgeon (*vulnerarius*), he immediately became popular. This happy state did not last. Arcagathus' vigorous use of the knife and cautery soon led to his being called executioner (*carnifex*). The cause of medicine appears to have been set back by public revulsion to his methods. In fact, about 100 years elapsed before we hear that another Greek physician (Asclepiades of Bithynia, ca. 100 B.C.) had taken up residence in Rome.

The coin we are examining, a denarius of the Acilia gens (family), was struck in Rome in 54 B.C. (see figure). The obverse shows the goddess Salus wearing a laurel crown, earrings, and a *torque* (necklace). Varro[5] tells us that Salus was of Sabine origin. Transplanted to Rome, she was associated with the general well-being (*salus publica*). In 302 B.C. a temple in her honor was erected near the Quirinal Hill by C. Junius Bubulcus.[6] During the late Republic, Salus became identified with her Greek counterpart Hygeia. With this came a change in meaning to the well-being of the emperor (*salus Augusta*), for whom annual prayers and vows (*vota*) were offered. Behind the head of the goddess appears the inscription SALUTIS.[1]

The reverse of the coin represents a statue of Salus which can, with

*Three notes on medical numismatics by the editor in chief of the *Bulletin* have appeared in previous issues: Medical numismatic notes I. *Bull. N.Y. Acad. Med.* 45:512-14, 1969; Medical numismatic notes II. The Montrose lunatic hospital. *Bull. N.Y. Acad. Med.* 45:637-39, 1969; and Medical numismatic notes III. The filtering-stone warehouse. *Bull. N.Y. Acad. Med.* 45:1124-25, 1969.

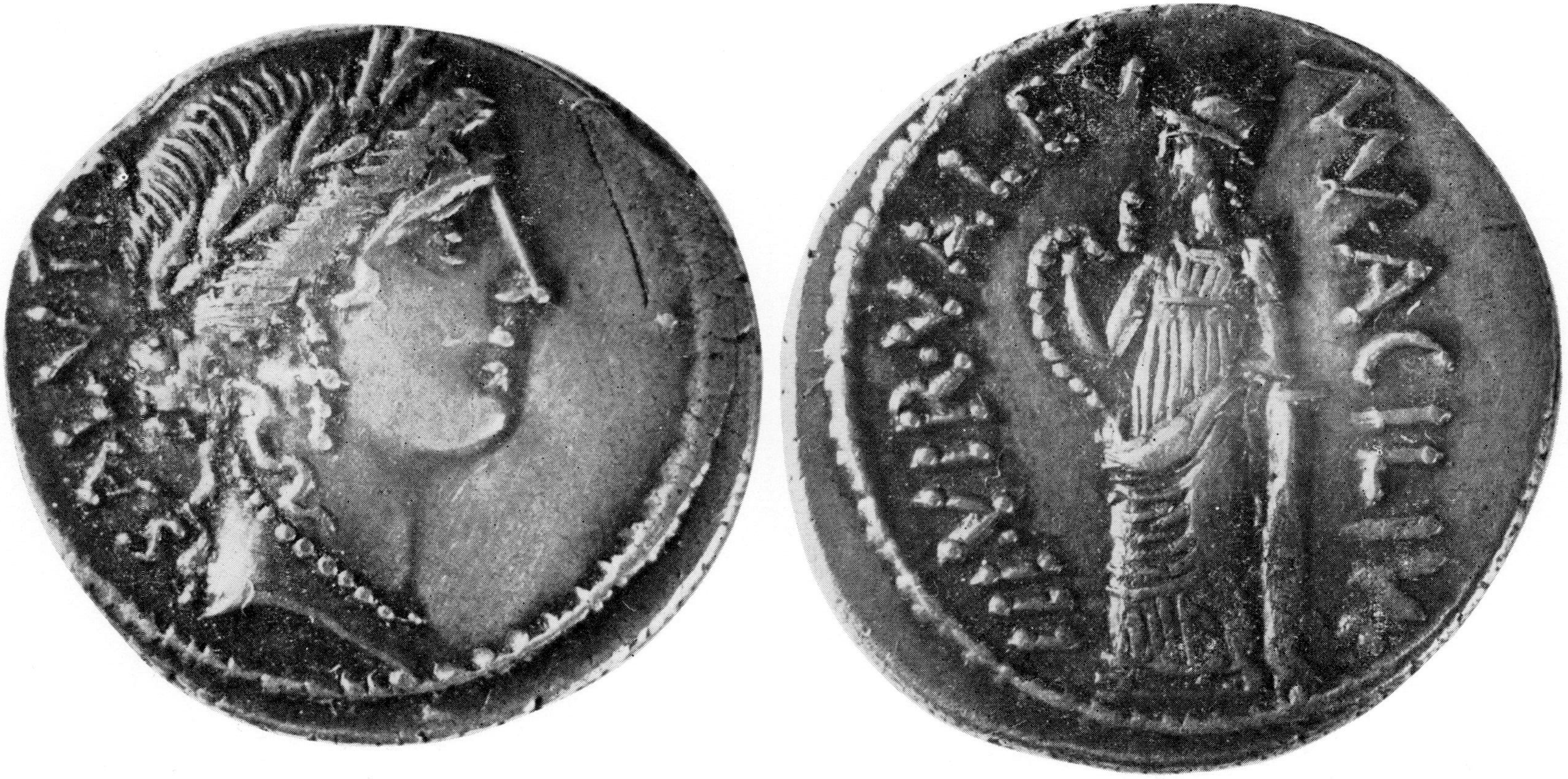

Roman denarius struck in 54 B.C. by a member of the Acilia family. Both sides depict the goddess Salus and commemorate the first doctor to come to Rome in 219 B.C. Obverse; reverse.

reasonable certainty, be identified according to Pliny[8] as the work of the Greek sculptor Niceratus; the statue stood in the Temple of Concord. Salus is depicted leaning on a column and holding a serpent in her right hand. The inscription is of considerable interest and reads M·ACILIUS III·VIR VALETV. It refers to the moneyer, Manius Acilius Glabrio, who became proconsul to Africa under Augustus. The abbreviation III·VIR refers to the board of three directors of the mint (*tresviri*) of which he was a member. It was usual for young men beginning their public careers to be given these posts. The tresviri were permitted considerable latitude in selecting the subject matter of the money they issued.[2] Hence it was usual to recall events associated with the family name—in this case, a contribution to the health and welfare of Rome.[3] VALETV appears to be an abbreviation for *valetudo* and is the word which most means health in the sense of freedom from disease. However, in certain contexts it can also mean ill health, in fact, military hospitals were called *valetudinaria*.

As Roman coins go, this one is unusually well documented. Although no direct reference exists in ancient writings to a connection between this coin and the ill-fated Arcagathus (did he go back to Greece?), there is enough information to support this supposition.

The coin is included in the numismatic collection of the New York Academy of Medicine, in the collection of the Numismatic Society, New York, N.Y., and in my private collection.

NOTES AND REFERENCES

1. Stevenson[7] lists various personifications: *Salus, Salus Augusta, Salus Exerciti, Salus Generis Humani, Salus Provinciarum,* etc. From this and other evidence we can surmise that Salus personified the broader connotation of welfare rather than "health" as we know it. The use of the word SALUTIS in the inscription is almost entirely restricted to coins of the *Acilia Gens*. On other coins (mainly of the empire) where Salus is depicted, the inscription reads SALUS.
2. The Romans were, perhaps, the most expert in understanding and utilizing the propaganda value of coins. Augustus has been shown by recent scholarship to have been unusually skillful at manipulating opinion, after the Battle of Actium and throughout his reign, by means of coins which had a vast circulation.
3. Babelon,[9] the outstanding expert on Roman republican coinage, confirms the prevalent opinion that the Acilia claimed to have introduced medicine to Rome and that they derived their name from the Greek ἀχέομαι, to heal.

4. Pliny: *Natural History,* XXIX, 6.
5. Varro: *On the Latin Language,* V, 74.
6. Livy: Book IX, 34.
7. Stevenson, S.M.: *Dictionary of Roman Coins.* London, 1889, pp. 713-16.
8. Pliny: *Natural History,* XXV, 4.
9. Babelon, E.: *Description Historique et Chronologique des Monnaies de la République Romaine,* vol. 1, pp. 100-07. Paris, 1885-1886. Reissued. Bologna, Forni, 1963.

Proceedings of the Eighth Meeting of the

CAREER SCIENTISTS OF THE HEALTH RESEARCH COUNCIL OF THE CITY OF NEW YORK

held at

THE NEW YORK ACADEMY OF MEDICINE

December 11, 1969

Officers and members of the
Health Research Council 452

Program of the meeting 453

Two Health Problems: One Solution
Mary C. McLaughlin 454

Abstracts of Presentations by Career Scientists . . . 457

Roster of Career Scientists 463

THE HEALTH RESEARCH COUNCIL OF THE CITY OF NEW YORK

JOHN V. LINDSAY, *Mayor of the City of New York*
BERNARD BUCOVE, *Health Services Administrator*
MARY C. MCLAUGHLIN, *Commissioner of Health*

Officers

COLIN M. MACLEOD, *Chairman*
JOHN V. TAGGART, *Vice Chairman*
GEORGE S. MIRICK, *Scientific Director*
MARION C. MORRIS, *Assistant Scientific Director*

MEMBERS

LEONA BAUMGARTNER
LARRY A. BEAR
ALBERT H. BOWKER
BERNARD BUCOVE
MARTIN CHERKASKY*
TIMOTHY W. COSTELLO
HOWARD REID CRAIG
EDWARD C. CURNEN, JR.*
J. FREDERICK EAGLE*
LUDWIG W. EICHNA*
MERRIL EISENBUD
J. HERBERT FILL
EDWARD E. FISCHEL*
MITCHELL I. GINSBERG
JACK R. GOLDBERG
WILLIAM T. GOLDEN
DEWITT S. GOODMAN*
LEO GOTTLIEB
FREDERICK O'R. HAYES
AUSTIN N. HELLER
MILTON HELPERN
DAVID M. HEYMAN
GEORGE K. HIRST
FRANK L. HORSFALL, JR.
GEORGE JAMES*
EDWIN D. KILBOURNE
MARY LASKER
RACHMIEL LEVINE
COLIN M. MACLEOD*
VAUGHAN MASON
MACLYN MCCARTY*
JAMES E. MCCORMACK
WALSH MCDERMOTT
MARY C. MCLAUGHLIN*
JOHN J. MENG
GEORGE S. MIRICK*
NORTON NELSON*
GERARD PIEL
HANS POPPER
CHARLES F. PREUSSE
MARIO A. PROCACCINO
FRANCIS D. ROGERS
BERTON ROUECHÉ*
OSCAR M. RUEBHAUSEN
DORIS SCHWARTZ
ROBERT J. SLATER
ROY C. SWAN*
JOHN V. TAGGART*
JOSEPH V. TERENZIO
HARVEY J. TOMPKINS
BETHUEL M. WEBSTER
ABRAHAM WHITE*

*Member of the Executive Committee

PROGRAM

JOHN V. TAGGART, *vice chairman,* The Health Research Council

DEWITT S. GOODMAN, *chairman,* The Association of Career Scientists

Guest Speaker

TWO HEALTH PROBLEMS: ONE SOLUTION

MARY C. MCLAUGHLIN
Commissioner of Health, City of New York

Career Scientist Presentations

1. PURIFICATION OF LUTEINIZING (LH) AND THYROID STIMULATING (TSH) HORMONES FROM HUMAN PITUITARY GLANDS
   B. B. SAXSENA, *Cornell University Medical College*
2. DEVELOPMENT OF AN ACTIVE TRANSPORT SYSTEM IN THE EMBRYONIC AVIAN ERYTHROCYTE
   H. J. CARROLL, *State University of New York Downstate Medical Center*
3. RHEUMATOID CELLS RESISTANT TO RUBELLA VIRUS
   A. I. GRAYZEL, *Montefiore Hospital and Medical Center*
4. THE IN VITRO FORMATION OF BILIRUBIN MONO AND DIGLUCURONIDE
   E. HALAC, JR., *New York University School of Medicine*
5. PHYSICAL CHARACTERISTICS OF THE DNA OF ADENOVIRUS TYPE 2
   W. DOERFLER, *The Rockefeller University*
6. ENZYME VARIANTS OF DPNH-METHEMOGLOBIN REDUCTASE IN HEREDITARY METHEMOGLOBINEMIA
   E. R. JAFFÉ, *Albert Einstein College of Medicine*
7. SELECTIVE EFFECTS OF CORTISONE ON THE EPINEPHRINE RESPONSIVE COMPONENT OF HEPATIC ADENYL CYCLASE
   M. W. BITENSKY, *New York University School of Medicine*
8. SURVEYS OF PSYCHIATRIC IMPAIRMENT IN WELFARE AND NONWELFARE CHILDREN
   T. S. LANGNER, *Columbia University School of Public Health and Administrative Medicine*
9. THE ROLE OF GUANIDES IN UREMIA
   B. D. COHEN, *The Bronx-Lebanon Hospital Center*

TWO HEALTH PROBLEMS: ONE SOLUTION*

MARY C. MCLAUGHLIN

Commissioner of Health of New York City
New York, N. Y.

IF you have been reading our newspapers—particularly the *Village Voice*—you are aware of the agitation that has arisen for the elimination of lead poisoning in children. This agitation is justified, for lead poisoning is a real public-health problem in New York City. May I tell you of some of our work on the problem, some of the complexities of it, and ask for whatever help you can give the Health Department on it.

When I joined the department nearly 20 years ago, my first major assignment dealt with lead poisoning. As a young, enthusiastic health officer, I did original epidemiological studies on this health problem: what and where it was, and what to do about it. As a result, we instituted a program to reduce this hazard; we had a case-finding campaign, with nurses, sanitarians, and laboratory workers assigned to it. We went out and found the children, arranged for them to be treated, and worked hard to prevent further cases.

Now, almost a score of years later, the problem remains unsolved. But for the first time I feel that we are in a position really to move things. Today, as you may know, we have 450,000 or more units of dilapidated housing, in which flaking paint can be peeled or chewed off by toddlers and eaten, or in which the paint falls off by itself. The presence of as little as 1% of lead in the old layers of paint—applied before lead-based interior paint was outlawed—can result in dangerously high levels of lead in the blood when lead is ingested by children.

No one would expect that any agency could wipe out this hazard overnight. To find safe housing for the occupants of these 450,000 units in New York City, while the old housing is refurbished or somehow made safe, is impossible. But something had to be done, and doing something always takes money; and no money was available. By pinching here and begging there, I was able to get together $150,000 for a crash

*Presented at the Eighth Annual Meeting of the Career Scientists of the Health Research Council of the City of New York held at the New York Academy of Medicine, December 11, 1969.

program. Everyone said "That's great!" But it was not great; it was just a stop-gap. It was not getting at the root of the problem.

It is one thing to diagnose critical blood-lead levels—0.06 mg. % or more per 100 cc. of blood—and another thing to correct the conditions that have caused it. The Health Code says that the commissioner may—note that it is "may" rather than "must"—force landlords to correct dangerous paint conditions. But here we get into the complexities of municipal administration—housing agencies, court battles, invisible and absentee landlords—plus actual technological problems of how to remove or cover the dangerous paint. We are working hard along all these avenues, but things still do not move fast enough. We are, however, going to obtain the convictions of some landlords.

There is no point, of course, in finding a case, "deleading" the child, and then sending him back to the same conditions. We are working on an interim housing program that includes a variety of foster-home organizations, but where can you find homes or halfway houses for 10,000 children and their families? We believe that we must try to keep families together. We are trying to obtain help from Medicaid on this interim housing program because it is very costly. So is the deleading treatment; it takes at least 10 days to two weeks to delead a child—always longer than you wish to keep a child from its family—often a child must be kept for months before a safe environment can be found.

Today it is estimated that there are 120,000 endangered children in New York City. At any one moment we might have 10,000 children with blood levels over 0.06 mg.%. Some will be symptomatic; some will not be. We can do 500 determinations of blood lead a week. We had high hopes for the testing of urine by means of (delta) amino levulinic acid, but the high number of false positives and false negatives has disappointed us. We are increasing our case-finding work in the so-called lead belts of the city. But all this takes money, and we have asked for $1.2 million in the coming fiscal year to mount an all-out attack. We are asking for another $500,000 for interim-care facilities.

A recent step forward was the development of a portable detection instrument which will make the job of pinpointing dangerous paint conditions much easier. The Health Research Council was the prime mover behind this. It funded a study by New York University of such an instrument, and now we have it. The tool takes a real burden off our laboratories by detecting as little as 1% of lead in old paint, even when the old layer of paint is buried under as many as 10 coats of lead-free paint.

This is where we could use your help. Getting a macrosample of blood for lead-level tests has always been difficult; no parent likes to see a nurse or doctor approaching the neck, arm, or leg of a tiny child in trying to obtain the amount of blood now needed for blood tests. What we need is a microtest–something that will show lead levels in a couple of drops of blood from a fingertip. If any of you are doing microtest work, or know someone who is, will you please have him give us the benefits of his thinking.

Another area in which we need help is in finding a qualified manager of the major lead-poisoning program we are planning. Neither I nor Dr. Donald Conwell nor Dr. David Harris can give this program full time; we need a mover-and-shaker who can pursue the problem on all fronts–medical, technological, legal, and political–to bring about a real solution. If any of you have such a man in mind, please let me know.

Now let us go from an unsolved problem to a solved one. Since the last epidemic of rubella in 1964 progress on this front has been phenomenal. Rubella is a first-degree public-health problem: in the 1964 episode more than 1,000 children were born with congenital defects, and it costs an estimated $200,000 to care for each child for the rest of its life. But now we have the tools to prevent another such outbreak. Here again the Health Research Council played an important part in testing new vaccines and making sure that vaccinated children could not infect older pregnant relatives. We selected 550,000 children–250,000 to be handled by our staff–in the lower school grades to receive immunization, and by the end of the year the Health Department will have vaccinated 300,000. If another epidemic of rubella strikes in 1971 or 1972, as had been predicted, we shall have accomplished our targeted goals, and it is to be hoped that we shall have cut effectively the transmission channels that have made epidemics possible in the past. We plan to extend this program to children of other ages as vaccine becomes available.

In the Health Department we feel that this is preventive medicine at its best, since we hope that we may have reduced heartbreak as well as a crushing burden in public support of malformed children resulting from rubella experienced during pregnancy in a large number of patients. So I am happy that, along with bad news, I can also bring you some good news.

Abstracts

*An asterisk indicates that the author is not a member of the
Association of Career Scientists

Selective Effects of Cortisone on the Epinephrine Responsive Component of Hepatic Adenyl Cyclase

M. W. Bitensky and V. Russell*

Department of Medicine
New York University School of Medicine
New York, N. Y.

Our previous work has provided evidence for separate epinephrine and glucagon responsive components of hepatic adenyl cyclase.† This included a demonstration of differences in the stability characteristics and centrifugal properties of the two enzymes and additive kinetics when saturating concentrations of both hormones were used in combination. Recent studies have added another distinguishing characteristic of the two hepatic enzyme systems. The administration of cortisone (7 days) in male or female 100 gm. Sprague Dawley rats produced more than an 80% fall in observable epinephrine responsive hepatic adenyl cyclase activity while the glucagon responsive component was not effected. ACTH had a similar effect in the intact animal but none in the adrenalectomized rat. Bilateral adrenalectomy or hypophysectomy were followed (within 48 hours) by a doubling in activity of the epinephrine responsive component of adenyl cyclase, and with no effect on the glucagon responsive component. Unilateral adrenalectomy had no effect on the activity of either enzyme. Adenyl cyclase activity was assayed in whole homogenate and purified membrane particle preparations; ATP 8-C_{14} was used as substrate, and the labeled product was isolated with descending TLC.

These data support the concept of two independent hepatic adenyl-cyclase systems and suggest that these enzymes are under separate genetic control.

†Bitensky, M. W., Russell, V., and Robertson, W.; *Biochem. Biophys. Res. Commun., 31*:706. 1968.

Development of an Active Transport System in the Embryonic Avian Erythrocyte

H. J. Carroll and R. D. Levere*

Department of Medicine
State University of New York Downstate Medical Center
Brooklyn, N. Y.

The deembryonated blastoderm of the chick, grown on an artificial medium, rapidly becomes a pure, phased culture of erythroid cells. We have employed this procedure to study the development of the energy-producing process for membrane transport of cations. Analysis for Na and K was performed on blastoderms (S1) which had grown in the shell for 24 hours after fertilization and which contained erythroid and nonerythroid cells. These ions were also measured in blastoderms of less than 5 somites grown for 24 (S2) and 48 (S3) hours on an agar-salt medium containing K, 5 mEq./l., and Na, 140 mEq./l. An active transport system for potassium (K pump) was thought to be present if K^{42} disappeared from the suspension medium and if this disappearance could be prevented by 10^{-5} M ouabain. Ratios of K:Na (mEq./l cell water) were 27:26 (S1), 49.0:41.5 (S2) and 57:37 (S3). Without ouabain the uptake of K^{42} (percentage of added isotope) measured 1.9 (S1), 11.8 (S2) and 13:3 (S3) in 90 minutes. With ouabain the figures were 2.5, 0.8, and 4.4. The data suggest that in the first 24 hours no cell in the chick embryo has a K pump. Thereafter the maturing erythrocyte apparently develops a ouabain-sensitive ATPase which participates in the process through which is established the high K:Na ratio which the mature erythrocyte of the chicken shares with most vertebrate cells.

The Role of Guanides in Uremia

Burton D. Cohen

Department of Medicine
The Bronx-Lebanon Hospital
New York, N. Y.

Among the precursors of urea, guanides have long been considered prominent candidates for the role of uremic toxins. One such substance, guanidinosuccinic acid (GSA) has been isolated from normal urine with a mean output of 10 mg. per day and rises in uremia to 60 mg. per day. It is recoverable from serum in uremia at a level of 2.5 mg. per 100 ml. and is totally dialyzable. It is identifiable in the serum of anephric patients and decreased in patients with combined renal and hepatic insufficiency. Intraperitoneal injections of arginine, citrulline, and aspartic acid in rats results in a prompt increase in excretion of GSA and, conversely, there is a total absence of urinary GSA in patients with arginine insufficiency. Finally, observations in uremic patients reveal a rise in serum levels of guanidinoacetic acid, a powerful repressor of the transamidinase responsible for the conversion of arginine to creatinine. It is suggested that GSA is the product of an alternative metabolic pathway for arginine when the normal pathway is blocked by nitrogen retention.

Studies have shown that the hemorrhagic diathesis associated with renal failure results from a qualitative platelet defect. This report demonstrates a decreased contribution of platelet factor 3 to prothrombin conversion when normal platelets are incubated with serum to which GSA is added and platelet aggregation can be inhibited by serum with GSA added. Electron micrography demonstrates that GSA reversibly blocks the central movement of platelet organelles induced by ADP, which suggests that the inhibitory action of GSA on the blood platelet is mediated through its influence upon ADP. It is speculated that GSA may function as an inhibitor, then, in a variety of ADP-dependent reactions in uremia.

Physical Characteristics of the DNA of Adenovirus Type 2

W. Doerfler

The Rockefeller University

A. K. Kleinschmidt*

Department of Biochemistry
New York University
New York, N. Y.

To carry the physical characterization of the DNA of human adenovirus type 2 (Ad 2) further, the following questions were asked: 1) Is there a unique distribution of sequences rich in adenine-thymine base pairs? 2) Is the gene sequence in the DNA of adenoviruses circularly permuted? The method of partial denaturation by heating the DNA in the presence of 12% formaldehyde and examination of the partially melted DNA molecules in the electron microscope was applied (Inman, R. B.: *J. Mol. Biol. 18*:464, 1966). The DNA of adenoviruses can be obtained in highly homogeneous form (Doerfler, W.: *Virology 38*:587, 1969), with more than 75% of its single chains intact. The mean length of Ad 2 DNA was determined in the electron microscope to be 10.96 ± 0.38 microns. Ad 2 DNA was heated to temperatures between 52° and 58° C. Regions of local denaturation, presumed to occur at sites rich in adenine-thymine base pairs, are clearly distinguishable. The size and location of these sites was measured in 113 randomly selected molecules heated to between 52° and 58° C. A unique pattern in the distribution of denaturation sites can be recognized. Denaturation occurs first (at 54° C.) in the region between 0.8 and 0.95 on the scale of fractional length (I in the scheme below); next between 0.5 and 0.6 as well as between 0 and 0.15 (II), at 55° C.; and finally at 0.4 and between 0.7 and 0.8 (III), starting at 57° C.). These data indicate that there exists a unique distribution of sites rich in adenine-thymine base pairs in Ad 2 DNA. The patterns obtained make it very unlikely that the gene sequence in Ad 2 DNA is circularly permuted and that a high degree of terminal redundancy exists.

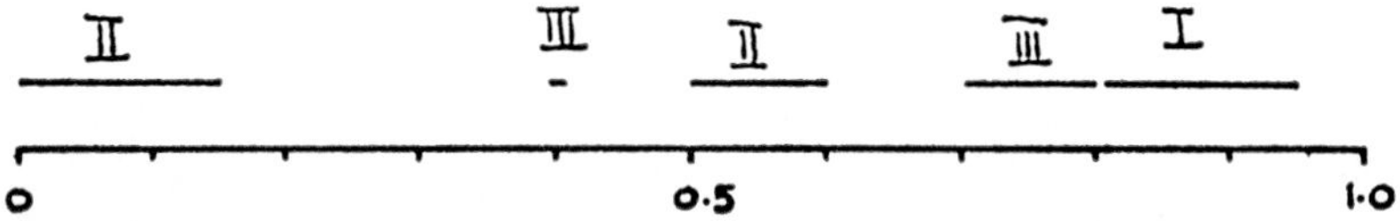

Scale of fractional length of the Ad 2 DNA molecule. The numbers I-III designate the order of appearance of denaturation sites as the temperature is increased.

Rheumatoid Cells Resistant to Rubella Virus

ARTHUR I. GRAYZEL AND CAROLYN BECK*

Departments of Medicine
Montefiore Hospital
and
Albert Einstein College of Medicine
New York, N. Y.

Rubella infections commonly cause an acute but limited polyarthritis. For this reason we have examined the replication of rubella virus in cells from explants of human synovial membranes. Synovial biopsies were obtained from patients with definite or classical rheumatoid arthritis who were undergoing reconstructive surgery. Nonrheumatoid synovial membranes were obtained from patients without inflammatory diseases undergoing surgery or from patients with chronic synovitis of a known cause (e.g., tuberculosis). Confluent monolayers of synovial cells were grown from explants of the membranes and each cell strain was subcultured 2 to 4 times before infection with rubella virus, strain F-8, at a multiplicity of 1-3 hemadsorption-negative particles per cell.

All 27 nonrheumatoid strains infected with rubella demonstrated marked cytopathic effects (CPE) by 12-14 days and usually died by 21 days, while none of the 16 rheumatoid strains demonstrated such changes even after several subcultures of the infected cells. Infectious rubella virus could be recovered from the nonrheumatoid cells showing CPE but no virus could be detected in the rheumatoid cells or medium. Neutralizing antisera against rubella prevented the development of CPE in nonrheumatoid cells. Data to be presented indicate that the resistance of rheumatoid cells to rubella virus is not mediated by interferon.

While the nature of the resistance is obscure, a noninterferon-mediated interference could reflect the acquisition of genetic information by the rheumatoid cells by virtue of a latent or defective virus rather than an alteration in their metabolic or immune function as a consequence of the disease.

The In Vitro *Formation of Bilirubin Mono and Diglucuronide*

E. HALAC, JR., P. DETWILER,* AND M. DIPIAZZA*

Department of Pediatrics
New York University School of Medicine
New York, N. Y.

Available techniques for the determination of bilirubin UDP-glucuronyl transferase (bil-UDPGT) activity do not distinguish between the formation of bilirubin monoglucuronide (bil-GA) or bilirubin diglucuronide (bil-GA_2). The nature of the products of the reaction requires a chromatographic analysis usually done after diazotization. Two recent reports indicate that the incubation of microsomes with bilirubin and necessary cofactors results in the synthesis of bil-GA, while it is known that most of the bilirubin present in bile is in the form of bil-GA_2.

We have examined the products of the bil-UDPGT reaction catalyzed by rat-liver microsomal fraction and the smooth and rough subfractions after dialysis against

EDTA. Our findings are: 1) the activity of rough microsomes (expressed in U./gm. liver or U./mg. protein) is higher in rough than in smooth microsomes; 2) smooth microsomes synthetize only bil-GA; 3) rough microsomes synthetize a mixture of bil-GA and bil-GA_2; 4) total microsomes synthetize bil-GA and bil-GA_2 in a proportion dependent on the relative activities of the two subfractions; 5) aged rough microsomes lose the capacity to synthetize bil-GA_2 when they can still synthetize bil-GA. These results lead us to believe that the formation of bil-GA_2 is dependent on at least two bil-UDPGTs. The enzyme that introduces the 2d GA mol would be localized in rough microsomes only.

Enzyme Variants of DPNH-Methemoglobin Reductase in Hereditary Methemoglobinemia

H. S. Hsieh* and E. R. Jaffé

Department of Medicine
Albert Einstein College of Medicine
New York, N. Y.

The enzymatic activity and electrophoretic migration of DPNH-methemoglobin reductase (DPNH-MR) in the RBC of 6 methemoglobinemic, 16 heterozygous, and 54 normal subjects were examined. In 22 instances activity was determined with both the methemoglobin-ferrocyanide (Hegesh) method and the diaphorase (Scott) method. Normal values were 2.86 ± 0.60 U/gm. Hgb. with the former method and $91 \pm 20 \Delta A \times 10^4/3.25$ mg. Hgb. with the latter. Both methods permitted a clear differentiation between normal subjects and homozygotes, although the correlation of activities with the two methods was not exact, and provided consistent results in obligatory heterozygotes. Starch-gel electrophoresis, *p*H 9.3, of DPNH-MR from the RBC of members of 7 families with significant methemoglobinemia (11-21% in homozygotes) revealed 5 variants with electrophoretic mobilities different from that of the normal. Hemolysates of RBC of 2 of 56 adults without methemoglobinemia were found to have two bands with DPNH-MR activity: one with normal mobility and one with more rapid migration. Family studies of these 2 subjects of Italian extraction demonstrated that this variant, which migrated to the same position as that of the single band observed in the hemolysate of another patient's RBC with very mild (3%) methemoglobinemia, were consistent with an autosomal mode of inheritance. In contrast to the other variants, this enzyme's function appeared to be less affected. The RBC of heterozygous subjects with this variant had a normal capacity to reduce nitrite-induced methemoglobin *in vitro* and the levels of DPNH-MR activity were normal. This investigation has demonstrated the genetic and biochemical polymorphism of hereditary methemoglobinemia associated with abnormalities in the DPNH-MR system. *(Supported by USPHS Grant AM-13698).*

Surveys of Psychiatric Impairment in Welfare and Nonwelfare Children

T. S. LANGNER, E. L. GREENE,* J. H. HERSON,* J. JAMESON,* AND J. A. GOFF*

Department of Epidemiology
Columbia University School of Public Health and Administrative Medicine
New York, N. Y.

Two major surveys of children in Manhattan have been completed and data are being analyzed. The initial survey involved a sample of 1,034 children randomly selected to represent a cross-section of Manhattan. The second survey focussed on 1,000 children in welfare AFDC homes. In both studies mothers were interviewed for approximately 2½ hours about given children between ages 6 and 18. Psychiatrists then evaluated each child's record and assigned impairment ratings and diagnoses. About 350 children were also given direct examinations by the psychiatrists. Preliminary results have indicated: 1) 12% of Manhattan children and 23% of Manhattan's welfare children were judged from two samples to have marked or severe psychiatric impairment; 2) Negro children, although as healthy at age 6 to 9 as white or Spanish-speaking children, ended up with the highest proportion of impaired children by the teens (14-18), and at this age their risk of impairment was the same as the risk of welfare children in general; 3) white children showed a decrease in impairment with increased age groups, while Negroes showed an increase with advancing age; 4) welfare children fought more with other children, showed more antisocial behavior, and were more anxious than low-income nonwelfare children.

Purification of Luteinizing and Thyroid-Stimulating Hormones from Human Pituitary Glands

B. B. SAXENA

Department of Medicine
Cornell University Medical College
New York, N. Y.

The purpose of this study was to isolate luteinizing hormones (LH) and thyroid-stimulating hormones (TSH) from human pituitaries for use in structural and radioimmunoassay studies. Ten thousand human pituitary glands were extracted to prepare a glycoprotein fraction containing follicle-stimulating hormones (FSH), LH and TSH. The glycoprotein was fractionated by ion-exchange chromatography on carboxymethyl Sephadex C-50. A fraction containing FSH was eluted by O.IM ammonium acetate-acetic acid buffer of *p*H 6.7. Subsequently, a fraction containing predominantly LH and TSH activities was eluted by the same buffer at *p*H 9.5. The *p*H 9.5 fraction was further purified by isoelectric focusing using carrier ampholytes in a sucrose gradient to avoid thermal convection during electrofocusing. The purified fractions of LH and TSH were freed of sucrose by ultrafiltration and lyophilized. The LH and TSH preparations containing, approximately, 9 NIH-LH-S1 and 5 NIH-TSH-S4 units, respectively, were obtained. The high degree of purity of these preparations was confirmed by polyacrylamide disc- and immunoelectrophoreses. In conclusion: LH from human pituitaries of potency significantly higher than those reported in the literature has been prepared.

Career Scientists of the Health Research Council of the City of New York*

The Council of the Association of Career Scientists of the Health Research Council of the City of New York
1969 - 1970

DeWitt S. Goodman, *Chairman* Richard M. Hays, *Secretary*

Councillors

Edward C. Franklin
David Schachter
Stanley Wallach

A

Al Askari, Salah, 7/1/64
Dept. of Urology
New York University School of Medicine

Asanuma, Hiroshi, 10/16/67
Dept. of Physiology
New York Medical College

August, Joseph T., 1/1/62
Dept. of Molecular Biology
Albert Einstein College of Medicine

Auld, Peter A. McF., 7/1/62
Dept. of Pediatrics
Cornell University Medical College

B

Bank, Norman, 10/8/59
Dept. of Medicine
New York University School of Medicine

Bassett, C. Andrew, 1/1/61
Dept. of Orthopedic Surgery
Columbia Univ. Coll. of Phys. & Surg.

Baum, Stephen G., 7/1/68
Dept. of Medicine
Albert Einstein College of Medicine

Becker, Frederick F., 7/1/62
Dept. of Pathology
New York University School of Medicine

Beller, Fritz K., 2/1/63
Dept. of Obstetrics and Gynecology
New York University School of Medicine

Benacerraf, Baruj, 1/1/61
Dept. of Pathology
New York University School of Medicine

Bennett, Dorothea, 7/1/63
Dept. of Anatomy
Cornell University Medical College

Berkovich, Sumner, 7/1/61
Dept. of Pediatrics
S.U.N.Y. Downstate Medical Center

Bernheimer, Harriet P., 1/1/64
Dept. of Medicine
S.U.N.Y. Downstate Medical Center

Bertles, John F., 7/1/62
Dept. of Medicine
Columbia Univ. Coll. of Phys. & Surg.

Bitensky, Mark W., 1/1/66
Dept. of Medicine
New York University School of Medicine

Blanc, William A., 1/1/63
Dept. of Pathology
Columbia Univ. Coll. of Phys. & Surg.

Bookchin, Robert M., 7/1/67
Dept. of Medicine
Albert Einstein College of Medicine

*With date of initial appointment and current affiliation.

Briehl, Robin W., 9/1/62
Dept. of Physiology
Albert Einstein College of Medicine

Brooks, Dana C., 7/1/65
Dept. of Anatomy
Cornell University Medical College

C

Caldwell, Peter R., 7/1/69
Dept. of Medicine
Columbia Univ. Coll. of Phys. & Surg.

Camerini-Davalos, R. A., 7/1/65
Dept. of Medicine
New York Medical College

Canfield, Robert E., 7/1/64
Dept. of Medicine
Columbia Univ. Coll. of Phys. & Surg.

Carroll, Hugh J., 7/1/65
Dept. of Medicine
S.U.N.Y. Downstate Medical Center

Chambers, Robert W., 1/1/62
Dept. of Biochemistry
New York University School of Medicine

Christian, Charles L., 7/1/61
Dept. of Medicine
Columbia Univ. Coll. of Phys. & Surg.

Cohen, Burton D., 7/1/65
Dept. of Medicine
The Bronx-Lebanon Hospital Center

Cohen, Morton I., 1/1/63
Dept. of Physiology
Albert Einstein College of Medicine

Coleridge, John C., 7/1/68
Dept. of Physiology
New York Medical College

Cooper, Louis Z., 7/1/67
Dept. of Pediatrics
New York University School of Medicine

Cox, Rody P., 7/1/62
Dept. of Medicine
New York University School of Medicine

D

Daly, Marie M., 7/1/62
Dept. of Biochemistry
Albert Einstein College of Medicine

Damadian, Raymond V., 7/1/68
Dept. of Medicine
S.U.N.Y. Downstate Medical Center

Darnell, James E., 7/1/65
Dept. of Biological Sciences
Columbia University

deHarven, Etienne P., 7/1/63
Dept. of Cytology
Sloan Kettering Institute

Del Guercio, Louis R., 7/1/65
Dept. of Surgery
Albert Einstein College of Medicine

Doerfler, Walter, 7/1/69
Dept. of Virology
The Rockefeller University

Dreizen, Paul, 4/1/63
Dept. of Medicine
S.U.N.Y. Downstate Medical Center

Drucker, William D., 7/1/62
Dept. of Medicine
New York University School of Medicine

E

Edelmann, Chester M., 7/1/69
Dept. of Pediatrics
Albert Einstein College of Medicine

Elsbach, Peter, 7/1/64
Dept. of Medicine
New York University School of Medicine

Enson, Yale, 7/1/61
Dept. of Medicine
Columbia Univ. Coll. of Phys. & Surg.

F

Feigelson, Philip, 10/8/59
Dept. of Biochemistry
Columbia Univ. Coll. of Phys. & Surg.

Feldman, Daniel S., 7/1/66
Dept. of Neurology
S.U.N.Y. Downstate Medical Center

Fox, Charles L., Jr., 7/1/62
Dept. of Surgery
Columbia Univ. Coll. of Phys. & Surg.

Franklin, Edward C., 7/1/63
Dept. of Medicine
New York University School of Medicine

Freund, Matthew J., 1/1/62
Dept. of Pharmacology
New York Medical College

Friedman, Eli A., 7/1/63
Dept. of Medicine
S.U.N.Y. Downstate Medical Center

G

Gerber, Donald A., 1/1/65
Dept. of Medicine
S.U.N.Y. Downstate Medical Center

Goldstein, Allan L., 7/1/67
Dept. of Biochemistry
Abert Einstein College of Medicine

Goodman, DeWitt S., 7/1/64
Dept. of Medicine
Columbia Univ. Coll. of Phys. & Surg.

Gordon, Edwin E., 1/1/61
Dept. of Medicine
New York University School of Medicine

Gottfried, Eugene L., 7/1/64
Dept. of Medicine
Cornell University Medical College

Grant, Lester Howard, 7/1/61
Dept. of Medicine
New York University School of Medicine

Grayzel, Arthur I., 7/1/63
Dept. of Rheumatology
Montefiore Hospital and Medical Center

Graziani, Leonard J., 7/1/67
Depts. of Pediatrics and Neurology
Albert Einstein College of Medicine

Greenbaum, Lowell, 7/1/65
Dept. of Pharmacology
Columbia Univ. Coll. of Phys. & Surg.

Grollman, Arthur P., 7/1/63
Dept. of Pharmacology
Albert Einstein College of Medicine

H

Haft, David E., 7/1/63
Dept. of Medicine
New York Medical College

Halac, Elias, Jr., 7/1/66
Dept. of Pediatrics
New York University School of Medicine

Hays, Richard M., 7/1/62
Dept. of Medicine
Abert Einstein College of Medicine

Heinemann, Henry O., 7/1/61
Dept. of Medicine
Cornell University Medical College

Herbert, Victor D., 7/1/65
Dept. of Medicine
The Mount Sinai School of Medicine

Hilton, James G., 7/1/60
Renal-Endocrine Section
St. Luke's Hospital

Hirschhorn, Kurt, 7/1/65
Div. of Medical Genetics
The Mount Sinai School of Medicine

Holt, L. Emmett, Jr., 2/1/61
Dept. of Pediatrics
New York University School of Medicine

Horwitz, Marshall S., 7/1/69
Dept. of Pediatrics
Albert Einstein College of Medicine

J

Jaffé, Ernst R., 7/1/61
Dept. of Medicine
Albert Einstein College of Medicine

James, Leonard S., 1/1/61
Dept. of Pediatrics
Columbia Univ. Coll. of Phys. & Surg.

Javid, Jamshid, 7/1/69
Dept. of Medicine
New York University School of Medicine

John, Erwin R., 7/1/64
Dept. of Psychiatry
New York Medical College

Josephson, Alan S., 7/1/63
Dept. of Medicine
S.U.N.Y. Downstate Medical Center

K

Kao, Frederick F., 7/1/61
Dept. of Physiology
S.U.N.Y. Downstate Medical Center

Karpatkin, Simon, 1/1/66
Dept. of Medicine
New York University School of Medicine

Kavaler, Frederic, 7/1/64
Dept. of Physiology
S.U.N.Y. Downstate Medical Center

Kaye, Gordon I., 7/1/63
Dept. of Surgical Pathology
Columbia Univ. Coll. of Phys. & Surg.

Kelly, William G., 7/1/64
Dept. of Pharmacology
Columbia Univ. Coll. of Phys. & Surg.

Kinney, John M., 1/1/65
Dept. of Surgery
Columbia Univ. Coll. of Phys. & Surg.

Knittle, Jerome L., 7/1/68
Dept. of Pediatrics
The Mount Sinai School of Medicine

Korein, Julius, 1/1/66
Dept. of Neurology
New York University School of Medicine

Krasnow, Norman, 1/1/64
Dept. of Medicine
S.U.N.Y. Downstate Medical Center

L

Lamm, Michael E., 1/1/66
Dept. of Pathology
New York University School of Medicine

Langner, Thomas S., 7/1/63
Dept. of Epidemiology
Columbia Univ. School of Pub. Health & Ad. Med.

Lee, Kwang S., 7/1/65
Dept. of Pharmacology
S.U.N.Y. Downstate Medical Center

Levine, Bernard B., 7/1/62
Dept. of Medicine
New York University School of Medicine

Levine, O. Robert, 7/1/62
Dept. of Pediatrics
Columbia Univ. Coll. of Phys. & Surg.

Lilly, Frank, 7/1/67
Dept. of Genetics
Albert Einstein College of Medicine

Lowenstein, Jerome, 7/1/67
Dept. of Medicine
New York University School of Medicine

M

MacLeod, John, 7/1/61
Dept. of Anatomy
Cornell University Medical College

Mahler, Richard, 7/1/68
Dept. of Medicine
New York Medical College

Mandel, Irwin D., 7/1/69
Dept. of Dentistry
Columbia Univ. Sch. of Dent. & Oral Surg.

Marcus, Donald M., 9/1/63
Dept. of Medicine
Albert Einstein College of Medicine

Marmur, Julius, 7/1/63
Dept. of Biochemistry
Albert Einstein College of Medicine

Marsh, Donald J., 7/1/64
Dept. of Physiology
New York University School of Medicine

May, Charles D., 3/1/61
Dept. of Pediatrics
New York University School of Medicine

McBride, Raymond A., 7/1/67
Dept. of Pathology
New York Medical College

McConnell, David J., 7/1/69
Dept. of Medicine
Columbia Univ. Coll. of Phys. & Surg.

Meikle, Thomas H., Jr., 7/1/69
Dept. of Anatomy
Cornell University Medical College

Miller, Orlando J., 7/1/61
Dept. of Obstetrics and Gynecology
Columbia Univ. Coll. of Phys. & Surg.

Moore, Cyril L., 7/1/68
Dept. of Biochemistry
Albert Einstein College of Medicine

Morrill, Gene A., 7/1/69
Dept. of Physiology
Albert Einstein College of Medicine

Morse, Jane H., 7/1/62
Dept. of Medicine
Columbia Univ. Coll. of Phys. & Surg.

N

Nagel, Ronald L., 7/1/69
Dept. of Medicine
Albert Einstein College of Medicine

Neu, Harold C., 7/1/65
Dept. of Medicine
Columbia Univ. Coll. of Phys. & Surg.

New, Maria I., 7/1/66
Dept. of Pediatrics
Cornell University Medical College

Nitowsky, Harold M., 7/1/67
Dept. of Pediatrics
Albert Einstein College of Medicine

Nussenzweig, Victor, 7/1/68
Dept. of Pathology
New York University School of Medicine

O

Oppenheimer, Jack H., 7/1/62
Endocrine Research Laboratory
Montefiore Hospital and Medical Center

Ovary, Zoltan, 1/1/61
Dept. of Pathology
New York University School of Medicine

P

Paulsen, Elsa P., 1/1/66
Guest Investigator
The Rockefeller University

Piomelli, Sergio, 7/1/64
Dept. of Pediatrics
New York University School of Medicine

Prince, Alfred M., 7/1/67
New York Blood Center
Community Blood Council of Greater N.Y.

R

Ranney, Helen M., 7/1/64
Dept. of Medicine
Albert Einstein College of Medicine

Rapaport, Felix T., 1/1/64
Dept. of Surgery
New York University School of Medicine

Reddi, Kutumba K., 7/1/67
Guest Investigator
The Rockefeller University

Ribble, John C., 7/1/62
Dept. of Pediatrics
Cornell University Medical College

Rieder, Ronald F., 7/1/69
Dept. of Medicine
S.U.N.Y. Downstate Medical Center

Rifkind, Richard A., 7/1/63
Dept. of Medicine
Columbia Univ. Coll. of Phys. & Surg.

Roheim, Paul S., 7/1/68
Dept. of Physiology
Albert Einstein College of Medicine

Rosen, Samuel M., 7/1/69
Dept .of Medicine
Albert Einstein College of Medicine

Rothenberg, Sheldon P., 1/1/65
Dept. of Medicine
New York Medical College

Ruben, Robert J., 7/1/66
Department of Otolaryngology
Albert Einstein College of Medicine

Rudick, Jack, 7/1/67
Dept. of Surgery
The Mount Sinai School of Medicine

S

Sandson, John I., 1/1/61
Dept. of Medicine
Albert Einstein College of Medicine

Saxena, Brij B., 7/1/69
Dept. of Biochemistry
Cornell University Medical College

Schachter, David, 7/1/61
Dept. of Physiology
Columbia Univ. Coll. of Phys. & Surg.

Siegel, John H., 7/1/66
Dept. of Surgery
Albert Einstein College of Surgery

Silber, Robert, 9/1/62
Dept. of Medicine
New York University School of Medicine

Simon, Eric J., 10/8/59
Dept. of Medicine
New York University School of Medicine

Sirlin, Julio L., 7/1/67
Dept. of Anatomy
Cornell University Medical College

Siskind, Gregory W., 1/1/66
Dept. of Medicine
Cornell University Medical College

Snyderman, Selma E., 1/1/61
Dept. of Pediatrics
New York University School of Medicine

Sobel, Edna H., 7/1/65
Dept. of Pediatrics
Albert Einstein College of Medicine

Soeiro, Ruy, 7/1/68
Dept. of Medicine
Albert Einstein College of Medicine

Song, Chull S., 7/1/67
Dept. of Medicine
The Rockefeller University

Southren, A. Louis, 1/1/63
Dept. of Medicine
New York Medical College

Speirs, Robert S., 7/1/61
Dept. of Anatomy
S.U.N.Y. Downstate Medical Center

Srinivasan, Supramaniam, 7/1/67
Dept. of Surgery
S.U.N.Y. Downstate Medical Center

Stracher, Alfred, 7/1/63
Dept. of Biochemistry
S.U.N.Y. Downstate Medical Center

Summers, Donald F., 1/1/66
Dept. of Microbiology
Albert Einstein College of Medicine

T

Tobin, Mark S., 1/1/63
Section on Hematology
The Brookdale Hospital Center

Turino, Gerard M., 7/1/61
Columbia Univ. Coll. of Phys. & Surg.
Dept. of Medicine

V

Valentine, Fred T., 7/1/69
Dept. of Medicine
New York University School of Medicine

Vande Wiele, Raymond L., 1/1/62
Dept. of Obstetrics and Gynecology
Columbia Univ. Coll. of Phys. & Surg.

Veith, Frank J., 7/1/65
Dept. of Surgery
Montefiore Hospital and Medical Center

W

Wallach, Stanley, 7/1/61
Dept. of Medicine
S.U.N.Y. Downstate Medical Center

Warner, Jonathan R., 7/1/65
Dept. of Biochemistry
Albert Einstein College of Medicine

Weber, Wendell W., 7/1/65
Dept. of Pharmacology
New York University School of Medicine

Weinstein, I. Bernard, 7/1/61
Dept. of Medicine
Columbia Univ. Coll. of Phys. & Surg.

Weiss, Harvey J., 9/1/69
Division of Hematology
The Roosevelt Hospital

Weissmann, Gerald, 1/1/66
Dept. of Medicine
New York University School of Medicine

Windhager, Erich E., 7/1/64
Dept. of Physiology
Cornell University Medical College

Winters, Robert W., 7/1/63
Dept. of Pediatrics
Columbia Univ. Coll. of Phys. & Surg.

Witkin, Evelyn M., 10/1/69
Dept. of Medicine
S.U.N.Y. Downstate Medical Center

Wittner, Murray, 7/1/65
Dept. of Pathology
Albert Einstein College of Medicine

Y

Yao, Alice C., 7/1/69
Dept. of Pediatrics
S.U.N.Y. Downstate Medical Center

THE DOCTOR TRAVELS WITH KARL BAEDEKER*

BRUNO GEBHARD

Director Emeritus
Cleveland Health Museum
Cleveland, Ohio

THE original Karl Baedeker was 27 years old when he published his first *Handbook for Travellers* in 1828. That his first guidebook on traveling along the Rhine was so successful is partly due to good timing, because in 1828 the Preussisch-Rheinsche Dampfschiffahrtsgesellschaft started regular trips between Cologne and Mainz. Neither Thomas Cook & Sons nor American Express were heard of at that time.

Through more than four generations the *Baedekers* have been famous for their dependability. As stated by A. P. Herbert: "For Kings and government may err—but never Mr. Baedeker." Karl Baedeker never described anything that he had not seen himself. There is a description of a tour he made from Pola to Fiume; he says, "This writer has made the trip at night and is, therefore, sorry that he cannot describe anything as he was asleep."

Karl Baedeker was unbelievably precise in everything he did. In Paris, at the cemetery of Père Lachaise (110 acres), which rates two stars, he spent eight hours one day and five and a half hours the next one in locating the graves and sarcophagi of famous men and women, such as Abelard (d. 1141), Héloise (d. 1163), Molière (d. 1673), Chopin, (d. 1827), and F. J. Gall, the phrenologist (d. 1825).

Baedeker was the first to select special objects and views of great interest, as well as reliable hotels, giving them one and very rarely two stars as a mark of commendation. One can easily argue about his rating system. Some of it is more or less timeless, as the double star for the Louvre, the Venus de Milo, Yellowstone National Park, St. Peter's, and the pyramids, but one might question the Morse Collection of Japanese pottery in the Museum of Fine Arts in Boston as rating a star.

The format and cover of the *Baedekers* have not changed for 100

*Presented at the annual meeting of the Ohio Academy of Medical History, Cleveland, Ohio, May 9, 1965.

years. The raspberry-red covers with gold lettering and marbleized edges, started in 1854, are well known. I have in my toy collection one of the famous oval *Nürenberger Spielzeugschachteln*, which contains about 40 figures of "A journey into the mountains." The set consists of a company of travelers, peasants of the mountain regions and, naturally, the mountains, and some trees. One of the travelers is on horseback and is holding the red-covered *Baedeker* in his hands, reading as he rides. There is the apocryphal story that at the funeral of Karl Baedeker (in 1858), a traveler happened to come along in the funeral procession with the red book in his hand. The handbook format was changed with the publication of Baedeker's *Autoführer*, after World War II.

Karl Baedeker's worldwide popularity in our days is well attested in many poems written about him. Among the best is a series of 12 *Sonnets to Baedeker* by David McCord, which appeared first in the New Yorker (April 23, 1932) and also in *A Subtreasury of American Humor*.[1] The first one reads:

My old companion on the beaten track,
Who brought me villages and bed and board,
Settled the day and laid me on my back
At inns whose tariffs I could not afford;
Sweet vade mecum of the Tuileries,
And audible in naves and barrel vaults,
Still smelling of an earlier Cheddar cheese,
Or blemished with red wines and English malts;
So I remember with what crafty charm
Of small italics and appropriate miles
Distinguished pages loosened a new swarm
Of ancient Ninevehs and distant Niles,
And played upon my mind as men at chess,
And sold me to American Express.*

Karl Baedeker made his first trip on a railroad in 1838 in Belgium. He writes in an enthusiastic letter to his father: "On the second of May I rode the railroad to Mecheln. The distance of six miles was traversed in three-quarters of an hour. A bell indicates the start and the *remorqueur* (locomotive) begins to groan and the wheels revolve

*Reprinted by permission: 1932, 1960, the *New Yorker Magazine*, Inc.

first slowly and then faster and faster, and then the train flies with its 23 to 30 coaches. What fun traveling is now."

The development of the European railroad system in the middle of the last century did much to promote what was then called "tourism." The "traveler," derived from travail (work), is replaced by "tour-ist" about 1850 and new words are coined, such as "sight-seeing." Thomas Cook started his first continental tour in 1856, and the sensation of the year 1869 was his "Conducted Crusade to the Holy Land for Middle-class People."

In 1844 Karl Baedeker published the first edition of *Switzerland*. By 1913 it had had 35 editions; in other words every second year there was a new up-to-date edition. All in all, at the beginning of World War I, nearly 50 different countries were covered in five different languages. The whole European continent, including Russia, also the Mediterranean Sea with parts of Northern Africa were covered. Baedeker ventured into India, Malaya, Siam, and Java with resulting guidebooks in 1914, but he never covered the Far East or the Australian continent. The United States and Canada each have a guidebook, but there is nothing on Central and South America.

Baedeker's style is basically one of precision and knowledgeability. It is sometimes dry as dust, but Bertrand Russell once said he had two models for his own style: Milton's prose and Baedeker's guidebooks. "The Puritan never wrote without passion," he said, "and the cicerone used only a few words in recommending sights, hotels, and restaurants. Passion was the voice of reason, economy the signature of brilliance."[2]

One usually does not read Baedeker for pleasure, but the quantity of incidental information that one may pick up is astonishing. In the *Baedeker* I own, published in 1869, on Mittel-Nord-Deutschland, the author mentions under Cassel, the monument erected even in his lifetime to Landgraf Friedrich II, and he states "*es darf nicht unerwähnt bleiben, dass von 1776-1784 fuer 22 Mill. Thaler 12,000 Landeskinder nach America an die Englaender verkauft wurden,*" which means "It must be mentioned that during the years 1776-1784 about 12,000 compatriots were sold to the British for 22 Million Thaler (dollars)."

Those who are interested in genealogy, especially that of their own family, will find surprises in looking through a Baedeker. In thumbing through Baedeker's *Das Generalgouvernement*—of that more a little later —I found mentioned Berthold and Matthias Stecker as *Stadtvoegte* (a kind of combination of city judges and city managers) active in 1250 in the city of Lemberg. This city, in what is now Poland, located in Galicia, had many families with German names, all listed by Baedeker. On my own family name I found in the volume on Austria the Gebhardsberg, named after St. Gebhard, born on August 7, 949, who was later a bishop of Constance. In 1964 Mrs. Gebhard and I went to see the Gebhardsberg, 1,965 feet high, which has a star because it "commands an extensive prospect, embracing the Lake of Constance, the valley of the Rhine and the snow mountains of Appenzell and Glarus." Unfortunately it was a rainy day and the view was limited; also the small church on the mountain, where St. Gebhard was born, was closed for renovation—so we shall have to try again.

I mentioned Baedeker's *Das Generalgouvernement*, published during World War II (1943) for the German army of occupation in Poland and the Ukraine. The historical introduction is a complete line-up for the "1,000 Year Reich of Adolf Hitler." I have never seen it listed in any catalogue.

With the single exception of this war publication, the *Baedekers* have the mark of "unimpeached authority"; this includes the introductory chapters dealing with the geography, history, politics, and language of each respective country. If you are looking for the *Gettysburg Address* Baedeker prints it in full[3] as the *Twenty Lines Address*, as it was known by contemporaries of Lincoln. By the way, the account of the Battle of Gettysburg was written by a Philadelphia newspaperman who was present at the battle as a special correspondent.

Any physician traveling with a *Baedeker* will always find something which is close to his professional interest. When necessary, any *Baedeker* is quite blunt and outspoken regarding cleanliness and convenience. About the state of affairs in northern Italy the book has this to say: "The popular idea of cleanliness in Italy is behind the age, dirt being perhaps neutralised in the opinion of the natives by the brilliancy of their climate."

As for the United States of 1909 he is not at all pleased with the public conveniences: "Public Conveniences are not usually provided in American cities, but their place is practically supplied by the lavatories of hotels, to which passers-by resort freely. Such public conveniences as do exist in New York and other large cities are disgracefully inadequate in number, size, and equipment."

Baedeker is up-to-date both with his *Travelbook* geared to railway travel and walking tours and also with his *Autoguides* (since 1957) for 10 European countries, but for the United States 1909 is the date of the latest edition, which has 824 pages, 33 maps, and 48 city plans. This book has been my steady companion during 30 years of travel in this country and is full of information that is still good. Baedeker suggests to visitors from England that "to enter into the spirit of American pastime, an Englishman need only to admire the gait of the trotting horse and to admire the merits of baseball."

Baedeker supplies an interesting glossary on words not usually familiar to the visiting Englishman, such as "two bits" and "sophomore."

He also touches on the Negro question: "Intimidation is rare, except in the Southern States, where it is still occasionally, though much more rarely than thirty years ago, practised upon the negroes."

For those interested in medical history the *Baedekers* are full of detailed information. The few occasions on which I talked with the late George Sarton were mainly consumed in exchanging tidbits about medical men and institutions we had found when we first came to this country in 1934. I learned from Karl that John S. Billings had been the director of the New York Public Library (p. 471), that the New York Academy of Medicine was originally the neighbor of the Century Club on West 43rd Street (p. 481), that Lenox Hill Hospital was the former German Hospital (p, 52). Here is what Baedeker tells us about the Rockefeller Institute (p. 54):

> At the foot of 66th St. is the Rockefeller Institute for Medical Research (Pl. I,4), endowed by Mr. John D. Rockefeller with $4,000,000 to promote discovery in medical science for the alleviation of suffering in man and animals (Dr. Simon Flexner, Scientific Director). It occupies part of the old Schermerhorn farm.

The statue of Dr. F. Marion Sims (1813-1883) was originally at 41st Street in Bryant Park—and so on. Have you heard of the "Sesrun Club," next to St. Luke's Hospital in New York? Baedeker gives the location—also the book reveals that "sesrun" is "nurses" spelled backward. Cemeteries always get much attention: here is his description of the Greenwood Cemetery in Brooklyn (p. 78):

> One of the most beautiful cities of the dead in America, rivalling Prospect Park in the charms of its undulating surface

and extensive views. It is 475 acres in extent. Carriages take passengers round the chief points for 25¢ each.

The principal (N.) entrance is in Fifth Ave. (cor. 25th St.; Pl. C. 6). The entrance gateway is an elaborate structure of brown stone, 142 ft. wide, with bas-reliefs and a tower 100 ft. high. Plans of the cemetery may be obtained here (10¢), showing the positions of the graves. Among the monuments of special interest, either from their subject or treatment, are those to the New York Volunteers (Section H), Roger Williams (p. 244; Sec. 130), De Witt Clinton (p. 92; 108), Elias P. Howe (the inventor of the sewing machine; H), S. F. B. Morse (p. 274; 25), Henry George (1839-97), the founder of the "Single Tax" movement (at the top of Ocean Hill), the magnificent mausoleum of John W. McKay, Horace Greeley (p. 39; 35), Henry Ward Beecher (p. 76; 140), Lola Montez, John Matthews (64), the Pilots (111), the Firemen (2), Peter Cooper (p. 42; 101), A. S. Scribner (160), James Gordon Bennett (107), Charlotte Canda (92), and the Brooklyn Theatre Fire Victims (N). One of the chief attractions of Greenwood is the beauty of the blossoming of the dog-wood (Cornus Florida) at the end of May or beginning of June.

Watering places and filtration plants are described in detail, as at Saratoga Springs or in Ocean Grove in New Jersey (p. 176). Of Ocean Grove he says:

> This extraordinary settlement, possible only in America, in which many thousands of persons, young and old, voluntarily elect to spend their summer vacations under a religious autocracy, which is severe both in its positive and negative regulations, is curious enough to repay a short visit. It is bounded by the sea on the E., by lakes on the N. and S., and by a high fence on the W.; and its gates are closed at 10 p.m. daily and all day on Sunday. The drinking of alcoholic beverages and the sale of tobacco are strictly prohibited, and no theatrical performances of any kind are allowed. No bathing, riding, or driving is permitted on Sunday. Innumerable religious meetings of all kinds are held daily, the chief place of assemblage being a huge Auditorium, which contains a very powerful organ and can hold 10,000 people. The annual Camp Meeting is the great

event of the season. Near the Auditorium is a large Model of Jerusalem. One section of the place consists solely of tents. The excellent bathing beach is skirted by a plank-walk, ¾ M. long.

On the same page Baedeker mentions Asbury Park—largely frequented by those who object to the religious management of Ocean Grove.

Baedeker dutifully records the places where historical personalities were born, lived, and were buried. In *Switzerland* you find information on the life of Paracelsus; in the volume on the United States there is an entry on page 165: "Philadelphia, Walnut St. N. 1524—the home of Dr. S. Weir Mitchell, the novelist"; today's tourist walking to Rittenhouse Square will be reminded of this by a bronze plaque. Describing sights in Baltimore, he says: "Dr. O. W. Holmes has remarked that three short American poems, each of the best of its kind, were all written at Baltimore (p. 204): viz., Poe's 'Raven,' Randall's 'Maryland, My Maryland' (melodie: O, Tannenbaum, O, Tannenbaum) and Key's 'Star-Spangled Banner.' "

Let us turn to Ohio, which is treated in the opening chapter of Section III, the Middle West, and more or less as a stopover on the way from Pittsburgh to Chicago (Columbus) or from Buffalo to Chicago, where *Baedeker* suggests the traveler stop at Cleveland. This city rates about four pages: the Hollenden Hotel gets a star. The book mentions the three-cent fare of the electric tramways, records seven places of amusement, one of which offers "first class vaudeville"; two others have the by-line "vaudeville and burlesque." No motion-picture houses are mentioned in this 1909 *Baedeker* on the United States.

Baedeker goes all out for Cincinnati, praises its location "finely situated on several terraces rising from the right (N) branch of the Ohio and surrounded by an amphitheater of hills 4-500 feet high." The book tells all about the district "Over the Rhine" and its inhabitants, becomes quite lyrical about Eden Park, which is starred, and the Art Museum; starred also are Spring Grove Cemetery and the zoo, which contains a fine collection of animals and is a favorite resort and restaurant; concerts are held there. The collection of Rookwood pottery is starred, and so is the suspension bridge across the Ohio River to Covington, Ky., built by John A. Roebling. A footnote "to the scientific traveler" says that Cincinnati is the most convenient locality from which to visit the famous Serpent Mound, which he describes in detail.

From a historian's viewpoint the volumes on Greece, Italy, Egypt, Palestine, and Syria are the most valuable, as the introductory chapters were written by outstanding scientists of the respective countries. I am sure the same can be said about the volume on India, which I have never seen; it is listed in a catalogue for 45 dollars.

Early editions of the *Baedekers* are difficult to get and have become collectors' items. The more contemporary ones mostly found their way into the hands of the general staffs of the armies involved in World War II. Some of these handbooks are still very useful for travelers, e.g., the volume on Russia, the eighth and last edition of which appeared in 1914, One of our best-known experts on Russia in this country states: "The 1914 *Baedeker,* despite two world wars, a revolution and the passage of nearly 50 years, continues to be the most accurate, reliable and handy companion of information for the traveler who is planning to go to Russia."

The Russians have copied Baedeker with a volume on Europe; a third edition was published in 1905. Not being able to read Russian, I do not know whether it is an honest Baedeker publication or a good facsimile of one. It is distinctive in that it includes photos of European sights. Baedeker never includes photos in his *Autoguides*; he uses charming pen-and-ink sketches, and older volumes carry engravings of mountain panoramas.

Traveling today—or shall we say tourism—has become a mass movement and is part of a recreational industry. The Grand Tour of the princely few in the 17th and 18th centuries has become possible for millions of young and old travelers. This has happened only in the last 40 years. In 1902 the Paris manager of American Express stated, "There is no profit in the tourist business as conducted by Thomas Cook & Son, and even if this were, this company would not undertake it."[4] The gentleman was quite wrong; American Express makes more than one million hotel reservations in Europe alone.

Traveling and trading have gone on since antiquity; pilgrimages and crusades followed in the early medieval days either on foot, or horseback, or wagon; regularly scheduled post coaches, an innovation of the dukes of Thurn and Taxis, made traveling easier, but steamboats, railroads, and airplanes made traveling possible for the masses. "Orientation for Educational Travel" is not an academic subject for international conferences trying to prove or disprove a well-known Spanish proverb, "The ass which goes abroad does not return a horse."[5]

Irwin Abrams, professor of history at Antioch College, Yellow Springs, Ohio, put it this way: "We don't want them [our traveling students] star-gazing à la Baedeker. We want them to use their own eyes and behold beauty on their own, to feel a thrill in coming upon the unexpected."[6] We agree only partly for, as Goethe says, "We see only what we know," and with that Karl Baedeker helps.

Guidebooks as we know them today have a 300-year history. One of the earliest is by James Howell, titled *Instructions for Forreine Travell*, published in William Harvey's time, in 1642.[7] Howell had traveled abroad for three years and four months in order to write his *Exact Survey of the Kingdomes and the States of Christendome*, meaning Continental Europe without Turkey. His book is in part a philosophy of traveling based on his observations, as shown in his opening chapter: "Of the Advantage and Preeminence of the Eye":

> . . . the Eare is not so authentique a witnesse as the Eye, because the Eye, by which as through a cleare christall casement, wee discerne the various works of Art and Nature, and in one instant comprehend halfe the whole Universe in so small a roome after so admirable a manner, I say the Eye having a more quick and immediate commerce and familiarity with the Soule (being the principall of her Cinq ports, and her Centinell . . .) taketh in farre deeper Ideas, and so makes firmer and more lasting impressions, conveying the object more faithfully (and clearly) to the memory, where it remaines afterward upon (lasting) record in particular topicall notes, (markes) and indelible characters.
>
> That one Eye-witnesse is of more validity than ten Auricular.

In his closing chapter, "What Course a Traveler Must Take After His Returning Home," Howell has this to say:

> For Forraine Travell oftentimes makes many to wander from themselves, as well as from their Countrey, and to come back mere Mimiques, and so in going farre, to fare worse, and bring back lesse wit, than they carrieth forth, they go out Figures (according the the Italian Proverb) and returne Cyphers.

His final admonition is this:

> An ingenious and discerning Traveller will disdaine this, and strive to distinguish 'twixt good and evil, 'twixt that which is tracefull, and what's phantastique, 'twixt what is to be followed,

and what's to be shunned, and bring home the best: Hee will strive to be rather Substance without shew, than shew without substance.

REFERENCES

1. White, E. G. and White, K. S.: *A Subtreasury of American Humor.* New York, McCann, 1941, pp. 1-701.
2. New Yorker Magazine, Dec. 9, 1961, p. 100.
3. Baedeker: *United States,* 4th ed., 1909, p. 195.
4. Hatch, A.: *A Century of Science, 1850-1950.* Garden City, N.Y., American Express 1950.
5. Abrams, I.: Orientation for Educational Travel. Presented at the European-North American Conference on Educational Travel and Exchange Programs, Cannes, 1965.
6. Antioch Notes, 42/6, III, 1965.
7. Republished in: *English Reprints,* Arber, E., ed. London, 1869.

ERRATUM

On page 268 of the *Bulletin* for April 1970 an illustration appears which the author and the editors accepted, on distinguished bibliographic authority, as a picture of Mozart as a boy. We are now informed by Professor Dr. Géza Roche of the Internationale Stiftung Mozarteum of Salzburg, Austria, that the illustration is a picture of Carl, Count Firmian.

SOME MEDICAL AND NONMEDICAL ITEMS IN BAEDEKER'S DESCRIPTION OF NEW YORK

For those who are fond of travel, Karl Baedeker's guidebooks have long been indispensable. Indeed, there are many old-timers who still prefer the old raspberry-red pocket-sized volumes to the newer version.

Not all of the conscientious thousands who have traveled, guidebook in hand, to the fjords of Norway or the bubbling asphalt of the Phlegraean fields have been aware of the fact that near the end of the 19th century the firm of Karl Baedeker at last recognized the United States. The Library of the New York Academy of Medicine possesses a copy of Baedeker's *The United States, with an Excursion into Mexico,* published in 1893. The title page bears the annotation "Leipsic: Karl Baedeker, Publisher. New York: Charles Scribner's Sons, 743-745 Broadway."

The guidebook was written by one Mr. J. F. Muirhead, M.A., "who has for several years taken part in the English editions of Baedeker's Handbooks, and has personally visited the greater part of the districts described." The introductory essays include not only the customary and usual information about money, hotels, and restaurants, but also *A Short History of American Politics* by John McMaster, *Constitution and Political Institutions of the United States* by the famous James Bryce (Lord Bryce), and *Physiography of North America* by the distinguished Nathaniel S. Shaler.

A section designated "Glossary" opens as follows: "The following short list of words in frequent use in the United States in a sense not commonly known in England may be found of service. The speech of the cultivated American, of course, varies little from the speech of the cultivated Englishman, and no misunderstanding is likely to arise in their verbal intercourse; but it will not infrequently be found that railway officials, cabmen, waiters, and the like do not know what is meant by the British equivalents of the following expressions." The list includes:

Bed-spread, coverlet, counterpane.

Biscuit, hot tea-rolls.

Block, square mass of building bounded by four streets.

Bright, clever.

Clerk, shopman.
Clever, good-natured.
Cracker, biscuit; also, in the Southern States, a poor white man.
Dumb, (often) stupid (Ger. *dumm*).
Horse-Car, tramway.
Pitcher, jug.
Prince Albert (coat), frock-coat.
Take out. An American takes a lady "out" to dinner, while an Englishman takes her "in."

Under "General Hints" the traveler is given some salutary advice: "The first requisites for the enjoyment of a tour in the United States are an absence of prejudice and a willingness to accommodate oneself to the customs of the country. If the traveler exercise a little patience, he will find that ways which strike him as unreasonable or even disagreeable are more suitable to the environment than those of his own home would be. He should from the outset reconcile himself to the absence of deference or servility on the part of those he considers his social inferiors. . . . The average Englishman will probably find the chief physical discomforts in the dirt of the city streets, the roughness of the country roads, the winter overheating of hotels and railway cars (70-75° Fahr. being by no means unusual), and (in many places) the habit of spitting on the floor; but the Americans themselves are now keenly alive to these weak points and are doing their best to remove them."

The excellent map of Manhattan surprisingly shows Broadway north of the Columbus Monument to be named the Boulevard. From 114th to about 120th Streets the map shows an open area containing the Bloomingdale Insane Asylum, Columbia University not yet having moved northward from 49th St. Central Park contains not only the Harlem Lake near its northeastern corner, but two large Croton Reservoirs. At the intersection of 103d Street and Fifth Avenue the map shows nothing but an oblong, indicative of housing.

In Baedeker's words "Fifth Avenue, the chief street in New York from the standpoint of wealth and fashion, begins at Washington Square . . . above 42nd St. it consists of handsome private residences, forming, perhaps, a more imposing show of affluence and comfort than any other street in the world. The avenue has been kept sacred from the marring touch of the tram or the elevated railroad, but it is traversed by a line of "stages" or omnibuses. . . . In 15th St. a little to the W. of Fifth Avenue, is the large building of the *New York Hospital*. . . . In *W. 43rd St.*, between Fifth and Sixth Avenues, are three handsome new buildings, completed in 1890-91. . . . Adjoining the Century Club is the *New York Academy of Medicine* . . . , a substantial and handsome edifice, with a front of reddish-brown stone, in a semi-Egyptian style. Beyond this are the extensive quarters of the *Racquet Club*." A dozen blocks farther north the old St. Luke's Hospital is described as a tasteful structure with two low campanile towers.

In describing the Park Avenue district the guidebook tells of the "large and conspicuous Armoury of the Seventh Regiment, the fashionable regiment of New York," the nearby Hahnemann Hospital, and—surprisingly—"the *Lenox* or *Presbyterian Hospital*, an effective building, extending back to Madison Ave." Beyond it to the north the old German Hospital is noted (nowadays called the Lenox Hill). Bellevue receives only half a sentence, and in fine print at that.

Other facilities recorded by Baedeker include baths, which "may be obtained at all the hotels (25 c.-75 c.) and large barbers' shops (25 c.)," and a respectable series of libraries, such as "*Mott Memorial Library* (medical), 64 Madison Ave. (11-9); *New York Hospital Library*, 8 W. 16th St. (medical). . . ."

Turning from indoor treasure to outdoor pleasure, Baedeker has this to say of our famous scenic attraction:

> The great promenade and open-air resort of New York is Central Park, occupying the centre of Manhattan Island, between 59th and 110th St. . . . The ground was originally a tract of swamp and rock, and its transformation into one of the most beautiful parks in the world is an important monument of American skill and perseverance. . . . The park is enclosed by a low cut-stone wall and has 20 entrances. The fashionable time for driving and riding is in the afternoon from 4 to 7, and the "Corso" here almost challenges comparison with that in Hyde Park.

Those who thought of venturing across the East River were told: "*Brooklyn* . . . is the fourth city of the United States in size and industrial interest, but it is so overshadowed by the proximity of New York as to bulk much less largely in the public eye than many smaller cities." A fair warning.

S.J.

CLIMATIC TREATMENT OF HYPOCHONDRIASIS

Among the diseases in which change of air is most frequently resorted to, there is none in which its beneficial influence is more manifest than in hypochondriasis, an affection so closely connected with morbid states of both the stomach and brain, that it is as frequently ascribed to one organ as to the other. But be its seat what it may matters little to the purpose of this work, since these viscera are so directly associated together that whatever affects either must react on both.

This state of chronic depression of spirits and morbid sensibility attended by deranged digestion, which is so intractable as regards its treatment by medicines, is nevertheless amenable to change of climate, and has been thus successfully dealt with for many centuries. The observation of the old physician who wrote on this subject upwards of 300 years ago, is still applicable to invalids of this class. Although our ordinary air be good by nature or art, yet it is not amiss to alter it. There is indeed no better physic for a melancholy man than travel, change of air, and variety of places.

In this disease the moral effects of travelling are not less marked than the physical, and both often result in a cure, after the ordinary resources of physic have been in vain exhausted. The primary action of "change of air" seems to consist in the improvement of the digestive functions, and is soon followed by a diminution of the nervous irritability.

The hypochondriacal invalid, who at home has probably been long accustomed to the anxious attentions of his family, or the patient services of his domestics, is, we will say, sent abroad at a mature age, for the first time, for change of climate, to a country of the language of which he is perfectly ignorant. On landing he goes to an hotel, where he is regarded as any other guest that pays his bill, and missing his accustomed comforts he fancies himself neglected. This might at first be considered an unfavourable position for such a person, but in reality it is the best that could be desired. For though usually the patient, at first, uses abuse and threats freely, or even resorts to blows, as I once saw an English valetudinarian do, with a Spanish servant, who in reply produced his albacete knife, and extorted an ample public apology for the insult; finding these means useless, the hypochondriac will perforce be obliged to curb his temper, and a more equable state of mind will thus gradually become habitual; while, at the same time, the attention of the patient will, by the change of scene, and the thoughts which the varieties of places and manners must occasion, be taken off for the time from their concentration on his own fancied, or even real, ailments.

In hypochondriasis, constant travelling for a few months will generally be found far more serviceable than a prolonged residence in any one place. It matters little where the tour be made, so that a complete change be accomplished; and, therefore, the further we remove from England the better.

A dry, bracing climate is that which is indicated, and a warm, humid atmosphere would in most cases be most prejudicial. In summer a tour in Switzerland or up the Rhine, may be tried with great prospect of success; and in winter the South of France, from Montpellier to Nice, or Italy, avoiding Pisa and Rome. In this complaint Naples is perhaps the best residence in Italy for a short time in winter or part of spring.

—Madden, Thomas M.: *On Change of Climate, A Guide for Travellers in Pursuit of Health.* London, Newby, 1864, pp. 56-58.

DISEASE IN NEPAL, 1819

On the whole I am inclined to believe, that the climate of the valley is healthful, although, immediately before our arrival, the inhabitants had been much troubled with fevers, and, for the first three months after our arrival, the whole of our native attendants were exceedingly sickly. The complaints to which they were chiefly subject, were fevers of the intermittent kind, and fluxes, attended with a very copious secretion of slimy matter, which, by the natives, is attributed to Bayu or wind; and which was brought on by very slight indulgences in eating. In the fevers emetics seemed much more efficacious than the cathartics which are usually employed at Calcutta; and, indeed, a dose of emetic tartar very frequently cut the fever short, as usual in temperate climates. The fluxes were not attended with much pain, and both these and the tendency in the bowels to the slimy secretions, seemed to require the frequent exhibition of spirituous bitters and small doses of opium. In such cases, I found the chirata tolerably efficacious, but I thought other bitters more powerful, especially the infusion of chamomile flowers, and the compound tinctures of Gentian and Peruvian bark. Our people probably suffered from having passed through the forest too late in the season; but the natives of Hindustan do not support a change of air, and on our first arrival they were not well provided with means to resist the weather, which to them was uncommonly cold.

I have seen no country where the venereal disease is so common as in Nepal, nor so generally diffused among all classes of the people, who are indeed very dissolute. During my stay I had application for medical assistance from all ranks labouring under the venereal disease; and I observed that the men did not consider it as extraordinary or shameful, when they found their wives afflicted with this malady. The dissolute manners of the inhabitants are carried to such a length, that a great many of the young men of rank, by the age of twenty-five, are debilitated, and have recourse to stimulants. The preparation of these forms a chief source of emolument to the medical men, and they are sometimes taken to a quantity that proves fatal.

Cutaneous disorders, and especially the itch, are also very common, and almost as prevalent as in Hindustan. The leprosy, in which the joints drop off, is as common as in Bengal; but in Nepal it cannot be attributed to the lowness of the country, nor to a fish diet, to which the people of Kathmandu have little or no inclination. Some of the persons afflicted with this horrid disorder, I found to be of considerable rank, and quite removed from the want of a nourishing diet. I am almost certain that this disease is not infectious, as I know an instance of a woman, who has lost all her toes and fingers, and who, in that state, has had a child, which she nursed. The child is two years old, and is very healthy. The natives consider the disease as hereditary, and allege that the child will become its victim.

The same kind of swelling in the throat that is common among the inhabitants of the Alps, prevails in Nepal, and, indeed, is frequently seen every where north from Patna. It might at first sight be supposed, that this disease does not derive its origin from the people drinking the water which came from mountains covered with perpetual snow, the cause to which in Europe it has been usually attributed. No water of this kind, however, flows through Nepal; for, although some of the inhabitants of the northern part of Bahar, who live near the Ganduki and Kausiki, drink the water springing from perpetual snow; yet by far the greater part of them drink the water of the various branches of the Vagmati, all of which arise in subalpine regions. It must, however, be observed, that the springs by which these rivers are fed may be supplied by the melted snow, which may sink into the earth of the Himalaya mountains, and not come to light till it reaches the lower hills.

Buchanan, F. H.: *An Account of the Kingdom of Nepal.* Edinburgh, Constable, 1819, pp. 71-73.

DANIEL DRAKE ON GEOGRAPHIC VARIATIONS OF DISEASE

That many physicians overrate the degree of variation from a common standard which the diseases of different countries present, I am quite convinced; but feel equally assured, that if the maladies of each country were studied and described, without a reference to those of any other, it would be found, if the state of medical science were equal to them, that the works thus produced would not be commutable, but that each would be better adapted, as a book of etiology, diagnosis, and practice, to the profession and people among which it was written, than to any other. *How much* better, would depend on the various identities and discrepancies which might exist between the countries thus compared. If their geological, hydrographical, topographical, climatic, social, and physiological conditions were nearly the same, of course their medical histories would be much alike; but if they differed widely in one or several of these conditions, a corresponding diversity would appear in the respective histories of all the diseases which admit of modification from causes referable to those heads.

Daniel Drake: *A Systematic Treatise . . . On the Principal Diseases of the Interior Valley of North America.* Cincinnati, Smith, 1850, page 2.

BULLETIN OF
THE NEW YORK ACADEMY
OF MEDICINE

VOL. 46, NO. 7 JULY 1970

THE PHYSICIAN AND THE COMMUNITY*

LAMAR SOUTTER

Dean
University of Massachusetts Medical School
Worcester, Mass.

IN consideration of the significant achievements of the New York Academy of Medicine in community affairs through its membership in general and particularly through its Committee on Medicine in Society and its Subcommittee on Social Policy for Health Care, it seems presumptuous of an outsider such as myself to discuss this subject. On the other hand medicine, like everything else nowadays, is changing rapidly, and the health needs and demands of society are increasing steadily, so perhaps it is timely to explore some of the new dimensions of the problem of what should be the physician's relations with his community, both as an individual and as a member of an organization.

Basically our present difficulties arise from the fact that the advances of medical science have enabled us to do much more for the sick at the same time that the population has enlarged enormously, particularly the poorer segments of it, with the result that the old system of health care is not geared to provide the many more services needed by more people. Then, too, our philosophy has changed. We are no longer satisfied with a high standard of health care for those with money and a

*Presented at the Stated Meeting of the New York Academy of Medicine, November 12, 1969.

lower one for those without it. The resounding statement of this Academy that "the availability of health services, as a matter of human right, should be based on health need alone, not on a tested ability to pay" is consonant with the thinking of the most advanced medical leaders of today. The report and studies of the staff of the Commission on the Delivery of Personal Health Services entitled *Community Health Services for New York City*, recently published, carries this statement in its opening sentence and quotes it in at least one other place.[1] The Academy expressed its determination as a challenge to all in the health fields, but it also has challenged itself to implement this concept with a new and higher level of community service.

We physicians have varying degrees of a sense of responsibility to society, and we fulfill our obligations variously both as individuals and through our medical organizations. What should we be doing as individuals in the cities where we work, and in our home communities if they are different? The most compelling force for participation in affairs in the community is the desire to serve society through the use of the skills which are particularly ours. This is reinforced by a concern with a growing need for more highly educated and trained people in the health professions. There are other reasons, however, for performing public services. If we go back 30 or 40 years we see the practicing physician performing his duty to the public by voluntary service in an outpatient department or in the charity wards of a hospital. The physician was satisfied, and the public was pleased with his service and held him in considerable esteem. He generally considered himself as separate from the rest of the community and independent of its affairs. We are all aware of the extensive deterioration of the physician's image in the public eye in the past 20 years. Collectively we physicians are regarded as rich, self-interested, and indifferent to public need. Our traditional withdrawal as individuals from community involvement is regarded as a sign of our disinterest in the welfare of society. A symptom of this feeling can be perceived in the selection of people to serve as members of the new health organizations. Whereas at one time a physician would have been sought to lead every such enterprise, nowadays he often is not, and in some instances no physician is asked to serve. The comprehensive health planning organizations in Massachusetts are a cardinal example of this. The guiding committees are almost devoid of physicians. In one large region of the state a group of businessmen banded together and tried to put a social worker in charge of the entire planning enterprise instead of someone in public health or a physician with some skill in this sort of planning. Doctors should be available and sought after for positions of leadership in most health organizations. We need a new image as concerned participators in community affairs and not just as purveyors of expensive services. In the next decade we shall be facing compulsory health insurance covering hospital costs and physicians' services. The form in which the public, through its elected officials, sets up this insurance program and its constraints upon the physician will depend in no small measure not only on how well we have served as doctors but also on how much interest we have shown in society as citizens.

How can and should the individual physician become involved in community affairs? The gamut of possible involvement is indeed very large, from joining health organizations such as the local tuberculosis society or the Visiting Nurse Service to acting as a trustee or advisor, or participating in local civil affairs and politics. There are, however, certain ground rules we need to know before we enter into any such endeavors. The first of these rules is that involvement means participation in the affairs of the organization, not just allowing one's name to appear on a letterhead. Hence we should assume only tasks in which we are thoroughly interested and intend to participate actively, and for which we have the competence to make a definite contribution. We should be sure that we can allot the necessary time to do justice to the job and give money if that is needed. Moreover, we probably should not take on a task which a paid worker can do as well or better. It is difficult to start becoming involved in community affairs but such involvement can be extremely rewarding.

Public spirited activities by organizations of physicians are nearly always in the field of health and, although such activities are undertaken in the interest of society, they seldom come to the notice of the public. I am not talking about hospitals that have a long-estabished relation between doctors and the community, but rather about the professional societies to which we belong. The many hours spent in recent years in the development of the Regional Medical Programs are a good example of this. The great wave of invested effort is hardly more than a ripple by the time it reaches the man in the street. Many of the activities of this Academy in the fields of drugs, automobile accidents, alcoholism, and a host of other problems are typical of public-spirited actions which seldom receive much popular recognition. New programs are now appearing and old ones are being changed in the health fields, which permits a wider scope of activities for our medical societies. Before going into any of these I should like to mention some thoughts on making such participation effective.

Voluntary organizations of physicians generally have stated purposes which govern their activities, but above all else their activities take place in their members' spare time. This means that their participation in community affairs is necessarily limited in scope and that they cannot furnish direct services for any prolonged period. One organization with which I have been associated became extremely concerned with the lack of professional services in a ghetto area and wanted to make an effort to supply some such services. There seems to be little understanding that the amount of such services required is very large and comprehensive. Supplying doctors and supporting staff falls far short of what is needed. The entire spectrum of the health and welfare needs of a ghetto community must be considered. It is not enough to provide good ambulatory care for a patient with a transient illness when the patient's basic problems of poverty, language difficulty, inadequate housing, malnutrition, and unemployment remain unsolved. It makes little sense to spend thousands of dollars arresting a case of tuberculosis and then return the patient to the same social conditions and exposure in which he acquired the disease. Supplying health and welfare care in a ghetto requires the expert services of professionals and participation by the local inhabitants. Such a community is no place for a job partly done. There is, however, a definite role which the interested medical association can play in this regard. The association can arouse public interest in seeing to it that services are provided; it can study what is needed and make recommendations; it can review accomplishments and suggest improvements. In short, if it acts as a consultant and makes its contributions in an advisory capacity, it can supply a needed service which no one else is apt to furnish and which a government agency can never do as well. Such agencies generally lack the skilled personnel which organizations such as medical societies or academies can muster and, further, they usually show little courage in carrying out their programs. Manpower is often a limiting factor in completing projects undertaken by societies despite initial enthusiasm. It is often difficult to find doctors who will work on an enterprise for a prolonged period. This means that it is often wiser to start a project which will run for a definite and limited period of time and then turn it over to someone else or discontinue it. Money, too, should be available, preferably someone else's money, such as that of the government or of a foundation. This renders the undertaking far more acceptable to the membership and sometimes makes the difference between approval and disapproval of a project. Finally, there is not much sense in entering upon a venture which some other organization, private or public, is already conducting, unless it is desirable to do so as an example for a limited period of time because of the failure of the other organization to do a satisfactory job.

Why should an association of physicians become involved in the health affairs of a community? I presented some of the reasons when I discussed the involvement of the individual physician. The need for our services is great and growing greater. Physicians should be the leaders in this field. If they are unwilling to give freely of their services, society will turn to others, and they will occupy an even less enviable position in the eyes of the public. Other nonmedical professional societies, as well as associations of businessmen and service organizations, are becoming more and more involved, and so should we.

Most of us want to do more for society. Often, however, we do not know where there is great need, particularly in the form of new problems demanding our help.

Perhaps the largest need in New York City at present is reorganization of the health services supported by the city. I have already mentioned the recently published report on Community Health Services for New York City.[1] Members of the commission which put it together are prominent laymen. Their chairman was Gerard Piel, publisher of the *Scientific American*, so probably the result of their efforts will be known as the Piel Report. The commission had a medical advisory committee of 14 prominent physicians, many of whom are members of this Academy. I assume that the conclusions and recommendations represent their ideas in a large measure. Probably most of you are more familiar with the recommendations than I am, so I shall mention only two as pertinent. The first is the consolidation of the health facilities and the services of the city that receive public support into a single unit, under which the system for the delivery of care would be divided into five regions, each based on a major teaching hospital or medical school. The next, which has important implications for the medical profession, is the creation of a public nonprofit corporation to take over the facilities and services which the city uses for the provision of care. There are a number of other important matters in this survey, but they are less related to the topic of this paper. The theme of the report, as mentioned before, is based on the Academy's stand that the availability of health services as a matter of right should be based on need alone.

In all of its years of service to the public, I doubt if the Academy has ever had a greater challenge than this report. Can the Academy work collectively and individually with the city now that the report has been approved, and can it help set up a comprehensive health-care system on a regional basis in the five boroughs? Can it be instrumental in guiding the public nonprofit corporation so that it runs the city hospitals and other facilities as they have never been run before to produce but one standard of health care in the city? I do not suppose that the report has provoked any great unanimity of opinion among physicians. I hope, however, that after due deliberation the substance of the recommendations or something close to them will be found to comprise a workable plan which doctors could endorse and sponsor and then, by working with the city and with other citizens, produce a health-care system for the people of New York City of which every citizen would be proud and which other large cities with similar unsolved health problems would hasten to emulate.

It is not possible to cover every health need in this community that a medical association might help to meet. Instead it might be more germane to give an example of a crying need which we as a profession have been prone to neglect. I mean the care of the chronically ill and the aged in nursing homes. These institutions have various names, and there are related institutions such as homes for the aged, convalescent homes, and so forth. Prior to 1930 there were very few nursing homes. When the Social Security Act of 1935 made public assistance funds available to the needy aged, nursing homes became a desirable place to put persons requiring some nursing care who could not, because of physical or mental illness or infirmity, care for themselves at home.

Let us see what has happened. In 1939 there were 1,200 nursing homes in the United States with a bed capacity of 25,000. By 1965 these had increased to 18,950 facilities of all types for care of the infirm or aged with a bed capacity of 760,441. Beds in nursing homes alone numbered 523,900.[2] The numbers are rapidly mounting throughout most of the country. In New York City there are about 9,400 beds in nursing homes and, until recently, despite a greater need, this figure has been fairly static.[3] The probabilities are that the number of beds will increase because of greater demand, more public funds for the aged, and an enlarging older population. In the country at large the average age of a nursing home patient is 80, and 70% of the patients are over 75. In 1950 there were 12 million people over 65. By 1960 there were 16 million, and it is projected that by 1970 this figure will rise to 20 million. In New York City it will reach 1 million this year. At present, 5% of those over 65 require bed space in a nursing home because they need some sort of nursing service. If this percentage is applicable to this city, 50,000 could need nursing-home care or the equivalent in 1970. The percentage of need is much greater for people over 80, of whom there will be 3,700,000 in the nation by 1970. To emphasize the size of the older element of the population it should be pointed out that there are presently 10,000 Americans over the age of 100.[4] The nursing home problem is a great one, not just because of numbers but because, by and large, the care in them is not very good, nor are such essentials as diet satisfactory. Some states such as Connecticut have improved the quality of care. That state conducts careful inspection of nursing homes. It also rates the services provided in them on a merit and demerit basis.[5] In 1963 New York City initiated a good code of regulations for proprietary nursing homes, to be enforced by the Board of Hospitals. How well this is done is hard to say. Most of the literature dealing with the subject presents statistical analyses rather than reports on the quality of care. The fact that New York State is the 31st state in the country in the quality of acceptable beds for patients requiring extended care per 1,000 people over 65 suggests that the quality is not very good, although better than in Massachusetts, which ranks 38th.

The medical profession must always be concerned about medical care, particularly when the care is poor. With the rapidly proliferating nursing homes providing the bulk of care for the chronically ill over 65, what was once a minor problem is now burgeoning into a major one that demands our concern. From the point of view of self-interest it should be pointed out that because of continued inflation, high taxes, and other drains on our resources, and because both New York State and federal statutes free children from the responsibility of supporting their indigent parents, every man and woman in this room who reaches the age of 80 will probably find himself in a nursing home unless he is extremely fortunate. The nursing home is not just for other people. It is also for us.

What is the quality of care in our nursing homes and what is actually needed? In the nation 87% of nursing homes are proprietary, 6% are voluntary, and 3% are publicly owned. In this city 58% are proprietary. As 72% of the patients are indigent, this means that the somewhat limited and static public funds allotted for their care, in addition to meeting this need, must leave a margin of profit for the proprietary home.[6] As a business enterprise the home must regard care of the patient as an item of expense which if extended will interfere with profit. Despite this alarming fact, some of the homes providing first-class care with very complete services are proprietary. Although many patients enter nursing homes because they cannot care for themselves at home, 56% enter after a period of short-term care in a hospital. They require continuing nursing care, medical attention, rehabilitation, mental and spiritual readjustment to new and not often pleasant surroundings, both occupational and recreational therapy, and preventive measures to avoid further disability. Hefferin, in a survey of the literature, described the following medical characteristics of nursing-home patients: 57% of them can be out of bed except for normal rest, about 57% can walk with or without support, 50% are disoriented at times, 20% have serious deficiencies of their hearing or sight, and 25% are incontinent.[7] Physicians' services are required by law to be available and used by proprietary nursing homes in this city. Elsewhere in the country this is usually not the case. Many a doctor, after bringing a patient successfully through an acute illness, regards his duty as discharged when the patient enters a nursing home. The nursing care itself is often quite inadequate. It is difficult, if not impossible, for many homes to meet the requirement of having 24-hour coverage by a skilled nurse and having at least one professional nurse on its staff. In fact, the majority of nursing homes cannot meet this minimal standard. Only a small percent of nursing-home personnel are registered nurses.

Even more difficulty is experienced in providing rehabilitative and therapeutic services. Most homes provide none. Some have them available but make no use of them unless the patient can pay an extra fee. What is the need for these services? In the first place, many of the patients entering nursing homes from hospitals will already have had some rehabilitation and may have had occupational therapy as well. The lack of therapy in the home can lead to a deterioration in the condition of such patients to the point of their becoming bedridden.

There are differences of opinion as to the effectiveness of rehabilitative services in nursing homes. It should be remembered, however, that even seemingly minor improvements are often very rewarding. The patient who can neither turn over nor feed himself becomes a much happier being when he is able to perform both these functions. Hackley has pointed out that in the nursing homes which do provide extensive rehabilitation services, 90% of the patients could be helped by them, 25% could reach the point of being discharged, 60% could be advanced to participation in the normal activities in the home, 5% could undertake some form of vocational training, and that experts in rehabilitation, speech or hearing therapy, vocational and recreational therapy can train nursing-home personnel to become skillful enough to provide these services on a continuing basis.[8] Mental illness and deficiencies are serious problems among the aged, yet only some large homes provide any mental care. The smaller ones will not list a mental defect as a diagnosis in order to avoid having to give therapy. The mental and spiritual adjustment of the patient to the nursing home comes at the time in life when he is least able to adjust to strange and uncomfortable surroundings. Nor is it made better by the fact that most clergymen, like most doctors, do not want to visit their parishioners in such places. To add to the problems, nursing homes head the list of places which are unsafe to live in because of the danger of fire. Every year a number of nursing homes burn down; usually the death of a number of occupants is recorded.[9]

In 1956 the Commission on Chronic Illness stated in regard to the institution for long-term care that "since the people it serves are so much at its mercy, the institution which cares for long-term patients must go to great lengths to serve them according to their needs."[10] As long as proprietary nursing homes are a business first and a facility for the care of patients second, this ideal will not be achieved. Should we be doing something about this situation? Certainly the traditional role of the physician is not just a compassionate concern for suffering. What makes us valuable to society is a willingness to provide active intervention. We could do much by studying the nursing homes in some depth, by making recommendations as to the improvement in the quality and diversity of services, and even providing a continuing inspection service. Or we could set up a model nursing home as an example to be widely publicized, copied, and later taken over by someone else.

Although improvement of the nursing home is one of the most important health problems needing our attention, there are many others in the community with which we could help if we looked for them. In this period of extensive social change the physician has a greater opportunity than ever before to provide valuable services to the public. I am sure that this Academy will in the future, as in the past, be in the forefront of those furnishing such services.

REFERENCES

1. Community Health Services for New York City: *Report and Staff Studies of the Commission on the Delivery of Personal Health Services.* New York, Praeger, 1969.
2. Eagle, E.: Nursing homes and related facilities: A review of the literature. *Public Health Rep. 83*:673-84, 1968.
3. Rogin, M., Goldfarb, A. E. and Turner, H.: Institutional care facilities for older people in New York City. *J. Mount Sinai Hosp. N.Y. 35*:358-70, 1968.
4. Hefferin, E. A.: Rehabilitation in nursing home situations: A survey of the literature. *J. Amer. Geriat. Soc. 16*: 296-313, 1968.
5. Foote, F. M.: Progress in nursing home care. *J.A.M.A. 202*:296-98, 1967.
6. Rogin, op. cit.
7. Hefferin, op. cit.
8. Hackley, J. A.: Instructing nursing home personnel in rehabilitation techniques. *Public Health Rep. 74*:989-94, 1959.
9. Eagle, E., op. cit., p. 681.
10. Commission on Chronic Illness: *Chronic Illness in the United States,* vol. 2: Care of the Long Term Patient. Cambridge, Harvard Univ. Press, 1956.

RESISTANCE TO SALMONELLA INFECTIONS IN INBRED MOUSE STRAINS*

DIETHELM H. BOEHME

Associate Professor of Pathology
Jefferson Medical College
Philadelphia, Pa.

Chief of Laboratory Services
Veterans Administration Hospital
Coatesville, Pa.

THE inbred mouse is usually selected as a model for experimentation in infectious disease under the hypothesis that genetic factors largely determine the equilibrium between invader and host. From the genetic viewpoint two aspects require consideration: first, the genetically controlled variation in pathogenicity of the invading organism and, second, the genetically controlled variation of the resistance of the host. Ideally, a single gene would be found which would determine a single resistance factor as, for instance, ability to phagocytize, production of opsonins, ability to reject or impede an invader by inflammation and formulation of granuloma, or anatomical and chemical organ factors that prevent penetration of an invader as, for instance, in the urinary bladder.

Provided that the invading organism is free of genetic variation, the genetic determinants of the host response can be analyzed, and two possibilities for this exist. When a single genetic factor determines resistance the susceptibility curve should show a bimodal or trimodal distribution, and the factor resistance should segregate among the offspring of resistant and susceptible hosts. By contrast, when several genes determine the outcome of an infection, the susceptibility curve would be expected to show a continuous distribution, and a clear segregation among the offspring will not be found.[1]

Only limited experimental evidence has been accumulated with inbred animal strains; instances in which resistance can be ascribed to a

*Presented at a combined meeting of the Section on Basic Medical Sciences and the New York City branch of the American Society for Microbiology, held at the Academy February 12, 1970.
This study was supported by the Veterans Administration, Washington, D. C.

single gene are rarer still. Although we must assume that the extensively investigated species differences in susceptibility to a wide host of infections are also genetic in origin, they have hardly been analyzed from this vantage point; this report, therefore, will deal with well-investigated examples of intraspecies differences.

Substantial work has been done concerning the susceptibility of mice to virus infections.[2, 3] Here, emphasis will be given to investigations carried out with the two mouse strains BSVS and BRVR, since they were also used in our investigations of *Salmonella typhimurium.* Originally, the mouse strain BSVS (bacteria susceptible, virus susceptible) and BRVR (bacteria resistant, virus resistant) was bred because of its resistance and susceptibility to the virus of St. Louis encephalitis and to *S. typhimurium.*[4] It was found later that the BSVS mouse was also susceptible to yellow fever virus, in contrast to the resistant PRI (Princeton) mouse. This difference was ascribed to a single pair of genes. The latter mouse, in addition, proved also resistant to other arboviruses of the "B" group.[5]

A similar result was obtained with West Nile virus; cultured splenic macrophages from strain BSVS contained significantly more viral organisms than cultures from macrophages taken from the resistant strain BRVR. An identical relation was observed when the susceptible mouse strain C3H was compared with the resistant strain PRI.[6, 7] This finding pertained not only to macrophages but also to kidney, brain, and lung cells. Its genetic nature could be ascertained by the back-crossing of C3H × PRI hybrids to C3H. The production of interferon was immaterial, since the susceptible BSVS mouse carried greater amounts of it in the brain than the resistant BRVR mouse. Injection of bone marrow or spleen cells from C3H mice into resistant PRI mice shortly after birth resulted in significantly elevated susceptibility to the West Nile virus.[8] Another mouse strain resistant to arbovirus "B" was developed through back-crossing and brother-sister mating, which resulted in the resistant C3HRV strain homozygous for the gene of resistance,[9] while at the same time it was congenic with the virus-susceptible parent strain.

Only recently, in VM mice, a gene was described which controls the incubation period with Scrapie agent ME-7.[10]

Cross-breeding of the progeny of Webster-Swiss × C57-BL6 F^1 hybrid mice resulted in a rabies-refractory strain. The refractory mice showed a significantly higher cellular level of ribonuclease when compared with the susceptible Webster-Swiss.[11] Also presumably genetically determined is the increased susceptibility of SWR-J and Webster-Swiss mice to the virus of lymphocytic choriomeningitis, a model in which C3H mice proved relatively resistant.[12]

Mice have also been employed in investigations of genetically determined resistance against parasites as, for instance, in the strain NMRI, which is endowed with resistance against *Plasmodium berghei*.[13, 14]

With respect to bacteria the two organisms most widely studied in genetic experiments have been *Mycobacterium tuberculosis* and *S. typhimurium*. The infection with tuberculosis was investigated thoroughly in the inbred rabbit strains C, FC, A, AD, and III, listed in increasing order of resistance. An important result of these studies was recognition of the fact that the infectious organism undergoes the same population changes in tissues as it would in the test tube: namely, a latent phase, a lag phase, a phase of logarithmic growth, a negative acceleration phase, a stationary phase and, finally, a phase of decline.

The main difference between the resistant and susceptible rabbit host consisted in the ability of the former to destroy more than one half of the inoculum in the lung during the latent phase whether it consisted of human or bovine tubercle bacilli. In contrast, the susceptible animal was entirely unable to reduce the number of infectious organisms during this phase. Further, the resistant animal was capable of accelerated drainage of the infectious organisms from the lung into the respective lymph nodes.[15] When the peritoneal macrophages of the resistant strain III were compared with those of strain TTC of lesser resistance and with those of the highly susceptible strain CaC, it was found that the resistant animals displayed higher metabolic activity toward certain substrates than the susceptible ones as, for instance, toward lactate, glucose-6-phosphate, glycerophosphate, glyceraldehyde-3-phospate, and acid phosphatase.[16, 17] In this connection it was also demonstrated that administration of L-triodothyronine or L-thyroxine could raise the level of native resistance to tuberculosis in a rabbit strain of intermediate resistance, i.e., TTC.[18]

Studies with *M. tuberculosis* have also been undertaken in mice. Inoculation of strain C57Bl-6 and Swiss with mammalian tubercle bacilli showed significantly longer survival of the Swiss strain. This difference also depended upon the age of the host at the time of injection. When the two strains were crossed, mice of the F^1 generation proved more resistant than either parent. This difference disappeared after repeated back-crosses in the fourth back-cross generation, in which the survival time was identical with that of the original parental strain.[19] The decisive importance of the genetic composition of the invading organism is well exemplified by the fact that the high virulence of the Vallée strain may wipe out all genetic differences in resistance observed with less virulent strains.[20]

Investigation into the susceptibility to Salmonella strains has been largely limited to *S. typhimurium*, mainly because of the substantial differences in susceptibility noted among various mouse strains when infected with *S. typhi* by various routes.[21]

The investigations employing the inbred mouse strains BSVS and BRVR were based on the observation that, apart from their susceptibility to and their resistance against the virus of St. Louis encephalitis, they behaved identically toward infection with *S. typhimurium*. During studies of the role of nutritional factors in this infection it was found that the infecting strain of *S. typhimurium* was not homogeneous but consisted of two distinct strains, one of which (RIA) was found to be avirulent both for the susceptible BSVS as well as for the resistant BRVR mice, while the second (SR-11) proved to be invariably lethal for the susceptible mice and, to a large extent, also for the resistant strain BRVR.[22, 23] In order to bring out fully the difference in susceptibility between BSVS and BRVR mice, a double-strain inoculation procedure was advised. This consisted of an intraperitoneal injection of 1,000 organisms of strain RIA, followed two days later by 100,000 cells of the virulent strain SR-11. When this experimental plan was strictly adhered to, all susceptible BSVS mice succumbed within three weeks, whereas more than one half of the resistant mice survived indefinitely.

The first experimental approach attempted to determine whether this difference in survival depended upon a difference of activity of the reticuloendothelial system.[24] While approximately the same magnitude of response was found in both mouse strains, the resistant mouse reacted with a somewhat delayed but protracted elevation of RES activity when measured with the carbon-clearance test.[25] By contrast, clearance activity in the susceptible BSVS mouse attained a peak almost immediately, only to drop off again with equal rapidity.[24] Carbon clearance may be considered an indirect gauge of RES activity since it determines the clearance of a standard dose of specially prepared India ink from the circulation of an infected animal.[26]

Further evidence of more potent RES activity in resistant BRVR mice consisted in their significantly greater increase in splenic weight under the influence of infection or of a variety of other antigens.

When RES activity was assessed as antibody production, titers of agglutinating antibody to RS-11 were found to be equal in the lymph nodes of both susceptible and resistant mice.[27] Also the formation of precipitating antibody against bovine serum albumin was equal in both strains.[28] When challenged with one or two intraperitoneal injections of pertussis vaccine, IgG production as determined by serum electrophoresis [29] and the time sequence of appearance of 19S or 7S antibodies was found equal. Ultracentrifugal analysis indicated, however, a quantitatively larger production of 7S antibody in resistant BRVR mice.

The virtual equality in antibody formation and the demonstrated differences in RES activity between the two mouse strains pointed to phagocytosis as the major factor determining their different response.

This is in keeping with the hypothesis advanced by others that opsonization is the prerequisite for effective phagocytosis of *S. typhimurium*. Inadequate opsonization would thus deprive the susceptible host of his most important means of resistance. Absence or inadequate formation of opsonins could be explained by the sharing of one or several antigens between host tissues and *S. typhimurium*,[30-33] a phenomenon subsequently designated as biological mimicry.[34]

We proposed that double-strain inoculation was well suited to test this hypothesis since it was found that the antigenic formulas of the two *S. typhimurium* strains RIA (avirulent) and SR-11 (virulent) were identical, i.e., 4, 12:i: 1.2 and, thus, conformed to the var. Copenhagen. The factors o1 and o5 were consistently absent in both strains; the only recognizable metabolic difference was that SR-11 fermented xylose while the avirulent strain RIA did not.[23] The respective endotoxins were extracted from both bacterial strains and by the cold phenol method.[33-37] At the outset it was reconfirmed that strain BSVS was susceptible and strain BRVR resistant when exposed to double-strain inoculation, as postulated. Infection with virulent *S. typhimurium* SR-11 alone resulted in the death of both resistant and susceptible mice. Both endotoxins, when given in high doses of 150 μg., reduced the survival rate in BRVR mice but failed to influence it in smaller doses. Further, pre-

TABLE I. BEHAVIOR OF INBRED MOUSE STRAINS BSVS AND BRVR TO VARIOUS ANTIGENS

Antigen	*BSVS*	*BRVR*
St. Louis encephalitis[4]	Susc.	Res.
Yellow fever[5]	Susc.	
West Nile[6]	Susc.	Res.
S. Typhimurium RIA/SR11 (double-strain inoculation)[22]	Susc.	Res.
Mouse brain[38]	Susc. (allergic encephalomyelitis)	Res.
Mouse testis[38]	Susc. (allergic orchitis)	Res.
Mouse muscle[38]	Susc. (allergic myositis)	Res.

treatment with the endotoxins, with pertussis vaccine, or with the endotoxin of *Salmonella abortus equi* failed to protect the susceptible BSVS mice. In the susceptible BSVS mice a nonlethal infection with avirulent *S. typhimurium* RIA could be converted into a lethal one through aftertreatment with the endotoxin of SR-11 but this did not happen in the resistant BRVR mice. Especially from this last experiment it was concluded that sharing of antigen could not explain the difference in susceptibility between the BSVS and BRVR mice[38] and was, in fact, contrary to the experience of others gained with a somewhat different model.[30]

The problem was further complicated by the observation that resistance and susceptibility applied not only to the infection with *S. typhimurium* but also to the administration with lyophilized mouse brain, testis, and muscle.[39] Assuming the existence of shared antigens, the finding of common antigenic components between these and other mouse tissues and *S. typhimurium* would have to be expected (Table I).

In a representative experiment, BSVS and BRVR mice were immunized against their own and the other strain's erythrocytes administered in Freund's adjuvant. Through examination by the double-diffusion technique it was observed that immune sera from BSVS mice against BSVS and BRVR erythrocytes showed one or two precipitation lines against lyophilized SR-11 or RIA bacteria. Precipitation lines were

TABLE II. SUMMARY OF RESPONSE DIFFERENCES BETWEEN BSVS AND BRVR MICE

	BSVS	*BRVR*
RES activity (carbon clearance)	Very rapid, limited	Slow, protracted
Antibody production against SR11, pertussis vaccine	equal	equal
Thymus weight	< 50 mg., unaffected by antigenic stimulus	90-120 mg., increases during antigenic challenge
Spleen weight	Rapidly increasing, max. 200 mg.	Slowly increasing, max. 450 mg.
Cross reacting RBC antigens RIA/SR11/	Present	Present

also observed with BRVR antisera directed against BSVS and BRVR erythryocytes; however, to a lesser degree.

In a second experiment antisera were produced in the rabbit against lyophilized mouse brain from BSVS and BRVR, and against BSVS and BRVR erythrocytes. These antierythrocytic sera were seen to react against saline-extracted mouse brain. Thus it appears that overlapping antigens might exist. Because of their presence in both resistant and susceptible mice, their actual significance remains a matter of conjecture.

When RES activity was tested with the carbon-clearance test after administration of brain, testis, or muscle[26] it corresponded to the activity observed following injection with *S. typhimurium.* Again, the resistant BRVR mice exhibited a slower, protected increase in RES activity, while BSVS mice showed a quick and limited rise in clearance.[39]

Investigation of the response to these tissue antigens confirmed further the quantitatively greater splenic weight gain in the resistant BRVR mice when compared with the susceptible BSVS mice. In addition, these studies revealed that the resistant mouse-strain BRVR had exhibited a slower protracted increase in RES activity, a significantly higher thymic weight, even in the untreated animal when compared with the susceptible strain BSVS. Stimulation with an antigen such as pertussis vaccine or brain resulted in an increase in thymic weight, but only in strain BRVR.

Histologically, the resistant mouse strain showed during the first half of the experiment a broad, subcapsular zone composed of large thymoblasts; this was absent in the susceptible strain BSVS. Increased thymoblastic activity could be confirmed in strain BRVR when dividing cells were labeled with tritiated thymidine.

In the spleen, proliferation of the follicles differed only quantitatively in the two mouse strains.

Summarizing our observations of the inbred mouse strains BSVS and BRVR (Table II), it might be stated that their susceptibility or resistance to *S. typhimurium* cannot be explained by one single factor which could be ascribed to a single gene. Of great importance was the phagocytic activity of the reticuloendothelial system, in particular of thymus and spleen. Tentative evidence for the existence of overlapping antigens between mouse erythrocytes, brain, and *S. typhimurium* were found, but this was insufficient to explain the different behavior of the two mouse strains.

REFERENCES

1. Allison, A. C.: Genetic factors in resistance against virus infections. *Arch. Ges. Virusforsch. 17*:280-94, 1965.
2. Lynch, C. J. and Hughes, T. P.: Inheritance to susceptibility to yellow fever encephalitis in mice. *Genetics 21*:104-12, 1936.
3. Webster, L. T. and Clow, A. D.: Experimental encephalitis (St. Louis type) in mice with high inborn resistance; A chronic subclinical infection. *J. Exp. Med. 63*:827-45, 1936.
4. Webster, L. T.: Inheritance of resistance of mice to enteric, bacterial and neurotropic virus infection. *J. Exp. Med. 65*: 261-86, 1937.
5. Sabin, A. B.: Genetic factors affecting susceptibility and resistance to virus diseases of the nervous system. *Proc. Assn. Res. Nerv. Dis. 33*:57-66, 1954.
6. Vainio, T.: Virus and hereditary resistance in vitro. I. Behavior of West Nile (E-101) virus in the cultures prepared from a genetically resistant and susceptible strain of mice. *Ann. Med. Exp. Fenn. 41*:1-24, 1963.
7. Vainio, T.: Virus and hereditary resistance in vitro. II. Behavior of West Nile (E-101) virus in cultures prepared from challenged back-cross and nonchallenged susceptible mice. *Ann. Med. Exp. Fenn. 41*:25, 1963.
8. Theis, G. A., Billingham, R. E. and Silvers, W. K.: Mechanism of natural resistance of mice to virus infection. *Virology 8*:264, 1959.
9. Gröschel, D. and Koprowski, H.: Development of a virus resistant inbred mouse strain for the study of innate resistance to arbo-V virus. *Arch. Ges. Virusforsch. 17*:379-91, 1965.
10. Dickinson, A. G., Meikle, V. M. H. and Fraser, H.: Identification of a gene which controls the incubation period of some strains of Scrapie agent in mice. *J. Comp. Path. 78*:293-99, 1968.
11. Enright, J. B., Frye, F. L. and Atwall, O. S.: Ribonuclease activity of peripheral leukocytes and serum in rabies-susceptible and rabies-refractory mice. *J. Histochem. Cytochem. 13*:515-17, 1965.
12. Oldstone, M. B. A. and Dickson, F. J.: Suspectibility of different mouse strains to lymphocytic choriomeningitis. *J. Immun. 100*:355-57, 1968.
13. Kretschmar, W.: Infektionsverlauf und Krankheitsbild bei mit Plasmodium berghei infizierten Mäusen des Stammes

NMRI. *Z. Tropenmed. Parasit. 12*:346-68, 1961.
14. Bafort, J. and Timperman, E.: Etude comparative d'une lignee de souris resistantes au *Plasmodium berghei. Tropen Medizin Parasit. 20*:74-80, 1969.
15. Allison, M. J., Zappasodi, P. and Lurie, M. B.: Host-parasite relationships in natively resistant and susceptible rabbits on quantitative inhalation of tubercle bacilli. *Amer. Rev. Resp. Dis. 85*:553-69, 1962.
16. Allison, M. J., Zappasodi, P. and Lurie, M. B.: Metabolic studies on mononuclear cells from rabbits of varying genetic resistance to tuberculosis. I. Studies on cells of normal noninfected animals. *Amer. Rev. Resp. Dis. 84*:364-70, 1961.
17. Lurie, M. B. and Dannenberg, A. M., Jr.: Macrophage function in infectious disease with inbred rabbits. *Bact. Rev. 29*:466-76, 1965.
18. Allison, M. J. and Gerszten, E.: Metabolic studies on mononuclear cells from rabbits of varying genetic resistance to tuberculosis. III. Studies on variation of thyroid function. *Amer. Rev. Resp. Dis. 86*:513-17, 1962.
19. Lynch, C. J., Pierce-Chase, C. H. and Dubos, R.: A genetic study of susceptibility to experimental tuberculosis in mice infected with mammalian tubercle bacilli. *J. Exp. Med. 121*:1051-70, 1965.
20. Grumbach, A. and Beer, H.: Tuberkuloseversuche an genetisch bekanntem Mäusematerial: Überlebensdauer von zwei homozygoten Mäusestämmen und der F-1-Generation ihrer Hybriden. 4. Mitteilung. *Acta Genet* (Basel) *12*:103-16, 1962.
21. Sacquet, E.: Contribution a l'étude de la sensibilité de diverses lignees de souris a l'inoculation de *Salmonella typhi. Ann. Inst. Past.* (Paris) *98*:880-86, 1960.
22. Schneider, H. A. and Webster, L. T.: Nutrition of the host and natural resistance to infection. I. The effect of diet on the response of several genotypes of musculus to *Salmonella enteridis* infection. *J. Exp. Med. 81*:359-84, 1945.
23. Schneider, H. A. and Zinder, N. D.: Nutrition of the host and natural resistance to infection. V. An improved assay employing genetic markers in double strain inoculation test. *J. Exp. Med. 103*:207-23, 1956.
24. Boehme, D. H., Schneider, H. A. and Lee, J. M.: Some physiopathological parameters of natural resistance to infection in murine salmonellosis. *J. Exp. Med. 110*:9-26, 1959.
25. Boehme, D. H.: The reticuloendothelial system and nonspecific resistance. *Ann. N.Y. Acad. Sci. 88*:172-83, 1960.
26. Halpern, B. N., Biozzi, G., Mène, G. and Benacerraf, B.: Étude quantitative de l'activité granulopexique du système SRE par l'injection intraveineuse d'enrc de Chine de particules de carbone de dimensions connues. *Ann. Inst. Pasteur 80*:582-604, 1951.
27. Hudack, S. S. and McMaster, P. D.: Agglutinin formation within the lymph nodes of resistant and susceptible mice. *Proc. Soc. Exp. Biol. Med. 31*:753-55, 1934.
28. Olitsky, P. K. and Lee, J. M.: The immunologic response of mice from stocks resistant and susceptible to acute disseminated encephalomyelitis. *J. Lab. Clin. Med. 45*:81, 1955.
29. Boehme, D. H. and Werdelin, O.: Response of the reticuloendothelial system to single and double IP injection of pertussis vaccine in inbred mouse strains. Reprinted from *Fed. Proc. 27*:1834, 1968.
30. Jenkin, C. R.: Heterophile antigens and their significance in the host-parasite relationship. *Advances Immun. 3*:351-76, 1963.
31. Jenkin, C. R. and Benacerraf, B.: In vitro studies of the interaction between mouse peritoneal macrophages and strains of Salmonellae and *Escherichia coli. J. Exp. Med. 112*:403-12, 1960
32. Jenkin, C. R.: An antigenic basis for virulence in strains of *Salmonella typhimurium. J. Exp. Med. 115*:731-43, 1962.
33. Jenkin, C. R. and Rowley, D.: The role of opsonins in the clearance of living and inert particles by cells of the reticuloendothelial system. *J. Exp. Med. 114*:63-373, 1961.
34. Zabriskie, J. B.: Mimetic relationships

between Group A streptococci and mammalian tissues. *Advances Immun.* *7*:147-88, 1967.

35. Westphal, O. and Lüderitz, O.: Chemische Erforschung von Lipopolysacchariden gramnegativer Bakterien. *Angew. Chem.* *66*:407-17, 1954.
36. Westphal, O., Lüderitz, O. and Bister, F.: Uber die Extraktion von Bakterien mit Phenol-Wasser. *Z. Naturforsch.* *7B*:148-56, 1952.
37. Fromme, I., Lüderitz, O., Nowotny, A. and Westphal, O.: Chemische Analyse von Lipopolysacchariden avs *Salmonella abortus equis*. *Pharm. Acta Helv.* *38*:391-400, 1958.
38. Boehme, D. H.: Response of inbred mice to virulent and avirulent *Salmonella typhimurium* and their endotoxins. *J. Reticuloendothel. Soc.* *3*:18-28, 1966.
39. Boehme, D. H.: Possibilities and limitations of production of autoimmune diseases in inbred mouse strains. *Path. Europ.* *2*:119-34, 1966 (contains comprehensive references).

STATEMENT*

ON

The Controlled Dangerous Substances Act of 1969 (S. 3246)

BY

THE NEW YORK ACADEMY OF MEDICINE

THE New York Academy of Medicine is an independent fellowship of physicians and scientists which for some time through its Committee on Public Health and other mechanisms has examined various aspects of the problem of drug use and abuse in our society.

On February 18, 1970, the Council of the Academy approved a statement on *Methadone Management of Heroin Addiction* prepared by the Committee on Public Health. In that statement the Academy called for enlightened legislation dealing with the treatment of the addicted and urged that a clear distinction be made between the medical and criminal aspects of drug use and abuse. In keeping with this approach, the New York Academy of Medicine wishes to record opposition to the general strategy adopted by the Controlled Dangerous Substances Act of 1969 (S. 3246). We consider this legislation to be a backward step.

Our general objection to the bill relates to its undue interference by the Department of Justice in the treatment of the sick and in medical research and education. The bill fails to distinguish between criminal and medical aspects of the drug problem. In the regulation of medical care and research too much power is given to the Department of Justice. Some of our specific objections are as follows:

1) In Title II of the bill the definition of "controlled dangerous substances" is scientifically unrealistic and administratively unwieldy.

2) The Department of Health, Education, and Welfare rather than the Department of Justice should be given the power to determine which pharmacological agents should be subject to legal regulation.

3) The Department of Health, Education, and Welfare rather

*Approved by the Committee on Public Health, March 2, 1970.
Approved by the Committee on Medicine in Society, March 2, 1970.
Approved by the Committee on Medical Education, March 12, 1970.

than the Department of Justice should be given the responsibility for sponsoring, approving, and conducting programs of research in drug use, an area in which the Department of Justice lacks competence.

4) The record-keeping and inspection requirements are unduly onerous and arbitrary. They threaten interference with responsible programs of research in drug use and abuse as well as in the care of patients.

The role of the Department of Health, Education, and Welfare in definition and treatment of, and in research into, problems of drug abuse should be strengthened. We strongly recommend appropriate legislation to assure this. However, for the above reasons we believe that the present thrust of S. 3246 is medically and scientifically unrealistic and that passage of this bill would represent an unwarrranted intrusion by the Department of Justice into the field of medical care and research, in which the department has no scientific expertise.

John L. Pool
President

March 13, 1970.

TREATMENT OF MALIGNANT TUMORS OF THE SALIVARY GLANDS*

JOHN CONLEY

Department of Otolaryngology
Columbia-Presbyterian Medical Center

Head and Neck Service
St. Vincent's Hospital

New York, N. Y.

SALIVARY-GLAND tumors have been of particular interest to clinicians and pathologists for the past 30 years, and significant advances have taken place in both their classification and their management. This is particularly true of parotid tumors, for which certain standardizations have been accomplished. Submandibular and minor salivary-gland tumors are much less frequent and have received less attention. There remain many aspects of the diagnosis and treatment of malignant tumors of all the salivary glands that require additional analysis and study.

Parotid Gland

The principal deterrents to the proper management of malignant tumors of the parotid gland are a lack of coordination of the microscopic classification to the operative technique and a genuine fear of advertent or inadvertent injury to the facial nerve. A grouping of these tumors according to their biological aggressiveness and according to the special surgical anatomy of the gland assists in clarifying this problem. Preoperative formal incisional biopsy for tumors of the parotid gland is unrealistic in general, and aspiration biopsy has proved inaccurate at times. A few shreds of tissue acquired by aspiration may not provide a completely accurate diagnosis in tumors which may have a pleomorphic pattern; a mutilating strategy based on such information could prove catastrophic.

The old-fashioned method of history-taking and physical examination will help to separate some of the malignant from the benign tumors. Indicative of malignancy are rapid growth, fixation, pain, ulceration, and facial-nerve paresis. Most of these indicate advanced disease

*Presented at a meeting of the Section on Otolaryngology, December 17, 1969.

or an undifferentiated neoplasm or both and must be considered as grossly unfavorable to the patient. It is obvious that a larger group of malignant neoplasms do not reveal their biological nature in their early stages and may present with all the clinical evidences of a benign tumor. The majority of these neoplasms are biologically low-grade and their true diagnosis is accomplished by surgical intervention. The basic type of surgical intervention is lateral lobectomy. This technique should resolve or assist in resolving the problem in the 75% of these neoplasms which prove to be benign. It will contribute to the resolution of the problem in another 5% and will point the way to an augmented ablative procedure in the remaining 20%. This may be accomplished at the time of the primary operation by frozen-section technique if the pathologist who will confirm this diagnosis is aware of the gravity of the problem and endorses a radical operation. If there is any doubt whatever in the mind of the pathologist or of the surgeon about proceeding under these circumstances, it is absolutely necessary to wait until the situation is clarified. It is unfortunate that not all neoplastic problems can be solved by either preoperative formal biopsy or frozen-section technique; it is precisely under these adverse circumstances that the surgeon must exert extreme caution.

Surgical Anatomy

The surgical anatomy of tumors of the parotid gland is a dominant feature in management. Although it is common to speak of the lateral lobe and the deep lobe of the parotid gland, there is no such clear-cut anatomical division. These areas simply represent various regions of the gland in respect to its general configuration and its relation to the facial nerve. All the glandular tissue lateral to the facial nerve is considered lateral lobe; the glandular tissue deep to the facial nerve is the deep lobe. The nerve trunks themselves form a sort of cleft in this portion of the gland. The gross bulk of the gland and the majority of tumors are located in the lateral lobe. This portion of the gland is surrounded by soft tissues and lends itself to block dissection. The deep portion of the gland is surrounded by bony structures and does not permit block resection.

The parotid gland has a rich network of intraglandular lymph vessels and lymph nodes which are determinant features in the spread of the malignant process inside the gland. Surgical compliance with this

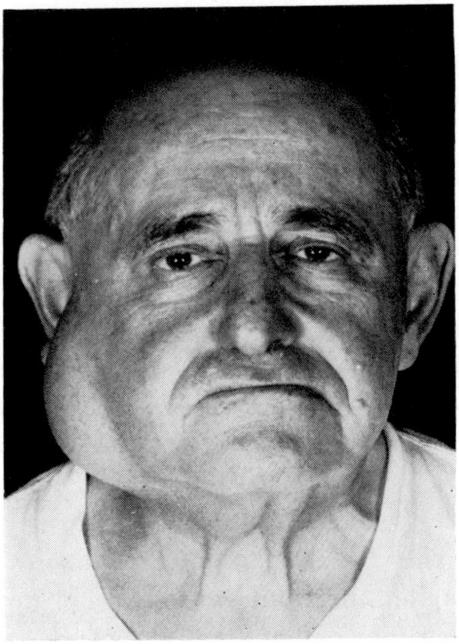

Fig. 1. Undifferentiated mucoepidermoid carcinoma of right parotid with early facial paralysis.

anatomical fact would favor a total parotidectomy. There is also a paraglandular collection of lymph vessels and nodes that connect with the drainage of the scalp, orbit, ear, and cheek. This paraglandular network connects with the intraglandular system and with the lymphatics of the neck. The latter anatomical features are important in planning the composite resection for undifferentiated malignant tumors of the parotid gland.

Classification

Primary malignant tumors of the parotid gland are divided into two groups for the purposes of management and prognosis. The clinical practicality of this classification identifies the neoplasms which have either a good or a poor prognosis. The group with a very favorable prognosis comprises the low-grade mucoepidermoid and certain varieties of acinous-cell type of adenocarcinoma. The group with the poor prognosis consists of squamous-cell cancer, all undifferentiated adeno- and mucoepidermoid cancers and, to a lesser degree, malignant mixed tumors (Figure 1). Adenoid cystic carcinoma belongs in the group with poor prognosis if surveillance is extended over a 10-year period; despite an initial favorable outlook it eventually overwhelms the patient by its pernicious effects.

It is realistic to state that the best chance for cure lies with the less aggressive tumors, but this should not become a license for inadequate surgery. It is also realistic to propose that all the malignant tumors with a poor prognosis should be treated initially by radical composite resection. A recognized exception to this may be debated in the elderly patient with an adenoid cystic carcinoma who could not accept the stress of a radical composite resection and in whom the life expectancy would be less than a strategic retreat with this persistent but often protracted neoplasm.

Secondary or recurrent malignant tumors of the parotid gland comprise a special group in which the prognosis routinely is reduced severely by seeding, implantation, disruption of normal anatomy, and the additional waiting period that permits the tumor to spread locally and to metastasize. Radical composite resection offers the best chance for control under these adverse circumstances.

Treatment

The surgical treatment of malignant tumors of the parotid gland comprises three basic techniques: total parotidectomy with preservation of the facial nerve, total regional resection (big-little operation), and radical composite resection (big-big operation).

There are variations on total parotidectomy with preservation of all or part of the facial nerve. These technical procedures are limited primarily to small low-grade mucoepidermoid and certain acinous-cell carcinomas in the lateral lobe or in the inferior portion of the lateral lobe. Under these circumstances, one may be justified in preserving the main trunk and the upper division of the facial nerve while carrying out a total parotidectomy. The deficiency in facial-nerve function is only 10% or 15% when the main upper segment is preserved. There is no need for nerve grafting under these circumstances. It is understandable that this technique is limited in its clinical application by an increased size in the tumor, by the position of the tumor that compromises the facial nerve, and by the aggressive biological nature of the tumor.

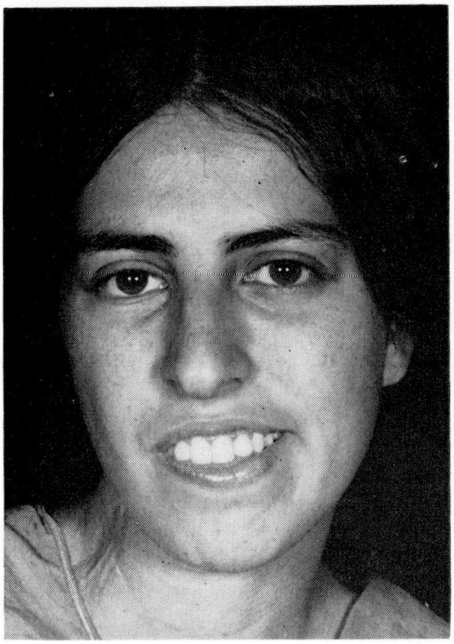

Fig. 2. Postoperative mucoepidermoid carcinoma of right parotid with facial nerve graft.

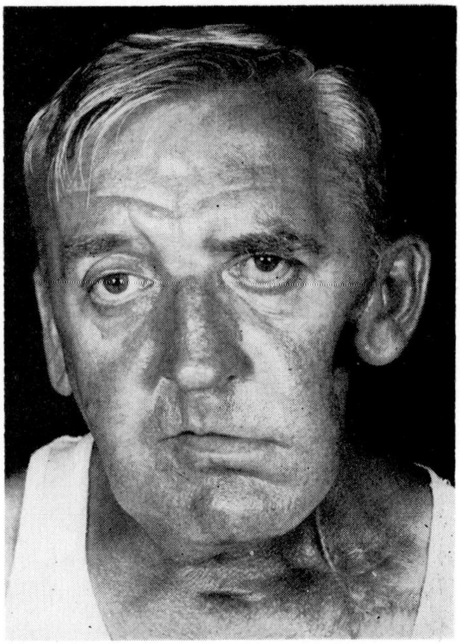

Fig. 3. Postoperative squamous-cell carcinoma; of radical resection of left parotid and lateral neck.

The regional radical parotidectomy is applied in the majority of medium-sized, primary, low-grade tumors consisting of low-grade mucoepidermoid and certain acinous-cell carcinomas. It may also be applied to small-to-medium malignant mixed tumors of the lateral lobe and to the special group of small adenoid cystic carcinomas in older patients. This operation, identified as the "big-little operation," consists in removing the total parotid gland with a cuff of normal tissue about it and also the immediate regional lymph-node systems. The cuff of normal tissue includes the platysma muscle laterally, a portion of the masseter muscle anteriorly, the posterior belly of the diagastric and stylohyoid muscles medially, a cuff of sternocleidomastoid muscle posteriorly with or without the tip of the mastoid, and the lymph nodes in the superior deep jugular and superior spinal-accessory regions. The facial nerve is included in the specimen but the hypoglossal and spinal-accessory nerves remain intact. The facial-nerve system is immediately rehabilitated with an autogenous nerve taken from the cervical plexus. There is approximately an 80% chance of some return of movement to the paralyzed face after an interval of approximately six months. Facial-nerve grafting should be considered an integral part of this operative technique (Figure 2).

The radical composite resection is generally applied to all high-grade malignant tumors, all tumors complicated by facial-nerve paresis, all large low-grade tumors, the majority of adenoid cystic carcinomas, and all recurrent malignant tumors. This operation, the "big-big operation," consists essentially of the classical radical neck dissection, but includes removal of the entire parotid gland, platysma muscle, masseter muscle, and posterior belly of the digastric and stylohyoid. It may also be extended to include the mastoid bone, ascending ramus of the mandible, and internal and external pterygoid muscle (Figure 3). In more extensive cases the ear, the skin of this region, and the infratemporal space may be added to the ablative technique .This great wound may have to be treated with regional chest flaps or free-skin grafts. Rhytidectomy and tarsorrhaphy are routine. Immediate autogenous-nerve grafting is not possible in many of these extensive procedures because of the magnitude of the wound. Nerves as long as 10 and 12 cm. have been anastomosed, however, with some return of facial movement.

Even though the operations reported in this review represent what might appear to be aggressive attacks on these neoplasms, local recurrence is not uncommon in the undifferentiated tumors and in the adenoid cystic carcinomas. It is therefore proposed that all tumors of the deep lobe and all undifferentiated tumors be given a full course of postoperative irradiation.

The cure rates under these circumstances would approximate 80 to 90% for the well-differentiated tumors, 30% for the undifferentiated tumors, 50% for the malignant mixed tumors, and 20% for the adenoid cystic carcinomas.

Malignant Tumors of the Submandibular Gland

The submandibular gland is a major salivary gland with a higher immunity against the development of neoplasia than the parotid gland, but paradoxically it has a higher relative incidence of malignancy over benignity. The most common afflictions of the submandibular gland are inflammatory disease and calculus.

In a review of 115 patients with tumors of the submandibular gland, 53% proved to be benign mixed tumors, and 47% proved to be malignant tumors. Seventy-four per cent of the benign tumors appeared in females, and 57% of the malignant tumors appeared in males. No tumors were present before the age of 10 and only 2% before the age of 20. The highest incidence of malignant tumors was in the fourth decade.

The predominant histologic types of malignant tumors were: adenocystic carcinoma (31%), mucoepidermoid carcinoma (31%), and adenocarcinoma (16%). Malignant mixed tumors and squamous-cell carcinomas were less common.

The presence of the mass in the submandibular area was the prominent sign in the malignant tumors. A small percentage of these patients manifested pain, ulceration, and dissemination of the cancer.

Surgical Anatomy

The regional surgical anatomy associated with the submandibular gland relates to the floor of the mouth, lingual nerve, the adjacent horizontal ramus of the mandible, the tongue, the myohyoid muscle, and the boundaries of the submandibular space. This anatomy, combined with the histologic nature of the tumor, determines the perimeters of resection.

The intraglandular lymph system is scanty compared with the parotid gland. The lymph vessels are small and there are no intraglandular lymph nodes.

Treatment

Management of malignant tumors of the submandibular gland contains a built-in deception, in that the predominant pathology in this region is inflammatory and the surgeon is frequently unprepared for the gravity of a malignant tumor. Seventy-five per cent of the 54 patients with malignant tumors had either a preoperative biopsy or an excision of the gland, and then were subjected to reoperation. Frequently the gland had been removed without frozen-section examination, and this frequently caused embarrassment and delay in the proper management of these tumors. Many surgeons preferred to hope that they had removed all of the malignant tumor, and elected to wait for further developments. If a tumor proved to be an infiltrative adenocarcinoma, an epidermoid carcinoma, or undifferentiated mucoepidermoid carcinoma there was usually local recurrence with fungation of the tumor and the development of noncontrolled growth (Figure 4).

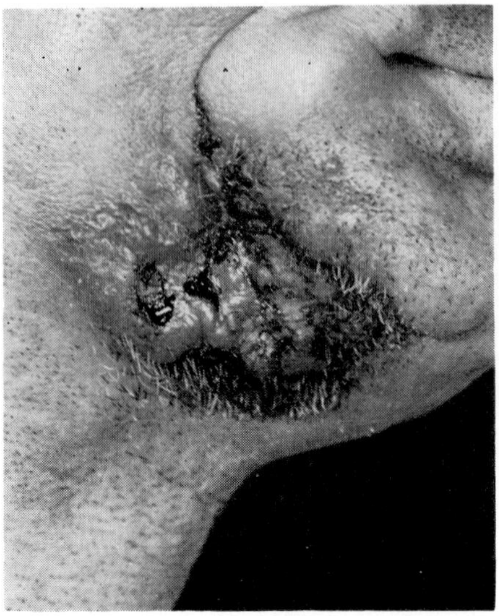

Fig. 4. Recurrent adenocarcinoma in right submandibular region.

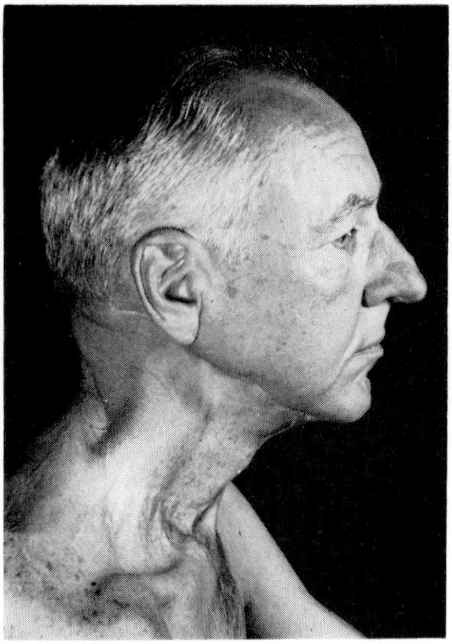

Fig. 5. This patient has had 19 operations for recurrent mucoepidermoid carcinoma over an interval of 15 years.

The general philosophy of management of these tumors is quite similar to that applied to the parotid gland. Small, well-differentiated tumors are handled by local resection in an attempt to procure a cuff of normal mucous membrane, floor of the mouth, myohyoid muscle, at times the rim of the mandible, the paraglandular areolar tissue, and the pre- and postvascular lymph nodes (Figure 5).

The classical composite resection, including lateral neck, floor of the mouth, horizontal ramus of the mandible, and small sections of tongue, is indicated for all undifferentiated tumors, high-grade adeno- and muco-epidermoid cancers and epidermoid carcinomas. Even though the adenoid cystic carcinoma enjoys a somewhat better prognosis in this region and in the parotid gland, its long-range pernicious effects are best handled by an initial wide, composite resection.

Each type of tumor in the submandibular area exhibited a different type of biologic behavior and a different prognosis. The adenoid cystic carcinomas produced a mortality rate of approximately 30% in five years; 11% of the patients lived with the disease up to 14 years; and 47% were free of disease for 3.4 years.

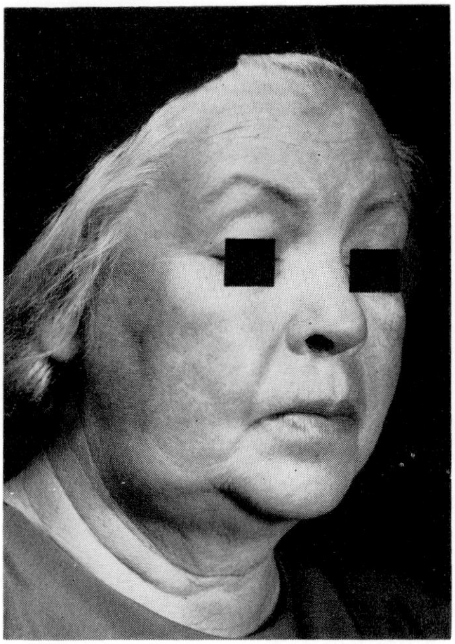

Fig. 6. Metastatic squamous-cell carcinoma in submandibular region from primary cancer in the vestibule of the nose.

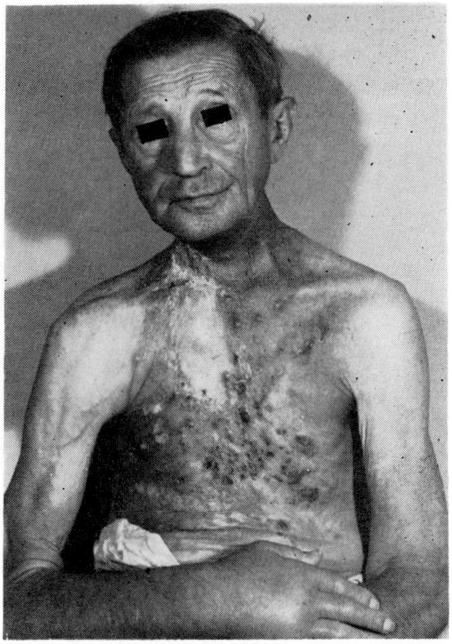

Fig. 7. Uncontrollable dermal spread of adenocarcinoma of the right submandibular gland.

In mucoepidermoid cancer slightly more than 70% of the patients were dead within two years, and only 17.6% survived five years. This tumor is obviously a much more aggressive variant than its counterpart in the parotid gland. All of the patients with adenocarcinoma were dead of tumor within two years. Malignant mixed tumors showed a mortality rate of 75%, squamous-cell cancer 50%, and undifferentiated carcinoma 66%. The majority of these tumors fell into the recurrent uncontrolled group, which emphasizes not only the gravity of all malignant tumors of the submandibular gland but particularly the gravity of those that have been mismanaged by inadequate primary resection (Figures 6 and 7).

Malignant Tumors of the Minor Salivary Glands

Tumors of the minor salivary gland present as a smooth, nonulcerating mass underneath the mucosa in the oral cavity, pharynx, or nasal cavity (Figure 8). They are about one fifth as common as tumors of the parotid gland, have a slight predilection for females, and occur most commonly during the fifth decade of life. In a review of 200 cases of

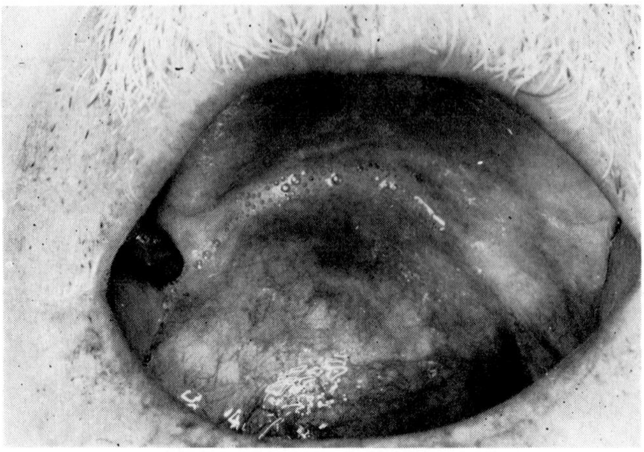

Fig. 8. Benign mixed tumor involving the entire soft palate.

minor salivary gland tumors 65% proved to be malignant. This definite escalation of malignancy from 25% for parotid tumors to 47% in submandibular tumors to 65% in tumors of the minor salivary glands alerts the clinician to the gravity of their management. Thirty-eight per cent of these tumors proved to be adenoid cystic carcinomas; the site of predilection was the region of the palate (Figure 9). It is interesting that approximately 18% of all the patients complained of pain or sensitivity in the region of the tumor and that in all of these instances the tumor proved to be adenoid cystic carcinoma. Fifty-eight per cent of the tumors that occurred in the region of the floor of the mouth, tongue, and alveolus proved to be malignant. In the buccal area, 65% were malignant and 50% were malignant in the nasal cavity.

These data immediately alert the surgeon to the fact that the majority of the tumors that arise from the minor salivary gland are malignant and that treatment should be designed along these lines.

Biopsy

It is certainly tempting for the surgeon to remove, as a minor office procedure done under local anesthesia, a small mobile accessible submucosal tumor. If this is done in light of the fact that 65% of these lesions will prove to be cancer, and that this technique should be considered no more than an excisional biopsy, then no harm has been done. Many surgeons are not acquainted with this high incidence of malig-

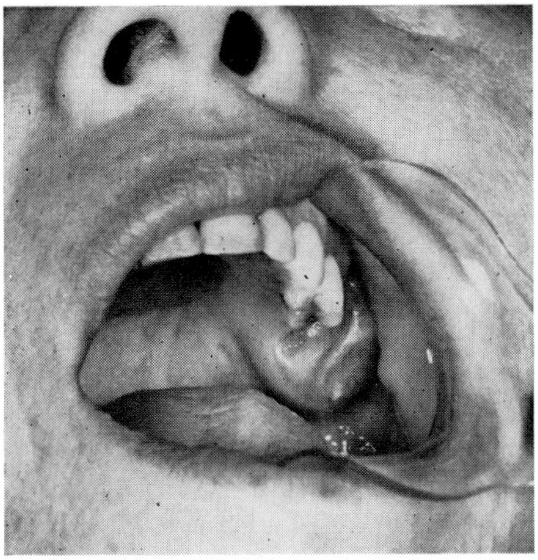

Fig. 9. Adenocystic carcinoma involving the left soft palate, alveolus, and pterygoid area.

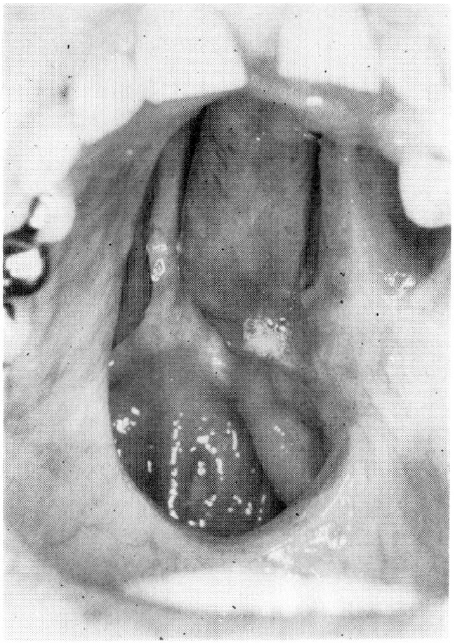

Fig. 10. Crippled palate following removal of adenoid cystic carcinoma of the palate.

nancy, however, and frequently prefer to wait to see what happens in the hope that they have removed all of the tumor.

If the tumors are larger or inaccessible and do not lend themselves readily to excisional biopsy, formal incisional biopsy is indicated in order that a definitive procedure may be planned. This alteration in proposing a preoperative biopsy under these circumstances seems justified by the fact that a routine operative technique for a group of tumors that are 65% malignant would be automatically upgraded, with the result that a disproportionate number would be overoperated. It is important to recognize deficiencies in this strategy. In a review of preoperative biopsies, 5% were misdiagnosed as benign and 9% were misdiagnosed as malignant. This combined error of 14% is disappointing but understandable in view of the fact that a biopsy specimen may not be totally representative of all the aspects of the neoplasm. When the tumor has been misdiagnosed as benign, an additional operation should be proposed. Although this deficiency in preoperative diagnosis weakens the general structure of preoperative planning, it does not destroy its basic value in the vast majority of instances. Frozen-section technique is found to be valuable in some instances but its applicability in tumors originating from the minor salivary gland is certainly more limited than its applicability in parotid tumors and submandibular tumors.

Surgical Anatomy

The surgical anatomy of tumors of the minor salivary gland relates primarily to the region involved. Since these tumors originate in the palate, floor of the mouth, alveolus, tongue, buccal mucosa, nasal cavity, pharynx, and lips, a specific and different surgical exercise is required in each instance (Figure 10). The difference between a radical ablative and conservative technique in these various regions is significant from a functional point of view, and even though all laboratory aids are used to secure the planning there will still be a small percentage of reversals and errors.

Treatment

One of the prime characteristics of all malignant neoplasms of salivary glands is local recurrence; in the instance of the minor salivary gland it was found that 40% of the patients had one or more local recurrences. The largest percentage of these occurred in the adenocystic carcinomas. It was surprising that 31% of these patients presented with metastases to the neck. The vast majority of these metastases appeared in individuals who had recurrent tumors and multiple unsuccessful surgical procedures, which suggested that repetitive surgical interventions enhance metastasis. Primary attack on the tumor was a monobloc resection of the primary site. Sixty-six per cent of the malignant mixed tumors responded favorably to this treatment, and 67% of the mucoepidermoid cancers responded favorably. Fifty-seven per cent of the adenocarcinomas were cured. Forty-two per cent of the patients with adenoid cystic carcinomas were free of neoplasm at five years, when 24% of the patients were living with neoplasm and 30% were dead of disseminated tumor; this again portrayed the chronic perniciousness of this tumor.

It is obvious from these data that the tumors which originate in the minor salivary gland are less aggressive, less infiltrative, and less undifferentiated than some of the other neoplasms considered and that they present the possibility of a more favorable course in management and prognosis.

THE NEW ROLE OF THE AUTOPSY IN THE COMMUNITY HOSPITAL*

ALFRED ANGRIST

Professor of Pathology
Albert Einstein College of Medicine
New York, N. Y.

THE RELATION OF THE AUTOPSY TO MEDICAL CARE

THE autopsy has an important function in the community hospital. It is the best available check on all medical care; it exposes and explains errors and forestalls their repetition; it teaches the house staff and the attending staff; it stimulates a deeper interest in scientific medicine and promotes investigation. It is the ultimate and penultimate in the care of patients. This much is certain: wherever the patient is the cynosure of effort in a hospital, there the autopsy is important and always will be.

The stimulus for obtaining autopsies differs in different hospitals; in many it is only the requirement of the Accreditation Commission for a minimum percentage, which corresponds to the hospital's residency programs. This requirement presumes, usually quite properly, that the higher the autopsy percentage the greater the interest of the staff, the better the teaching program and, ultimately, the better the care of the patient. The trouble is that this quantitative index, without qualitative considerations, can be self-defeating. The crass percentage figure equates a careful meticulous dissection, plus thorough follow-up, including microscopic, bacterial, biological, biochemical investigations and other specialized studies–histochemical, cytochemical, and immunological–with the "quick-look-see" procedure, wherein a body is opened and some organs are examined externally manually only, and few or no tissue sections are made. No quality control exists as to the autopsy from the standpoint of approval and accreditation.

The proposed abolition of the requirement of a minimum autopsy percentage may have some advantages if a quality control, in the form of a careful evaluation of the scientific caliber of the autopsy as an

*Presented at the Monmouth Medical Center, Long Branch, N. J., April 1, 1970.

investigative procedure and teaching instrument, were to be substituted for the bald percentage figure. This change might then promote further improvement of the autopsy procedure and thus make it still more meaningful.

Effect of New Stress on Care of the Patient

The community hospital is becoming more important for present and future medical care. Greater emphasis is being placed upon medical care and upon earlier application of the recent advances in medicine to the patient. The community hospital is the direct link to the patient for such improved total care. The community hospital is the last bastion that assures the physician the opportunity and capability of giving to the patient specialized comprehensive care properly coupled with personalized medical service, whether government intrudes further or socialized medicine supervenes. In the recent past, research has received primary consideration. We do not imply that research should not be supported; rather a proper perspective demands that the pragmatic care of the patient receive a high priority.

With the coming of government-financed regional programs and the expansion of insurance coverage, the good community hospital can make it possible for the physician to deliver good private care to all. Thus the good community hospital can and will again be the training ground for practitioners and specialists as it used to be. As a community effort the hospital should have a broad base of support; to deserve this support it must give good scientific care. The hospital must attract qualified interns and residents; it must have an adequate well-trained and experienced staff caring for patients. Thorough and good medical care, i.e., full and comprehensive personal care of all patients, must receive due recognition, equivalent to the rewards and kudos given scientific experimental research and productive publication. Such improved care of patients embraces clinical research also.

The Place of the Autopsy in the New Medical Era

With efforts directed more toward the patient, the role of the autopsy changes too. The autopsy gains new stature and does this by virtue of its own potential and its own contribution. If autopsies are done properly, then each becomes a catalytic stimulus and an incentive to obtain more autopsies; a healthy cycle of interest in the autopsy follows. This is a better incentive than a required fixed minimum percentage figure.

The Monmouth Medical Center should be commended for its appreciation of the future role of the autopsy in the medical scene. In developing this beautiful and functional autopsy suite you are taking a definite step to meet this new direction of effort in medicine and in giving the highest priority to the care of the patient. With such total care as an objective, you must succeed in making Monmouth Medical Center an even better institution, i.e., a more scientific one and a more stimulating one for all. Many associated benefits will follow naturally. I wish you every success in this endeavor.

The Future of Laboratory Medicine

How does this change of focus affect laboratory medicine? Several courses are open to the community hospital. It can go "the way of all flesh" and stress the relevant in relation to cost only. This attitude denies broad scientific study of the patient beyond the direct and immediate need. This attention to only the proximate need of the patient soon becomes pragmatic symptomatic care only, with loss of perspective for what constitutes scientific progressive medicine. A community hospital can have it so; it can then boast of an efficient profit-making venture, with all care reduced to the minimum.

With this myopic approach, the autopsy would naturally lose any new relevance. There is no financial reward in the autopsy. If the autopsy is done properly it will always be a costly procedure for which no equivalent return is made. In most communities today nothing is allowed for this deficit expenditure. Are such hospitals, which denigrate the autopsy, offering an enlightened service to patients and physicians? Will the community thus hampered ultimately have increasingly progressive medical care? Will it attract good interns and residents? Will the staff be stimulated by the joys of science and medicine, by the satisfaction of pinpointed accurate diagnoses, and the rewards of properly directed and up-to-the minute effective therapy? Will the institution be satisfied with the balanced budget only? Will the doctors be content with their own financial gain as their own reward?

Regrettably some laboratory directors would just as soon forget the autopsy; they rationalize that they are employing their morphological training in surgical pathology. In contrast with the autopsy, surgical pathology is a profit-making operation with the advantage of more apparent immediate tangible benefits to the living patient. But can surgical pathology be divorced from the autopsy and remain scientific? Will medical and surgical knowledge be extended thereby? Will the next patient who comes to that hospital with a similar illness gain thereby? Will as many questions be answered and as many errors corrected? Will the community benefit from such a static approach? Will the exponential benefits of stimulating scientific medicine be lost, with all that this implies for medical care?

The Future Role of the Pathologist and the Autopsy

Finally, where does the pathologist fit into this new direction in medicine, with its better balance of profits and closer orientation to the care of the patient as an individual and to the health of the whole community? The pathologist is best suited to be the laboratory administrator; at least he possesses the broad and general scientific background which good laboratory administration requires. His training gives him this advantage. He must also develop the managerial skills; here too proper special training can help. Modern clinical laboratory service requires directors who have broad knowledge, even though at times it is only superficial; admittedly this is quite different from the former approach in depth in morphology at the autopsy and the biopsy.

As laboratory director, the pathologist can organize and administer an effective autopsy service, along with the rest of the service functions. A well-organized autopsy service can transform the community hospital and make it even more effective than the medical college in giving better, more realistic medical training to students, interns, and residents, and in maintaining the alertness of the hospital staff—all this with better care to the patients. The laboratory director can show his managerial skill by developing a program which utilizes each and every autopsy maximally for teaching, for training, for investigation, and for research, so that the full benefits from the autopsy can accrue to all in the institution. Automation can be extended to the recording of observations, the preparation of permanent records and entries for utilization by the computer, and for photorecording, both gross and microscopic. The autopsy service will then become more attractive and, as its benefits extend beyond the department of pathology to the institution and the community, it will become ever more important.

Without the autopsy, the laboratory director becomes a laboratory manager only; with the autopsy he remains a physician and a pathologist. The autopsy will always remain in the domain of the pathologist, a personalized service which he alone can render. This too needs organization and proper techniques of management, from the acquisition of the consent to the completion of all studies in depth, with the utilization of all special facilities and all subspecialty skills, including computers. The achievement of meaningful educational presentations to all levels of the staff is the final reward. It is all a question of adequate organization of personnel for study of the autopsy, just as it is for all clinical laboratory service.

Orienting the Organization of the Autopsy Service to the New Era

This new orientation for the autopsy to this renewed interest in the patient begins with proper physical facilities. This you have now created here. Then follows the need for proper staff in the autopsy room. I want to emphasize the need for trained mortuary personnel who can assist with the manual parts of the autopsy procedure. Having a pathologist saw a skull to remove the brain is demeaning and represents a waste of specialized skill and is the ultimate in disorganization. Trained dieners soon become aware of the legal problems of identification, the complexities of the autopsy law, and the importance of attitudes in the community. Without capable permanent mortuary personnel there is no continuity, for all interns and residents come and go. Good mortuary personnel obtain the cooperation of the undertakers by assisting them in every way possible in the performance of their function for the community. Qualified help in the autopsy room is imperative if the study of autopsy pathology is to grow. Such personnel help with the preservation of tissues, with the preparation of photographs and cultures, and with special studies. If proper mortuary staff is available, residents will not be driven away from the specialty, a serious present predicament. It is all a question of organization and management. In all this, financial support can be helpful.

The pathologist is no longer the only important student of disease, as of old. Nowadays he is often more the organizer of laboratory services; this important function demands much of his energy and time. Other physicians and other scientists in each community are also students of disease. Specialized clinicians are often better prepared to solve many medical problems; they require their own laboratory studies and appropriate facilities for probing for new knowledge on their own. The laboratory director must help them in such commendable efforts.

The Role of the Clinical Pathologist in the New Era

The care of the patient today also requires more and better clinical pathology in all its subdivisions, from urinanalyses to viral studies, and it includes all aspects of surgical pathology, neuropathology, genetics, cytology, microbiology, immunology, blood banking, virology, mycology, biochemistry, isotopology, hematology, studies in coagulation, blood-protein partitions, laboratory endocrinology, and all the many special studies, as indicated. It is unrealistic to believe that one clinical pathologist can be expert in all these special fields or, to quote Oliver Goldsmith, "and still the wonder grew that one small head could carry all he knew." It is not the presumption of "knowing it all" that justifies the position of the clinical pathologist so much as his ability to make all required specialized knowledge available to the patient and the physician, i.e., to organize those with the specialized knowledge to supply the need.

The outstanding clinical pathologist today in the community hospital is not the one who knows more procedures or can do them faster or even better; though it is still desirable that he be knowledgeable in many if not all of the wide range of subjects embraced by clinical pathology. Also it is preferable that he be expert in at least one narrow field. The latter specialization is recommended to assure his status as a contributing member of the laboratory team and to make certain that he is respected by the laboratory staff and the community of physicians. Finally, however, his reputation and his contribution to medical care in the community will rest on how well he can organize space, equipment, and qualified people in all categories—from porters and technicians of all grades and kinds, to the advanced supervisors and M.D.'s and Ph.D.'s. He is a *laboratory manager* who recognizes the needs of laboratory service in medical care and can develop the logistics to meet that need properly. He has this important administrative function.

The laboratory director has the responsibility to see that all the advantages of medical ethics are not lost in the kaleidoscopic changes that are overtaking laboratory medicine. He must assure uninterrupted service for the patient and his doctor; as a corollary this includes the development of training programs at all levels. The good laboratory director is an individual who not only has the managerial skills but also the personality traits that promote the respect, devotion, and loyalty of his colleagues and can inspire them to be concerned personally with the welfare of the patient. He must be able to unite the laboratory group into a cooperative team to be effective and productive in meeting the challenge of providing increasingly better service.

Laboratory Service is Big Business

Clinical laboratory effort today is *big business*, and this accounts for the fact that big business is coming into the field and doing it rapidly and in a big way. Many prominent drug and chemical companies are making large investments in purchasing clinical laboratories. Big business has always recognized managerial skills. In fact the "new nobility" in medicine will be comprised of such managers, whether laboratory directors, hospital superintendents, or other administrative functionaries in the health field. They will replace the pure research workers, the recent "nobility" in medicine. It is significant that many research workers with large grants have often really been managers as much as they have been inspired and creative investigators. Increased productivity and publication are the goals of the research worker. Many were unidirectional in their efforts and gave higher priority to the esoteric than to the pragmatic, often blind to the needs of the patients and the community. The better they were as research workers the further they were from the patient; in fact freedom from care for the patient was, and to a less extent still is, a status symbol.

With the present change in priorities and with coming financial support to promote the new direction of effort toward helping the patient, those who care for the patient will once again obtain better recognition and reward. Appreciation of the good clinician and the brilliant diagnosis will return, and with it the comprehensive, personal care of the patient. Appreciation of the good autopsy analysis will again be an important component of this new direction of medical care.

Obtaining the Full Benefits of the Industrial Revolution

With clinical pathology now a big business the big money has come, with all its troubles. Automation in the laboratory has compounded the effects of specialization—which already has changed all medicine. With its many benefits have come all the trials and the anguish of the industrial revolution; and in the laboratory this has come to pass altogether too rapidly and with greater impact. Thus far relatively little of the savings of automation has been transmitted to the patient. Some of the gains, as an illogical matter of policy, have been used to cover deficit operations in other departments of the hospital. The trouble then is that the laboratory director and staff are blamed for the persisting high cost of care. The benefits of automation, now reflected in larger and often inordinate profits from the laboratory, must be diverted directly to the immediate lowering of costs to the patient.

To achieve the full benefits of the industrial revolution in laboratory medicine—and these can be considerable indeed—we require the full capabilities of American management with its genius for organization. Automation requires expensive equipment, and this compels the sharing of such equipment. Automated equipment now available will do 600 blood sugars per hour—each on only 0.02 cc. of serum—accurately and with all quality controls. The Swedish autochemist costs half a million dollars. We need only bring enough tests to the machine; unless we do just that, the new technology cannot be exploited; no one hospital can use its full capacity. The problem is one of management and of logistics, not one of pathology or chemistry. Economic forces of this kind are promoting *regionalization* of laboratories, so that one central laboratory will take care of the needs of many institutions and all the physicians of the community. In essence, this is part and parcel of the present tendency toward regionalization in the organization of all medical care.

May I close with the admonition so true for all medicine in general and for laboratory medicine in particular: stand still and you are soon far behind! What you are doing is more than just taking a step forward; it is a big stride upward to a higher level of medical care, with the assurance of continuing progress. As the first instance of such an adjustment to the new era with its high priority given to patient care, you may well be making history in medical education and medical care.

SUMMARY

The recent high priority now given to care of the patient gives added importance to the autopsy and to the pathologist. Specialization has given us the equivalent of the industrial revolution in medical care. In the laboratory automation has been added to the consequences of ever-increasing subdivision of specialties to accelerate and magnify the effects of the industrial revolution, with all its attendant benefits and drawbacks. The high cost and potential capacity make sharing of equipment and personnel by regionalization imperative in order to exploit modern technology fully. To obtain the total benefits of automation for the patient and physician, regionalization of laboratory medicine will therefore probably come before the regionalization of the rest of medical care. In this new era laboratory service and the autopsy require reorientation, particularly with respect to procedures and techniques. The autopsy has always been an instrument of control of medical care and of progress in medicine, and it can come into its own on its own with this renewed emphasis on care of the patient.

NEEDED: A HEALTH CONSUMERS' ORGANIZATION*

GREER WILLIAMS

Assistant Professor of Preventive Medicine (Communications)
Tufts University School of Medicine
Boston, Mass.

THIS inquiry might well begin with the anecdote about my neighbor, a lawyer, who jogs to keep his heart healthy. Jogging by itself does not content him, so he also jogs his bloodhound on a leash; further, he picks up and deposits in a brown bag the empty beer cans he finds by the road. The dog, large, clumsy, and useless, one morning succeeded in tripping up his master, who pulled up lame and in pain, with a strained Achilles tendon. Hopping along home, my friend called the local orthopedic surgeon. The doctor's secretary answered and said she could give my friend an appointment in one month. "If I had had the foresight to know one month ago that I was nearly going to break my leg today," said my friend, "I would have made an appointment," and hung up. He thereafter resorted to home remedies and, after a few days on a crutch, was able to walk normally again.

Perhaps my remarks should be entitled, "Hurry, Doctor, If You Don't See Me Soon, I'll Have to Get Well Without You." In any event, I think this story fairly well characterizes the health-care plight of American people in their less-than-fatal experiences. Not only the poor and the elderly find it difficult to get medical care the way they would like it and when and where they need it. Many of us have our own anecdotes about difficulties in getting medical attention where purchasing power is not a problem.

If we had as much trouble obtaining groceries, gasoline, electricity, water, or other so-called essentials of modern, civilized life, I am sure the republic, even under a Republican administration, would be in a state of revolt.

As a longtime lay medical writer, I for many years have pondered why public and private efforts to provide reasonably good health

*Presented at a meeting of the Subcommittee on Social Policy for Health Care, Committee on Medicine in Society, January 30, 1970.

services, preventive and therapeutic, fall so far short of the mark. As we know, such services in recent years have been getting farther and farther from what we used to call adequate and now call optimum. I have in turn blamed the individual competence of physicians (we always have had a shortage of *good* doctors), a lack of knowledge, a failure to apply knowledge, the American Medical Association (AMA) and the private profession's well-established economic motivations, the self-centeredness and aloofness of medical academicians, the timid, fumbling attempts of bureaucratic government to do better, and the antisocial and partisan interests of politicians. Eventually I realized that it was a mistake to look for a villain. Probably we all deserve a share of the blame, whether medical doctors or word doctors; but blaming one another does not solve the problem.

I have finally come to the conclusion, not alone, of course, that the general failure of the medical and other health professions and their institutions to meet people's needs lies, in essence, in the low priority that people themselves assign to medical care as an approach to better health. Another somewhat different way of saying this is that there are quite a number of things we value more than protection of our health. For example, it is now pretty clear that the attack and death rates from certain diseases could be considerably reduced by diet, exercise, and the abandonment of cigarettes. But how many will impose this much self-discipline? How many will put long-term ahead of short-term objectives? My neighbor is in a small minority, I think, in his willingness to accept the hardship of jogging to avoid a possible later pain in his chest. On the other hand, is it significant that, although he is active in such public affairs as conservation, he did not become interested in the availability of medical service before he needed it? Generally speaking, who does?

On this occasion I want to look at the question from three viewpoints that may suggest where the answer lies, although I cannot profess to know how to produce the answer; its realization would require a rationalism and activism of which none of us health consumers, so far, appears capable. The first viewpoint concerns the nature of voluntary health movements in this country; the second will contemplate who cares about health care and how much; the third considers present strategy under the heading—Do We (or Don't We) Want National Health Insurance?

The Nature of Voluntary Health Movements

If one examines the history of our leading national voluntary health organizations, he will find a curious fact: that while these organizations are commonly thought of as citizens' movements or campaigns, and while they frequently involve a great deal of lay participation and involvement, and usually depend for their success on this characteristic of mass appeal and support, the original inspiration, initiative, and leadership has tended to come from physicians. In other words, the germination is not directly and primarily that of consumer demand; rather, it constitutes professional recognition of a need and then mobilization of support.

I shall have to dispose of some notable exceptions. One of the first and most effective health crusaders in this country was Dorothea Dix, a school teacher. A New England-bred personification of righteous indignation, Miss Dix did not need an organization, though she did receive much help from physicians and politicians. Her consumers were the pauper insane who, in the mid-19th century, were consigned to jails and poorhouses. For 40 years she traveled through the United States exhorting state legislatures to establish state hospitals. She was a one-woman national health and welfare agency, and more persuasive than most. Twenty states established hospitals as the direct result of her efforts. Tragically, the state hospital system that evolved became a dumping ground for the mentally ill. This was not what Miss Dix had in mind. Her model was the moral-treatment hospital, the earliest version of the therapeutic community.

Clifford Beers, also a layman, founded the National Committee for Mental Hygiene in 1908. Since 1950 this organization has been called the National Association for Mental Health. Beers was a discharged mental patient and author of *A Mind that Found Itself*. He interested William James, Dr. Adolf Meyer, Dr. William H. Welch, and others in the humanitarian reform of mental institutions. Dr. Meyer suggested the name "mental hygiene" for the organization. The movement, having fallen under the spell of the early eugenicists and child psychologists, shifted its emphasis from Beers' concern, the care and treatment of the hospitalized psychotic, to the pursuit of positive mental health via mental-health education and child guidance. For many years the committee was led by its medical director, Dr. Thomas W. Salmon and then, for many more years, by Dr. George S. Stevenson. Beers suffered recurrences of his manic-depressive psychosis throughout his life. He remained, in effect, a mental patient. As it evolved, the National Committee for Mental Hygiene was completely dominated by psychiatrists; it was not until quite recent times that it acquired the dynamics of the more typical citizens' movement, with laymen playing an active part in building support of professional services. I can illustrate what I mean by citing the National Association for Retarded Children, founded in 1950, which was started by parents of mentally retarded children. Lay members of the association outnumber professionals about 50 to 1. This organization quickly outran the National Association for Mental Health, as shown by the fact that it raises more than twice as much money from the public.

There are some other voluntary health organizations with strong lay origins. Planned Parenthood-World Population, Inc., with its claim to the world's first or second biggest health problem, depending on how you rate population against war and pollution, was started in 1916 as the National Birth Control League by a woman willing to go to jail for her convictions—Mrs. Margaret Sanger. This organization, like the National Easter Seal Society for Crippled Children and Adults, appears to have created a happy blend of lay and professional influences. The crippled-children movement was started nationally in 1921 by a layman named Edgar F. (Daddy) Allen.

I am not overlooking the strong lay character of such organizations as the National Safety Council, United Cerebral Palsy Association, National Multiple Sclerosis Society, National Cystic Fibrosis Research Foundation, and National Council on Alcoholism. Nor, above all, am I overlooking the National Foundation for Infantile Paralysis, now the National Foundation-March of Dimes, founded by one lawyer, Franklin D. Roosevelt, while he was president (1938), and directed by another, Basil O'Connor. This foundation has enjoyed more criticism and more success than any other, I imagine. It is the only national voluntary health organization that can claim to have eradicated a disease by popular subscription. The National Foundation was the primary source of support for the research and development of the Salk vaccine; it also supported the Sabin vaccine. These two vaccines, we know, ended the threat of poliomyelitis in the United States and wherever else they have been effectively applied.

Having said all this, in the form of a disclaimer, I still credit the rise of the voluntary health movement in the United States mainly to the vision of doctors of medicine. The first national voluntary organization was the National Tuberculosis Association. Dr. Lawrence F. Flick was the guiding light in founding its precursor, the Pennsylvania Society for the Prevention of Tuberculosis in 1892. One of the prime movers of the national association was Dr. S. Adolphus Knopf. This organization, highly successful in its sale of Christmas Seals, had the good fortune to ride a 150-year downward curve in mortality from tuberculosis, a decline in recent times reinforced by specific treatment.

It was Dr. Prince A. Morrow who got the forerunner of the American Social Health Association off the ground in its long and trying campaign against syphilis, gonorrhea, and prostitution, as the Society for Social and Moral Prophylaxis. Known from 1914 on as the American Social Hygiene Association, it was headed for many years by Dr. William F. Snow.

Dr. Wendell C. Phillips founded the American Society for the Hard of Hearing in 1919. Doctors were prominent among the founders of the National Society for the Prevention of Blindness, first in England and then in the United States.

Dr. Thomas D. Cullen in 1913 launched the American Society for the Control of Cancer, the forerunner of the American Cancer Society. Cullen had the help of fellow surgeons in the American Gynaecological Society. The object of this group was to collect information and educate the public about cancer. The founders were 10 physicians and five laymen. In the modern version of this sharply focussed, hard-hitting organization—it has probably given us more intimations of mortality than any other like group—its direction is equally divided among physicians and laymen.

Physicians and scientists founded the American Diabetes Association and were prominent in the Arthritis and the National Kidney foundations. Dr. Lewis I. Connor and Dr. Haven Emerson started the first organization against heart disease in New York City in 1913. This became the American Heart Association, incorporated in 1924 by a group of cardiologists. In modern times the Heart Association's membership has included about three physicians and scientists for every four related professionals and lay volunteers.

At the end of a four-hour interview, Dr. John Enders remarked to me, "The only thing I am finally sure of in biology is individual variation." May I add one other thing we can be sure of: the human tendency to look at diversity and yearn for unity. Complexity confuses and fatigues us; in the end we want to put everything together. In 1921 the National Health Council was formed as a coordinating agency for voluntary health organizations. It was primarily an organization of health professionals and has remained so. It is now made up of 19 voluntary health agencies and 32 agencies that fall into a professional or other membership category. It is hard to identify a real live consumer in this group, though we must recognize that many health professionals and health administrators represent consumer blocs and do have their interests at heart.

In their 1945 study, *Voluntary Health Agencies*, Selskar M. Gunn and Philip S. Platt said that "the practical achievements of the Council have fallen far short of the early hopes. The Council has not developed leadership in important cooperative health planning that called for action; it is has not brought about joint financing of national health agencies; nor has it brought the several agencies or movements any nearer to unification. It has seldom spoken with the voice of authority on health matters. . . ."

I regard these remarks less as fault-finding than as a definition of the problem of special interests and "splinteration," known in other contexts as the American Way. The fundamental characteristics of a categorical health movement are a capacity: 1) to identify with a given problem; 2) to reach out and offer help to people with this problem; and 3) to join with others of like mind in seeking a solution of this problem.

It is true, as the National Health Council points out, that its member organizations include millions of citizen volunteers, people who contribute their time and their talents, all the way from sitting on the board of trustees down to working in a back ward. But the leadership has come mainly from health professionals and, by and large, the laymen have been content to let the professionals speak for them.

Gunn and Platt saw this: "It is notable that as scientific discoveries enabled us to control and eventually to eliminate certain specific diseases, physicians, usually specialists, took the lead in organizing group efforts for the attack. In research and in treatment, as well as in guidance of education, members of the medical profession have shown the way and have borne the heat and toil of the day-by-day advances."

The degree of cooperation and action that can be achieved when professionals and laymen—providers and consumers, in the modern idiom—in some instances, doctors and patients—find common cause in a specific problem is one of the wonders of democratic society. Such groups have exerted tremendous pressures on the public and the government, which is usually expected to carry out in massive ways what the voluntary agencies can undertake only on a demonstration basis. Nevertheless the source of the categorical agency's strength and success—a combination of personal and professional interest and high motivation to do something specific—is also a source of weakness and failure when it comes to achieving progress across a broader base, as in developing health-care services that combine many targets.

Obviously it is just as hard for people with a special interest to identify with the system as a whole as it has been for medicine in an age of specialization to maintain a whole-man approach. Smart people tend to keep on doing what they find they can do well; this process has put our specialized agencies in the position of competing with one another for manpower, for money, and for facilities; it leaves the public, as Dr. Leona Baumgartner has said, with a medical-care system made up of "bits and pieces."

Rationally it would seem desirable for a voluntary health agency to emphasize the building of a broad base of comprehensive health services in each community and region. For example, the heart, cancer, and mental-health movements have as big a stake in the primary-care base and a comprehensive system as do the public and the health professions in general. Irrespective of the disease, this is where case-finding begins; where early detection, secondary prevention, and health education should begin. Illness, as we know, is first seen not as a labeled disease, but as a complaint or a disturbance, a sign or a symptom. To look at cancer or mental illness not as a center of interest but as a piece of the action in health manpower, organization, and system, however, is to lose the power of the specialized appeal, it seems. As both categorical agencies and professional specialists often say about the rest of the health enterprise, "That's not our business."

The question remains: Whose business is it? How do we develop community health leverage? Or can we?

Who Cares About Health Care?

Health-care leaders are having trouble adjusting to the unpleasant realization that President Richard M. Nixon and quite possibly the silent majority assign a much lower order of importance to health care as a human right than do those of us who personally or professionally concern ourselves with the sick or the dying.

You do not find anything about health in the United States constitution. The revolutionary judgment that health care—meaning preventing illness as well as treating it—is an essential service that must be readily available to all first received statutory recognition during a period (1963-1967) when Congress passed more major health legislation than at any time in its history. This phenomenon was a fortuitous, opportunistic response to two compelling stimuli—liberal grief over the assassination of John F. Kennedy and the landslide for Lyndon B. Johnson. The Democrats were in power. It has been said, doubtless by a Democrat, that the difference between Democrats and Republicans is that the one party emphasizes human, and the other, economic, values. President Nixon, however, also talks about improving the "quality of life."

Surely there is some economic evidence for assuming that people see medical services as essential to the good life, for in 1969 Americans spent about $60 billion for such services, public and private, or about 6.5% of gross national product. This represents a fivefold increase from $12 billion in 1950. Nevertheless, this increase in costs, as we well know, did not represent any commensurate increases in services.

Finding service of the kind you need, when and where you want it, is more a game of hide and seek than an easy exercise of a human right. The *patient* is correctly named. To get good medical care, a person needs 1) the determination to find a competent doctor and to cover whatever time and distance lies between them, 2) a disease that interests this doctor, 3) sufficient personal appeal to win acceptance, and 4) an ability to pay the bills.

Almost everyone, liberal or conservative, now agrees that there is a marked shortage of physicians, dentists, and nurses; that our medical-care system has gaps and deficiencies; that the poor, black and white, are medically neglected; that primary-care services (the first place to which a family turns) are, if not totally lacking, scattered, inattentive, and overworked.

Likewise, no one disputes that medical care constitutes a special economic problem. The assembled doctor and hospital bills in any major illness sometimes equal the price of a cabin cruiser, ski chalet, or trip around the world. The statistics are persuasive: medical care costs are increasing twice as fast as the cost of living. Demand outruns supply, and the sick consumer has little choice. He must buy the service he can get.

President Richard M. Nixon himself stipulated the problem last July when he said: "We face a massive crisis in this area, and unless action is taken both administratively and legislatively within the next two or three years, we will have a breakdown in our medical care system which could have consequences affecting millions of people in this country."

That is plain enough. What confuses professionals is that health care is not on the president's high-priority list. It took him six months to appoint an Assistant Secretary of Health and Scientific Affairs, the No. 1 federal health administrator. It took a year to get a 1969-1970, hold-the-line health budget through Congress, not counting the presidential veto delay because of uninvited increases. As a result, many medical education and care programs were consigned to an "approved-but-not-funded" category, and new applications were delayed.

The president ignored health care in his State of the Union speech to Congress. After peace, as a No. 1 goal, he gave priorities to such problems as stopping inflation, enforcing the law, cleaning up the environment, abolition of hunger and poverty, and decentralization of government powers. He asked for large budgets against crime and pollution. His emphasis on reduced federal spending in other directions means opposition to substantially increased federal aid in developing the health resources of the country; to do this would require moderately large spending programs (but nothing like war, antimissile defense, or space research).

A new question now intrudes itself on our attention. Having made the choice of living with a "massive crisis" rather than actively pursuing its resolution, has the administration adopted a policy of devaluating health care's importance to our quality of life? Equally significant, does such a policy reflect public opinion?

Because of the pressures of the nuclear threat, population, pollution, the "ugly American war," civil violence, and youthful defiance, has our democratic society reached a time when it wishes to abandon its most fundamental value: the individual's right to live? Is it ready to agree with totalitarian ideologies that a given life is relatively cheap and meaningless? Should we bother to try to save every baby and old person when we so obviously have more than we can love or support?

The silent majority and some noisy minorities do not appear sensitive to these kinds of values. I doubt that many share the heavy mood of impending doom that pervades our university medical centers. True, medicine is crisis-minded. We have scared up one health crisis after another for as long as I can remember; that is quite long. But now John Platt, biophysicist, finds us in "multiple crises, a crisis of crises all at one time." In *Science* (November 28, 1969), Platt presents a table classifying United States and world problems and crises by estimated time of arrival and intensity. In a scale headed "total annihilation," as a Grade 1 crisis, health problems such as cancer and heart disease, smoking and drugs, artificial organs and transplanted hearts rank no higher than Grades 5 to 7. Administrative management, slums, participatory democracy, racial conflict, transportation, neighborhood ugliness, and crime all are assigned a higher order of importance. "We are," Platt states gloomily, "in the gravest danger of destroying our society, our world, and ourselves in any number of different ways before the end of the century."

Since man is nothing if not hopeful, it is almost a necessity to react to such a pessimistic statement by making light of it. Nonetheless the mood is widely shared among health professionals; I happen to agree with it and with Gerard Piel, who sees us all as victims of "a mindless power system."

On the other hand, we have learned to test the cry of "Ouch" by asking what hurts. American biomedical scientists have received about $10 billion in National Institutes of Health support of their research in the last 20 years. This largesse, a hitherto politically popular policy, crested at $1.2 billion in 1968. By then other costs (to some extent, the costs of killing people) caused the government to have economic second thoughts in its quest for the good life. Compulsively honest critics, recalling that federally-supported medical research had been advertised and sold on the promise of mass life-saving, looked at the results. There were some good ones, mainly in prevention and treatment of infectious diseases. But the annual death rate had stopped dropping in 1954; more people were dying of chronic diseases than ever before. It also became apparent that by living longer people were acquiring more opportunities to become sick. For example, the average terminal illness in old age has been estimated as 29 months!

Health propagandists, long the subject of scientific in-group distrust, came under quiet political scrutiny for raising too many unfulfilled hopes. Health bureaucrats became preoccupied with cost-benefit analyses; they found methods of measuring health too crude to prove anything. Health-science buffs became anxious about whether they had been worshipping a false god.

One possible source of depression among biomedical scientists, therefore, may be a basic insecurity, complicated by some ambivalence, arising from the decerebrate way our government makes and carries out policy. Federal support, mainly for research, has increased from a small fraction to well over 50% of total medical-school expenditures since 1950. Only in the last five years has Congress accepted the commensurate need to stimulate the training of more health workers to apply the knowledge coming out of research. This aid, coming too little and too late to produce a balanced effort thus far, has been tied to expansion of student enrollment. This has put financially needy schools under pressure to over-extend themselves. The government was guilty of irrational planning and distortion in its early neglect of medical education, and now is playing off education against research support.

The president, unlike some predecessors, cannot be accused of playing politics with health. He is not playing at all. He seems to have preferred the threat of institutional destitution for schools simultaneously being called on to meet the nation's medical manpower needs.

For some people this is not mere administrative rhetoric. Cutting off funds actually means cutting short their lives. For instance, persons with complete kidney failures can be kept alive and well indefinitely by hooking their blood circulation to an artificial kidney (hemodialysis) two or three times a week. The only problem is that it costs $10,000 or more a year for treatment. Not many can afford that much. The head of a state kidney program in Boston told me he can accept only one out of five applicants. "Is that all you can save?" I asked. "No," he said, "we could treat three out of every five we see." This physician is placed in the position of signing a death warrant for 40% of his patients. Case histories show that these people die with the feeling their fellow man has let them down.

A dollar value has been placed on human life whether we like it or not. I know of places where sick blacks seeking medical care are asked by the doctor or hospital if they have the money to pay, in cash; if they do not have it, they are rejected. All that remains to be done is for the president to appoint a study commission to determine the exact value of life. Lives will have to be graded, of course—poor, rich, white, black, very important persons, not so important. It is a matter of common observation that public hospitals treat patients in accordance with their class. If you are brought in as an accident victim, your chances are better if you are well-dressed, clean, young, and do not smell of alcohol.

Professors of preventive medicine have talked bravely of "the coming revolution in medicine." They emphasize what often is lacking, such as family and home care, vigorous case-finding and follow-up, and a comprehensive system of moving patients through general to specialized services, from a community health center or a community hospital to a university medical center and back again, as needed. Every study available shows that from 20 to 80% of hospital patients would not need to be there, at a cost to them of $50 to $100 a day, if appropriate community services were available.

Unfortunately our prophets of a better day do not say who is going to lead this revolution. They leave the impression that the public is demanding these changes and that doctors and hospitals are not responding too well. As a matter of fact, Richard M. Bailey, economist, suggests that the present system of medical care has evolved in rather precise recognition of the fact that not many people associate their health with doctors and hospitals. You might say that we have a healthy urge to stay away from them. People have to be really sick, alarmed, or helpless before they see the pressing need for having adequate medical care available. Our doctors and hospitals are nicely adjusted to this viewpoint. They tend to prefer the more serious, more dramatic, more challenging disease problems, provided they can do something about them. A doctor gravitates, in short, toward meeting crises in the role of hero.

People seem to know, or behave as if they knew, the sources of their good health. Epidemiologists long have pointed out that medical care—care of the sick—is only one factor and probably not the most important one in the historic rise of life expectancy. Good food, good hous-

THE SEVEN LEADING ITEMS FOR WHICH PURCHASING POWER IS EXPENDED

1. Food (including tobacco and alcohol)	23.2%
2. Housing	14.4
3. Household operation	14.1
4. Transportation	13.4
5. Clothing (including accessories and jewelry)	10.3
6. Medical care	7.2
7. Recreation and travel	7.0

ing, sanitation, hygiene, health education, immunization, safer living and working conditions, reduced stress, all have contributed.

The way people spend their money gives clear evidence of what they want most. In 1969 American consumers distributed their purchasing power among the seven leading items shown in the accompanying table.

These items reflect middle-class values. Yet the poor, who have more than their share of ill health, do not see their needs much differently. When Dr. H. Jack Geiger established the Tufts-Delta Health Center in Mound Bayou, Mississippi, under the Poverty Program, spokesmen for the black population said: "This is nice, to have the health care, but we need other things more."

The list became extensive. It began with enough to eat and moved on to roofs that did not leak and fuel to keep people warm and then to the lack of automobiles and gasoline to run them, shoes for the children so they could walk to school in winter, and jobs that paid a living wage. Improved health can be more of a social and economic than a medical problem.

Such words come as unkind cuts to those—I am one—who would like to see a greater national, as well as private, investment in resources for direct prevention of disease and for scientific and humane care of the sick. But we might as well face the fact, as President Nixon seems to have done, that this kind of upgrading of services is not going to take place until the American public actively demonstrates a desire for them.

It is too much to expect a Republican president to lead a medical revolution when we remember that even Franklin D. Roosevelt did not mention health when he spoke of the Four Freedoms. So far there has been no *health* march on Washington in quest of a *fifth* freedom—freedom from illness. Health-consumer leadership and organization are lacking. Some Democratic senators and congressmen have taken the lead, but they often have been short-sighted and badly advised. The logical course of action is clear enough, however difficult to achieve. Politicians obligingly point out that pressure moves them; when pressures come from all directions, as they often do, politics tends to move in the direction of the most pressure, provided it appears overwhelming and opposition can be neutralized. Organized medicine, hospitals, and voluntary health organizations with special interests (cancer, heart, and so on) have lobbyists. They have some influence, but are easily identified as special pleaders.

The general health consumer lacks a large vocal organization to work in his behalf, to pressure the government and the providers. Big labor unions do an effective job but, like everybody else's, their interests tend to be narrowly channeled. Their large-group method of negotiating and bargaining nonetheless sets the pattern for a health-consumers' organization. "We are convinced that our greatest pressure is as a buyer," says Thomas G. Moore, director of the California Council for Health Plan Alternatives, a union of unions formed to negotiate health benefits. In contrast, we have seen only a spattering of small, citizen confrontations with health institutions; these express isolated goals.

The health consumer is not only a buyer but a voter. To paraphrase Bismarck on the subject of war and generals, health is too important to be left to the doctors. It is also too important to be left to the politicians. In the course of federal, regional, and community planning efforts, much has been made of the need for more consumer representation. It is liberal health professionals who talk this way mainly. But who listens? More to the point, who cares? As yet there is not much evidence that the public listens to health professionals, or cares. Until it does it cannot expect much more from our health services than it now receives.

Do We (or Don't We) Want National Health Insurance?

If, as has been said, a camel is an animal designed by a committee, then that many-splintered mansion, American medical care, is a system designed by a committee of camels. Its characteristics of professional and institutional self-centeredness, of performing as passive producer of services actively sought by its consumers, of regarding the needy people it does not see as not its business, have been repeatedly criticized from industrial, engineering, managerial, social, and economic viewpoints. Reciting well-known complaints is hardly worthwhile here, except to note that Dr. Robert H. Ebert has called medicine "one of the last of the push-cart industries."

What brings me to this rhetorical boil are the clear indications that national health insurance—now also called universal health insurance (UHI)—is becoming topical again, and is almost certain to be a presidential campaign issue in 1972. President Nixon so far has obliged by leaving the subject to the Democrats, presumably recognizing it as their baby. *Medical World News* predicts "the bloodiest battle yet." What disturbs me is that events may prove Santayana right when he said: "Those who cannot remember the past are condemned to repeat it." It would seem that, all because a Republican and economic conservative is in the White House, some of our best Democrats are about to forget everything they learned, or should have learned, in the past quarter of a century.

The first alarming sign was the formation, toward the end of 1968, of a Committee for National Health Insurance, headed by Walter Reuther, Mrs. Mary Lasker, Whitney M. Young, Jr., and Dr. Michael E. DeBakey, all veterans of national health politics. As people get older, fewer things surprise, much less horrify them. A health veteran myself, I admit faint horror at this new focus of attention, and some surprise at how fast various parties got on the bandwagon. The charge was led by Senator Edward M. Kennedy and later joined by the medical deans; the Association of American Medical Colleges passed a resolution approving UHI "in principle." I should have thought the deans would ask Mr. Reuther to help them with their first order of business—developing medical manpower resources for family care.

I see no objection to UHI *in theory*—it works in countries where public interests have more muscle than private interests. But a storm of talk about it in the foreseeable future will only complicate—if not effectively obstruct—progress in the present intricate effort to meet neglected needs and to try to get local medical doctors connected with large medical centers for consultation with patients and continuing education. The success of ongoing regional and community health planning depends not only on increased federal aid, but on finding points of agreement among differing viewpoints, and on finding ways in which providers and consumers, private and public, can work together—on negotiation, not confrontation. This, in fact, has been called "creative federalism," using financial incentives to catalyze joint and cooperative planning. Congress enacted the enabling legislation in 1965 and 1966, using concern about heart disease, cancer, and stroke as a point of entry. These programs, one of the health bureaucracy's better ideas, are likely to be the first casualties in political cross fire over UHI.

I agree with Dr. Roger O. Egeberg, assistant secretary for Health and Scientific Affairs: "We are not ready for anything of this kind in this country." And with Robert H. Finch, secretary of Health, Education, and Welfare, who points out that the nation does not have the service capacity to meet the demands that UHI would generate. It is a matter of record that their chief, President Nixon, is opposed to big spending programs with centralized federal controls, and Republican opposition to such legislation is therefore a foregone conclusion.

Senate committee hearings on various UHI approaches and alternatives are expected this spring. All relate to the recognized weaknesses and limitations of Blue Cross, Blue Shield, and other voluntary forms of health insurance. Eighty-five per cent of the population has some kind of third-party protection on medical expenses, but these cover only 33% of the costs. The hospital-sponsored Blue Cross has been an enormous help to millions of hospitalized people in the last 30-odd years, but its general effect has been inflationary, due to its inability to control excessive use, price-hiking, and quality of service.

The American Medical Association (AMA), which has been fighting "socialized medicine" for 50 years, is sponsoring a bill that would allow $150 to $400 income tax credits against voluntary health insurance premiums paid by persons who make less than $5000 a year, and credits of $37.50 to $100 to those who make more than $10,000 a year. Persons who pay no income tax would get this limited insurance free. This proposal incorporates most of the drawbacks of voluntary plans without meeting the basic problem of delivering comprehensive health care.

The Reuther proposal is much the same as the Wagner-Murray-

Dingell bill that during the Truman Administration received some public attention, mostly from the AMA and organized labor. The AMA spent several million dollars lobbying against the bill. Its belligerence, like that of a moose at bay, its carelessness with facts, and general public-be-damned attitude set a new low in public-relations methods. Its agents, Whitaker & Baxter, told me at the time: "We show them the Devil and lead them to the altar." The Devil is a bureaucracy-based, Social Security-type system of paying medical bills out of an employer-employee-shared payroll tax and general tax funds. Almost everyone would be eligible for all kinds of personal health services. Presumably standards and controls would be imposed. It is simply good business to have specifications and accountability.

A UHI system, when phased in by age groups, could be expected to cover the majority of private-consumer expenditures for medical care (now $40 billion) plus a major part of federal and state expenditures (perhaps $10 billion) and take off from there, as costs increased. Unquestionably, UHI would increase people's health-care purchasing power tremendously.

Compulsory-health-insurance proponents claim full awareness that this financing mechanism will not bring people all the medical care they need or want without an expansion of health manpower and reorganization of the service delivery system. Indeed, the Reuther plan asks that the proposed Office of National Health Insurance Administration be allocated adequate funds for support of education, training, facility construction, organizational development, and demonstration programs, to assure the availability of services as rapidly as possible.

Let us set aside the question of whether medical schools and teaching hospitals; dental, nursing and social work schools; and junior colleges training technical aides would like to see the priority and destiny of their programs controlled by a government insurance office. An even more curious feature of the Reuther plan is that capital investment in plant, production, and distribution is made subordinate in organization to paying doctor and hospital bills—to stimulating an already-existing, now further-accelerated market for scarce personal health services. Supply comes later—much later considering the time it takes to train health professionals. It has taken American medical schools 20 years of strenuous effort to increase their annual production of physicians from 5,000 to 8,000, against an estimated need for almost twice 8,000.

This demand-first, supply-later approach, while seemingly designed to produce chaos and disappoint consumers, is not a planning accident or oversight. It pursues the theory known as "pressuring the system" or, in translation, how to move the old medical elephant. The desire for some such leverage can be appreciated by anyone familiar with the history of foot-dragging among both medical faculties and private practitioners in facing up to the manpower shortage and the obsolescence of medicine's small-business-man practices.

In his report to President Harry S. Truman on the nation's health in 1948, Oscar Ewing said: "It is clear that the Nation must greatly increase its investment in education for all the health professions if we are to produce the manpower needed for health and medical services." Some universities began to build new medical schools and expand old ones in the 1950's, but the AMA did not admit the existence of the physician shortage until 1967!

The system pressurers have good intentions, but their technique, basically one of confrontation, tends to be counter-productive. What it gains in political appeal it loses in rationality. Its frequent application to government health policy has distorted, diverted, and damaged the whole health enterprise. University leaders are well aware of this, but, being federal grantees, have been fairly quiet about it.

The underlying fallacy, I think, comes from misconstruing medical care as free enterprise. By virtue of being uninformed in economics and the social sciences and by thoughtless reiteration, conservative private practitioners are sure they are engaged in free enterprise. The system pressurers likewise seem to assume this.

Free enterprise has certain characteristics not found in medical practice. The primary one is an open market, where the consumer is free to buy or not to buy, and sellers move to meet public demand in competition with one another. If unregulated, prices rise when goods are scarce and drop when they are abundant; profit derives not only from a higher price but from an ability to mass-produce goods of attractive quality at the lowest possible cost.

A sick patient does not have a free choice; he must buy what service is immediately available and compete with other patients for attention. The provider is free to select his patients and set his price, generously or selfishly.

Meanwhile competition among doctors is rigidly limited by the opportunities of young men and women to become physicians. The number encouraged to seek medical education is not much different now from what it was 20 years ago. Roughly, of 20,000 applicants each year, 10,000 are rejected for lack of student places, although the American Association of Medical Colleges acknowledges that 33 to 50% of those rejected are qualified. Medical-school space for these 3,500 to 5,000 is lacking.

The longtime policy of medical faculties and the AMA Council on Medical Education, the medical school accreditation body, maintains this input bottleneck. It is done in the interests of high-quality education, or what I have described elsewhere as the Doctrine of the Chosen Few. The American medical profession evolved into a guild type of monopoly after Abraham Flexner, in 1910, set out to raise doctors' competence—sorely needed—by putting inferior medical schools out of business. Paradoxically, this movement suited the aspirations of both medical academicians and local practitioners (who despised one another) and also the early health crusaders who hoped to eradicate diseases and reduce the need for doctors. It was not foreseen that the need would increase—that as medical science advanced, people lived longer, and the population increased, the demand for medical care would rise.

To pressure such a rigid, restrictive, professionally elite, economically royal system for study and treatment of disease by increasing the mass' power to purchase its services is as apt to lead to conflict, waste, and poor care as it is to expansion of capacity to serve—unless *preceded* by a rationally-planned, long-range plan of capital development for the expansion of manpower and system. This includes a major investment in allied professional and subprofessional health workers who would act as service expanders.

Our health history is flagged with warnings. Due to the politicians' weakness for doing what is popular and hopefully noncontroversial, government health policy since Truman largely has been directed to stimulating public demand and increasing purchasing power. Briefly, the most spectacular effort has been $10 billion in grants to medical centers for biomedical research, an exciting and wholly desirable quest for knowledge. With the help of the press, however, this effort has oversold the public on the possibility of medical miracles—new "cures for death"—while people keep on sickening and dying from the various "dread diseases." The eventual outcome we are observing now has been disenchantment and economic backlash.

The research money has kept the medical schools alive and growing —growing more interested in research and less interested in their primary mission of training practicing physicians, more interested in the laboratory than community service. So interpreted, the acts of Congress have contributed to the sharp decline of interest in family practice and to the generally slow pace of medical-manpower development.

Another example is the Hill-Burton hospital construction program, a great success story in providing hospital beds for sick Americans through a matching program totalling nearly $10 billion. Some 3,700 communities have been able to build hospitals and nursing homes. But this was a bricks-and-mortar proposition, unconcerned with providing brains, hands, or system, with the result that many hospitals or hospital wings long stood vacant for lack of staff; some still have closed-off wards. Review of noble efforts is a thankless task, but we must note that the Hill-Burton program favored rural hospital construction during an era in which needy people were moving into the inner city, now a medical-disaster area.

Together with Blue Cross, Hill-Burton made it possible for hospitals to do in the most expensive way what might be done more cheaply by keeping patients at home, provided the ambulatory services were available and insured. As Hospital Consultant Anthony Rourke once said: "A built bed is a filt bed."

Medicare, a combination of federal subsidy and voluntary insurance for the aged, was a presidential campaign issue in 1960. Millions of elderly people organized, raised their voices, and voted for Johnson in 1964. The AMA contributed its usual verbal violence in another expensive campaign against a federally based program, but this time it was overpowered and beaten by act of Congress in 1965. Included in the Medicare legislation was Medicaid, a federal-state matching, state-administered program paying medical bills for the poor. Medicare has been a moderate success, though costing much more than expected. Medicaid has been a scandal, in the use-and-abuse column, in red tape, and skying costs. Together, these programs now cost about $10 billion a year, or more than 75% of the federal health budget.

Noting that medical bills are rising almost twice as fast as the cost of living, and that doctors angrily resist any effort to control quality or cost of their services, Rashi Fein, economist discusses the consequences in timid government policy: "After a bruising political battle to enact Medicare and Medicaid, government extended a hand of friendship to the medical community . . . by signing a blank check. . . . The medical community was gracious and accepted the offer. And prices—discretionary prices—rose. Did we expect to change the whole financial structure and have prices stay the same? There was, after all, a whole history of behavior under Blue Cross and Blue Shield . . . a history of fee increases paid for by insurance companies (and ultimately the consumer) because the physician and others could more readily raise their fees to that impersonal thing called an insurance company than to the individual patient. But that history was forgotten or ignored."

Will it be again? Will this "unfortunate experience," acknowledged by Dr. Isadore S. Falk, principal architect of the Reuther plan, and blamed on lack of manpower and system, remain in view in the heat of battle, when the AMA once more mobilizes against "socialized medicine"? The fight will be about insurance. Manpower and system meanwhile may be neglected.

The mistake the UHI crusaders seem to be making is both one of logic and tactics. Tactically, to propose a federally controlled medical-care system to the private medical profession is a bit like the Japanese attack on Pearl Harbor—it was an effective way to unite Americans in total defense of their country. The logic does not take into account the low interest the public commonly exhibits in comprehensive health-care services. Indeed, the public often has to be educated to use what is available. It has been observed that financing mechanisms largely or wholly eliminating the economic barrier to medical care do not consistently stimulate either demand or supply. Sweden, as a case in point, is often cited both for its superior mortality rates and its presumably related payment system (the government reimburses the patient for 75% of all medical costs). Yet Swedes visit their doctors only about half as much as do Americans. What has occurred in Sweden, as in Great Britain, Germany, and in the United States, is an overutilization of hospital beds in the absence of enough manpower and more appropriate and less costly services in the community. Medicare and Medicaid increased purchasing power without considering what would be available for purchase; it thereby increased the demand for hospitalization and the opportunity for a largely closed and already overloaded system to increase its charges.

The Nixon administration's proposed budget for health rose from \$13.2 to \$14.9 billion from fiscal 1970 to 1971, about 78% of the \$1.7 billion increase coming from the continued spiral in Medicare and Medicaid costs. It does not take a Ph.D. in economics to appreciate that, in a period of attempted deflation, the more the federal government spends on the purchasing of services the less it can spend on expansion and improvement of these services.

Agitation for universal health insurance at this time, in my opinion, sets a new record for short-sightedness. I say this in full recognition that the mistakes made in the past, a la Santayana, are themselves hard to exceed.

It is also worth noting, finally, that—President Nixon's apparent conviction to the contrary—federal investment in expansion of health-care resources—increased supply—should in the long run prove anti-inflationary. In the short run, the president has inherited an inflationary national policy in health from the Democrats and has continued to pursue it.

Conclusion

I have identified questions, as I said that I should, without coming up with satisfactory answers. Perhaps what I am implying is that when we must depend on politics to determine action on health plans, there is no satisfactory answer. The vital pressure point, I am convinced, lies in the organization and action of actual consumers, in keeping with that well-worn cliché: "When the public speaks, the public will be heard." In its personal and categorical interests, you might say the public has spoken and has been heard; it also has been exploited and misled.

I should like to see the rise of a general health-consumers' organization, but I do not quite see what will motivate it or who will lead it. And, if it did come into being, I do not quite see how it would accomplish what should be done, for what should be done is rational and objective, whereas public appeal and political pressures spring from emotional and subjective sources. More and more I am persuaded by the words of Walt Whitman: "It is provided in the very essence of things that from any fruition of success, no matter what, shall come forth something to make a great struggle necessary."

TOLLUND MAN AND OTHER BOG BURIALS

The map of Europe reveals that large areas of bog are to be found in Denmark (especially in Jutland) and in northern Germany. In these regions the encroachment of vegetation has converted lakes into deposits of peat. By geologic standards the alteration is regarded as relatively rapid. To this process the comparatively shallow glacial lakes are quite susceptible; and the regions just mentioned were all subject to glaciation during the Pleistocene epoch.

The peat bogs thus created are filled with vegetable debris, which forms an acid soil highly favorable to the preservation of human soft tissues. Accordingly, some of the most interesting discoveries in human paleontology have been made in the bogs of northern Europe. The number of these cadavers (the so-called *Moorleichen*) is estimated at somewhat less than 700, of which 166 are from Denmark.

In 1950 in a peat bog at Tollund, near Silkeborg in the Danish peninsula of Jutland, a singularly well-preserved human cadaver was found.[1] It is remarkable not only because of the relatively good condition of the soft tissues but also because of the startling lifelike appearance of the face (see accompanying figure).

The cadaver is that of an adult male. It was found under about seven feet of peat and was lying on its right side, with lower limbs drawn upward toward the torso. One hand was placed immediately above the knees, the other was near the chin.

The body was unclothed, except for a pointed sewn hat made of fur and a belt made of hide. Around the neck there was a tightly fastened rope made of hide and formed into a noose. This rope had produced deep linear impressions at the side of the neck and under the chin; the knot had left no mark. The rope was a meter long and its free end had been cut off sharply. These facts signified that the man had been hanged and then cut down. Since the cervical vertebrae were decalcified, confirmatory roentgen evidence of vertebral damage could not be obtained.

The well-preserved intestinal tract contained the remains of a meal

1. Thorvildsen, K.: *The Tollund Man.* Fred Mallett, transl. Silkeborg, Silkeborg Museum, 1962. 16 pp.

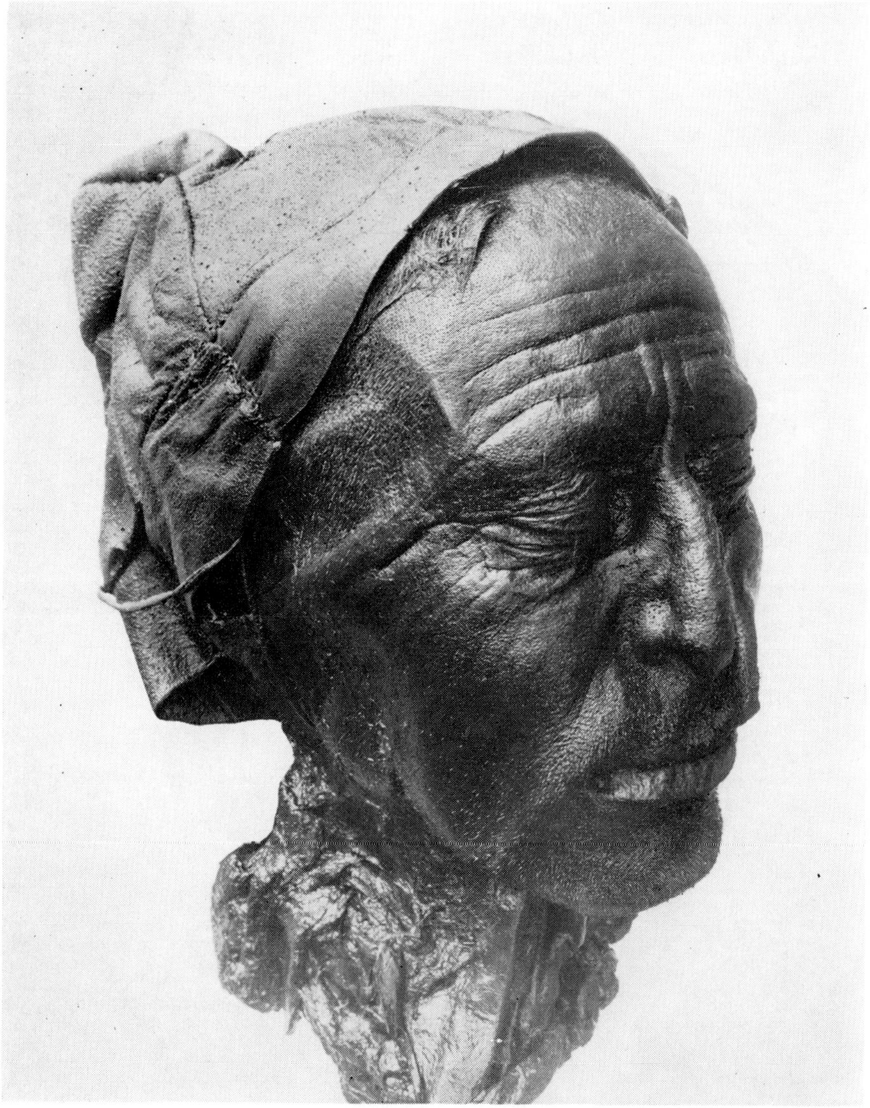

Head of Tollund Man.
Reproduced by courtesy of the National Museum, Copenhagen, Denmark.

eaten between 12 and 24 hours before death. It consisted of a sort of porridge containing such vegetable materials as barley and flaxseed. There were no residues of meat. It was inferred that death had occurred during the winter.

The cadaver of Tollund Man is dated at 1-200 A.D. In the opinion of Thorvildsen,[2] on whose account these notes are based, Tollund Man and a cadaver found nearby in a peat bog at Grauballe were victims of ritual manslaughter, the alternative possibility being that they were criminals and were executed.

There are several passages in the *Germania* of Tacitus (ca. 98 A.D.) which throw light on the death of Tollund man, without being fully decisive; one of these is quoted by Thorvildsen.[3] There are also a few smaller Tacitean fragments that deserve consideration, since Tollund man is thought to have lived at a time not very distant from that in which Tacitus wrote.

The Roman historian says of the German tribes as a whole that many men who had survived a war terminated their disgrace with a noose,[4] i.e., cowardice in battle might be punished by hanging. Any large punishment such as capital punishment, imprisonment, or even a blow, might be administered only by priests.[5]

Tacitus also remarks that when the death penalty was exacted, the manner of its imposition differed according to the crime. Traitors and deserters were hanged from trees, whereas cowards and persons of vicious habits were plunged in the mud of marshes with a hurdle on their heads.[6] If trees were customarily used for hanging, it is reasonable to infer that Tollund man was hanged on solid ground and was later thrown or buried in the bog where the body was found. We may add this inference to the collection of observations made by the archaeologists.

From another statement in the *Germania*[7] it is apparent that among the Germans—with whom Tacitus includes the inhabitants of Holland, Denmark, and Sweden—the dead were usually cremated.[7]

Finally, in telling of tribes that lived in and about the peninsula of Jutland, Tacitus says that in general they worshipped a divinity called

2. Thorvildsen, op. cit., pp. 14-15.
3. Tacitus, *Germania* 40; Thorvildsen, op. cit., pp. 14-15.
4. Tacitus, *Germania* 6.
5. Tacitus, *Germania* 7.
6. Tacitus, *Germania* 12. The use of a hurdle to add ignominy to punishment is also mentioned in Livy, I. 51. 9.
7. Tacitus, *Germania* 27.

Nerthus or Mother Earth—*in commune Nerthum, id est Terram matrem colunt*—and believed that she intervened in the affairs of human beings.[8] It is therefore probable, as Thorvildsen believes, that Tollund Man was sacrificed to this divinity. If Tacitus is right in stating that capital punishment could be inflicted by the priesthood only, the distinction between judicial and sacerdotal execution must have been tenuous.

Addendum. Since the above was written I have received the volume by P. V. Glob, *The Bog People; Iron-Age Man Preserved*, translated into English by Rupert Bruce-Mitford.[9] In this clear and well-written account the reader will find much additional information.

S.J.

8. Tacitus, *Germania* 40.
9. London, Faber and Faber, 1969, 200 pp., 76 illus., 2 maps.

EFFECTS OF THE AMERICAN REVOLUTION

I shall first mention the effects of the military, and, secondly, of the political events of the revolution. The last must be considered in a two-fold view, accordingly as they affected the friends, or the enemies, of the revolution.

I. In treating of the effects of the military events, I shall take notice, first, of the influence of *actual* war, and, secondly, of the influence of the military life.

In the beginning of a battle, I have observed *thirst* to be a very common sensation among both officers and soldiers. It occurred where no exercise, or action of the body, could have excited it.

Many officers have informed me, that after the first onset in a battle they felt a glow of heat, so universal as to be perceptible in both their ears. This was the case, in a particular manner, in the battle of Princeton, on the third of January, in the year 1777, on which day the weather was remarkably cold.

A veteran colonel of a New England regiment, whom I visited at Princeton, and who was wounded in the hand at the battle of Monmouth, on the 28th of June, 1778 (a day in which the mercury stood at 90° of Fahrenheit's thermometer) after describing his situation at the time he received his wound, concluded his story by remarking, "that fighting was hot work on a cold day, but much more so on a warm day." The many instances which appeared after that memorable battle, of soldiers who were found among the slain without any marks of wounds or violence upon their bodies, were probably occasioned by the heat excited in the body, by the emotions of the mind, being added to that of the atmosphere.

Soldiers bore operations of every kind, immediately *after* a battle, with much more fortitude than they did at any time afterwards.

The effects of the military life upon the human body come next to be considered under this head.

In another place I have mentioned three cases of pulmonary consumption being perfectly cured by the diet and hardships of a camp life.

Doctor Blane, in his valuable observations on the diseases incident to seamen, ascribes the extraordinary healthiness of the British fleet in the month of April, 1782, to the effects produced on the spirit of the soldiers and seamen, by the victory obtained over the French fleet on the 12th of that month; and relates upon the authority of Mr. Ives, an instance, in the war between Great Britain and the combined powers of France and Spain, in 1744, in which the scurvy, as well as other diseases, were checked by the prospect of a naval engagement.

The American army furnished an instance of the effects of victory upon the human mind, which may serve to establish the inferences from the facts related by Doctor Blane. The Philadelphia militia who joined the remains of General Washington's army, in December, 1776, and shared with them a few days afterwards in the capture of a large body of Hessians at Trenton, consisted of 1500 men, most of whom had been accustomed to the habits of a city life.

These men slept in tents and barns, and sometimes in the open air, during the usual colds of December and January; and yet there were but two instances of sickness, and only one of death, in that body of men in the course of nearly six weeks, in those winter months. This extraordinary healthiness of so great a number of men, under such trying circumstances, can only be ascribed to the vigour infused into the human body by the victory of Trenton having produced insensibility to all the usual remote causes of disease.

Militia officers and soldiers, who enjoyed good health during a campaign, were often affected by fevers, and other diseases, as soon as they returned to their respective homes. I knew one instance of a militia captain, who was seized with convulsions the first night he lay on a feather bed, after sleeping several months on a matrass, or upon the ground. These affections of the body appeared to be produced only by the sudden abstraction of that tone in the system, which was excited by a sense of danger, and the other invigorating objects of a military life.

The NOSTALGIA of Doctor Cullen, or the *home-sickness*, was a frequent disease in the American army, more especially among the soldiers of the New England states. But this disease was suspended by the superior action of the mind, under the influence of the principles which governed common soldiers in the American army. Of this General Gates furnished me with a remarkable instance in 1776, soon after his return from the command of a large body of regular troops and militia at Ticonderoga. From the effects of the nostalgia, and the feebleness of the discipline which was exercised over the militia, desertions were very frequent and numerous in his army, in the latter part of the campaign; and yet during the *three weeks* in which the general expected every hour an attack to be made upon him by General Burgoyne, there was not a single desertion from his army, which consisted at that time of 10,000 men.

The patience, firmness and magnanimity, with which the officers and soldiers of the American army endured the complicated evils of hunger, cold and nakedness, can only be ascribed to an insensibility of body produced by an uncommon tone of mind, excited by the love of liberty and their country.

Before I proceed to the second general division of this subject, I shall take notice, that more instances of apoplexy occurred in the city of Philadelphia, in the winter of 1774-5, than had been known in former years. I should have hesitated in recording this fact, had I not found the observations supported by a fact of the same kind, and produced by a nearly similar cause, in the appendix to the practical works of Doctor Baglivi, professor of physic and anatomy at Rome. After a very wet season in the winter of 1694-5, he informs us, that "apoplexies displayed their rage; and perhaps (adds our author) some part of this epidemic illness was owing to the universal grief and domestic care, occasioned by all Europe being engaged in a war. All commerce was disturbed, and all the avenues of peace blocked up, so that the strongest heart could scarcely bear the thoughts of it." The winter of 1774-5 was a period of uncommon anxiety among the citizens of America. Every countenance wore the marks of painful solicitude for the event of a petition to the throne of Britain, which was to determine whether reconciliation, or a civil war, with all its terrible and distressing consequences, were to take place.

The apoplectic fit, which deprived the world of the talents and virtues of Peyton Randolph, while he filled the chair of congress, in 1775, appeared to be occasioned in part by the pressure of the uncertainty of those great events upon his mind. To the name of this illustrious patriot, several others might be added, who were affected by the apoplexy in the same memorable year. At this time a difference of opinion upon the subject of the contest with Great Britain had scarcely taken place among the citizens of America.

II. The political events of the revolution produced different effects upon the human body, through the medium of the mind, according as they acted upon the friends or enemies of the revolution.

I shall first describe its effects upon the former class of citizens of the United States.

Many persons, of infirm and delicate habits, were restored to perfect health, by the change of place, or occupations, to which the war exposed them. This was the case in a more especial manner with hysterical women, who were much interested in the successful issue of the contest. The same effects of a civil war upon the hysteria, were observed by Doctor Cullen in Scotland, in the years 1745 and 1746. It may perhaps help to extend our ideas of the influence of the passions upon diseases, to add, that when either love, jealousy, grief, or even devotion, wholly engross the female mind, they seldom fail, in like manner, to cure or to suspend hysterical complaints.

An uncommon cheerfulness prevailed every where, among the friends of the revolution. Defeats, and even the loss of relations and property, were soon forgotten in the great objects of the war.

The population in the United States was more rapid from births during the war, than it had ever been in the number of years since the settlement of the country.

I am disposed to ascribe this increase of births *chiefly* to the quantity and extensive circulation of money, and to the facility of procuring the means of subsistence during the war, which favoured marriages among the labouring part of the people. But I have sufficient documents to prove, that marriages were more fruitful than in former years, and that a considerable number of unfruitful marriages, became fruitful during the war. In 1783 the year of the peace, there were several children born of parents who had lived many years together without issue. . . .

Rush, Benjamin: *An Account of the Influence of the Military and Political Events of the American Revolution upon the Human Body*. In Medical Inquiries and Observations, 5th ed., vol. 1., pp. 128-32. Philadelphia, Carey, 1818.

Just Published —

EPSTEIN, C. **$6.95**

INTERGROUP RELATIONS FOR POLICE OFFICERS. IX, 194 pages, (1962) Reprint 1970

Also Available —

KOOS, EARL L. **$6.00**

THE HEALTH OF REGIONVILLE. XIV, 177 pages, 21 illus. (1954) Reprint 1967

McKEOWN, THOMAS **$5.25**

MEDICINE IN MODERN SOCIETY. 324 pages, illus., maps. 1966

MALLORY, F. B. **$13.50**

PATHOLOGICAL TECHNIQUE. 434 pages, illus. (1938) Reprint 1968

HAFNER PUBLISHING COMPANY

DEPT. A — BOX 2000

DARIEN, CONN. 06820

Over 5 million prescriptions already filled at Macy*s

All 13 Macy Prescription Centres satisfy your patients with efficient professional service

- You may phone in your patients' prescriptions (except for narcotics, amphetamines, and barbiturates).
- Your patients may charge their prescriptions on their Macy Shopping Accounts or C-T Plans.
- Your patients may have their prescriptions delivered anywhere free of extra charge.
- We serve your patient with a full line of convalescent and diabetic needs.

Macy's Herald Square, OX 5-4400
Macy's Parkchester, TA 8-7000
Macy's Jamaica, OL 7-9000
Macy's Flatbush, UL 6-5000
Macy's Roosevelt Field, PI 6-8200
Macy's Huntington, AR 1-3000
Macy's White Plains, WH 6-5015
Macy's New Haven, Conn. 624-9271
Macy's Bay Shore, MO 5-8400
Macy's Queens, AR 1-9100
Macy's Colonie, 459-1950
Macy's New Rochelle, 633-7700
Macy's Smith Haven, 724-4900

BULLETIN OF
THE NEW YORK ACADEMY
OF MEDICINE

VOL. 46, NO. 8 AUGUST 1970

NINETEENTH CENTURY WOUND MANAGEMENT OF THE PARTURIENT UTERUS AND COMPOUND FRACTURE: THE SEMMELWEIS-LISTER PRIORITY CONTROVERSY*

OWEN H. WANGENSTEEN

Regents Professor of Surgery
University of Minnesota Medical School
Minneapolis, Minn.

THE mid-19th century was a period of exciting ferment for medicine. The significant contributions of Vesalius[1] (1543) and Harvey[2] (1628) had much importance for the advance of anatomy, pathology, and physiology. However, their impact upon practical medicine and surgery was miniscule contrasted with the biological revolution that emerged after the discoveries of Pasteur,[3] which lit the way for Lister's (1867-1875) great impress upon surgery.[4] Koch's (1878-1882) development of cultural methods[5] gave birth to experimental microbiology, making assessment of bacterial virulence possible. When Koch demon-

*Presented at a meeting of the Section on Historical Medicine, December 10, 1969.
These studies were supported by Public Health Service Research Grant No. 1 RO1-LM-00050-03 of the History of Life Sciences Study Section, National Institutes of Health, Bethesda, Md., and by the Alice M. O'Brien Foundation and the Frederick and Margaret L. Weyerhaeuser Foundation, St. Paul, Minn.

strated his plate cultures at the International Medical Congress in London (1881), Pasteur is said to have rushed forward with the exclamation: "*C'est un grand progrès!*"[6] Ehrenberg's[7] monograph of 1838 had depicted and described bacteria but pragmatic clinicians took no note of them. Henle's[8] *Von den Miasmen und Kontagien* (1840) shifted the explanation of disease transmittal from "pestilential emanations" from bogs and swamps to microbial origin, though the designation "microbe" had to wait another 36 years.

Semmelweis'[9] astute inference, stemming from the death of his obstetrical colleague, Jakob Kolletschka (1847), was highly significant for understanding of the nature of puerperal fever, its transmittal, and its prevention. It is a unique example of penetrating insight without parallel in the history of medicine.

It is the purpose of this presentation to survey the practices of this period from 1847 to 1880 with special reference to the management of the wounds of compound fracture and of the parturient uterus. Examination of the contributions to practical wound management during this period will provide evidence that sheds light on the long-standing controversy between Semmelweis and Lister concerning priority of discovery.

Infection Still Challenges the Surgeon

Acceptance of antiseptics and asepsis did not eliminate the threat of infection in surgical procedures. Complete asepsis in operations is still to be achieved. During the lifetime of younger members of this audience, systemic chemotherapeutic and antibiotic agents virtually eliminated cellulitic infections. However, the less threatening staphylococcus of my training days is today the bête noire of hospitals and surgeons.

Over the centuries, before sulfanilamide and antibiotics became available, a number of promising young physicians lost their lives from fingerpricks sustained during work. Hunczkovsky (1798), Kolletschka (1847), Semmelweis (1865), and Curt Schimmelbusch (1895) were snuffed out in this manner. Dr. William Murray (1926), our professor of ophthalmology, pricked his finger during a myringotomy for otitis media. In desperation his arm was amputated but he died a few days later. One of my contemporaries, Lucy Wilder, a graduate student in anatomy, working with a culture of streptococcus, let a drop fall on her forearm. She suffered a scratch at the site while injecting a rabbit. A few days later she died of septicemia. Even today the problem of infection follows the surgeon like his shadow and is a significant factor in most deaths after operation.

Antisepsis in many of its aspects extends back into antiquity. In the history of ideas, the microscope and techniques of growing and staining bacteria and using heat to destroy them contributed more to the surgeon's ability to cope with infection than all prior practices.

Elective Operations before Antisepsis

Theodoric, bishop of Cervia, and Henri de Mondeville, 13th-century surgeons, had striven for primary union of contaminated wounds.[10] Any compromise with this objective has been frowned upon by many historians of surgery. Yet in studies of the story of amputation it was noted that pre-Listerian surgeons such as Edward Alanson (1782), Vincenz von Kern (1809), Robert Liston (1837-1841), and A. Carl von Burow (1859-1873), all of whom left the wound open, achieved a rate of success unmatched until the arrival of aseptic surgery at the beginning of the 20th century.[11] Likewise Cl. Pouteau (1760) and William Cheselden (1723) and a few other skilled operators who performed lithotomy and left the perineal wound open to be washed by urine achieved records not surpassed until the aseptic era.[12] The explanation came only when Theodor Billroth (1865) showed that granulating wounds were far less susceptible than fresh wounds to invasive pyogenic organisms.[13]

Perusal of the literature of intestinal obstruction indicates that long before the days of antiseptic surgery, some surgeons had a record of accomplishment with external strangulated hernia and internal strangulation that deserves study. Astley Cooper, who was quite restrained in recommending operation for strangulated hernia, tried having the patient carried about the ward in the inverted posture over the shoulders of a strong ward attendant, hoping thereby for spontaneous reduction.[14] He recommended enemas of tobacco and suggested that surgeons who neglected this procedure did not appreciate its merit.[15] Yet a thorough search of Cooper's text indicates that his mortality of 42% for surgical relief of strangulated hernia in the first quarter of the 19th century was not grossly in excess of that of modern-day surgeons performing intestinal resection for that condition. Obviously

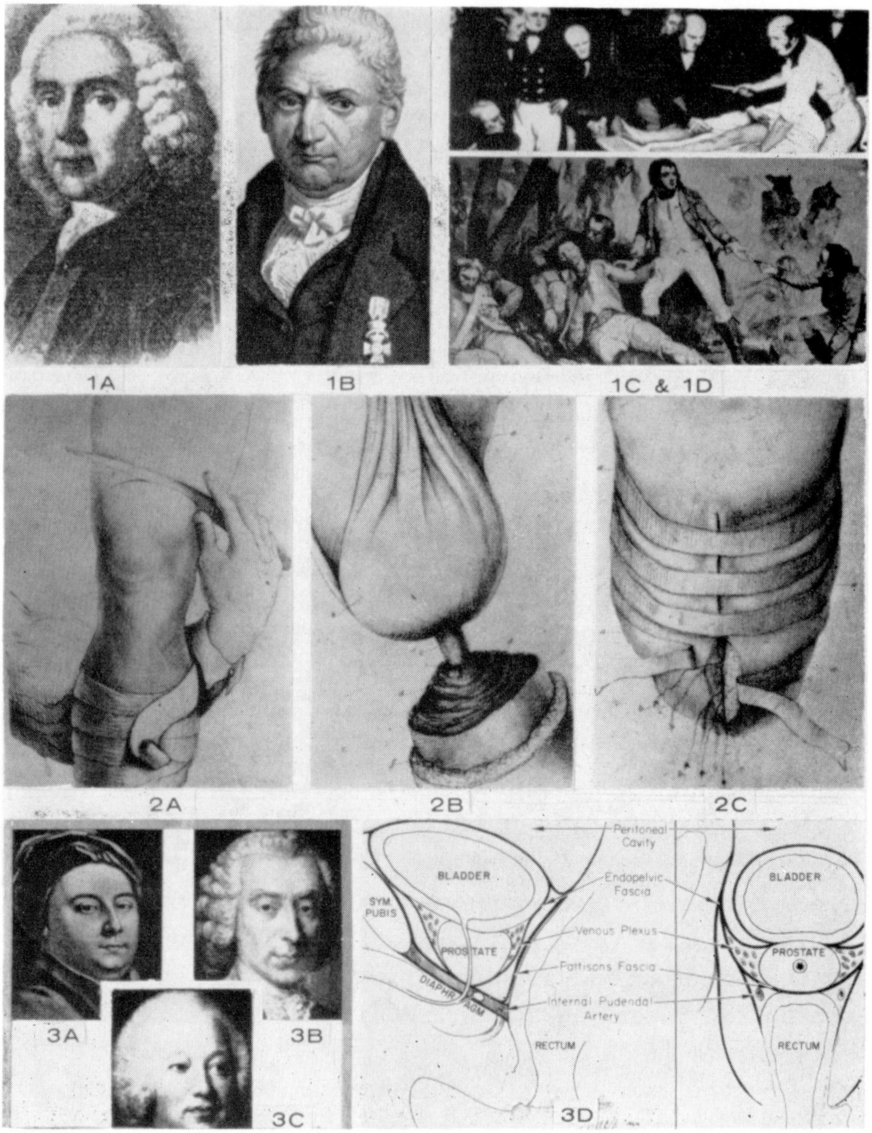

Figs. 1-3. *Eighteenth and nineteenth century amputation.* 1*a*. Monro, *b*. von Kern, *c*. Liston. *d*. Larrey. Fig. 2. Charles Bell's sketch of thigh amputation. Fig. 3. *Heroes of perineal lithotomy*. *a*. Cheselden. *b*. Pouteau. *c*. Louis. *d*. Anatomy of perineal lithotomy operation.

surgeons are not yet as alert as they should be to the threat of intestinal strangulation.

Some French surgeons more than two centuries ago in the heyday of the Royal Academy of Surgery had successes with internal strangulation which would surprise if not startle today's specialist. The only difference is that the French surgeon, after excising the dead bowel, left the adjacent viable open ends in the wound. Moreover, he occasionally was able to reestablish intestinal continuity by mobilizing and approximating the two stomas in the wound.[16] All this, mind you, before the days of anesthesia and antisepsis!

Intestinal resection obviously is a far more delicate operation than excision of an ovarian cyst. Yet ovariotomy (1809) had to await the pioneering courage of Ephraim McDowell of Danville, Ky.[17] His innovation came 75 years after intrepid French surgeons had dealt successfully with internal intestinal strangulations. The reasons for this long hiatus are not easy to find, but aspiration of ovarian cysts frequently provided temporary relief and could be repeated. Puncture through the rectum was done occasionally in the hope that the cyst would be permanently drained, a rather dangerous expedient, as subsequent events demonstrated.

Pre-Listerian Antiseptic Wound Practices

The long history of surgery is replete with accounts of the use of various agents now known to have antiseptic qualities. The wise men of the East brought gold, frankincense, and myrrh to the Christ child,[18] token gifts of great worth in that day. Myrrh and spirits of wine or alcohol and vinegar were favored in wound management by many surgeons. No surgeon, however, followed a course in which trials were made with consecutive use of a single medium now known to be antiseptic.

Turpentine stands out prominently as one of the most effective agents and one which early enjoyed wide use. John Woodall spoke of it often as good wound therapy in his *Surgeons Mate* (1655).[19] Matthaeus G. Purmann (1699) used turpentine with other ingredients in the management of compound fractures,[20] as did Johann von Muralt (1691).[21]

Other agents which have proved on assessment to have demonstrable antibacterial activity are alcohol, ammonium chloride in combination with alcohol, vinegar or turpentine, ferric chloride, balsam of Peru, creosote, and zinc chloride. The story is too long to tell here but a number of surgeons, especially in the mid-19th century, documented series of cases in which such antiseptic agents were used with surprising and gratifying success in wound management. Lemaire[22] and Déclat[23] in Paris had anticipated Lister in the use of phenol, but unfortunately recommended it for many types of wounds, making critical assessment difficult. What the agents actually did was not understood until the germ theory of disease and the pathogenicity of bacteria became generally known.

Hippocrates' management of fractures has a modern ring. For compound fractures he advocated keeping the wound moist, and he placed a goatskin beneath the extremity in order to carry fluid away from the wound. He also used pitch cerate (turpentine) and wine dressings,[24] practices, says Malgaigne, that were continued by Celsus, Galen, and Avicenna. Malgaigne[25] relates that Ambroise Paré was a keen advocate of water irrigation for many types of wounds, including compound fracture,* an attitude shared by two later celebrated French military surgeons, Pierre-François Percy and Dominique-Jean Larrey of Napoleon's army.[28]

Henry Yates Carter (1792-1795), the Englishman, employed dressings soaked in a solution of vinegar and 3% ammonium chloride (sal ammoniac) for severe wounds and compound fractures. Occasionally he added 6% turpentine. Of 8 patients with severe wounds or compound fractures, in which the wounds were left open and treated in this manner, only one died, from shock, attending an accident which had severed the upper thigh and scrotum.[29, 30]

A unique effort was made by Jules Guyot (1835) to assess the effect of warm air upon wounds. For this purpose he built a square box into which he admitted air at temperatures of 30 to 40° and as high as 70° C. Preliminary experiments with the method were made on wounded rabbits. Jean-Edouard Laborie, an associate who participated in the experiments, reported 64 survival trials on 30 rabbits. Guyot concluded that the hot air had a beneficial influence on the wounds. Professor François Magendie, who had followed the study,

*Malgaigne admitted difficulty in defining the word "irrigation."[25] Perusal of Malgaigne's *Paré* would suggest that Paré more often used water dressings than irrigation.[26] The Pravaz syringe first became available in 1851. Three centuries after Paré, Billings related that when inducted as a surgeon in the Union Army (1861) he brought along a hypodermic syringe. It was in constant use, for no other surgeon had one.[27]

asked Professor Gilbert Breschet to try the method at the Hôtel Dieu. Observations were begun late in 1833 upon four patients with chronic ulcers. The first was submitted to a 36-hour trial with warmed air to the leg wound at an old fracture site; the oppressive heat, the patient insisted, damaged his lungs. The lesions of the three other patients apparently were all improved by the treatment. Laborie (1838) reported Guyot's observations in some detail "in the interest of science," believing the method had real merit.[31, 32]

During this same period, irrigations of cold water as devised by Bérard were being used enthusiastically in several Paris hospitals for compound fractures and other surgical wounds.[33, 34]

Macartney of Dublin (1836) recommended evaporation of water over a flame as an anti-inflammatory device in the management of all wounds, including compound fractures and battle injuries, noting that the vapor directed through a tube to the wound thwarted suppuration.[35] Vincent Nivet (1838) reported continuous water irrigation of the wound in compound fractures. Of nine patients treated in this manner, two died, a mortality of 22.2%.[36]

One of the most celebrated proponents of water dressings was Robert Liston. He "rode his hobby of water-dressing in the treatment of wounds rather hard," reminisced Erichsen in a fine account of Liston's successful open-wound therapy of the stump after amputation. "It was," says Erichsen, "the perfection of lightness compared with a poultice; the perfection of cleanliness contrasted with ointments. . . ."[37]

John Crowther (1802) wrote of the prevention of gangrene in compound fracture by a method, he said, that had been practiced with the greatest success by his ancestors near Halifax since time immemorial, being handed down from father to son. In his report Crowther related observation of 98 fractures from April 28, 1789, to October 5, 1800, of which 28 were compound; in none was there any evidence of gangrene. The same success, Crowther states, attended the practice of his two brothers William and Robert over many years.

It was the custom of the Crowthers to place "a large quantity of black basilicon ointment, made with tar instead of pitch, to be liquefied in an iron earthern pot, and made hot, then put into it with all dispatch a large pledget of tow, sufficient if possible to cover the whole wound, so as totally to exclude all external air." If one pledget was not sufficient to cover all the lacerated parts, another was applied. The tow was dipped into the hot ointment, then placed directly over the wound. John Crowther next put on a roller-bandage dressing moistened with vinegar. For later dressings smaller amounts of hot basilicon were used. When purulent discharge occurred during convalescence the dressing was applied cold. Such moist bandages were continued until the inflammation abated.[38]

Baron Larrey (1824) implanted styrax into the wounds of compound fractures. Styrax is an ingredient of compound tincture of benzoin, which is an effective antibacterial agent. Larrey applied linen coated with styrax, then compresses soaked in wine or in camphorated vinegar as a dressing over the wound, and immobilized the extremity in a splint. A many-tailed Scultetus bandage was next crossed many times in an oblique direction over the fracture area. This dressing was changed only once or twice during the entire period of treatment.

Larrey relates, "a dozen subjects of the Guard were treated in this manner in our hospital from 1821 to 1824 uniformly and successfully." He cites two instances of his cavalrymen who fell from their horses, suffering severe compound fractures of the leg. With extension and a liberal dressing of styrax and compresses of camphorated vinegar, amputation was avoided and the fractures mended.[39]

When Larrey (1766-1842) wrote this (1824), his illustrious war years were behind him. In earlier days he had been a strong protagonist of early amputation for fracture by gunshot and had severed as many as 200 limbs in a 24-hour period, an occurrence which provoked the Scottish military surgeon H. Home Blackadder (1818) to accuse him of "operative mania."[40] Great as was Larrey's fame as a military surgeon, he obviously did not have sufficient influence later to win Parisian civilian surgeons over to his conservative therapy. Why his suggestion or a variant thereof was not tested in some of the large Paris hospitals is a mystery. Moreover, in recounting his management of battle wounds (1830), Larrey made no allusion to his important paper of 1824.[41]

In his monograph on subcutaneous surgery, Adams (1857) cites the unusual record of success of the late Mr. Edward Bennion, of Oswestry in Shropshire, who treated compound fractures regularly with compound tincture of benzoin.* After reduction of the fracture, Bennion

*Sampson Gamgee (*On the Treatment of Wounds and Fractures: Clinical Lectures*, 2d ed., London, Churchill, 1883, p. 125) mentions Adams' reference to Bennion but incorrectly dates Adams' publication as 1867 instead of 1857.

soaked a large piece of lint in compound tincture of benzoin and encased the bandaged extremity in a splint, which remained untouched for a month if there were no symptoms. Adams added that Bennion's unusual success* with compound fractures was well known in that area.[42]

Bryant (1876), using a compound tincture of benzoin, treated 14 consecutive cases of compound fracture at Guy's Hospital without a death.[43] In 1861 Bryant had noted that mortality from compound fracture in the prior 20 years at the same hospital was 38.3%; for those treated conservatively it was 27.1%.[44]

A quest for information on the management of compound fractures in published monographs in the first three quarters of the 19th century proved very disappointing. This challenging facet of wound management seems to have been avoided studiously. The texts of Alexis Boyer (1805), Pierre-Joseph Desault (1817), Astley Cooper (1832), Lonsdale (1838), Guillaume Dupuytren (1847), and J. F. Malgaigne (1859) are virtually bare of helpful suggestions concerning compound fractures. Great surgical historian that he was, Malgaigne overlooked the significant contributions of Crowther (1802) and Larrey (1824).

A monograph with the promising title, *Mémoire sur cent fractures compliquées guéries*, by Jolieu (1843) offers little useful information. Several of the fractures described were compound. The author occasionally alludes to washing the wound. However, he usually avoids saying what the wash was. In one instance (p. 52) it was tincture of myrrh which, if it contained as much alcohol as the tincture currently available, would certainly have been a good antiseptic. In one case that went on to amputation because of gangrene, the amputation wound was dressed with *baume de Arceus*, of which the active agent is turpentine.[45]

Paré had barely escaped amputation for a compound fracture of the leg,[46] as did Pott two centuries later (1755).[47] Larrey's report of 1824 documents the beginning of a reaction against primary amputation for compound fracture in civilian practice,† yet amputation continued to be the order of the day in the Crimean War (1854-1856), our

*Charles Talbot of the Wellcome Institute of the History of Medicine turned up this item: "In the *Oswestry Advertiser* for 8 April, 1869, the following notice appears: 'In another column we record the death of Dr. E. D. Bennion. . . . He was perhaps best known as the son of the celebrated Dr. Edward Bennion whose fame for surgical skill extended over this and many neighboring counties.' "

†In a Paris thesis of the Listerian era, Biencourt (1873) said that, "Larrey and [Auguste] Bérard had changed the treatment of compound fracture completely."[48] If the practices of Crowther (1802), Larrey (1824), and Bennion (1857) had been adopted by the profession, Biencourt's statement could have been significant.

own Civil War (1861-1865), and the Franco-Prussian War (1870-1871). In the Russo-Turkish War of 1876-1877, in the hands of a young Russian military surgeon, Carl Reyher, extensive debridement and antiseptic wound management succeeded in replacing primary amputation.*[49, 50]

Anesthesia was a great boon to both patients and surgeons in the reduction of fractures and dislocations. Caldwell of Louisville (1838) reported successful reduction of a compound fracture of the thigh by bleeding 24 to 26 ounces, until the patient became limp. When traction was applied no muscular resistance was encountered. Caldwell placed a firm roller bandage dressing over the fracture site.[52]

Lister and Compound Fracture

A force necessary to drive a splintered bone through the muscular and cutaneous integuments obviously must be a great force, resulting almost invariably in heavy contamination of the wound. The risk attending incised wounds in the preantiseptic era was measured almost solely by the surgeon's standard of cleanliness. The mortality of simple fractures was minimal, that of compound fractures was always large. It was to this type of wound that Lister applied his carbolic-acid dressing. In his first series of 11 cases there were two compound fractures of the femur, one of which ended fatally.† The others were mainly compound fractures of the leg, undoubtedly the most frequent variety. One of these resulted in amputation; the ultimate fate of the patient was not stated.[6] Also, in 1867, in a Paris thesis, de Ségogne wrote of the application of alcohol to wounds. He mentions six patients with compound fractures treated with alcohol dressings without mortality, the first in 1864, the others apparently in 1867. In addition he tells of one of La Peyronie's patients (prior to 1747) treated successfully with local applications of coal tar and brandy. Lister's discernment of the origins of the hazard in open fracture is missing in de Ségogne's account.[56]

*Puschmann (1889) relates that "Schmucker (1738) saw a patient at the Hôtel Dieu in Paris who underwent bilateral thigh amputation for simple fracture"![51]

†Boyer (1808),[53] Banner (1843)[54] and Huguier (1856)[55] alluded to the greater mortality of compound fractures of the lower extremity, contrasted with similar fractures in the arm or forearm; the reasons are not entirely clear, but soft-tissue injury is undoubtedly one factor. In the first edition (1826, p. ix) of his monograph on the *Application of Lunar Caustic,* Higginbottom asked if the eschar produced could thereby "reduce the case to the state of a simple fracture"?, a question repeated in the second edition of 1829. In the third edition (1865), Higginbottom stated (p. 5): "The eschar from the nitrate of silver excludes the atmospheric air from the wound and so reduces the dangerous circumstance of compound fracture to that of a simple fracture, the wound being healed by the first intention."

Statistics

Florence Nightingale (1859) lamented that statistical materials were woefully incomplete.[57] The same could well be said of the results of operations. Accomplishment was so poor for most operations that surgeons were reluctant to publish their over-all experience. One can read through large tomes on fracture and find bare mention of the results in compound fractures. Great surgeons such as Liston, William Fergusson, and John Erichsen wrote monographs and discussed problems philosophically without providing an assessment of their own experiences.* Said Sir James Paget in 1862, "Every surgeon has lost a large proportion of his patients after those operations [hernia tracheotomy, and trephining]: but the operations themselves are very rarely the cause of death; the worst that can be said of them is that they do not always save lives. For myself, I have, as yet, scarcely lost a case in true consequence of either of these operations; yet nearly half of those cases that I have operated on for hernia have died, and more than half after tracheotomy, and nearly all after trephining. But these were deaths after operations; not because of them."[58]

Said Volkmann (1877), "It is not everyone who has the courage of my friend, Professor von Nussbaum, who . . . has not hesitated to put in print that of sixty-four thigh amputations performed in military and civil practice combined, during the sixteen years immediately preceding the introduction of antiseptics, he had only saved seven cases (89% mortality). After Nussbaum's admission, it is very easy for me to acknowledge that my own results were very little better. But now, since introduction of the antiseptic method of treating wounds, I get more successful cases in a single year than during the whole of my surgical career."[59] Acceptance by a few distinguished Continental surgeons—Danish, German, and Swiss—of the antiseptic management of compound fractures was the beginning of the end of stubborn resistance to Lister's practices though opposition lingered for almost a decade in high places in England and the United States.

*Alexander Miller, in his "Inquiry into the average mortality in Lithotomy cases" (1831, pp. 8-11), complained that reliable hospital statistics were rarely available. Marcet (1819, p. 24) wrote: "it is scarcely credible that in the largest hospitals of London, St. Bartholomew's, St. Thomas', Guy's and the London Hospital, no regular or at least no ostensible records of the cases of lithotomy . . . should be preserved." (*An Essay on the Chemical History and Medical Treatment of Calculous Disorders.*)

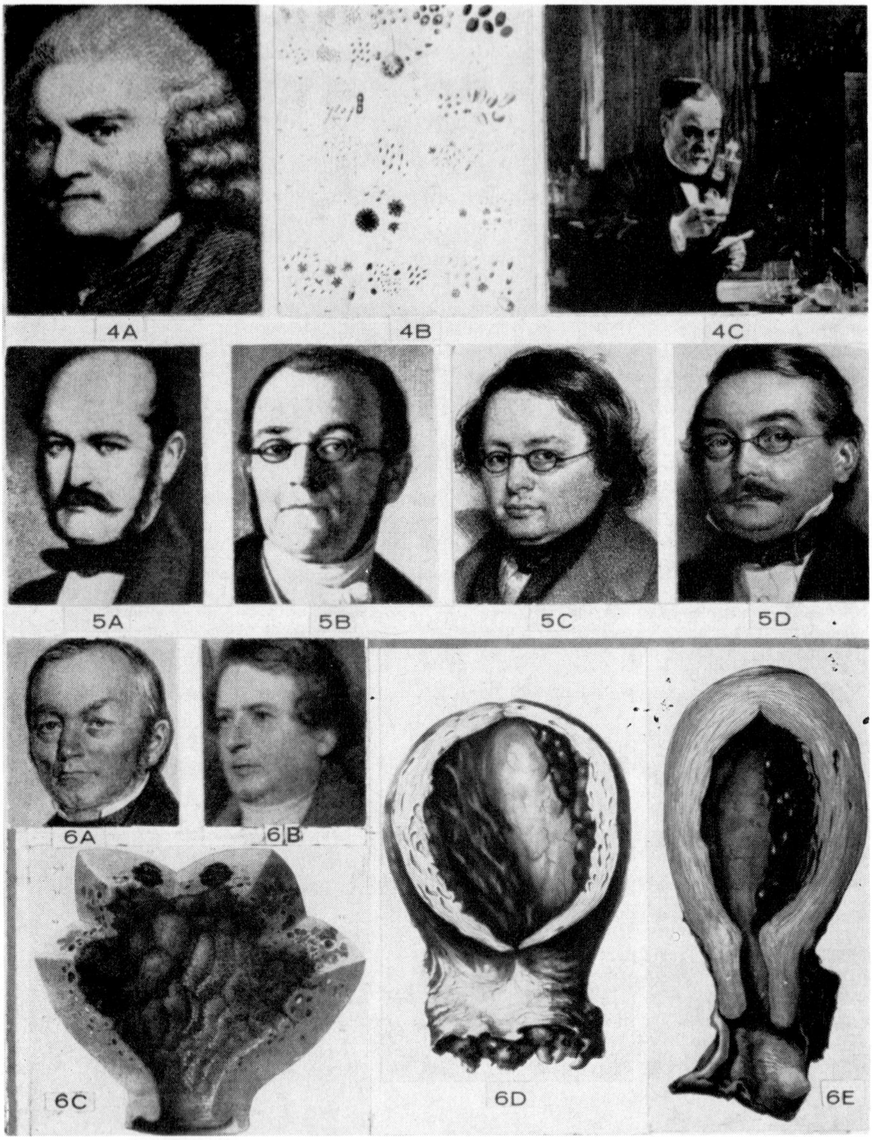

Figs. 4-6. *Puerperal fever.* 4*a*. Pringle, author of "antiseptic." *b*. Bacteria (Ehrenberg, 1838). *c*. Pasteur, who labeled streptococcus as cause, 1879. 5*a*. Semmelweis. *b*. Rokitansky. *c*. Skoda. *d*. von Hebra. 6*a*. Klein. *b*. Rosas. *c*. Gangrenous uterus, 4th day. *d*. Uterine wound after delivery. *e*. Normal uterine involution, 3d day.

Puerperal Fever

It is strange that large works on surgery often fail to mention puerperal fever, yet the post-partum uterus provides a big fresh raw wound. On basis of measurements provided by Lea (1910), the area can be said to be approximately 900 sq. cm.[60] A more recent evaluation by Kehrer (1952) is in general agreement: the placental attachment, the segment of greatest denudation, constitutes about one third the area.[61] This large wound is obviously a fertile source for bacterial implantation. The analogy, therefore, between wounds of the parturient canal and surface wounds is an acceptable parallelism and gives Semmelweis a significant place in the history of wound management.

Among the first to recognize the similarity between surgical wound infections and puerperal fever were Pouteau (1760) and Kirkland (1774).*[62] "Attentive examination" of the cadavers of women dead of puerperal fever revealed to Pouteau "ravages of an erysipelatous-like inflammation."[63] It remained, however, for James Simpson (1851-1856) to give this thesis articulate expression, an observation that apparently escaped Lister.[64, 65]

It is to be recalled that in mid-May, 1847, Semmelweis introduced into the obstetrical services at the Allgemeines Krankenhaus at the University of Vienna a technique that made an amazing impact upon the incidence and mortality of puerperal fever. As Semmelweis relates (1861), he instituted a plan of hand washing with warm soap and water, followed by thorough washing in chlorine solution until the hands became slippery. "Hands so treated," said Semmelweis, "are completely disinfected." He said further: "The carrier of decomposing materials is not alone the examining finger, but all situations and materials which are unclean and which come in contact with the patient's parturient canal." These agents too, Semmelweis insisted, must be similarly disinfected before use (p. 103). To this category Semmelweis assigned "instruments, bed cloths, sponges and washbasins, etc., etc." (p. 269).

The death of his colleague, Kolletschka, from a fingerprick sustained during a dissection performed on a patient dying of puerperal fever prompted Semmelweis to institute the chlorine hand-washing technique. Semmelweis' assessment included a study of the mortality

*Thomas Nunneley in a *Treatise on Erysipelas* (1841) emphasized the similarity of puerperal fever and erysipelas.

statistics for parturient women at the hospital. He found that between 1784 and 1823 the annual death rate was less than 1%, but that between 1822 and 1824, when medical students began to participate regularly in post-mortem dissections while on obstetric call, there was a significant rise in maternal mortality.

In the beginning Semmelweis stressed the importance of the surgeon's hands and fingers transporting putrescent materials from the dissection of fresh cadavers, many of which represented deaths from puerperal fever. However, having observed that puerperal fever was transmitted also from the lochia of a woman dying of cancer of the uterus and subsequently from a patient with purulent infection of the knee, Semmelweis in his publication of 1861 (p. 59) included decomposing animal-organic matter of whatever source (from utensils, instruments, linen), "living organisms" as sources of infection. Semmelweis rightly concluded that puerperal fever is not contagious save by contact with a source of infection or infected materials (pp. 103, 269). He also stated that such decomposed animal-organic material can be communicated by anatomists, surgeons, and patients on surgical stations (p. 106).

Semmelweis concludes his monograph (p. 537) by saying that in the not distant future the only instances of puerperal fever would occur through self-infection. Then he adds, "If I shall be denied the privilege of seeing with my own eyes the conquest of puerperal fever, the conviction, that sooner or later this thesis will find acceptance, will cheer my hour of death."[66]

One feature which distinguished the Semmelweis era (1847-1849) from the Listerian (1867-1878) was the change in status of the biological sciences. By the time of Lister, microscopy and cultural methods were beginning to be accepted by pathologists and clinicians, thus heralding the birth of the science of microbiology, to which the brilliant and consecutive labors of Pasteur (1862-1878), Koch (1878-1882), and others, lent great impetus.

When Semmelweis instituted chlorine hand washing as a routine procedure for the accoucheur, bacteria had been described by Ehrenberg (1838),[7] but for most clinicians his work had no meaning. Carl Rokitansky, in whose institute Semmelweis did his dissections, had at first abjured the microscope, as had John Hunter.*[67] Rokitansky's

*Rosas, who with Klein deprived Semmelweis of his appointment at the University of Vienna (1849), was a vigorous opponent of microscopy. His pupils could pursue microscopic studies in ophthalmology only behind locked doors.[68]

neglect of the microscope in his multivolume treatise on pathology (1842-1846) evoked severe censure from Virchow (1846). Had Rokitansky counseled Semmelweis to examine microscopically the lochia of parturient women, he probably would have observed the organisms which Ehrenberg depicted and which Pasteur later (1879) labeled as the cause of puerperal fever.[69] Yet Pasteur's announcement did not find ready acceptance amongst obstetricians in Paris.

Fleetwood Churchill (1849) collected the writings of several British students who wrote about puerperal fever before 1800.[70] Gordon (1795) recognized the relation of the attendant accoucheur to the origin of the disease but did not indicate how the contagion was conveyed, presumably on the accoucheur's raiment. He believed that if he could see the patient within the first 12 hours, there was an excellent chance of cure–the remedy was bleeding of 20 to 24 ounces and purgation![71]

Collins' brilliant work at the Dublin Rotunda Hospital* in reducing the incidence of puerperal fever by strict sanitary measures including fumigation of the obstetrical wards is especially noteworthy. Whitewashing all woodworks, including floors, walls, and ceilings with chloride of lime gave the hospital an air of cleanliness. Collins' low mortality record of maternal deaths, 0.54%, was the envy and goal of all obstetricians.[72] Collins, however, was unaware of how the contagion of puerperal fever was communicated. Since he was a 19th century obstetrician, his name was not included in Churchill's review, nor was that of Oliver Wendell Holmes (1843) who, like Gordon, recognized that the physician conveyed the infection. Holmes advised physicians to wash their hands in chloride of lime *after* visiting patients suffering from puerperal fever.[73]

In a very perceptive and painstaking effort Erna Lesky, professor of the history of medicine at the University of Vienna, has dissected the events leading up to Semmelweis' dismissal.[74] It was not simply a matter of difference between the pupil Semmelweis and his superior, Johann Klein, but more realistically a power struggle in the faculty between the old and the new. Johann L. Böer, Klein's preceptor and predecessor,

*Semmelweis had planned to work in the Rotunda obstetrical wards before his dismissal in Vienna (pp. xxvii and xxx).[66]

was deposed in 1822 from his position as chief of the University Obstetrical Service, to be replaced by Klein.*[75]

The crafty maneuverer, Anton E. von Rosas, professor of ophthalmology, and Klein represented the old; Rokitansky, who was dean of the faculty, J. Skoda, F. von Hebra, Carl Haller, Ernst Brücke, Dlauhy, Johann von Dumreicher, and others, the new. The year 1848 marked the coming of a revolution in Europe that extended from the Baltic to the Mediterranean, and the decision of the Ministry of Education in Vienna may have represented in part an entrenchment against innovation. In any case, in retrospect, the fact that Klein and Rosas, two undistinguished members of a great faculty, could offset the judgment and recommendations of Dean Rokitansky and a brilliant staff, defies understanding.

The Semmelweis-Lister Controversy: Priority of Discovery

Since publication of a brief paper on Preludes to Lister in 1965,† the centennial of Lister's first trials with phenol and compound fractures, I have continued to study the question of who was the inventor of antiseptic surgery. Pringle (1753) showed that putrefaction in small dead animals could be prevented by immersing the bodies in dilutions of mineral acids.[76] Semmelweis anticipated and *prevented* wound sepsis by the use of an antiseptic, chlorinated lime. His perceptive intuition is the more remarkable in that the germ theory of disease was still latent and had not been subjected to the test of trial and controversy. His cleansing and antiseptic treatment of the accoucheur's hands protected the parturient against infection and became the first overt systematic application of the antiseptic principle. Semmelweis' practice was antisepsis in the true sense.‡ Joseph Lister's was an attempt to control existing infection by the application of an antiseptic, carbolic acid, to the wound, a technique which has since been abandoned in favor of wound excision and revision.

*Boer employed the phantom rather than the cadaver to teach students the technique of delivery. He was conservative in his methods and followed the expectant plan of noninterference during descent of the unborn infant upon the mother's pelvic floor as opposed to the French school that favored instrumental delivery.[68] Boer has often been referred to as the founder of modern obstetrics. Semmelweis apparently had no direct contact with Boer, but probably was influenced by his teachings.

†Wangensteen, O. H.: Preludes to Lister and the interdependence of the sciences. *Surgery 58*:931-34, 1965.

‡Dr. Glenn E. Bartsch, associate professor of biometry, University of Minnesota, subjected the maternal mortality rates of the first Vienna Obstetrical Clinic (1784 to 1848) to statistical analysis. In the year 1819 and in the entire period from 1823 to 1846 the maternal mortality was excessively high, exceeding 3.66%. In the years 1847 and 1848, the maternal mortality was strikingly lower, 2.98 and 1.28% respectively. The test for Extreme Values indicates that these data have a high level of statistical significance ($p > .01$).

It has been said that Lister discovered antisepsis. Those who disaffirm this often suggest that he introduced a new principle; Lister himself called it the antiseptic principle. Of course, he did neither. Pringle (1750) coined the word "antiseptic."[77] Semmelweis (1847) recognized the mode of transmission of contagion and employed a solution of chlorinated lime to *prevent* puerperal fever, disinfecting all material likely to come in contact with the parturient's vaginal tract. Auguste Nélaton (1852-1864) had used alcohol in major elective surgery with considerable success.[11] What Lister did do was to introduce the scientific method in examining the effectiveness of a succession of antiseptic agents in wound management. Lister's test case was a good one, viz., compound fracture.

Who Is the Discoverer?

When the priority of discovery is debated, three items bear upon the issue: 1) Who first showed the way? 2) Continuance of the practice. 3) The influence of the discovery upon contemporary practice.

Semmelweis' insistence on disinfection of the accoucheur's hands and of all materials likely to come in contact with the large raw wound of the parturient uterus is a practice that is continued up to the present time. His shrewd assessment of the nature of contagion and puerperal fever has rarely been matched in medicine.

Lister's work had a more far-reaching significance for surgery. His first attack upon wound contamination was application of carbolic acid to the wound and efforts to minimize contamination from the air (carbolic-acid spray), accompanied by sterilization of the surgeon's hands and instruments with phenol.

Dakin's solution (Semmelweis' chlorine wash) found wide usage in World War I and the ensuing period until the arrival of sulfonamides. Lister's method of placing antiseptics in wounds has almost completely disappeared. Such chemical agents, while destroying bacteria, also damage tissues. Debridement is today the accepted remedy for compound fractures; it is complemented by forceful irrigation with saline solution (an old method) and administration of a broad-spectrum antibiotic. Long before Friedrich (1898)[78] demonstrated the efficacy of wide excision of an infected area when done within six hours, Reyher (1878) showed the value of extensive debridement of battle wounds. The surgery of World War I served to reemphasize this technique.[50]

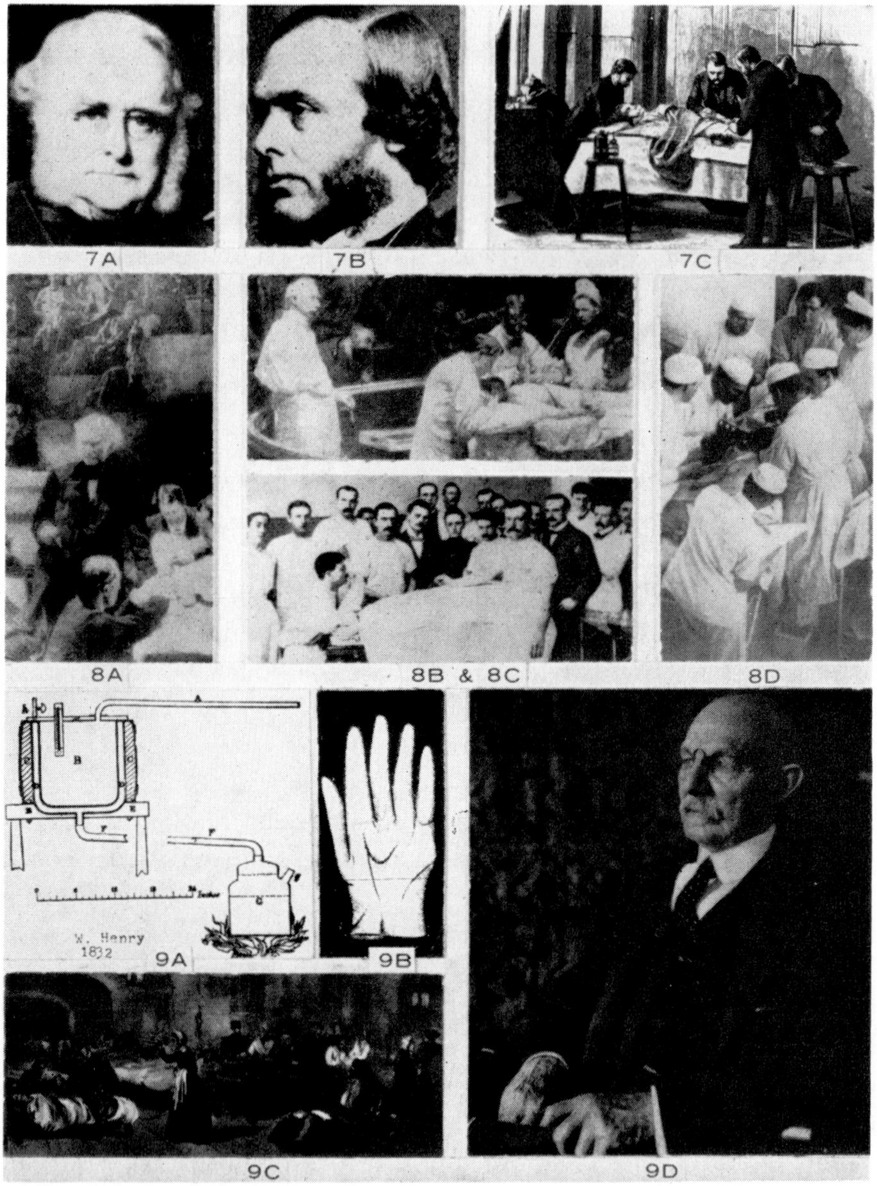

Figs. 7-9. Surgery progresses. *7a.* Spencer Wells, 1864. *b.* Lister, who used phenol in open fractures, 1867. *c.* Operation in Lister's clinic, ca. 1870. *8a.* Gross. *b.* Agnew, 1889. *c.* Kelly, *d.* Halsted operating, 1904. *9a.* Henry, sterilization. *b.* Forster, rubber gloves, 1878. *c.* Florence Nightingale, Crimea. *d.* Halsted.

Recent studies have shown that topical application of antibiotics in wounds does lessen the hazard of wound infection, but whether it is superior to systemic administration of antibiotics is questionable. The most effective agent, however, is adequate wound debridement.*

The medical world of Semmelweis' day was not ready to accept contamination of the accoucheur's hands as the source of puerperal fever. In this sense, the genius of Semmelweis was his own nemesis: he was too impatient with criticism which he felt was unwarranted and was reluctant to publish.† Semmelweis had already demonstrated that when the lochia from women with puerperal fever was placed in the vagina of female rabbits directly following delivery, sepsis did not occur if chlorinated lime also was introduced into the rabbit's vagina.[79]

Mayer (1862) found "vibrios" in the vaginal canal of multiparous women who complained of burning and itching of the vulva.[80] In May 1865 Mayrhoefer was able to demonstrate the presence of microorganisms in the lochia of women with puerperal fever.[81] Späth‡ (1864), at first an opponent of Semmelweis, noted the low mortality amongst *Gassengeburten* ("alley births," patients who delivered before reaching the hospital) was influenced by the success of Semmelweis' program of preventing contact infection and capitulated to his practices.[82]

Announcement of Discovery versus Proof of Its Validity

Is it the discoverer's responsibility, beyond the announcement, to effectuate adoption of the principle he advocates? In the view of the public, this would appear to be the situation. I need allude only to Edward Jenner and smallpox vaccination and to Jonas S. Salk and Albert Sabin, famed for their work with vaccination for poliomyelitis. Nobel Prize committees, on the contrary, are more likely to trace the story to the person who made the telling observation which eventuated in the conquest. For their method of demonstrating how the poliomyelitis virus could be cultivated, John F. Enders and his colleagues, Frederick C. Robbins and Thomas H. Weller, were cited by the Nobel Prize

*After a long operation and following resection procedures in the alimentary canal, excision of the soft tissues in the wound edges, including skin and fat of the subcutaneous tissues, will probably eliminate more bacteria in a few seconds than can be achieved by any other means. A controlled trial would soon determine the validity of this suggestion.

†The *Aetiologie* (1861) provides good evidence of Semmelweis' lack of skill in writing.

‡The story of Vienna obstetrics and obstetricians from the founding of the University (1365) and the establishment of the first chair in obstetrics (1754) is well told by Isador Fischer in *Geschichte der Geburtshilfe in Wien* (1909).

Committee (1954) before the work of Salk and Sabin had shown conclusively the effectiveness of the vaccination program. For demonstration of the utility of angiographic techniques, the Nobel Committee awarded the prize in 1956 to D. W. Richards and André F. Cournand but also reached back to Dr. John Forssmann (1929), who had made the first heroic cardiac catheterizations upon himself and thus demonstrated the potential of the method.[83]

Empiricism almost invariably precedes the scientific approach, as witnessed by use of antiseptic agents by many surgeons over centuries to lessen the threat of suppuration in wounds. In the time of Semmelweis, the existence of bacteria was known but their relation to disease and to wound infections had not yet been clarified. Long after the germ theory of disease found almost universal acceptance, some surgeons were still asking: "How can bacteria possibly do any harm? We all live surrounded by them and they do not seem to hurt us. Why are they hazardous in wounds?"[84]

There is usually an anachronistic relation between empirical discovery and factual objective evaluation. A host of researchers from various disciplines today, including surgeons, are struggling in an empirical manner to resolve the problem of tissue rejection in transplantation. Perhaps someone doing empirical trials will stumble upon a fruitful method. The surer approach, however, is factual validation of the nature of rejection and the mode of preventing it.

It is a great thing to be able to press a button and in an instant produce light. What an intricacy of effort and sophistication goes into the conversion from darkness to light and of ignorance to understanding! Such is the story of aseptic surgery, the product of a number of contributions from many disciplines.

Lister's Avowed Ignorance of Semmelweis' Work

Godlee (1917) has written a very sensitive and penetrating biography of his uncle, Lord Lister, including a nice account of Semmelweis' work. He quotes from a 1906 letter of Lister to Dr. Weckerling: "When in 1865 I first applied the antiseptic principle to wounds, I had not heard the name of Semmelweis and knew nothing of his work."[85] This is indeed a strange statement from a person who had been a student of the problem of inflammation since the middle 1850's. As Erna Lesky (p. 41) has remarked, "Scarcely ever had a discovery attained such quick publicity as did that of Semmelweis."*[74] Hebra,[86,87] Skoda,[88] and Haller[89]† all read papers announcing Semmelweis' important work (1847-1850) and Semmelweis himself appeared twice before the Vienna Medical Society to discuss his methods.[90]

The Englishman D. H. F. Routh, who had been a student in Vienna, returned to London and gave a paper on Semmelweis' doctrines before the Royal Medical and Chirurgical Society in November 1848. An abstract of his communication appeared the next month in the *Lancet.* The paper was published in the society's *Transactions* in 1849. Reviews of Routh's paper appeared in other English publications and in America and Scotland.[91]

Arneth (1851), a friend and colleague of Semmelweis in the Vienna Clinic, went to Paris,[92] Edinburgh,[93] and Ireland to announce the importance of Semmelweis' discovery. He later moved to Moscow, where he took a leading part in the discussions (1863) of Semmelweis' work at meetings of the St. Petersburg Medical Society.[75] The Irish surgeon E. W. Murphy published Semmelweis' findings in the Dublin *Quarterly Journal of Medical Sciences.*[94] In fact, in 1862 Semmelweis submitted a brief summary of his work, "On the Origin and Prevention of Puerperal Fever," which appeared in the *Medical Times and Gazette* (June 7, 1862, pp. 601-02), and was reprinted in *Braithwaite's Retrospect* in 1863 (vol. 46, pp. 150-53). In 1864 a review of Späth's report on the mortality of puerperal fever in Vienna appeared in the *British Medical Journal,* which alluded to the significant work of Semmelweis.[82] It would have taken very little effort for someone with a professed keen interest in inflammation and who, like Semmelweis, appreciated the identity of surgical and puerperal fever, to acquaint himself with the effective prophylaxis devised by Semmelweis for thwarting infections of any large wound of the parturient uterus.

Wieger of Strasbourg (1849) published his favorable experiences with the Semmelweis method. He concluded by saying, "Semmelweis acquainted an English obstetrician with his technique who said that on his side of the channel the technique was not new and that all his

*It is abundantly clear from Lesky's account (p. 215) that many members of the Vienna faculty appreciated the great significance of Semmelweis' discovery. Leopold Auenbrugger's discovery (1761) of percussion had gone unnoticed by Vienna's first medical faculty, an oversight which Skoda, Hebra, Rokitansky, and Haller felt strongly should not be repeated in the instance of Semmelweis. Whenever, before or since, have colleagues struggled so valiantly and sympathetically, even though ineffectually, to alert a profession to a great discovery?[68]

†In a presentation before the Pathology Section of the Vienna Medical Society, February 23, 1849, Haller,[89] adjunct director of the Vienna Allgemeines Krankenhaus, indicated that the mortality from puerperal fever on the First Obstetrical Service had been reduced more than 80% by Semmelweis' introduction of chlorine antiseptic methods.

colleagues changed their clothes when leaving the hospital!"[95]

In the French Academy of Medicine the Semmelweis thesis of the origins of puerperal fever was roundly debated in sessions from February 23 to July 6, 1858.[96] However, trial, not debate, is the proper manner in which to resolve a question of this kind.

When Klein, professor of obstetrics, died in 1856, Carl Rokitansky together with Dumreicher, professor of surgery, and Dlauhy, professor of public health, and Skoda, professor of medicine, urged the recall of Semmelweis for appointment to the chair of obstetrics in the University of Vienna; the recommendation of this distinguished committee was ignored. It is a tragic story reflecting intrigue and lack of vision. History does have a way of repeating itself.[74]

Lister and James Syme's eldest daughter, Agnes, were married in April 1856. A goodly portion of their honeymoon was spent abroad and they returned to Edinburgh in October. They had passed two weeks in Vienna, where Rokitansky, who had been a guest in Lister's home many years before, returned Lister's hospitality generously. The young Listers were entertained in Rokitansky's home and Rokitansky spent three hours and a quarter, Godlee relates, in showing Lister and other visitors his museum.[85] Lister, an accomplished microscopist, had begun his studies (1855) on the early stages of inflammation. Rokitansky also had taken to microscopy since his censure by Virchow (1846). Lister's visit to Vienna was made about the time that Rokitansky and others of the Vienna faculty were urging the appointment of Semmelweis as Klein's successor. Can it be that Lister in his two weeks in Vienna and in intimate conversations with Rokitansky did not hear the name of Semmelweis? The Medical Faculty undoubtedly was still buzzing over the controversy about Semmelweis' appointment. It would have been strange indeed for an ambitious young surgeon interested in inflammation not to have heard of Semmelweis and his work.*

It is proper that Semmelweis be recognized as the discoverer of the role of antiseptics in preventing wound infection. It is fitting to honor Lister as the leader whose careful study of the influence of antiseptics on compound fractures lent meaning to the provocative work of Pasteur for surgery. The coordinated contributions of a number of disciplines brought asepsis into being and greatly extended the realm of surgery.

*The *British Medical Journal* (August 26, 1865, p. 215) considered Semmelweis' death important enough to mention.

Transition to Asepsis

Practicing physicians long harbored patronizing attitudes toward paramedical scientists who dabbled in medical research. The physician-experimentalist Claude Bernard said to the chemist Pasteur at a meeting of the French Academy of Medicine that "when a doctor enters a room, he always looks as if he were going to say, 'I have just been saving a fellow man!"[97] When the zoologist Fritz Schaudinn announced discovery of the *Treponema pallidum* from a chancre as the cause of syphilis (1905) at a meeting of the Berlin Medical Society (*Berl. Klin. Wochensch* *42*:729-34, 1905), the presiding officer Ernst von Bergmann remarked, "The discussion is closed until our attention is called to the next announced cause of syphilis." A certain skepticism is a healthy quality, but the history of wound management is replete with doubting Thomases who, as members of commissions or adjudicating committees, obstructed and retarded the progress of surgery between the time of Semmelweis and Lister.

After his first publication in 1867, a series of important papers emanated from Lister's pen and clinic. Lister abandoned carbolic acid and the carbolic spray and explored a succession of other antiseptics. In 1907, 14 years after his retirement at Kings College Hospital, Lister prepared a powder-wound dressing of "the double cyanide of mercury and zinc" to which he added rosalane (Rosanilide) as a dye.[98] Rosanilide has recently been demonstrated to be a very effective antiseptic.

As early as October 1868, trials of carbolic acid in compound fractures were begun in Leipzig.[99] Just Lucas-Championnière interrupted his medical studies in Paris in 1868 to observe Lister in Glasgow. He returned to Paris full of enthusiasm, and by persistent effort gradually won support from French surgeons.* Influenced by commissions whose verdict was "not proved" (1864, 1866), French surgeons had earlier rejected Auguste Nélaton's alcohol soaks for elective surgery, as well as J. Lemaire's and G. Déclat's use of carbolic acid for wounds.[11] It was Lister's methodical consecutive labor that carried the day. However, 10 years were to elapse before his work gained enthusiastic endorsement from Volkmann of Halle, Germany (1877).[59] Gradually resistance lessened and aseptic surgery came with the work of Pasteur

*See unsigned obituary of "Just Lucas-Championnière" (*Brit. Med. J. 2*:1186, 1913).

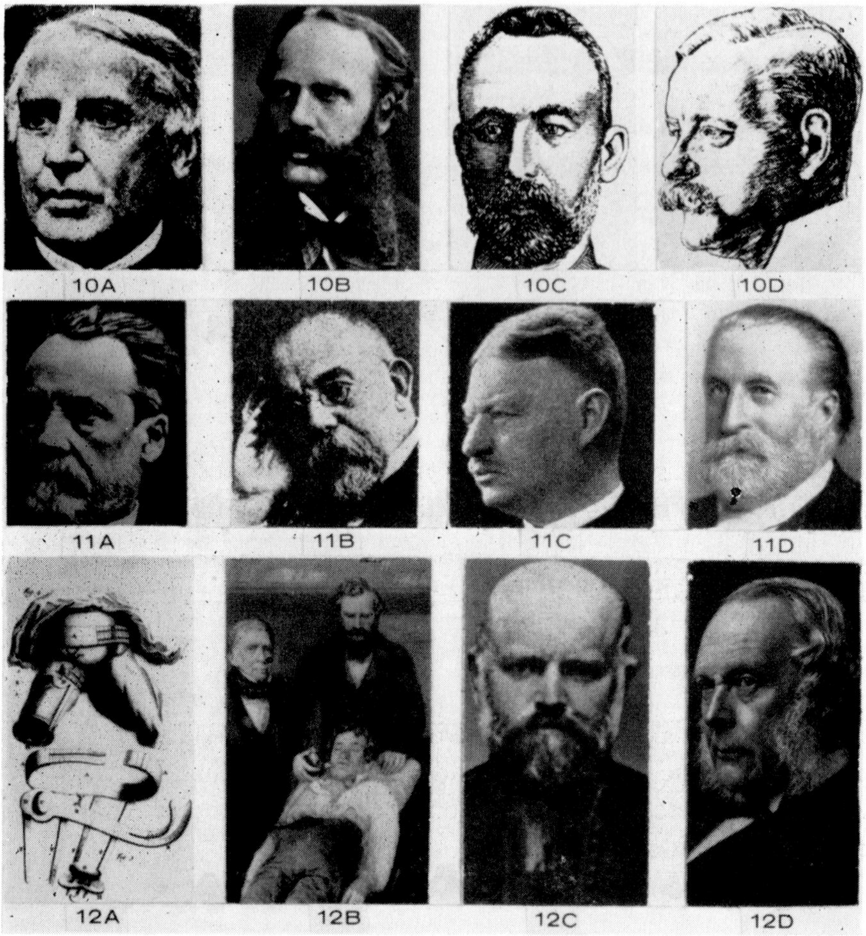

Fig. 10. *Contributors to advance of surgery. a.* Nélaton, alcohol soaks in elective surgery (1852-1864). *b. Volkmann,* protagonist of Lister. *c.* Reyher, debridement in military surgery, 1878. *d.* Friedrich, proved value of debridement, 1898. Fig. 11. *Beginnings of asepsis. a.* Pasteur, 1878. *b.* Koch, cultured bacteria, 1878. *c.* Neuber, 1883, implemented asepsis in surgical practice. *d.* Bergman, demonstrated value of asepsis. Fig. 12. *Great innovations and innovators. a.* Tourniquet, Petit, 1718. *b.* Anesthesia, 1846. *c.* Semmelweis, demonstrated hazards of unclean hands in wounds, 1847. *d.* Lister, confirmed value of antiseptics for wounds, 1867.

(1863-1879), John Tyndall (1877), and Koch (1878). Their discoveries were put to clinical test by Neuber (1883),[100] von Bergmann (1891),[101] and Schimmelbusch (1892).[102] Mikulicz initiated the wearing of face masks (1894) to reduce droplet infection of the wound from the nose and mouth of the surgical team[103] and Halsted followed with rubber gloves* (1890-1897).[105] Thus the mystery of wound suppuration was finally unraveled and its threat to surgeons and their patients lessened. Erysipelas and parotitis, though no longer rampant in surgical wards, continued as an occasional postoperative complication until sulfanilamide and the antibiotics arrived to rid hospitals permanently of their hazards.

It is a long and thorny trail, from the microscopists Athanasius Kircher (1658) and Antonj van Leeuwenhoek (1696) to the contagionists Francisco Redi (1671) and Lazaro Spallanzani (1765), to the biologists Theodor Schwann (1836) and Matthias J. Schleiden (1838), and the histologist Jacob Henle (1840). The significant work of these biologists preceded the surgeon-actors' appearance in the drama but apparently were without meaning to the myopic physicians and surgeons of the mid-19th century. Thomas Trotter in 1806 wrote scornfully of the "relicts of the old animalcule" hypothesis of contagion.† Wound infection became intelligible only when Pasteur marshalled patrols of vibrios onto the scene and was followed by Koch with battalions of bacteria of demonstrated virulence.

A function of the educator is to recognize a man of promise before the world proclaims him. The discerning discoverer, Semmelweis, made a significant assessment on a few facts that were meaningful to him but he failed to persuade other workers. In this unbelieving world, the anachronistic observer with a message, born before his time, as this account reaffirms, encounters suggestions of sympathetic acceptance for his ideas only in retrospect, not in prospect.

Summary

From this recital it is apparent that many antiseptics enjoyed wide usage extending back through the Middle Ages to Hippocrates. However, proof of the efficacy of such management was missing until

*Thomas Forster had taken out a patent for a surgical rubber glove in 1878. Sir Thomas Watson (1842) and William Acton (1848) had devised rubber gloves for the protection of the hands of anatomists and surgeons.[104]

†Quoted in Scott, H. H.: *History of Tropical Medicine.* London, Arnold, 1942, vol. 1, p. 29.

Semmelweis established the antiseptic principle of preventing wound infection in the parturient uterus denuded of its epithelium. Collins of the Dublin Rotunda Hospital had achieved equally good results in the prevention of puerperal fever by maintaining high standards of cleanliness in his hospital. He failed to note, however, that the accoucheur's hands were the principal source of conveying the contagion.

A few surgeons who expounded the practice of leaving the wound open in the management of contaminated wounds and in elective surgery (amputation and perineal lithotomy) had achieved low mortality rates not equaled until aseptic surgery came at the turn of the century.

Lister's application of carbolic acid to compound fractures turned the tide against primary amputation for compound fracture, an attitude further strengthened by Reyher's demonstration of the utility of early debridement in gunshot injuries during the Russo-Turkish War of 1876-1877.

Antiseptic management of wounds has disappeared. Of all antiseptic agents, the hypochlorites employed by Semmelweis survived the longest and had a rebirth of interest for surgeons in World War I.*

In my opinion the question of priority for having introduced the antiseptic principle of wound management is not a contest between Lister and Lemaire or Déclat, who preceded Lister in the use of phenol for contaminated wounds. It is more a question of how to divide the laurels properly between Semmelweis, the discoverer who showed the way, and Lister, whose consecutive studies convinced surgeons and the medical profession that antiseptic management of compound fracture obviated primary amputation while minimizing the risk. Crowther (1802) used wound dressings of hot tar with striking success in the management of compound fracture. Larrey (1824) and Bennion (1857) had startling results with benzoin in the management of compound fractures before Lister. The profession took no serious note, however, of these significant contributions.

Our profession hails Semmelweis and Lister and their durable contributions for mankind. The honor can be shared without loss to either. Semmelweis had only a sharp perception to guide him. Pasteur was

*Fifty years ago balsam of Peru enjoyed wide usage in the management of chronic infections and ulcers. It is somewhat strange to learn that its use is being once more considered. In his current monograph on *Fractures* Böhler (1966) recommends its application together with limited debridement for compound fractures.[106] Dr. Jander found that the addition of 1% formalin to balsam of Peru made it an effective antibacterial agent.[107]

Lister's guiding light. Antisepsis was only a preliminary victory in an ongoing battle against wound infection. The adulation of a grateful people, accorded Pasteur and Lister, is well deserved; but who in the history of medicine, guided only by a discerning flash of insight, has made so significant a discovery as Semmelweis? Certainly his name merits placement high on any list of mankind's great benefactors.

Asepsis, the product of a number of disciplines, extended the borders and the safety of surgery considerably. Antibiosis has made additional gains possible. Total conquest of the problem awaits future research and clinical trial.

Conclusion

What significance have this inquiry and recital for us?

In the history of surgery, perhaps no wounds have been so badly managed as those of compound fracture. The disability occasioned by a broken bone and an open wound undoubtedly urged many a surgeon to meddlesome interference. Certain it is that if Crowther's suggestion (1802) or Larrey's (1824) had been tested by any of the distinguished authors of monographs on fracture of the first half of the 19th century, amputation for compound fracture would have ceased to be routine long before the Russo-Turkish War of 1876-1877. That Semmelweis' warning of the threat of infection communicated by unclean fingers had meaning only for wounds of the parturient uterus indicates how slowly the significance of useful information is absorbed, understood and communicated within a discipline. It is definitely the business of authors to know of prior suggestions and progress originating within their discipline. That they fail to interpret and relate advances in other disciplines to their own is understandable and emphasizes the current need for interdisciplinary research and improved communication to which attention has previously been drawn.[108] Certain it is that lessons of the past, besides imparting useful information, can help to light the way for today's inquiring wayfarers.

Acknowledgments

I have had invaluable help from my wife, Sarah D. Wangensteen, research associate in medical history. Mr. Dennis Hammond, research assistant, and Mrs. Jacqueline Smith helped with study of the literature of compound fractures and of puerperal fever. To many librarians at the University of Minnesota and at the National Library of Medicine I am beholden for patient and competent assistance. Mr. Martin Finch, director of the Department of Medical Art and Photography, University of Minnesota, skillfully arranged the illustrative materials.

With permission of the publishers, several of the photographs are reprinted from references 11, 12, and 40. Figures 5 and *6a* and *b* are from Erna Lesky.[74] Figure *6c* is from J. Cruveilhier, vol. 1, book 4, plate 6 (1829-1835). Figures *6d* and *e* are from A. W. Lea (1910), plates 3 and 4.

REFERENCES

1. Vesalius, A.: *De humani corporis fabrica.* Basel, I. Oporinus, 1543.
2. Harvey, W.: *De motu cordis.* Frankfort, W. Fitzer, 1628.
3. Pasteur, L.: Mémoire sur les corpuscles organisés qui existent dans l'atmosphère. Examen de la doctrine des générations spontanées. *Ann. Sc. Nat. 16*:5-98, 1861.
   Idem.: Recherches sur la putrefaction. *C. R. Acad. Sc. Paris 56*:1189-94, 1863.
   Idem.: La théorie des germes et ses applications à la médecine et à la chirurgie. *C. R. Acad. Sc. Paris 86*:1037-43, 1878.
4. Lister, J.: On a new method of treating compound fracture, abscess, etc., with observations on the conditions of suppuration. *Lancet 1*:326, 357, 387, 507; *2*:246, 1867.
   Idem.: On the antiseptic principle in the practice of surgery. *Brit. Med. J. 2*:246, 1867.
5. Koch, R.: Die Ätiologie der Milzbrand-Krankheit, begründet auf die Entwicklungsgeschichte des Bacillus Annthracis. *Cohn's Beitr. Bioligie Pflanzen 2*:277-310, 1876.
   Idem.: *Untersuchungen über die Aetiologie der Wundinfectionskrankheiten.* Leipzig, Vogel, 1878.
6. Garrison, F. H. *An Introduction to the History of Medicine,* 4th ed. Philadelphia, Saunders, 1929, p. 579.
7. Ehrenberg, C.: *Atlas von vier und sechsig Kupfertafeln.* Leipzig, Vos, 1838.
8. Henle, J.: Von den Miasmen und Kontagien und von den miasmatischkontagiösen Krankheiten. In: *Pathologische Untersuchungen.* Berlin, Hirschwald, 1840, pp. 1-82.
9. Lesky, E.: *Ignaz Philipp Semmelweis und die Wiener medizinische Schule.* Verh. XIX, int. Kongr. Geschichte der Medizin Basel, 1964. Basel, Karger, 1966, pp. 347-53.
10. Nicaise, E.: Mondeville et le traitement des plaies au XIVe siècle. *Rev. chir. 14*:64-65, 1894.
11. Wangensteen, O. H. and Wangensteen, S. D.: Military surgeons and surgery, old and new: An instructive chapter in management of contaminated wounds. *Surgery 62*:1105, 1113-115, 1967.
12. Wangensteen, O. H., Wangensteen, S. D. and Wiita, J.: Lithotomy and lithotomists: Progress in wound management from Franco to Lister. *Surgery 66*:949, 1969.
13. Billroth, T.: Beobachtungs-Studien über Wundfieber und accidentelle Wundkrankheiten. *Arch. klin. Chir. 6*:444, 1865.
14. Cooper, A.: *The Anatomy and Surgical Treatment of Abdominal Hernia.* From: 2d London ed., Key, C. A., ed. Philadelphia, Lea & Blanchard, 1844, p. 82.
15. Cooper, A.: *A Series of Lectures on the Most Approved Principles and Practice of Modern Surgery: Principally Derived from the Lectures Delivered by Astley Cooper,* Jones, C. W., ed. 1st Amer. from 2d London ed.

Boston, Ewer, 1823, p. 285.
16. Wangensteen, O. H.: Historical aspects of the management of acute intestinal obstruction. *Surgery 65*:363-83, 1969.
17. McDowell, E.: Three cases of extirpation of diseased ovaria. *Eclect. Repert.* (Philadelphia) *7*:242-44, 1817.
18. Matt. *2*:11.
19. Woodall, J.: *The Surgeons Mate or Military & Domestique Surgery.* London, Bourne, 1655, pp. 46, 52, 159.
20. Purmann, M. G.: *Chirurgia curiosa.* London, Browne et al., 1706, pp. 214-215.
21. Fischer-Defoy, W.: Die Behandlung der Frakturen in Deutschland am Ende des XVII. Jahrhunderts. *Muenchener med. Wochenschrift* (Part 2) *56*: 2018-19, 1909.
22. Lemaire, J.: *Du coaltar saponiné désinfectant énergique, arrêtant les fermentations.* Paris, Germer-Baillière, 1860.
23. Déclat, G.: *Nouvelles applications de l'acide phénique.* Paris, Baillière, 1865.
24. Hippocrates: *The Genuine Works,* Adams, F., transl. London, Sydenham Soc., 1849, vol. 2, p. 60.
25. Malgaigne, J.-F.: *De l'irrigation dans les maladies chirurgicales.* Concours thesis. Paris, Lecaplain, 1842, pp. 5-13.
26. Paré, A.: *Oeuvres complètes.* J.-F. Malgaigne, ed. Paris, Baillière, 1840, vol. 2, pp. 334-335.
27. Garrison, F. H.: *John Shaw Billings: A Memoir.* New York, Putnam, 1915, p. 20.
28. Cahours: Des irrigations continues dans les fractures comminutives des membres. *Bull. gén. thérap. méd. chir. 72*:114-16, 1867.
29. Carter, H. Y.: Case of a compound fracture of the leg; with remarks. *Med. Facts Observ. 2*:1-25, 1792.
30. Carter, H. Y.: An account of the good effects of a solution of sal ammoniac, in vinegar, employed, as a topical application, in cases of lacerated wounds. *Med. Facts Observ. 6*:66-85, 1795.
31. Guyot, J.: Premier mémoire sur l'influence thérapeutique de la chaleur atmosphérique. *Arch. gén. méd. Paris 8*: 273-307, 1835.
32. Laborie, J.: De l'application de l'air chaud, comme moyen thérapeutique, dans le traitement des grandes plaies, d'après le procédé de M. Jules Guyot. *Bull. gén. thérap. méd. chir. Paris 15*: 155-66, 1838.
33. Bérard, A.: Mémoire sur l'emploi de l'eau froide comme antiphlogistique dans le traitement des maladies chirurgicales. *Arch. gén. méd., Paris 7*: 5-34, 317-27, 1835.
34. Godin, A.: Observations d'irrigations continues d'eau froide; recueillies dans le service de M. A. Bérard. *Arch. gén. méd. Paris 1*:343-58, 1837.
35. Macartney, J.: Observations sur la guérison des plaies sans inflammation. *Mem. Acad. roy. méd. Paris 5*:64-67, 1836.
36. Nivet, V.: Mémoire sur l'emploi des irrigations continues d'eau froide dans le traitement des fractures compliquées. *Gaz. méd. Paris 6*:36-43, 49-53, 1838.
37. Erichsen, J. E.: Liston and water-dressing. *Lancet 1*:65, 1879.
38. Crowther, J.: A successful mode of preventing gangrene in compound fractures; as practised by Messrs. William, Robert and John Crowther, in the West Riding of Yorkshire. *Med. Phys. J.* (London) *7*:307-10, 1802.
39. Larrey, D.: Mémoire sur une nouvelle manière de réduire ou de traiter les fractures des membres compliquées de plaies. *J. compl. dict. sc. méd. 20*: 193-200, 1824.
40. Wangensteen, O. H., Smith, J. and Wangensteen, S. D.: Some highlights in the history of amputation reflecting lessons in wound healing. *Bull. Hist. Med. 41*:105, 1967.
41. Larrey, D.: *Clinique de l'Hôpital du Gros-Caillou. Rapport chirurgical sur les dernières journées de juillet 1830.*
42. Adams, W.: *A Sketch of the Principles and Practice of Subcutaneous Surgery.* London, Churchill, 1857, pp. 15-17.
43. Cases of compound fracture in which the wounds were closed with com-

presses soaked in compound tincture of benzoin (under the care of Mr. Bryant). *Lancet 2*:747, 1876.
44. Bryant, T.: Contributions to the subject of compound fracture; being an analysis of 302 cases. *Med.-chir. Trans. 43*:20-28, 1861.
45. Jolieu, J.: *Mémoire sur cent fractures compliquées, guéries.* Paris, Baillière, 1843.
46. Paré, A.: *The Workes of That Famous Chirurgion Ambrose Parey,* Johnson, T., transl. London, Cotes & Young, 1634. Reprint, New York, Milford House, 1968, pp. 582-90.
47. Pott, P.: *Chirurgical Works . . . ed.* [*with*] *a . . . Life of the Author . . . by James Earle.* London, Johnson et al., 1790, pp. 14-16.
48. Biencourt, L.: *Considérations sur le traitement des fractures compliquées de plaie . . .* Thesis. Paris, 1873, p. 14.
49. Reyher, C.: Die antiseptische Wundbehandlung in der Kriegschirurgie. In: *Volkmann's Sammlung Klinischer Vorträge* (Chirurgie, no. 30) pp. 1207-62, 1878.
50. Reyher, C.: Ueber primäres Debridement der Schusswunden. In: International Medical Congress, *Transactions* (London) *2*:587-97, 1881.
51. Puschmann, T.: *Geschichte des Medicinischen Unterrichts von den ältesten Zeiten bis zur Gegenwart.* Leipzig, Veit, 1889, p. 313.
52. Caldwell, T. L.: Case of compound fracture of the thigh, successfully treated. *Med. Examiner 1*:504-06, 1838.
53. Boyer, A.: *The Lectures of . . . upon Diseases of the Bones, Arranged . . . by A. Richerand. . . .* 2 vol. in 1. 1st Amer. ed. Farrell, M., transl. Philadelphia, Humphreys, 1805, pp. 21, 22.
54. Banner, J. M.: A report of the cases of fractures of the larger bones of the extremities . . . *Edinburgh Med. Surg. J. 59*:6-13, 1843.
55. Huguier: [discussion reported] *Bull. Soc. Chir. Paris 16*:302, 1856.
56. de Ségogne, E.-R.: *De l'emploi de de l'alcool dans le pansement des fractures compliquées des plaies.* Thesis. Paris, Parent, 1867, pp. 35-55.
57. Nightingale, F.: *Notes on Hospitals.* . . . London, Parker & Son, 1859, pp. 1-2.
58. Paget, J.: The address in surgery. *Brit. Med. J. 2*:157, 1862.
59. Volkmann, R.: Abstract of a clinical lecture on the treatment of compound fractures. *Med. Times Gaz. 2*:561, 1877..
60. Lea, A. W.: *Puerperal Infection.* London, Oxford Univ. Press, 1910, p. 41.
61. Kehrer, E.: *Anatomie und Physiologie der Schwangerschaft in Biologie und Pathologie des Weibes. Handb. Frauenheilkunde und der Geburtshilfe,* 2d. ed. Berlin, Urban & Schwarzenburg, 1952, vol. 7, pt. 1, pp. 354-55.
62. Kirkland, T.: *A Treatise on Child-bed Fevers . . .* London, Baldwin & Dawson, 1774, pp. 73-74.
63. Pouteau, C.: *Mélanges de chirurgie.* Lyon, Regnault, 1760, p. 182.
64. Simpson, J. Y.: Some notes on the analogy between puerperal fever and surgical fever. *Monthly J. Med. Sc. 11*:414-29, 1850.
65. Simpson, J. Y.: *Obstetric Memoirs and Contributions.* Philadelphia, Lippincott, 1856, vol. 2, pp. 17-25.
66. Semmelweis, I. P.: *Die Aetiologie, der Begriff und die Prophylaxis des Kindbettfiebers.* Reprinted from 1861 ed., with introduction by Alan F. Guttmacher. New York, Johnson Reprint, 1966.
67. Hunter, J.: *Works of . . . , with Notes,* Palmer, J. F. ed. London, Longman et al., 1835, vol. 3, p. 60.
68. Lesky, E.: *Die Wiener medizinische Schule im 19. Jahrhundert. Graz,* Böhlaus, 1965, pp. 215-19, 227.
69. Pasteur, L.: [communication on puerperal fever] *Bull. l'Acad. méd. 8*: 271-74, 1879.
70. Churchill, F., ed.: *Essays on the Puerperal Fever and Other Diseases Peculiar to Women. . . .* London, Sydenham Soc., 1849, pp. 470-72, 479-81, 489.
71. Gordon, A.: *A Treatise on the Epidemic Puerperal Fever of Aberdeen.* London, Robinson, 1795, pp. 63-65, 84-85, 92.
72. Collins, R.: *A Practical Treatise on*

Midwifery, Containing the Result of Sixteen Thousand Six Hundred and Fifty-Four Births. . . . Philadelphia, Haswell et al., 1838, pp. 192-93.
73. Holmes, O. W.: The contagiousness of puerperal fever. *New Eng. Quart. J. Med. Surg. 1*:518, 1843.
74. Lesky, E.: Ignaz Philipp Semmelweis und Wiener medizinische Schule. In: *Osterreichische Akademie der Wissenschaften, Philosophisch-historische Klasse.* Wien, Böhlaus, 1964, vol. 3, pp. 23-89.
75. Sinclair, W. J.: *Semmelweis: His Life and His Doctrine.* Manchester, Univ. Manchester Press, 1909, pp. 27, 80-81, 156, 259.
76. Pringle, J.: *Observations on the Diseases of the Army. . . .* London, Millar, 1753, appendix, pp. 309-403.
77. Pringle, J.: Some experiments on substances resisting putrefaction. *Phil. Trans. Roy. Soc. London 46*:487, 1749-1750.
78. Friedrich, P. L.: Die aseptische Versorgung frischer Wunden. . . . *Arch. klin. Chir. 57*:300-09, 1898.
79. Skoda, J.: Vortrag . . . eine der wichtigsten Entdeckungen im Gebiete der Medicin. *Sitzungsberichte der kaiserlichen Akademie der Wissenschaften. Mathematisch-naturwissenschaftliche Classe* (Part 2), pp. 168-82, 1849.
80. Mayer, L.: Über die pflanzlichen Parasiten der weiblichen Sexual-organe in ihrer praktischen Bedeutung. *Monatsschr. f. Gebúrtsk. 20*:9-15, 1862.
81. Mayrhoefer, C.: Zur Frage nach der Aetiologie der Puerperalprocesse. *Monatsschr. f. Geburtsk. 25*:124-129, 1865.
82. Späth, J.: Historische Ueberblicke der Vorkommnisse im Wiener Gebärhause seit 1784 bis 1863, mit besonderer Berücksichtigung der Puerperal-Erkrankungen. *Wiener med. Wochenschr. 14*:164-67, 1864.
Idem.: Mortality in the Vienna Lying-in Hospital. *Brit. Med. J. 1*:476-77, 1864.
83. Sourkes, T. L.: *Nobel Prize Winners in Medicine and Physiology, 1901-1965.* London, Abelard-Schuman, 1966, pp. 315-22, 330-41.
84. Hiller, A.: Ein experimenteller Beitrag zur Lehre von der organisirten Natur der Contagien und von der Fäulniss. *Arch. klin. Chir. 18*:697, 1875.
85. Godlee, R. J.: *Lord Lister.* London, Macmillan, 1917, pp. 53-58, 141.
86. Hebra, F.: Höchst wichtige Erfahrungen über die Ätiologie der in Gebäranstalten epidemischen Puerperalfieber. *Ztschr. der kais. kön. Gesellschaft der Aerzte zu Wien,* (Part 2) *4*:242-44, 1847.
87. Hebra, F.: Fortsetzung der Erfahrungen über die Ätiologie der in Gebäranstalten epidemischen Puerperalfieber. *Ztschr. der kais. kön. Gesellschàft der Aertze zu Wien,* (Part 1) *5*:64-65, 1849.
88. Skoda, J.: Über die von Dr. Semmelweis entdeckte. . . . *Ztschr. der kais. kön. Gesellschaft der Aertze zu Wien 6*:107-17, 1850.
89. Haller, C.: Protokoll der Sektion für Pathologie; Sitzung am, Feb. 23, 1849. *Zeitschr. kais. kön. Gesellschaft der Aerzte zu Wien.* Jg. 5, Bd. 1, p. LV, 1849.
90. Gyory, T.: *Semmelweis' Gesammelte Werke. . . .* Jena, Fischer, 1905, p. 600.
91. Routh, D. H. F.: On the causes of the endemic puerperal fever of Vienna. *Lancet 2*:642-43, 1848; *Amer. J. Med.* Reviews in: *Sc. 17*:509-10, 1849; *Edinburgh Med. Surg. J. 75*:244-51, 1851.
92. Arneth, F. H.: Note sur le moyen proposé et employé par M. Semmelweis [*sic*]. . . . *Ann. d'hygiène pub. méd. légale 45*:281-90, 1851.
93. Arneth, F. H.: Evidence of puerperal fever depending upon the contagious inoculation of morbid matter. *Monthly J. Med. Sc. Edinburgh 12*:505-11, 1851.
94. Murphy, E. W.: Puerperal fever. *Dublin Quart. J. Med. Sc. 24*:1-30, 1857.
95. Wieger, F.: Des moyens prophylactiques mis en usage au grand hôpital de Vienne contre l'apparition de la fièvre puérperale. *Gaz. méd. Strasbourg 9*:97-105, 1849.
96. *De la fièvre puérperale: De sa nature et de son traitement: Communications à l'Académie impériale de médécine.* . . . Paris, Baillière, 1858.

97. Vallery-Radot, R.: *The Life of Pasteur. . . .* New York, Doubleday, Doran, 1928, p. 226.
98. Lister, J.: Note on the double cyanide of mercury and zinc as an antiseptic dressing. *Brit. Med. J. 1*:795, 1907.
99. Berthel, C. F.: *Die antiseptische Behandlung der complicirten Fracturen mit Carbolsäure.* Thesis. Leipzig, 1870, p. 4.
100. Neuber, G.: *Anleitung zur Technik der antiseptischen Wundbehandlung und des Dauerverbandes.* Kiel, Lipsius Tischer, 1883.
101. Bergmann, E.: [visit to Bergmann's clinic] Tenth International Medical Congress, vol. 1, 1891, pp. 318-20.
102. Schimmelbusch, C.: *Die Anleitung zur Aseptischen Wundbehandlung.* Berlin, Hirschwald, 1892.
103. Mikulicz, J.: Das Operieren in sterilisierten Zwirnhandschuhen und mit Mundbinde. *Zentralbl. Chir. 24*:713, 1897.
104. Randers-Pehrson, J.: *The Surgeon's Glove.* Springfield, Ill., Thomas, 1960, p. 15.
105. Halsted, W. S.: Ligature and suture material . . . also an account of the introduction of gloves. . . . *J.A.M.A. 60*: 1123-24, 1913.
106. Böhler, L. *The Treatment of Fractures.* New York, Grune, Stratton, 1966, p. 2310.
107. Jander: Experimentelle Untersuchungen über bakterienfeindliche Eigenschaften des Perubalsams. *Arch. klin. Chir. 90*: 529-42, 1909.
108. Wangensteen, O. H.: Role of medical history as incentive to scholarship and spur to interdisciplinary research. *Mayo Clinic Proc. 42*:345-49, 1967.

CURRENT CONCEPTS OF THE PATHOGENESIS AND MANAGEMENT OF ASTHMA*

MICHAEL H. GRIECO

Director, Allergy and Infectious Disease Division
Department of Medicine
St. Luke's Hospital Center

Assistant Clinical Professor of Medicine
Columbia University College of Physicians and Surgeons

New York, N. Y.

ASTHMA is usually divided into two basic types, extrinsic and intrinsic. These terms were used initially in 1864 by Salter.[1] Extrinsic or atopic asthma refers to disease resulting from environmental antigenic exposure. Intrinsic or infective asthma refers to disease not associated with exposure to exogenous allergens. The differentiation between extrinsic and intrinsic asthma is important in treatment and prognosis. The characteristics of each type are outlined in Table I. In this presentation I shall review some important developments affecting current concepts of the pathogenesis and management of asthma.

Pathogenesis

EXTRINSIC ASTHMA

IgE. The target cells are considered to become sensitive to a specific antigen by virtue of having fixed to their surface a special class of antibody, usually designated as reaginic or skin-sensitizing antibody. These antibodies are virtually undetectable by standard serologic methods; until recently they were studied exclusively by passive sensitization of human skin as first described by C. Prausnitz and H. Küstner. Over the years human reaginic activity has been ascribed to almost every class and type of immunoglobulin. The most important advance in the study of allergic disease has been the demonstration by Kimishige and Teruko Ishizaka,[2] at the Children's Asthma Research Institute in Denver, Colo., that most reaginic activity is contained in a previously undescribed class of immunoglobulins, IgE. Original studies that sug-

*Presented at a meeting of the Section on Medicine, April 28, 1970.

TABLE I. CHARACTERISTICS OF EXTRINSIC AND INTRINSIC ASTHMA

Characteristics	*Extrinsic*	*Intrinsic*
1. Genetic influence	Present	Variable
2. Age of onset	<35	<5, >35
3. Hay fever	Frequent	Infrequent
4. Skin sensitizing antibody	Usually present	Absent
5. Sputum	Eosinophils	Eosinophils PMN leukocytes Bacteria
6. Associated infection	Secondary	Primary
7. Intractable asthma	Uncommon	Common
8. Death	Rare	More frequent

gested that skin-sensitizing antibody is IgA were due to undetected IgE which migrated close to IgA on Sephadex G and DEAE cellulose chromatograms. The important step was the demonstration that rabbit antisera to reagin-rich serum which had been absorbed against gammas A, G, M, and D (empty antiserum) was able to precipitate reagin. Immunoelectrophoresis demonstrated a gamma 1 precipitin band between the reagin-rich fraction and the empty rabbit antiserum. This precipitin band combined with radioactive allergen derived from ragweed extracts on radioimmunoelectrophoresis. Qualitative and quantitative correlation of IgE antibody with skin-sensitizing activity was followed by structural studies of the immunoglobulin obtained from two patients with IgE multiple myeloma characterized by absence of bony lesions and plasma-cell leukemia.[3,4] These properties are summarized in Table II. It is now clearly established that anti-IgE serum linked to insoluble immunoabsorbents will remove the reaginic antibody from sera.

IgE has been demonstrated on human leukocytes and tissue mast cells by the ability not only of antigens but also of anti-IgE serum to release histamine *in vitro* and in skin. More recently, Ishizaka et al. demonstrated with ^{125}I anti-IgE the presence of IgE on basophilic leukocytes by autoradiography of the cells.[5] There was no standing of neutrophils, eosinophils, lymphocytes, or erythrocytes. Experiments designed to determine the mechanism of histamine release in IgE activity showed that whole anti-IgE molecule (8S) dimer and 5S F ab

TABLE II. IgE GLOBULIN

Molecular weight	196,000
Sedimentation coefficient	7.9 S
Carbohydrate content	11%
Sulfur-containing amino acids	Large amount of methionine & cystine
Light chain	Lambda, kappa
Heavy chain	Epsilon, E
Normal serum level	100-1300 ng./ml. (mean of 250 ng./ml.)
Heat	Labile (effect skin binding)
Complement fixation on aggregation	No
Passive sensitization	Monkey lung, skin Human lung, skin, leukocytes

TABLE III. MEASUREMENT OF IgE ANTIBODY TO SPECIFIC ALLERGENS

Radioallergosorbent[9]
Red-cell-linked antigen antiglobulin[10]
Radioimmunodiffusion assay (RID)
Histamine release after passive sensitization of monkey or human tissue

dimer fragment both induced release, while 3.5 monomer did not. This suggests that bridging of cell-bound IgE molecules may be the initiating step in the release of the chemical mediator from sensitized cells.

Serum IgE levels average 250 ng./ml. in the normal as measured by radioimmunodiffusion (RID assay) and radioimmunosorbent techniques. Sixty three % of patients with allergic asthma as compared to 5% of patients with nonallergic asthma have been found to have elevated levels of serum IgE globulin.[6] Elevated levels have also been found in Ethiopian children infected with ascaris worms.[7] Using a double antibody immunoassay, Gleich et al.[8] confirmed the presence of elevated levels of IgE in allergic individuals.

By means of fluorescent antibody techniques, IgE-forming cells have been found in tonsils, adenoid tissues, bronchial and peritoneal lymph nodes, the Peyer's patches of monkeys, and the mucosal tissues of the nose, respiratory system, stomach, small intestine, and rectum. In addition, IgE antibody to specific allergens as measured by several

Table IV. BRONCHOCONSTRICTOR AND BRONCHODILATOR AGENTS

Bronchoconstriction	*Bronchodilation*
histamine	theophylline
SRS-A	
bradykinin	
acetylcholine	B_2 adrenergic stimulators

techniques listed in Table III has been detached not only in serum[9, 10] but also in nasal washings and sputa from allergic patients.[11-13]

The protective role of IgE in respiratory secretions is currently under investigation.

Thus, the role of IgE as reagin appears to be firmly established. We shall now move on to the next step, the chain of events leading to the release of clinical mediators.

Release of chemical mediators from the target cells (Table IV). Ishizaka as noted earlier has demonstrated that only the basophilic leukocyte had demonstrable IgE globulin attached. The circulating basophil is functionally similar to the mast cell which is located beneath the respiratory mucosa and exists also in other tissues. These cells contain granules rich in histamine, probably bound ionically to either heparin or protein. The release of histamine from human lung and human leukocytes has been studied.[14] The technique of histamine release from leukocytes is based on the observation of Katz and Cohen[14] in 1940 that the addition of antigen to the whole blood of a patient allergic to that antigen led to the release of histamine from the formed elements of the blood into the plasma. As presently employed, the system utilizes washed, isolated peripheral leukocytes suspended in a serum-free buffer. The fluorometric determination of histamine is outlined in the following tabulation. About half the blood histamine is apparently contained in the basophils; the rest reside in the eosinophils and neutrophils. Leukocytes may be obtained from naturally sensitive donors or the cells of normal donors may be sensitized *in vitro* by a brief exposure to allergic serum followed by washing. The chief virtue of this model system is that each of the elements of the reaction-target cell, sensitizing antibody, blocking antibody, and antigen is subject to experimental manipulation. The most extensive studies with this system have been conducted by Lichtenstein, Osler, Levy, and Norman.[15]

TECHNIQUE OF THE RELEASE OF HISTAMINE FROM LEUKOCYTES.

leukocyte	+	antigen	→	extraction in acid aqueous layer
		or		
suspension		10% TCA (total release)		OPT conjugation measure fluorescence at 450 mu with activation at 360 mu

Important factors in the antigenic release of histamine from leukocytes include 1) calcium; 2) *p*h (7.3 to 7.4 optimal); 3) ionic strength (0.14 to 0.16 optimal); 4) temperature (37° C. optimal); 5) antigen concentration; 6) cell number; and 7) lag period of 30 seconds.

The release of histamine can be inhibited by the following: 1) removal of calcium; 2) heating to 45°C.; 3) chilling to 4°C.; 4) unsubstituted fatty acids such as dodecanoate; 5) iodoacetate; 6) 5% human-serum albumin; 7) inhibition of glycolysis by nicotinamide, fluoride, 2-deoxyglucose; and 8) inhibition by both methylxanthines and catecholamines.[16] Theophylline, the most active of the methylxanthines, is an inhibitor of phosphodiesterase which destroys 3′5′ cyclic AMP; epinephrine and isoproterenol activate an adenyl cyclase which generates cyclic AMP from ATP. Thus both classes of compounds *cause an increase in the intracellular cyclic AMP* level with inhibition of the release of histamine. As will be discussed later, this same increase of ATP in bronchial smooth muscle cells may be associated with bronchodilation.

Studies of the release of histamine from leukocytes in immunization have led to three significant observations. First, cell sensitivity, defined as the concentration of antigen required for the 50% release of histamine with the cells suspended in normal serum or buffer, is decreased in children but only rarely in adults.[17, 18] In the study of Sedan et al.[17] the cells of children in the control group became more sensitive to antigen. In the 18 treated children cell sensitivity decreased and in three children the cells became unreactive. Second, blocking antibody (IgG globulin) titer, defined as the reciprocal of the dilution required to inhibit histamine release by 50% is increased. This is the same classic antibody described initially by Cooke et al.[19] as a thermostable blocking antibody in passive transfer studies. Third, reagin titers, defined as the dilution of serum that passively sensitizes a set of normal leukocytes to release 50% of the histamine, increase acutely. This confirms the studies of Sherman and Connell, who have demonstrated the acute rise followed by decreasing titers over two to four years.[20]

These observations provide a firm rationale for the beneficial effects of injection therapy, which has been practiced clinically since 1911.

The leukocyte histamine release reaction is not cytotoxic but a secretory reaction. The cells remain motile under phase contrast microscopy, do not release potassium, and there is no evidence for complement requirement. The intracellular enzymatic steps leading to the release of histamine remain to be elucidated although the serine esterases have been implicated from organophosphorus inhibition studies.[21]

Slow-reacting substance of anaphylaxis (SRS-A) refers to an acidic, lipid, soluble, proteolytic-resistant mediator which contracts smooth muscle more slowly than histamine. Initially isolated by Feldberg and Kellaway from the perfusion of guinea pig lung with cobra venom,[22] this substance has also been isolated from allergic guinea pig, rabbit, monkey, and the asthmatic lung in man. Usually, assay involves the contraction of guinea pig ileum in the presence of an antihistamine, antiserotonin, and atropine.

Although the cell source in humans is unknown, it has been isolated from guinea pig and rat leukocytes.[23] As might be expected, monkey-lung fragments passively sensitized *in vitro* with human serum rich in IgE antibody release both histamine and the slowly reacting substance of anaphylaxis upon specific challenge with allergen or IgE, which strongly suggests the release of both mediators following IgE and allergen interaction.[24]

Serotonin (5-hydroxytryptamine) is not a bronchoconstrictor of isolated human tracheal chains[25] and is also not contained within human mast cells. This mediator is not likely to be involved in human asthma. Although the decapeptide, kallidin I (bradykinin), does initiate bronchoconstriction in the asthmatic lung when administered by aerosol,[26] this has not been isolated from human asthmatic lung after allergen challenge. However, kallikrein is released from guinea pig lung during anaphylaxis.[27] Allergic persons who have received a local challenge with ragweed antigens have been found to have increased levels of bradykinin in their nasal secretions.[28] Kinins have also been demonstrated in the perfusate of skin challenged by allergens to which the patient is sensitive[29] and have been reported as increasing tenfold in the blood of a patient experiencing an acute asthmatic attack.[26] Of the long-chain, unsaturated, oxygenated fatty acids referred to as protaglandins, only PGF_{2a} has been found in the human lung and none has been implicated in bronchoconstriction.[30]

Cellular hypersensitivity to clinical allergens as reflected by pollen-induced lymphocyte transformation in hayfever subjects indicates the presence of a sensitized thymus-dependent cell population.[31] The cells also give rise to positive machrophage and leukocyte migration-inhibition tests *in vitro* and delayed-type skin tests *in vivo*. The role of these cells in the pathogenesis of bronchial asthma is uncertain.

Intrinsic Asthma, the Beta-Adrenergic Blockade Theory

Our attention is now directed to the bronchial smooth muscle. The hypothesis that asthma is due to a functional imbalance of the autonomic nervous system was proposed by Eppinger and Hess[32] in 1917 when they presented their concept of vagotonia and suggested that asthma might be due to excessive cholinergic activity. Experimental support for this hypothesis has been inconclusive. An important advance in the study of the autonomic nervous system was introduced in 1948 by Ahlquist,[33] who proposed that the variable actions of epinephrine and other drugs could be accounted for if two sets of receptors, alpha and beta, were present in or near end organs affected by these substances. Beta-adrenergic stimulation, as defined by the effects of isoproterenol and the effects of beta-adrenergic receptor-blocking drugs such as propranolol, is associated with relaxation of bronchial smooth muscle, myocardial stimulation, and peripheral vasodilation. Alpha-adrenergic stimulation, as defined by the effects of drugs such as methoxamine and the effects of alpha-adrenergic receptor-blocking drugs such as phenoxybenzamine, is associated with peripheral vasoconstriction but not with bronchial or direct myocardial effects.

A series of investigations in animals has led Szentivanyi and others[34, 35] to the hypothesis that partial beta-adrenergic blockade is a cause of bronchial hypersensitivity in humans. Normal mice sensitized with an injection of *Bacillus pertussis* demonstrate a 30- to 300-fold increased sensitivity to histamine and a 20- to 50-fold increased sensitivity

TABLE V. FEV_1 CHANGES RESULTING FROM 20 MG. OF INTRAVENOUS PROPRANOLOL

FEV_1

	Control (ml.)	*Propranolol preatropine (% change)*	*Atropine (% change)*	*Propranolol postatropine (% change)*
N.N.	652	—17.9	+31.3	+30.7
B.C.	2036	—18.1	+31.0	+34.5
D.C.	345	———	severe respiratory distress	———
E.C.	1125	—13.0	+32.9	+20.7
P.H.	657	—29.5	+46.9	+68.0
Mean	1118	—19.6	+35.5	+38.5
	p = 0.01	p = 0.01	p> 0.2	

to serotonin. In nonimmunized mice treated with dichloroisoproterenol, a beta-adrenergic blocking agent, a similar hypersensitivity to the effects of histamine and serotonin developed.

The beta-adrenergic theory of human bronchial asthma has been reviewed extensively by both Szentivanyi[36] and Reed.[37] The beta-receptor theory states that excessive irritability of the bronchial tree is the fundamental abnormality in asthma and that the cause of the excessive irritability is a diminished responsiveness of the beta adrenergic receptors of the bronchial glands, smooth muscle, and mucosal blood vessels. This has been proposed as an explanation for the triggering of bronchoconstriction by a large variety of nonallergic stimuli such as infection, psychic factors, inhalation of cold air, nonantigenic dust fumes, and aerosol histamine or methacholine.

While it is likely at the present time that partial bronchial beta-adrenergic blockade is present, either as a primary or secondary abnormality, studies from our laboratory have failed to demonstrate metabolic or cardiovascular abnormalities.[38-40] Recent studies in our laboratory have been concerned with the mechanism of bronchoconstriction resulting from beta-adrenergic blockade with 20 mg. of propranolol given intravenously. FEV_1 significantly decreased 19.6% in four asthmatic subjects; in a fifth severe respiratory distress prevented recording of further respiratory measurement. Atropine aerosol resulted in a rise of FEV_1 to 35.5% above controls and prevented a propranolol-induced decrease of this measurement (Table V). These observations

TABLE VI. FEV_1 CHANGES RESULTING FROM 50 MG. OF INTRAVENOUS PRACTOLOL

FEV_1

	Control (ml.)	*Practolol (% change)*
N.N.	725	+ 7.2
B.C.	2119	+43.3
D.C.	345	— 0.9
E.C.	1352	+20.7
P.H.	657	+31.4
G.B.	958	— 6.0
Mean	1026	+19.3
	p = 0.1	

support a previous suggestion by Macdonald et al. that a *cholinergic* mechanism may be responsible for propranolol-induced bronchoconstriction.[41] Previously atropine was shown to block bronchoconstriction associated with pulmonary embolism, aerosol methacholine, dusts, citric acid aerosol, hypoxemia, occasional cases of exercise-induced asthma, placebo allergens, and nasal and nasopharyngeal irritation with silica particles. Cholinergic efferent pathways may be responsible for asthmatic reactions to nonallergic factors such as infection, which may alter bronchial beta-adrenergic activity or sensitize cough receptors.

Ahlquist's designation of adrenergic receptor systems has been augmented recently by the differentiation of beta receptors into $beta_1$ and $beta_2$ by Land et al.,[42] $beta_1$ for lipolysis and cardiac stimulation and $beta_2$ for bronchodilation and vasodepression. Practolol, a selective $beta_1$ antagonist, failed to reduce the FEV_1 in six asthmatic patients recently studied (Table VI). While it would appear premature to propose a definitive classification of subtypes until more information is available on a greater number of species and organs, the bronchial receptor can be temporarily considered as a $beta_2$ subtype. Although it is unclear whether partial bronchial beta-adrenergic blockade is the primary defect in intrinsic asthma leading to bronchoconstriction to both allergic and nonallergic stimuli, it is certain that the hypothesis is leading to a greater understanding of the role of the autonomic nervous system in this disease. As with numerous other hormones, it is believed that cyclic AMP[43] is the second messenger that mediates the bronchodilation resulting from $beta_2$-adrenergic stimulation.

MANAGEMENT

The numerous modalities available for the treatment of mild, moderate, and severe bronchial asthma will not be discussed here. Instead, I should like to emphasize only a few important considerations.

The cyclic AMP system. Cyclic AMP (adenosine 3', 5'–monophosphate or cyclic adenylate) is now recognized as a second messenger mediating a variety of hormonal effects, including those of catecholamines. The formation of cyclic AMP from ATP is catalyzed by adenyl cyclase, which is located in the cell membranes. Cyclic AMP, which leads to glycogenolysis and lipolysis, is associated with both inhibition of leukocyte-histamine release in basophil and relaxation in bronchial smooth muscle. Corticosteroids presumably act by enhancing the catecholamine-induced release of adenyl cyclase in cell membranes of bronchial smooth muscle cells while methylxanthines such as theophylline block the inactivation of cyclic AMP by AMP phosphodiesterase. Thus asthma may represent a disease that involves a lesion at the level of cyclic AMP in bronchial smooth muscle. The weak bronchodilation effect of cyclic AMP on tracheal rings is consistent with this concept.

Catecholamines. Three points are worthy of note. First, isoproterenol, a potent bronchodilator, does produce significant hemodynamic side effects. In a study in our laboratory,[39] significant increases of cardiac output and decrease of peripheral resistance was noted for 15 to 30 minutes after aerosolization of 1-500 of the drug for 15 minutes. Although Powles et al.[44] have suggested combining practolol with isoproterenol to block unwanted tachycardia and palpitation, this can also be accomplished by the use of drugs that act predominantly as beta$_2$-adrenergic agonists such as isoetharine and salbutamol.[45] The latter represents a new class of drugs with long action resulting from resistance to catechol-o-methyl transferase.

Second, the hypoxemia characteristic of moderate to severe asthma is aggravated by isoproterenol, aminophylline, or epinephrine in about 50% of patients who show a further decrease in PaO_2 of 5 mm. Hg or more, accompanied by an increase of alveolar-arterial oxygen-tension gradient. This is presumably caused by a reversal of preexisting, compensatory pulmonary vasoconstriction and consequent uneven ventilation-perfusion ratios. The net effect of catecholamine therapy probably

TABLE VII. PRESSURIZED CATECHOLAMINE AEROSOLS

Isoproterenol	*Mg./inhalation*
Vapo-N-iso	0.070
Mistometer	0.125
Medihaler-iso	0.075
Duo-Medihaler	0.160
Medihaler-iso forte	0.440
Epinephrine	
Medihaler-epi	0.150
Isoetharine	
Bronkometer	0.350

benefits the patients despite the documented decrease in arterial oxygen tension.

Third, since 1966 when Keighley described three asthmatic patients who developed delayed severe airway obstruction following the use of aerosol isoproterenol,[46] pressurized catecholamine aerosols have been suggested as a cause of increased mortality from asthma.[47, 48] Paradoxic bronchoconstriction from isoproterenol may result from the conversion in the body to 3-methoxyisoprenaline, a weak beta-adrenergic antagonist.[49] Human bronchial tissue contains catechol-o-methyl transferase, hence it is possible that some of the inhaled isoprenaline is O-methylated in the bronchi to form 3-methoxyisoprenaline. It is important to note the wide differences in concentration of catecholamines per pressurized nebulizer inhalation to evaluate potential overuse of nebulizers (Table VII).

Methylxanthines. Theophylline, the most commonly used methylxanthine, requires at least a level of 10 ng./ml. plasma to be effective The recently developed theophylline hydroalcoholic compounds have the advantage over the previous preparations of rapid absorption following oral administration. These include:

Theokin elixir – Calcium salicylate theophylline
Brondecon – Choline theophylline
Lixaminol – Theophylline ethylenediamine
Quibron – Theophylline free
Elixophylline – Theophylline free

Disodium chromoglycate and diethylcarbamazine. Altounyan, aware of the antispasmodic activity of the chromone, khellin, examined the effect in experimental asthma of one of its analogues, disodium chromoglycate. He induced asthma in himself by the inhalation of mixed pollen antigens and observed that the prior inhalation of disodium chromoglycate prevented the reduction in FEV_1 associated with subsequent antigen challenge.[50] Several reports have now appeared describing the apparent efficacy of this drug in *extrinsic* asthma. Orange and Austen[51] have demonstrated that pretreatment of rats with disodium chromoglycate inhibits the homocytotropic antibody-mediated release of histamine from the peritoneal mast cells of the rat. Conversely, pretreatment with diethylcarbamazine (hetrazan), a drug noted to relieve intractable bronchospasm associated with tropical eosinophilia, inhibits the release of SRS-A from the peritoneal polymorphonuclear leukocytes of the rat by thermostable antibody. Both drugs appear to act intracellularly to block formation or release of mediators. Drug trials are underway at present throughout the United States to determine the role of disodium chromoglycate, administered as a powder to the bronchial tree in the treatment of extrinsic asthma.

REFERENCES

1. Salter, H. H.: *On Asthma: Its Pathology and Treatment.* Philadelphia, Blanchard & Lea, 1864.
2. Ishizaka, K. and Ishizaka, T.: *Characterization of Human Reaginic Antibodies.* Proceedings Sixth Congress of the Int. Ass'n. Allergology. Montreal, Nov. 5-11, 1967.
3. Stanworth, D. R., Humphrey, J. H., Bennich, H. and Johansson, S. G. O.: Inhibition of Prausnitz-Küstner reaction by proteolytic-cleavage fragments of a human myeloma protein of immuno-globulin class E. *Lancet 2*:17-18, 1968.
4. Ogawa, M., Kochiva, S., Smith, C., Ishizaka, K. and McIntyre, O. R.: Clinical aspects of IgE myeloma. *New Eng. J. Med. 281*:1217-220, 1969.
5. Ishizaka, K., Tumioka, H. and Ishizaka, T.: Presence of γ E and γ G molecules on human leukocytes. Abstract, 26th Annual Meeting, American Academy of Allergy, New Orleans, La., Feb. 16-18, 1970.
6. Johansson, S. G. O.: Raised levels of a new immunoglobulin class (IgND) in asthma. *Lancet 2*:951-53, 1967.
7. Johansson, S. G. O., Mellbin, T. and Vahlquist, B.: Immunoglobulin levels in Ethiopian preschool children with special reference to high concentrations of immunoglobulin (IgND). *Lancet 1*: 1118-20, 1968.
8. Gleich, G. J., Averbeck, A. M. and Swedland, H. A.: Concentration of IgE in serum of normal and allergic individuals. Abstract, 26th Annual Meeting, Amer. Acad. Allergy. New Orleans, La., Feb. 16-18, 1970.
9. Wide, L., Bennich, H., and Johansson, S. G. O.: Diagnosis of allergy by an in vitro test for allergen antibodies. *Lancet 2*:1105-07, 1967.
10. Coombs, R. R. A., Hunter, A., Jonas, W. E., Bennich, H., Johansson, S. G. O.,

and Panzani R.: Detection of IgE (IgND) specific antibody (probably reagin) to castor bean allergen by the red-cell-linked antigen-antiglobulin reaction. *Lancet 1*:1115-18, 1968.

11. Tse, K. S., Wicher, K. and Arbesman, C. E.: The effect of immunotherapy on IgE antibodies in nasal secretions and serum of ragweed-sensitive patients. Abstract, 26th Annual Meeting, Amer. Acad. Allergy, New Orleans, La., Feb. 16-18, 1970.
12. Arbesman, C. E., Tse, K. S. and Wicher, K.: Antibodies to ragweed in external secretions. Abstract, 26th Annual Meeting, Amer. Acad. Allergy, New Orleans, La., Feb. 16-18, 1970.
13. Newcomb, R. W. and Ishizaka, K.: Human γE in sputum and nasal fluids. Abstract, 26th Annual Meeting, Amer. Acad. Allergy, New Orleans, La., Feb. 16-18, 1970.
14. Katz, G. and Cohen, S.: Experimental evidence in histamine release in allergy. *J.A.M.A. 117*:1782-88, 1941.
15. Lichtenstein, L. M. and Norman, P. S.: Human allergic reactions. *Amer. J. Med. 46*:163-73, 1969.
16. Lichtenstein, L. M. and Margolis, S.: Inhibition of *in vitro* histamine release by the catecholamines and methylxanthines. *Science 161*:902-06, 1968.
17. Sadan, N., Rhyne, M. B., Mellits, D. E., Goldstein, E. O., Levy, D. A. and Lichtenstein, L. M.: A study of clinical and immunologic parameters in children receiving immunotherapy for ragweed hayfever. *J. Allergy 41*:116-24, 1968.
18. Pruzansky, J. J., and Patterson, R.: Histamine release from leukocytes of hypersensitive individuals. *J. Allerg. 39*:44-50, 1967.
19. Cooke, R. A., Barnard, J. H., Hebald, S. and Stull, A.: Serological evidence of immunity with co-existing sensitization in a type of human allergy (hayfever). *J. Exp. Med. 62*:733, 1935.
20. Connell, J. T. and Sherman, W. B.: Changes in skin-sensitizing antibody titer after injections of aqueous pollen extract. *J. Allerg. 43*:22-32, 1969.
21. Becker, E. L.: Enzymatic mechanisms in complement-dependent chemotaxis. *Fed. Proc. 28*:1704-09, 1969.
22. Feldberg, W. and Kellaway, C. H.: Liberation of histamine and formation of a lysocithin-like substance by cobra venom. *J. Physiol.* (London) *94*:187-196, 1938.
23. Stechschulte, D. J., Austen, K. F. and Bloch, K. J.: Antibodies involved in antigen-induced release of slow reacting substance of anaphylaxis (SRS-A) in the guinea pig and rat. *J. Exp. Med. 125*:127-47, 1967.
24. Ishizaka, T., Ishizaka, K., Orange, R. P. and Austen, K. F.: The capacity of human immunoglobulin E to mediate the release of histamine and slow reacting substance of anaphylaxis (SRS-A) from monkey lung. *J. Immun. 104*:335-43, 1970.
25. Mongar, J. L. and Schild, H. O.: Cellular mechanisms in anaphylaxis. *Physiol. Rev. 42*:226-70, 1962.
26. Herxheimer, H. and Stresemann, E.: The effect of bradykinin aerosol in guinea pigs and in man. *J. Physiol.* (London) *158*:38, 1961.
27. Jonasson, O. and Becker, E. L.: Release of kallikrein from guinea pig lung during anaphylaxis. *J. Exp. Med. 128*:509-22, 1966.
28. Dolovich, J., Back, N. and Arbesman, C. E.: Presence of bradykinin-like activity in nasal secretions from allergic subjects. *J. Allerg. 41*:103-13, 1968.
29. Michel, B., Russel, T., Winkelmann, R. K. and Gleich, G. J.: Release of kinins during wheal and flore allergic skin reactions. *J. Clin. Invest. 47*:68, 1968.
30. Bergström, S.: Prostaglandins: Members of a new hormonal system. *Science 157*:382-91, 1967.
31. Brostoff, J. and Roitt, I. M.: Cell-mediated (delayed) hypersensitivity in patients with summer hayfever. *Lancet 2*:1269-71, 1969.
32. Eppinger, H. and Hess, L.: *Vagotonia. A Clinical Study in Vegetative Neurology,* 2d ed. New York, Nervous and Mental Diseases, 1917.
33. Ahlquist, R. P.: Study of adrenotropic receptors. *Amer. J. Physiol. 153*:586-96, 1948.
34. Szentivanyi, A., Fischel, C. W. and Talmadge, D. W.: Adrenaline mediation

of histamine and serotonin hyperglycemia in normal mice and the absence of adrenaline-induced hyperglycemia in pertussis-sensitized mice. *J. Infect. Dis. 113*:86, 1963.

35. Fischel, C. W., Szentivanyi, A. and Talmadge, D. W.: Sensitization and desensitization of mice to histamine and serotonin by neurohumors. *J. Immunol. 89*:8, 1962.

36. Szentivanyi, A.: The beta adrenergic theory of the atopic abnormality in bronchial asthma. *J. Allerg. 42*:203-32, 1968.

37. Reed, C. E.: Beta adrenergic blockade, bronchial asthma and atopy. *J. Allerg. 42*:238-42, 1968.

38. Grieco, M. H., Pierson, R. N., Jr. and PiSunyer, F. X.: Comparison of the circulatory and metabolic effects of isoproterenol, epinephrine and methoxamine in asthmatic subjects. *Amer. J. Med. 44*:863-72, 1968.

39. Pierson, R. N., Jr. and Grieco, M. H.: Isoproterenol aerosol in normal and asthmatic subjects. *Amer. Rev. Resp. Dis. 100*:533-41, 1969.

40. Grieco, M. H. and Pierson, R. N., Jr.: Cardiopulmonary effects of methacholine in asthmatic and normal subjects. *J. Allerg.* In press.

41. Macdonald, A. G., Ingram, C. G. and McNeill, R. S.: The effect of propranolol on airway resistance. *Brit. J. Anesth. 39*:919-26, 1967.

42. Land, A. M., Arnold, A., McAuliff, J. P., Ludwena, F. P. and Brown, T. G.: Differentiation of receptor systems activated by sympathomimetic amines. *Nature 214*:597-98, 1967.

43. Sutherland, E. W., Robison, G. A. and Butcher, R. W.: Some aspects of the biological role of adenosine 3′, 5′—monophosphate (cyclic AMP). *Circulation 37*:279-306, 1968.

44. Powles, R., Shinebourne, E. and Hamer, J.: Selective cardiac sympathetic blockade as an adjunct to bronchodilator therapy. *Thorax 24*:616-18, 1969.

45. Tattersfield, A. E. and McNicol, M. W.: Salbutamol and isoproterenol. A double-blind trial to compare bronchodilator and cardiovascular activity. *New Eng. J. Med. 281*:1323-26, 1969.

46. Keighley, J. F.: Iatrogenic asthma associated with adrenergic aerosols. *Ann. Intern. Med. 65*:985-95, 1966.

47. Speizer, F. E., Doll, R. and Heaf, P.: Observations on recent increase in mortality from asthma. *Brit. Med. J. 1*:335-39, 1968.

48. Inman, W. H. W. and Adelstein, A. M:. Rise and fall of asthma mortality in England and Wales in relation to use of pressurized aerosols. *Lancet 2*:279-85, 1969.

49. Paterson, J. W., Conolly, M. E., Davies, D. S. and Dollery, C. T.: Isoprenaline resistance and the use of pressurized aerosols in asthma. *Lancet 2*:426-29, 1968.

50. Altounyan, R. E. C.: Inhibition of experimental asthma by new compound-disodium cromoglycate "Intal." *Acta Allerg. 22*:487, 1967.

51. Orange, R. P. and Austen, K. F.: Prospects in asthma therapy; disodium cromoglycate and diethylcarbamazine. *New Eng. J. Med. 279*:1055-56, 1968.

THE ORIGINS OF MODERN SCIENTIFIC THINKING

GREGORY I. ALTSCHULLER

Consultant in Medicine
The Roosevelt Hospital
New York, N. Y.

MEDICINE always has had and always will have two aspects: one scientific and the other clinical, in the broadest sense of the words. In different periods of history one or the other has dominated the mind of the medical man but both aspects have always been present.

Speaking of the origins of modern scientific thinking implies, therefore, also discussing the origins of scientific medicine. Some of the great natural philosophers of ancient Greece, as well as some of the outstanding scientists of modern times, have been physicians who contributed greatly both to physical sciences and to medicine. However, specific problems of medicine, important as they are and however closely they are connected with the development of scientific thinking, will be discussed only briefly in this essay.

Richard Mead, M.D. (1673-1754), physician to Sir Isaac Newton and physician-in-ordinary to King George II of England, was one of the most prominent and successful physicians in London, widely known for his professional skill and his literary reputation and respected for his kindness and generosity. He was a protégé of Dr. John Ratcliff, who presented him with his famous gold-headed cane as a token of respect and friendship.[1]

Dr. Mead lived at the time when somewhat primitive iatrochemical and iatrophysical theories impressed the minds of many leading medical men. He belonged to a small group of English physicians who at the very beginning of the 18th century attempted to apply the methods and principles of mathematics and of physical science to medicine. He acquired knowledge of these methods and became an ardent adept of the iatrophysical school while studying medicine in Padua and Leyden.[2] However, he avoided the most extreme theories of his teacher, John Pitcairn, representative of the iatromathematical school in England, although in his paper on "Mechanical Account of Poisons" (1702)

Dr. Mead tried to explain the action of poisons as the effect on the stomach of "small knives and daggers" he had observed under his microscope. In his later works he attempted to explain the influence of celestial bodies on the course of various diseases by gravitational attraction, by variations in the atmospheric pressure, and by similar factors. His ideas about the importance of quantitative mathematical methods as applied to medicine are best expressed in the following passage:

> . . . It is very evident that all other Methods of improving Medicine have been found ineffectual by the Stand It has been at these Three or Four thousand years, and since late Mathematicians have set themselves to the study of It, Men do already begin to talk so Intelligibly and Comprehensively even about abstruse Matters that it may be hoped in a short time, if Those who are designed for this Profession, are early, while their Minds and Bodies are Patient of Labour and Toil, initiated in the Knowledge of Numbers and Geometry, that Mathematical Learning will be the Distinguishing Mark of a Physician from a Quack, and He, who wants this necessary Qualification will be as ridiculous as One without Greek or Latin.[3]

Even if this enthusiastic prediction has not come true in the past 200 odd years, ours is the age of computers, and we are coming rather close to the ideas of Dr. Mead.

What are the characteristics of modern science? Without making any attempt at an accurate definition, we might summarize them as follows. Modern science is characterized by a desire to discover the laws of nature. These laws must be of general order and few, the tacit assumption being, as in ancient Greece, that there exists in nature an *order* and that nature loves simplicity ("*natura simplicitatem amat*"). All laws of nature must be expressed in mathematical language, and qualities must be replaced by quantities. Numbers and measurements are the basic tools of modern science, and deduction is combined with induction.[4]

Newton's universal law of gravitation is of such a general order. Since the time of Newton two important forces have been added to the force of gravity: the *electromagnetic force*, known since the time of Michael Faraday, and the *intra-atomic*, *nuclear force*, which became known in the 20th century. James C. Maxwell's field theory, first described in his paper "A Dynamical Theory of the Electromagnetic Field" (1865),[5] gradually replaced the older Newtonian concept of force and became one of the most important discoveries of modern physics. It led to Albert Einstein's theory of relativity and to his concept of a four-dimension continuum that forms the world of events.[6] In its final development matter and field became only two forms of energy which differ quantitatively but not qualitatively.[7]

Modern physicists accept the force of attraction that holds things together, such as the force of gravity and a centrifugal force which causes the expansion of the universe or the repulsion of particles with an opposite electrical charge.

Of great importance is the use of models and experiments instead of the simple observation of nature. Niels Bohr's model of the atom and the double helix as the model of DNA described by James D. Watson and Francis H. C. Crick are examples of the use of models in modern science. Experiments are the most important tools in modern scientific research, whether the laws of nature are discovered on the basis of experiments, as in Newtonian theory or, as in the epistemological approach of Einstein and other modern scientists, an experiment proves or disproves theoretical concepts deduced by the scientist from certain a priori assumptions.

The results of his theoretical investigations are applied by the modern scientist to problems of practical importance. This last point is the one which makes such a great difference between the work of ancient natural philosophers and of modern scientists.

In ancient Egypt, as well as in Babylon and Assyria, there was a highly developed technology but no science in the proper sense of the word. Pyramids were built, and also temples, an elaborate system of roads, mines on the Sinai Peninsula, and endless canals on which the very life of Egypt depended. In medicine hundreds of detailed prescriptions—some empirical, others rather magical—were recorded in papyri. A perfectly organized hierarchy of physicians existed that would gladden the heart of the 18th century professor Johann Peter Frank, famous author of the *System einer vollständiger medicinischer Polizey*. There was a Chief of the Secrets of Health, the Guardian of the Imperial Anus, and a whole network of inspectors, supervisors, and superintendents of various ranks who controlled the activities of thousands of physician-specialists; each took care of only one part of the body. In addition to these there were ordinary physician-magicians.[8]

But behind this imposing structure there was very little knowledge of pathology, very little rational theory. Physiology begins when man enters into speculations about the significance of three basic substances essential to life: air and food, both coming from the outside world, and blood within the body itself. The only rational pathology created by ancient Egypt was the theory of *WeHeDuW*, or *perittoma* in its later Greek version, related to the universal observation of the decay of all organic matter. It was probably based on the observation that the decomposition of a corpse starts in the large intestine. The decay of organic matter produces heat and odor. In the body of a sick man this decay or the process of putrefaction produces a pyogenic principle *WeHeDuW* which can pass into the bloodstream and cause fever and rapid pulse. Thus a state of pyemia is created which, if not treated properly, endangers health and life. Before the poisonous residues are absorbed into the bloodstream, they must be removed by enemas or purges or, later, by bloodletting. The Egyptian idea of putrefaction of the ingested food in the intestine as the major etiological principle of most illnesses was taken over by the Cnidians, still later elaborated by Galen,[9-11] and became the logical basis for bloodletting, which dominated therapeutics for centuries, until the beginning of the 19th century. The wide use of enemas and purges known to the Egyptians and to many African tribes since time immemorial could also be rationalized by physicians on the basis of the theory of *WeHeDuW* or *perittoma*. It is interesting to note that the absorption of poisonous matter from the intestines with advancing age was believed to be an inescapable process, which led eventually to the destruction of the body.[12, 13]

The theory of *WeHeDuW* seems to be the only rational pathological idea created by the Egyptian physicians. The Egyptians and Babylonians knew much more about astronomy through millennia of observation of the movements of celestial bodies. They knew, for instance, the difference between the calendar year and the solar year. They had a very cumbersome system of mathematics based on the decimal system but with separate symbols for the numbers 1, 10, 100, 1000, and so on. All this had been all-important for the practical pragmatic minds of the Egyptians. But there was very little theoretical basis for this knowledge.

In ancient Greece science had existed as a rational system from the time of the Milesians, but technology was completely neglected. The reason for this basic difference between the two cultures is complex and probably can be best understood as a result of the difference between the pragmatic mind of the Egyptian and the philosophical, contemplative mind of the Greek. The ancient Greek wanted to understand the world and the laws of nature but saw no need for any change or improvement which required manual work unworthy of a man of intelligence. In the words of Aristotle: ". . . It is owing to their wonder that men both now begin and at first began to philosophize. . . . They wondered originally at the obvious difficulties, then advanced little by little and stated difficulties about the greater matters and the phenomena of the sun and of the stars and about the genesis of the universe. And the man who is puzzled and wonders thinks himself ignorant. . . . Therefore, since they philosophized in order to escape from ignorance, evidently they were *pursuing science in order to know*, and not for any *utilitarian end*. . . ."[14]

It was left to man of the late Renaissance and of the 17th century—adventurous, daring, free from the chains of scholasticism—to try to understand the laws of nature in order to tame nature, to exploit and to conquer it. Scientific, rational thinking was then first applied to day-to-day problems of practical importance, and out of this new-found union of science and technology was born the enormous progress of both modern scientific thinking and of modern technology.

But long before this union occurred the great minds of ancient Greece had laid down the foundations of rational scientific thinking and, for the first time in the history of mankind, they tried to replace *mythos* by *logos*. They tried to discover the general laws of nature and they tried to explain the discrepancy between the unity of the cosmos and the plurality of sense-observed phenomena, between the eternal orderly movements of celestial bodies and the chaotic movements of sense-objects on earth.

Deduction was their main tool in analyzing observed phenomena, and only gradually did the quantitative approach to nature replace the old qualitative approach. But the endeavor to exploit nature, to apply the new discoveries to practical problems, to apply science to technology, was alien to them.

These limitations of ancient science are important. But without the cosmologists of Miletus, without the atomists and Anaxagoras, there would have been no foundation on which to build modern science.

SCIENCE AND THE EVOLUTION OF LANGUAGE

Replacing quality by quantity, replacing poetical descriptions of events by mathematical formulas had been a great step forward. It gave man a powerful tool for understanding nature and the laws of nature. But it required the growth of rational logical thinking instead of the mythical explanation of observed facts. The truth of logical thought can and must be investigated, and it can and must be accepted by all once proved right. Mythical truth is always *revealed* as such and must be accepted without any proof or argumentation.

It is obvious that the development of rational ideas requires a certain degree of linguistic development. The appearance of new scientific concepts and terms is the result of the evolution of language. It took almost five centuries, from the time of Homer to Plato and Aristotle, before the basic concepts of science and philosophy and abstract terms and concepts such as infinity, space, velocity, continuum, matter, force, and time evolved gradually in ancient Greece. It is a very long way from *the* horse of the hero of Homer to a concept of *a* horse, an abstract term. Words change their meaning. The "psyche" of Homer meant only a vital force which leaves the body when a man dies. The psyche as soul, as a thinking and feeling principle, appeared much later. The "aether" meant to Empedocles the most rarified substance, the fill of the universe. It was the Fifth Substance for Aristotle, identical to *pneuma* for the Stoics, and again something quite different to Galen, to René Descartes, to Newton, to the scientists of the 19th century or to Einstein and his followers.[15-18]

The same is true of mathematical thinking. It is a long way from natural and rational numbers or even from the irrational numbers of the Pythagoreans to the invention of analytical geometry by Descartes or of calculus by Leibnitz. The Romans simplified the cumbersome system of the Egyptians by using fewer symbols (X, C, D, M) and, to a very limited degree, the place-value property. But only with the Indo-Arabian system in the second half of the first millennium A.D., when the integer zero was introduced with the full use of the place-value property, did a real development of mathematics become possible.

The ancient Greeks had a fully developed system of logical thinking and of philosophical concepts but their mathematics remained rather primitive.

Science and the Rise of the Individual

Homer lived in the ninth century B.C., about two generations before the time of King David and King Solomon of Biblical tradition. The world of Homer was that of heroes dominated by deities. Homer sang to the courts of Achaean princes, and the heroes of Homer's epics had all the characteristics of an ideal warrior: courage, magnanimity in victory, dignity in defeat. The hero was fearless and strong, an ideal of a man close to the image of the Homeric gods. But his knowledge of things was deceptive, and his fate was in the hands of gods who had the complete knowledge of things. And both men and gods had to obey the forces of time and fate.[19]

The attitude of men toward the acquisition of knowledge gradually changed. Xenophanes (ca. 540 B.C.) taught that man could acquire knowledge, though incomplete, not as a gift of gods but by his own industry and perseverance. He denied the existence of anthropomorphic gods. For him there was only one God, "who sees all over, thinks all over and hears all over" and who had a real knowledge of things. The knowledge of man would always be partial, but whatever knowledge he could acquire, he would gain only by a long seeking.[20-22]

Alcmeon (500 B.C.), the greatest of the pre-Hippocratic physicians, belonged to the same philosophical school of Croton in southern Italy that is connected with the names of Xenophanes and Pythagoras. He was probably the first known to practice anatomical dissections and to make experiments on animals. He was the first to state that the brain and not the heart is the seat of the senses and of the intellect. He described the optic nerves and their crossing and he assumed that the optic nerves conduct the perception of light into the brain. The function of the brain, Alcmeon thought, is to transmit the sense of perception, to recollect, and thus to lead to the acquisition of knowledge. Only conjecture based on facts born out of perception may lead, according to Alcmeon, to some knowledge of invisible reality. Thus he introduced the concept of induction as a way to acquire knowledge.[23, 24]

In his medical teachings Alcmeon was very close to the basic ideas of Pythagoras, and to Alcmeon we owe the fundamental principles of humoral pathology. Health, he believed, is a state of perfect harmony, disease is a disturbance of this harmony, and cure is the return to the original state of harmony. Many of the ideas of the Hippocratic school can be traced to this great physician of Croton.

Man slowly asserted his right to be independent from the whims of anthropomorphic gods. Archilochus was born about 650 B.C. at Paros, son of a nobleman and a slave girl. He moved from Paros to Phasos and there took part in the wars against the Greek invaders from the mainland. He fought in many wars and belonged to the type of mercenary soldiers who served in the armies of Pharaoh Psammetichus I and who helped him to liberate Egypt from the Assyrians. Archilochus was a soldier and a poet. He saw war without any illusions; he saw in it not only heroic deeds but also blood, suffering, and cruelty. Instead of the glorification of heroes he sang about the naked realities of war. Not the gods but man was the center of his attention.[25]

And then came Sappho of Lesbos and Anacreon, who asserted themselves in their lyrics as human beings and emphasized the reality of human passions, of love and hate. The beautiful monodic songs of Sappho are the revolt of individualism against the chains of hesiodic theogony. Man wanted to think for himself and to know and to feel reality.[26, 27]

About 700 years before the birth of Sappho, in the middle of the 14th century B. C., a spiritual revolution took place in Egypt at a time when the country was ruled by the young Pharaoh Ikhnaton, a dreamer and philosopher, "the world's first idealist and the world's first individual." It was a revolt of a dreamer against the powerful priesthood and against centuries-old tradition. Ikhnaton introduced the worship of a new supreme god, Aton, that was a new name for the old sun-god Re. Temples were built and new rituals and symbols were created. Hymns were written which resemble closely the psalms of King David. Ikhnaton insisted on "living in truth," and in the religion, the art, and in the poetry of his time one observes the passionate desire to see and understand the realities of life instead of an idealization of the world of the dead.[28] Beautiful love songs appeared; they are preserved in the papyri and many of them are surprisingly similar to the Song of Songs of the Bible. They were recently recreated from learned translations of egyptologists by outstanding American and Russian poets.[29, 30]

But Ikhnaton, philosopher and spiritual reformer, could not defend his kingdom against the forces of external and internal enemies. After his death (1358 B.C.) the short-lived Egyptian spiritual revolution came to an end, the new temples were destroyed, and the old traditions and the old way of life were restored by the combined forces of the priesthood and powerful courtiers. A decline of the empire followed and only after years of stagnation in art and economics was the orderly organization that Egypt had once enjoyed gradually brought back.[31]

The spiritual revolution in Egypt ended with the death of Ikhnaton. The outburst of individualism in Greece in the seventh century B.C., which had been the result of a centuries-long process of evolution of language and thought helped to clear the way for the rational approach to nature. The revolt of the individualism that had been spearheaded by the Greek lyrics of the seventh century B.C. seems to have much in common with a similar movement that took place in Western Europe at the end of the 16th and the beginning of the 17th centuries. The Elizabethan poets and musicians (Thomas Morley, John Wilbye) began to write madrigals in which they used not only translations of the sonnets of Petrarch and Tasso but folk songs and love songs known to the man in the street, somewhat like the rock songs of our time. At the same time a group of young musicians and poets (the Camerata) gathered in a back room of a palace in Florence and discussed passionately the new creative art later called by the traditionalists "baroque," a derogatory term meaning ugly, irregular. The operas of Claudio Monteverdi were written then. In them the man on the stage was not submerged in the majestic polyphony of the early Renaissance but spoke and sang about his sorrows and passions and joys. The same revolt spread all over Europe. About 20 years later John Milton, long before writing his *Paradise Lost*, published his tracts on divorce and the famous *Areopagitica* in defense of freedom of the press. The teleologically oriented philosophy of the Middle Ages changed gradually and gave way to a new philosophy and a new science. Copernicus in the early 16th century proved by mathematical reasoning that the earth is not the center of the universe; the immensity of the universe was soon proved, contrary to medieval religious and philosophical teachings. And then, in 1687, the young Isaac Newton wrote his brilliant *Principia* in which he proved that the same laws of nature govern the movements of the stars, the sun, the moon, and sense objects on earth.

The revolt of individualism in Europe, once started, continued to grow and can be traced in the birth of the English novel and in the creation of sonata-form with its conflict of human passions brought to perfection by Haydn, Mozart, and Beethoven; it dominated music until our time. The baroque movement in art and science led the way to Cartesian philosophy and to the mathematization of science by Galileo Galilei, Newton, and Leibnitz. The development of modern science began in the 17th century and never stopped.

The Early Milesians

The birth of rational philosophy in Greece took place in the city of Miletus, founded by Ionian settlers soon after the Dorian invasion of the Greek mainland.[32] Miletus very early became the center of a lively trade with its eastern neighbors and with Egypt. In the course of time these commercial ties brought cultural influences. And two medical schools, the cradles of Hippocratic and Asclepiadic medicine, were founded on the tiny islands Cos and Cnidos off the shores of Miletus.[33]

The three great Milesians—Thales, Anaximenes, and Anaximander—all tried to solve the basic problem which is still puzzling the theoretical physicist today: What is the nature of matter? For the first time in the history of mankind they attempted to solve the problem by rational methods outside the realm of religion, myth, and magic. How is one to explain the unity of the universe and the plurality of the sense-perceived world? What is real and what is only an illusion? In our time Pierre Teilhard de Chardin, the late theologian, philosopher, and scientist, devoted the first chapter of his book *The Phenomenon of Man* to this problem of unity and plurality.[34] The explanation given by the Milesian philosophers might seem naive to us; primordial matter was water for Thales, air for Anaximenes, and *arche* for Anaximander, substance without limits, ageless and eternal. But the approach of these thinkers was radically different from that of Homer or Hesiod. Ocean for Homer was a mythical unity—the origin of men and gods. To Thales water was the water we see and drink, which becomes ice and vapor. If for Homer the rainbow was a bridge walked by the messengers of the gods, for Anaximenes it was a result of "the beams of the sun falling on the thick, condensed air." This was not yet a scientific discovery but a first attempt at a rational explanation of an observed natural phenomenon. And the statement of Anaximenes that the plurality of sense-objects was caused "by the virtue of rarefication and condensation of air in different substances" was a first attempt to substitute quantity for quality.[35]

Anaximander, another Milesian, wrote that all life comes from the sea and that the present forms of animals including man are the result of their evolving through a process of adaptation to the environment: "Living creatures arose from moist element as it was evaporated by the sun. . . . Man was like another animal, namely as a fish in the beginning, he was born from animals of another species. . . . While other animals quickly found food for themselves, man alone requires lengthy period of suckling. Hence had he been originally as he is now, he would never have survived."[36]

Anaximander was not a precursor of Charles Darwin, but nevertheless his was the stroke of intuition of a genius. He was the first to use models and drawings while explaining the movements of the stars to his pupils.

What fascinated these first natural philosophers was the striking discrepancy between the majestic order and constancy of the movements of celestial bodies and the chaotic changes observed daily in the sense-perceived world.

This discrepancy led Parmenides, the great philosopher of Elea, to whom Plato owed so much, to speak of all observed changes as pure illusion and to accept as real only the unchangeable, motionless eternal Being: "What is—is uncreated and indestructible for it is complete, immovable and without end. . . . Nor was it ever, nor will it be, for now it is, all at once, a continuous one. . . ."[37] This discrepancy led Leucippus to state that nothing occurs by chance but there is a reason and necessity for everything.[38] The idea of order in nature and of causality had been the basis of the philosophical quest of the first Milesians and still is an assumption accepted a priori by every scientist: "Without the belief that it is possible to grasp the reality with our theoretical constructions, without the belief in the inner harmony in our world, there could be no science. This belief is and always will be the fundamental motive for all scientific creation."[39]

Empedocles and the Pythagoreans

Thales, Anaximenes, and Anaximander taught the monistic theory of the universe. Primordial eternal matter had been for them either water, air, or an "eternal Being." It was Empedocles of Akragas who first broke with this monistic tradition. For him the eternal elements, unchangeable and indivisible, are four, not one, and the plurality of sense-objects results from the endless variety of combinations of those four primordial elements: "For all of these (fire and water and earth and air) are equal and alike in age . . . and nothing comes into being besides these, nor do they pass away. . . . For out of these spring all things that were and are and shall be—trees and men and women, beasts and birds and the fishes that dwell in the waters, yea and the gods that live long lives and are exalted in honors. For there are these alone, but running through one another, they take different shapes—so much does mixture change them. . . ."[40]

These four "roots" of all things were identified with the cold, the hot, the moist, and the dry. And the four elements of Empedocles remained the basis of scientific medicine and of humoral pathology for the next two thousand years. To Hippocrates they became black bile, yellow bile, blood, and phlegm, and they can be traced in one form or another in the writings of Galen and Avicenna and in the writings of all great medical men to the end of the 17th century. The four elements of Empedocles were eternal and equal parts of primordial matter. The same four elements in Plato's *Timaeus* became not substances but geometrical forms which become matter only when put together.[41] Much later, with the acceptance of Aristotelian metaphysics, they became not equal but different in their dignity and value, and the lighter elements, air and fire, were considered *nobler* than earth and water.

This number 4 had been borrowed by Empedocles and Alcmeon from Pythagoras and his school. The Pythagoreans formed a secret society with a complicated ritual, strict rules of behavior, and a belief in the transmigration of the soul and in reincarnation.[42] Aside from the mystical elements in their teachings, the essence of the cosmos to the Pythagoreans was numbers. Numbers were for them spatial concepts; the number 1 represented a point; 2, a line; 3, a plane, and 4, a solid. All things are numbers and can be properly expressed only in numbers. The quality of musical pitch corresponds to a measurable length of a string and therefore can be replaced and explained by a mathematical formula. Thus the harmony of the sounds depends on a proper choice of numerical values, and the harmony of the spheres depends on the eternal harmony of the heavens.[43]

To the pythagoreans the number 4 and all even numbers were unlimited and all odd numbers were limited. A whole allegorico-metaphysical philosophy developed later on the basis of this theory of numbers. Numbers became symbols. The number 3 represented a man, and 2 a woman, so that marriage could logically be said to be represented by number 5. Great minds of the 16th century were preoccupied with this mystery of numbers. In England in 1570 John Dee maintained in his address *To the Unfained Lovers of Truthe* that the universe consisted of "Numbrings."[44] Galileo wrote once in terms almost Platonic that ". . . philosophy is written in that vast book which stands forever open before our eyes, I mean the Universe, but it cannot be read until we have learned the language and become familiar with the characters in which it is written. It is written in mathematical language and the letters are triangles, circles and other geometrical figures without which means it is humanly impossible to comprehend a single word. . . ."[45]

Pythagoras knew irrational numbers too, such as the square root of 2; his pupils called them "devoid of logos." They knew that irrational numbers are squeezed between the integers and that this confinement can be narrowed indefinitely and that *reality can be approached only through approximation.* The pythagoreans kept this knowledge secret for about 200 years, until their society declined completely. Archimedes in the third century B.C. used this principle in calculating the famous "pi," the ratio of the circumference of a circle to its diameter, by inscribing and circumscribing regular polygons with ever-increasing numbers of sides. Pythagoras applied numbers to the sensory world and to the cosmos in general; he replaced qualities by quantities as does modern science.[46]

Plato divorced numbers from all sense-perceived objects and applied them to the world of ideas or forms. His authority made impossible any real progress in the quantitative analysis of the sensory world for nearly 2,000 years. Similarly the authority of Aristotle, who firmly believed in the immobility of the earth, made it impossible for the scientists of many generations to accept the heliocentric theory of earth movements taught by Aristarchus of Samos as early as 270 B.C.[47]

It seems, however, that in the 20th century we are again approaching the platonic teachings of the relation between the world of ideas and the sensory world. The elementary particles of Plato's *Timaeus* were in the final analysis not substances but mathematical forms. The only mathematical forms available at that time were such geometrical forms as regular solids and triangles. In modern quantum theory there can be no doubt that the elementary particles will also be mathematical forms but of much more complicated nature.[48] Matter and energy are expressed by the modern theoretical physicist in the form of mathematical abstractions, and the network of these abstractions becomes the only reality, not unlike the platonic world of ideas in contrast to which the sense-perceived world becomes a pure illusion.

Empedocles introduced not only the four fundamental elements as the building blocks of nature but he was the first to introduce the concept of force as the cause of the movements of matter. He recognized two forces, which he called Love and Strife. In using these poetical terms he wanted to indicate that one force brings things together, whereas the other pulls them apart: "At one time it grew to be only one out of many; at another, it divided up to be many instead of one. . . . And these things never cease continually changing places, at one time all uniting in one through *Love*, at another each borne in different directions by the repulsion of *Strife*."[49] We might replace his terms by concepts more familiar to us: attraction and repulsion. The centrifugal force of Huygens and the force of attraction which became the starting point that led to the discovery of the great law of gravitation by Newton are quite similar to the two forces of Empedocles, who in the fifth century B.C. came so close to the ideas of the great men of the 17th century A.D.

Some other statements of Empedocles show the greatness of his intuition. He stated that light as it propagates through space requires time to reach the observer. One of the late commentators, Philoponus, described his opinion as follows: "Empedocles said that light is a streaming substance which, emitted from the source of light, first reaches the region between earth and sky and from there comes to us; but we are not conscious of this movement, because of the speed." Thus for the first time the idea of the velocity of light had been clearly expressed.[50, 51]

More than 2,000 years later Galileo in his *Dialogues Concerning Two New Sciences*, first published in 1637, expressed the opinion that . . . "the familiar bit of experience is that sound, in reaching our ear, travels more slowly than light; it does not inform me whether the coming of the light is instantaneous or whether, although extremely rapid, it still occupies time. . . . The fact that the speed of sound is as high as it is, assures us that the motion of light cannot fail to be extraordinary swift. . . ." And Galileo proceeds to devise a method by which one might accurately ascertain whether ". . . The propagation of light is really not instantaneous."[52] His method, while logically correct, could not be properly applied with the primitive experimental techniques of his time. However, about 50 years later Olaus Roemer, the Danish astronomer, proved in 1675 that the velocity of light is finite. He used astronomical observations to calculate the speed of light, contrary to the terrestial method suggested by Galileo. By observing the revolutions of the first satellite of Jupiter at the different positions of the earth on its orbit around the sun, Roemer calculated the velocity of light to be 308,000 kilometers per second, or very close to what we know it to be.

His calculations were checked and found to be correct by the greatest authority of the time, Huygens.[53] Much later, with the refinement of the experimental technique, Armand H. L. Fizeau confirmed his result by terrestial experiments as did Albert A. Michelson in the 20th century.[54]

Empedocles taught that air has the properties of a body or matter; this was an entirely new concept.[55] But much more important for the further development of science and medicine was his theory of the "shedding of particles" by all objects. Those particles or "effluences flow from all things that have come into being." The infinitesimal indivisible particles enter our sense organs and are the true basis of sensation, vision, and smell. Perception is due to the meeting of an element in us with the same element outside. This takes place when the pores of the organ of sense are neither too large nor too small for the "effluences" which all things are constantly emitting. However, Empedocles believed that hearing is produced when the air moved by the voice sounds inside the ear.[56]

The idea of the emission of particles had been fully developed by the atomists, especially by Democritus, whose "atoms" were really "effluences." To Democritus the only reality consisted of atoms and the void; this led him to distinguish between the real or primary qualities and the secondary qualities. Galen quotes Democritus as saying ". . . all the qualities of the things perceived by us result from collision of the atoms. In reality there no white, no black, no yellow, or red, or bitter or sweet. . . . Colors exist by convention, sweet by convention, bitter by convention, in truth nothing exists but the atoms and the void." And in another fragment: ". . . Senses give us no information about the reality but only the interplay of atoms."[57]

Johannes Kepler, who lived at the time of the revival of pythagorean and neoplatonic ideas and of platonic geometrical atomism, but long before the atomism of Democritus and Epicurus became common knowledge, thought ". . . that knowledge offered the mind by the senses is obscure, contradictory and untrustworthy. The real world is a world of quantitative characteristics only, the differences are differences of numbers alone."[58] Somewhat later Galileo, who even more than Kepler believed in the mathematical foundation of nature, insisted, contrary to the vague theories of the Pythagoreans, that exact mathematical methods must be applied to studies of nature. The reality of the universe is geometrical; the ultimate characteristic of nature, the primary qualities, are those of which certain mathematical knowledge is possible: number, figure, position, magnitude, motion. All other qualities are subjective. ". . . I think that these tastes, odors, colors . . . on the side of the object in which they seem to exist are nothing else but mere names, but hold their residence solely in the sensitive body. . . ."[59]

This and similar opinions which are so close to the statements of Democritus led, a few decades later, to the Cartesian dualism. Still later, at the very end of the 17th century they were fully developed by John Locke. Locke, the first of the English empiricists, famous author of *An Essay concerning Human Understanding*, philosopher, and physician, was a close friend of Dr. Thomas Sydenham and a contemporary of Dr. Richard Mead. Locke also accepted fully the Newtonian concept of nature as essentially mechanical in its dynamics and corpuscular in its structure. He believed that all our knowledge is based on perception and that ". . . perception is the first operation of our intellectual faculties and the inlet of all knowledge in our minds." The objective cause of perception is direct or indirect contact with the object, and Locke distingushed between the real or primary qualities such as solidity, extension, figure, and motility and the secondary qualities which are "in truth nothing in the objects themselves but powers to produce various sensations in us by their primary qualities. . . . For it being manifest that there are bodies and good store of bodies each whereof are so small that we cannot by any of our senses discover either their bulk, figure, or motion . . . and that the different motions and figures, bulk and number of such . . . insensible particles of matter . . .

affecting the several organs of our senses, produce in us the different sensations which we have from the smells and the colors of the bodies. . . ."[60]

The materialistic philosophy of Locke was fought violently by his younger contemporary, George Berkeley, who for philosophical and religious reasons denied the very existence of the external world. However, Locke's theory of the working of the human mind, opposed in England by Berkeley and later by David Hume,[61] had been further developed in France by the French sensualists and by Etienne B. de Condillac, whose famous expression "penser c'est toujours sentir" defines best the views of that school.

The ideas of Condillac (1715-1780) were systematized about 20 years after his death by a group of outstanding medical men: M. F. X. Bichat, Pierre J. G. Cabanis, Philippe Pinel, and François Magendie—all well known in the history of medicine. Radical analytical empiricism characterized the methods of these thinkers, who later became known as the Ideologues and whose strictly materialistic philosophy in many aspects resembled the philosophy of Locke.[62]

The Shedding of Particles and the Miasmatic Pathogenesis of Diseases

Another aspect of the theory of the empedoclean shedding of particles and of the democritean emission of atoms was the miasmatic theory of the pathogenesis of infectious diseases. The word miasma had been used as a medical term since the time of Hippocrates but in the course of centuries it changed its meaning many times. To Hippocrates "miasma" meant some vaguely defined contamination of the air; when air spoiled by miasma is inhaled "men turn sick." Galen, who wrote extensively about miasmas, connected them with the concept of putrefaction and spoke of "putrid miasmas" that flow in the air and are the cause of fever and disease in those who are susceptible.[63] The authority of Galen kept the concept of putrid miasmatic effluvia alive for centuries long after the existence of an invisible *contagium animatum vivum* was postulated as a cause of disease in human beings, animals, and even plants by Girolamo Fracastoro, who wrote in 1546 that "the contagium of putrefaction goes from one body to another whether adjacent or distant," and that "these seeds *(seminaria prima)* have the faculty of multiplying and propagating rapidly." Girolamo

Fracastoro, one of the greatest scientists of the 16th century, expressed ideas very close to the theories of modern pathology and epidemiology.[64] However, a miasmatic etiology of major epidemic diseases—of cholera, typhus, yellow fever, and plague—in its more modern version had been accepted and passionately defended up to the second half of the 19th century by the majority of the most prominent European physicians.[65] Austin Flint, in the fifth edition of his *Treatise on Principles and Practice of Medicine*, written in conjunction with William H. Welch and published in 1881, i.e., on the very threshold of the new bacteriological era, wrote, "that infectious diseases may or may not be communicable by means of contagium. If communicable—it is a communicable infectious disease. If not communicable, it is an infectious, miasmatic disease."[66] The ancient concept of miasmatic propagation of diseases, which originated in the works of ancient Greek scientists, disappeared forever from the pages of the medical textbooks in the bacteriological era. But in 1888 Dr. Louis Smith, clinical professor of children's diseases at Bellevue Hospital Medical College in New York City, still believed that most children "developed diphtheria by inhaling infectious sewer gas."[67]

The Atoms and the Void

The rational scientific thinking of the Greek natural philosophers reached its heights in the two opposite schools of thought represented on one side by the atomists and on the other side by Anaxagoras and later by the stoics. The ideas of both schools are of great significance and are closely related to the development of modern scientific concepts of matter, space, and force.

The atomists, whose main representative was Democritus, one of greatest geniuses of the ancient world (460-370 B.C.), also included Leucippus (ca. 460 B.C.), Epicurus and his school (341-270 B.C.) and, finally, the Roman poet T. Lucretius Carus (d. 55 B.C.).

The world of the atomists, with a few differences between the teaching of Democritus and of the epicureans, consisted of an infinite number of invisible and indivisible atoms of various sizes and shapes which moved constantly in a void or vacuum. The matter of which the atoms are made is uniform or, as stated by Aristotle: "the nature of them all is, they say, the same, just as if each one separately were a piece of gold. Matter is eternal . . . nothing can be created out of nothing nor can it be destroyed and returned into nothingness."[68-70] This is a sort of law of conservation of matter, and it was first postulated by Parmenides of Elea, who was born at the end of the sixth century B.C. and was still alive in 449 B.C. when he conversed with the young Socrates in Athens.[71] He wrote: "What is, is uncreated and indestructible; for it is complete, immovable and without end. . . . Nor was it ever nor will it be; for now it is, all at once and continuous one. . . ."[72]

The atoms of Leucippus and Democritus move perpetually in the infinite void, overtake each other and collide; ". . . some of them rebound in random directions, while others interlock because of the symmetry of their sizes, shapes, positions, and arrangements, and remain together. This was how compound bodies were begun."[73] However, the atomists never explained what force causes the movements of the atoms. They accepted it as a fact as they postulated the existence of atoms.

Epicurus modified slightly the teachings of Leucippus and Democritus by introducing the concept of the weight of atoms, which according to Democritus differed only in their shape and size. However, both agreed on the existence of a void ". . . because unless there is a void . . . there can not be *many*, since there is nothing to keep them apart. . . ." The atoms of Epicurus move through the void with equal speed "nothing colliding with them. For neither will the heavy move more quickly than the small and light . . . nor again the small more quickly than the great having their whole course uniform when nothing collides with them either." This conclusion based on pure deduction is very close to the famous law of inertia of Galileo, who wrote that an "undisturbed body continues to move uniformly in a straight line or remains at rest." Galileo also discovered terrestrial acceleration and thus cleared the way for Newton's law of gravitation and for the newtonian concept of mass as different from weight. Galileo was first to make motion the object of exact mathematical study.[74]

Mathematical analysis was unknown to the ancients. The absolute determinism of Democritus did not explain the creation of the world. Epicurus admitted spontaneous deviation of the atoms from their predetermined course in the void and by this act of the "free will" of the atoms explained the possibility of their collision as the starting point of the creation of matter.[75]

If we replace the size and the shape of the atoms by their atomic weight and allow the absolute void of Democritus to be filled with an extremely rarefied matter (the ancients called it ether; for the Stoics it was *pneuma*),[76, 77] we arrive at the theory of matter and the universe that was valid and was taught in physics and chemistry to the very end of the 19th century.

Democritus stated emphatically that the atoms, the fundamentals of nature, are not perceptible to the senses. The senses give us only the interplay of atoms. It is impossible to know how each thing is in reality.

All sensation depends on the contact of atoms of various shapes with our organs of sense. However, perception varies with the state of the body of the perceiver: "For this reason one kind of atom sometimes produces the opposite sensation while the opposite produces the original one."

Epicurus modified this complete negation of the values of our sensations. Three hundred years later Lucretius summed up the opinion of Epicurus in the following sentence: "You will find that the concept of truth was originated by the senses and that the senses cannot be rebutted. . . . If they are not true, then reason in its entirety is equally false."[78]

For the atomists all qualities were replaced by quantities. How can one explain the infinite variety of sense-perceived objects? Democritus, as quoted by Aristotle, gave a brilliant analogy as an explanation of the plurality of the sensory world: atoms are like letters of the alphabet, per se they are devoid of quality or meaning. But letter-atoms acquire meaning when combined into syllables and words. Change one letter in a word and its meaning is changed. Change one atom in a combination of atoms and the properties of the matter are changed. What is true for the letters is also true for the atoms. "Tragedy and comedy are both composed of the same letters."[79-81]

Pythagoreanism, Atomism, and the Birth of Modern Science

Atomism in all its various forms, as the geometrical atomism of Plato's *Timaeus* or as that of Democritus, Epicurus, or the Roman poet Lucretius, together with the revival of pythagoreanism, became the most important major link between the ancient Greek philosophers and the great minds of the 16th and 17th centuries, who created the foundations of modern science and technology. Plato's *Timaeus* attracted attention and fascinated the medieval thinkers as early as the 11th century, when Aristotle was still known only as the author of books on logic. Toward the end of the Middle Ages Aristotelian philosophy and metaphysics with its teleology, its strict homocentrism and geocentrism, and its attitude to nature as mainly qualitative, with logic and not mathematics as the real key to knowledge, united in the minds of medieval men with the Christian theology. However, the platonic ideas of the world as fundamentally geometrical, simple, and harmonious—together with the pythagorean theory of the importance of numbers—remained a powerful counterpart of the dominant Christian and Aristotelian philosophy. All or almost all of the medieval thinkers were deeply religious. But once the world is accepted as essentially geometrical and quantitative in the platonic and pythagorean sense, a mathematical approach to knowledge is legitimate and is not in conflict with the basic teachings of religion.

At the very end of the Middle Ages Nicholas of Cusa (1401-1464), a theologian, a cardinal since 1448, a man deeply interested in platonic philosophy as well as in mathematics and in physical science, wrote that "number is the first model of things in the mind of the Creator" and that "knowledge is always measurement." He insisted on quantitative measurements of time and weight, with the use of a balance for physical, physiological, and even mathematical investigations. His book on philosophy bears a curious title *De Docta Ignorantia* (the learned ignorance); in it he wrote about the relativity and imperfection of human knowledge.[82, 83] Nicolaus Copernicus, who was born 10 years after the death of Nicholas of Cusa, lived in a time of great cultural, economic, and social upheaval when many conflicting, strange, and radical ideas had to be faced by intelligent men in Western Europe. Copernicus studied mathematics and astronomy at the University of Cracow and early accepted the pythagorean doctrine of numbers and the geometrical atomism of Plato. He spent several years in Italy and, while studying mathematics under Domenico Maria de Novara, professor of astronomy in Bologna, became dissatisfied with the orthodox, ptolemaic theory of the movements of celestial bodies. In Padua he studied medicine with Girolamo Fracastoro. In 1504 he returned to Germany. The revolutionary idea that dominated his thinking all his life matured slowly but by now he was certain that he could offer a better, simpler, and more harmonious explanation of the movements of the earth and the planets than did the followers of Ptolemy. He postulated the diurnal rotation of the earth around its axis and annual motion of the earth around the sun. By doing so he was concerned only with giving a more accurate and simpler explanation of the observed facts by replacing the 80 ptolemaic epicycles by his 34. However, by placing the sun in the center of the universe instead of the earth and by reviving the heliocentric theory of Aristarchus of Samos that was familiar to him, Copernicus met intense opposition both on theological and scientific grounds. He worked on his great book *De Revolutionibus* all his life, and it was published in 1541, two years before his death.[84] Copernicus was helped in writing it by a young mathematician, Rhaeticus, who stayed with him as a devoted student and admirer. One may doubt whether the great book of Copernicus would have been written if this young and talented mathematician and devoted disciple had not stayed with the aging genius and helped him to accomplish his work.

The heliocentric theory of Copernicus had been understood and accepted in his time by few but was bitterly criticized by many. Melanchthon wrote about this "Sarmatian (Slavic) astronomer who moves the earth and fixes the sun." And Martin Luther spoke with disdain of "the fool who will overturn the whole art of astronomy." Aristotelian philosophy dominated the minds of a majority of intelligent people of his time to whom daily experience proved beyond any doubt the immobility of the solid, massive, and stable earth.[85]

However, about 50 years later the great revolutionary idea of Copernicus was seized and fully developed by a young genius, Johannes Kepler (1571-1630).

As a young man Kepler had been impressed by the importance of the sun in the heliocentric system of Copernicus. In 1593, while still a student in Tübingen, he wrote that "the sun alone by virtue of its dignity and power is suited for this motive duty and worthy to become the home of God himself not to say the first mover."[86] For the rest of his life Kepler was involved in the mystical implications of the neoplatonic and pythagorean theories of numbers and in the allegorical symbolism of celestial bodies. To the platonics the universe was fundamentally geometrical, and Kepler accepted fully the geometrical atomism of Plato's *Timaeus:* God created the world in accordance with the principles of perfect harmony;[87] real knowledge is mathematical; and knowledge acquired through the senses is deceptive and unreliable. However, Kepler above all else was a brilliant mathematician, and within the framework of the neoplatonic and pythagorean philosophy of numbers he searched constantly for new harmonies of the universe, primarily for the mathematical harmonies of the movements of celestial bodies. Kepler endeavored to verify the harmonious simplicity of the world of Copernicus by exact mathematics, never disregarding as irrelevant the deviations between the observed facts and the results of pure deduction.

Very important and fortunate for the great discoveries of Kepler were those of one of the greatest astronomers of his time, Tycho Brahe; irritable, arrogant, and full of prejudices, he despised and distrusted all the calculations and conclusions of Copernicus. Yet he admitted young Kepler, an admirer of Copernicus and his heliocentrism, as an assistant to his observatory and his workshop near Prague, where he lived in semiexile.[88]

There, for a year and a half, until the death of Brahe, Kepler was able to obtain full knowledge of Brahe's methods and observations; after the death of his master, he was able to use the enormous factual material collected by Brahe during almost 40 years of patient and precise astronomical observation.

Kepler, after years of incessant work, found new mathematical harmonies in his three famous laws of planetary motion. But pythagorean mysticism dominated his mind, as did platonic geometric atomism. As late as 1619 in his book *Harmonices Mundi,* while describing his third law of planetary motion which he called the "harmonic law," Kepler discussed in great detail the "music of the spheres" and made a serious attempt to express it in the form of musical notation.[89-92]

A deeply religious man, Kepler nevertheless firmly defended the right of the philosopher or scientist to seek the truth about the real nature of the world. "In theology," wrote he, "to be sure, the force of authorities is to be weighed; in philosophy, however, that of causes. . . . Worthy of sainthood is the dutiful performance of moderns who, admitting the meagreness of the earth, yet deny its motion. But truth is more saintly for me, who demonstrate by philosophy, without violating my due respect for the doctors of the church, that the earth is both round and inhabited at the antipodes and of most despicable size and finally is moved among the stars."[93]

Kepler's great and voluminous book, *Astronomia Nova,* remained unnoticed and was read by only a few scientists, partly because of its poor latinity and unclear style. However, it was accepted enthusiastically by Galileo, then a young professor of mathematics in Padua.

Galileo was born in 1564 and was a contemporary of Kepler, with whom he maintained a lively correspondence for many years. His philosophy, like that of Kepler, was essentially pythagorean and platonic, and geometric atomism was the basis of his theory of matter. However, the mysticism of pythagoreanism had much less importance for him than for Kepler. Even long before the atomism of Democritus and Epicurus became well known through the writings of Pierre Gassendi, Galileo adopted some of the concepts of the atomic theory of matter. Nature to him was geometrical and mathematical because God was a geometrician in his labors, and "matter consists of infinite number of small indivisible units (atoms)." In his search for an explanation of the events of nature, Galileo asked "How?" instead of "Why?" and he patiently applied exact mathematics and experiments in his studies of motion. The philosophical and theological problems of the "ultimate cause" or of the creation of the world were all-important to him,[94] but he wrote cautiously that "considerations of this kind belong to a higher science than ours. We must be satisfied to belong to that class of less worthy workmen who procure from the quarry the marble out of which, later, the gifted sculptor produces those masterpieces which lay hidden in this rough and shapeless exterior."[95] He had boundless admiration for his predecessors, for Aristarchus and Copernicus, but he turned his attention from the movements of celestial bodies to the motions of the objects on earth, which became the object of exact mathematical studies and painstaking experiments. The problems of terrestrial dynamism led him to the discovery of the law of inertia, to the concept of acceleration, and to the refutation of the Aristotelian theory of motion. However, mass to Galileo was still equivalent to weight; it was Newton who first expressed mass in terms of force, and force in terms of mass, in his law of gravitation.

By the middle of the 17th century pythagoreanism had lost the influence it had had in the preceding century. With great progress in new branches of mathematics the geometrical platonic approach to nature gave place to algebraic analysis. But atomism as taught by Democritus and particularly by Epicurus became familiar as never before to the philosophers and scientists through the work of Gassendi, whose *Syntagma Philosophicum* appeared in 1649. One of the chapters of this fruit of his life-long studies was titled *De Atomis* and subtitled *Quid dicatur atomus et qui illius assertores* ("what is the atom and who are those who accept it").

Gassendi devoted his attention almost exclusively to the atomism of Epicurus and Lucretius. Unlike Kepler and Galileo, he did not apply atomism—whether geometrical or that of Epicurus—to new discoveries. His was an erudite, not a creative mind, and he oscillated all his life between the teachings of the atomists and the tenets of Christian theology. A stubborn defender of atomism, he characteristically stated that the heliocentric theory of Copernicus would be the best if it did not contradict the teachings of the Church.

Whatever his limitations, Gassendi was the first in modern times to defend atomism openly and to make the atomism of Epicurus known and popular.[96]

Newton's corpuscular atomistic theory of matter was the last in the long line of revivals of the theory of matter of Democritus by the founders of modern science. Newtonian theories had a very great impact on the development of science in general and of physics in particular for about 200 years. Not until the very end of the 19th century had Newtonian classical physics been gradually replaced by new theories based on new ideas and confirmed by new experiments. The ideas of atoms and the void were replaced by the concept of the continuum.[97]

Anaxagoras and the Stoics

Anaxagoras was born about 488 B.C. and died in 428 B.C., the year Plato was born. He was one of the founders of the continuum theory of matter. In many respects his ideas were a logical development of the pluralistic theory of Empedocles, as opposed to the monism of the first Milesians. But, contrary to Empedocles and the atomists, he postulated an absolute continuum of matter. To Anaxagoras matter consisted of an infinite number of infinitesimal, invisible, and indivisible particles, real and eternal—each particle containing something of everything, unlike the atoms of Democritus. Any finite object is made up of an infinite number of these infinitely small particles (Anaxagoras called them "seeds"), and the stream of these invisible building blocks of matter makes the continuum the substrate of all objects and also the "fill of the universe." Our sense perception is too weak to allow us to know the truth, "visible existences are only the sight of the unseen," but sensations prove the existence of physical reality.

The continuum of Anaxagoras was a dynamic and active concept, not the immovable unchangeable eternal *one* of Parmenides. And the infinite variety of sense objects was to him the result of endless combinations of an infinite number of particles and not of combinations of a finite number of atoms which differ from one another only by their shapes and sizes.

Of even greater importance than his theory of matter was Anaxagoras' concept of *force* which causes the movements of everything, a concept of a dynamic organic force which he called "mind" (*nous*). This force differs from matter because it is incorporeal, it cannot be perceived, and it can be known only by the effect it exerts on matter.

This "cosmic mind" of Anaxagoras permeates everything: it is the source of changes in the universe, of all motion as well as of static order. There is a complete analogy between the mind of the individual, be it man, animal, or even a plant, which as an organizing principle controls the functioning of the living organism, and the cosmic mind which controls the whole universe, as it is the embodiment of the idea of natural law which governs the ordered behavior of physical reality. This cosmic mind of Anaxagoras is not unlike the dynamic force of modern physics which we call energy. It seems that in his concept of matter and of the unifying dynamic cosmic force Anaxagoras was much closer than the atomists to the 20th century theories of modern physicists.[98, 99]

Many years after the death of Anaxagoras his rational materialistic approach to natural philosophy was severely criticized by Plato in the *Laws*. In the 10th book of his *Laws* Plato wrote: ". . . when you and I argue that there are Gods and produce the sun, moon and stars as Gods or divine beings, if we would listen to the aforesaid philosophers we should say that they are earth and stones only which can have no care at all of human affairs. . . ."[100] And in another statement: "All that moves in the heaven appears to them to be full of stones and earth and other soulless bodies which dispense the causes of the whole cosmos."

Anaxagoras was the first scientist who tried to apply the same approach to the explanation of terrestrial and celestial phenomena. His attempt was naive and primitive. Two thousand years later Newton's universal law of gravitation proved in exact mathematical terms the identity of the laws which govern the movements of objects both on earth and in the heavens.

Anaxagoras had been accused of atheism and sentenced to life imprisonment. Pericles, his pupil and friend, saved him from prison, and Anaxagoras was exiled to a small island on the eastern shores of the Mediterranean. He died there at the age of 70, respected and beloved by many.

The theory of the continuum and the denial of the existence of the void was also the basic concept of the physics of the Stoics. Their main representatives were Zeno (332-262 B.C.), Chrysippus (280-207 B.C.), and Poseidonius (135-51 B.C.). To the Stoics the cosmos was a single harmonious organism governed and united by *pneuma*, the "spirit" which makes the whole world a single unit. The Stoics postulated the existence of *pneuma* as a kind of primordial matter very similar to the soul, which fills the universe, both objects and the space between objects. In the words of a late commentator, "Chrysippus . . . supposes that the whole of nature is united by the pneuma which permeates it and by which the world is kept together and is made coherent and interconnected."[101]

The denial of the void and the assumption of a continuum led the Stoics to the wave theory of the propagation of physical phenomena contrary to the theory of the atomists: "The air is not composed ot particles, but it is a continuum which contains no empty spaces. If it is struck by an impulse it rises in circular waves proceeding in straight sequence to infinity, until all the surrounding air is stirred, just as a pool is stirred by a stone which strikes it. But whereas in this latter case the movement is circular, the air moves spherically." And in another statement quoted by a late commentator: "We hear because the air between the voice and the hearer is struck and expands in spherical waves which reach our ears. . . ."[102]

Newton, in the English edition of his *Opiticks*, published in 1704, about 2,000 years after Anaxagoras and the Stoics, accepted the main principles of the ancient atomists, i.e., the existence of the atoms and of the void. He also accepted, with certain reservations, the existence of ether as "a most subtle spirit which pervades and lies hid in all gross bodies." This subtle substance which, according to Newton, might be of various degrees of rarity and density, fills the universe; it is inside matter and outside it. Newton's theory of light was atomistic and corpuscular. To him the rays of light were very small particles emitted from luminous objects which hit other objects. In other words, matter hits matter.[103, 104]

Robert Hooke, one of the founders of the Royal Society of London, and soon after him Huygens, one of the greatest mathematicians of his time, taught that light consists of spherical waves which hit the particles of ether and cause thus an infinite number of secondary waves: "Light takes time for its passage . . . it spreads, as sound does, by spherical surfaces and waves, for I call them waves from their resemblance to those which are seen to be formed in water when a stone is thrown in it. . . ." (quoted by Einstein).[105] This is a theory of a continuum that denies the existence of the void accepted by the atomists and Newton. And thus Newton, the atomist, and Huygens, the teacher of the continuum, repeated in the 17th century the controversy that existed in 500 B.C. between the atomism of Democritus and the theories of Anaxagoras and the Stoics.

It seems that today there are still two accepted ways of explaining the nature and the propagation of light: one corpuscular, in the form of the photons of the quanta theory, and the other based on the wave theory of light.

The evolution of scientific thought is a part of the general evolution of culture. In any period of history man's search for an explanation of observed natural phenomena depends on the interrelation of the fundamental theological and philosophical assumptions and on the degree and refinement of the experimental technique which exists at this particular time. The short-lived spiritual revolution in Egypt in the 15th century B.C. created new ideas and new attitudes toward nature and art; even after it came to a sudden end, it continued to influence generations of medical men. The pythagoreans and their theory of numbers as well as the atomism of ancient Greece had enormous influence on the development of modern science in the 16th and 17th centuries and played a major role in replacing the medieval scholastic, Aristotelian philosophy of man's relation to the universe by cartesian and newtonian rationalism and the mathematization of science and nature.

Fundamental religious and philosophical assumptions and postulates are always the background of the search for scientific truth, and they define the direction this search will follow. The concept of the four basic elements of Empedocles which replaced the monistic theory of the early Milesians had been in turn denied by the atomists, who on the basis of pure deduction postulated the existence of invisible and indivisible atoms and of the void. The atomistic theory of matter and newtonian classical physics dominated scientific thinking until the end of the 19th century, but then new philosophical assumptions, a new dynamic concept of space and time, gradually destroyed the very foundation of newtonian physics, and the growth of technology and the refinement of experimental techniques broke down the indivisible atom and led to the search for subatomic particles as ever-elusive elementary building blocks of matter, and finally to the dissolution of the very concept of matter into a continuum of fields and energy.

The philosophical and scientific revolution of our time is just another step in the never-ending search for truth which started thousands of years ago in ancient Greece.

REFERENCES

1. MacMichael, W.: *The Gold-Headed Cane,* 5th ed. London, Kimpton, 1923, pp. 39-110.
2. MacMichael, W. and Hawkins, F.: *Lives of British Physicians.* London, Murray, 1830, pp. 155-167.
3. Rotblat, J., ed.: *Aspects of Medical Physics. The First International Conference on Medical Physics,* Harrogate, 1965. London, Taylor & Francis, 1966, pp. 4-5.
4. Carnap, R.: *Philosophical Foundations of Physics.* New York, Basic Books, 1966. pp. 105-114.
5. Bork, A. M.: Maxwell and the vector potential. *Isis 58*:210, 1967.
6. Holton, G.: Einstein, Michelson and the crucial experiment. *Isis 60*:160-167, 1969.
7. Einstein, A. and Infeld, L.: *The Evolution of Physics.* New York, Simon & Schuster, 1950, pp. 255-260.
8. Sigerist, H.: *A History of Medicine,* vol. 1: *Primitive and Archaic Medicine.* New York, Oxford Univ. Press, 1951, pp. 320-324.
9. Galen: *De Methodo medendi.* Liber XI, cap. 8, Kühn, C. G., ed., 10. Leipzig, Cnobloch, 1823-1831, p. 753.
10. Galen: *De Sanitate tuenda.* In: Op. cit., Liber 1, cap. 3. Kühn, 6, p. 8.
11. Galen: Op. cit., cap. 12. Kühn, C. G., ed. 6 pp. 63-64 ff.
12. Steuer, O. and Saunders, J. B. de C. M.: *Ancient Egyptian and Cnidian Medicine.* Berkeley, Univ. Calif. Press. 1959, pp. 21-30.
13. Saunders, J. B. de C. M.: *The Transisition from Ancient Egyptian to Greek Medicine.* Lawrence, Kansas, Univ. Kansas Press, 1963, pp. 20-30.
14. Aristotle: Metaphysics, In: *The Basic Books of Aristotle,* McKeon, R. ed. New York, Random, 1941, book 1, chap. 2, 982-b, p. 692.
15. Galen: *De Plenitudine Liber,* cap. 3. Kühn 7, p. 522-525.
16. Wilson, L. G.: Erasistratus, Galen and the Pneuma. *Bull History Med. 33:* 293, 1959.
17. Snell, B.: *The Discovery of the Mind.* New York, Harper, 1960, pp. 228-245.
18. Einstein, A. and Infeld, L.: Op. cit., pp. 183-185.
19. Auden, W. H.: In: *The Portable Greek Reader.* New York, Viking,

1948, pp. 17-24.
20. Burnet, J.: *Early Greek Philosophy,* 4th ed. London, Black, 1930, p. 119.
21. Snell, B.: Op. cit., pp. 139-143.
22. Copleston, F. S. J.: *A History of Philosophy.* New York, Doubleday, 1962, vol. 1, part 1, p. 65.
23. Castiglioni, A.: *A History of Medicine.* New York, Knopf, 1941, pp. 135-137.
24. Snell, B.: Op. cit., pp. 146-147.
25. Snell, B.: Op. cit., pp. 46-54.
26. *The Portable Greek Reader,* op. cit., pp. 499-501.
27. Snell, B.: Op. cit., pp. 55-57.
28. Seton, L.: *The Art of the Ancient Near East.* New York, Praeger, 1961, pp. 175-185.
29. Pound, E. and Stock, N., transls.: *Love Poems of Ancient Egypt.* New York, New Directions, 1962.
30. Akhmatova, A. transl.: *Lirika Drevnego Egypta.* Moscow, Khudozhestvennaia Literatura, 1966.
31. Breasted, J. H.: *A History of Egypt.* New York, Bantam, 1964, pp. 297-319.
32. Bury, J. B.: *A History of Greece.* New York, Modern Library, pp. 56 ff.
33. Sudhoff, K.: *Kos and Knidos.* Muenchen, Verlag der Muenchner Drucke, 1927, pp. 285-300.
34. de Chardin, T.: *The Phenomenon of Man.* New York, Harper, 1965, pp. 39-44.
35. Burnet, J.: Op. cit., pp. 73-77.
36. Burnet, J.: Op. cit., pp. 70-71.
37. Burnet, J.: Op. cit., pp. 174-175.
38. Burnet, J.: Op. cit., p. 340.
39. Einstein, A. and Infeld, L.: Op. cit., p. 313.
40. Burnet, J.: Op. cit., p. 209.
41. Plato: *Timaeus.* Lee, H. D. P., transl. New York, Penguin, 1964, pp. 31, 67-68.
42. De Vogel, C. J.: *Pythagoras and Early Pythagoreanism.* Assen, Netherlands, Van Gorcum, 1966 chaps. 2 and 3, pp. 20-51.
43. Helm, E. E.: The vibrating string of the pythagoreans. *Scientific American 217*:92-104, 1967.
44. Patrides, C. A.: The numerological approach to cosmic order during the English renaissance. *Isis 49*:394.
45. Burtt, E. A.: *The Metaphysical Foundations of Modern Physical Science,* rev. ed. London, Routledge & Kegan Paul, 1932, p. 64.
46. Sambursky, S.: *The Physical World of the Greeks.* London, Routledge & Kegan Paul, 1960, pp. 26-46.
47. Sambursky, S.: Op. cit., pp. 70-71 and 207-208.
48. Heisenberg, Werner. *Physics and Philosophy.* New York, Harper, 1962, pp. 71-72.
49. Burnet, J.: Op. cit., pp. 207-208.
50. Burnet, J.: Op. cit., p. 239.
51. Sambursky, S.: Op. cit., p. 20.
52. Galileo, G.: *Dialogues Concerning Two New Sciences,* Crew, H. and de Salvo, A., transls. New York, Dover, 1954, pp. 42-43.
53. Sagnac, P. and de Saint-Leger, A.: *Peuples et Civilisations.* La Preponderance Française, 2d ed. Paris, Presses Univ. France, 1944, pp. 286-287.
54. Einstein, A. and Infeld, L.: Op. cit., p. 96.
55. Burent, J.: Op. cit., p. 229.
56. Burnet, J.: Op. cit., pp. 247-249.
57. Galen, C.: *De Elementis ex Hippocrate,* Liber 1, cap. 2. Kühn, 1, p. 415-419.
58. Burtt, E. A.: Op. cit., pp. 56-57.
59. Galileo, G.: *Discoveries and Opinions of Galileo. The Assayer.* St. Drake, S., transl. New York, Doubleday, 1957, p. 274.
60. Locke, J.: An Essay Concerning Human Understanding. In: *The Empiricists.* New York, Doubleday, 1961, pp. 26-33.
61. Berkeley, G.: *The Principles of Human Knowledge.* New York, Meridian, 1963, pp. 81-96.
62. Rosen, G.: The Philosophy of Ideology and the Emergence of Modern Medicine in France. *Bull. Hist. Med. 20*: 328, 1946.
63. Galen: *De Differentiis Febrium.* Liber 1, cap. 6. Kuhn, 7, pp. 289-290.
64. Castiglioni: Op. cit., pp. 455-459.
65. Ackerknecht, E.: Anti-contagionism between 1821 and 1867. *Bull. Hist. Med. 22*:562-593, 1948.
66. Flint, A.: *A Treatise on the Principles and Practice of Medicine,* 5th

ed. Henry Lee's Sons, 1881, p. 98.
67. Rosen, G.: *A History of Public Health.* New York, M.D. Publications, 1958, pp. 287-90.
68. Aristotle: *De Caelo.* Bk. 1, chap. 7, 276a, op. cit., p. 412.
69. Aristotle: *De Generatione et Corruption,* bk. 1, chap. 1, 314a and bk. 1, chap. 7, 325a. Op. cit., pp. 470 and 497.
70. Sambursky, S.: Op. cit., pp. 111-113.
71. Copleston, F. S. J.: Op. cit., p. 65.
72. Burnet, J.: Op. cit., pp. 174-175.
73. Sambursky, S.: Op. cit., p. 113.
74. Sambursky, S.: Op. cit., 162-163.
75. Lucretius: *On the Nature of Things,* chap. 2. Munro, H. A. J. transl. New York, Doubleday, 1960, pp. 37 ff.
76. Galen: *De Plenitudine Liber,* cap. 3. Op. cit., p. 525.
77. Sambursky, S.: Op. cit., p. 134 ff.
78. Lucretius: Op. cit., pp. 104-05.
79. Aristotle: *De Generatione et corruption,* bk. 1, chap. 1, 315b. Op. cit., p. 473.
80. Aristotle: *Metaphysics,* bk. 1, chap. 4, 985b. Op. cit., p. 697.
81. Burnet, J.: Op. cit., p. 336, footnote 4.
82. Burtt, E. A.: Op. cit., p. 43.
83. Sarton, George: *Six Wings. Men of Science in the Renaissance.* Indiana Univ. Press, 1957, pp. 77-78.
84. Burtt, E. A.: Op. cit., pp. 24-39.
85. Sarton, G.: Op. cit., pp. 55-62.
86. Burtt, E. A.: Op. cit., pp. 48 ff.
87. Kepler, J.: *Harmonices Mundi,* liber. 5, cap. 3, pp. 299, 308. In: *Gesammelte Werke,* Casper, M., ed. Muenchen, Beck'sche, 1940, vol. 6.
88. Sarton, G.: Op. cit., pp. 66-67.
89. Helm, E. E.: Op. cit., pp. 97-98.
90. Kepler, J.: *Harmonices Mundi,* liber. 5, cap. 4. In: op. cit., 316.
91. Burtt, E. A.: Op. cit., p. 58 and footnote 45.
92. Kepler, J.: Concerning the more certain fundamentals in astrology. Meywald, E., transl. *Amer. Astrol.* July, pp. 7-12: August, pp. 17-23, 1941.
93. Kepler, J.: *Astronomia Nova.* In: *Gesammelte Werke,* op. cit., vol. 3, pp. 33-34.
94. Burtt, E. A.: Op. cit, pp. 87 ff.
95. Galileo, G.: *Two New Sciences,* op. cit., p. 194.
96. Rochot, B.: *Les Travaux de Gassendi (1592-1655) sur l'Epicure et sur l'Atomisme.* Paris, Librairie Philosophique J. Vrin, 1944, pp. 168.
97. Heisenberg, W.: Op. cit., pp. 59-70.
98. Sambursky, S.: Op. cit., pp. 190-91.
99. Gershenson, D. E. and Greenberg, D. A.: *Anaxagoras and the Birth of Scientific Method.* New York, Blaisdell, 1964, pp. 5-26.
100. Plato: In: *The Works of Plato. The Laws.* Jowett, B. transl. New York, Tudor, 1948, p. 454.
101. Sambursky, S.: Op. cit., pp. 134 ff.
102. Sambursky, S.: Op. cit., p. 138.
103. Newton, I.: *Opticks.* London, Smith & Walford, 1704, Definition 1 and pp. 138 ff.
104. Newton, I.: *Philosophiae Naturalis Principia Mathematica,* Liber 3, edi. ultima. Amsterdam, 1714, pp. 484 ff.
105. Einstein A. and Infeld, L.: Op. cit., pp. 110-111.

STATEMENT*

ON

The Federal Drug Abuse and Drug Dependence, Prevention, Treatment and Rehabilitation Act of 1970 (S. 3562)

BY

THE NEW YORK ACADEMY OF MEDICINE

In March of this year the New York Academy of Medicine approved a statement objecting to the passage of "The Controlled Dangerous Substances Act of 1969" (S. 3246) by Congress on the basis that the bill was "medically and scientifically unrealistic" and that its passage "would represent an unwarranted instrusion by the Department of Justice into the field of medical care and research," in which field the Department of Justice has no expertise.

On March 9, 1970 a bill entitled the "Federal Drug Abuse and Drug Dependence Prevention, Treatment and Rehabilitation Act of 1970" (S. 3562) was introduced by Senator Harold Hughes of Iowa. Unlike the former bill, S. 3562 approaches treatment, education, and research in drug use from a realistic viewpoint and is in line with responsible medical practice. Moreover, it places the responsibility for organizing and administering the program in the Department of Health, Education, and Welfare rather than in the Department of Justice. This delegation is proper and in line with the views of the Academy as outlined in the March 13th statement.

Accordingly, the Committee on Public Health endorses S. 3562 as a progressive and realistic first step toward the solution of a most serious problem.

*Approved by the Committee on Public Health, April 27, 1970.

THE MOUTH AS AN INSTRUMENT HOLDER

Not many months ago the editorial page of the *Bulletin* was devoted to the discussion of a drawing by Rembrandt that had been exhibited during a tercentenary celebration at the Royal Museum in Stockholm.[1] The drawing shows a seated man and several attendants, one of whom, a woman, is apparently applying a cloth to the patient's face, as if to wipe away tears or blood. Another attendant is standing and holds in his mouth what appears to be a slender knife. The gloomy scene is customarily designated "The Eye Operation." If this interpretation is correct, the procedure depicted may be a couching for cataract, since the operation of extraction had not yet been introduced.

In the discussion of Rembrandt's drawing, attention was called to the fact that the surgeon apparently was holding the knife in his mouth; a few fragments of modern reminiscence were added, suggesting that this method persisted into the recent past. In response to the editor's request for additional information, Dr. Owen H. Wangensteen of Minneapolis kindly called attention to several passages in the surgical literature. These are cited in two of Dr. Wangensteen's recent historical studies. [2,3]

When the original texts mentioned by Dr. Wangensteen are excerpted and cumulated, we receive a varied yet curious coherent impression of old-time surgical method.

H. F. Le Dran, the famous 18th century French surgeon, wrote as follows of lateral perineal lithotomy:

> The ligatures being thus applied [to immobilize the patient], I introduce the staff into the bladder . . . and feel for the stone. . . . The staff being rightly placed, I take the knife from the assistant who holds the instruments, *and put it in my mouth;* then pressing the beak of the staff against the rectum, I feel the

1. Rembrandt's "Eye Operation." *Bull. N.Y. Acad. Med. 45*:1396-98, 1969.
2. Wangensteen, O. H., Wangensteen, S. D. and Wiita, J.: Lithotomy and lithotomists: Progress in wound management from Franco to Lister. *Surgery 66*:929-52, 1969. See esp. page 938.
3. Wangensteen, O. H., Smith, J. and Wangensteen, S. D.: Some highlights in the history of amputation reflecting lessons in wound healing. *Bull. Hist. Med. 41*:97-131, 1967. See esp. pp. 108, 110, and footnote 35 on p. 112.

> curvature of it through the perinaeum. The incision ought to terminate an inch and a half below where we feel the bottom of the curvature.[4]

Apparently Le Dran's use of his mouth as an instrument-holder was a matter of convenience and perhaps also of time-saving. It will be observed that Le Dran's surgical work was done a century later than the scene depicted by Rembrandt.

The old practices continued into the 19th century, as is evident from an anonymous reminiscence of Robert Liston (1794-1847):

> The manner in which he handled the knife had in it something remarkable. . . . As a lithotomist he has never been surpassed. . . . In more complicated operations, when he wished to use both hands, he saved much time by holding the knife in his mouth, instead of entrusting it to an assistant or laying it down—a habit he was led to adopt from having carefully watched the manner in which the butchers of Edinburgh rapidly separated different joints of meat.[5]

A later author in the series mentioned by Dr. Wangensteen is the distinguished Halsted, who discussed a presentation by Dr. Thomas M. Markoe as follows:

> Dr. William S. Halsted thought that it would be difficult in a given case to know just what to attribute a bad result to, with the imperfect antiseptic technique at present existing even in our best New York hospitals. . . . He had repeatedly observed ligatures handed to the operator from the mouth of the interne. . . .[6]

Halsted's comment exemplifies clearly the way in which the new science of bacteriology had provided insight into the errors of traditional practices.

---

4. Le Dran, H. F.: *The Operations in Surgery of Mons. Le Dran,* 3d ed. Gataker, T., transl. London, Hitch and Hawes, 1757, pp. 233-34. Italics added.

5. Anonymous: Heroes of medicine. Robert Liston. *The Practitioner,* n.s. *10*:546-49, 1899.

6. Halsted, W. S.: Discussion of presentation by Thomas M. Markoe on recurring carcinoma of the arm. *N.Y. Med. J. 40*:497, 1884.

An additional retrospect was provided by W. W. Keen (1837-1932) of Philadelphia, whose experience spanned the Civil War and World War I. In his essay *Military Surgery in 1861 and 1918*[7] Keen says:

> It can easily be understood how and why we surgeons in 1861-65, utterly unaware of bacteria and their dangers, in our ignorant innocence committed grievous mistakes which nearly always imperilled life and often actually caused death. . . . If there was any difficulty in threading the needle we moistened it with (as we now know) bacteria-laden saliva. . . .

Keen's essay, from which this excerpt was taken, is memorable as a concise and impressive summary of the technical progress that a distinguished surgeon had witnessed during a very long lifetime.

S. J.

7. Keen, W. W.: Military Surgery in 1861 and in 1918. *Ann. Amer. Acad. Polit. Social Science 80*:11-22, 1918; see p. 14.

THE PHRENOLOGIST DISCUSSES FRIENDSHIP

I WAS requested to take, for my collection, a cast of the head of a lady who was, as they told me, the model of friendship. I took her cast, more out of kindness than in the expectation of making any discovery, and I endeavoured to get a correct one. On examining this head, I found two great prominences, constituting the segment of a sphere, by the side of the organ of the love of offspring. As, up to that time I had never seen these prominences, which however were evidently formed by the brain, and exceedingly symmetrical, I considered them as a cerebral organ: but what were the functions of this organ?

In order to get some general view on this point, I inquired of all the friends of the lady, respecting her qualities and faculties. I attempted to learn of the lady hereself, what propensities and faculties she believed she possessed. All united in confirming what had been told me, that she had an invincible attachment to her friends. Although her fortune, at different periods, had experienced great changes, and by degrees she had passed from poverty to honors, her feelings for old friends had never changed. This characteristic trait struck me. The idea occurred to me, that the disposition to friendship might also be founded in a particular cerebral organ. This opinion acquired with me a still greater degree of probability, as the prominences, that I had observed on the head of the lady, were placed immediately above the organ of physical love, and by the side of that of the love of offspring, and these three sentiments have some analogy with each other. Whatever may be the difficulty of making exact observations in man, on the organ in question, and on its functions, the idea, that attachment and friendship depend upon a particular cerebral organ, acquired by a degree of probability almost equal to certainty.

From GALL, F. J. *The Influence of the Brain on the Form of the Head*. Lewis, W., Jr., transl. Boston, Marsh, Capen, Lyon, 1835, vol. 3, pp. 299-300.

BULLETIN OF
THE NEW YORK ACADEMY
OF MEDICINE

VOL. 46, NO. 9 SEPTEMBER 1970

ANNUAL MEETING
OF
THE NEW YORK ACADEMY OF MEDICINE

*THE RESPONSIBILITY OF THE NEW YORK ACADEMY OF MEDICINE IN THE COMMUNITY**

JOHN L. POOL

President
The New York Academy of Medicine
New York, N. Y.

It is the president's duty to report to the Fellowship the events of the past year and it is a pleasure to bring you the more than usual activities of the past year on this warm spring evening. We seem to have made a good choice in moving from the blizzards and transit strikes of January to the welcoming weather of April for this Annual Stated Meeting. The physical facilities in which we exist have needed major effects just to keep even: namely, re-covering the roof, which had started to leak, waterproofing the enormous east wall of the building, and development of more stack space in the library. We are coming to the end of such stack space and must look for other means to house continuing enlargement of our precious collection of books, pamphlets, and medical journals. The most visible improvement of the year has been the refurbishing and air conditioning of conference rooms on the second floor, which also provides more flexibility. The addition of a high-speed dumbwaiter allows more areas where dinners and receptions can be

*Presented at the annual meeting of the New York Academy of Medicine, April 29, 1970.

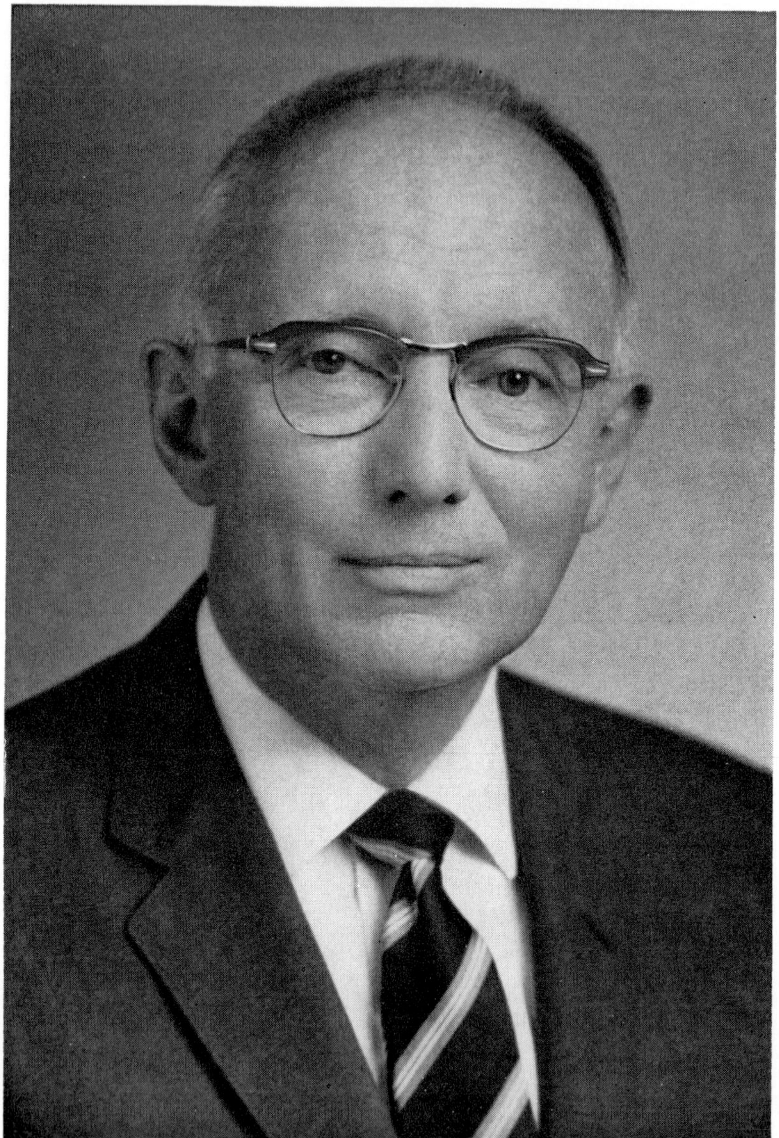

JOHN L. POOL, M.D.

readily handled, and this is a growing trend among the sections, the affiliated societies, and other groups using the Academy building. The finances, one must remember, are based on an endowment which provides over 95% of the cost of running our operation, and the endowment is the result of generosity from Fellows and other friends of the Academy. The only government participation in our operation is tax abatement and support of some activities of the library. The increase in dues needed this last year by increased cost-of-living expenses has been well received by the Fellowship and a particularly happy new program has been the remittance of all dues for 30-year members. There has been much appreciation. The associate-membership group is growing, particularly stimulated by the development of the new section in biomedical engineering and the proposed development of discourses between lawyers and physicians, library workers, and physicians. Our developing interest in teaching programs for paramedical personnel should add other groups to our associate Fellowship.

There remains, I am sure, in our immediate future the need for a campaign for additional funds, the purpose of which will be to give better current and pension status to our staff, to maintain the building in the loving style of 1926 when Dr. Samuel W. Lambert, the 1927 and 1928 president said, "The New York Academy of Medicine is not a local medical group. It has become a national institution. This building is an asset of which we may be proud, but it is also a liability which calls for more expenditures now and in the future."

Our facilities are being increasingly and adequately used, particularly the smaller rooms. The use of Hosack Hall by physician groups has diminished over the last decade. At the same time its use by paramedical and community-minded groups, many of them lay and student in character, has increased so that we can extend the maximum availability of our facilities to the health professions in the concepts of today.

Committee Activities

The Library. During this year some close looks have been taken at the actual reader use of the library facilities. A Saturday afternoon survey, for instance, has demonstrated 30 to 40 people reading and browsing and studying. Few of these are actually physicians, but our facilities are far from limited to Fellows and library subscribers. We welcome the opportunity to provide scientific information and stimulus to responsible students and investigators of all sorts. New publications of the year include the author catalogue, which costs over $2,000.00 for 43 volumes, and just now the first volume of the projected 34-volume subject catalogue has come out at approximately the same cost. The value of the collection is such to other librarians that the Academy should make a profit on these expensive volumes. This year also there has been some experimentation in computer retrieval and electronic communication, which are growing areas of competence, and the library has remained the hub of medical libraries in the state, in the metropolitan area, and as a backup for medical-school and hospital libraries in this area, being particularly useful, we believe, to medical students in the schools a few blocks to the north and south of us. Janet Doe, the librarian, said in 1950, "The possession of an outstanding accumulation of the scientific literature brings with it a certain moral obligation to see that its resources are accessible to all who need them. It has extended its general services as far as seems justifiable on a free basis. It has developed very special services most of them free. Furthermore, it has believed wholeheartedly in the practice of mutual help among libraries as the surest way to advance the interests of all. By assistance to and from each other the ability of all libraries to give better service has been increased." Twenty years later this statement is very true. The physical growth of the library poses a real problem in space. The selection and maintenance of volumes and journals requires maximum selectivity and reevaluation of library goals. We cannot possibly maintain every single medical publication in world literature or, if we were nonselective, even in English-language literature or United States publications; therefore we must be motivated to maintaining that element of current publication which forms the broadest base for reference work in the medical sciences. We need to concentrate not on the esoteric but on the broadest possible representational material to back up the hospital and medical-school libraries. Library sciences are in a state of change due to the electronic and duplication facilities, though the latter cause more wear and tear on the printed page than simple reading! We must come to the forefront by experimentation and cooperation with other libraries in bringing adequate, rapid, and needed reference material to the working medical scientist with the least waste, motion, and expense.

Public Health. This year has brought forth scholarly and pertinent works with the approval of the president and the council on *The Present Status of Abortion Laws*, *Methadone Management of Heroin Addiction*, and a revised manual on autopsy protocol for New York City: this latter in collaboration with the Health Services and United Hospital Fund. Studies are in progress on how to grapple with the marijuana problem in this urban area, the control of lead poisoning, and other public-health matters.

Medical Education. The knotty problem of continuing education for the physician is receiving continuing study and investigation in the hope of systematizing the welter of information coming at us from all sides on this subject. Across the country this year there have been many conferences and all kinds of advice but few national organizations aside from the Academy of General Practice have a firm, insistent program of continuing education for their membership. We are grappling with the policy matters of how to engage the physician in continued study, conferences, attendance at meetings, and the question of relicensure. Furthermore, we must come to grips with the relation of the community physician and the hospital-based physician in an effort to bring them closer to each other and to bring their separate knowledge to each other. The medical assistant, what he is, what he can do, how he can be used within the legal safeguards of patient, hospital, and doctor, and the future place of all paramedical personnel are other matters under current investigation. Our 17 sections are showing a mean attendance of 125. The new area of bioengineering seems off to a useful start with discussions of electronic devices for control of the heart rate, the computerization of physical examinations. The urology section honored with the Valentine medal this year the four pioneers in renal transplant: John Hartwell Harrison, David Milford Hume, John Putnam Merrill, and Joseph Edward Murray.

Medicine in Society. This group has been the spearhead and the goad in our studies attempting to relate the physician to the rapid current changes in the social fabric. Many discussions have been held, some supported by a grant from the Ford Foundation and published in the *Bulletin* and subsequently in independent reports. There have been task forces in various areas, and one of particular importance is concerned with ambulatory care. There is an ongoing study reviewing, with the New York Urban Coalition, the Morrisania Youth and Service Center, the relations of the center to the needs of that neighborhood, to the community physicians, and to the local hospital as well.

Many of the activities stemming from the committees become, in the end, activities of the whole Academy, and our director has been particularly skillful in bringing the talents of executives and Fellows from many disciplines in the Academy membership to bear on specific problems. An outstanding event of the year in such a category, led by the Committee on Medicine in Society, has been the spring Health Conference held this month, attended by some 700 active workers in the field, entitled *Community Participation for Equity and Excellence in Health Care.* At this conference the attitudes and words of community workers were relevant, informative, and resilient. Everyone working on panels and speeches seemed open and receptive to the points of view of others, allowing an active exchange of information and attitudes between physicians who, after all, are the ones actually delivering health care and the leaders of communities, especially of deprived communities, who are the recipients most in need of improved health care today. The neutral atmosphere of the Academy seems to have been extraordinarily maintained over the decades, and I think it was well demonstrated at this conference. The doctor's position in the community was discussed there, and varied points of view on the subject were given equal time, so to speak, and the result was, as Ralph Waldo Emerson said and is now engraved on the wall at Hunter College—"We are of different opinions at different hours but may always be said to be at heart on the side of truth." It was no small achievement to have so many diverse viewpoints expressed.

This year has seen perhaps more involvement in the public sector than in some time past. For instance, the position paper that would place abortion under the general provisions of the Medical Practice Act of the various states was not only made known to Governor Nelson A. Rockefeller and the members of the state legislature but also was accompanied by supporting letters from the Academy indicating that this was an Academy-wide position. The Academy is also taking a stand on the controversial drug-control bill in Congress, feeling it to be medically and scientifically unrealistic and an unwarranted intrusion by the Department of Justice into the field of medicine where that department does not have competence.

In the matter of revised control of health matters in this city, with particular attention to the health-and-hospital corporation: the Academy has made public our position that leadership in health matters should not be in the hands of executives whose administrative skill has been developed in other fields, no matter how competent such men may be in matters of finance and administration. There has been developed a discussion with administrators in the city health services that we hope will be fruitful to the city management faced with the colossal task of revitalizing city hospitals and developing community health centers and should also prove of benefit to the best care of the patient by the individual physician, thereby providing the city administration with the many facets of special health knowledge and experience available to physicians alone.

These events of the year again and again bring to the fore the difficulties of the professional man in his obligation as a citizen. The Academy as such represents a cross section, one might say, of the doctors in the broad metropolitan area. It may be a special cross section because Fellowship is attractive to those physicians interested in the public weal, in continuing medical education, and in the beauties of a medical library. In the current changing medical climate we have a vital role as a repository of medical knowledge, as a meeting ground where physicians of particular skill and extensive experience in special problems can work out statements on the major health problems of the day that have the authenticity of knowledge, wisdom, and compassion, and where conferences can attract the best minds of the country. Just the same, the Academy cannot in these times rest at this point, but must increasingly, I believe, make its knowledge and position available and known to the profession at large, to our political leaders, and to the public we serve.

There is so much that physicians have done in this country and, perhaps, especially in this city, to further mankind's knowledge of disease process, its cure, and its prevention, that one is readily startled when doctors are subject to continued criticism because they are not accomplishing enough today. The government is in the business of medicine, and the financial commitments of the past decade show that government is here to stay. The continuing discoveries and sophistication of patient care costs more year by year, and the better recompense of paramedical personnel also escalates. To quote Dwight Wilbur, "We have reached the point where there is one physician for every eighteen in the allied health services. The problem for us is how to exert the kind of leadership which will result in effective patient and community care. What we must avoid above all else is the care of a patient by a committee rather than by an individual." Dr. John R. Tanner recently said, in summarizing a conference held at the New York Academy of Sciences on education in the health-related professions, "We are advised to be flexible and innovative, but in closing this meeting let us be reminded that the absolute basis of all medical care begins with intimate relation of the patient to his physician. We must maintain this relationship in all our planning and in our search for efficiency, for if it falters, all the efforts of all the nurses, all the technicians, all the therapists, and all the administrators may be a team effort in futility."

So I say the climate of the times points to a current great need to bring the quality of medical care to the highest level and to an equal level for all citizens, without lowering the best treatment now available to many but not to the whole population. The doctor presumably tries, patient by patient who seek out his service, to give the best that is in him, but this is not enough. He must show care, sensitivity, and humility to the needs of all the people and to the needs of all the people for health matters all the time. In other words, the ordinary physician can no longer accept as adequate his former belief and training that public-health matters belong in the compartment of the public-health physician, and that the practicing doctor's responsibility started and ended with removing the appendix or treating heart failure or acute pneumonia. The physician is certainly not guiltless. The financial reward of the private practitioner is adequate, maybe too adequate, and the fact that the doctor has been, so to speak, on a pedestal in the public eye makes him especially subject to criticism when it is discovered that some physicians, regardless of how small a percentage, have been venal in their response to Medicare and Medicaid laws. It is not enough that we be like other men. We have an obligation to be like Caesar's wife. The matter of continuing medical education is also a moral issue that must concern the physician and society. We have not come to grips with it. Finally, the habitual separation of the average physician from activities as a citizen in the community needs to be altered if he is to retain or perhaps regain a leading part in the delivery of quality care to all. Again, it is not enough for us to be content with one patient-one doctor relations. We must find time, and take time—perhaps from our leisure—to aid government at all levels in the organization and delivery of health care for all citizens.

UNIVERSAL HEALTH INSURANCE*

NELSON A. ROCKEFELLER

Governor
State of New York
Albany, N. Y.

I FEEL very strongly that two basic essentials in life—particularly for young people—are education and good health. If a person today has a good education and good health, the opportunities are just unlimited. There have been prejudices and restrictions, but I think these are being overcome.

On the other hand, if the individual does not have either one or the other of these, I think we as a society have to take a share of the responsibility in seeing that they get them.

In education I think we have been out in front, as a state, in meeting our responsibilities.

But now we face the problem of providing good health and good medical care for all our citizens. Dr. John L. Pool has expressed this as a goal of your Academy, and it certainly has been one of mine. The issue is how to achieve it.

You men of medicine have created the know-how to provide every American with a level of medical care unmatched anywhere in the world. But the financing and delivery of that care is an uneven patchwork that deprives all too many people of medical attention in their time of need. This matter has concerned me for a long time. I started out in 1931 as a member of the Westchester County Board of Health, so I have been in the public-health area a long time.

I also had the privilege of serving as President Dwight D. Eisenhower's Undersecretary of Health, Education, and Welfare, and one of the things that most disturbed me at that time was that 3% of the people in this country were being bankrupted by catastrophic medical costs each year.

We worked out an agreement at that time with the insurance companies to set up a reimbursement pool to provide coverage for such

*Anniversary Discourse, presented at the annual meeting of the New York Academy of Medicine, April 29, 1970.

catastrophic medical-care costs. This was a compromise plan of the companies because we had introduced a bill in which the federal government would have set up a reinsurance pool of its own.

The president withdrew that bill when the insurance companies agreed to set up the pool. But after he withdrew the bill, the companies forgot the pool, so that plan never got off the ground.

When I became governor one of the first things I did was to set up a group to study the advisability of statewide Universal Health Insurance. The conclusion reached at that time was that for one state alone to do this would be very difficult because of the adverse competitive position its business would be placed in with those in other states. With the mobility of industry and business today the relative costs of doing business in one area of the country or another is a very sensitive factor. If industry in one area incurs higher costs this can drive it away.

In 1960 I took the idea of Universal Health Insurance for people over 65 to the National Governors' Conference where we won approval of the concept. So I have been speaking out on this idea now for years.

By 1965 the federal government finally adopted an over-65 plan in the form of Medicare and also passed Title 19, better known as Medicaid.

We in New York State, since the time of Al Smith, have been aiding the medically indigent. So we were in a position, when Title 19 was passed, to take advantage of it. We read the law very carefully and then found out what we could get in the way of assistance from the federal government and passed laws that corresponded.

As a goal Medicaid was fine, but as a means of financing it was a disaster. Many local communities had to double their real-estate taxes in order to pay for it. So Congress next year cut the Medicaid Program way back and we had to do likewise. We had to take 1,200,000 persons off the eligiblity rolls in New York State.

And we have been in a situation where, ever since, in the implementation of this law, we have had financial and administrative confusion. What is more, Medicaid has been an important factor in the rising costs of hospital care, because it has overloaded the system.

I believe very strongly that national Universal Health Insurance is the answer. It would provide the key to a genuine system of health care available to all, a system that this country now lacks. Universal Health Insurance at the federal level would mean that no one would ever be denied medical care because of a lack of personal resources.

Universal Health Insurance also gives beneficiaries a direct say in the prudent management of the system because they are paying into it. It would not interfere with the customary doctor-patient relation and it would be built on our existing well-defined base of private and non-profit health-insurance operations. By having a nationwide system, no state would be at a competitive disadvantage because of the added cost to employers and employees.

But instead of Universal Health Insurance, all we have from the federal government thus far is Medicaid and Medicare, with state and local matching funds. Passage of these bills is symptomatic of our whole piecemeal approach to the problem in medical care today.

Now we are in a difficult period of transition. We are somewhere between the hands-off role that government used to play in medicine, and a well-thought-through, comprehensive, over-all approach to the financing and delivery of medical care for all our people. We are caught up in a hodge-podge system that is difficult for the medical profession, difficult for government, and difficult for patients.

We seem to have backed into this dilemma on a step-by-step basis, and the result is that we do not have a delivery system adequate to meet the needs at reasonable cost. We have not produced a good comprehensive plan. And by dealing with only part of the problem, such as partial financing of this care, we have aggravated problems in other areas, such as the delivery of the care.

For example, Medicare and Medicaid have been enormously helpful to those in need of care who were fortunate enough to be covered. But they have also overloaded the present medical-care system in many places. This situation has been exacerbated by inflation and by the lack of any real control over hospital costs. We have no control because the interpretation of the law in Washington is that we have to pay "reasonable costs" but have no right to question the hospitals' figures.

As a result, a semiprivate room in a hospital in this city that averaged about $11 a day 20 years ago, cost $61 last year. This year the average could go to $70. We even have one hospital where the costs are over $140 a day. And we have to pay it.

If there is one lesson we have learned, it is that we cannot solve the health-care problem simply by pouring more money into our present system. We must put just as much effort into improving the total system—from educating enough doctors to building enough of the right kind of hospitals—if we are going to meet our present medical needs.

Throughout these years of discussion and debate concerning Universal Health Insurance, we have taken a series of steps to help meet our health care needs in the state.

We began the first state program for licensing and regulating hospitals by the State Health Department, established a state loan program to modernize badly outdated hospitals and voluntary hospitals, and state loans to build badly needed nursing homes.

We established regional hospital-planning councils to avoid the overbuilding and duplication of services that send hospital costs sky high; and we started new state research institutes for kidney and heart diseases. We doubled the state's support for cancer research at Roswell Park Memorial Institute. We began a ghetto medical program and provided special state aid that is allowing hospitals to train 115 new doctors a year—the equivalent of a whole new medical school.

In addition, we have built a brand new medical school at Stony Brook and a major health center at Buffalo.

But proud as we are of these efforts, I am convinced that in the absence of federal action we owe our people universal health protection on a state level. I say, quite confidently, that the Universal Health Insurance bill advocated this year was one of the finest measures ever placed before a deliberative body in this country. That does not mean they passed the bill; they did not.

When we started talking about this bill, private companies in this state were paying $580 million in premiums for health insurance for their employees. This year they are up to $1,200,000,000 in premiums for their employees. The bill we proposed would have added only $200,000,000 to private corporate expenditures for premiums.

We worked out this program after extensive discussions with top leaders in medicine, hospitals, the insurance business, and labor.

The bill we proposed would have extended a basic benefit policy to all employees and their families who have no health insurance and to those who have inadequate coverage. It would have preserved freedom of choice and permitted the use of private health insurance rather than a program run by government.

Futher, this plan recognized what I mentioned before—that we cannot just deal with the payment mechanism. We have to improve the delivery system, too. And so we included in our universal health proposal an excellent beginning toward that goal.

What we proposed was legislation that would have enabled physicians to provide group medical practice on a prepayment basis or to form corporations affiliated with insurance companies or hospitals. Our present laws unduly restrict this kind of modern practice.

More and more persons who are concerned with health care, in medicine and out, see this kind of prepaid group arrangement as a much needed supplement to the present health-care system. It would help to extend care to those areas where it is not available. This arrangement could also provide greater freedom of choice among different forms of practice—and I have been told that group practice works best where solo practice is also available.

I am convinced that you and other doctors throughout the state will ultimately recognize that Universal Health Insurance is desirable for your own best interests as well as the interests of the people. I say this because I am convinced that Universal Health Insurance is an idea whose time has come. If anything, it is overdue. If this concept is not adopted soon, this country will begin to move, in my opinion, toward socialized medicine. And if we do not develop a sound insurance system we are going to get something which will come from Washington, and which I think everybody will regret.

Many leading medical men, respected and revered in the profession, hold themselves aloof from this question, of questions such as this; they regard them as political rather than professional matters. But we need your leadership. We need your knowledge and wisdom. We need you to make the system work.

Let me emphasize once more—money is not the whole answer. But the combination of prepayment with an encouragement of group practice and other innovations in providing medical care can go far toward turning our present patchwork system in this period of transition into a real system for financing and delivering health care.

It is my earnest hope that this distinguished group will lend its enormous prestige and influence to the cause of Universal Health Insurance and a more comprehensive system of health care.

You have been part of the advance that has truly achieved miracles in modern medicine. Now let us work together to place these benefits within the reach of all our people.

I do not think there is any difference in our objective. It is a difference only in means and methods. And I really feel that we need to work together—those in government, those in public health, and you who have devised the means of achieving these goals—to achieve a sound solution. In my opinion, if we do it on an insurance basis then we shall not be taking away research funds or any other funds coming directly from government. I think that the individuals who are the beneficiaries, the corporations, should contribute jointly.

PRESENTATION OF THE ACADEMY PLAQUE TO JAMES BURNS AMBERSON, M.D.*

DICKINSON W. RICHARDS

Department of Medicine
Columbia University College of Physicians and Surgeons
New York, N. Y.

A GREAT teacher is rarer by far than a scientist or a clinician of equal distinction. He also contributes more to his profession, and so to all the world.

A teacher in medicine, moreover, must possess in great measure the abilities of all three: teacher, scientist, and clinician. All these things are superlatively true of James Burns Amberson, the man whom we honor on this occasion with the New York Academy of Medicine Plaque.

Born in Waynesboro, Pa., he received his B.A. degree at Lafayette College and his M.D. at Johns Hopkins. He was for three years physician and then physician in chief at the Loomis Sanatorium. In 1927 he joined the staff of the Bellevue Hospital Tuberculosis Service under Dr. James Alexander Miller, himself a distinguished physician and teacher as well as leader in the affairs of the Academy.

In 1938, on Dr. Miller's retirement, Dr. Amberson became director of the service now named the Bellevue Chest Service. This institution, already known throughout the country and the world as a clinical and teaching center, advanced remarkably under Dr. Amberson's leadership in excellence and in the opportunities offered to physicians of all ages and at all stages of training.

The key, of course, to all this has been Dr. Amberson himself, whose way of teaching is deceptively simple; it concentrates on the direct examination of the patient, use of the x ray, and basic laboratory data. Dr. Amberson marshals and evaluates the evidence in masterly fashion, his diagnostic skill exceeded only by his primary concern for his patient's welfare.

*Presented at the annual meeting of the New York Academy of Medicine, April 29, 1970.

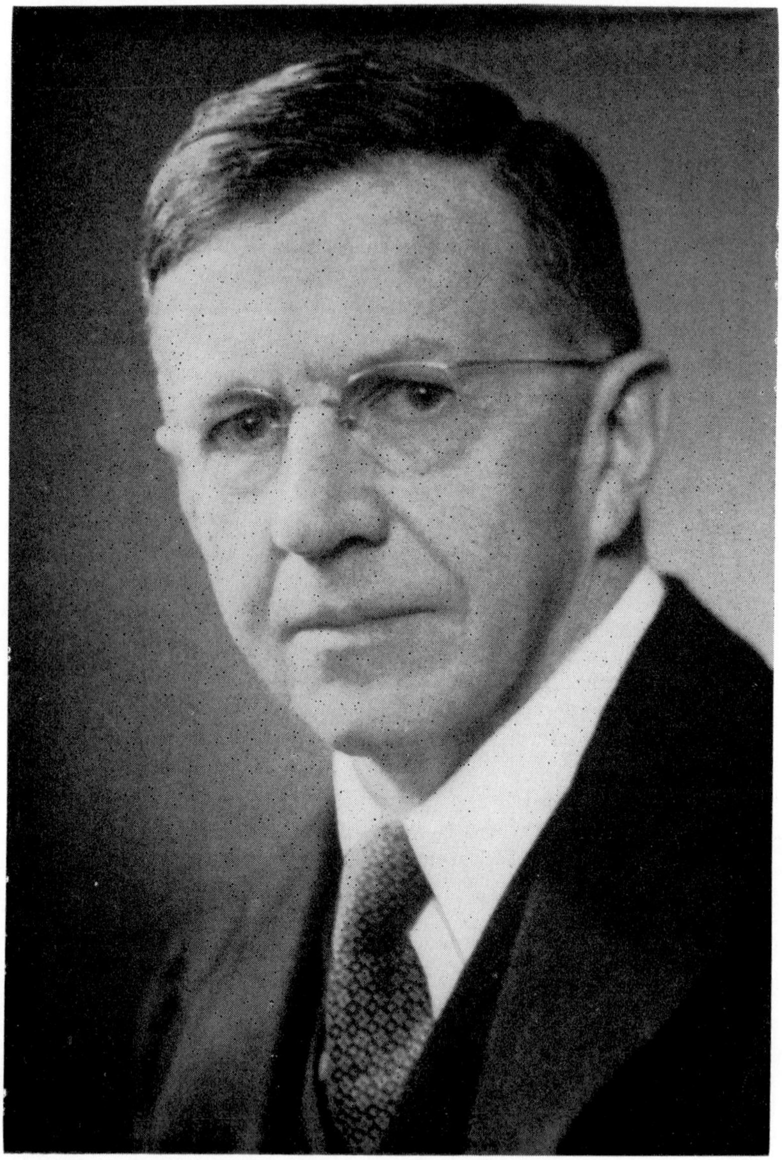

James Burns Amberson, M.D.

In guiding his students and staff he is considerate and discerning, and they look to him with all confidence. It has been my privilege to be one of these, and later in my capacity as director of the First Medical Division next door to the Chest Service at Bellevue, to work in close association with him for nearly 20 years.

Unlike Julius Caesar, the good that Dr. Amberson has done lives after him. He has two enduring monuments. The first is the great number of his students over all these years who look to him as their teacher, guide, and friend. The second is the Bellevue Chest Service itself. Having gone recently through a complete change of management, as our business friends say, it continues with all its vitality and enthusiasm. It is about to give a dinner, incidentally, for Dr. Amberson, in celebration of a certain anniversary of his. If I were to say what anniversary, you would not believe it, so I shall not say it. Dr. Amberson has received many awards and honors, but I do not need to mention these.

The New York Academy of Medicine Plaque is given particularly for contributions and service to the Academy. Dr. Amberson has given most generously of his time and interest to Academy affairs. He was a member of the Council on Medical Education for two terms; has been on the Committee on Public Health since 1952; on the By-Laws Committee; was vice president of the Academy at various times for a total of five years; and has just completed five years as a trustee. But the number of his positions still does not measure the quality of his service. At least in my memory, which goes back a long way, it seems as though every time a problem comes up in which differences of opinion are most violent, personal feelings most abraded, and the political situation on edge, Dr. Amberson turns up as chairman of the committee to deal with it, and somehow the problem is always resolved with reason and judgment and with agreement and even good feeling on all sides.

Dr. Amberson: to you as a great teacher and clinician, as a distinguished member of our profession, and as our colleague in the service of the Academy, it is my very great privilege to present the New York Academy of Medicine Plaque for the year 1970.

PRESENTATION OF THE ACADEMY MEDAL TO HARRY EAGLE, M.D.*

ALFRED GILMAN

William S. Lasdon Professor and Chairman
of Pharmacology
Albert Einstein College of Medicine
New York, N. Y.

I AM greatly flattered to be chosen to give the citation for the 1970 award of the Academy Medal. At the outset, I must confess that I am moonlighting, for it would take at least three scientists to describe adequately the achievements of the recipient, Dr. Harry Eagle, as will soon be apparent. And any one of these achievements would qualify him for the award that he so richly deserves.

Harry Eagle was born in New York City in 1905. As an infant he showed his precociousness by moving himself and his family to Baltimore, a city in which he was destined to spend many but by no means all of his productive years, for Harry Eagle is truly peripatetic, both geographically and, if the term applies, scientifically. He received his A.B. and M.D. from Johns Hopkins University in 1923 and 1927 respectively, after which he interned and, for the next three years, he was an instructor in the Department of Medicine at his alma mater.

His first research interests were in immunology, both basic immunological mechanisms and, particularly, the serology of syphilis, a subject to which he made many fundamental contributions for a period of 23 years. His scientific curiosity drew him to Harvard for the year 1932-1933 where, as a National Research Council Fellow, he became interested, under the influence of the late Dr. E. J. Cohn, in the mechanisms of blood clotting. He then went to the University of Pennsylvania and spent three years as assistant professor of microbiology. His papers during this period dealt with the serology of syphilis and the fundamentals of coagulation. In the latter field he was the first to demonstrate that the clotting mechanism depended upon a complex series of enzymatic reactions. He was 30 years ahead of his field.

In 1936 Harry Eagle became a commissioned officer of the U.S.

*Presented at the annual meeting of the New York Academy of Medicine, April 29, 1970.

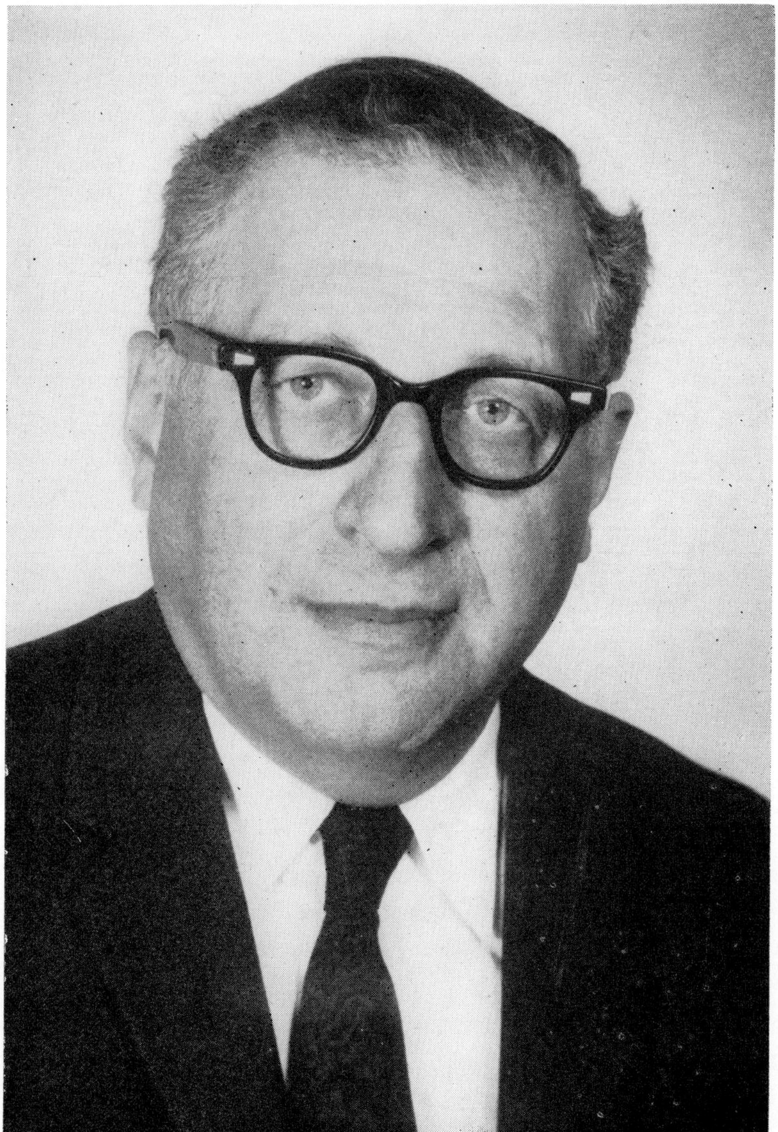

Harry Eagle, M.D.

Public Health Service. His reasons for accepting this post were compelling. He was the first such officer to receive an unrestricted assignment with the liberty to pursue his own research interests. He became director of the Venereal Disease Research Laboratory and Laboratory of Experimental Therapeutics, U.S. Public Health Service, and Johns Hopkins School of Hygiene and Public Health, a position he was to hold for 12 years. Harry Eagle's interests now turned to the chemotherapy of syphilis, trypanosomiasis, and leishmaniasis. He became a true pharmacologist in the days when the tools of chemotherapy were very crude indeed, namely compounds of arsenic, bismuth, mercury, and antimony. The host was almost as vulnerable as the parasite to these chemotherapeutic blunderbusses. Undaunted, he worked out the basic mechanisms of the actions of these drugs on both parasite and host, introduced new chemotherapeutic agents, and combined both basic and applied research. In those days, the treatment of syphilis was long and protracted, alternating between courses of arsenicals and either bismuth or mercury for a period of at least one and one-half years. There was an aphorism at the time: "A night with Venus and a lifetime with Mercury." Harry Eagle decided to do something about this sequence; I am referring of course to the lifetime with Mercury. He initiated a study on the intensive treatment of syphilis—probably his only effort that was not crowned with success because penicillin came on the scene, and arsenic and mercury became obsolete.

You can guess the next chapter in Harry Eagle's scientific career. He now turned his attention to penicillin and, in a brilliant series of papers published between 1944 and 1954, established basic concepts of chemotherapy that are as valid today as when first proposed. One of my most vivid memories is the presentation of this work made by Harry Eagle at the Combined Staff Conference of the Columbia University College of Physicians and Surgeons. The standing ovation he received from students and staff was most unusual.

In 1947 Harry Eagle moved to the National Institutes of Health, Bethesda, Md., where he occupied a number of important research and administrative posts. In 1955 he again changed his area of research; he now worked in cell biology, specifically cell and tissue culture. He realized that the crude media then in use precluded the type of studies he wished to pursue. Therefore he meticulously determined the amino acid, vitamin, and mineral requirements necessary for the growth of cells in culture, and Eagle's medium became famous throughout the world. With this powerful tool Eagle now embarked upon a series of quantitative studies on the pathways of amino-acid and nucleic-acid metabolism of cells in culture and, more important, the examination of their function and regulation. He is now engaged in the investigation of the biochemical basis of malignancy; he proceeds by studying the interactions in tissue culture between normal and malignant cells, their biochemical differences, and the metabolic changes that occur when a normal tissue culture becomes malignant by the application of oncogenic viruses. Many questions have already been answered. Surely if the mysteries of malignant growth and its control are ever to be solved, it will be by the methods that have been initiated by Harry Eagle and that are now in the hands of cell biologists the world over,

Dr. Eagle's accomplishments have received such wide recognition that to list his honors and awards as well as his activities on the national scene is impractical. However, I am happy to make one more remark about his scientific career. In 1961 he left the National Institutes of Health to become professor and chairman of the Department of Cell Biology at the Albert Einstein College of Medicine. He is now the professor and chairman of the Division of Biological Sciences. His impact on the school can be appreciated only by those who have had contact with him. Suffice it to say that the quality of his teaching is equal to that of his research.

If I have been too long in my presentation, blame the recipient and not the speaker. It is one thing to dabble in many areas of science, it is another to become successively a leader in each of the fields of immunology, hematology, pharmacology, microbiology, and cell biology. I very much fear that in an attempt to cover the gamut of Harry Eagle's achievements, full justice has been afforded to none.

Despite his many honors, I am sure the medal he is about to receive will be one he will cherish most highly.

STANDING COMMITTEES OF THE ACADEMY—1970

The President and the Director of the Academy are ex officio members of all committees

COMMITTEE ON ADMISSION

George R. Merriam, Jr., *chairman*
Arthur H. Aufses, Jr., *secretary*

E. Lovell Becker
Quentin B. Deming
Vincent J. Fontana
Schuyler G. Kohl
Robert S. Litwak
S. Arthur Localio
Louis R. Orkin
Myron S. Roberts
Melvin B. Watkins
Aaron O. Wells

COMMITTEE ON LIBRARY

Ralph L. Engle, Jr., *chairman*

Frank B. Berry, *emeritus*
Edgar M. Bick
Eric T. Carlson
Paul F. Cranefield
George E. Daniels
Carlo Henze
John R. Herman
Saul Jarcho
Samuel W. Lambert, Jr.
Albert S. Lyons
Aubre de Lambert Maynard
William B. Ober
Rulan Rawson
Bronson S. Ray
Blair O. Rogers
Morton D. Schweitzer
Hilton H. Stothers
Joseph A. Tamerin
Walter A. Wichern
Adrian W. Zorgniotti

Thomas Bassler, *librarian*

COMMITTEE ON PUBLIC HEALTH

William J. Eisenmenger, *chairman*
Alfred E. Fischer, *vice chairman*

J. Burns Amberson
Henry Aranow, Jr.
William A. Bauman
Otto E. Billo
Abram Blau
William Henry Button, Jr.
McKeen Cattell
Henry I. Fineberg
Arthur A. Fischl
Arthur V. Greeley
Frederick C. Green
Harry J. Greene
Leonard L. Heimoff
William M. Hitzig
Wilbur B. Hurlbut
Henry L. Jaffe
Robert W. Laidlaw
Norton M. Luger
Mark J. Markham
Richard L. Masland
S. W. Moore
Eugene Moskowitz
Equinn W. Munnell
Theodore W. Oppel
Jean P. Papps
Bernard J. Pisani
Guy F. Robbins
George M. Saypol
Robert J. Slater
Harvey J. Tompkins
Peter Vogel

By invitation
Mary C. McLaughlin

Emeritus
George Baehr
Milton J. Goodfriend
Oswald R. Jones*
Asa L. Lincoln
Howard A. Patterson
Beverly Chew Smith
Maximin De M. Touart

Arthur J. Lewis, *executive secretary*

*Deceased

STANDING COMMITTEES OF THE ACADEMY—1970 *(continued)*

COMMITTEE ON MEDICAL EDUCATION

George G. Reader, *chairman*
Edward E. Fischel, *vice chairman*

Alfred Angrist
Hugh R. K. Barber
Ernest L. Becker
Joseph G. Benton
Albert M. Betcher
Donald J. Cameron
Michael M. Dacso
Douglas S. Damrosch
Robert C. Darling
John A. Downey
J. Frederick Eagle, Jr.
Robert E. Eckardt
Jose M. Ferrer
David Harris
S. G. Hershey
Henry D. Janowitz
M. Ralph Kaufman
Patricia L. Kendall
Donald S. Kornfeld
Abraham L. Kornzweig
William S. Langford
Carroll M. Leevy
David Lehr
Michael J. Lepore
J. Lowry Miller
Pablo Morales
Carl Muschenheim
George R. Nagamatsu
Blair O. Rogers
Albert C. Santy
Morris Schaeffer
Arthur G. Ship
Leonard V. Smiley
Max L. Som
Marvin Stern
Isidore Sternlieb
Phillip D. Wilson, Jr.
Robert L. Wolf
William I. Wolff
Harry M. Zimmerman

Honorary emeritus
Clarence E. de la Chapelle
Leo Mayer
Rustin McIntosh
Milton J. Raisbeck
Paul Reznikoff
Isidore Snapper

Robert S. Goodhart, *executive secretary*

COMMITTEE ON MEDICINE IN SOCIETY

John M. Cotton, *chairman*
Irving Graef, *vice chairman*

Norton S. Brown
Duncan W. Clark
William Cooper*
John W. V. Cordice, Jr.
Edwin F. Daily
Murray Dworetzky
William W. Field
Alfred M. Freedman
Maxwell L. Gelfand
Carl Goldmark, Jr.
Sidney M. Greenberg
August H. Groeschel
Carlo E. Grossi
Harold D. Harvey
Philip E. Henig
John L. S. Holloman, Jr.
Louis Leiter
Mack Lipkin
David Lyall
Henry B. Makover
Marvin E. Perkins
S. David Domrinse
Joseph Post
Willard C. Rappleye
J. Beall Rodgers
Leonard S. Rosenfeld
Frank A. Seixas
Carl H. Smith
Samuel Standard
Milton Terris
Edward Tolstoi
George M. Wheatley
Herbert B. Wilcox, Jr.
Byard Williams

Emeritus
Harry S. Altman

Marvin Lieberman, *executive secretary*

*Deceased

Other Committees—1970

EDITORIAL BOARD

SAUL JARCHO, *editor in chief*

CHARLES A. RAGAN, JR., *chairman*
RALPH W. GAUSE
FRANK L. HORSFALL, JR.
J. LAWRENCE POOL
ROBERT J. SLATER
FRANK C. SPENCER
STUART S. STEVENSON
FREDERICK G. ZAK

COMMITTEE ON ART

ALBERT C. SANTY, *chairman*

JOHN L. CONLEY
MEYER M. MELICOW

COMMITTEE ON REVISION OF BYLAWS

JOHN MADDEN, *chairman*

JARVIS COFFIN
FRED METTLER
JAMES J. SMITH

COMMITTEE ON PHYSICAL FACILITIES

ROBERT E. LEVY, *chairman*

FRANK B. BERRY
HOWARD REID CRAIG
FRANK GLENN
SAMUEL W. LAMBERT
ALBERT SANTY
JAMES E. THOMPSON

SALMON MEMORIAL COMMITTEE

FRANCIS J. BRACELAND, *chairman*

KENNETH E. APPEL
DAVID LEVY
WILLIAM LHAMON
LAWRENCE C. KOLB
H. HOUSTON MERRITT
FREDERICK C. REDLICH

OFFICERS OF SECTIONS

1969-1970

SECTION ON ANESTHESIOLOGY AND RESUSCITATION

SARAH JOFFE, *chairman* JOSEPH ARTUSIO, JR., *secretary*

SECTION ON BASIC MEDICAL SCIENCES

MORRIS SCHAEFFER, *chairman* MARION E. WILSON, *secretary*

SECTION ON BIOMEDICAL ENGINEERING

PHILIP D. WILSON, JR., *chairman* ERWIN R. TICHAUER, *secretary*

SECTION ON DERMATOLOGY AND SYPHILOLOGY

CHARLES P. DEFEO, JR., *chairman* WILBURT B. HURLBUT, *secretary*

SECTION ON HISTORICAL MEDICINE

BLAIR O. ROGERS, *chairman* JOHN M. CONVERSE, *secretary*

SECTION ON MEDICINE

MICHAEL S. BRUNO, *acting chairman*

SECTION ON NEUROLOGY AND PSYCHIATRY

ARTHUR ZITRIN, *chairman* FLETCHER H. MCDOWELL, *secretary*

SECTION ON OBSTETRICS AND GYNECOLOGY

BENEDICT B. BENIGNO, *chairman* MYRON GORDON, *secretary*

SECTION ON OCCUPATIONAL MEDICINE

ROBERT E. ECKHARDT, *chairman* THEODORE E. ALLEN, *secretary*

SECTION ON OPHTHALMOLOGY

J. GORDON COLE, *chairman* IRA S. JONES, *secretary*

SECTION ON ORTHOPEDIC SURGERY

KENNETH C. FRANCIS, *chairman* GEORGE B. AMBROSE, *secretary*

SECTION ON OTOLARYNGOLOGY

JOSEPH R. RONGETTI, *chairman* WILLIAM F. ROBBETT, *secretary*

SECTION ON PEDIATRICS

JEAN PAKTER, *chairman* PETER R. SCAGLIONE, *secretary*

SECTION ON PHYSICAL MEDICINE AND REHABILITATION

MILTON LOWENTHAL, *chairman* EDWARD J. LORENZE, *secretary*

SECTION ON PLASTIC AND RECONSTRUCTIVE SURGERY

BERNARD E. SIMON, *chairman* WILLIAM P. WHALEN, *secretary*

SECTION ON SURGERY

W. GRAHAM KNOX, *chairman* WILLIAM METCALF, *secretary*

SECTION ON UROLOGY

PABLO MORALES, *chairman* HARRY GRABSTALD, *secretary*

OFFICERS OF AFFILIATED SOCIETIES

THE HARVEY SOCIETY

JOHN V. TAGGART, *president* ELLIOTT F. OSSERMAN, *secretary*

THE NEW YORK PATHOLOGICAL SOCIETY

RAFFAELE LATTES, *president* SHELDON SOMMERS, *secretary*

NEW YORK ROENTGEN SOCIETY

DAVID H. BAKER, *president* SAMUEL H. MADELL, *secretary*

STATEMENT

ON

Implementation of the New York State Abortion Law*

BY

THE COMMITTEE ON PUBLIC HEALTH

OF

THE NEW YORK ACADEMY OF MEDICINE

There is much confusion at present concerning the implementation of the New York State Law regarding medical abortion, which becomes effective July 1, 1970. Many committees have been meeting to draw up guidelines in an attempt to implement the law in a manner consistent with medical practice of the highest quality.

The Committee on Public Health of the New York Academy of Medicine has also considered this matter and has reviewed the recommendations of the Advisory Committee on Obstetrics and Gynecology of the New York City Health Department. At its meeting on June 1 the Committee on Public Health endorsed the Health Department recommendations.

In addition, the Committee on Public Health believes that the following observations are appropriate to ensure proper implementation:

1) There is an anticipated scarcity of hospital beds in New York City for patients requesting elective abortion. At present such abortions should be hospital based (on either an inpatient or outpatient basis) and should be performed as early in the course of pregnancy as possible to ensure high-quality medical care and to minimize complications. Management is more complicated after the 12th week of pregnancy.

2) For the present, priority should be given in New York City to women residing within the city or to previous patients of New York City physicians because of the over-all shortage of beds, as well as for

*Approved by the Executive Committee, May 25, 1970.
Approved by the Council of The Academy of Medicine, May 27, 1970.
Approved by the Committee on Public Health, June 1, 1970.

the need to have facilities available for patients with diagnostic and therapeutic problems of an emergency nature.

3) No physician or other person or hospital should be required to perform or participate in a medical or surgical procedure which may result in the termination of pregnancy.

4) Adequate financing from both the public and private sectors should be available to provide adequate space, qualified physicians, and nursing staff, as well as necessary equipment.

The Committee on Public Health affirms the need for adequate facilities and qualified personnel. The Committee also feels strongly that medical care of high quality should not be sacrificed in the resolution of the many problems that may arise.

THE BATTERED-CHILD SYNDROME: PARENTAL MOTIVATION, CLINICAL ASPECTS

Gabriel V. Laury

Instructor
Department of Pediatric Psychiatry
Columbia University College of Physicians and Surgeons
New York, N. Y.

Malnutrition, bruises, scars, black-and-blue marks, burns, and old or recent fractures may not be accidental but part of the battered-child syndrome. During the past few years there has been growing concern over the battered child, and many reports on the subject have appeared in the lay press as well as in medical journals. With increasing frequency radio and television programs too are now focusing on the topic. Legislators throughout the country more and more are trying to protect these juvenile victims by making compulsory the reporting of cases of child abuse. In New York State, for instance, 11 professional groups that include physicians and nurses must submit written reports within 48 hours in cases of child abuse. A statewide registry is kept up-to-date to help detect recidivists. Lately there has been an increasing incidence of reports of maltreatment of children under three years of age, even of babies under six months. Kempe et al. in 1962 related the results of a United States survey of hospitals and law-enforcement agencies. They found that within a year 749 children had been overtly mistreated. Of this number 78 died and 114 suffered permanent damage to the brain.[1] It seems, however, that the number of unreported cases of tortured and battered children far exceeds the reported ones.[2] Indeed, professionals are often reluctant to consider this diagnosis and even more so to report such cases. A 1966 survey involving 179 physicians revealed that 25% of them would not report suspected battering.[3] According to De Francis, who studied 662 cases of physical abuses of children, the father was responsible in about 38% of the cases, the mother in about 29%, and both in 5%. The parents were of all ages, and their social origins varied "from the poorest slum areas to some country-club districts."[4] According to these reports there are more battering fathers than mothers. Many of these mothers are quite masculine in appearance and demeanor and their husbands correspondingly passive and retiring.[5] For infanticides, statistics reveal that mothers outnumbered fathers by three to one.[6]

Many normal parents go through periods of deep-seated hostility toward their child. In a momentary fit of rage they may feel the impulse to act against him in an abusively hostile and aggressive way, and fear that they may lose control over themselves. Rheingold came to the conclusion that the wish to kill her offspring is present in normal mothers.[7] However, the vast majority of parents succeed in checking their impulses and controlling themselves, and do not batter their children. Yet in some cases abuses do occur. It can be a single, nearly accidental attack on a child or it can be on a constant basis, day in and day out. The performer of the isolated battering often feels apologetic, perplexed, and very guilty. The chronic battering individual on the other hand, has grown accustomed to and blasé about his cruelty. When confronted with his acts he feels concern for himself but shows generally little guilt or remorse for his actions. There can be complete denial of any knowledge of inflicted trauma to the child and convincing pretension of complete innocence.[8]

Some parents manage to leave the "dirty work" of battering their children to somebody else, or the child is led into hurting himself in "preset accidents." This "battering by proxy" is quite common. The mother asks the cruel father to punish her child, or leaves it to an older sibling, a selected baby sitter, or a neighbor. In an institutional setting, an employee may suggest to a group of children to gang up against his victim. This subtler form of battering conveniently absolves anyone of guilt and of legal consequences.

Finally, there are children who, out of some hard-to-explain masochistic urge, provoke beatings over and over again. They seem to bring it on themselves.[9]

When interviewed, abusive parents usually try to explain their acts by giving "good reasons." Further contacts with them often reveal underlying motives of which they are unaware. I shall review below some apparent reasons and underlying motivations for the battering-parent's pattern and present a few clinical illustrations.

Apparent Reasons

Some parents claim that they beat their children for their own good, and feel that their abuses are only a justified punishment. This carries the implication of magically beating strength, decency, knowledge, and good behavior into the victim. Yet we have to keep in mind that some parents believe, in good faith, in the efficacy of a "good" beating. It may be hard to differentiate admissible punishment from real abuse. Caffey, who has been studying battered children for over 25 years, notes, "It is not fully appreciated that the line between an ordinary spanking and a serious injury or even fatal injury may be a very fine one indeed. Often this difference is a matter of pure chance."[10] The beating is done regardless of the age of the child. In 1966 Rorsch reported that a quarter of the 100 mothers she studied started spanking their children before the age of six months.[11] Two centuries ago Rousseau had already written, "the child is punished for faults before he knows anything about them and even before he is able to commit them."[12]

John was a five-year-old boy who was thrown against the wall and sustained multiple fractures. The father had wanted to punish him for being lazy and was "only trying to make a man out of him."

Other children are maltreated on account of their behavior, that is, for the parent's sake. The adult indignantly reports that the child "likes" to scream for no good reason, that he does not "want" to let him sleep, that he "succeeds" in making him angry, and obviously "enjoys" wetting and soiling. He is also a feeding problem, refuses to behave, and "tries hard" to prevent his parents from sexual intercourse by entering the bedroom at the crucial moment. He is a competitor who wilfully tries to monopolize and take over love, time, and attention. The dependent little child is thus seen as an antagonistic and powerful adult who has to be dealt with as such.

Mothers may also blame the child for their sagging bosoms, for the loss of shape of their hips, for their obesity, wrinkles, varices, and frigidity. This attitude is often encouraged by what is found in the lay press and folklore about the children's destructive effects: grey hair is due to worries caused by children; long-lasting hemorrhoids, caries, or even the loss of teeth are caused by pregnancy. Not to mention those who believe that they would have had an exciting professional career if they had not been tied down by their children. All these beliefs may influence the parents who "get even" with the culprits, the children.

Another motivation for battering is the parent's feeling that the child has failed to meet expectations. In effect the child can disappoint them in two ways. Either because he is abnormal or because he is not ideal.

In the first subgroup are the children with brain damage, mental illness, or retardation. They are "disciplined," that is, maltreated, because they are "lazy, stubborn, cannot sit still, do not want to obey or listen." Yet all these traits may be consequences of their condition and thus beyond their control. The battering may only worsen their psychopathology by increasing their feelings of frustration and rejection, and by diminishing their self-esteem. A similar pattern can also occur in the case of physical defects.

Mrs. S. had always been a loving and devoted mother to Richard, her four-year-old son. When it finally occurred to her that he was retarded she became enraged and severely bit him.

In the second subgroup we find the child whose only fault is not to be the "ideal" dreamed of by his parents, who had assumed that the child merely existed for their convenience and pleasure; they wanted him to do their "thing," and anxiously to await praise when showing him off. This attitude is readily encouraged by some vulgarizing, pseudomedical magazines which constantly emphasize the concept of the perpetual "bundle of joy." The child is expected to bring only happiness to the family and is invariably destined for the brightest future. (For example, the vogue of toddler's sweatshirts with the inscription "Harvard, Class of '85" and such jokes as "my son the doctor.") When the real child does not live up to such fanciful expectations some parents act out their profound disllusions against the 'bad" offspring and may then abuse him.

Ralph was a seven-year-old boy who was mercilessly beaten by an overly ambitious father for not being at the top of the class. As beatings did not improve the boy's scholastic performances the father took him to a psychiatrist to cure him of his laziness. The physician had psychometric evaluations done and the results showed that the boy was clearly a borderline mental defective. It took several interviews with the father to dissuade him from beating the child for not being the genius he had hoped to have.

Some parents abuse a child because they feel that he is not really theirs. Indeed quite frequently the battered child is unwanted, a foster or adopted child; he was deserted or not legitimized by the father, or came from a previous marriage, or was felt to be sired by somebody else.[13] This is closely related to the retaliatory aspect of child battering. In order to get even with the spouse, one parent makes him suffer through the suffering of his children. The slaying of the children by

Medea was used in Greek mythology to punish the unfaithful father.

Pseudointellectual rationalizations have been used for battering children. Individuals will go from physician to physician, from friend to friend until they finally find excuses for what they are doing to the child. One mother would constantly leave her infant alone, outside in a baby carriage, because the pediatrician had said that he should have plenty of fresh air. Whenever neighbors would worry about the safety of the baby, who was trying actively to get out of the carriage and already had fallen on his head with loss of consciousness, the mother would announce from the house, "the doctor told me he needs fresh air, he should know." The same mother would let the child scream for hours without coming to his rescue because she had been told that it was good for his lungs. She would let the child lie for hours in his vomitus "by order" of her doctor. In fact her physician had only said that she should not worry about vomiting but, conveniently for her, he had not spelled out that "kids-should-not-be-left-lying-in-their-vomitus."

Mrs. P. had been told and believed that kids need to have initiative, should not be watched all the time, and that anyway they heal fast, and she used to leave her son Francis unattended for hours. At age five he was hit by a car while crossing a major thoroughfare alone. He sustained multiple fractures and subsequently developed signs of brain damage. The mother was much surprised to find out that there were physical and psychiatric sequels to the accident. She spent the following years suing insurance companies. Meanwhile she continues to disregard the safety of her son, who by this time had started to play with the hunting rifles his father had left hanging on the wall.

Sadistic or psychopathic parents or parental substitutes may gain satisfaction from the suffering of the child. In Victor Hugo's *Les Misérables*, one of the heroines is the pathetic child Cosette, who was exploited and abused by a sordid couple, had to slave from early morning to late at night, was mercilessly beaten for any minor infraction, and was finally sold to a stranger. "Cosette ran upstairs and downstairs; washed, brushed, scrubbed, swept, ran, tired herself, got out of breath, lifted heavy things and did the hard work. No pity; a ferocious mistress, a malignant master. She was nearly eight years old but one would barely have thought her six. Her skin showed through her ragged clothes here and there, and black and blue spots could be distinguished which indicated the places where her bosses had touched her."[14] We have witnessed several similar cases where exploitation was coupled with battering, to which Hugo's description still applies. In other instances the adults obtain sexual gratification from inflicting the suffering. They feel quite safe, as the child may not be believed, nor is he capable of retaliation. More than once have we seen children who were cruelly abused until they "willingly" submitted to the sexual whims of grown-ups. In this case the beatings were used to coerce the child into homo- or heterosexual acts.

Jean, age 12, was brutally beaten by her stepfather because she refused to have intercourse with him. When she ran away, she was brought back by police. She attempted suicide three times, and only when comatose from an overdose of insulin was she taken seriously and finally separated from her stepfather.

Some battering parents are mentally sick, and the child may become part of their distorted reality and delusional system. A paranoid parent may thus view his child as part of his persecuting environment and then feel justified in retaliating against him. Such a parent may also be an alcoholic or may suffer from epileptic automatism. It is quite interesting to note at this point that some parents may reveal their pathology only when dealing with their children. Such parents may have gone through life as "normal" persons, and the child psychiatrist is the first to conclude justly that they are mentally sick.

Bizarre reasons, in the absence of mental illness, are given at times by parents. The following case is one of starving four little girls, three, four (twins), and five years old; the brutal handling of them in this case was secondary in importance.

Clara, a four-year-old girl, "was not doing well." Her parents called an ambulance to take her to the hospital where she was pronounced dead on arrival. The post-mortem examination confirmed the clinical impression of starvation. Her three sisters were then admitted to the hospital for observation. They were cachectic, underdeveloped, but alive. They had marks on the lower part of their body "suggestive of the battered-child syndrome," as stated on the admission note. When the mother was asked to come to visit her surviving daughters on the ward, she said she could not, as she had to buy a black veil for the funeral. Her only comment on the death of her child was that "she had a voracious appetite." Afterwards she added that everybody in the family ate adequately and went on describing in detail the well-balanced meals she would serve regularly. The three siblings, while hospitalized, ate voraciously and rapidly gained weight. Both parents appeared well fed and in no financial distress. The mother showed unconcern about the death of her child and the severe emaciation of the three others. Two and a half years earlier one of the sisters had been taken to the same hospital for an "accident" in which her abdomen sustained a large second-degree burn. At that time the diagnosis of "partial neglect" had been established.

Finally, in some cases no evident motivation can be found. The incriminated parent professes surprise at his own acts, invokes his "short fuse," and calls it an accident. This type of behavior seems less destructive to the child's emotional integrity. The parent is not considered all bad, all rejecting, and all cruel, and a warm relation with the child still remains possible. In many cases, in fact, it is very difficult to differentiate volitional from accidental battering even after repeated interviews with the parents.

Frank was the apple of the eye of well-to-do, warm, and loving parents. Yet one day he sustained a broken nose, black eyes, a dislocation of his thumb and a fracture of the wrist, after being assaulted by his father. The latter acknowledged, with deep regret, having committed the assault but was unable to give any motive. Similarly in a survey of 83 children victims of homicides there was a "disturbing 10% of cases in which the assailant was not overtly psychotic nor was there any apparent motive for what appeared to be a completely senseless crime."[6]

Underlying Motivations

Whereas the apparent reasons are the ones the parents give for their behavior, further probing usually reveals underlying motivations of which they are mostly unaware.

Some parents compensate for the frustrations and tensions of daily life by beating an innocent and conveniently weak victim. Figuratively, the child is selected to become the sponge for the parent's excessive hostility.[15] The parents who are afraid to grow up, that is, to assume adult responsibilities and to behave maturely, resent the child whose very existence forces them into this unwanted role. Other parents are still looking for somebody to help them and love them when a child comes into the picture. Not only is the child unable to play the expected role, but he loudly requires to be taken care of by his parents. Such frustrations and stress may account for the abuse. In some instances the battering parent imitates unwittingly his own battering parent. One who has never been loved as a child is unable to love his children. Or cruelty becomes a displaced revenge for their own parent's cruelty.[9, 16] In one study of parents who abused their offspring there was a constant history of their having been raised in the same manner which they were now repeating in rearing their own children.[17] Mass media such as newspapers, radio, television, and movies often convey the message that violence and cruelty are justified under certain circumstances. Such media may thus contaminate the mind and insidiously influence the behavior of susceptible parents. Finally, quite often, the child becomes the scapegoat, the one responsible for an untimely or unhappy marriage, for the lack of social life, and for the disappearance of the romanticized "good old days" when one was young, beautiful, happy, and without obligations.

Often children may be looked upon as evil possessions because they inadvertently remind the parent of their own wicked thoughts in childhood or at the present time. Or the mother may hate her child because he renews the memory of her hated lover, husband, or parent; in his veins runs their "bad blood."

On the other hand, it is no secret that some mothers gain satisfaction from parenthood only when their children are sick or helpless. This makes the mother feel omnipotent again. To beat the child makes him weak and sick; she then feels needed and will take care of him. This is even more true if the child is abused by the father; it enlarges the need for mother's magical protection. In some rare cases, the parent may feel that he punishes himself by hurting someone he loves, i.e., his child.

The underlying motivations are multiple; in actuality each case is different and has its own dynamics. Often many sessions with the parents and the child are needed to elicit them.

Other Clinical Illustrations

John, a five-year-old boy, was severely abused by his mother, and his teacher had noticed that he arrived covered with fresh bruises every morning. The mother claimed that he was bad, nasty, misbehaved, and used foul language. Whatever the reason, she used to beat him daily when alone with him in the house. The child was the product of a previous marriage. The mother had remarried, and her second husband had accepted him. The boy was a constant reminder to her of many things she wished to forget. Years earlier her own mother had warned her against marrying her first husband, but the warning had been ignored, and a few months after the marriage her mother had died without having talked to her again. About the same time her husband had abandoned her while she was pregnant with John. By beating the child she was taking revenge on—in fact, beating—the first husband, who was out of reach. Deep down, she would fantasize that the father could hear his son's screams and would suffer. In this case, the beating had a much deeper and more complex motivation than the mere punishment of questionable behavior. Involved were husband-wife, daughter-mother relations. The aggression was directed at her husband.

Mr. R. would brutally beat his son because the boy was undisciplined. The couple had been childless for years, and Mr. R. had always been convinced that his wife was sterile. When at their physician's suggestion, artificial insemination was tried and found successful, the father was forced to acknowledge that he was the sterile partner. The child, ever since his conception, always represented a living insult to his "father's" virility. Thus a basic motivation for the father's aggressive behavior stemmed from the circumstances surrounding the child's birth.

Conclusion

The child-battering syndrome may have many motivations. Some battering appears to be only incidental, and at times no reason at all can be found. In most cases parents claim that they beat their children for "good reasons," which often have themes of punishment, retaliation, or rejection. Further probing, however, reveals that the underlying motivations for attacking the child are multiple and often unknown to the parent. They usually reflect deeper seated hostility in the parent, which may pertain only tangentially to the child. This hostility usually is directed at the environment or at the parent himself.

REFERENCES

1. Kempe, C. H. et al.: The battered child syndrome. *J.A.M.A. 181*:17-24, 1962.
2. Bleiberg, N.: The neglected child, *N. Y. J. Med. 65*:1880-86, 1965.
3. Silver, L. et al.: Child abuse laws: Are they enough? *J.A.M.A. 199*:65-68, 1967.
4. De Francis, V.: Child abuse. Children's Division, Amer. Humane Ass., Denver, Colo., 1964.
5. Galdston, R.: Observations on children who have been physically abused. *Amer. J. Psychiat. 122*:440, 1965.
6. Myers, S.: The child slayer. *Arch. Gen. Psychiat. 17*:211-13, 1967.

7. Rheingold, J. C.: *The Fear of Being a Woman; A Theory of Maternal Destructiveness.* New York, Grune & Stratton, 1964.
8. Fontana, V.: The neglect and abuse of children. *N. Y. J. Med. 64*:215-24, 1964.
9. Laury, G. and Meerloo, J. A. M.: Mental cruelty and child abuse. *Psychiat. Quart. 41*:203-54, 1967.
10. Caffey, J. Diagnosis of Traumatic Injury to Children. *J. Pediat. 67*:1013, 1965.
11. Rorsch, B. M. The abused child. *Med. Tribune,* Apr. 2, 1966.
12. Rousseau, J. J.: *Emile.* Boyd, W., transl. New York Teachers College, Columbia Univ., 1965.
13. Tabibian, Y.: Les enfants victims de sevices. *Med. Hyg. 272*:861, 1969.
14. Hugo, V.: *Les Misérables.* New York, Modern Library, 1960, p. 338.
15. Wasserman, S. The abused parent of the abused child. *Children 14*:5, 1967.
16. Silver, L. et al.: Does violence breed violence? *Amer. J. Psychiat. 126*:404, 1969.
17. Helfer, R. and Kempe, C. H.: *The Battered Child.* Chicago, Univ. Chicago Press, 1968.

DEFUNCT AND DYING DISEASES*

BERNARD STRAUS

Professor of Medicine
New York Medical College
Bird S. Coler Hospital
New York, N. Y.

Some will allow no Disease to be new. Others think that many old ones are ceased; and that such which are esteemed new, will have but their time.

SIR THOMAS BROWNE

DISEASES are mortal and seem to have a life of their own. They are born, flourish for a time, and then die. Many have a distinct morbidity but linger on in a weakened, unhealthy state and with an obviously poor prognosis. Some die suddenly and others fade away. What happened to them? A few were authentic diseases which disappeared for reasons unknown. Some fell victims to advances in medical science, I am happy to say. Much has been said of the diseases of medical progress, but not enough concerning diseases which have been eliminated because of medical progress. Some disorders simply reflected mistaken notions or misinterpretations which have been corrected as a result of greater understanding of the pathogenesis and mechanisms of disease.

Disease and death are blood brothers in a relation in which formerly the first represented a dynamic process and the latter an end point. We have seen in our own time a change in which disease has been characterized increasingly by an end point and death has lost its finality. Even the very definition of death, for which we once had an easy answer, is now a subject of controversy, confusion, and soul-searching. Definition retains its philosophic relevance but not its simplicity, and it has become important for our clinical practice. Our concepts of disease, however, remain dynamic and subject to revision and change. The ebb and flow of specific diseases, which sometimes have a beginning and increasingly have an end, is the subject of this discourse.

*Presented at a meeting of the Section on Historical Medicine, May 27, 1970.

This will be no nostalgic threnody to dubious diseases of the ancients. We are concerned here only with diseases which have persisted to modern times, beginning roughly about the turn of the century. Before then too many nondescript and fanciful notions existed concerning a variety of disorders to concern us here. They are of interest, to be sure, but belong among the incunabula of medicine.

The Virginal Love Sickness

What did happen to chlorosis, "the green sickness," for example? The name was due to the greenish-yellow color of the affected girls. The disease was also known as the love sickness because love, presumably unrequited, was believed to be an etiologic factor. Chlorosis had a long life beginning in 1520, when it was described as a disease of virgins, until about 1912 when it virtually disappeared. It was interred with a rather belated obituary by W. M. Fowler in 1936.[1] This disorder was believed to be a primary or "essential" anemia "occurring in young girls due in part to hereditary influences, neurosis, ovarian insufficiency, autointoxication or 'copraemia'." It was thought to be a result of absorption of poisons–leucomaines and ptomaines–from the large bowel. Alternatively it was ascribed to the wearing of tight corsets.[2] Not too long before its demise, it became clear that the green sickness was an iron-deficiency anemia caused by malnutrition with an inadequate intake of iron aggravated by infections, overwork, and poor sanitary conditions. Sir William Osler was aware that iron depletion was a characteristic feature of the disorder and that iron was a specific in the treatment of this condition. Curiously, he states, "It is a minor matter *how* the iron cures chlorosis. . . . Iron is present in the faeces of chlorotic patients before they are placed on any treatment so that the disease does not result from any deficiency of available iron in the food."[3] Since chlorosis was due to a deficiency of iron, and as this deficiency is not uncommon today, why do not the girls turn green any more? We probably shall never know.

The current best seller by John Fowler entitled *The French Lieutenant's Woman,* which discusses some events of 1867, mentions the green sickness. Fowler relates that the doctor was called to "look at" an unfortunate maid, and pronounced the diagnosis green sickness. The maid was subjected to the wrath of her mistress because she had neglected one Tuesday to water the ferns in the second drawing room!

She narrowly escaped condign punishment by the discovery that she had fainted twice as a result of her illness. For treatment, Dr. Grogan recommended that she be moved out of the maids' dormitory and be given a room with more light. Her superior took upon herself much of the special care the chlorotic girl needed. Unfortunately we are not told what the special care or other treatment was.

As many gardeners know, chlorosis survives as a disease in green plants. Affected plants turn yellow or white. The treatment is adding iron chelates to the soil.

Little Fees and Fevers

Another disease that has vanished was known as febricula, meaning a little fever. This was also related to ephemeral fever which, indeed, both have proved to be. Presumably it was one of the little fevers that Oliver Wendell Holmes referred to when he announced, "Little fevers (and little fees) will be gratefully accepted." The name is so unfamiliar that it would seem to have been defunct for a long time. In fact, it was treated with respect, but some suspicion, as late as 1927 by Horace S. Baldwin, the contributor to the chapter on this disease in the first edition of Cecil's *Textbook of Medicine*.[4] Its lingering agony persisted until 1947 in the 16th edition of Christian's *Principles and Practice of Medicine*.[5] The author devoted a page to the disease with the statement that he preferred the term fever, cause unknown, instead of febricula or ephemeral fever. Much before this, however, febricula as an entity had fallen into disfavor.

Febricula referred to a fever of slight duration which was probably due to a variety of causes. According to Osler, a febrile paroxysm lasting for 24 hours and disappearing completely is spoken of as ephemeral fever. "If it persists for three, four or more days without local affection, it is referred to as febricula." Several groups were described: those which represented abortive types of typhoid fever, measles, or scarlet fever; those which developed with dyspepsia or following the drinking of stale beer; and those which follow exposure to foul odors or sewer gas. A variety of symptoms are described which will not be recited. However, the treatment suggested by Osler has a quaint virtue, the efficacy of which in a self-limited disorder certainly cannot be challenged: "Rest in bed, a laxative, and a fever medicine containing nitrate of potash and sweet spirits of nitre."

Does anyone know what sweet spirits of nitre is (are, were!)? I shall pass on the results of my research. They are nothing more nor less than an alcoholic solution of ethyl nitrite. I did not pursue my investigations to discover what these sweet spirits actually did as none of my pharmacology texts had even a passing reference to this drug. I am quite certain, however, that it is a potent antidote for stale beer.

As suspected by astute clinicians, febricula was not a specific disease but included a variety of infections which have since been more clearly defined and delineated. Many presumably were mild viral infections of the respiratory tract. The attribution of illness to stale beer, foul odors, and sewer gas was not uncommon at one time; it recalls the ancient role of the different humors and the frequent references to miasmas or noxious emanations of nondescript character.

Miasmas, Megrims, and the Vapors

For a long time these were cavalierly dismissed as implausible or imaginary. We have come full circle, however, for our present concern with pollutants and environment is, of course, related to these very miasmas or noxious emanations, although these are no longer so vague and nondescript. The miasmas were quite different from a condition known as the "vapors." This latter term has been obsolete for so long that it appears only occasionally in the form of a humorous literary allusion or a piece of memorabilia.[6] It is mentioned in Beaumarchais' *Marriage of Figaro* where Susanna refuses the contessa's medication for the vapors on the ground that they affect the nobility, not mere servants. The vapors referred to hypochondriasis or depression, and for a long time no fashionable lady could be without them at convenient periods. Related to the vapors were the megrims, which referred to lowness of spirits as from headache or general physical disturbance; the "blues," or morbid or whimsical states of feeling. Megrim was also a corruption of migraine. The megrims persist in veterinary medicine where it refers to a sudden attack of sickness in a horse at work, when he reels and either stands still for a moment, dull and stupid, or falls to the ground insensible. These attacks are often periodic but are most frequent in warm weather.

Probably related to the vapors and the megrims was the swoon. In the Victorian era swooning was de rigeur at appropriate intervals for all proper ladies. Some vile obscenity such as "darn" was enough to induce it. At least, this was the polite fiction which was widely held. Recent publications highly esteemed by devotees of pornography such as *My Secret Life—Diary of a Gentleman of Fashion* suggest that not all the swooning ladies of that period were quite so proper. At any rate the swoon is definitely no longer in fashion, and is fast disappearing. I am confident that all self-respecting members of the Woman's Liberation Movement would disdain swooning as sexploitation of the second sex. In fact, it is conceivable that even such a reprehensible four-letter word as hell would be unlikely to provoke a swoon in a modern maid.

The Sweating Sickness

An interesting infection that seems to have disappeared was known as miliary fever or the sweating sickness—not to be confused with miliary tuberculosis. This disease was characterized by fever, profuse sweats, and an eruption of miliary vesicles. Severe cases were characterized by delirum, high fever, profound prostration, and hemorrhage. The death rate was usually high, death often following in a few hours after the onset of the disease, which occurred in epidemics in Europe, including England, during the 15th and 16th centuries. An epidemic occurred in France as late as 1907. What it was is not clear. Could it have been malaria? This is not very likely because skin lesions are not common in any form of malaria. Whatever it was, we probably shall never know, for it has vanished into limbo.

Shoddy fever was a disease that affected workers on initial exposure to the grinding of rags. It was characterized by attacks of chills and fever. It has disappeared with technological progress and we shall never know what it really was. It may have been related to byssinosis, which is caused by the inhalation of cotton dust. The latter, however, is accompanied by wheezing and shortness of breath as prominent symptoms.

Another infectious disease, noma or gangrenous stomatitis, has virtually disappeared as a result of better hygienic conditions, improved nutrition, and antibiotics. Ludwig's angina, which once was a dread disease, has retreated into history probably for the same reasons. Quinsy, or the quinsy or quinsy sore throat, is a traditional name for peritonsillar cellulitis or abscess. Formerly very common, it is seen infrequently at present, in large part because of antibiotic therapy or tonsilectomy. Erysipelas, which was once a common infection, has decreased greatly in frequency and severity, probably due to penicillin and other antibiotics. Spirochetal bronchitis was once regarded as an important disorder. It was of dubious authenticity and in any case seems to have died quietly.

The Mysterious Thymus

The thymus gland was once termed an organ of mystery and several strange diseases were associated with it. Status thymicolymphaticus had a long tenure as a disease entity. It is now clear that this was an imaginary disorder. It was believed to be an inherited diathesis characterized by an enlarged thymic gland and a tendency to general lymphoid hyperplasia. One author waxed expansive and stated that the skin of patients with this condition "is extremely fine and smooth and they have beautiful pink complexions." Attacks of cyanosis, unconsciousness, convulsions, and sudden death were also features of the alleged disorder. Treatment with x ray or thymectomy was recommended for those who did not die suddenly. Walter Timme, the contributor of the chapter on Diseases of the Thymus Gland in Cecil's first edition, stated that as a result of his efforts to recognize this condition during life, "It is now established that most of these patients do not die."[4] According to this author, the disease was caused by what he called, with a certain degree of hubris, Timme's multiglandular syndrome or the thymus-suprarenal-pituitary syndrome, or status hypoplasticus. A rather variegated list of symptoms, physical findings, and chemical alterations were described, all of which were quite vague. The author concluded his description of the patients by saying severely: "In respect to behavior, they remain children. They follow the path of least resistance, shirk responsibility and lack the ability to concentrate. Consequently, they are apt to feel inadequate and inferior." Of the treatment, he advised, the less said the better, but sodium iodide (2 to 5 gr. daily) was only one of a variety of remedies. X-ray treatment was also recommended for the cure of the enlarged thymus. This treatment of the thymus in infancy probably contributed to the late development of cancer of the thyroid in some patients.

Timme's multiglandular syndrome was short-lived. Status thymicolymphaticus survived for many years but is now dead. It is of interest that the cause of sudden death in infants is still mysterious and the search continues.

Thymic asthma was a related disorder. A large thymus which supposedly produced symptoms of pressure in the upper mediastinum accompanied by dyspnea was thought to be the cause. Prompt treatment with x ray and, in some cases, thymectomy were said to cure the condition. This disease too has disappeared into oblivion.

Yet another imaginary disorder was Pende's syndrome, or hyperfunction of the thymus. It was described in 1928 as a congenital condition resulting in adiposity, genital dystrophy, and retarded mental and somatic development. This disease has disappeared utterly, a victim to medical progress and greater understanding of the thymus. An equally bizarre disorder described by Timme and memorialized briefly in Cecil's celebrated first edition was something he called pineal myopathy. The syndrome was characterized by progressive muscular weakness with or without atrophy, by mental precocity, and by the presence of a pineal shadow in x rays of the skull. Timme reported four cases of this type, all of which had apparently been cured by ingestion of pineal substance (dried gland, gr. 1/5, three times a day), and other glandular medication—the nature of which, alas, was not specified. In several other instances the progress of the disease was arrested and remained stationary for several years as a result of treatment, but by far the greatest number of patients (about 34) continued to fail although, he added, perhaps more slowly. For this no solemn requiem need be held. It is enough to say that it was a nondisease which has passed from the medical scene. Probably René Descartes' notion that the pineal gland was the seat of the soul had as much to recommend it.

Sic Transit . . . .

As anyone who has interviewed applicants for internship knows, the name of William Osler has lost a good deal of its magic and its meaning. The very name of this charismatic physician evokes blank expressions from many young physicians despite his numerous contributions. William Osler said so many things that were right and wise that we can only marvel when we come upon his description of catarrhal jaundice. According to Osler, who followed the description of the European pathologists, catarrhal jaundice was due to swelling and obstruction of the terminal portion of the common duct. It was thought to be an extension of a gastroduodenal catarrh, and the process was believed to be most intense in the pars intestinalis of the duct which projects into the duodenum. "The mucus membrane is swollen, and a plug of inspissated mucus fills the diverticulum of Vater and the narrower portion just at the orifice, completely obstructing the flow of the bile." This was an accepted doctrine until about a generation ago. How strange all this seems now when, with the wisdom of hindsight, we realize that most of the cases of catarrhal jaundice were cases of infectious hepatitis. Osler's treatment was homely but had the virtue of being addressed to the presumed condition.

He recommended that "the patient should drink freely of the alkaline mineral waters of which Vichy is the best. Irrigation of the large bowel with cold water may be practised." The cold was supposed to excite peristalsis of the gall bladder and ducts and thus aid in the expulsion of the mucus. Osler adds with a certain diffidence and his usual insight: "This practise has been followed in my wards for several years, but I cannot speak warmly of the results." Many years later another authoritative source stated with greater assurance than wisdom, "Catarrhal jaundice is never fatal."[4] Recently I was surprised to hear acute infectious hepatitis referred to as "cat fever" by a physician no more venerable than myself. This, of course, is not to be confused with cat-scratch fever.

Ptosis and Ptomaines

A disease with a long and questionable history is visceroptosis. It has finally been tenderly laid to rest. This malady included the various subdivisions, such as gastro-, colo-, hepato-, and nephroptosis. As late as 1927 three pages were devoted to this disorder in Cecil's first edition. It was suggested that visceroptosis should be suspected when a person with the characteristic habitus and a neurasthenic cast of mind complains of a variety of abdominal symptoms. The author seemed suspicious of the condition, did considerable hedging, and obviously was approaching the modern view.

The neuralgias were once ubiquitous. They have largely disappeared and at present only trigeminal neuralgia seems to retain any status. Most of the other neuralgias have become quite disreputable. It is somewhat startling to learn that acupuncture, which we associate with the Orient and Europe, was recommended in this country as a treatment for neuralgia. Aquapuncture, the injection of distilled water under the skin, was also recommended.[3] This latter form of treatment, I understand, still has a vogue in this country for the treatment of a variety of psychosomatic ills by "injection specialists."

Essential gastrorrhagia at one time was a perfectly respectable diagnosis. This form of gastric hemorrhage was said to be much more common in women than in men and was believed to represent vicarious menstruation. It was also alleged that in certain cases it followed "some derangement of the general visceral nervous systems with disturbance of the regulating influence of the neighboring organs upon the general circulation." If this sounds suspiciously like verbigeration to anyone, let him not be too top-lofty. Today's words of pregnant wisdom are tomorrow's gobbledygook.

Ptomaine poisoning had a long and dishonorable history before it was exposed as a fraud. Ptomaines and their close relations, the leucomaines, were considered to be highly poisonous putrefactive alkaloids resulting from the bacterial decomposition of protein foods. It has become quite clear that most forms of food poisoning are due to bacterial or viral infections. The remainder are due to chemical contamination. This has been demonstrated so conclusively that the term ptomaine has disappeared from the medical lexicon although it is still used widely by the laity.

Athlete's Heart

Athlete's heart is a concept that has changed materially since the turn of the century. Osler originally thought that it was a form of aortic incompetence. He alleged that aortic incompetence was found so often in "strong, able-bodied men among the working classes," without any history of rheumatism or special febrile diseases with which endocarditis is commonly associated that other conditions must be sought to explain its frequency. Of these, unquestionably, strain is the most important, he thought—not a sudden, forcible strain, but a persistent increase of the normal tension to which the segments are subject during diastole of the ventricle. This increase in tension was due primarily to heavy and excessive use of the muscles. So often is this form of heart disease found in persons devoted to athletics, he declared, that it is sometimes called "athlete's heart." Alcohol was considered a second important factor, and was stated to raise considerably the tension in the aortic system. A combination of these two causes is extremely common, he thought. This concept of the cause of athlete's heart and aortic incompetence was abandoned gradually. However, the idea that cardiac hypertrophy was due to continued exertion and resulted in "athletic heart" persisted for many years but is now forgotten. By 1927 Cary Eggleston, writing in Cecil's first edition, stated that the prolonged, excessive physical exertion required of professional athletes and certain classes of laborers has been thought to cause hypertrophy and chronic myocardial damage. Studies by Gordon, Levine, and Wilmaers* on a series of marathon runners failed, however, to reveal cardiac enlargement, even in men who had engaged in the most vigorous physical effort for many years. Eggleston stated that it seems probable that physical exertion alone does not cause myocardial damage in the absence of infection, vascular changes, or other disease. That effectively ended the illusory concept of "athletic heart." It became a nondisease and has disappeared from the medical scene.

The possibility that aortic insufficiency may result from a ruptured cusp following sudden, violent exertion, is still valid however. Severe physical strain may result in rupture of a valve or of chordae tendinae or, rarely, of a right or left papillary muscle. These may affect not only valves diseased by rheumatic, syphilitic, or atherosclerotic disease but also normal valves.

Myocarditis

In the early part of this century chronic myocarditis was a popular diagnosis which comprised a mixed bag including most cardiac diseases which were not clearly valvular. With advances in our knowledge and the increasing use of the electrocardiograph, it became apparent that many cases of coronary arteriosclerotic heart disease had been included in the term chronic myocarditis. Soon the latter term became an invidious one, and coronary heart disease was applied to most adult patients with nonvalvular heart disease. As our knowledge has progressed, we have begun to recognize a number of different types of primary myocardial disease or cardiomyopathies. Fiedler's myocarditis, which has had a long and respected history, was originally described as an acute, isolated myocarditis. It is a rare condition which has a sudden onset with chills, fever, and precordial pain. It is accompanied by dyspnea, tachycardia, cardiac dilation, and other manifestations of heart failure.

*Cited by Cecil, R. L. and Kennedy, F., eds. *A Textbook on Medicine,* 1st. ed. Philadelphia and London, Saunders, 1927, p. 1015.

Careful study of the original case description suggests that Fiedler's myocarditis, too, represented a heterogeneous group rather than a distinct entity. Reluctantly we must part with this convenient pigeonhole and include Fiedler's with the cardiomyopathies of unknown origin, although some would designate it as acute, idiopathic myocarditis.

Presbycardia or the Senile Heart

Does age alone cause failure of the heart? Does presbycardia or senile heart disease exist? Both William Dock and Tinsley Harrison have been proponents of the concept. It has been alleged that there are occasional instances of heart failure in the elderly, carefully observed during life and at autopsy in which coronary disease, hypertension, valvular disease, anemia, thyrotoxicosis, etc., have been excluded and histologic examination reveals no structural myocardial disease. It is stated that these represent myocardial failure caused by senile heart disease alone.[7] Clinical findings, however, are not sufficiently distinctive to delineate a syndrome or justify a name. Moreover, with so many old people, it is surprising that more old hearts or patients with presbycardia should not be found. Presbycardia remains a possibility but primary myocardiopathy of undetermined origin would seem to be a more accurate designation.

Chacun a Son Gout

At one time saturnine gout was commonly diagnosed, especially in England. This is lead gout or gout caused by an association with lead poisoning. Sir Alfred B. Garrod believed that workers with lead were especially prone to gout. In 30% of his hospital cases the patients had been painters or lead workers. In this country saturnine gout has been a great (and questionable) rarity and has been forgotten in the text books. It apparently was defunct or obsolete. Recently, however, a case report appeared entitled Saturnine Gout that represents a revival of the entity.[8] The authors believe that saturnine gout is a secondary form of gout probably associated with chronic lead nephropathy, and they suggest a causal relation. Talbot, on the other hand, declares that the widespread use of this heavy metal and the low incidence of gout among exposed workers suggests no causal relation.[9] However, in 1969 Ball and Sorensen described 37 cases of saturnine gout secondary to prolonged consumption of moonshine whiskey contaminated with lead. They performed studies of renal function that show that lead nephropathy produces a severe depression of uric-acid clearance resulting in hyperuricemia. Thus lead acts by specifically inhibiting the tubular secretion of uric acid causing a secondary form of gout.[24] In an accompanying editorial comment, Klinenberg calls saturnine gout a moonshine malady.[25] From having been at death's door, the disease may be considered revived and more clearly defined.

Another rheumatic disorder, palindromic rheumatism, created a great stir when it was first described by Hench and Rosenberg in 1941.[10] It owed some of its popularity to the titillating name which falls trippingly from the tongue and has the piquancy of obscurity. Palindromic is simply the Greek for "returning" or "recurrent." The disorder is characterized by multiple febrile attacks of acute arthritis and periarthritis with pain, swelling, redness, and the disability of one or more joints. Attacks are sudden in onset and disappear rapidly in a few hours or days. The joints of the fingers are sites of predilection. There is little or no constitutional reaction. Each attack is usually followed by a complete remission with no residual disability. Laboratory tests are normal and roentgen examination is unrevealing. Salicylates are not helpful but treatment with gold has been useful in some patients. After the initial flurry of excitement created by the original report, palindromic rheumatism continued to be relatively viable but relegated to obscurity until 1966, when Mattingly published a report of 20 patients with typical palindromic rheumatism studied during a 10-year period from 1955 to 1965.[11] He found more than half the patients developed signs and symptoms of a low-grade polyarthritis with erosive changes in the joints. Of the 10 patients without radiological changes, four had a rheumatoid factor and two others had transient subcutaneous nodules. Chrysotherapy appeared to suppress the acute attack but toxic side effects were common and relapses frequent. Palindromic rheumatism, Mattingly concluded, is probably an episodic, prodromal, or atypical form of rheumatoid arthritis. Some patients never develop permanent joint damage and the prognosis is generally better for these patients than for those with classical rheumatoid arthritis. With this report certain misgivings previously entertained by others were awakened, and the disease has sustained a rapid decline. It exists as a rare and obscure variant but has lost its independence. While it has not disappeared, it has subsided into relative obscurity. Palindromic rheumatism is probably one of the uncommon variants of rheumatoid arthritis although its relation to the latter condition is still controversial.

TAO: The Smoking Sickness

Thromboangiitis obliterans was first described as an entity in 1908 by Leo Buerger. For 50 years it held a secure and unchallenged place in our lexicon of diseases. Since then it has entered into a serious decline. TAO, as everyone knows, is an obliterative vascular disease affecting men between 20 and 45 years of age. Most of those affected are Jews and almost all are smokers. The blood vessels of the extremities are primarily involved although those of the heart, mesentery, kidney, and brain are sometimes affected as well. The disease produces a panphlebitis resulting in obstruction and the development of a collateral circulation. Intermittent claudication and superficial migratory phlebitis are characteristic features. Severe pain occurs at rest from ischemic neuritis or ulceration. Calcification of the vessels is not seen on x-ray examination.

After a long period of full acceptance some preliminary misgivings began to be voiced. In 1960 a full-scale assault on TAO was launched by Weissler et al. under the title, "A Critical Evaluation of Thromboangiitis Obliterans. The Case Against Buerger's Disease."[12] These investigators pointed out that in the 1950's no patients were seen at the Beth Israel Hospital in Boston in whom a diagnosis of Buerger's disease could be made with certainty. They examined the clinical records of all patients with peripheral arterial occlusive disease admitted to the hospital from 1928 to 1956. Pathological examination was done of all amputated limbs, and superficial vein biopsies and autopsy material were obtained from patients with onset of arterial insufficiency before the age of 45. Analysis by age and sex was done of an unselected series of hearts studied by a special injection and dissection technique from 1936 to 1945, and a series of leg amputations was examined by a special injection and dissection technique from 1949 to 1957. A group of unselected venous biopsies was also studied. Finally, examination of a small special group of private outpatients with peripheral arterial or venous disease was done. The investigators concluded that the disease originally described by Buerger is indistinguishable from atherosclerosis, systemic embolization, or peripheral thrombosis singly or in combination. They state that the assumption that a specific arterial disease in association with a specific clinical syndrome exists when arterial obstruction is present in patients with the type of phlebitic reaction described by Buerger goes far beyond the available facts. Under these circumstances they assert with finality "thromboangiitis obliterans cannot be considered an entity in either the clinical or pathologic sense and we therefore recommend that the term be discarded." A rather acrimonious debate promptly ensued. McKusick et al. made a study of cases in the Orient and did arteriographic and histopathologic studies of cases in Baltimore.[13] They found that Buerger's disease of classic type occurs relatively frequently in Korea and Japan despite the rarity of atherosclerosis and of thromboembolic disease. The arteriographic findings in Buerger's disease, particularly the involvement of the arteries of the upper extremities and the focal changes, they believe, are distinctive. They also are of the opinion that characteristic histopathologic changes are demonstrable and declare that Buerger's disease is a distinct clinical and pathologic entity. While this controversy has been raging the disease seems to be quietly disappearing for reasons unknown. Wilkins recently declared that the number of patients with TAO has decreased remarkably in the past few decades. "Whether this is secondary to a decrease in an etiologic infectious agent, such as rickettsiae or fungi or to the fact that the disease is not a separate entity cannot be definitely decided at present,"[14] and Stead affirms that there is little doubt that most of the patients diagnosed in the past as having thromboangiitis obliterans had atherosclerosis.[7] It is evident that the lifeblood of this disease is ebbing. However, we are loath to part with it and view its approaching demise with a certain tempered regret. TAO was an excellent object lesson for many years on the evil of smoking. Of course it is true that bronchogenic carcinoma of the lung is an even more potent and convincing brief against tobacco.

Debate on Hemochromatosis

The traditional view that idiopathic hemochromatosis is an hereditary disease has had a determined assault made upon it by Richard A. MacDonald. Not true, says MacDonald, who quotes the formidable Virchow in behalf of his thesis as follows: "If one surveys the almost immeasurable number of diseases which have been held to be hereditary, it soon becomes obvious that the habit of doctors of recognizing the hereditary character of certain diseases has changed almost according to fashion. An inclination in this direction has always existed, as the assumption of heredity protects against any further mental efforts concerning the cause of the condition." This represents a determined onslaught bolstered by a sacred cow but hardly calculated to win friends. What is MacDonald's argument? It is that *hereditary* hemochromatosis is a nondisease. Hemochromatosis is an acquired disease which is not a single entity with a single cause and course of development but a condition produced by the coexistence of two factors, one of excess iron and a second of nutritional, especially folic-acid deficiency, usually associated with the development of cirrhosis. The cirrhosis is not related to the iron accumulation. The latter is a result of increased ingestion or parenteral administration. Chronic alcoholics are susceptible to the development of hemochromatosis because they often suffer from malnutrition and develop cirrhosis due to the alcohol. They may ingest wine or other forms of alcohol that contain iron. Transfusion hemochromatosis is a result of excess iron administered in blood or as iron. The cirrhosis develops for reasons unknown. Possible causes for the cirrhosis are malnutrition, alcoholism, hepatitis (viral), biliary obstruction, and chronic vascular congestion. Pancreatic damage, dietary alterations, and hematologic diseases, all of which are especially common in chronic alcoholics, may affect absorption of iron. In answer to the objection that hemochromatosis occurs in nonalcoholics too, MacDonald says that nonalcoholics may have the same factors in their environment, especially iron intake in medications, and folic-acid deficiency. He does not believe that a satisfactory familial occurrence has been demonstrated.

Resisting valiantly in defense of the hereditary concept of hemochromatosis, William H. Crosby dismisses malnutrition as a cause. He cites evidence that most patients with the disease are not malnourished. He rejects alcoholism because abuse of alcohol is common while hemochromatosis is rare. Also in some series as many as 50% of patients are total abstainers. He concedes that alcohol may be contributory but not a primary cause in the pathogenesis of the disease, and states that abuse of alcohol may accelerate the accumulation of iron by further impairment of a genetically disordered mechanism for control of iron balance. Thus with alcoholism a compensated case of hereditary hemochromatosis might decompensate. Similarly he suggests that an excess of dietary iron may provide critical stress on an abnormal system. Crosby lumps the MacDonald thesis with the now discredited but not forgotten argument of Mallory, who related hemochromatosis to copper ingested with contaminated whiskey. Both iron-contaminated wine and copper-contaminated whiskey are necessary in excessively large amounts to have epidemiologic credibility. Crosby makes due reference to the fact that Mallory was indiscreet enough to include Cooley's anemia with copper-induced iron-loading diseases, and to suggest that Cooley's anemia is hemochromatosis in the child. He then brings *his* big gun into play by quoting the great George H. Whipple, who commented as follows: "We do not propose to join in the debate relative to copper as the cause of liver cirrhosis and hemochromatosis, but we do feel that these cases of thalassemia give no support to this thesis and actually exclude copper as a cause of this particular pigmentary abnormality. If copper is the cause of the pigmentation of the viscera, then it is also the cause of the bone abnormalities and the peculiar anemia with splenomegaly, as these conditions always develop together in the same child. Also copper must injure the Mediterranean people and trail families like a bloodhound." Decisively and even loftily, Whipple then delivers the coup de grace from on high by adding, "It does not seem necessary to pursue the argument."

If Crosby's inclusion of the mighty Whipple's Olympian thunderbolt seems perilously close to annihilation by analogy, you are invited to make the most of it. Chalmers acts as referee in the debate remarking on the complete divergence of views of the two protagonists. He then implies cautiously that both may be right and suggests judiciously that further evidence is needed.[15] This resolution recalls the story of bickering disputants who went to see a wise man to settle their argument. "Oh, wise man," said the first, "I know whereof I speak, assuredly the earth is round as a ball." The sage pondered and replied, "You are right." The second man then said, "On the contrary, this I know beyond dispute—the earth is flat as a pancake." The wise man thought deeply and then delivered his dictum, "Ah, you are right." Another who had hung on the words of the learned man then exclaimed, "Oh wise one, surely both cannot be right." "My friend," replied the sage, "You too, are right."

Has hereditary hemochromatosis been dealt a mortal blow? No, but it can hardly be said to be alive and well and living in tranquility. As between the venerable Virchow and the formidable Whipple, I hope I may be permitted, without being accused of chauvinism, to side with Whipple, who is alive and well, and living in Rochester, I am glad to say.

The Case of Histiocytosis X

The constant war between the lumpers and the splitters is neatly illustrated by the strange case of histiocytosis X. Back in the halcyon days of the 1930's, certain bone diseases of the histiocytic or reticulo-endothelial system had been grouped as metabolic disorders. These were the lipidoses or lipoid histiocytoses including Gaucher's disease, Niemann-Pick's disease, and Hand-Schüller-Christian's disease. Early in the 1940's W. T. Green and S. Farber, Henry L. Jaffe and Louis Lichtenstein, S. Otani and Ehrlich, and others described eosinophilic granuloma of bone whose pathologic features closely resembled those of Schüller-Christian's disease. It was also shown that Letterer-Siwe's disease (variously termed aleukemic reticulosis, nonlipoid histiocytosis, and reticuloendotheliosis) bore a strong resembance to both Schüller-Christian's disease and eosinophilic granuloma. These three conditions are nonfamilial and show no racial predilection. Histologically, Schüller-Christian's disease, Letterer-Siwe's disease, and eosinophilic granuloma are inflammatory granulomata. The essential lipoid histiocytoses, Gaucher's and Niemann-Pick's diseases, are inherited metabolic disorders and storage diseases. It seemed important to differentiate or split these from the inflammatory, nonfamilial histiocytic diseases. These three entities, it had been suggested, are closely related. The pathologic processes are similar and the clinical manifestations show a considerable degree of overlapping. In a paper published in 1948 entitled *Metabolic and Inflammatory Histiocytosis* I concluded that Hand-Schüller-Christian's disease, Letterer-Siwe's disease, and eosinophilic granuloma of bone represent clinical syndromes that are variations of the same basic disorder which might collectively be lumped and termed inflammatory histiocytosis. The familial lipidoses including Gaucher's and Niemann-Pick's I separated from the former and called metabolic histiocytosis.[16] I had become a splitter *and* a lumper!

The term inflammatory histiocytosis was not a particularly good one etymologically, although it was the best I could do at the time.

It never attracted much favor and it died quietly. In 1953 Lichtenstein, who had done some of the original work in this area with Henry L. Jaffé, hit upon the name histiocytosis X, because the etiologic agent was unknown. Under this designation he integrated eosinophilic granuloma of bone, Letterer-Siwe's disease, and Schüller-Christian's disease as related manifestations of a single nosological entity.[17] This name soon became popular and gained wide acceptance. It seemed that the lumpers had won the day. But not for long. After a period of about 16 years during which histiocytosis X held almost undisputed sway the splitters returned to the fray. In 1969 Lieberman et al. analyzed 82 cases and concluded that there was no justification for the current theory that eosinophilic granuloma of bone, Hand-Schüller-Christian's disease, and Letterer-Siwe's disease represent component parts of a single nosologic entity. They believe that the term histiocytosis X is unnecessary and may lead to therapeutic errors.[18] The basis for their conclusions is too detailed and involved to go into in this discussion but the assault is serious and the prognosis for the disease must be guarded. Must we bid histiocytosis X a fond farewell? We await with eagerness the next chapter in the mystery of this malady.

Jod-Basedow

As all good Germans know, Basedow's disease is exophthalmic goiter or vice versa. Some unpleasant sticklers for accuracy and minutiae may point out that Robert J. Graves preceded Basedow and that Caleb H. Parry preceded Graves. But no matter—what is Jod-Basedow? It is iodine-induced hyperthyroidism, and it occurred as a complication when iodine was given for endemic goiter. I use the past tense because such hyperthyroidism no longer occurs. Some experts even question whether it ever did happen. The evidence, however, is good that patients and animals, including dogs and rabbits, with goiters, will develop hyperthyroidism if given enough iodine. This was well known at the end of the last century and many experienced clinicians observed the relation. Why has this disease became defunct? One explanation which comes to mind is that this condition was an early iatrogenic disease. Iodide in the form of potassium iodide was a very popular remedy at one time and was given frequently for a variety of ills—sometimes in large amounts. It is possible that iodide stimulates excessive formation of thyroid hormone by nodules or paranodular tissue of goiters which have become autonomous. Iodides have lost their popularity and hence Jod-Basedow has become defunct as a complication of our therapy. However, in 1954 Stanbury et al. reported that they had administered 1,500 μgm. of iodine to each of three human beings with goiters associated with iodine deficiency. In one patient lasting hyperthyroidism developed. In two it did not.[19] Therefore, iodine reduces the hyperplasia and excessive vascularity and function of the thyroid in hyperthyroidism and stimulates the activity of the thyroid in endemic goiter. Iodine is a cause and a cure, although the latter is temporary.

Planned Obsolescence

I shall not dwell on familiar diseases which are in a state of decline as a result of medical discoveries. But surely mention at least should be made of typhoid fever, which is now so rarely seen in the United States. Twenty-seven pages were devoted to this disease in Cecil's first edition and only three and one-half in the last. Most young physicians have never seen a case. Galloping consumption or tuberculous pneumonia has almost vanished. It certainly rarely gallops. Poliomyelitis has become a rarity. Whooping cough and diphtheria are no longer threats in this part of the world. Mastoiditis is almost a thing of the past. Undulant fever is most unusual in this country, although it is common in Mexico and some other countries. There are other such diseases. To these and many others we bid a glad farewell.

A serious iatrogenic disease was retrolental fibroplasia. This cause of blindness has been almost eliminated since it was discovered that a high content of oxygen in the incubators of premature infants was the cause. In another area is a problem which has not yet been entirely resolved. Otomycosis has been a controversial disorder for some years. Recently it was alleged to be a myth, only to be revived two years later and declared to be a genuine entity.[20, 21]

Finally, there are several diseases whose present reality is indisputable but which have disappearing features. Disappearing bone disease is a strange disease of the skeleton of unknown origin in which the bones seem to melt away. The vanishing diabetes mellitus syndrome of Houssay follows the development of pituitary insufficiency as a result of destruction of the gland by tumor or necrosis. Remission of diabetes mellitus results and insulin is no longer required. Hypoglycemic cerebral manifestations appear; they vary from semistupor to coma with absence of classical signs of hypopituitarism. Recently spontaneous disappearance of diabetes mellitus was reported in a patient who had symptoms suggesting a collagen disease. The diabetes had been insulin-resistant for 10 months. This is the second reported case of spontaneous disappearance of insulin-dependent diabetes.[22] In this group are cases of leukemia in which the leukemia has disappeared following the development of tuberculosis.[23]

L'Envoi

We do not mourn the diseases of yesteryear. We bid them good riddance and God-speed. But there will be no dearth of diseases. We exchange new ones for old. Almost as fast as one disease is conquered new ones are discovered and sometimes created. The balance is clearly on the credits side, and it is a fact that many of the old scourges, real or imaginary, are gone or are vanishing.

Acknowledgment

I thank Drs. Magdalena R. Berenyi and Joseph B. Rogoff for helpful suggestions.

REFERENCES

1. Fowler, W. M.: Chlorosis—An obituary. *Ann. Med. Hist. 8*:168, 1936.
2. Wintrobe, M. M.: *Clinical Hematology,* 6th ed. Philadelphia, Lea & Febiger, 1967.
3. Osler, W.: *The Principles and Practice of Medicine,* 1st ed. New York, Appleton, 1892.
4. Cecil, R. L.: *A Textbook of Medicine,* 1st ed. Philadelphia, Saunders, 1927.
5. Christian, H. A.: *Principles and Practice of Medicine,* 16th ed. New York, Appleton-Century, 1947.
6. Scarlett, E. P.: The vapors. *Arch. Intern. Med. 116*:142, 1965.
7. Harrison, T. R. et al., eds.: *Principles of Medicine,* 5th ed. New York, McGraw-Hill, 1966.
8. Ehrlich, G. E. and Chokatos, J.: Saturnine gout. *Arch. Intern. Med. 118*:572, 1966.
9. Talbot, J. H.: *Gout,* 2d ed. New York, Grune & Stratton, 1964.
10. Hench, P. S. and Rosenberg, E. F.: Palindromic rheumatism. *Proc. Mayo Clinic 16*:808, 1941.
11. Mattingly, S.: Palindromic rheumatism. *Ann. Rheum. Dis. 25*:307, 1966.
12. Wessler, S., Ming, S-C., Gurewich, V. and Freiman, D. G.: A critical evaluation of thromboangiitis obliterans. *New Eng. J. Med. 262*:1149, 1960.
13. McKusick, V. A.: Buerger's disease: A distinct clinical and pathologic entity. *J.A.M.A. 181*:93, 1962.
14. Beeson, P. B. and McDermott, W.: *Textbook of Medicine,* 12th ed. Philadelphia, Saunders, 1967.
15. Ingelfinger, F. S., Relman, A. S. and Finland, M.: *Controversy in Internal Medicine.* Philadelphia, Saunders, 1966.
16. Straus, B. Metabolic and inflammatory histiocytosis. *Amer. J. Med. 5*:245, 1948.

17. Lichtenstein, L.: Integration of eosinophilic granuloma of bone, "Letterer-Siwe Disease," and "Schuller-Christian Disease" as related manifestations of a single nosologic entity. *Arch. Path. 56*:84, 1953.
18. Lieberman, P. H., Jones, C. R., Dargeon, H. W. K. and Begg, C. F.: A reappraisal of eosinophilic granuloma of bone, Hand-Schuller-Christian syndrome and Letterer-Siwe syndrome. *Medicine 48*:375, 1969.
19. Stanbury, J. B. et al.: *Endemic Goiter.* Cambridge, Mass., Harvard Univ. Press, 1954.
20. Kingery, F. A. J.: The myth of otomycosis. *J.A.M.A. 191*:129, 1965.
21. McGonigle, J. J. and Jillson, O. T. Otomycosis: An entity. *Arch. Derm. 95*: 45, 1967.
22. Bruce, D. H., Bernard, W. and Blackard, W. G.: Spontaneous disappearance of insulin-resistant diabetes-mellitus in a patient with a collagen disease. *Amer. J. Med. 48*:268, 1970.
23. Heinle, R. W. and Weir, D. R. Morphologic obliteration of chronic myeloid leukemia by active tuberculosis. *Amer. J. Med. Sc. 207*:450, 1944.
24. Ball, G. V. and Sorensen, L. B.: Pathogenesis of hyperuricemia in saturnine gout. *New Eng. J. Med. 280*:1199, 1969.
25. Ibid. Klinenberg, J. R.: Editorial. Saturnine gout: A moonshine malady, p. 1238.

THE RELEVANCE OF THE KAISER-PERMANENTE EXPERIENCE TO THE HEALTH SERVICES OF THE EASTERN UNITED STATES*

Ernest W. Saward

Medical Director
The Permanente Clinic
Portland, Ore.

In preparing this discussion I wondered how widespread the concept might be that our manner of organizing medical care should be considered a local or regional phenomenon. The wide-ranging discussion about the availability and accessibility of contemporary medical care and its high costs seems to be topical not only throughout the United States, but in all Western industrialized countries.

I propose to divide this presentation into five parts. I shall give, first, a brief description of the Kaiser-Permanente organization, although I know you are all fairly familiar with it; second, a discussion of some of the trends that seem to prevail in medical care; third, a description of how the Kaiser-Permanente system relates to these trends and with what results; fourth, a brief examination of what differences there may be between the urban East and the urban West; and, last, some brief comments on why prepaid group practice of the Kaiser-Permanente type has not spread rapidly into the urban East and elsewhere.

It seems redundant to describe the Kaiser-Permanente system to this audience. However when I have not done so in the past questions have reflected the lack of base-line information. Our system evolved from the premises that Dr. Sidney Garfield put into practice in the 1930's. Kaiser-Permanente has a particular dynamism that we believe relates to the *manner* of organization and not to the place or to the person. In the past I have stated that we have a "genetic code"; by this I have meant a set of linkages of the organizations that make up the Kaiser-Permanente system which, if significantly altered, result in a nonviable or sick program. I used this term originally about the time

*Presented at a meeting of the Subcommittee on Social Policy for Health Care of the Committee on Medicine in Society, February 26, 1970.

James D. Watson and Francis H. C. Crick received their Nobel Prize for demonstrating the structure of DNA and its influence on the building of cells, and the words were on my mind for that reason. It has led to much discussion since (and, I must say, to much derision) about the existence of any such thing as a genetic code for the organization of successful prepaid group practice. It certainly was not intended to imply that a genetic code allows for no variation, for indeed there are three billion viable extant examples of the human genetic code.

The Kaiser-Permanente plan has significant variations in each region and, whenever representatives from these regions gather, the variations are emphasized, but the similarities are overwhelmingly dominant. A number of new programs have been started in the last few years, often at eminent institutions of learning, some of which have paid close attention to the manner of interorganizational relations, and we are observing the results with great interest.

To begin with, the program must be sponsored by a nonprofit organization. In the last few months we have seen what amounts to a prospectus of a stock offering presented by entrepreneurs interested in conducting such an organization on a profit-making basis. Although our culture is changing rapidly I believe that ethical considerations should discourage any such idea.

Another fundamental premise is that the organization should be self-sustaining. Grants may be necessary to get such a program started; but they should be capable of amortization once the program is operating successfully. Membership payments for certain groups may have to come from taxes, but this in no way impairs the concept of the *program* as self-sustaining. The other side of the coin is that the program should not be called upon to effect large charitable benefits. The members who together are paying the costs of the program should not be taxed involuntarily for this purpose any more than the rest of the population.

Since the basic principles of the program are well known and oft-repeated, I shall describe them only briefly.

The first principle is the prepayment of monthly dues to mutualize the cost of medical care. The program is community-rated. There are many ways to have dues paid; Medicare, Medicaid, and Office of Economic Opportunity (OEO) groups have been adapted to the Kaiser-Permanente program with varying degrees of difficulty; that is, difficulty for the administrators, not for the members. The coverage and the services provided must be comprehensive.

The second principle, group practice, means to us independent and autonomous medical groups which make contracts with the Kaiser Health Plan. All income is pooled. Members of the groups are full-time specialists, and they all practice in the group facilities.

The third principle is that of having medical-center facilities: a hospital and ambulatory clinical center where all services are available and are coordinated with neighborhood primary-care clinics situated in peripheral areas. All facilities use a single medical record, and all administrative services are unified. Today this is called "regional planning"; 25 years ago it was called integration and convenience of services for the members.

The fourth principle is voluntary enrollment. Since every individual must choose the program, obviously there must be an alternate choice; if there is not, we do not offer our program. There are no 100% groups. Neither employer nor union may choose the plan for all members, and there must be a periodic exercise of choice.

The fifth principle is capitation payment. The medical group is paid an annual capitation, as are the hospitals that serve the program. We believe that such budgetary systems lead to different motivation in the providers than fee-for-service or reimbursement of costs. When broadly comprehensive services are arranged and equal coverage of all types of services is provided, and when physicians have fiscal responsibility for services, a different pattern of use prevails.

This, then, is a thumbnail sketch of the concepts underlying the Kaiser-Permanente program.

A number of trends occur in medical care that greatly affect the expectations and attitudes of the public. This is, of course, but part of a pattern of changes that have been brought about by science and technology, by greater degrees of education both formal and informal, by more effective informational media, and also by the vastly greater affluence of most members of society, despite the sharp contrasts in income that still exist. The belief that medical care has a great deal to offer underlies its definition as a basic human right. This is the basis of the current and ever-increasing interest of the consumer in participation in the organization of medical care.

At the beginning of this century medical care was sought only in crises. It is still sought largely in an episodic manner but certainly no longer only in crises. More and more, health maintenance is taken seriously. For several decades health educators have advocated the benefit of periodic health examinations. Only a very small fraction of the public responded in the past. Today there is far greater confidence in science and technology; there is greater affluence; and there is health insurance in which larger numbers are participating. An attempt is being made to cope with this huge demand by automated multiphasic testing for its sparing of physicians. However, it is as yet unclear whether, like the sorcerer's apprentice, we have started something without understanding how to control it.

The trend toward expanded technology is clear and need not be elaborated here. The problems of medical manpower—not only as to quantity but also as to new kinds and new uses—have been well publicized because of their great importance. The continued and, I believe, irreversible trend toward specialization among physicians is likewise manifest. There are significant developments in assessing the quality of medical practice, in giving greater access to medical care through regional planning and controlling costs through similar planning, and in bringing the kinds of management skills that first came to our attention in the medical-care field in the U.S. Department of Defense 10 or 15 years ago.

If these are the trends of medical care in the United States, how does the Kaiser-Permanente plan fit them? Insofar as the plan matches these trends it has relevance—not to any special region but to the entire country. Public expectations have been met. It is seen at once that there is a system and an institution organized for the delivery of health services. If the public is to have an effective voice in the kinds of services it receives it must relate to some kind of organized setting, to an institution that will be responsive and in which it may participate in arranging these vital and personal health services.

Each personal physician in the group relates to others in a team function. The patient values his relation with his personal physician and relies on him, as does any patient. However, he understands at once that there is great value in the unit medical record and that all his radiographs and laboratory findings, from whatever specialist, are all recorded in the same chart, whether he has been an ambulatory or a bed patient. The services are available to him 24 hours a day thanks to the team concept. The patient knows that if he requires service in the middle of the night and his personal physician is not at hand the unit medical record will serve as a relevant background by which to judge the new emergency. Here is easy access, comprehensiveness, and continuity. One does not have to search for it; it is there already.

The technical facilities, the equipment, and the specialists who use them can be as great as the demographic base will support. In the group setting the new types of health professionals can be used effectively. There is a proper framework of control and a scale of operations to make their use feasible, as well as a budgetary method of payment that provides economic incentives to integrate every effective health professional into the medical team. The techniques of contemporary management can be readily brought to bear upon the delivery of health services because organization and scale make possible system planning, budgeting, cost-benefit analysis, and the use of a computer. Innovation in systems has great rewards. The cumulative effect of these many savings from better-designed systems reduces the cost of health care. Comprehensive coverage and the organization of comprehensive services ensures that in this framework the appropriate service will be used.

The trend toward audit of the quality of medical care is more readily carried out by the organized group. First, there is the selection of the members of the group. These are departmentalized and under the control of the chiefs of service. A unified medical record is used for all services and the work of any member of the team is constantly visible to colleagues. The system of auditing is essentially the same for outpatients and inpatients.

Public acceptance of this program is perhaps the best test of its relevance. Every subscriber has a voluntary choice and must exercise it annually. Please remember that we are not just insuring these persons—we are providing medical services—and to do this we must create the clinics and hospitals, find the physicians, nurses, and other kinds of health personnel in the right amount, in the right place, and at the right time. In each geographic area where the program exists there has been heavy involvement in the creation of these facilities for medical care and a constant process of planning and replanning the organization of services in response to needs. Therefore, throughout extensive periods of time in each of the different regions, membership in the program has been closed to new groups because facilities could not be built as rapidly as the demand grew. Despite this the program has grown from 30,000 members in early 1946 to half a million in 1955, to a million in 1962, and to 2 million in 1969. Whether we shall be able to double that total again in a few years depends on factors as far removed from the manner of the organization of health services as the money supply and interest rates, for to double the total again would involve a capital investment of over 300 million dollars at current construction costs.

Perhaps equally illustrative of public acceptance and on a scale more readily managed is an analysis of the Federal Employees Health Benefits Program. The government makes a health-insurance contribution for each federal employee, but a significant amount of the health-insurance premium must be deducted from the salary of the employee. The method of enrollment prohibits solicitation. Information on the programs available comes through material prepared and distributed by the personnel office of the government. Because of its comprehensiveness the Kaiser program—though it does save families significant out-of-pocket costs—does not have low premiums. So when the choice is made it is not between a low-premium Kaiser plan and a high-premium plan.

Of the five plans offered federal employees in Portland, where I am most familiar with the program, not only do most employees choose the Kaiser program, but this program is chosen by almost as many as the other four programs combined. Each successive open enrollment has recorded a larger number of persons who have chosen this program. This, we feel, is a significant evaluation. I might also add that the utilization of hospitals by these federal employees in the Portland region follows the national pattern of prepaid group practice that charges a significantly reduced amount of usage. For the most recent year for which we have figures (1968) the utilization rate of nonmaternity hospitals is essentially half that of federal employees enrolled in other programs.

The Federal Employee Health Benefits Act of 1959 may serve as an interesting model for a national health insurance plan. This act provides for standards of comprehensiveness, noncancelability, and review. It involves competitive underwriting and hence is less inflationary. With the periodic choice of competing programs and partial self-payment by payroll deduction there are inherent incentives favoring the most effective program. This "experiment" has been applied to 8 million persons and is well accepted in its 10th year.

I think it worthwhile to reiterate our experience with hospitalization under Medicare Part "A" in Portland. The national rate is approximately 3,600 acute-care general hospital days per 1,000 patients per annum. Those Medicare patients on the Portland program use half this number, less than 1,800 days; and I might add that the figure for those 75 years of age and over is only 2,200 days.

Our experience with the OEO population served by the program in Portland is comparable to utilization in our community-rated program despite an extensive outreach and transportation service. We have found the OEO program well adapted to our community-wide service. The greatest injustice of the current health scene, the inequality of access, is abolished for all enrolled.

Having briefly reviewed the Kaiser-Permanente system, the trends in health services in the United States and how the Kaiser-Permanente system adapts to and fits them and, having noted the results, I come at last to the question of how this system is relevant to the eastern urban areas of the United States. Let me hasten to say that I have no intimate knowledge of these areas although I was born and raised and had all my schooling and residency training here and although my parents have lived here all their lives. I have now only the visitor's view of the many strikes that cause so much public inconvenience and of the performance of the Long Island Railroad. Most of the ingredients for a successful program such as ours seem present in all of the large Eastern cities. Our membership is based on the employed population much as is the income tax and Social Security tax of the federal government. The attitudes and expectations of health care of the Eastern urbanite, as revealed by all the public information media, seem typical of other sectors of the country.

There are, however, some legislative and regulatory difficulties to be overcome in the East. I am no expert on the law, but I understand that in New York State the insurance commissioner does not allow the pooling of funds for hospitalization with funds for medical services, although there is a bill in one of the state legislative committees at the present time intended to correct this narrow view of health financing. In Pennsylvania permission was given to carry out a prepaid group practice program within the past year, but only in a restricted manner. Just a few years ago the Supreme Court of the State of New Jersey struck down the restrictive regulations in the law there. Dr. I. S. Falk and his colleagues fought a vigorous battle a few years ago in the state legislature of Connecticut against a law that empowers only a particular program to function in that state. And only 10 years ago restrictions in the state of Ohio were removed by legislation that permitted the Community Health Foundation program to function in Cleveland.

On the West Coast the legislative background is quite different. The program was already in operation there before special interests had time to think of restrictive legislation.

The Kaiser-Permanente program has withstood the tests of cultural transplantation fairly well. Oregon is very unlike California. It is much like New England but without any similar historical sense of the 17th or 18th centuries. The city of Portland is called "The Old Lady of the Willamette"—not without reason. Many years ago it was said that if the program worked there it will work anywhere. It does indeed work there. Ten years ago there was great doubt that the program could make the transcultural jump to Honolulu with its very different population. It not only did so but is now locally regarded as part of the concept of "aloha." When the program was introduced into Cordoba, Argentina, in 1962, once again the cry arose, "We're different. It won't work here." It did and does work, and exactly to the extent that it follows the genetic code. In 1963 in Cleveland there was the same cry, "We're different." The success of the program there speaks for itself.

Another interesting difference between East and West Coast urban areas is the more comprehensive coverage of ambulatory services generally prevailing in the West; hence the larger fringe-benefit payments to health and welfare trusts for this purpose. Prepaid group practice programs started in certain East Coast cities have encountered difficulty in having the premiums covered by such contributions because of the low local level of comprehensiveness. Kaiser's existence as a competitive factor in the West Coast market for 25 years may have played an etiologic role in this difference.

I have frequently encountered individuals with unrealistic expectations of the program. In Portland we have demonstrated thoroughly over the past three years that an indigent population can be integrated with the dues-paying health-plan membership to produce a true community program. It is highly questionable, however, whether the program can be sustained for a massive indigent population alone.

Physicians are attracted to a career commitment to the program when they see it is a broad community program. They are reluctant to accept any label from people they serve, whether it be an employer, union, poverty group, or any other group. If the membership is broadly representative of the community and has freely chosen the program over realistic alternatives, then physicians will be attracted to it on the basis of the kind of medical care it provides.

If the Eastern urban areas are viewed in this light the Kaiser-Permanente program is applicable. If the experience in Cleveland is regarded as Eastern enough, it validates this impression.

This brings us to the last of my topics: the question of why the Kaiser-Permanente program has not spread rapidly all over the country.

First, let me state the obvious fact that the program has grown in an exponential manner and, at the same time, has had to provide the facilities for its rapidly increasing membership; in doing so it has needed all its talents as well as all the capital and manpower available. The growth on the West Coast has by no means reached a plateau. Therefore, the question my be rephrased, "Why hasn't prepaid group practice spread to the Eastern cities?"

Aside from the legislative and regulatory restrictions previously discussed, there are three cardinal reasons: membership, money, and manpower. The enrollment of a membership base for such a program takes time to create, and this initially is a very slow process. To create the kind of integrated facilities, hospital-based with outlying neighborhood centers and staffed by a broad range of specialists, requires the support of a large membership. A mature system is attractive and has a constant growth in dual choices. But a small initial membership will not support such a program. One needs an enrollment mechanism that overcomes this prolonged period of inadequate membership. The national Blue Cross organization has been quite perceptive about this, and if it is not handicapped by restrictive regulation, as indeed it seems to be, it could cooperate in providing a dual choice within the Blue Cross enrollment. This could rapidly become a significant method of initiating prepaid group practice for the delivery of medical care. Certainly a national health insurance could conceivably be created in a form that would enhance the enrollment process in this kind of system with the previously mentioned Federal Employees Health Benefits Act as a partial prototype. However, I must add that this national insurance plan could not easily be so created if it were written in the form of the Medicare Law;

for the Title 18 regulations, at least in the way they are being administered, take little cognizance of the dynamics of prepaid group practice and its budgetary system of payment.

All the newly started programs are having significant problems with enrollment. Until a better solution is found for this prolonged initial period there will be no epidemic of prepaid group practice.

The other problems are certainly worth noting but less serious. Money is required, capital for the ambulatory facilities that make group practice a practical reality and for initial costs. While it is desirable to have the program control a hospital—and it must be at least hospital-related—it does not require the creation of a new hospital. But for fully integrated functioning, an integrated management and administration of all the medical-care facilities is desirable.

The last difficulty to overcome—the professional manpower shortage—is specifically characteristic of the national problem. We have a highly inflationary sellers' market for physicians' professional services. One must provide balanced comprehensive services in a program of this kind. There are a number of specialties in medicine for which the annual supply seems to bear little relation to demand. The imbalance in the supply of the various medical specialties is a significant handicap to the organization of comprehensive services.

There is one further problem that affects the spread of prepaid group practice in the United States: the sponsorship of such programs. The sponsorship of the Kaiser program was unique, and its eminent success ensures the continuity of a distinguished board of directors. It is essential that the program represent no special interest group in the community. Recently its sponsorship by distinguished universities has been salutary, but it is doubtful that this can be a general pattern. How such programs should be sponsored, and by whom, and with what capabilities seems to be an unresolved dilemma of the consumer movement.

In summary: the Kaiser-Permanente program, an eminent success as demonstrated by its public acceptance in those metropolitan areas where it now exists, seems to be readily applicable to fulfilling the public's expectations in Eastern urban areas. But it must first overcome restrictive legislation and regulatory barriers; it must solve the problem of significant communitywide enrollment to initiate such a program; it must have sources of capital available to create the initial group facilities and to cover starting expenses; it must compete in an inflationary sellers' market for professional manpower; and it must find able, representative, community sponsorship that understands the program and will dedicate itself to this cause. Not only must it do these things, but it must do them all at the same time. The timing of each factor must be precise or money and morale will evaporate. It is possible that answers will be found in the established mechanism of the Blue Cross or in that of some other dominant carrier in a given area. It is also possible that the spread of organized delivery systems of this type awaits universal entitlement through a national health insurance; but here one must see to it that such developments are permitted by the act and not prohibited, as they were, in effect, under Medicare.

ASSURING STABLE AND EFFECTIVE FINANCING OF LOCAL HEALTH SERVICES: THE ROLE OF INTERGOVERNMENTAL GRANTS-IN-AID*

JAMES F. KELLY

Assistant Secretary, Comptroller
Department of Health, Education, and Welfare
Washington, D.C.

I have never relished the idea of speaking to physicians about how to manage the health affairs of the nation. On the other hand, I hope that my participation can make some contribution to the worthwhile effort you people are making in grappling with the social problems in the health field.

I know of no more important subject that faces the nation, and I am firmly convinced that we are in a crisis that is shown in the manifestations of public concern and in the evidences of a lack of public confidence in a system which, not many years ago, we proudly considered the greatest system that had ever been created to take care of health. One wonders what has happened that makes the newspapers, on their front pages, stress the breakdown in health and the inadequacy of the health system.

We are really not dealing with the question of having lost ground; rather, we are dealing with a greater awareness of where we have been, where we are, and where we ought to be. I believe that the shortage of doctors would have been an acute problem even if the Medicare and Medicaid programs had not been enacted.

People are not any less healthy than they were before the enactment of Medicare and Medicaid; people are not any unhappier or unhealthier than they were before the advent of the large expansion of Blue Cross and Blue Shield and other prepayment plans. Rather, there are more people that can compete for limited services, and a much sharper division is drawn. It is much clearer today than it was just a few

*Presented at a meeting of the Subcommittee on Social Policy for Health Care of the Committee on Medicine in Society, March 26, 1970.

years ago that there is a tremendous disparity in the distribution of health services and that the accessibility is just not equitably distributed throughout the nation.

Today we have an alarmed, concerned nation. The nation says the situation is not fair, that it is not right, and that something must be done about it. A whole series of actions were begun to try to do something about the situation, and everything done had a tendency to sharpen the issues, to bring to light and to focus on some of the problems that were inherent in the system but not so apparent.

Certainly, the shortage of manpower has been known for a long time in the health professions, but now it is acutely felt by the general population. The disparity in the distribution of health services also has long been known to the health professions. All sorts of efforts have been made to try to resolve the problem. The expansion of the emergency rooms in hospitals to handle outpatients and the heavy dependence upon the foreign graduates of medical schools in coping with problems in the center cities are evidences of attempts to deal with this problem. When resources were made available through Medicare and Medicaid, it became very clear that those who were poor, irrespective of resources made available to them, did not have access to the same level and quantity of medical care.

The federal government has made a series of strides in trying to remedy the situation. Sometimes it looks as if we have ridden off in all directions at the same time. How are we going to stabilize this activity? How are we going to bring it into a more rational and stable arrangement than has existed in prior years?

Until about 10 years ago the health system of our nation was built upon a relatively clear distinction between public health and private health. Public health dealt with problems then called sanitation and now called environmental: problems of communicable disease areas that were a threat to a large segment of society.

As health scientists had successes in these fields and conquered them, they moved into other areas of unmet needs. I think that the development of our American medical research capability is one of the great monuments to governmental achievement. We recognized the need to expand support to the National Institutes of Health (NIH), and over a period of 15 years we went from what was a relatively piddling sum of less than $50 million to today's expenditures of one and one-quarter billion dollars for both biomedical research and training.

The results have been greatly beneficial. The significance of the accomplishments of the NIH has been recognized in almost every walk of life. An important aspect is that the NIH did not simply develop a federal capability; it created and supported a system of research throughout the United States. This system was relatively stabilized although it had many growing pains and problems in its development. One of the areas that was frequently the concern of policymakers was the question of using the research dollar to develop manpower and to support more than just research. It was asked if this was rather a backdoor arrangement for the support of education.

Hence the government undertook the task of modifying and correcting that weakness through the development of a health-manpower program, the purpose of which was to increase the supply of physicians, nurses, and other health-professional and allied health personnel. At the same time the government gave support to the medical schools in trying to cope with the shortage of physicians and other health manpower. This administration has selected as one of its highest priorities the increase of manpower in order that the system will not be retarded by shortages.

The task of preventing such shortages is most difficult. A substantial amount of money is required for the development of health manpower, the construction of facilities, the support of medical schools, and aid to students. This year, for example, there was an attempt to develop a program intended to increase the number of physicians by offering 10 million dollars to medical schools to increase their first-year enrollments by 1,000 students.

The funds thus far have been able to stimulate only 560 new positions even though the entire 10 million dollars has been expended. The cost of medical education, as you all know, is stupendous. It is an area which is going to require the concerted effort of the health professions, of educators, of state, local, and federal governments to find better ways of increasing the supply.

The federal government has undertaken a mission of trying to find out how to improve the delivery system. How does one improve the distribution and accessibility of available resources without loss of quality? How does one bring about a more economical arrangement for the provision of health services? As you know, health care fits into that portion of our total economy which is called service; but service in the health field, unlike that in any other field, has not shown increased productivity on the part of the workers involved, as it has, for example, in manufacturing.

When the Department of Health, Education, and Welfare (HEW) was created, the average hospital employed 184 employees for every 100 patients. The figure today is about 274 employees for every 100 patients. This, of course, registers as a decrease in the productivity of manpower. Moreover, approximately 80% of all costs of health services represent manpower costs. As a result, if we cannot find a way to bring about more effective utilization of manpower, we are not going to find a way to control costs.

The belief of the administration is that the health program has not developed a systematic organization for the provision of national services and that there is need of a system that will eliminate unnecessary competition and duplication of equipment and services.

The department is persuaded that it must build a methodology into the health system that will provide incentives for improving management and performance; that it should not proceed on the basis that cost reimbursement alone will produce the desired results. An office has been established within HEW's Health Services and Mental Health Administration for research and development in health services funded at a level of approximately $60 million dollars.

Further steps are being taken. The department has requested Congress to strengthen the legislative base for the Regional Medical Program, the Comprehensive Health Planning and Services Program, and the Health Services Research and Development Program by clarifying their common objectives and by treating these as a unity. You may recall that in 1966 Congress enacted the Partnership for Health Program, which undertook to make planning funds available to states and localities. These planning funds were somewhat different from those normally made available. They were not program-planning funds; instead, they were designed to ascertain what the needs were, who had responsibility for meeting these needs, and what pertinent methods could be employed.

Thus the planning was to be at a broader level than planning how to spend federal funds; it was aimed at trying to find through both state and areawide planning how to fulfill health needs. The funds were made available to the states and to localities throughout the states in a way that gave local officials substantial discretion as to how to use the funds.

Prior to this enactment almost all of the funds for health that were available to states and localities from the federal government were highly categorized. Funds were made available for tuberculosis, venereal disease, heart control, cancer control, and for mental-health activities. Under the Partnership for Health Act, however, the block grant was made available to a state for use at its own discretion in dealing with its problems and in establishing relative priorities for the needs of a particular area and community.

There was widespread concern when this law was enacted over the possibility that it might result in decreased appropriations. There was the fear that once the legislator no longer had to decide whether to increase or decrease funds for tuberculosis, venereal disease, or heart control and dealt instead with a general over-all pattern he would no longer be interested in supporting those programs and activities. Fortunately, this has not occurred. Congress has approved substantially all of the funds requested by the administrations since 1966. Actually, each year the appropriation has been slightly larger than that of the preceding year; in fiscal year 1971 $90 million dollars will be available, 18 million dollars more than in the preceding year.

A companion part of the Partnership for Health Act, in addition to the formula-grant area, is that of funds for special projects. These funds support individual demonstration and service-related projects throughout the United States that are approved at a federal level rather than through the states. I believe, though, that there are no exceptions to the general policy that each project will be coordinated with statewide planning, and therefore that the projects will have been funded with concurrence of state and local health officials.

These project funds, as well as the contract funds that were also available to health services and mental health, had previously been very distinctly categorized. There were project grants for tuberculosis, venereal disease, kidney dialysis, cervical cancer, and for other individual health programs.

There is now a strong tendency to phase out the support of these individual categorical-support projects. One would leave to the states under the block grant the responsibility for fulfilling these needs and would use the project-grant mechanism in a more innovative manner. Instead of being a disease-oriented category, each would be socially oriented. A substantial amount of the project funds during this next year will be used for family planning; there will be a phase-out of the support of individual projects in the area of tuberculosis; there already has been a substantial phase-out of the projects that were developed in the area of renal dialysis. There is also a phasing out of the chronic disease projects in heart, stroke, and cancer control.

The funds for individual project grants will be very greatly increased, and the increase will be used for new purposes. One purpose will be to develop new neighborhood health centers as a part of the program of improving the health-delivery system and of trying to provide health services in centers where they do not now exist.

HEW will assume responsibility for 30 million dollars worth of neighborhood health centers now operated by the Office of Economic Opportunity (OEO), which will continue to provide health services to neighborhood health centers, but it will do so only in the sense of being purely innovative. When the centers have been relatively stabilized and have proved their purpose, they either will be phased out or continued in operation under the jurisdiction of HEW. Fifteen such projects will be transferred on July 1, 1970, and we shall have a task force charged with the responsibility for identifying the fifteen.

A companion piece of legislation enacted in the same year, in 1966, was the Regional Medical Program, which came from a task force headed by Dr. Michael DeBakey of Houston, Texas. The approach of this program was almost the opposite of the approach of the Partnership for Health Program. Rather than make the state and local governmental officials members of the planning body, with state and local health departments as the implementing bodies for the use of public funds, the Regional Medical Program moved out of the public sector and into what I suppose you could call a combination of the health-educational sector and the private health sector.

It was a theory under which one could improve the delivery of health services by radiating the knowledge being acquired and practiced at the teaching hospital out to all community hospitals and all the schools of medicine. This approach would tie together the skills, the capability, and the improvements which were developing in the system, and it would make continuing education an organized reality in the health sector. Now we have 74 regional medical programs in the United States that cover substantially the entire population.

These regional medical programs now have resources of about 68 million dollars. They are programmed at 74 million dollars by the end of this year, and at 94 million dollars for fiscal year 1971. Roughly, they are the size of the grant programs that go to the states under the Partnership for Health Program.

Many fear that the two programs are on a collision course. They fear that we have given the responsibility for heart, stroke, and cancer in the regional medical programs to the academic and private health sectors to plan and develop; and that we have given the responsibility for planning the total health services to the states and local governments. They say that there is no viable apparatus for coordination of the two programs.

Dr. Roger Egeberg, assistant secretary for Health and Scientific Affairs, and Dr. Jesse Steinfeld, surgeon general, are persuaded that the two programs can be made fully compatible, so that they will complement each other and help to fulfill our total needs. As I have already mentioned, those officials have proposed legislation which has just gone to Congress to develop these programs further. Their plan removes from the Regional Medical Program the limitation that its resources must be devoted to heart, stroke, cancer, and related diseases, and makes its funds noncategorical, that is, available for all health programs.

Drs. Egeberg and Steinfeld recommended that we treat the several programs as companion pieces of legislation by appointing a single national advisory committee for the programs. All policies developed by this committee would work together to establish a sort of triparty arrangement under which the administrators for the Partnership for Health Program, the administrators of the Regional Medical Program, and the administrator of the Center for Health Services Research and Development would work as a single team. The research component would utilize both the Partnership for Health Program and the Regional Medical Program as the testing grounds for the methods of improving and perfecting the system of delivery in order to make it more accessible, more effective and efficient, and more economical.

The public involvement in the total health sector has undergone a very substantial change as a result of Medicare and Medicaid. The total health budget of the nation is about 60 billion dollars, with 25% in the federal sector and 33% in the public sector. In other words, about 8% of the health budget is in the state and local government area, 25% in the federal area, and 66% in the private sector of our economy.

Hence, if we are to have an effective health program, there must be a partnership arrangement. We must find a methodology that brings together into cohesion and a cooperative working relation the health professionals, the health institutions, the health-educational system, the health-financing mechanism, health insurance, prepayment programs, the state governments, local governments, and the federal government. It is a challenge which I think the American people have put before us. If we do not respond to it, some undesirable and unfortunate decisions and choices will have to be made to satisfy the consumer more fully.

I feel confident that we can create an effective health program. As if to accommodate us at this session, the secretary of HEW issued a statement only yesterday on the financing of health. The statement outlines actions that he proposes to take with respect to Medicaid and Medicare that would improve the distribution of benefits and the accessibility of health care, decrease the cost of health care, and start in motion what he hopes will be a chain reaction to build incentives into the system. These incentives are designed to maintain high quality and to increase effectiveness without contributing to continually spiralling costs.

As you know, until now health services have risen at an annual rate twice that of the cost-of-living index. At present the costs of hospital services are still rising at 13%, double the rate of the cost of living. This situation is giving tremendous concern to everyone in the field. It concerns the people who establish rates under hospital policy, who establish rates for part B Supplementary Services, who establish the tax rates for Social Security to cover the cost of services, and who are seeking appropriations from general funds. They are all faced with these costs.

The objectives of the secretary's proposed legislation are to take hospitals out of after-the-fact reimbursement for costs associated with Medicare patients and to work out instead a system of negotiation in advance of the rate at which services will be provided. The hospitals take the risk; and if they can improve the management of the services, they get the benefit of it. Thus the incentives would move them in the direction the administration would like them to go.

Fees would be established on the same basis that was proposed six months or a year ago in connection with Medicaid, that of using the prevailing rates—now at the 75th percentile. Then the growth in those fee schedules would be restrained to a rate that corresponds to the related aspects of the cost-of-living index. In addition to wages there are some other elements in the cost-of-living index that would serve as guides. In this way the growth would be at the same rate as that of the economy but no more rapid.

The legislation would rule that persons and institutions that have abused or defrauded the system would become ineligible as participants.

The principal new element in the statement released by the secretary, however, deals with the question of comprehensive health services for a per capita fee. This concept permits the patient to pay for his total health services at a fixed price, and it assures him of total comprehensive service, including preventive and curative care. Secretary Robert H. Finch refers to this feature as paying for being kept well.

It is recognized that this whole program cannot be accomplished in one year. On the other hand it is believed that it will develop over a period of years as a method of gaining a more systematized management of a health-service system. As you know, there are about 5 million people now covered by such plans. The Social Security Administration would contract with people who organize such a plan. The plans would ensure that first they would fulfill a total comprehensive health service and, second, that the rate charged would be lower than the cost of the provision of services under Medicare by the traditional methods now being used.

The person covered by Social Security would be able to make his own choice as to whether he wanted to go under the plan and whether he wanted to continue under the arrangement. If the person went into the plan and was not satisfied with it, he could drop out of it.

In connection with Medicaid, the legislation proposes to increase federal participation in the cost of ambulatory and outpatient health services to stimulate their greater use. It would decrease federal participation in extended care, that is, care beyond 90 days in nursing homes and in mental-health institutions. It does not eliminate federal participation but it diminishes it as an incentive to states to increase their utilization of reviews and to emphasize that they are to try to minimize the overutilization of facilities.

Also, there is recognition that the Medicaid program was designed as a health program but that it is sometimes used as a program for custody rather than as a health service. The new program would try to minimize the extent to which Medicaid serves in that capacity.

With all the programs that have evolved, those that have been mentioned, and the many others—such as the maternal and child health, the crippled-children's program, and special programs for migrants—the administration set out shortly after it took office to try to find a method of improving its management of the responsibilities which the public sector had assumed. It sought to clarify the relations that exist between the federal government and the grantee community (states, localities, hospitals, universities, and nonprofit institutions). A whole series of efforts are under way. While we cannot go very deeply into them on this occasion, they are worthy of identification because I believe that over the next two years some fairly substantial changes will be made in how the federal government conducts its business.

Each of the individual programs of the department has been designed and developed to fit a specific need; therefore the programs have been tailored by people concerned with that need, rather than by people concerned with the total array of activities that we conduct. We have just about driven the states' authorities into complete confusion and frustration.

I was introduced on a platform in Minneapolis recently by the vice president of the University of Minnesota, who bragged about the marvelous computer they had installed to handle all of their financial and statistical reporting. This official said it fulfilled every need except filing the reports required by HEW, something no computer could do.

We are setting out to try to resolve the problem. Two of our plans require legislation. The first is for consolidation of programs. It is difficult to get legislation enacted that merges programs, since the various programs all have vested interests. The government has found that in connection with reorganizing, one cannot change cabinets, create cabinets, or consolidate independent agencies because of these vested interests; hence the Reorganization Plan was enacted.

This plan is a system whereby the president can develop a reorganization plan and send it to Congress, which cannot change it. Congress can either allow the organization to come into being within 60 days or can veto it or vote it down. The president proposes to do the same thing on program consolidation. This would give him the authority to submit plans which would consolidate programs that could be voted down. If Congress does not vote against such proposals within 60 days they become law. There are many ramifications on some of the technicalities, such as how various matching formulas are pieced together. Nevertheless, if Congress will enact this legislation, it will go a long way toward decreasing the tremendous number of programs we have now. This plan would move us away from the process of making appropriations by category and moving it to a broader basis.

The second effort the president made was to submit to Congress a simplification act which has as one of its principal purposes the ability to join fund projects. Where one recipient, such as a Community Action Agency, a hospital, or a university, is engaged in one broad undertaking and has funds from 8, 10, or 15 sources, all of which effectively contribute to it, we could appoint a single federal manager to operate the project. The manager would be permitted to modify the requirements of each program and each agency in order to have a single set of requirements associated with the undertaking.

Some of the legislative requirements that might impede doing this could be waived. We have several demonstration projects underway now to find out how to use this method if Congress enacts the legislation. The prospects of enactment look relatively good.

A third step the president has taken which requires Congressional legislation was his request that Congress enact a revenue-sharing proposal. This proposal is designed to recognize the need for increased resources for public services at the local and the state levels. It is based on the conviction that the federal government could better achieve its purpose by making funds available on an unrestricted basis. It would utilize the categorical programs for innovation, for leverage, and for change; but basic public services would be decided upon by state and local officials. One could call such financing the broadest possible categorical grant because revenue sharing would require a maintenance of effort so that there would be additional funds for additional services, required to be spent for public services.

If enacted it should relieve substantially some of the pressures now felt by state and local governments, since they would decide how much of the revenue they shared was for education, for health, and whatever. The president proposed one half billion dollars for the first half year after enactment, with estimates rising to 5 billion dollars.

In addition to these actions that require legislation by Congress, the administration has initiated, with HEW in the forefront, a series of efforts. First, we have task forces in eight different areas identifying potential program consolidations that we shall recommend to Congress if and when we can consolidate our programs.

Second, we are reviewing every federal program that involves a state formula grant with a requirement for a state plan. The review of the state plans involves identifying the intended use of the funds. The plans really tend to identify the basic organizations, eligible expenditures, methods of appointing people, etc., and are not plans for the fulfillment of the plan. Many historical data that persons are spending much energy in developing and reviewing do not seem to be furthering the programs. It would appear that we are going to have a much more simplified approach to state formula-program plans, and to state plans.

Third, we have under way a massive approach concerned with how to process the requests for grants we receive—tens of thousands of applications for project grants for the many programs administered by HEW. Each program has developed a different approach and methodology by which to perform its job—the design of the application, what must be associated with it, where it goes in the organization, who does what with it. A staff of analysts is now trying to develop process-and-flow charts for every step of that process, in order to develop the shortest process possible, one which will produce the most effective decision making, that will do it more rapidly, and that will impose to a lesser degree on the applicant.

Another effort under way is an attempt to identify all of the requirements that we impose on a grantee, to see if we cannot make those requirements more nearly uniform. In a given university one finds that in one program we are concerned with salaries and appointment procedures while in another we are not. Some programs require prior approval and others do not. Some require that purchases of equipment be made in the name of the federal government and some do not.

There is a tremendous array of requirements. We have a very

competent management firm working for us; it is identifying and putting into a computer every requirement established for every program. The plan will make it possible by computer analysis to provide data on each grantee, on any particular kind of program, on any management system, on any policy requirement. We shall be able to evaluate the requirements as to which are best and to substitute them for those that now exist.

Fifth, we are engaged in a study of how to improve the quality of the management of the grantee. We are faced with the serious problem that in order to fulfill the mission of HEW we must assist the citizens that live in every community, the students that attend every university, and the patients in every hospital. We cannot afford to take the position of the Department of Defense, that it is competitive in determining who receives appropriations: for example, whether to give the contract to one firm or another. If one of them does a poor job, the contract is terminated, which cannot be done in many of our programs. It is very difficult, for example, for us to take money out of New York and give it to New Jersey.

Where we have problems of mismanagement and poor or inadequate management, it does not behoove us to sever connections with the grantees. Rather, we have a responsibility to bring operations up to an acceptable level of management. We tend to marshal our resources for technical assistance in the areas where most money is spent. There is some evidence that these areas have the best managers and that we should be devoting our energies to those that have the poor managers, whoever they may be, to help them improve.

We have therefore endeavored to develop a test that will identify the objectives of good management in each area. On the basis of self-evaluation, it will stimulate the grantee community, including the local health departments, the state health departments, the hospitals, the colleges, universities, and nonprofit institutions to evaluate their own management against those objective standards and to identify the actions they should take to improve it.

We shall review what they have done, reach our conclusions, and classify the grantees. We hope to do this in a way that will relieve excellent managers of some of the burdens of their relations with the federal government. Such relief could be in the area of prior approval requirements, with some of the reporting requirements also waived. In this way the grantees will benefit by being identified as good managers.

On poor managers we shall impose special requirements on future grants that are more restrictive or that require greater technical assistance. In some cases grants would not be awarded until the managers reached acceptable levels of efficiency. This procedure would be preferable to ruling that the grantee does not satisfy our requirements and that therefore his patients, the citizens, or the students are not to benefit from the federal program.

This approach offers an opportunity for us to work with the grantee community in a way that will be mutually advantageous and from which the public will benefit greatly.

As illustrated by the various efforts I have described to you, the administration hopes to improve our American system of health-care delivery. Further, in partnership with all of you, and with hospitals, state and local health agencies, and the consumer, the department is confident it will find ways to assure stable and more effective financing of the health services.

DISCUSSION OF THE PAPER BY JAMES F. KELLY: "ASSURING STABLE AND EFFECTIVE FINANCING OF LOCAL HEALTH SERVICES: THE ROLE OF INTERGOVERNMENTAL GRANTS IN AID"*

ALANSON WILLCOX

Retired General Counsel
Department of Health, Education, and Welfare
Washington, D.C.

I BELIEVE that a lawyer's comment on anything said by Mr. Kelly would be pretty much of an anticlimax.

I was a little surprised to hear Mr. Kelly speak of negative changes in productivity, and to hear him give the increase in personnel in hospitals as an example. I wonder whether the increase in personnel has, in terms of actual delivery of health care, been offset or more than offset by the improvement in the quality and techniques of the service.

How much really effective planning has yet come out of the Partnership for Health Act and the statewide and areawide planning that act contemplates? This planning has been slow in getting started, at least in most states and cities, and I am impressed by the difficulty of the process, particularly with the participation of consumers that is required—by how much the groups responsible for the planning will have to educate themselves before they can make any constructive contributions.

But let me turn to some questions within a lawyer's competence. Until a few years ago the federal grant was of almost no concern to the legal profession except to those few of us who had to advise public officials what they could and could not do under particular statutes. Lawyers, like many other people, tended to feel that federal grants were like private charity and that it would be unseemly to quarrel with a grantor—one does not bite the hand that feeds one, and so on.

*Presented at a meeting of the Subcommittee on Social Policy for Health Care of the Committee on Medicine in Society, March 26, 1970.

This attitude has changed very radically in the last few years, largely because the Office of Economic Opportunity (OEO) has been supporting a widespread system of legal services for the poor. Since a large proportion of programs supported by federal grants are designed for the benefit of the poor, these programs began to be challenged in many of their provisions, and the courts have accepted those challenges and dealt with many of them. The Supreme Court held a year or so ago that the exclusion of newly arrived residents from a state public-assistance program was unconstitutional, and it held later that terminating benefits to a public-assistance recipient without a hearing was also unconstitutional. There have been many cases in the lower courts that challenged various aspects of public-welfare programs, educational programs, and other forms of benefits. These challenges involve not only the racial issue; there has been quite a radical change, for instance, in the universities and schools on the extent to which the administrators can censor speeches on campus or discipline students, and there are new requirements for hearings and other procedural safeguards.

Several publications report developments in these areas of the law, and every month there is a long list of new cases and new decisions; there are always some of these in the health field. The health field is perhaps less concerned with what is going on in the courts than is welfare or education or housing, but it is not unconcerned by any means.

Let me illustrate by focusing on one area that has concerned me a good deal: the local-project grant set up to serve a limited group of people. How are those people selected, and how does one justify the fact that other persons who live nearby and who are just as needy do not receive the benefit given to the favored group? This problem is accentuated if, as in some of these health projects, you draw rigid lines and say that if a person lives on one side of the street he gets service, but if he lives on the other side of the street he does not. That may be statistically convenient but it seems difficult to justify in terms of equal treatment. What has always troubled me most in this connection is the use of a control group as much like the beneficiaries as possible, to whom are denied the benefits merely for purposes of comparison.

We are going to need a good deal of thinking about this sort of problem. There has been no challenge thus far, to my knowledge, to any health program or any similar program on this basis, but I should be rather surprised, with all the legal service available, if some such challenge does not develop before very long. I expect that the courts will recognize the need for experimentation and demonstration, and that they will be tolerant of some inequities that are inherent in this process, but I hope that health-service areas can be set up without quite such rigid boundaries. One thing that bothers me even in demonstration programs is that they go on year after year: after a while the justification that you are experimenting or demonstrating begins to wear thin. And the people who are on the outside looking in may have a complaint to which the courts will listen.

These issues require consideration. Moreover, many other areas in health services may be vulnerable to attack. The Court of Appeals in the District of Columbia recently directed a hospital there to perform an abortion that its staff had refused to perform. The residents-in-training in the big municipal hospital in Los Angeles have brought a suit against the hospital to require it to curtail its admissions because they claimed it was so overcrowded they could not give decent medical care, pointing out that other mechanisms are available to the welfare department for the care of persons in private hospitals.

These are problems that a few years ago could hardly have arisen in court. Anybody who was doing good for the public was generally thought to be free to do so on the terms he thought best, just as a private philanthropist is. This is no longer true, and it is necessary in devising these programs to take some account of what the legal rights are, both of those persons who are included and, perhaps before long, also of those persons who have been excluded.

There is one other legal development I want to discuss briefly. For the last few years, particularly in the OEO, there have been occasional complaints about what was alleged to be high-handed action on the part of the agency in terminating a grant, in refusing to renew it, or in other aspects of administration. The concern of the legal profession which, as I say, has become very active on the substantive end of grants and the rights of grantees, has more recently been extended to a concern with grant procedures: how decisions are made; how the money is handed out; whether there is discrimination; whether there are fair procedures on termination of grants; and other matters of this sort.

The Administrative Conference of the United States—a body set up by Congress that was slow in getting started but is now organized and doing business—has the responsibility to survey, study, and make recommendations on all aspects of federal government procedure. It is composed of able men; it includes most of the academic leaders in the field of administrative law, many government lawyers, and many private practitioners. Fortunately, unlike earlier efforts in this direction, it is a permanent body and so does not have to move at any predetermined speed.

The American Bar Association has also become interested in this question; last autumn it held a two-day conference in Washington on the subject of procedures in discretionary grants, particularly grants focused on urban problems. The conference was surprisingly well attended and engendered vigorous discussion. Now the administrative-law section of the American Bar has created a special committee on discretionary grant procedures.

There are some enthusiasts who want to lay down meticulous rules for every step in the grant process. I believe that the Administrative Conference will be wise enough to make haste slowly and to eschew precipitate and sweeping recommendations; I hope that the American Bar will be a little more restrained than it has sometimes been in making recommendations.

There are some legitimate grievances to consider. Mr. Kelly commented on the difference between grants of the kind the Department of Health, Education, and Welfare makes and government-procurement activities, in which the rights of the vendors are carefully guarded by law. Yet some grants are quite similar to contracts both in function and in operation—when, for example, the government goes shopping for a grant applicant to do something it wants done—and the question is fairly asked: Why should the grantee have so much less protection than the contractor? Competitive bidding seems generally quite inappropriate to a great program, yet in cases of this kind why should potential competitors be excluded? Have we adequate machinery to ensure that all would-be applicants know of the availability of grant funds, and of the terms and conditions on which grants may be awarded? If not, I should say, there is a just complaint. Does the staff of a granting agency help applicants to put their papers in approvable form, and is this assistance equally available to all? What happens when a grantee, charged with wasting the granted funds, disputes the charge? Should he have the same right to an administrative hearing that a contractor has, and perhaps to court review?

The law of grants-in-aid, both substantive and procedural, is under scrutiny today as never before, and I should like to close by inviting you, the receivers of grants, to join in the scrutiny. If we are to make the grant process both fairer and more effective we must see it as it is seen by those on the receiving end. Courts tend to respect professional opinion in fields other than the law, and so too, I am sure, will the Administrative Conference. So I urge you, and other groups like yours, to be ready to participate in discussing the grant process and to help guide that discussion into constructive directions.

HOSPITALS DEPICTED IN OLD MAPS AND PANORAMAS (I)

THE second World War stimulated the advance of many branches of science and of many branches of medicine, including epidemiology and public health. These advances were not only substantive but also methodological. It is not surprising, therefore, that the mapping of disease increased rapidly in scope and effectiveness.

Medical cartography has now existed long enough and progressed far enough for a retrospect to be profitable. But as yet we possess only a few scattered facts and a few rudimentary opinions as to the way in which this highly sophisticated cultural product may have originated. The subject is beginning to attract the attention of historians; the essay by Stevenson[1] is evidence of this trend.

At the present stage of inquiry it is necessary to distinguish between medical maps—those which present any subject of medical interest—and maps of disease, which constitute a much smaller category. It appears that the latter are the newer and perhaps represent a specialized form of the distributional, economic, and agricultural mapping that gained currency during the last few decades of the 18th century.

Aspects of these early developments were recently reviewed in a historical periodical.[2] Attention was called to the work of a Russian scholar, O. B. Shkurlatov, who referred to a map or picture of Kiev (1683), which was said to show hospitals or hospices, in addition to churches and monasteries. This implies that a systematic search of old city maps and old panoramic views might disclose details of medical interest.

Those who visit the Norwegian city of Bergen, well known for its culture and for the courage of its inhabitants, are likely to see an old panoramic picture, sometimes titled simply *Bergen,* or *Berga Noorwegiae*. This map is seen in the windows of shops and in public places such as hotel lobbies. A piece of the attractive design also serves to decorate the ticket that the traveler receives on paying his admission

1. Stevenson, L.: Putting disease on the map: The early use of spot maps in the study of yellow fever. *J. Hist. Med.* *20*:226-61, 1965.
2. Jarcho, S.: Yellow fever, cholera, and the beginnings of medical cartography. *J. Hist. Med.*, *25*:131-42, 1970.

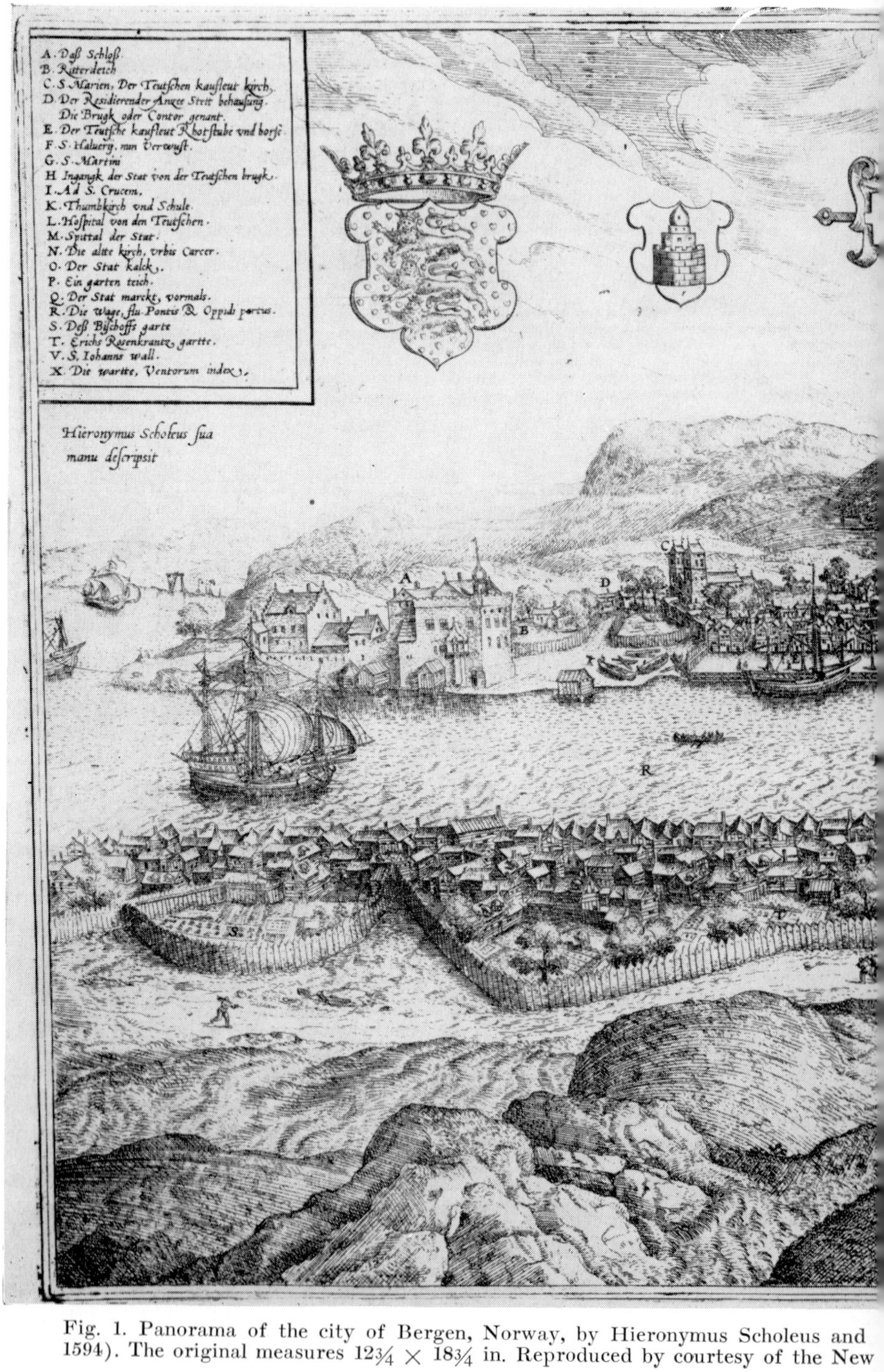

Fig. 1. Panorama of the city of Bergen, Norway, by Hieronymus Scholeus and
1594). The original measures 12¾ × 18¾ in. Reproduced by courtesy of the New

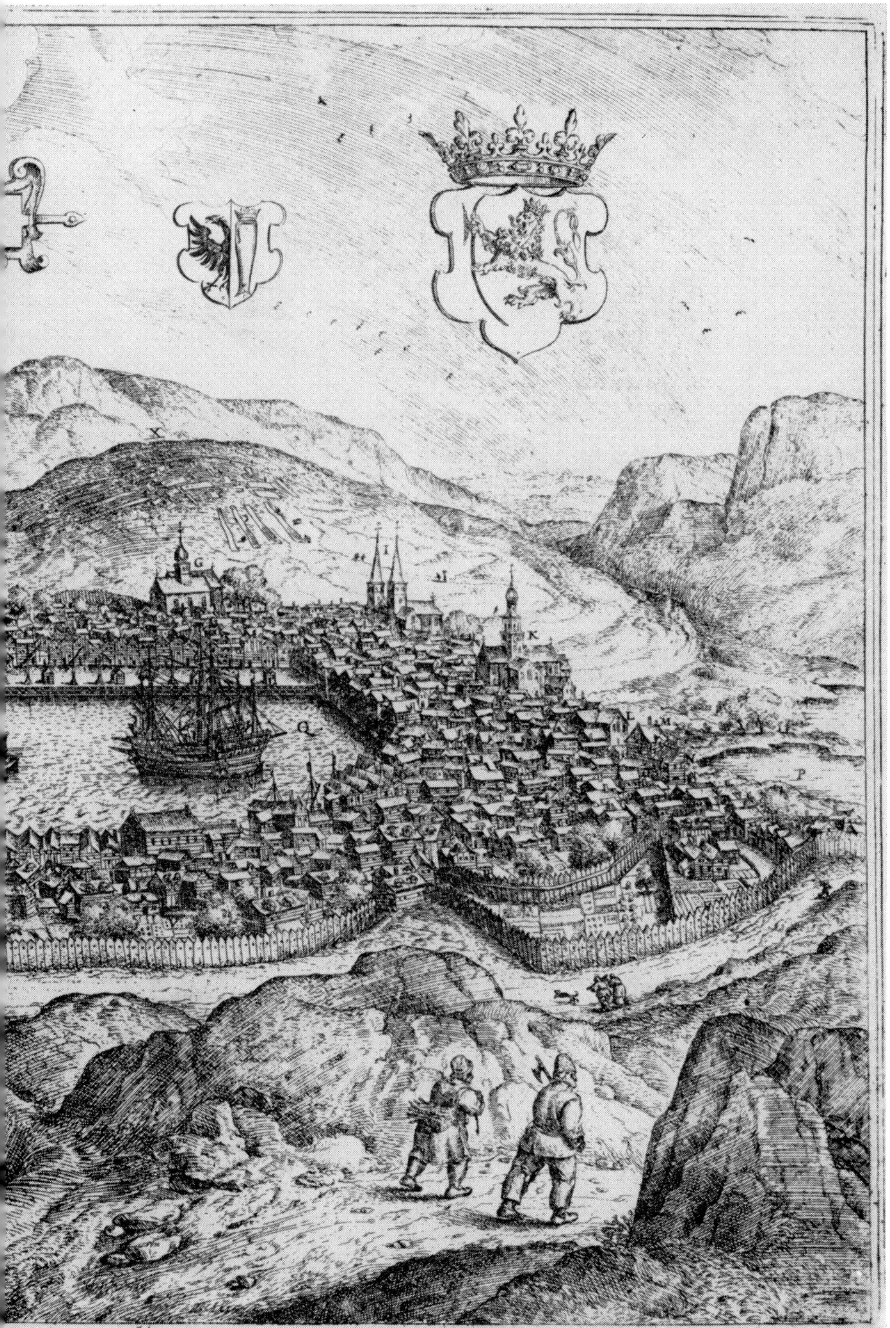

erg, from Georg Braun's *Civitates Orbis Terrarum,* Cologne 1572-1618, (vol. 4,
Library.

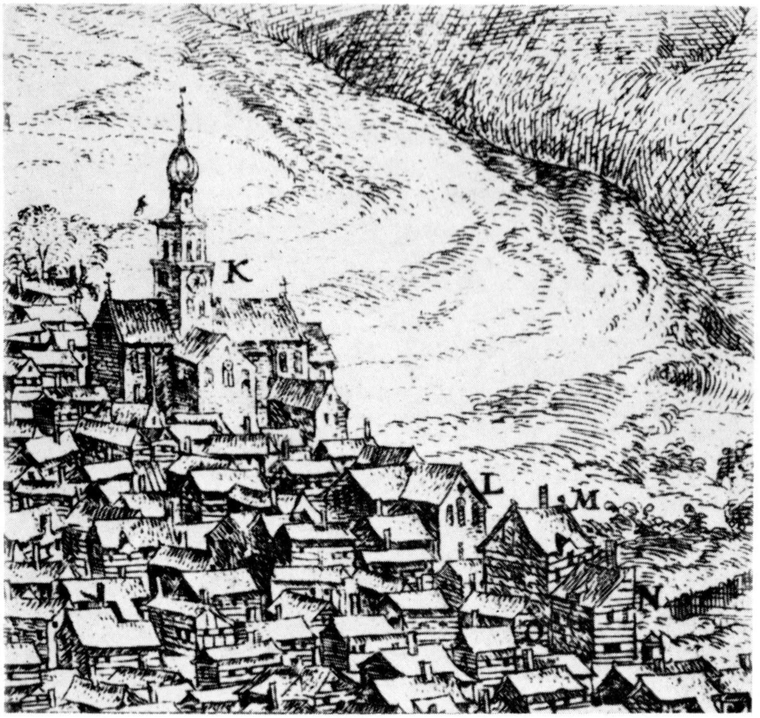

Fig. 2. Enlarged detail of Scholeus-Hogenberg map of Bergen, 1594 (see Figure 1). *L* indicates the German Hospital. *M* indicates the City Hospital. Reproduced by courtesy of the New York Public Library.

fee at the Rosenkrantz Tower, which overlooks Bergen harbor.

Mr. S. Bonge of the Universitetsbiblioteket at Bergen kindly identified the map as the work of Hieronymus Scholeus, draughtsman, and Franz Hogenberg, engraver.[3] The original appears in Braun, G.: *Civitates Orbis Terrarum.* Cologne, 1572-1618, volume 4 (1594), plate 37. (Facsimile reprint, 6 vols. in 3, Amsterdam, Theatrum Orbis Terrarum, 1965.) It is reproduced (Figure 1) by courtesy of the New York Public Library.

In the upper left-hand corner of the map is a table of symbols, in which can be read:

L Hospital von den Teutschen

M Spittal der Stat

3. Mr. Bonge kindly sent the author an article by Prof. Hallvard S. Bakken, which discusses the history of the map. Bakken, H. S., Scholeus-stikket. *Bergens Tidende,* Sept. 3, 1960.

These two establishments, the hospital for Germans and the city hospital, are depicted in the right central portion of the map (see enlargement, Figure 2). Presumably these hospitals, especially the German hospital, reflected the activities of the Hanseatic League. Additional information may be obtained from an essay contributed by G. Armauer Hansen,[4] the famous leprologist.

The classic history of cartography by Bagrow and Skelton[5] makes no mention of Hieronymus Scholeus. Information obtained from Swedish sources[6] is virtually limited to the fact that he contributed views of Bergen and Stockholm to Braun's collection.

Bagrow and Skelton refer to Georg Braun (Joris Bruin) as having published several editions of Münster's well-known map of Germany and as having collaborated with the engraver Frans Hogenberg (1535-1590) and other Flemish craftsmen in the production of *Civitates Orbis Terrarum.*

Additional representations of hospitals are to be found in a book on medieval leprosy by Prof. V. Møller-Christensen.[7] This author points out that in Scandinavia lepers were treated in special hospitals under the patronage of St. Jørgen (Saint George).[8] These establishments were often located outside the walls of cities and are so portrayed in old maps and panoramas, such as those of Copenhagen[9] and Visby.[10]

These observations indicate that old city maps, city plans, and panoramas can be made to yield information of medical importance and perhaps contain the origins of modern medical cartography.*

S. J.

4. Hansen, G. A. and Lie, H. P.: Die Geschichte der Lepra in Norwegen. *Lepra 8* (suppl.): 314-40, 1909; see esp. p. 317.
5. Bagrow, L.: *History of Cartography.* Revised and enlarged by R. A. Skelton. Cambridge, Harvard Univ. Press, 1964, pp. 186 and 234.
6. Andersson, K.: Hieronymus Scholeus. In: *Svenskt Konstnärs Lexikon.* Malmö, Allhems, 1967, vol. 5, p. 79.
7. Møller-Christensen, B.: *Ten Lepers from Naestved in Denmark; A Study of Skeletons from a Medieval Danish Leper Hospital.* Copenhagen, Danish Science Press, 1953.
8. See also Danielssen, D. C. and Boeck, W.: *Traité de la Spédalskhed.* Paris, Baillière, 1848, pp. 133, 136.
9. Møller-Christensen, op. cit., Figure 18a, p. 38.
10. Møller-Christensen, op. cit., Figure 18b, p. 38.

*The author thanks Mrs. Maude Cole of the New York Public Library and Mrs. Richard North for their assistance.

OPINIONS OF THE AMERICAN ABORIGINES

Among the Americans, as well as other uncivilized nations, many of the rites and observances which bear some resemblance to acts of religion, have no connection with devotion, but proceed from a fond desire of prying into futurity. The human mind is most apt to feel, and to discover this vain curiosity, when its own powers are most feeble and uninformed. Astonished with occurrences, of which it is unable to comprehend the cause, it naturally fancies that there is something mysterious and wonderful in their origin. Alarmed at events of which it cannot discern the issue or the consequences, it has recourse to other means of discovering them, than the exercise of its own sagacity. Wherever superstition is so established as to form a regular system, this desire of penerating into the secrets of futurity is connected with it. Divination becomes a religious act. Priests, as the ministers of Heaven, pretend to deliver its oracles to men. They are the only soothsayers, augurs, and magicians, who profess the sacred and important art of disclosing what is hid from other eyes.

But, among rude nations, who pay no veneration to any superintending power, and who have no established rites or ministers of religion, their curiosity to discover what is future and unknown is cherished by a different principle, and derives strength from another alliance. As the diseases of men, in the savage state, are (as has been already observed) like those of the animal creation, few but extremely violent, their impatience under what they suffer, and solicitude for the recovery of health, soon inspired them with extraordinary reverence for such as pretended to understand the nature of their maladies, and to be possessed of knowledge sufficient to preserve or deliver them from their sudden and fatal effects. These ignorant pretenders, however, were such utter strangers to the structure of the human frame, as to be equally unacquainted with the causes of its disorders, and the manner in which they will terminate. Superstition, mingled frequently with some portion of craft, supplied what they wanted in science. They imputed the origin of diseases to supernatural influence, and prescribed or performed a variety of mysterious rites, which they gave out to be of such efficacy as to remove the most dangerous and inveterate maladies. The credulity and love of the marvellous, natural to uninformed men, favoured the deception, and prepared them to be the dupes of those impostors. Among savages, their first physicians are a kind of conjurers of wizards, who boast that they know what is past, and can foretell what is to come. Incantations, sorcery, and mummeries of diverse kinds, no less strange than frivolous, are the means which they employ to expel the imaginary causes of malignity; and relying upon the efficacy of these, they predict with confidence what will be the fate of their deluded patients. Thus superstition, in its earliest form, flowed from the solicitude of man to be delivered from present distress, not from his dread of evils awaiting him in a future life, and was originally ingrafted on medicine, not on religion. One of the first, and most intelligent historians of America, was struck with this alliance between the art of divination and that of physic, among the people of Hispaniola. But this was not peculiar to them. The *Alexis*, the *Piayas*, the *Autmoins*, or whatever was the distinguishing name of their diviners and charmers in other parts of America, were all the physicians of their respective tribes, in the same manner as the *Buhitos* of Hispaniola. As their function led them to apply to the human mind when enfeebled by sickness, and as they found it, in that season of dejection, prone to be alarmed with imaginary fears, or amused with vain hopes, they easily induced it to rely with implicit confidence on the virtue of their spells, and the certainty of their predictions.

Whenever men acknowledge the reality of supernatural power and discernment in one instance, they have a propensity to admit it in others. The Americans did not long suppose the efficacy of conjuration to be confined to one subject. They had recourse to it in every situation of danger or distress. When the events of war were peculiarly disastrous, when they met with unforeseen disappointments in hunting, when inundations or drought threatened their crops with destruction, they called upon their conjurers to begin their incantations, in order to discover the causes of those calamities, or to foretell what would be their issue. Their confidence in this delusive art gradually increased, and manifested itself in all the occurrences of life. When involved in any difficulty, or about to enter upon any transaction of moment, every individual regularly consulted the sorcerer, and depended upon his instructions to extricate him from the former, as well as to direct his conduct in the latter. Even among the rudest tribes in America, superstition appears in this form, and divination is an art in high esteem. Long before man had acquired such knowledge of a deity as inspires reverence, and leads to adoration, we observe him stretching out a presumptous hand to draw aside that veil with which providence kindly conceals its purpose from human knowledge; and we find him labouring, with fruitless anxiety, to penetrate into the mysteries of the divine administration. To discern, and to worship a superintending power, is an evidence of the enlargement and maturity of the human understanding; a vain desire of prying into futurity, is the error of its infancy, and a proof of its weakness.

From this weakness proceeded likewise the faith of the Americans in dreams, their observation of omens, their attention to the chirping of birds, and the cries of animals, all which they suppose to be indications of future events, and if any one of these prognostics is deemed unfavourable, they instantly abandon the pursuit of those measures on which they are most eagerly bent.

Robertson, William: *The History of America*, 10th ed. London, Strahan, 1803, vol. 2, pp. 204-09.

BULLETIN OF
THE NEW YORK ACADEMY
OF MEDICINE

VOL. 46, NO. 10 OCTOBER 1970

New York Heart Association

CONFERENCE ON GLOMERULONEPHRITIS*

Held at The Waldorf-Astoria
New York, N.Y., January 27, 1970

Introduction

IN this conference on glomerulonephritis it might be interesting to turn time back for a moment and consider the original description of nephritis, which has been referred to as Bright's disease. Two of the original cases described by Richard Bright represent two forms of glomerulonephritis. While Bright was given credit for the original description of kidney disease as we know it today, he in reality described the morbid anatomy and not the histology. His collaborator, Bostock, a clinical chemist, pointed out that the urine of these patients was coagulable and that patients with Bright's disease had an elevated urea and a hard pulse.

Figure 1 is a histological section taken from the kidney of Mary Brooks, a 24-year-old woman who had a five-year history of anasarca; on chemical analysis her blood contained 15 grains of urea per 1,000 grains of serum. The albumin was decreased according to Mr. Bostock. On careful drying there were only 15 grains of albumin and the nor-

*Publication of the proceedings of this *Conference on Glomerulonephritis* is supported in part by the Eaton Laboratories Division of the Norwich Pharmacal Co., Norwich, N.Y.

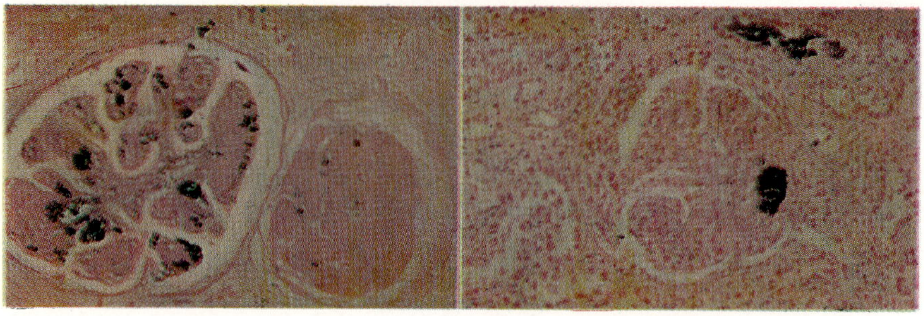

Fig. 1 Fig. 2

Fig. 1. Hematoxylin and eosin stain of kidney tissue of Mary Brooks. These alterations are compatible with the diagnosis of chronic glomerulonephritis.

Fig. 2. Hematoxylin and eosin stain of kidney tissue of Edward M. These alterations are compatible with the diagnosis of acute glomerulonephritis.

mal value was between 80 and 100. This microphotograph reveals a pattern of glomerulonephritis not unlike that which you will hear about on this occasion. The dark staining material is lead oxide, which was used by Bright as a preservative for the kidney. The tissue reveals marked fibrosis of the interstitial tissue with scarring in hyalinized glomeruli.

Figure 2 is the kidney of Edward M., a sailor who took ill in the Straits of Gibraltar and was autopsied at Guy's Hospital in 1827. The interstitial tissue was edematous, and crescents in the glomeruli are noted. This tissue is compatible with the diagnosis of acute glomerulonephritis. (We are indebted to the Department of Pathology of Guy's Hospital Medical School for the tissue sections and permission to publish this material.)

So in reality we are not dealing with a disease which is new to the medical profession, but rather one which was described more than 150 years ago. In this conference our emphasis will be on the pathogenesis and treatment of glomerulonephritis.

It is a pleasure for me to recognize the contribution of the members of the Scientific Committee which planned this conference, Dr. Jacob Churg, Dr. John H. Laragh, Dr. Jerome Lowenstein, Dr. Kurt Stenzel, and Dr. Gerald Turino, and to thank the officers and staff of the New York Heart Association who made the conference possible.

E. Lovell Becker, M.D.
Chairman, Planning Committee

GLOMERULONEPHRITIS: CLINICAL ASPECTS*

David P. Earle

Professor and Chairman, Department of Medicine
Northwestern University-McGaw Medical Center
Chicago, Ill.

Patients with glomerulonephritis present many fascinating clinical problems related to proteinuria, edema, biochemical abnormalities, and other manifestations. These topics are considered later in this symposium. I shall, therefore, limit my discussion to clinical problems related to the diagnosis and to the natural history of the several glomerular diseases.

Glomerulonephritis is a broad diagnostic term, hardly more useful than the term "Bright's disease." The label "glomerulonephritis" has been applied indiscriminately to a number of different diseases, of different etiologies and different pathologies. These diseases have different prognoses, and different responses to treatment.

The long-term painstaking correlation of the clinical course of different glomerular diseases, with the pathology as revealed by serial renal biopsies, has gone a long way to improve our definition of the natural history of some of these diseases. As I believe Drs. Jacob Churg and Robert T. McCluskey will agree, the mutual interest of pathologists and internists is essential. Much of what I have to say is based on joint work performed with Dr. Robert Jennings and his colleagues in our Department of Pathology. Since Drs. Churg and McCluskey will thoroughly review the pathology of glomerular diseases, I shall not stress this aspect. However, I hope that you will accept the various classifications I shall discuss, and recognize that adequate renal biopsies were obtained in every case included in this report.

Acute Nephritis

Several etiologies of acute nephritis are shown in Table I. Poststreptococcal acute glomerulonephritis, a well-defined disease, is usually

*Presented at a *Conference on Glomerulonephritis* held by the New York Heart Association at The Waldorf-Astoria, New York, N. Y., January 27, 1970.

This study was supported in part by Public Health Service Research Grants HE 07057 from the National Heart Institute and FR 0048 from the Division of Research Facilities and Resources, Bethesda, Md., and from the Otho S.A. Sprague Memorial Institute, Chicago, Ill.

TABLE I. ETIOLOGIES OF ACUTE NEPHRITIS

1) B-Hemolytic streptococcal infection
2) Subacute bacterial endocarditis
3) Pneumococcus lobar pneumonia
4) Staphylococcal infections
5) Viral infections
6) Miscellaneous infections
7) Focal glomerulitis
8) Associated with systemic diseases
9) Caused by drugs or toxins

the first etiology to come to mind.[1] Acute glomerulonephritis with either focal or diffuse glomerular lesions may occur in the course of subacute bacterial endocarditis.[2]

Pneumococcus lobar pneumonia also has been reported as an antecedent to acute nephritis,[3] but most of the cases in the literature were described before the availability of antistreptolysin titers. I have yet to see a patient with pneumococcus pneumonia and acute nephritis who did not also have increased streptococcal serum antibodies.

Staphylococcus infections from time to time are incriminated as an etiologic factor in acute nephritis. Recently two patients were described in which no evidence for associated streptococcal infection existed.[4] However, staphylococcal etiology must be rather uncommon.

Viral infections are said to cause acute nephritis from time to time. Infectious mononucleosis, hepatitis, and other viruses have been described as being associated with acute nephritis. I do not doubt that some viral infections are associated with acute nephritislike syndromes. Often this association appears to me to be the result of overenthusiastic interpretation of thick histologic preparations of renal biopsies. However, there are several circumstances where acute nephritis does follow viral infections. We studied an outbreak of hemorrhagic nephritis at Great Lakes Naval Training Station more than 10 years ago, at a time when the base was on penicillin prophylaxis.[5] A number of recruits were admitted with gross hematuria. They all were associated with pharyngitis, which was demonstrated unequivocally not to be of streptococcal etiology. The acute nephritis cleared rapidly. This is probably the same disease described in New York City more than 40 years ago by Dr. George Baehr, who labeled it "benign hemorrhagic acute nephritis."[6]

Over the years investigators have proclaimed the association of a wide variety of infections with acute nephritis, usually on inadequate evidence. Sometimes syndromes resembling acute nephritis, or at least the abrupt onset of hematuria and abnormal urine, are found on renal biopsy to be associated with focal glomerulitis. Hypertension, edema, and other signs of acute nephritis are rarely found in focal lesions.

A number of systemic diseases such as systemic lupus erythematosus and arteritis may be associated with the syndrome of acute nephritis. Nor should we forget the possible association of drugs and toxins with this syndrome.

Glomerular Lesions

I promised not to go very deeply into pathology, but it is important to recognize that glomerular lesions may be distributed either diffusely or focally. Focal glomerulitis refers to the condition in which some glomeruli are diseased and others are normal. In contrast, when parts of glomeruli are diseased and other parts of the same glomeruli are normal, the distribution is said to be local. For purposes of the subsequent discussion of focal glomerular lesions, both focal and local distributions are considered under the term focal.

In poststreptococcal acute glomerulonephritis the glomerular lesions are diffuse and all are of the same age. Endothelial-cell proliferation and polymorphonuclear leukocytes contribute to the typical hypercellularity. In severe instances necrosis of some glomerular loops may occur and may lead to adhesions, while epithelial crescents appear to be a response to fibrin or its degradation products. The lesions may be primarily proliferative or primarily exudative; usually both features are present.

The glomerular capillary basement membrane appears normal by light microscopy. However, electron microscopy and immunofluorescent studies reveal deposits on the epithelial side of the membranes.

As poststreptococcal acute proliferative glomerulonephritis subsides, the peripheral capillary loops open up. The residual hypercellularity is confined to the mesangial area, which also contains an increased amount of basement membranelike material. The peripheral capillary loops and the basement membranes still appear normal. After six weeks,

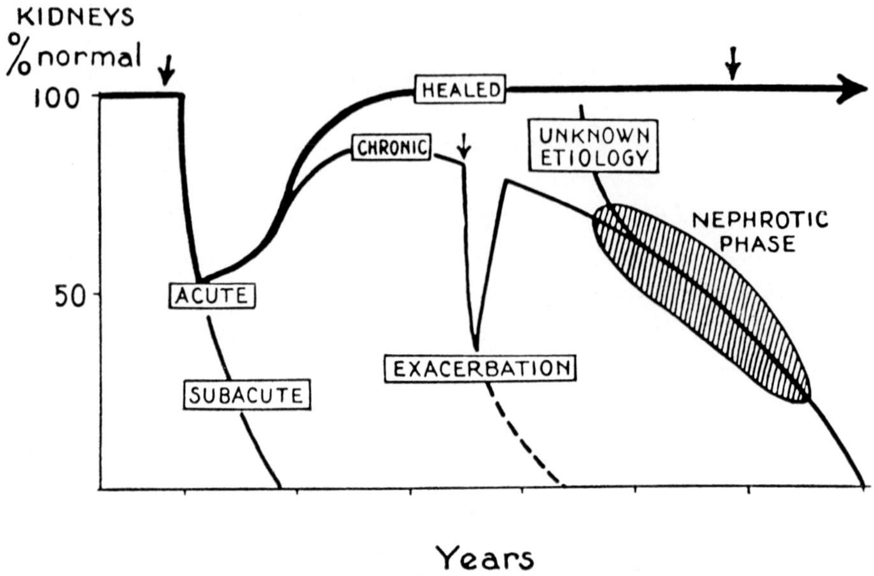

Natural history of diffuse glomerulonephritis. Arrows indicate group A hemolytic streptococcus infections. Dashed line below "exacerbation" indicates that a few exacerbations are followed by rapid progression of renal functional impairment, perhaps analogous to the relatively uncommon subacute course subsequent to an initial attack of acute glomerulonephritis. Modified from: GLOMERULONEPHRITIS by David P. Earle, Jr., in *Disease-a-Month.* Copyright, 1956, Year Book Medical Publishers, Inc. Reproduced by permission.

even by electron microscopy, the peripheral basement membranes appear normal, although the mesangial areas may remain abnormal for several years.

In contrast, membranous glomerular lesions are diffuse. Here, depending on the disease, deposits appear on either the epithelial or endothelial sides of the membrane, or both. Eventually the membrane itself becomes involved and thickened. Ordinarily the rest of the lobule remains normal and shows little or no proliferative change. Mixed membranous and proliferative lesions occur and probably represent a different disease or diseases.

Natural History of Poststreptococcal Glomerulonephritis

A concept of the natural history of poststreptococcal glomerulonephritis is shown in the accompanying figure.[7] This was constructed about 20 years ago, and I see little reason for changing it. I shall use this diagram as a framework for discussion of some aspects of the natural history of poststreptococcal acute glomerulonephritis.

The arrows indicate streptococcal infections. The glomerular filtration rate is the most convenient reference for the diagram. In this instance, the filtration rate has fallen to about 50% of normal. However, poststreptococcal acute glomerulonephritis may occur in any degree of severity. Some instances may be so mild that the patient does not even know he has the disease, which can be detected only by the alert physician who does serial urinalyses at the appropriate times.

How often the subclinical form of acute nephritis occurs is not known. It is a difficult diagnosis to establish. A large epidemic of acute nephritis associated with cutaneous infections is under study in Trinidad.[8, 9] We have studied the families of patients admitted to the hospital with acute nephritis. For the three overt cases we have been able to establish the diagnosis of subclinical acute nephritis in only one. Ordinarily, I should expect that mild subclincal cases would outnumber overt cases. Perhaps we do not visit the families frequently enough. These are not proposed as accurate statistical data. Perhaps we should just say that it is hard to find subclinical acute nephritis even when sought.

As shown in the figure, several outcomes of acute glomerulonephritis are possible. A small percentage of these patients will die, probably much less than 1%. A subacute clinical course is illustrated in the figure. I have seen records of such patients, but in our personal experience this is an extremely rare course following proved poststreptococcal acute nephritis. In fact, when a patient follows this course the disease usually turns out not to be poststreptococcal acute glomerulonephritis.

The glomerular lesions in the majority of patients with poststreptococcal acute nephritis will heal, especially in children and in victims of epidemics. In our Trinidad studies, involving mostly children, the number of patients who have abnormal urine two and three years after their acute nephritis is less than 1%. Of these, we have established the diagnosis of proliferative chronic diffuse glomerulonephritis in only two or perhaps three persons.

Observations such as this have led Rammelkamp[10] and perhaps some of the speakers at this conference to believe that poststreptococcal acute nephritis is not an antecedent of chronic glomerulonephritis. However, in sporadic cases in adults, we believe that we have followed a number of patients whose initial attack of poststreptococcal acute nephritis unequivocally has failed to heal. Further, several such patients have had exacerbations with subsequent streptococcal infections. An exacerbation is an exact replica of the initial acute attack, but it occurs in a patient with chronic glomerulonephritis. Usually renal function returns to its former level after an exacerbation. Exacerbations do not appear to increase the rate of progression in chronic glomerulonephritis. In the absence of hypertension patients with poststreptococcal chronic glomerulonephritis do quite well. They may go 20 to 40 years before renal function decreases to levels that produce symptoms.

Once the lesion has healed, second attacks of acute nephritis are very unusual. This probably reflects the lasting immunity induced by specific M types of streptococci and the relatively few M types associated with nephritogenicity. However, cutaneous infections apparently are associated with the ready emergence of new M types, many of which also appear to be associated with nephritogenicity. In Trinidad, for instance, over a five-year period five separate peaks in the epidemic were associated with a different M type of streptococcus.[11]

This turmoil in skin streptococcus affords a greater opportunity for second attacks, and this already has been reported in rural areas around cities in the southeast United States.

In the figure the nephrotic phase is illustrated as developing toward the end of the course of chronic glomerulonephritis. A special line in the figure reminds us that the majority of patients with the nephrotic syndrome do not have poststreptococcal diffuse proliferative glomerulonephritis. And probably no more than a quarter of patients with chronic diffuse proliferative glomerulonephritis ever develop the nephrotic syndrome.

We have studied[12] a group of 35 patients with chronic nephritis who on renal biopsy were found to have had diffuse proliferative glomerulonephritis similar to the lesions seen in patients who had acute diffuse glomerulonephritis that failed to heal. At least two thirds of these had an onset of acute nephritis that followed infections that could be streptococcal in origin.

Analysis of Type 12 serum antibodies in the serum of this group of 35 patients revealed that one third were positive.[12] Studies in other renal diseases, or in the general population, reveal Type 12 antibodies in only 10 to 12%. Some of these patients also had the nephrotic syndrome. However, the majority of instances of the nephrotic syndrome represent other diseases.

Table II. CHRONIC GLOMERULONEPHRITIS

1)	Diffuse proliferative—poststreptococcal: early latent, chronic, active, terminal
2)	Diffuse membranous
3)	Mixed membranous and proliferative: lobular, progressive, hypocomplementemic (?)
4)	Focal: membranous, proliferative, or mixed
5)	Associated with other diseases: amyloid, diabetes, systemic lupus erythematosus, periarteritis, etc.
6)	Familial nephropathy

Chronic Glomerulonephritis

Different types of chronic glomerulonephritis are listed in Table I. Chronic diffuse proliferative glomerulonephritis has already been discussed. Diffuse membranous glomerular lesions appear to represent a fairly homogeneous group, and perhaps even a single disease. I shall discuss the natural history of this later.

Some patients with chronic nephritis are found on renal biopsy to have mixed membranous and proliferative lesions. Some investigators call this membranoproliferative glomerulonephritis. Other labels include lobular glomerulonephritis and rapidly progressive chronic glomerulonephritis. This also may represent a group of diseases that West has labeled hypocomplementemic glomerulonephritis.[13] I shall not say much about it, because our group has studied only five such patients. In any case, these instances are quite different from the classic diffuse proliferative disease and from diffuse membranous glomerular lesions. The question mark in Table II represents the uncertainty that all investigators are talking about the same or different diseases under these labels.

Since renal biopsies have become available, one of the most common findings in patients with persistently abnormal urine has been focal glomerular lesions. These may be membranous, proliferative, or mixed. This probably is not a homogenous group. The natural history of this will be discussed later.

Chronic glomerular lesions also may be associated with any number of systemic diseases or other general diseases such as amyloid, diabetes, and systemic lupus erythematosus. Familial nephropathy should be kept in mind in patients who appear to have chronic glomerulonephritis. These patients may have episodes of gross hematuria, sometimes in association with infection. This condition, I believe, is a fairly common

TABLE III. NEPHROTIC SYNDROME: CAUSES

1) Lipoid nephrosis—synonym "nil disease"
2) Membranous—diffuse, focal
3) Proliferative—diffuse, focal
4) Mixed membranous and proliferative
5) Others: amyloid, diabetes, renal vein thrombosis, allergy, drugs, etc.
6) Rarely, if ever—pyelonephritis and nephrosclerosis

TABLE IV. THIRTY-FIVE ADULTS WITH THE NEPHROTIC SYNDROME

Glomerular lesion	*Number of patients*	*Present number with progressive disease*	*Number dead*
Lipoid nephrosis	9	0	2*
Membranous	7	4	4
Proliferative	14	8	4
Mixed	5	5	4
Totals	35	17	14

*See text. Reproduced by permission from Earle, D. P., Jennings, R. B. and Bernik, M. A consideration of the histopathological basis for the nephrotic syndrome. *Prog. Cardiov. Dis.* 4:48-69, 1961.

cause of abnormal urine and renal insufficiency. In the Chicago area we now have at least seven families with familial nephropathy. Most of these were diagnosed as chronic glomerulonephritis by their physicians.

NEPHROTIC SYNDROME

Some of the different diseases that may be associated with the nephrotic syndrome are listed in Table III. The nephrotic syndrome is not a disease, but will occur in any renal disease in which enough albumin is lost in the urine to lower the serum albumin to the extent that edema ensues. It is associated with a number of different lesions. Nephrosis, lipoid nephrosis, or no glomerular lesion by light microscopy all refer to the same disease. Hereafter it will be called lipoid nephrosis. This is a common cause of the nephrotic syndrome in childhood, but it also occurs in adults.

Membranous glomerular lesions, either diffuse or focal, are commonly associated with the nephrotic syndrome. Not commonly associated are chronic proliferative glomerular lesions. The nephrotic syndrome also may be associated with a number of other diseases, some of

TABLE V. OUTCOME OF DIFFUSE MEMBRANOUS GLOMULAR LESIONS

*Outcome**	*Number of patients*	
Remission	9	Urine became normal in 6
No change	3	2 died of myocardial infarction
Deterioration	24	12 died (2 of myocardial infarction), 11 currently have azotemia or uremia

*Remission = disappearance of proteinuria, normal renal function.
No change = proteinuria in excess of 4 gm. per day, persisted; renal function did not decrease.
Deterioration = proteinuria persisted, renal function declined.

which are listed in Table III. Rarely, if ever, will pyelonephritis and nephrosclerosis have sufficient proteinuria to result in the nephrotic syndrome.

Table IV, taken from an earlier paper,[14] illustrates developments in 35 adults with nephrotic syndrome. All patients had adequate renal biopsies. Of the nine patients listed as having lipoid nephrosis, one had died and one had progressive renal failure at the time this paper was written. Even with these patients included, the prognosis is better than for the membranous and proliferative groups.

These old data are presented to illustrate a mistake which we believe is very instructive. In the group with lipoid nephrosis only two patients failed to respond to moderate doses of steroids. Clinically, these patients appeared no different from the others in this group. And in both the initial renal biopsy was interpreted as lipoid nephrosis. Unfortunately, electron microscopy was not available to us at that time.

One patient began to develop renal insufficiency after two years, and was dead at three years. Repeat renal biopsies near the onset of renal insufficiency and at autopsy showed diffuse membranous glomerular lesions. The other patient died after five years of a progressive downhill course, and at autopsy showed diffuse membranous glomerulonephritis.

At first we thought that these were instances of lipoid nephrosis that progressed into membranous glomerulonephritis. However, this was quite unlike our previous and subsequent experience with lipoid nephrosis in adults. Thus, Dr. Jennings restudied the initial biopsies. He obtained excellent evidence that we had made a mistake. The initial biopsies revealed that both patients had had diffuse membranous

TABLE VI. TWENTY-THREE PATIENTS WITH FOCAL GLOMULAR LESIONS

Type of lesion	*Number of patients*	
Glomular scars and RBC in Bowman's space and/or tubules	5	All have normal rental function 4 to 11 years after onset
Membranous	3	2 died 8 and 13 years after onset; 1 has azotemia
Proliferative	10	3 died; 6 have persistent urine abnormalities; 1 is normal
Mixed membranous and proliferative	5	4 have hypertension; 2 are on chronic dialysis

lesions from the beginning. We again can state that all our adult patients with lipoid nephrosis have responded to steroid therapy.

Diffuse Membranous Glomerular Lesions

Our experience in 36 patients with diffuse classical membranous glomerular lesions is summarized in Table V. All patients were followed to death, or for at least five years, and some of them longer. Nine patients underwent remissions, and in six the urine became normal. These nine, the three who had no change, plus a number of other patients—a total of 24—were treated with steroids. The response to steroids in this group of patients was so slow that it was difficult to ascribe with assurance the good outcome to steroid therapy with the exception of one patient who had a prompt and dramatic response. Of those not treated, none had a spontaneous remission. However, most of these patients were not treated because of the advanced stage of their disease.

Of this group 14 have died, four of myocardial infarctions at relatively young ages. The over-all prognosis of this group is not good. At the time of the last study 20 of the 22 who have not died had significant reduction in renal function. The rate of decline of renal function was variable, but glomerular filtration rates were reduced within three years of onset in 19 of the 36 patients. But in another four, from 8 to 17 years was required before renal function began to deteriorate. In contrast, patients with chronic diffuse proliferative glomerulonephritis may go for 25 to 45 years before they get into trouble.

Of the entire group of 36, serum complement was reduced in only one.

Focal Glomerular Lesions

The outcome in 23 patients with focal glomerular lesions is summarized in Table VI. Many of these patients were described in greater detail in an earlier paper.[15] These patients were also followed to death, or for at least four years. They all had adequate renal biopsies. During the time these patients were studied another 51 patients with focal glomerular lesions were seen who were lost to follow-up, or were followed for less than four years. The two groups did not differ clinically or in the distribution of type of lesions.

One group of patients with focal glomerular lesions had intermittent gross hematuria. In five of these renal biospy showed nothing but red blood cells in Bowman's space or in tubules with some glomerular scarring. Four of these are well. One still has abnormal urine but has not developed progressive decrease in renal function. In several the gross hematuria was associated with infections. The disease, whatever it is, appears benign.

Focal membranous lesions were found in three, two of whom have already died, although the course was not rapidly progressive. The survivor has azotemia.

In the proliferative group the disease in three has cleared while a trace of proteinuria continues in one. Three have died, and the others have developed hypertension or some degree of renal insufficiency. Very few of these patients were treated with steroids. No beneficial effects were noted when steroid therapy was tried.

In this group of patients with focal glomerular lesions a transient decrease in serum complement was noted in one. Three patients appeared to have some unknown systemic disease.

Another group of patients had focally distributed mixed membranous and proliferative glomerular lesions. The course of these patients has been fairly rapidly downhill. Two are already on dialysis, the others have impairment of renal function, and some have developed hypertension.

Summary

A variety of glomerular lesions are associated with acute and chronic renal diseases. Some of these diseases follow fairly predictable courses, and some have fairly uniform histologic appearance. We can establish diagnostic labels for many, but in most we have no good idea as to what the real etiology is. We do not even know what the natural histories of many of them are.

REFERENCES

1. Seegal, D. and Lyttle, J. D.: Anti-streptolysin 0 titer of the serum in acute glomerulonephritis. *Proc. Soc. Exp. Biol. Med., 31*:211, 1933.
2. Baehr, G. and Lande, H.: Glomerulonephritis as a complication of subacute streptococcus endocarditis. *J.A.M.A. 75*:789, 1920.
3. Seegal, D.: Acute glomerulonephritis following pneumococcic lobar pneumonia. *Arch. Intern. Med. 56*:912, 1935.
4. Tu, W. H., Shearn, M. A. and Lee, J. C.: Acute diffuse glomerulonephritis in acute staphylococcal endocarditis. *Ann. Intern. Med. 71*:335, 1969.
5. Bates, R. C., Jennings, R. B. and Earle, D. P.: Acute nephritis unrelated to group A hemolytic streptococcus infection. *Amer. J. Med. 23*:510, 1957.
6. Baehr, G.: A benign and curable form of acute nephritis. *J. Amer. Med. Assn. 86*:1001, 1926.
7. Earle, D. P. and Seegal, D.: Natural history of glomerulonephritis. *J. Chron. Dis. 5*:3, 1957.
8. Poon-King, T., Mohammed, I., Cox, R., Potter, E. V., Simon, N. M., Siegel, A. C. and Earle, D. P.: Recurrent epidemic nephritis in South Trinidad. *New Eng. J. Med. 277*:728, 1967.
9. Potter, E. V., Moran, A. F., Poon-King, T. and Earle, D. P.: Characteristics of B-hemolytic streptococci associated with acute glomerulonephritis in Trinidad, West Indies. *J. Lab. Clin. Med. 71*:126, 1968.
10. Rammelkamp, C. H., Jr.: The Streptococcus and Chronic Glomerulonephritis. In: *Controversy in Medicine.* Ingelfinger, F., Relman, A. and Finland, M., eds. Philadelphia, Saunders, 1966, p. 342.
11. Earle, D. P., Poon-King, T., Potter, E. V., Finklea, J. F., Sharrett, E. R. and Ortiz, J.: Streptococcal skin infections and epidemic acute nephritis in Trinidad. *Trans. Amer. Clin. Climat. Assn.* In press.
12. Earle, D. P. and Jennings, R. B.: Poststreptococcal Glomerulonephritis. In: *Ciba Symposium on Renal Biopsy.* Wolstenholme, G. E. W. and Cameron, M. P., eds. London, Churchill, 1961, p. 156.
13. West, C. D., Winter, S., Forristal, J., McConville, J. M. and Davis, N. C.: Evidence for *in vivo* breakdown of BIC-globulin in hypo-complementemic glomerulonephritis. *J. Clin. Invest. 46*:539, 1967.
14. Earle, D. P., Jennings, R. B. and Bernik, M. B.: A consideration of the histopathologic basis for the nephrotic syndrome. *Progr. Cardiov. Dis. 4*:148, 1961.
15. Earle, D. P. and Jennings, R. B.: Focal glomerular lesions. *Trans. Amer. Clin. Climat. Ass. 72*:24, 1960.

PATHOLOGY OF GLOMERULONEPHRITIS*

JACOB CHURG

Clinical Professor of Pathology
Mount Sinai School of Medicine
New York, N. Y.

THE morphological features of glomerulonephritis were established by post-mortem examination during the second half of the 19th and the first half of the 20th centuries.[1] In the last 20 years much additional information has been obtained from renal biopsies by means of a variety of newer histologic techniques such as thin sectioning, special stains, electron microscopy, and immunofluorescence microscopy.[2, 3] This information has improved our understanding of the structure of the kidney, of the nature of the pathologic processes in the glomerulus, and of the interrelations between the various forms of glomerulonephritis.

The structure of the normal glomerulus is well known and is discussed in detail in the standard textbooks of histology. For our purpose it is sufficient to note that the glomerulus has three structural components: the Bowman's capsule, the capillary walls, and the mesangial stalk. Each component consists of cells and intercellular material represented by basement membranes and mesangial matrix. The structural components enclose two spaces: the Bowman's or urinary space and the blood space of the capillary lumina.

Glomerulonephritis is characterized by a striking increase in the number of cells and in the amount of intercellular material in one or more of the structural components but especially in the mesangium and in the Bowman's capsule. Other "inflammatory" changes also occur, such as exudation of leukocytes, thrombosis of the capillaries, and necrosis of the glomerular tuft. A special feature of glomerulonephritis is deposition in various parts of the glomerulus of proteins derived from blood plasma, such as gamma globulins, complement, and fibrinogen.

*Presented at a *Conference on Glomerulonephritis* held by the New York Heart Association at The Waldorf-Astoria, New York, N. Y., January 27, 1970.

This study was supported by Public Health Service Research Grant AM-00918 from the National Institute of Arthritis and Metabolic Diseases, Bethesda, Md.

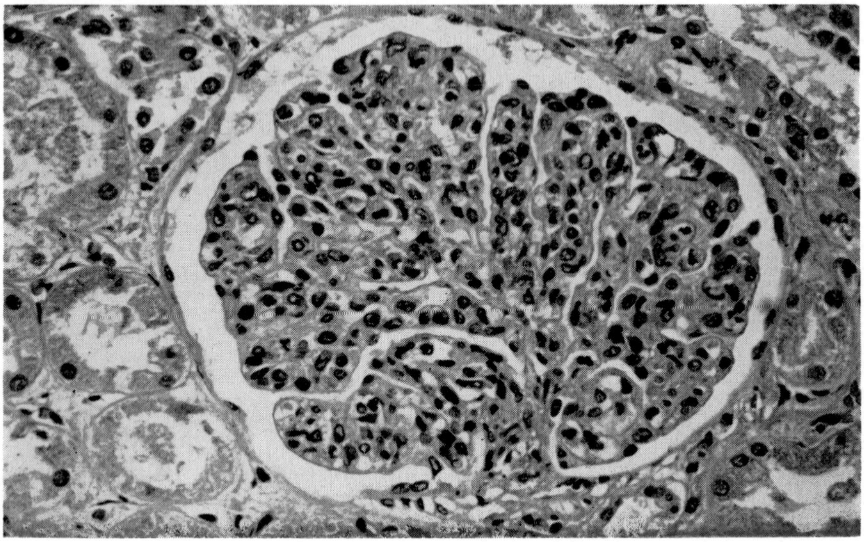

Fig. 1. Diffuse proliferative glomerulonephritis. There is marked increase in the number of cells, most of them mesangial. A small number of polymorphonuclear leukocytes is also present. Most of the capillary lumina are compressed. ×350

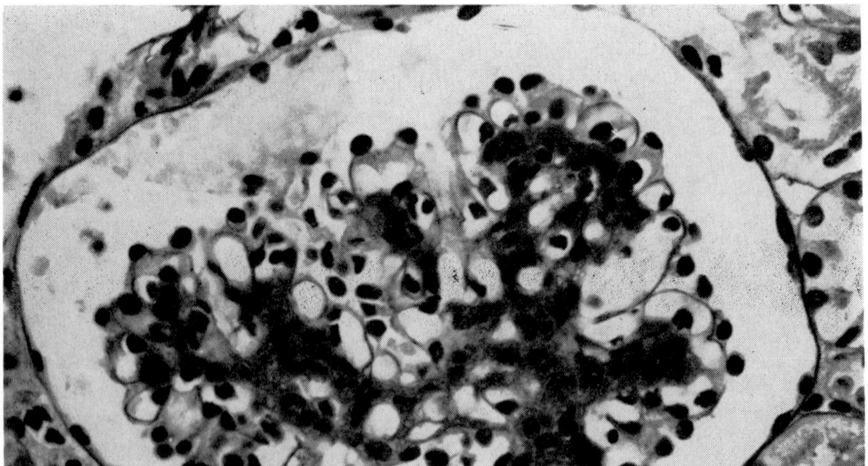

Fig. 2. Resolving diffuse glomerulonephritis. Increased number of cells and some matrix are present in the mesangial stalk. The capillaries are present. ×560

Traditionally glomerulonephritis is divided into two types: diffuse, where 90 to 100% of glomeruli are involved, and focal, where only some glomeruli and usually only parts (segments) of these glomeruli are affected. This division is not absolute since focal glomerulonephritis may progress to diffuse and, on the other hand, resolving diffuse glomerulonephritis may be apparent in some glomeruli only.

Diffuse Glomerulonephritis

Proliferation of mesangial cells occurs in most varieties of glomerulonephritis but is especially characteristic and striking after a streptococcal or other infection. This process is often given the name of acute proliferative glomerulonephritis. However, "acute" is a clinical term; to the pathologist the disease should be called *diffuse proliferative and exudative glomerulonephritis* (Figure 1). The cells multiply rapidly, expanding the mesangium, which may enlarge to many times normal size. The capillary lumina are compressed by the pressure of the mesangial cells and also by swelling and perhaps by some proliferation of the endothelial cells. A variable number of polymorphonuclear leukocytes is found in the capillary lumina, the mesangium, and the urinary space. In the more severe cases the mesangium invades the capillary wall so that some of the proliferating cells lie between the basement membrane and the endothelium. A small amount of mesangial matrix may be laid down early in the disease, which adds to the size of the mesangium. Rarely do thrombi form in the capillary lumina. On occasion the epithelial cells of the Bowman's capsule also participate; they form crescents of variable size. All these processes may combine to obstruct completely the flow of blood in the glomerulus and to produce renal failure. However, in many instances cellular proliferation remains mild and tends to regress rapidly. Generally there is little correlation between the severity of the anatomical and the clinical manifestations except that renal failure is much more apt to occur when severe morphological changes are present.

The major contribution of both electron microscopy and immunofluorescence microscopy was the demonstration of protein deposits in the capillary walls. These deposits are localized between the epithelium and the basement membrane in the form of isolated dome-shaped or flame-shaped structures, often called "humps." They consist of, or at least contain, gamma globulins, complement, and some fibrinogen.

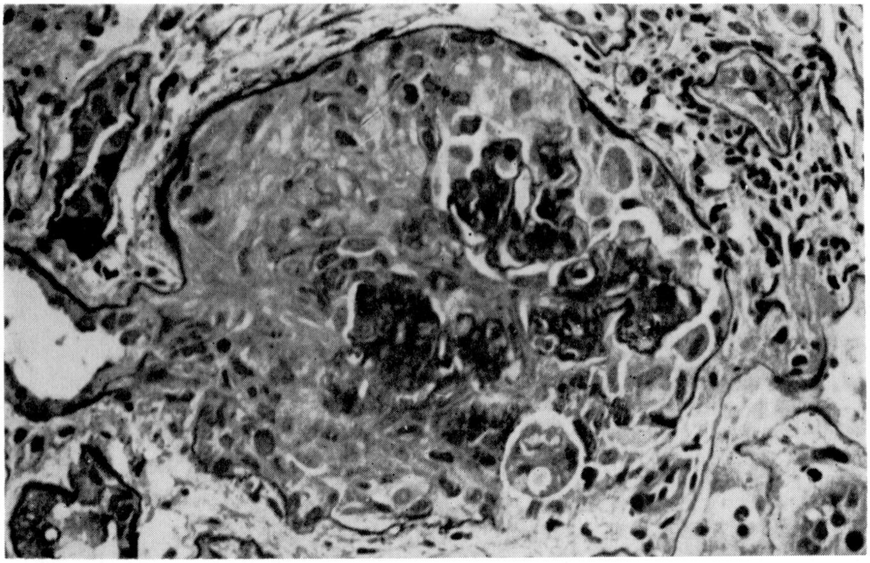

Fig. 3. Rapidly progressing (extracapillary) glomerulonephritis. The urinary space is filled by a large fibroepithelial crescent. The compressed capillary tuft is represented by small dark areas toward the center and the right side of the glomerulus. ×410

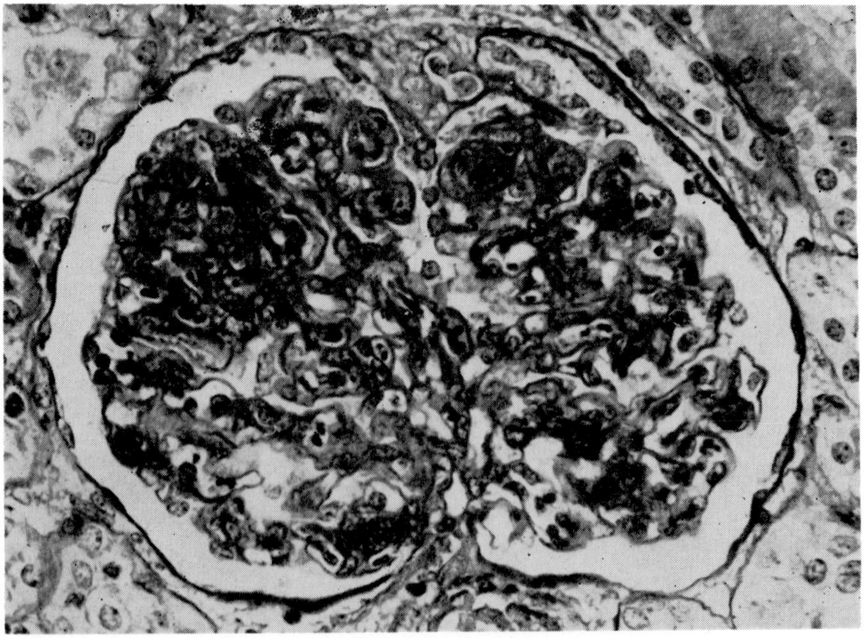

Fig. 4. Chronic membranoproliferative (mesangiocapillary) glomerulonephritis. The mesangial areas are enlarged and contain cells and dark-staining matrix. ×430

There is also some evidence that they contain material derived from streptococci, possibly in the form of antigen-antibody complexes.

As is well known, the great majority of patients—80 to 85% of children and a somewhat lower percentage of adults—recover completely. In some patients recovery takes several months or even several years, with persistent proliferation of mesangial cells in the stalk (Figure 2) and gamma globulin deposits. These changes gradually diminish and the symptoms abate. In other instances a few glomeruli are severely damaged and continue to leak protein until they become completely obsolete. This represents "healing with a defect." Relatively few patients, perhaps 10% of children and 20% of adults, progress to chronic glomerulonephritis. A small percentage, perhaps no more than 5%, used to die in acute failure, either renal or cardiac, but this number has decreased with the advent of dialysis.

Rapidly Progressive Glomerulonephritis

Another form of proliferative glomerulonephritis, less common but much more serious, is characterized by multiplication of the cells of the Bowman's capsule with formation of large crescents and compression of the capillary tufts. Proliferation of the mesangial or endothelial cells is much less conspicuous and is often entirely absent. This disease may also occur after an infection, streptococcal or otherwise, but usually has no known antecedents. It is known to clinicians as *rapidly progressive or malignant glomerulonephritis* and to pathologists as *extracapillary glomerulonephritis* (Figure 3). Proliferation of the epithelial cells is accompanied by deposition of a supporting framework. This at first consists of fibrin, later of material that resembles basement membranes, and finally of collagen. Epithelial crescents are thus converted into fibrous masses. If seen early, the disease is often focal, but it rapidly becomes diffuse. Clinically, it may be associated with a number of entities or syndromes, such as Goodpasture's syndrome, Henoch-Schoenlein purpura, or periarteritis nodosa. However, it is often "idiopathic." Prognosis is always grave because of the rapid obliteration of the glomeruli.

Electron microscopic findings are not specific, but immunofluorescence shows linear deposits of gamma globulin along the capillary basement membranes. These appear to be located on the endothelial side of the basement membrane.

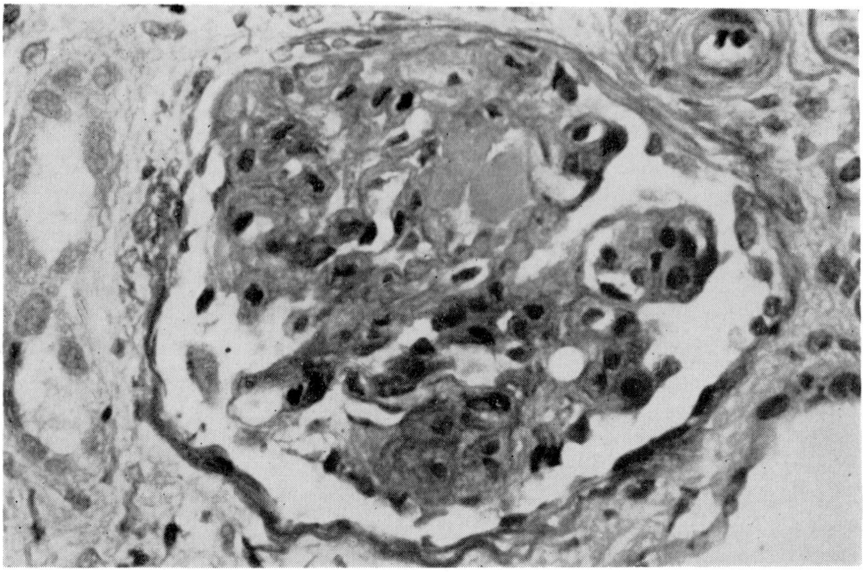

Fig. 5. Chronic sclerosing glomerulonephritis. The glomerulus is largely replaced by mesangial matrix (dark staining) and hyalin (lighter staining). A small number of cells can still be identified. ×560

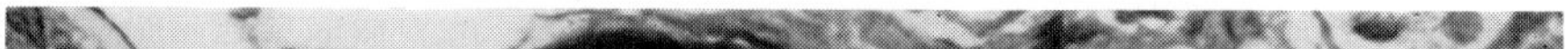

Fig. 6. Focal glomerulonephritis. A segment of the glomerular tuft on the right side shows proliferation of cells, sclerosis, and hyalinization. ×560

Chronic Glomerulonephritis

Transition of diffuse proliferative glomerulonephritis from the acute into the chronic stage is marked by the increasing presence of intercellular substances, such as mesangial matrix and collagen. In the earlier (subacute) phase of the chronic stage the quantity of these substances is about equal to that of cells (proliferative and sclerosing glomerulonephritis). Later the cells are replaced progressively by the intercellular material (sclerosing glomerulonephritis) until the glomeruli are converted into acellular nodules ("end-stage" glomerulonephritis). This process is accompanied by atrophy of tubules, interstitial fibrosis, and inflammation and also by sclerosis of arteries and by hypertension.

It is well established that in the great majority of cases of chronic glomerulonephritis there is no evidence of preceding acute glomerulonephritis. It is probable that in some patients the acute attack has been inapparent or has been forgotten. However, in most patients the disease appears to be chronic from the beginning and has no known etiology.

The newly formed mesangial matrix and the proliferating cells expand the mesangial stalk, though at first they do not obliterate the capillaries. In some instances the lobular centers are markedly enlarged (*lobular glomerulonephritis*). In the more severe cases, mesangial cells and matrix invade the capillary walls growing between the endothelium and the basement membrane. Deposits of protein within this newly formed mesangial layer, or between the basement membrane and the endothelium, further increase the thickness of the capillary walls. This form of the disease is known as membranoproliferative glomerulonephritis. However, the basement membranes are not actually thickened and a better name for the disease would be mesangiocapillary glomerulonephritis (Figure 4). Expansion of the lobular centers and thickening of the capillary walls are but two aspects of the same process and usually occur together.

Fibrocellular and later fibrous crescents are often seen in chronic glomerulonephritis, but they are relatively uncommon in the lobular and membranoproliferative forms.

In the sclerosing or "end-stage" glomerulonephritis most of the cells have disappeared and the glomeruli consist mainly of mesangial matrix, collapsed capillary basement membranes, and protein (hyaline) deposits (Figure 5). A variable number of fibrous crescents may also be present.

Diffuse sclerosing glomerulonephritis is usually the result of a previous diffuse proliferative and sclerosing disease, but it may also represent the terminal stage of a focal glomerulonephritis.

Focal Glomerulonephritis

Focal glomerulonephritis is characterized by a limited involvement of the kidney that affects, at least initially, only small segments of some glomeruli. The glomerular lesions are somewhat similar to those of diffuse glomerulonephritis except that they are limited in scope. The affected part of the glomerular tuft shows proliferation of mesangial, endothelial, or epithelial cells and, later, increased amounts of intercellular material. This represents focal proliferative glomeruonephritis. A more severe form of the same disease is called focal necrotizing glomerulonephritis. Here thrombosis and necrosis of the capillaries is usually accompanied by prominent epithelial crescents.

Proliferative and necrotizing focal glomerulonephritis is seen in many systemic diseases involving the kidney, such as systemic lupus erythematosus, periarteritis nodosa, Henoch-Schoenlein purpura, subacute bacterial endocarditis, and Goodpasture's syndrome. However, in some instances the disease appears to be purely renal. Focal glomerulonephritis in its acute stage may progress into diffuse glomerulonephritis. On the other hand, the lesions may heal, possibly by resolution but more often by focal sclerosis or scarring. Such scarring is usually accompanied by the formation of adhesions between the affected segment of the tuft and the Bowman's capsule (Figure 6).

Another form of focal glomerulonephritis is manifested from the very beginning by segmental sclerosis together with cell proliferation. Crescents may overlie the sclerotic areas. Progression of the disease consists of involvement of increasingly larger areas in the glomerulus and involvement of glomeruli which were initially spared. The end stage of this process may be indistinguishable from the diffuse sclerosing glomerulonephritis.

REFERENCES

1. Bell, E. T.: *Renal Diseases*, 2d ed. Philadelphia, Lea & Febiger, 1950.
2. Heptinstall, R. H.: *Pathology of the Kidney*. Boston, Little, Brown. 1966.
3. Becker, E. L.: Structural Basis of Renal Disease. New York, Evanston, Ill., and London, Hoeber Medical Division, 1968.

EVIDENCE FOR IMMUNOLOGIC MECHANISMS IN SEVERAL FORMS OF HUMAN GLOMERULAR DISEASES*

ROBERT T. McCLUSKEY

Professor and Chairman
Department of Pathology
School of Medicine
State University of New York at Buffalo
Buffalo, N. Y.

It is now well established that there are two major forms of immunologically induced glomerular disease, namely, immune complex disease and antiglomerular basement membrane antibody (anti-GBM) disease. Both forms have been studied extensively in experimental models and both have been recognized in human glomerular diseases.

In order to provide a background for the understanding of the diseases in man some of the salient features of the experimental models will first be reviewed (Unanue and Dixon,[23] McCluskey and Vassalli[16]). Immune complex diseases may be defined as diseases in which the lesions, which occur principally in glomeruli, are due to the deposition from the circulation of antigen-antibody complexes (immune complexes). The glomerular lesions can be referred to as immune complex glomerulonephritis or nephritis. Complexes that contain any one of a variety of antigens can produce glomerular disease and, in all instances, they localize in glomeruli for reasons not related to the immunologic specificity of the antibody. The mechanisms leading to glomerular localization of complexes are not entirely understood; ultimately localization depends on the size of the complexes which cause them to be trapped along the basement membrane or in mesangial regions. However, it is clear that other factors influence localization, including vasoactive amines which are released in the circulation as the result of the presence of immune complexes (McCluskey and Vassalli[16]).

The first form of immune complex diseases studied experimentally was acute serum sickness. This is usually produced in rabbits by a single intravenous injection ("one shot") of a large amount of foreign serum

*Presented at a *Conference on Glomerulonephritis* held by the New York Heart Association at The Waldorf-Astoria, January 27, 1970.

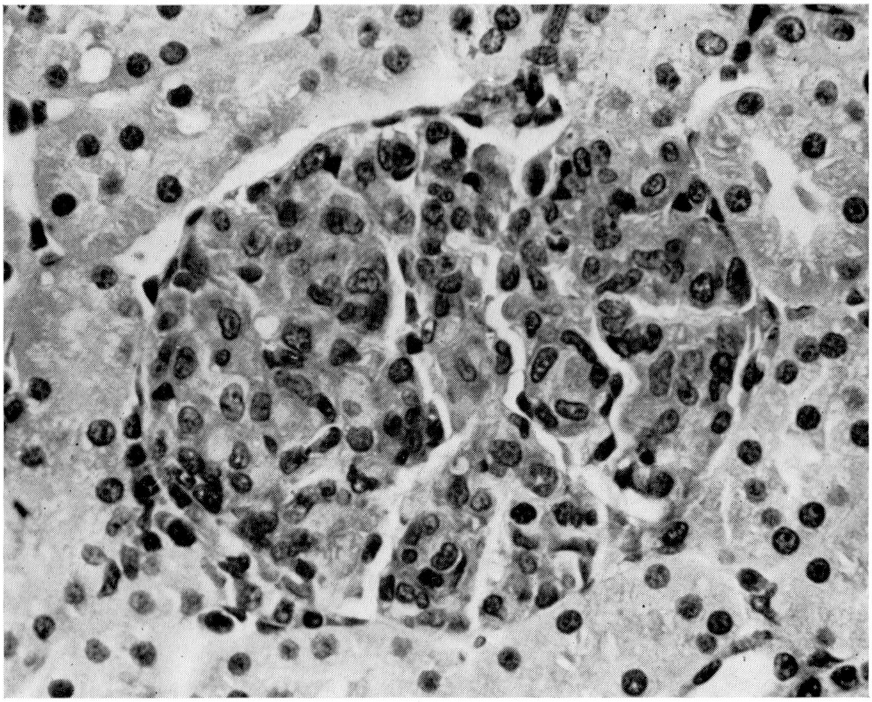

Fig. 1. Glomerulus from a rabbit with acute serum sickness. There is considerable swelling and proliferation of endothelial and mesangial cells (H & E). Reproduced by permission from: McCluskey, R. T. and Vassalli, P. Experimental Glomerular Diseases. In: *The Kidney*. New York, Academic Press, 1969.

or foreign plasma protein, commonly bovine serum albumin (BSA). Several days after the injection the rabbit begins to produce antibodies against the injected protein. When these are first released into the blood there is still a high level of antigen there, and for this reason soluble antigen-antibody complexes are formed. Most of these are quickly removed from the circulation by the cells of the reticuloendothelial system, within which they are rapidly degraded. However, in some rabbits fairly substantial amounts are deposited over the course of several days in glomeruli, where they usually lead to acute diffuse glomerulonephritis (Figure 1) and focally within arteries where they produce a necrotizing arteritis. The glomeruli are usually rather uniformly involved, but sometimes focal necrotizing changes are seen. Within the affected glomeruli, antibody, antigen, and components of complement are generally demonstrable by immunofluorescence as sparse, scattered,

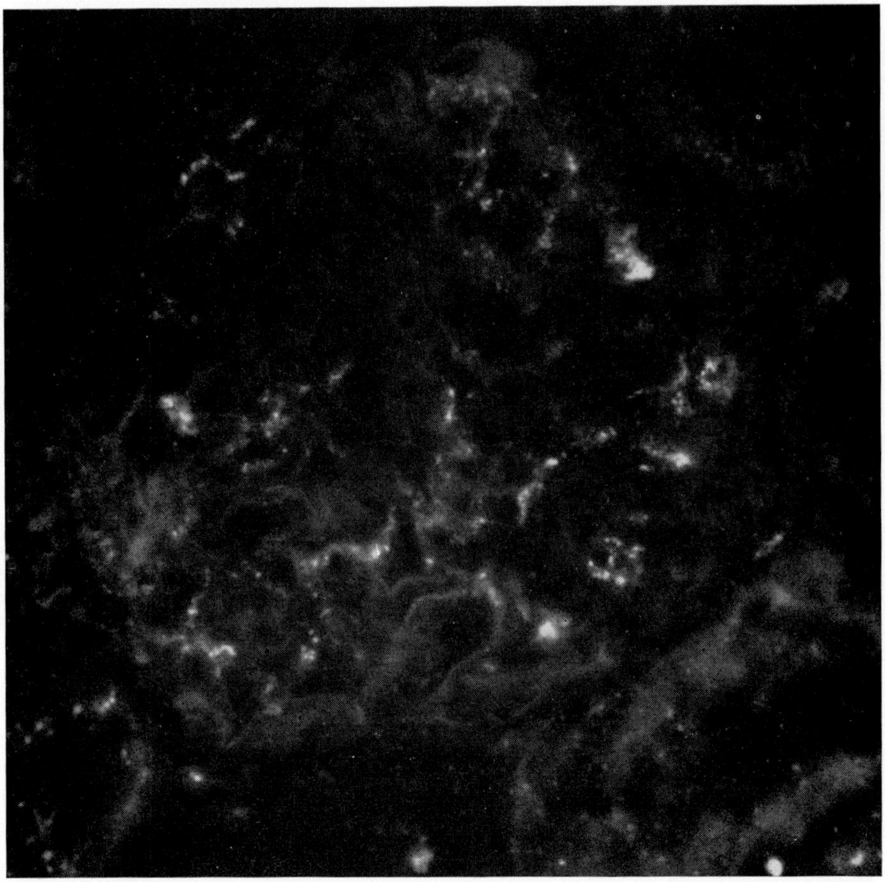

Fig. 2. Immunofluorescent section of glomerulus from rabbit with acute serum sickness stained for gamma globulin. Granular deposits are present focally along the basement membrane and in mesangial regions. Reproduced by permission from: McCluskey, R. T. and Vassalli, P. Experimental Glomerular Diseases. In: *The Kidney,* New York, Academic Press, 1969.

granular deposits in mesangial regions and along the basement membrane (Figure 2). By electron microscopy the immune complexes can sometimes be seen as dark granular deposits, often on the epithelial side of the basement membrane. In rabbits with acute serum sickness the glomerular lesions heal rapidly provided no further injections of antigen are given.

Other types of glomerular lesions may be produced by giving rabbits daily intravenous injections of smaller amounts of foreign plasma protein for many weeks or months (chronic serum sickness) (Dixon, Feldman,

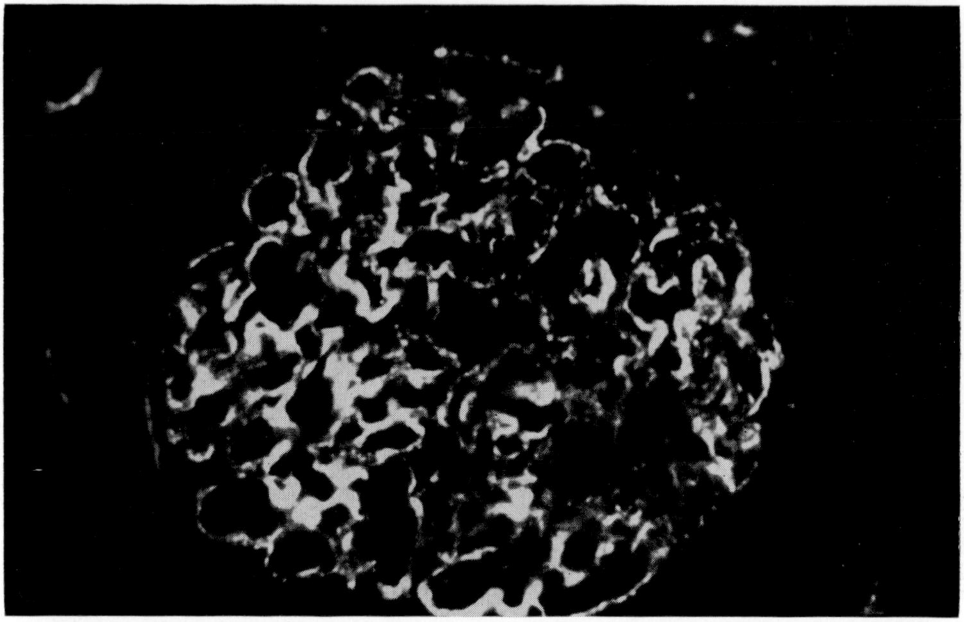

Fig. 3. Immunofluorescent findings in glomerulus of animal with chronic immune complex disease (Heymann's nephrosis). Finely granular deposits of gamma globulin are seen all along the basement membranes. Kindly provided by Dr. John Klassen.

and Vazquez[4]). Some rabbits treated in this way produce antibody in such amounts that each injection of antigen leads to the formation of soluble complexes in the circulation, which persist for at least several hours. After weeks or months of daily injections most such rabbits develop chronic glomerular lesions characterized by diffuse thickening of glomerular capillary walls caused principally by numerous, large deposits of immune complexes, usually along the epithelial side of the basement membrane (Figures 3 and 4). In many of these rabbits, proliferation of glomerular cells and neutrophil infiltration are inconspicuous or absent. However, in other rabbits proliferation of mesangial cells with accentuation of lobular structure and increased mesangial matrix are predominant features of the glomerular lesions (Germuth et al.[7]). Thus a wide variety of morphologic varieties of glomerular lesions may be produced by immune complexes deposited from the circulation. Probably this depends on many factors, including the species, the amount of deposition, the time during which complexes are deposited, varying capacity of different complexes to produce tissue damage, and precise

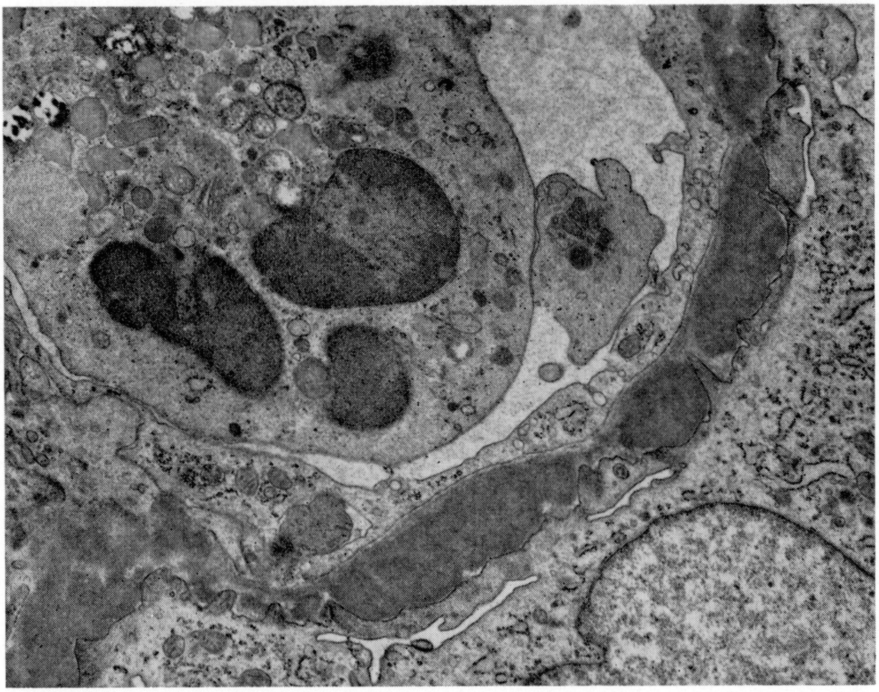

Fig. 4. Electronmicrograph of glomerulus from rabbit with chronic serum sickness. Broad, electron-dense deposits are seen along the outer surface of the basement membrane. Figure, kindly provided by Dr. Joseph D. Feldman, is reproduced by permission from: McCluskey, R. T. and Vassalli, P. Experimental Glomerular Diseases. In: *The Kidney*. New York, Academic Press, 1969.

localization of complexes within glomeruli. In addition, secondary pathogenic mechanisms which come into play undoubtedly influence the type of glomerular reaction; these include the effects of neutrophils, the coagulation system, and probably many others (Unanue and Dixon;[23] McCluskey and Vassalli[16]).

Aside from foreign serum proteins another type of exogenous antigenic material which has been shown to be capable of inducing immune complex disease is material of viral origin (Dixon and Oldstone[5]). Thus it has been found that mice injected at birth with lymphocytic choriomeningitis virus develop a glomerular disease with granular accumulation of gamma globulin and complement; gamma globulin eluted from the glomeruli displays antiviral activity, and hence it presumably represents antibody deposited in the form of immune complexes containing viral antigen. Of particular interest is the fact that these mice may exhibit no severe manifestations of viral disease other than chronic immune complex disease affecting glomeruli. Although, as discussed later, several human glomerular diseases appear to be caused by immune complexes containing bacterial antigens no entirely satisfactory experimental model of such a disease has been described.

Still another type of immune complex disease is that produced by complexes formed of autoantibody and circulating autologous antigen (autologous immune complex disease). The best-studied model of this type is that first described by Heymann et al.,[11] who reported that rats given repeated intraperitoneal injections of homologous kidney extracts plus adjuvant develop a chronic glomerular disease manifested by the nephrotic syndrome. The glomeruli show little histologic change, but electron microscopy reveals numerous electron-dense deposits along the epithelial side of the basement membrane; by immunofluorescence numerous finely granular deposits of immunoglobulin and complement are seen (Figure 3). Although it was first thought that this represented a classical form of autoimmune glomerulonephritis, i.e., a disease caused by an immunological attack against an antigen normally present in glomeruli, the glomerular damage has been shown to result from the deposition of circulating immune complexes. Its pathogenesis can be summarized as follows (Glassock et al.[8]). The immunizing procedure with homologous renal tissue in adjuvant results in the formation of *auto*-antibodies directed against an autologous antigen normally present in renal tubular epithelium. This antigen normally is released continuously in small amounts into the circulation, where it forms complexes with the autoantibody, which then deposits in glomeruli, as any type of complex is prone to do. The fact that the antigen is a normal constituent of the kidney is irrelevant from the point of view of pathogenesis. Presumably any autologous material which is released into the circulation and against which autoantibody formation can be induced could be the antigen involved in autologous immune complex disease.

Aside from experimentally induced immune complex diseases there are several spontaneous forms seen in animals commonly used for experimental purposes. The most thoroughly studied is the disease seen in NZB/W and related strains of mice. The great majority of NZB/W mice spontaneously develop a severe glomerular disease which bears many morphologic similarities to lupus nephritis. The glomeruli show deposits of gamma globulins and complement which are usually most

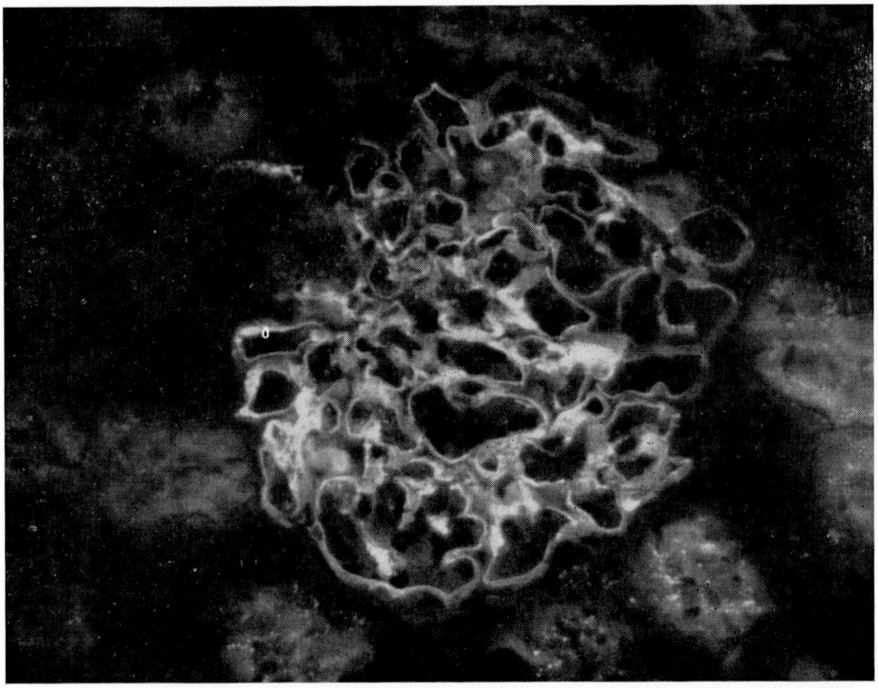

Fig. 5. Immunofluorescent pattern of staining for gamma globulin in animal with anti-GBM disease. There is completely continuous ("linear") staining along the basement membrane. Reproduced by permission from: McCluskey, R. T. and Vassalli, P. Experimental Glomerular Diseases. In: *The Kidney*. New York, Academic Press, 1969.

conspicuous in mesangial regions and on the endothelial side of the basement membrane. It has been found that the deposits represent immune complexes that contained antinuclear autoantibodies and nuclear antigens (Dixon, Oldstone, and Tonietti[6]). In other words the glomerular disease is an example of autologous immune complex nephritis. The etiology of the disease is unknown, but interestingly it has been shown that various viral infections will accelerate the appearance of antinuclear antibodies and of the glomerulonephritis (Dixon, Oldstone, and Tonietti[6]).

The second major type of immunologically induced glomerular disease is caused by antibodies directed against constituents of the glomerular basement membrane (anti-GBM disease). Two basic models have been described, one due to heterologous anti-GBM antibodies (Masugi or nephrotoxic serum nephritis) and the other by autoantibodies (autoimmune anti-GBM glomerulonephritis). The latter form is obviously more pertinent to the pathogenesis of spontaneous glomerular disease. Autoimmune anti-GBM glomerulonephritis was first described by Steblay,[20] who reported that sheep injected with heterologous glomerular basement-membrane preparations plus Freund's adjuvant often develop a severe, rapidly progressive glomerulonephritis characterized by proliferative and sclerosing changes with numerous conspicuous crescents. A highly characteristic feature is seen by immunofluorescence; it consists of an entirely smooth, continuous ("linear") accumulation of gamma globulin and complement along the basement membranes in all glomeruli (Figure 5). By electron microscopy dark deposits are either inconspicuous or absent. Studies of gamma globulin eluted from such glomeruli have shown that it is indeed anti-GBM antibody. In addition anti-GBM antibodies may be found in the circulation (Rudofsky and Steblay;[19] Lerner and Dixon[14]), and their titer is frequently elevated after bilateral nephrectomy; this indicates that they are being removed continuously from the circulation by fixation in glomeruli.

Based on observations of experimental models a summary may now be given of the features by which immune complex disease and anti-GBM diseases can usually be recognized. Immune complex diseases are characterized by irregular deposits of immunoglobulins (chiefly IgG) and complement and, when known, of antigen. Although the pattern of granular subepithelial deposits has been emphasized as most typical of immune complexes they may be seen in a variety of patterns along either side of, or within, the basement membrane and in mesangial regions. Nevertheless in all instances they are discontinuous deposits. In addition, electron microscopy of immune complex nephritis reveals dark granular deposits corresponding to sites where complexes are found by immunofluorescence. In contrast, anti-GBM disease is characterized by completely continuous "linear" accumulation of gamma globulin along the glomerular basement membranes. Although occasionally the deposits of immune complexes are so contiguous or so finely granular as to give a somewhat continuous pattern, under high power some granularity can always be discerned (Figure 3).

Turning to the situation in man: it can now be stated with assurance that both major forms of immunological glomerular diseases occur. Immune complex disease appears to be considerably more common than anti-GBM disease.

Glomerular diseases which on the basis of available evidence appear

TABLE I. HUMAN GLOMERULAR DISEASES APPARENTLY CAUSED BY IMMUNE COMPLEXES

1) *Diseases of known etiology*
   a) Poststreptococcal glomerulonephritis
   b) Glomerulonephritis associated with other bacterial infections: staphylococcal?; pneumococcal?; syphilis?; bacterial endocarditis?
   c) Glomerulonephritis associated with malaria
2) *Glomerular diseases associated with systemic diseases of unknown cause*
   a) Lupus nephritis
   b) Nephritis with anaphylactoid purpura
   c) Nephritis in periarteritis nodosa?
   d) Nephritis in idiopathic "mixed" cryoglobulinemia?
3) *Primary glomerular diseases of unknown cause*
   a) Membranous glomerulonephritis
   b) Membranoproliferative glomerulonephritis
   c) Chronic sclerosing glomerulonephritis?
   d) Unclassified glomerular diseases?
   e) IgA IgG nephropathy (Berger)[3]

to be forms of immune complex nephritis can be considered under three groups (Table I): 1) diseases of known etiology, 2) systemic diseases of unknown etiology, and 3) diseases of unknown etiology affecting only glomeruli. In the first group (Table I) the most important disease is poststreptococcal glomerulonephritis, which in most respects is faithfully reproduced in the model of acute ("one-shot") serum sickness. Histologically acute poststreptococcal glomerulonephritis is usually characterized by diffuse swelling and proliferation of endothelial and mesangial cells and by variable degrees of neutrophil infiltration. Although this picture closely resembles that seen in acute serum sickness, this alone would not provide impressive evidence of a common type of pathogenesis. However, the immunofluorescent and electron microscopic studies usually reveal the characteristic features of immune complex disease, namely, granular accumulation of immunoglobulins and complement along the basement membrane, and less often in mesangial regions, and electron-dense deposits, typically along the epithelial side of the basement membrane (humps). The immunofluorescent findings not only provide evidence for an immune complex basis but appear to eliminate the possibility that the glomerular disease is caused by anti-GBM antibodies. This mechanism has been suggested because there are cross-reacting antigens contained in streptococci and glomerular basement membranes. There has been disagreement as to whether streptococcal antigens are demonstrable within glomerular deposits, but at least two groups have reported their presence (Andres et al.;[1] Treser et al.[22]).

On the basis of these considerations the probable sequences of pathogenic events can be summarized as follows. During the streptococcal infection some streptococcal material is liberated in fairly large amounts into the circulation and, several days later, as specific antibodies are released, circulating complexes are formed with the streptococcal material. Substantial amounts of complexes are deposited in glomeruli during the course of several days but not thereafter. This scheme would account for the fact that poststreptococcal glomerulonephritis reaches its maximal intensity early (McCluskey and Baldwin[15]) and thereafter resolves until in most if not in all cases complete recovery ensues. However, granting the general validity of this scheme a number of questions remain, notably the peculiar efficiency of certain types of Group A streptococci to produce immune complex nephritis and the relatively long time required in many cases for recovery, in comparison with acute serum sickness.

Aside from poststreptococcal glomerulonephritis certain other unusual types of glomerulonephritis are associated with bacterial infection and on the basis of admittedly scanty evidence can probably be considered as immune complex diseases. These include rare cases of acute diffuse glomerulonephritis in association with staphylococcal infections and, possibly, pneumococcal infections, glomerulonephritis that occurs in patients with bacterial endocarditis and, possibly, the glomerular lesions in some patients with syphilis.

Another glomerular disease of known etiology that is presumably an immune complex disease is a form of chronic proliferative glomerulonephritis associated with malaria. Further, there is evidence that malarial antigenic material is present in glomerular deposits (Ward and Conran[24]).

The second group of presumed immune complex diseases (Table I) are those that occur in patients with certain systemic diseases of unknown cause. The most important of these is lupus nephritis. Although the etiology of systemic lupus erythematosus (SLE) is unknown, there is now abundant evidence that the glomerular lesions are due to immune complexes deposited from the circulation. This interpretation is supported by immunofluorescent observations of irregular, often granular,

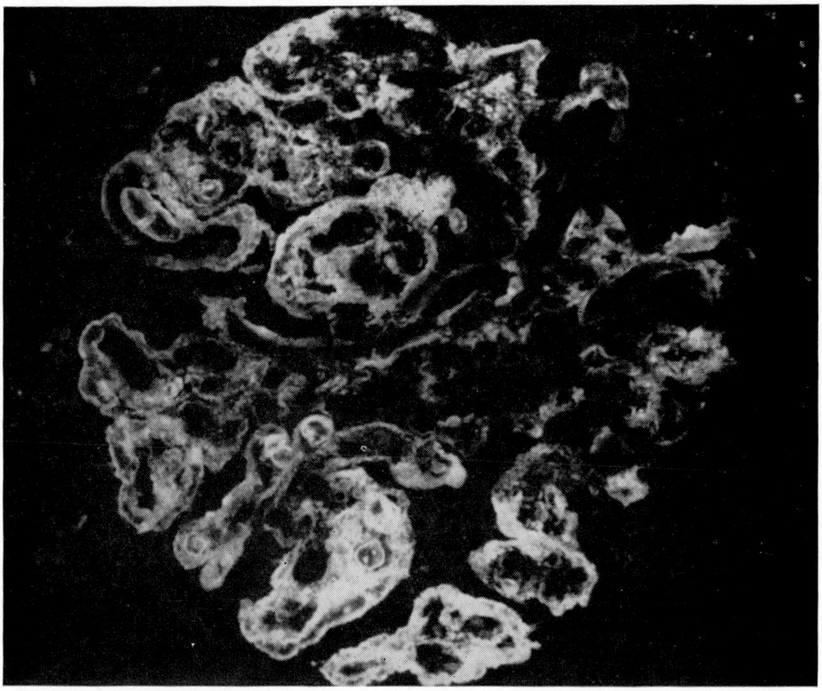

Fig. 6. Glomerulus from a patient with lupus nephritis stained for gamma globulin. There are markedly irregular deposits along the basement membrane and in mesangial regions. Reproduced by permission from: McCluskey, R. T. Immunopathologic Mechanisms in Human Renal Disease. Int. Convoc. on Immunol. Buffalo, N.Y., 1968. Basel, München, New York, S. Karger, 1969, pp. 300-12.

deposition of immunoglobulins and complement along the basement membrane and in mesangial regions (Figure 6) as well as by the finding by electron microscopy of dense, granular deposits in these locations. Further and more conclusive evidence has been provided by studies which have shown that both DNA antibody and DNA antigen can be identified within glomeruli (Krishman and Kaplan;[13] Koffler, Schur, and Kunkel[12]). Thus the complexes in glomeruli are composed of autoantibodies and autologous antigens, and lupus nephritis can be considered to be a form of autologous immune complex disease. The evidence obtained so far indicates that DNA anti-DNA complexes are the major if not the only complexes of pathogenetic significance. Why this is so is not clear and, in view of the numerous autoantibodies in SLE, it would seem likely that there would be the opportunity for the formation of a variety of complexes. The peculiar significance of DNA may be related to the fact that, unlike most autologous antigens against which autoantibodies are formed in SLE, it gains access to the circulation (Tan et al.[21]). Whether this occurs as the result of tissue damage or is a normal process is not known.

The glomerular lesions in patients with anaphylactoid purpura may also be caused by immune complexes, although the evidence is not conclusive and rests primarily on the finding of irregular deposits of immunoglobulins and complement in glomeruli. Nothing is known about the antigen presumed to be present in the deposits.

Another systemic disease of unknown etiology in which glomerular lesions occur and which may represent an immune complex disease is periarteritis nodosa (PAN). Considerable impetus for this belief came from observations that the arterial lesions closely resemble those of acute serum sickness. In addition immunoglobulins are demonstrable in some cases within the arterial and glomerular lesions in PAN. However in other cases immunoglobulins are absent, and further observations are needed to determine whether PAN is indeed an immune complex disease. Nothing is known of the possible antigen involved; the evidence relating the disease to drug hypersensitivity is not impressive (Baldwin and McCluskey[2]).

Finally, another systemic disease with glomerular lesions which may be caused by immune complexes is a recently described idiopathic condition characterized by a distinctive cryoglobulin and a syndrome consisting of purpura, arthralgia, weakness and, sometimes, glomerular disease (Meltzer et al.[18]). The cryoglobulin is composed of IgG and IgM; the latter has rheumatoid activity. The glomerular lesions which have been seen in patients studied so far can be classified as diffuse proliferative glomerulonephritis. Both IgM and IgG have been demonstrated in glomeruli as irregular deposits along the basement membrane. Assuming that the cryoglobulins are in fact immune complexes, this may be another example of autologous-immune complex disease.

In the third category of human glomerular diseases presumed to be immune complex diseases are several conditions of unknown cause which affect only glomeruli (Table I). At present these can be classified only on morphologic grounds (although certain clinical correlations exist), and even on morphologic grounds the classification of many of these diseases (almost all of which are included under the broad heading of glomerulonephritis) is not satisfactory.

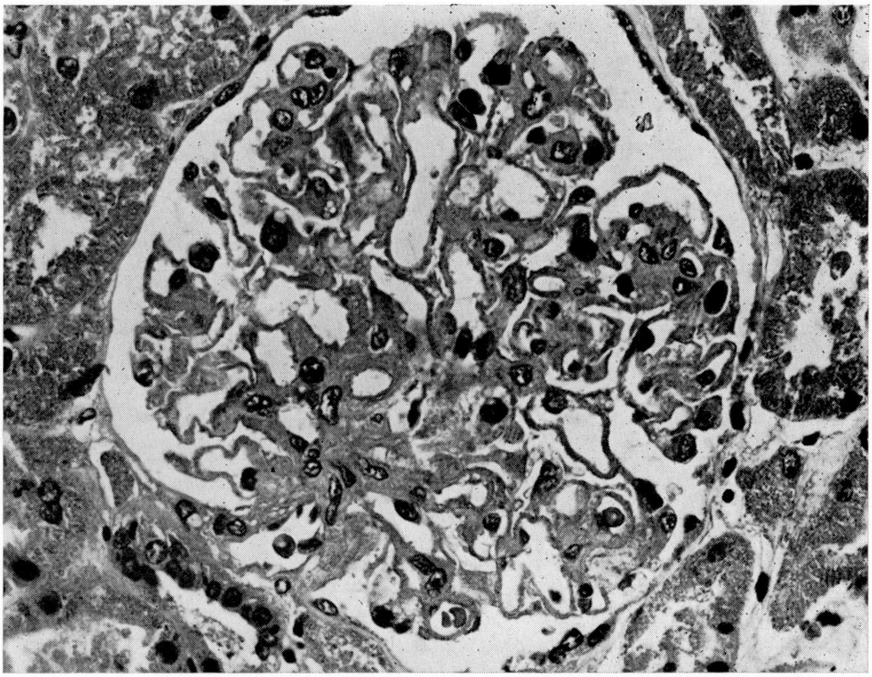

Fig. 7. Glomerulus from a patient with membranous glomerulonephritis. There is thickening of capillary walls which in places can be seen to have a granular appearance. H & E.

The first condition in this group is most often referred to as membranous glomerulonephritis (or membranous nephropathy). The patients are usually adults who present with the nephrotic syndrome, which follows a chronic course that occasionally remits and that sometimes ends in renal failure. The histologic picture is typical; all glomeruli show uniform thickening of capillary walls without significant proliferation or other changes (Figure 7). By immunofluorescence (Figure 8), granular deposits of immunoglobulins and complement are seen all along the basement membrane in all glomeruli (McCluskey et al.[17]). These correspond to electron-dense deposits along the epithelial side of the basement membrane. The resemblance of the lesions of membranous glomerulonephritis to those of certain forms of experimental chronic serum sickness and experimental autologous-immune complex disease (Heymann's nephrosis) make it seem almost certain that it is a form of chronic immune complex disease. However, there is no in-

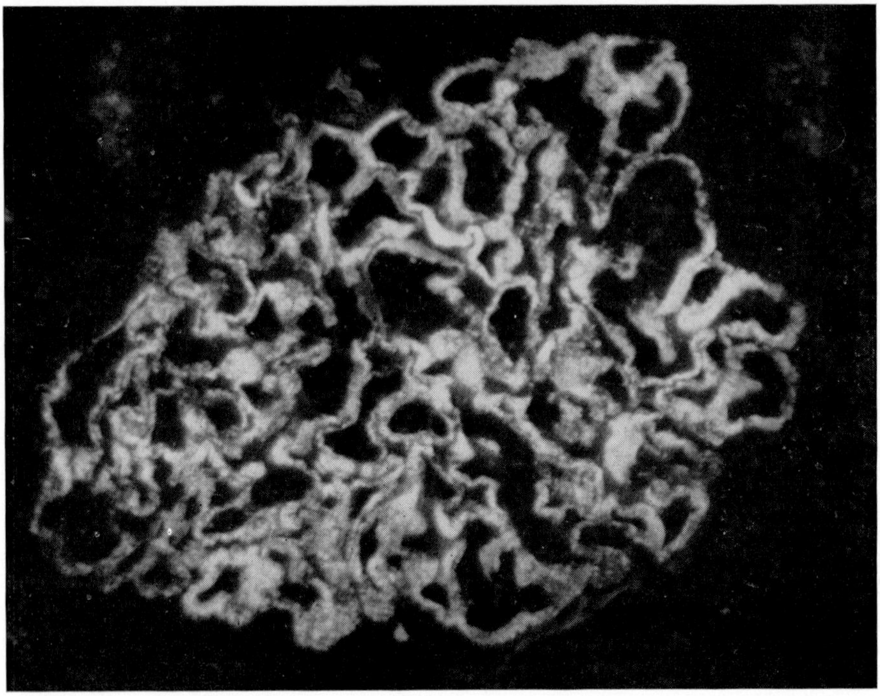

Fig. 8. Immunofluorescent picture in membranous glomerulonephritis. Granular deposits of gamma globulin are seen all along the basement membrane.

formation about the nature of the putative antigen, which could be either exogenous or endogenous. Further, the antigen need not be the same in all cases, since from experimental studies it is clear that complexes that contain different antigens may produce the same morphologic picture.

The other primary glomerular lesions, which represent a fairly well-defined morphologic entity and which appears to be an immune-complex nephritis is now generally classified as membranoproliferative glomerulonephritis (which appears to include lesions classified as lobular glomerulonephritis or chronic diffuse proliferative glomerulonephritis). The patients are often older children, adolescents, or young adults who usually present with the nephrotic syndrome, often with hematuria. They follow a chronic course which usually terminates in uremia. Some of the patients have low levels of serum complement, and these have been described as hypocomplementemic nephritis (West et al.[25]).

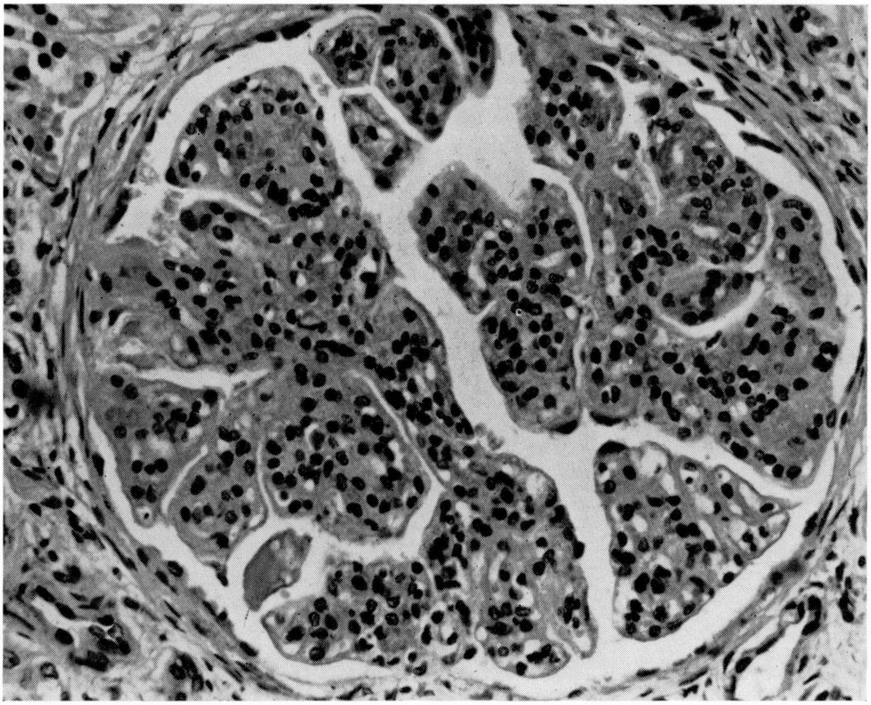

Fig. 9. Membranoproliferative glomerulonephritis. Marked mesangial hypercellularity is seen, associated with lobular accentuation and increase in mesangial matrix. All the glomeruli were similar to this one. H & E.

Histologically membranoproliferative glomerulonephritis is characterized by diffuse, fairly uniform proliferation of mesangial cells with increase in mesangial matrix (basement membranelike material) and increased lobulation (Figure 9). The capillary loops may show thickening or reduplication. By electron microscopy electron-dense deposits are found usually along the endothelial side of the basement membranes and in mesangial regions. Immunofluorescence shows irregular accumulations of immunoglobulins and beta 1C (sometimes only the latter), corresponding to the electron-dense deposits (Figure 10). Although membranoproliferative glomerulonephritis is perhaps not as faithfully reproduced in experimental models as membranous nephritis, the salient features have been seen in some rabbits with chronic serum sickness (Germuth et al.[7]). Assuming it is a form of immune complex disease nothing is known of the antigen, and the comments made in connection with membranous glomerulonephritis are relevant here. Although

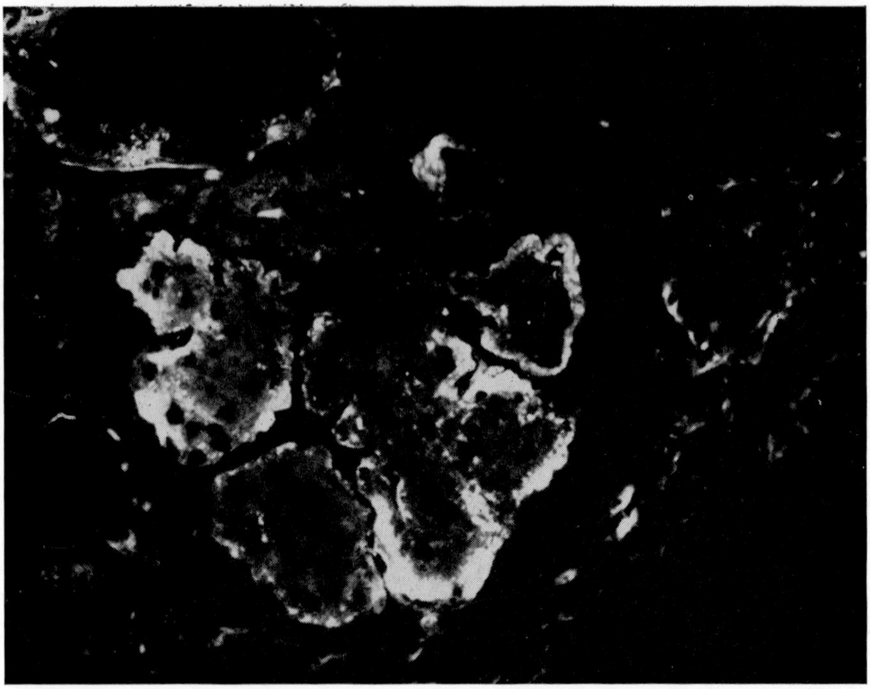

Fig. 10. Immunofluorescent pattern of gamma globulin in membranoproliferative glomerulonephritis. Broad or granular deposits are present along the basement membrane.

it has been suggested that membranoproliferative glomerulonephritis is at least in some instances a poststreptococcal disease there is, in my opinion, no substantial evidence favoring this view.

A somewhat less well-defined condition in which there is only scanty evidence for an immune complex basis is chronic sclerosing glomerulonephritis (end-stage kidney in chronic atrophic glomerulonephritis). Typically the patients are found to have urinary abnormalities and hypertension; subsequently they develop chronic progressive renal failure, or are seen for the first time in uremia. The past history does not indicate acute glomerulonephritis or the nephrotic syndrome. The kidneys are small and finely granular. Most of the glomeruli are hyalinized, although some may show only focal sclerosis and compensatory hypertrophy. Irregular tubular atrophy, interstitial fibrosis, and arterial and arteriolar sclerosis are also typical. In most instances immunoglobulins are not found in glomeruli; however, some of the incompletely sclerosed glomeruli occasionally contain irregular, sometimes granular deposits of immunoglobulins and complement. The significance of these findings is not always clear; although they may well represent immune complexes, the possibility that the gamma globulin is nonspecifically stuck in damaged glomeruli cannot be excluded. Further, it seems likely that chronic sclerosing glomerulonephritis represents the final pathway for a variety of diseases, only some of which may be immunologically induced.

In addition to the conditions just discussed there are a variety of glomerular diseases which cannot be satisfactorily classified, even on morphologic grounds, especially when only renal biopsy material is available for study. A variety of glomerular abnormalities are seen in such cases, including irregular proliferative and sclerosing changes. Undoubtedly many of these cases are classified simply as chronic glomerulonephritis or focal glomerulonephritis (a term which includes many morphologic types of glomerular disease, only some of which, as described by Heptinstall[10] are well defined). However it seems preferable to put them into a category simply referred to as unclassified glomerular disease. In some such cases scattered deposits of immunoglobulins and complements are found but, as in chronic sclerosing glomerulonephritis, their significance cannot be determined and it may be that in some instances the diseases are caused by immune complexes and in others not.

Available evidence provides no support for the concepts that diabetic glomerulosclerosis or amyloidosis are immune complex diseases (although the stimulus for the production of amyloid may be immunological. Further studies are needed to elucidate the role of immunologic mechanisms, if any, in patients with familial nephritis.

Before leaving immune complex diseases, mention should be made of a recently described condition which may represent a form of immune complex disease and which may possibly be a disease entity. This is a condition described by Berger,[3] which is characterized by accumulations of IgA and IgG, predominantly in mesangial regions. The patients studied so far have presented with hematuria, which often recurs. Only mild proteinuria is found and, except for one patient, renal insufficiency has not developed. There are no characteristic histologic features: in some patients the glomeruli appear normal; in others irregular mild proliferative or sclerosing changes are found. The characteristic findings are demonstrable by immunofluorescence: large irregular deposits of IgA, and usually of IgG also, are seen, predominantly in mesangial regions. In contrast, in most other forms of immune complex disease IgG is the predominant immunoglobulin and IgA is usually not found, except in some patients with anaphylactoid purpura or lupus nephritis. In the condition under discussion electron microscopy shows electron-dense deposits in mesangial areas. There is no information as to the etiology (or etiologies) of this condition or, assuming it is a form of immune complex disease, the antigen. It has no satisfactory name: Berger's disease probably cannot be used since without French pronunciation, it could be confused with thromboangiitis obliterans. Berger himself refers to the condition as nephropathy with mesangial IgA-IgG deposits. Probably most cases of this condition have been classified as focal glomerulonephritis, although it is not suggested that most lesions classified as focal glomerulonephritis will turn out to be instances of IgA-AgG nephropathy.

It should be emphasized that although the resemblance of several forms of primary glomerular disease to certain experimental models strongly supports the interpretation that they are immune complex diseases, final proof will depend upon the demonstration that the glomerular deposits contain antigen and specific antibody. Beyond that it is necessary to establish how the antigen induces antibody formation and why it is present in the circulation so as to form complexes.

The second major category of immunologically determined glomerular disease (anti-GBM disease) has also been definitely shown to occur in man, but diseases of this type are certainly considerably less common than immune complex diseases. Two morphologic forms have been well studied, namely, the glomerular disease seen in patients with Goodpasture's syndrome and in patients with a condition now most generally referred to as rapidly progressive glomerulonephritis (often classified pathologically as subacute glomerulonephritis). Both conditions are characterized clinically by rapidly progressive renal failure and pathologically by severe proliferative and necrotizing glomerular lesions, with many conspicuous crescents. Goodpasture's syndrome differs only in having lung hemorrhage in addition to the other findings. Immunofluorescence shows the completely smooth, continuous ("linear") accumulation of immunoglobulins and complement which is so characteristic of anti-GBM disease. Further, studies of gamma globulin eluted from glomeruli have shown that it is, in fact, anti-GBM antibody. A word of caution is in order concerning "linear" staining for gamma globulin since this is encountered in some patients who do not appear to be suffering from anti-GBM disease. This has been seen especially in patients with diabetes and lupus, but also in other diseases and even in normal glomeruli. It appears to be more of a problem with autopsy than biopsy material. The explanation for this finding is not clear. Aside from immunofluorescent studies of renal tissue, the diagnosis of anti-GBM disease may be made by demonstrating circulating anti-GBM antibodies. Because of the finding in experimental animals that circulating antibodies are frequently not demonstrable unless both kidneys are removed there is a tendency to believe that it is futile to search for them. However circulating anti-GBM antibodies have been found in some patients prior to nephrectomy and this approach to diagnosis is definitely indicated.

Although the pathogenesis of the glomerular lesions in most patients with Goodpasture's syndrome and rapidly progressive glomerulonephritis has been shown to be due to anti-GBM antibodies, the etiology of these conditions is unknown, that is, it is not known what initiates the formation of autoantibodies.

Finally, it remains to be determined whether all cases (or nearly all) of rapidly progressive glomerulonephritis are due to anti-GBM antibodies and whether anti-GBM antibodies are ever responsible for less serious forms of glomerular disease than those described so far.

REFERENCES

1. Andres, G. A., Accinni, I, Hsu, K. C., Zabriskie, J. B. and Seegal, B. C.: Electronmicroscopic studies of human glomerulonephritis with ferritin conjugated antibody. Localization of antigen-antibody complexes in glomerular structures of patients with acute glomerulonephritis. *J. Exp. Med. 123*:399, 1966.
2. Baldwin, D. S. and McCluskey, R. T.: Renal Involvement in Systemic Lupus Erythematosus, Periarteritis, Nodosa, Scleroderma, and Cryoglobulinemia. In: *The Structural Basis of Renal Disease*, Becker, E. L., ed. p. 428, New York, Harper and Row (Hoeber), 1968.
3. Berger, J.: IgA glomerular deposits in renal disease. *Transplant. Proc. 1*:939, 1969.
4. Dixon, F. J., Feldman, J. D. and Vazquez, J. T. Experimental glomerulonephritis. The pathogenesis of a laboratory model resembling the spectrum of human glomerulonephritis. *J. Exp. Med. 113*:899, 1961.
5. Dixon, F. J. and Oldstone, M. B. A.: Lymphocytic choriomeningitis: Production of antibody by "tolerant" infected mice. *Science 158*:1193, 1967.
6. Dixon, F. J., Oldstone, M. B. A. and Tonietti, G.: Virus induced immune-complex-type glomerulonephritis. *Transplant. Proc. 1*:945, 1969.
7. Germuth, F. G. Jr., Senterfit, L. B. and Pollack, A. D.: Immune complex disease. I. Experimental acute and chronic glomerulonephritis, *John Hopkins Med. J. 120*:225, 1967.
8. Glassock, R. J., Edgington, T. S., Watson, J. I. and Dixon, J. F.: Autologous immune complex nephritis induced with

renal tubular antigen. II. The pathogenetic mechanism. *J. Exp. Med. 129*:573, 1968.
9. Gutman, R. A., Striker, G. E., Gilliland, B. C. and Cutler, R. E.: The Glomerulonephritis of Staphylococcal Endocarditis with Hypocomplementemic—An Immune Complex (Abs.). Third Annual Meeting, Amer. Soc. Nephrology. 1969, p. 25.
10. Heptinstall, R. H.: Focal Glomerulonephritis. In: *Pathology of the Kidney.* Boston, Little, Brown, 1966, p. 315.
11. Heymann, W., Hackel, D.B., Harwood, S., Wilson, S. G. F. and Hunter, J. L.P.: Production of nephrotic syndrome in rats by Freund's adjuvants and rat kidney suspensions. *Proc. Soc. Exp. Biol. Med. 100*:600, 1959.
12. Koffler, D., Schur, P. H. and Kunkel, H. G.: Immunological studies concerning the nephritis of systemic lupus erythematosus. *J. Exp. Med. 126*:607, 1967.
13. Krishman, C. and Kaplan, M. H.: Immunopathologic studies of systemic lupus erythematosus. II. Antinucleus reaction of gamma globulin eluted from homogenates and isolated glomeruli of kidneys from patients with lupus nephritis. *J. Clin. Invest. 46*:569, 1967.
14. Lerner, R. A. and Dixon, F. J.: Transfer of ovine experimental allergic glomerulonephritis (EAG) with serum. *J. Exp. Med. 124*:431, 1966.
15. McCluskey, R. T. and Baldwin, D. S.: Natural history of acute glomerulonephritis. *Amer. J. Med. 35*:213, 1963.
16. McCluskey, R. T. and Vassalli, P.: Experimental Glomerular Diseases. In: *The Kidney.* Rouiller, C. and Muller, A. F., eds. New York, Acad. Press, 1969.
17. McCluskey, R. T., Vassalli, P., Gallo, G., and Baldwin, D. S.: An immunofluorescent study of pathogenic mechanisms in glomerular diseases. *New Eng. J. Med. 274*:695, 1966.
18. Meltzer, M., Franklin, E. C., Elias, K., McCluskey, R. T. and Cooper, N.: Cryoglobulinemia. II. Cryoglobulins with rheumatoid factor activity. *Amer. J. Med. 40*:837, 1966.
19. Rudofsky, U. and Steblay, R. W.: Studies on autoimmune nephritis in sheep. II. Passive transfer of nephritis in sheep by plasma. *Fed. Proc. 25*:659, 1966.
20. Steblay, R. W.: Glomerulonephritis induced in sheep by injections of heterologous glomerular basement membrane and Freund's adjuvant. *J. Exp. Med. 116*:253, 1962.
21. Tan, E. M., Schur, P. H., Carr, R. I. and Kunkel, H. G.: Deoxyribonuleic acid (DNA) and antibodies to DNA in the serum of patients with systemic lupus erythematosus. *J. Clin. Invest. 45*:1732, 1966.
22. Treser, G., Semar, M., Sagel, I., Ty, A. and Lange, K.: A Specific, Type Independent, Nephritogenic Antigen in The Streptococcal Plasma Membrane in Acute Glomerulonephritis. Third Annual Meeting; Amer. Soc. Nephrology, 1969, p. 69.
23. Unanue, E. R. and Dixon, F. J. Experimental glomerulonephritis: Immunologic events and pathogenic mechanisms. *Advances Immun. 6*:1, 1967.
24. Ward, P. and Conran, P.: Immunopathology of renal complications of simian malaria and human quartan malaria. *Milit. Med. 134*:1228, 1969.
25. West, C. D., McAdams, A. J., McConville, J. M., Davis, N. C. and Holland, N. H.: Hypocomplementemic and normocomplementemic persistent (chronic) glomerulonephritis, clinical and pathologic characteristics. *J. Pediat. 67*:1089, 1965.

GLOMERULONEPHRITIS: PEDIATRIC ASPECTS*

WALLACE W. MCCRORY

Professor and Chairman
Department of Pediatrics
The New York Hospital-Cornell Medical Center
New York, N. Y.

GLOMERULONEPHRITIS covers a very broad group of disorders of varied etiology about which we still have much to learn.

The advances in our understanding of the pathogenesis and natural history of these diseases in the past two decades have occurred through two areas of investigation stimulated in part by the development of renal transplantation. The two aspects concern our better understanding of the immunopathogenesis of nephritis and its treatment. We now face a new frontier in the sense that heretofore the diagnosis of glomerulonephritis has been essentially an academic exercise in the labeling and sorting of syndromes, but there has been no specific intervention that could alter the course of the disease.

The possibility now exists that there may be one or more mechanisms basic to the progression of the disease and hence for the capacity to intervene if we can get a clear diagnosis early enough to intervene in some types of glomerulonephritis. Therapeutic efforts in immunosuppression and prevention of abnormal clotting are now of greatest interest in this regard. If we are to use either of these approaches we need to apply them in types of nephritis where the risk of undesirable side effects will be clearly outweighed by the potential benefits. In the case of typical acute glomerulonephritis we are dealing with a disease that is usually fairly benign in terms of its immediate mortality and its long-term morbidity.

I propose to concentrate on the acute manifestations of nephritis because these are the most easily recognized clinically, and because this disease is most likely to bring the patient to the physician at a time when intervention may still be of benefit. By the term acute glomerulonephritis, as has already been pointed out here, we mean a disease of

*Presented at a *Conference on Glomerulonephritis* held by the New York Heart Association at The Waldorf-Astoria, New York, N.Y., January 27, 1970.

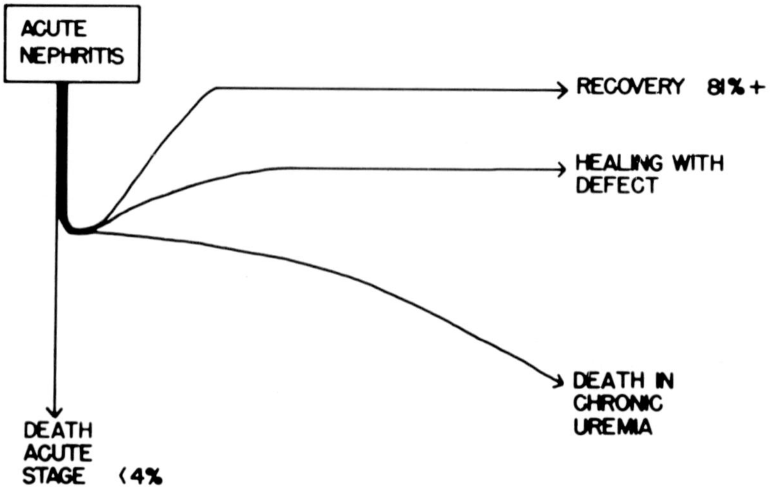

Course of acute glomerulonephritis in childhood

multiple etiology. This is a disease that predominantly affects the young. The maximum age incidence would be found between five and ten years of age. In this group it is usually a benign disease, both in terms of acute mortality and morbidity and as judged by the frequency of the evolution of chronic nephritis as a sequela. That chronic nephritis frequently evolves from acute glomerulonephritis is still believed by some but this is a matter of considerable controversy.

There are only a limited number of reliable long-term follow-up studies of the outcome of acute glomerulonephritis. We have reviewed these[1] and have recently reported our own data based on five-year follow-ups that cover the period 1942 to 1962. The status of our patients at two and five years after onset confirmed the reports in the literature that documented the low incidence (less than 5%) of chronic nephritis as a sequela of poststreptococcal acute glomerulonephritis. The outcome (see accompanying figure) can be summarized as follows: the great majority (more than 90%) will become clinically well and normal by measurement of endogenous creatinine clearance, ability to concentrate urinary solutes, quantitative measurement of protein, and excretion of red and white cells. A small number (5 to 10%) will become "active," which means clinically well but with minimal proteinuria or microscopic hematuria and normal renal function. These patients are classified into three states after five years: 1) they will ultimately recover; 2) they will recover with a defect, that is, with evidence of persistent minimal proteinuria and impaired solute-concentrating ability but otherwise with normal renal function, and they will be clinically well with biopsy findings that show two populations of nephrons, the majority normal with some focal areas of glomerular scarring and fibrosis that ultimately obliterate the affected nephrons; and 3) they develop chronic nephritis with progressive reduction in renal function. The latter course was observed in only two of 73 cases followed for five years. We had one instance of what has been called subacute or rapidly progressive nephritis in which renal function showed progressive deterioration following the acute onset and never returned to normal. We have not observed a case in which quantitative urinalysis was found to be normal and in which the patient subsequently demonstrated signs of chronic nephritis or the nephrotic syndrome. Some authors have claimed that such a latent form exists in which the patient appears clinically well but ultimately progresses to chronic nephritis. We have not observed this course in any of our patients, and we believe that this course is a misnomer in patients whom we classify as active but not recognizably so unless quantitative examination of urine protein and sediment is done serially. The term latent is also used by pathologists for patients who show signs of histological activity of glomerulonephritis by biopsy without clinical or laboratory signs of activity. Since healing of the renal lesion may require a longer time than the clearing of laboratory signs of the disease the latter definition lacks supporting clinical documentation by long-term follow-up at present and should be dropped. The low incidence of chronic nephritis we have reported is confirmed in recent studies that employed renal-biopsy studies at onset; it thus appears valid. Contrary to the experience of Dr. David P. Earle, we did not find the nephrotic syndrome to be a significant late complication of children, although it was seen in association with the acute attack in eight children, of whom six recovered completely.

One of the more important aspects of this problem now being more critically examined involves the certainty with which one can identify patients with nephritis as having poststreptococcal glomerulonephritis.

Reported differences in the frequency of acute mortality and in the frequency of late occurrence of chronic glomerulonephritis between adults and children have been subjects of great interest. Children may follow a more benign course than adults, but these presumed differences

TABLE I. CAUSES OF ACUTE RENAL FAILURE

1) Acute (poststrep) glomerulonephritis
2) Acute nephritis with anaphylactoid purpura
3) Thrombotic microangiopathy with hemolytic anemia and uremia
4) Gram-negative sepsis with D.I.C.
5) Drug toxicity
   Hepatorenal (carbon tetracl.)
   Hemolytic (salicyclates)
6) Metabolic disorders
   Oxalosis
   Hyperuricemia
7) Prerenal azotemia—shock, dehydration

TABLE II. RENAL FAILURE: NEW YORK HOSPITAL, 1954-1969

Diagnosis	*No.*	*Died*	*%*
Acute glomerulonephritis	17	3	17
Hemolytic-uremic syndrome	10	5	50
Thrombotic thrombocytopenic purpura	1	1	100
Obstructive uropathy	2	2	100
Prerenal uremia	8	3	37
	38	14	40

may also reflect different etiologies for acute nephritis. The excellent outcome we have reported applies only to poststreptococcal nephritis. Is the same disease more serious in the old than in the young or is the etiology different? The latter possibility, I think, seems more likely.

It is now apparent that the severity of the initial damage to renal function judged by the development of acute renal failure (oliguria or anuria) and its duration does correlate with histopathologic evidence of severity and death in the acute stage or failure to recover subsequently.

The causes of acute renal failure in children are shown in Table I. The most frequent cause of acute renal failure in children admitted to the pediatric service at the New York Hospital in the last 15 years was acute glomerulonephritis (Table II). The second most frequent cause was the so-called hemolytic uremic syndrome, a clotting disorder that involves small blood vessels associated with thrombosis and that especially involves the glomerular capillaries in children and causes acute non-immunologic hemolytic anemia. This condition can and should be distinguished from acute glomerulonephritis and has a much higher acute

TABLE III. RENAL FAILURE IN CASES OF ACUTE NEPHRITIS: NEW YORK HOSPITAL, 1954-1969

	No.	%
Total cases	128	100
Oliguria	17	13
(< 350 Ml./M ²S.A./day)		
N.F.U.	4	24
Recovered	7	42
Active	3	17
Anuria	3	17
Died	3	2.3

mortality rate (10 to 50%). This disorder apparently is only rarely a cause of acute nephritis in the adult.

The mortality rate in acute renal failure varied in accordance with the cause, as shown in Table II. In patients with acute nephritis that we have followed the only deaths in the acute stage were in those who developed oliguria.

In prerenal uremia, by which we mean renal failure that is not due to primary renal disease, it is not always easy to distinguish this from acute glomerulonephritis. The mortality rate is less than that of the hemolytic-uremic syndrome but higher than that of acute glomerulonephritis.

The development of oliguria in older patients is considered a serious complication. There have been statements in the literature to the effect that recovery, once a patient is anuric, is unusual in adult subjects. A recent report by Leonard et al.[2] reports that oliguria that occurs in adults with proved poststreptococcal nephritis has a relatively good outlook (90% recovered) while patients with oliguria and nonstreptococcal acute glomerulonephritis had a very high mortality (10% recovered).

The exact definition of oliguria becomes important because differences in outcome can arise if there are differences in the definition of oliguria. In our series (Table III), the definition of oliguria is 350 cc. per meter of squared surface area per day. I do not say that is the best definition but according to it we had 17 patients (13%), and the three patients who died had developed anuria. The over-all mortality rate in this series was low (2.3%), as was the mortality rate in patients with oliguria (17%).

Dr. John Lewy of Chicago[3] has followed 14 children with more severe renal failure due to poststreptococcal nephritis, each of whom had an output of less than 100 cc. for two days or more, or anuria; 8 of the 14 recovered, and 6 died (43%). The mortality rate, then, does increase with oliguria as one defines the increasing evidence of renal failure.

Studies of the correlation of clinical course and renal histology strongly suggest that the severity of the renal functional derangement at onset will correlate with the mortality and the later morbidity. The differences in the acute mortality rates in children and adults can be explained partly by differences in the etiology of acute nephritis.

We have already observed this in the nephrotic syndrome. If one classifies the causes of the nephrotic syndrome in any large group of patients more than 30 years of age, few of them will be found to have what we call "minimal-change" disease. In any large group of nephrotics under 10 years of age, 70% will be found to have minimal-change disease. I think I heard Dr. Earle say that an adult with minimal-change disease responds to steroids much as does the child with minimal-change disease. The differences in response to steroids between the child and the adult with the nephrotic syndrome relate to differences in the frequency of its etiology.

We should always be quite certain of the pathological diagnosis before we attempt new modes of treatment. It is obvious that the diagnosis must rest on more than clinical grounds and should include histopathology and serologic and coagulation studies if we are to clarify this aspect further. The attention we focus on initial diagnosis is important because the outcome of the disease can be predicted to some degree. If we are to intervene, we need to define the patients in danger.

A second point to be kept in mind in the argument over whether chronic glomerulonephritis ever evolves from poststreptococcal nephritis is one that concerns the pathogenesis. I believe that there is evidence that this does occur, and that the proof of the argument to the contrary rests on others. However, instead of considering only that the disease causing it may be different in children and adults when we find that a complication occurs in less than 5% of the group in danger, it certainly is reasonable to suggest that this may be caused by differences in the host.

Dr. Robert T. McCluskey discussed the rabbit foreign-protein experimental models of nephritis. As I remember the study, a small number

TABLE IV. DIAGNOSIS OF ACUTE GLOMERULONEPHRITIS

1)	History of infection
2)	Hematuria, proteinuria, RBC casts of sudden onset
3)	Serological signs of recent streptococcal infection
4)	Edema, hypertension $> 50\%$
5)	Mild anemia HB > 8 gm%
6)	Mild reticulocytosis $< 10\%$
7)	Platelets normal
8)	Decreased serum complement
9)	Elevated sedimentation rate
10)	Renal biopsy confirms

(about 5%) of the rabbits went on to develop the progressive form of glomerulonephritis, and they were poor producers of antibody. Patients thus afflicted could have less than the normal capacity for the production of antibody or different immunologic competence. We should bear in mind this possibility when considering the cause of an unusual disease with a low incidence; factors in the hosts (our patients) must be examined before we can answer some of these questions of pathogenesis.

Since acute glomerulonephritis in the child can have numerous causes it is useful to review its differential diagnosis. At the present time the approach we use to establish the diagnosis with greatest certainty is the one outlined in Table IV. It is very important to ascertain whether there is a history compatible with recent streptococcal infection, because the absence of this means one may be dealing with one of the nonstreptococcal disorders, in which case the course is quite unpredictable. We believe it is important to look for serological signs of streptococcal infections in every patient; for this we use the ASLO (antistreptolysin-O) Titer. In view of the Japanese report of a proved epidemic of poststreptococcal nephritis in which, apparently, the streptococcus had no capacity for the production of streptolysin, it may be necessary to do more than just measure the ASLO titer; some attempt at serological identification of the preceding streptococcal infection is necessary. By our standards, anemia of significant degree, or reticulocytosis, is not found in typical poststreptococcal acute glomerulonephritis, and one must look for a second complication. I think the value of the rest are self-evident.

We also have a coagulation laboratory and a coagulation expert looking over our shoulders. I find it difficult to understand all of the factors

Table V. EVIDENCES OF INTRAVASCULAR COAGULATION

			Normal
1) Thrombocytopenia			150-200,000 m.[3]
2) Low fibrinogen	—	(I)	200-400 mg.%
3) Low prothrombin	—	(II)	80-120%
4) Proaccelerin	—	(V)	— +
5) AHF	—	(VIII)	— +
6) Fibrin breakdown products			+
7) No excessive fibrinolysis, euglobulin clot lysis time normal			
8) Abnormal bleeding			
9) Increased RBC destruction			

relating to laboratory evidences of active intravascular coagulation, but we found it useful to carry out a coagulation-screening program (Table V) in treating children who presented with severe acute glomerulonephritis. We are turning up increasing evidence of increased fibrinolytic activity and products of the breakdown of fibrin in acute nephritis. Thrombocytopenia is very unusual. Very low levels of fibrinogen would suggest that intravascular coagulation may be occurring. When both of these occur, one may be dealing with what we call the hemolytic uremic syndrome rather than uncomplicated acute glomerulonephritis; anticoagulant therapy may be indicated. The big question here, of course, is whether anticoagulant therapy can be of any value in acute nephritis with renal failure. In our experience this therapy has not been of value in patients who are already in renal failure. The proof of this opinion, I think, will be obtained only when one has good laboratory evidence of clotting abnormalities and can intervene early, before renal failure has developed.

REFERENCES

1. McCrory, W. W. and Shibuya, M.: Acute glomerulonephritis in childhood: Long-term follow-up. *New York J. Med. 68*:2416, 1968.
2. Leonard, C. D., Nagle, R., Striker, G. E. and Scribner, B. H.: Oliguric acute glomerulonephritis. I. Clinical features. Amer. Soc. Nephrology, Third Annual Meeting, Washington, D.C., 1969. Abstracts, p. 39.
3. Lewy, J., Cruz, H. and Metcoff, J.: Acute Renal Failure and Some Renal Functions in Acute Glomerulonephritis. In: *Acute Glomerulonephritis.* Metcoff, J., ed. Boston, Little, Brown, 1967, p. p. 342.

CONFERENCE ON GLOMERULONEPHRITIS*

Closing Morning Discussion

DAVID P. EARLE, *Moderator*

Professor and Chairman
Department of Medicine
Northwestern University Medical Center
Chicago, Ill.

DAVID S. BALDWIN AND CHESTER M. EDELMANN, JR.

DR. DAVID P. EARLE. In addition to the participants who have presented papers thus far two speakers will give brief discussions on two of the presentations. Dr. David S. Baldwin, associate professor of medicine, New York University School of Medicine, New York, N.Y., will discuss my paper, and Dr. Chester M. Edelmann, Jr., professor of pediatrics, Albert Einstein College of Medicine, New York, N.Y., will then comment on Dr. Wallace W. McCrory's paper on pediatric aspects.

DR. DAVID S. BALDWIN. I should like to make a few comments based on our own experience during the past 10 or 15 years, during which we also have studied a variety of glomerular diseases. We utilized the renal biopsy technique.

In general, our experience pretty closely corresponds with Dr. Earle's. However, there are a few points that bear emphasis, and perhaps a few in which our experience differs somewhat from his.

Many of you may wonder what all the wrangling is about, and why we have become so deeply involved in this attempt to classify glomerulonephritis. We face many problems in classification, principally because we have been restricted to a pathologic basis for classification rather than to etiologic considerations.

However, we must give credit to the percutaneous renal biopsy, for prior to the use of this technique the various diseases that we have discussed this morning were all considered forms of a single entity, "glomerulonephritis." Having had the opportunity now to study pa-

*Held by the New York Heart Association at The Waldorf-Astoria, New York, N. Y., January 27, 1970.

tients early in the course of their disease and to observe histologic changes prior to the end-stage kidney, we have been able to recognize a variety of different diseases formerly included in the all-inclusive term of glomerulonephritis. This, then, is a good beginning.

We still have a major problem to solve: to determine the nature of the disease or diseases which lead to the most common type of end-stage kidney, the disease in which the patient presents simply with urinary abnormalities or with hypertension and renal failure, with no history of an edematous or nephrotic stage. Such a disease progresses over the course of a few years, sometimes a great many years, to atrophic kidneys and terminal renal failure. None of the entities that we have discussed this morning appears to progress in this way. We should realize that we are still left with a major problem: the nature of the disease that leads to the classic vest-pocket, atrophic, end-stage kidney.

To return just briefly to a few of the entities that Drs. Earle, Churg, and McCrory discussed, I might comment on our experience at New York University.

First, poststreptococcal glomerulonephritis. Although we may argue about whether chronicity occurs at all in this disease, I think we can all agree that poststreptococcal glomerulonephritis rarely leads to chronic renal disease. This constitutes a major advance in our thinking about glomerulonephritis. Although poststreptococcal glomerulonephritis might be the most common among the diseases that we have discussed here it certainly is one of the least important diseases in terms of chronic renal failure. We ourselves have never documented progression to chronic renal failure in a patient who showed recovery or improvement from the initial stage. We have seen death occur in the initial stage, so-called subacute or persistently active acute glomerulonephritis, that leads to death in a few weeks or months. However, in our patients who have survived the initial stage, we have not seen chronic disease develop. Even if such progression should prove to occur, and I think it does from what Drs. Earle and McCrory have reported, this must be a very rare occurrence.

In addition, our experience differs somewhat from Dr. Earle's in that we have not observed exacerbations after an initial attack of acute glomerulonephritis. In fact, we are not really sure that they ever occur. By exacerbation we mean a reinfection with the beta-hemolytic streptococcus that causes a recrudescence of the original pathologic process.

We have seen the nephrotic syndrome occur in acute nephritis. In our experience it occurs early as part of the acute stage, and we cannot agree with the diagram which Dr. Earle showed us, which indicates the appearance of the nephrotic syndrome years after the onset of the disease and after a period of remission. We believe that patients who present with the nephrotic syndrome will prove to have one of the other lesions described here: membranous or membranoproliferative, rather than a sequela of acute poststreptococcal glomerulonephritis.

Let us turn now to a few comments about membranous nephritis. Our experience is very similar to Dr. Earle's in this condition. Of all the diseases discussed this morning besides acute nephritis, where we seem to know something about etiology, membranous nephritis is the best defined entity. Histologically it is very well defined, and the clinical features give support to our concept that this probably is a nosologic entity. All of our patients with membranous nephritis have had the nephrotic syndrome. Most of our patients have followed a course characterized by persistent heavy proteinuria and progressive renal failure. Terminal renal failure develops after periods ranging from as little as two years to as long as 10 or 15 years. Perhaps one patient in six shows a spontaneous remission. As regards management of membranous nephritis I think we should interpret remissions differently from Dr. Earle, who has said that following treatment with steroids, remissions were induced after many months or a few years of disease. We have seen remissions occur at the same intervals after onset of the disease. However, we have not used steroids because our early experience indicated that these patients did not respond to steroids. We have seen spontaneous remissions occur without the use of steroids. Dr. Earle's failure to observe remissions in patients who were not given steroids may be explained by the fact that he did not use steroids in patients who had renal failure and advanced disease. These are the very patients in whom one would not expect to observe spontaneous remissions. We have some patients who are living up to seven or eight years and who have not yet developed renal failure, but the majority have progressed to some evidence of glomerular insufficiency.

Turning now to a few comments on focal glomerulonephritis, it should be stressed that focal is a poorly defined type of glomerular disease. We ourselves use the term only when we see focal proliferation. Dr. Earle included also patients with focal scars, focal membranous changes, and combined focal membranous and proliferative changes. We probably all agree that these various focal lesions represent a variety of different glomerular diseases. We have seen the nephrotic syndrome rather frequently in patients with focal proliferative glomerulonephritis; the prognosis in these patients has not been consistently poor. A fair number of the patients with nephrotic syndrome have responded to steroids and have had temporary remissions. However, in general, our experience with focal nephritis has not been good. The majority of our patients, after periods of observations of about five years, have had renal failure.

The important point is that patients with focal glomerular lesions probably represent the group who eventually develop the typical atrophic end-stage kidney. It is evident that acute glomerulonephritis and membranous nephritis could not account for the atrophic end-stage kidney on either clinical or histologic grounds. However, patients who have focal disease and only urinary abnormalities could easily be in the beginnings of a disease or diseases which eventually progress to end-stage kidney disease without antecedent clinical acute nephritis or an edematous stage.

Finally, a word about what is now called membranoproliferative glomerulonephritis. We have referred to this form of nonpoststreptococcal glomerulonephritis as chronic diffuse proliferative, but we shall now go along with the others and use the term membranoproliferative. It may be helpful to change the name because this is not a stage of acute diffuse glomerulonephritis. We have observed this important disease more frequently than Dr. Earle indicated he had. I think he said he had seen only five patients with this condition during the period of his study. We have seen as many patients with this lesion as we have with membranous nephritis. Membranoproliferative glomerulonephritis is one of the commonest causes of nephrotic syndrome in the adult population. The prognosis is uniformly bad. These patients appear usually with the nephrotic syndrome and hematuria and, over the course of two to five or six years, go on to chronic renal failure, still edematous and nephrotic. This is a disease for which no therapy seems to be effective, steroids or immunosuppressives, and is by no means a rare cause of irreversible renal failure.

We have made some progress in our understanding and classification of glomerulonephritis. However, we must be aware of the fact that until we can classify glomerular diseases etiologically, we shall still be confused about the nature and the natural history of many of the conditions that we have discussed on this occasion.

DR. DAVID P. EARLE. As predicted, there obviously is not common agreement on all points. Dr. Edelmann, Jr., will be the next discussant.

DR. CHESTER M. EDELMANN, JR. I should like to comment first that it has been somewhat surprising to me—and gratifying—that a group of internists, pediatricians, and pathologists appear to have as much agreement concerning renal disease as has been evidenced this morning.

At the risk of being somewhat redundant, I should like to make some observations on the course of acute glomerulonephritis in children as compared to that in adults. I think that many of the apparent differences we used to talk about have now been resolved. There has been agreement in the past that the great majority of children with acute glomerulonephritis go on to complete recovery. There has been agreement also that in some instances nephritis may be so severe, with so many nephrons irreversibly damaged, that complete recovery is not possible. The disease in these children is readily identifiable soon after its onset. The point on which there has been considerable difference of opinion is whether children appear to recover clinically, only to have a subclinical or subacute course with insidious development of chronic glomerulonephritis that appears in renal failure when the children are adults 10 or 20 years later. As recently as 1965, at the *Seventeenth Annual Conference on the Kidney* sponsored by the National Kidney Foundation, which was devoted to acute glomerulonephritis, the opinion was expressed that such a course does occur and that many or even most adults with chronic glomerulonephritis have their disease as a consequence of an apparently benign episode of acute glomerulonephritis in childhood. I think it is of great importance to note that the idea of this sequence, long challenged by pediatricians, is now being relinquished by internists as well.

The question has been raised here of the nature of the relapses that are observed in the course of recovery from acute glomerulonephritis. Very commonly we see an abrupt increase in hematuria and proteinuria in a child who had appeared to be recovering uneventfully. The exacerbation often is associated with a viral respiratory illness, and only rarely with recurrent streptococcal infection. The entire episode usually is short-lived; the child quickly returns to his previous state and continues to show progressive improvement. We have no idea of what the mechanism of this relapse is or why it is so often associated with intercurrent respiratory infection, but we have learned not to be concerned about it since we have never observed it to be followed by a worsening of the disease.

The great nonspecificity of acute glomerulonephritis bears emphasizing. Let me make it clear that I am referring now to the *clinical syndrome* of acute glomerulonephritis, characterized by an abrupt onset of hematuria, proteinuria, hypertension, edema, and azotemia. This syndrome is observed most commonly after streptococcal infection. However, there is no specificity in the clinical features, other diseases may manifest with the identical clinical syndrome, and the course of these diseases may be quite different from poststreptococcal glomerulonephritis. Therefore, in order to manage the patient knowledgeably and to give meaningful information with regard to prognosis it is extremely important to use all available tools to establish the precise nature of the underlying disease. For this purpose, a renal biopsy often is necessary.

If a patient has all the characteristic features of acute poststrepococcal glomerulonephritis, with mild to moderately severe disease clinically, transiently depressed serum complement, and evidence of streptococcal infection, one is probably certain enough of the diagnosis to defer renal biopsy in anticipation of complete recovery with return of the urine to normal. However, in severe cases, in patients who do not exhibit all the typical features of the disease, or in instances in which recovery does not seem to take place as rapidly as expected, a renal biopsy can be of immeasurable value in establishing diagnosis, predicting outcome, and in the hope of someday permitting the institution of specific therapy. Much of the confusion regarding the natural history of acute glomerulonephritis stems from making this diagnosis solely on the basis of clinical criteria and then interpreting incorrectly the progression of what is in fact a different disease. Thus we have identified by biopsy a number of children with various chronic diseases who otherwise would have been considered to represent insidious progression of acute to chronic glomerulonephritis.

The ability to examine renal tissue and to make a pathological classification has been of inestimable value in advancing our understanding of renal disease. An example of this is the nephrotic syndrome. Working with a number of clinics, we have been conducting a cooperative study of the nephrotic syndrome in children under the direction of Dr. Henry L. Barnett. We have now studied almost 200 children from the onset of disease. Renal biopsies are examined by several pathologists who are unaware of the course of the patients' disease. In the course of the study the pathologists have developed a classification of the various histologic types of disease that may underly the nephrotic syndrome. With this classification we are now able to predict with an extremely high degree of accuracy which child will respond to steroid therapy and which will not, with obvious prognostic implications. Of particular interest is a group of children, almost 10% of the total, whose biopsies revealed focal sclerosis. Each of these children has had severe morbidity or mortality. Some of them probably would have been diagnosed previously as "minimal change" or "nil" disease because of a failure to appreciate the significance of the focal lesions. In addition it is recognized that a biopsy may fail to contain these lesions, as in one child whose biopsy was interpreted as showing minimal change, but in whom autopsy examination shortly thereafter demonstrated focal disease.

Rarely is pure membranous nephropathy observed in children with the nephrotic syndrome, as discussed by previous speakers, The course in children appears to be about the same as in adults. It may go on to complete clinical remission, with or without treatment, but our experience has been that the renal lesions progress inexorably, despite apparent clinical improvement.

Previous speakers have referred to the entity membranoproliferative or hypocomplementemic glomerulonephritis. It is of interest that this condition appears to vary considerably in its prevalence in different parts of the country. In certain areas it comprises a higher percentage of all children with renal failure whereas in the New York area it is extremely uncommon. There is probably an important clue in this wide geographic variation, but at the moment we are not able to offer an explanation.

I conclude with a word about therapy, which has been discussed very little here. Avoiding the question of the possible benefit of adrenocortical steroids in patients with the nephrotic syndrome, there is very little that we seem to accomplish in children with glomerulonephritis (with the exception of lupus) with steroids, other cytotoxic or immunosuppressant drugs, or heparin. Many patients appear to improve after administration of one of these drugs. But many do so without treatment. I take this opportunity, therefore, to make a plea for cautious interpretation of uncontrolled data, and for the performance of more controlled clinical trials, which have been almost nonexistent in the field of renal disease, since this is the only means by which the efficacy of any therapeutic agent can be established.

Dr. David P. Earle. As moderator I have the advantage of making further comments. We appreciate Dr. Baldwin's remarks, which explain so clearly our concern and interest in accurate classification.

The example of response of lipoid nephrosis to steroid therapy is a good one. When patients with the nephrotic syndrome are treated without accurate diagnosis, as has been done in some prospective studies, the results are really quite meaningless. However, when the diagnosis is accurately known, response of patients with the nephrotic syndrome to therapy can be predicted in many instances. Lipoid nephrosis responds very well to steroid therapy.

The problem of whether acute poststreptococcal glomerulonephritis becomes chronic is of more than academic interest. Much emphasis is placed these days on prevention of disease. But it is difficult to prevent a disease unless the cause is known.

Streptococcal acute nephritis could be prevented by eradication of streptococcal infection. But the question is: Would this eliminate chronic glomerulonephritis? Even in areas where large numbers of such cases occur a prophylactic campaign against the streptococcus probably would have little effect on the incidence of chronic renal failure, since so few cases in children and epidemics become chronic. I say this even though I may be the only speaker here who has data to show that poststreptococcal acute nephritis may become chronic. This occurs mostly in sporadic cases in adults. Prevention of chronic nephritis in this group would be almost impracticable under current circumstances.

May I comment on the point that we have variations among investigators in their ideas on the incidence of membranoproliferative glomeulonephritis. The variations undoubtedly result from variable histologic criteria for differentiation of diffuse proliferative lesions with some mesangial changes from lesions that have basement membrane lesions together with active endothelial thickening.

In regard to exacerbations: they are not very common, but we do see them. On an anecdotal basis, I can quote patients whom we observed in their first attack of acute nephritis, whose disease failed to heal, and in whom we subsequently observed exacerbations. In one which proved to be associated with a streptococcal infection, renal biopsy showed typical acute changes superimposed on typical chronic changes. Subsequently, another exacerbation in the same patient followed a proved A_2 attack of influenza. Renal biopsy at that time showed no specific acute changes.

I emphasize that we made no claim that steroid therapy affected the membranous glomerular lesion. I was careful to say that the response was so slow that we could not be sure that treatment was doing anything. But every now and then more dramatic responses suggested some cause and effect. An adequate prospective study is still necessary.

I have one comment to make on Dr. Wallace W. McCrory's remarks about the ASO titer in acute glomerulonephritis, with regard to the Japanese study. Dr. McCrory said that ASO titers did not increase in many cases. We can confirm this. In our Trinidad studies, all patients with acute nephritis at first had good ASO increases. At present very few patients have significant ASO responses. However, they all do have good antihyaluronidase (AH) responses.

AN OVERVIEW OF NEPHRITIS*

JOHN P. MERRILL

Associate Professor of Medicine
Harvard Medical School
Boston, Mass.

A number of factors, I think, account for our marked interest in glomerulonephritis in the past five years.

First, both Dr. John Dosseter and I, in contradistinction to Dr. Wallace W. McCrory, have found that glomerulonephritis is far and away the most frequent cause of the need for transplantation. Obviously it is to our interest to do something about this disease.

Second, the similarity that has been pointed out between experimental models and syndromes in man has been shown to be relevant in a number of areas, particularly those in which experimental immune complex disease appears to be the basis for the renal lesion.

One can cite lupus nephritis, as others have done. We have seen a case of syphilitic nephrosis resembling complex disease. Penicillamine nephritis and probably malaria nephrosis all are examples in man of serum immune complex disease.

Then again, as has been pointed out, the use of new techniques, such as immunofluorescent microscopy, the delineation in man of basement membrane antigen and antibody, refinement of electron microscopy, and improved use of renal biopsy have all been helpful factors.

Last but certainly not least in my opinion has been our ability to do prospective studies of nephritis in man through the perhaps unfortunate observation of the recurrence of glomerulonephritis in renal isografts in man, that is, in grafts between identical twins. And now we have observed glomerular lesions and the clinical course thereof, which resembles that of the naturally occurring disease that recurs in a considerable number of renal-isograft recipients whose donors are not twins.

With all these refinements, however, I think the picture has become

*Presented at a *Conference on Glomerulonephritis* held by the New York Heart Association at The Waldorf-Astoria, New York, N. Y., January 27, 1970.

more exciting and more complex and, if anything, less clear at the moment. For instance, we still have the problem in terminology already mentioned. It is difficult for one man, I think, to know exactly in all instances what kind of lesion another man is describing. Further, although in the full-blown classic experimental lesion "lumps and bumps" and the linear distribution of antibody are quite clear in the models of Dr. Frank Dixon, the changes reported by light microscopy, and even by electron microscopy in the same models, are by no means completely reproducible; thus the clear pictures that we see are nice as illustrations, as focuses, as models, but we must not forget that they are not the same in every animal.

This certainly is increasingly true in man. As already mentioned in this conference, the lesions recognizable by conventional microscopy may vary considerably even with the same antigenic stimulus. For instance, if I administer a foreign serum protein to produce complex disease the type and extent of the lesion will vary with the route of administration of the antigen, the amount of antigen, the potency of the antigen, and particularly with the response of the individual animal to the antigen. Another factor is the number of doses of antigen administered.

The rabbit, in which many of the standard tests were done, is notorious for the varied degree of response it will have to any antigen administered by the same route, and by the same technique.

I suppose that the same thing is true in man. Of course none of these factors can be controlled in man, which may be the reason that we cannot specifically label a disease as related to a specific antigen in man.

Further, it must be stressed that certainly in complex disease, and possibly in antiglomerular-basement-membrane disease, the resulting syndrome depends not upon the amount or distribution of the antigen-antibody combination but upon the sequence of events which follows the deposition of complex or of specific antibody.

This, I think, is a point that has not been sufficiently emphasized. If one produces an antibody reaction to an antigen in experimental animals and stops there, one has the antigen and the antibody, but there may be no disease. It is the sequence of events that follows this combination that is important: the activation of the complement sequence, the production of leukotoxic factors, and the subsequent role of the polymorphonuclear leukocytes which move in and release lysosomes and proteolytic enzymes, increase vascular permeability, and denude the basement membrane so that platelets then aggregate upon it. The platelets in turn favor the deposition of fibrionogen and, ultimately, fibrosis or sclerosis.

It has been shown experimentally, as I have already mentioned, that the amount and the distribution of the immune complexes in the experimental disease have no relation to the activity of the lesion. Recently a group in Chicago has shown similarly that in lupus nephritis in man there is no relation between the activity of the nephritis and the amount and distribution of the immune complexes.

Therefore I think that in the future we must look a little further than simply into the antigen-antibody reaction in the totality of immune phenomena. We must consider the whole sequence of events that follows the deposition of antibody upon basement membranes, or the deposition of complexes within it. All of these may modify both the histological and clinical picture, certainly the frequency with which nephritis occurs after exposure to any nephritogen. For instance, there is no precise relation between the detection by immunofluorescent techniques of immunoglobulin (IgG) and the activity of the disease.

The role of IgG is becoming increasingly complex, as is the clotting problem. The deeper one goes the more factors one finds. We now recognize that there are four subgroups of IgG, and that the one which is deposited specifically may be the important one in determining the reaction that ensues. For example, IgG No. 2 appears to be less active in the complement fixation than Nos. 1, 3, and 4, and clinical studies by Dr. Edmund Lewis in our group have shown that where IgG 2 was predominantly deposited there seemed to be less of an inflammatory process.

However, again there was no consistent pattern in the deposition of any of these components of IgG in any of the different kinds of nephritis which have been described here. This splitting up of antibody globulin per se is important, not only because this problem is important in nephritis but because, as Dr. Guy Voisin in France has shown, subgroups of IgG, the same that we are using, will produce entirely different kinds of antibody. One fraction will produce cytotoxic antibody, an antibody that kills cells, and another fraction of the same immunoglobulin will produce enhancing antibody—which favors the growth of cells, particularly cancer cells. This is what we must consider. We must study these results and learn more about them. In others words, as our tools become sharper, the problem becomes more difficult to solve.

The role of the renal biopsy has been stressed adequately. While the discussion of it has been extremely helpful some errors have been made, in my opinion, in interpreting what renal biopsies can do for us. This in part is due to errors of sampling. Focal lesions do occur. Since all glomeruli in our experience are seldom affected equally, sampling errors must exist. I have a slide I like to show to students which pretends to illustrate tissue from a patient before he was treated and after he was treated. Actually it is the tissue from the same patient at the same time, in which deeper or corticomedullary glomeruli look considerably better than do the cortical glomeruli. This sort of thing can lead to misinterpretation.

Then again, cytologists, clinicians, and pathologists are afflicted with difficulties in communication which have not yet been overcome in spite of conferences, international and national, and committees on nomenclature.

One tends to do sequential renal biopsies and follow the progress of the disease by biopsy and to talk about the fact that "the biopsy shows improvement." A biopsy done last week cannot show improvement because it is fixed in formalin. Perhaps the next biopsy will show glomeruli that look better than the first one, but I am not sure that this necessarily tells you the lesion is healing as well as some other parameters may indicate.

It is well known, as already mentioned, that the histological picture obtained on sequential biopsies might be exactly the same in the full-blown nephrotic syndrome as it is in the same patient who has no clinical evidence of renal disease.

This has been most recently documented in two cases of renal-amyloid disease in which the patients had the full-blown nephrotic syndrome and were cured; they had no proteinuria after treatment of the underlying disease. Yet in both cases the amyloid persisted histologically, insofar as one could tell, in the same distribution and in the same amount.

What we see in a biopsy, I believe, is the battlefield after the battle is over; we are counting dead soldiers rather than recording progress of the action, which is what we want to consider. Anyone who has attempted to estimate the renal function of the patient from a renal biopsy should be well aware of this.

In our own group we tend to do an initial open-wedge biopsy because we do a great many immunofluorescent studies. We do electron microscopy and several stains for light microscopy. Once a week a group of clinicians, immunologists, pathologists, and coagulation experts meets to go over the evidence in hand. We attempt to make some kind of judgment from the first biopsy with all the material we have and then, as far as treatment goes, to follow the patient by the clinical parameters. Is his creatinine clearance improving? What is happening to his serum complement? Is his excretion of protein decreasing? Are his glomeruli becoming more selective in the type of protein they excrete? In this way we are not just studying him by looking at the 15 glomeruli of the biopsy but at several million glomeruli.

Although things do not appear as simple as they might from the original animal model, we are learning from the differences: for instance, that the route of administration of antigen may be as important in man as in the experimental model.

We know, for instance, that poststreptococcal nephritis is certainly associated with complex disease in most instances. It is probably correct that streptococcal antigen in these complexes has been identified by several investigators, notably by Drs. Beatrice Seegal and Kurt Lange. But it is also interesting to note, as Dr. David P. Earle mentioned, that the production of antibody to streptococcus does vary in diseases; it depends upon whether the streptococcus invades by the pharyngeal or the respiratory route or by the skin—which suggests again, perhaps, the importance of the route of administration of the antigen.

In addition to these factors in complex disease, something that has always confused me has been the wealth of literature that points out clearly that in man there is a cross reaction between products of the hemolytic streptococcus and glomerular basement membrane, and that one can absorb out antibodies produced against streptococcus protein by incubating them with glomerular basement membrane.

This suggests that not only deposition of antigen-antibody complexes but perhaps cross-reacting antibodies, antibodies against streptococcus, will cross-react with glomerular basement membrane. This possibility may be important; it has yet to be proved.

The role of the virus in the production of renal lesions has been extremely interesting. The evidence that this occurs in man is very slim. I think this is because our tools are not yet sharp enough to elicit sufficient evidence to prove it. Patients with chicken pox and infectious mononucleosis may develop nephritis.

The animal models are exciting because they tell us much about the possible way in which viruses may cause nephritis in man. We can say that there are a number of spontaneous models for nephritis in the animal, such as nephritis of the Aleutian mink, and that in all cases that have been studied the disease is a complex disease. Where the antigen is known in all of these, the antigen is always a virus or a part of it.

There is a lupuslike syndrome that occurs spontaneously in certain hybrid mice, of which approximately 60 to 70% die two to six months after they are born. The disease resembles lupus in man in every respect. The animals have hemolytic anemia. They have proteinuria. They have complex deposits that one can see. Apparently this is the result of deposition of DNA, probably of viral origin. The interesting thing is that if you challenge these animals with lymphocytic choriomeningitis virus when they are very young, they develop the lesion much earlier and die in a much higher percentage. Even more important to me is the fact that the parents of these hybrid mice, which do not have the disease very often, if challenged with the same virus, very often develop the same disease, which occurs spontaneously in hybrids. This suggests to me that it is indeed very much like the clinical syndrome of lupus, that such a viral etiology for nephritis-complex disease perhaps may be important in man. Other than this, however, we have no real evidence for this supposition.

The words "autoimmune diseases" have been applied to nephritis for a good many years but again, as already pointed out at this conference, we did not have a good model for autoimmune disease until quite recently. Dr. Ray Steblay, in experiments on sheep did indeed develop what is a true autoimmune disease. By this I mean that he made animals produce antibody to their own kidneys. If this can be done in sheep by immunizing them with renal fraction and adjuvants in the right way, the disease they get is autoimmune disease, for one can take antibody circulating in the plasma of a sheep, transmit it to another sheep, and the other sheep acquires the disease.

The interesting thing is that experimenters did not know this until they excised the kidneys of the first sheep, because they did not find any antibodies in the serum while the kidneys were in place. Once the kidneys were excised the sponge that soaked up the antibodies disappeared and the antibodies now had no place to go. They floated around in the serum and could be harvested and given to the next animal, which would then develop the disease. By the way, this kind of disease produces the linear kind of distribution of immunofluorescent globulin that Dr. Robert T. McCluskey has mentioned.

This, too, has a parallel now, at least in one instance in man. We had a patient with rapidly progressive nephritis and linear distribution of globulin on his own kidneys. This patient had no antibodies in his serum at the time we did bilateral nephrectomy prior to transplantation. However, following removal of both his kidneys, which we do routinely before transplanting a normal kidney, antibody to glomerular basement membrane appeared in the serum very much as it does in the sheep after nephrectomy. We found that when these antibodies were incubated with normal kidney slices they would indeed attach to the glomerular basement membrane. Even more important, when a transplanted kidney was put into such a patient these antibodies disappeared from his serum and linear immunoglobulin fluorescence appeared on his own kidney. Presumably the same antibody globulin that disappeared from the serum now attached to his own kidney. Even more important, if only to confirm this supposition, is the fact that Dr. Dixon and his group were able to elute from the patient's damaged kidneys antibodies which, when injected into monkeys, reproduced the nephritis.

Thus in one patient we do have evidence that autoimmune disease occurs, and that its occurrence is associated with antibodies against the patient's own glomerular basement membrane, which causes the disease.

The deposition of immunoglobulin in a linear fashion on glomeruli has been demonstrated adequately in another disease in man: Goodpasture's disease. As you know, Goodpasture's disease involves not only the kidney but the lung; this too has its parallel in the experimental model. Many years ago Dr. Howard Goodman pointed out that if one produced antikidney antibodies in animals one could absorb out some of the antibodies with lung, spleen, and placenta. Thus antikidney antibodies do cross-react with other tissues, presumably in Goodpasture's disease, with the lung.

Again, however, it is not quite as simple as that. We have seen one patient with typical Goodpasture's disease, i.e., hemorrhagic nephritis, pulmonary hemorrhage, and renal failure, who both by immunofluorescence and electron microscopy had not the linear disease that one would expect but "lumpy-bumpy" or complex disease. Further, the Wisconsin group reported eight patients in whom typical antiglomerular basement-membrane staining was present as well as staining of human alveolar septa. However, of these eight patients three had no pulmonary disease. Thus presence of antibody per se is not necessarily followed by the disease.

Finally, a concept that Dr. McCluskey has introduced seems to me especially important: autologous immune complex diseases or autoimmune complex diseases during which the patient produces immune complexes by reason of immunization, either with a fraction of his own kidney or an antigen similar enough to his own tissues to cause the latter may continue to stimulate antibodies and thus to form complexes. Thus a complex is formed which produces complex disease in the kidney. This, I believe, is particularly important because it is the kind of thing we see frequently in the glomerular lesion of kidney transplants (certainly a classic example of the way in which one may immunize a patient is by transplanting a kidney into him). We are finding a considerable number of glomerular lesions in our transplant patients, and a good many of these appear to be complex disease, which suggests again a parallel in man to the animal model.

And now a word about complement. I mentioned earlier that complement activation is the first step in the chain of reactions after the antigen-antibody combination, which has many reactions, any or all of which may cause nephritis.

The finding of low-serum complement levels in acute disease or in hypocomplementemic nephritis, as Dr. Clark West has called it, suggests that the complement is low because it is being withdrawn from the serum and put on the kidney. We know that that is not why the complement is low. In our own transplantation patients and in patients with low complement disease at Children's Hospital, Boston, Mass., it appears that complement is low not because it is being pulled down but because in some way its synthesis of it is being suppressed. In other words, one must look at this condition as a dynamic situation, not simply a static one. Net turnover of complement is important.

Further, as Dr. Clark West himself has pointed out, the complement is probably low in his patients not, again, because it is being withdrawn from the serum and being put on the kidney, but because there exists in the serum a specific inhibitor or lytic agent for one factor of complement. What this has to do with the disease per se we do not know.

Certainly in the experimental model the deposition of complement has an important role. I am especially interested, as I know Dr. McCluskey is, in the role of fibrinogen and the deposition of fibrin because, again, it is not proteinuria or hematuria that kills the patients; it is not even antigen-antibody combinations that cause the disease: it is what happens afterward. What kills the patient is sclerosis of the glomeruli of fibrosis, with destruction of functioning units.

Immunofluorescent studies of our own group and of those of Dr. McCluskey have shown very clearly that the deposition of fibrinogen is very common in glomerular lesions, no matter what their cause. Dr. William Braun of our group several years ago showed a good correlation between the activity of nephritis, the rejection of transplants, and the finding of split products of fibrin in the urine. More recently a group from Wisconsin has shown the same thing: they correlated activities of the disease in acute nephritis with the presence of fibrin split products in the plasma.

The major problem, however, seems to be: What makes the disease progress after the initial insult? Dr. Dodge, quoted early in this symposium, has recently suggested that progressive disease is simply an exacerbation of the disease in persons with preexisting renal lesions. I am not sure that this is true. One possibility for continued activity is that cross-reacting antibodies are developed upon exposure to the hemolytic streptococcus. These antibodies then react with glomerular basement membrane to cause the lesion of nephritis.

Since basement membrane, as we know, is constantly being liberated in urine—sometimes in plasma—this surge, as it were, of antigen may elicit a countersurge of antibody, as has been shown in lupus, and may produce repeated insult with fibrinogen deposition, with healing by fibrosis and, ultimately, with death of the nephron and of the patient.

We do not know that this occurs in progressive nephritis in man. However, we do know that it occurs in patients with a transplanted kidney.

Dr. Ronald Guttmann in our laboratory has utilized a rat model that illustrates this kind of thing very nicely. If one transplants a kidney between two rats whose histocompatibility difference is very small, a slowly rejecting kidney is obtained. In this slowly rejecting kidney transplant the principal lesion is a lobular type of glomerulonephritis.

Thus the rat that is slowly and constantly rejecting the transplanted kidney or the foreign antigen manifests a progressive destruction of his glomeruli which histologically is indistinguishable from the naturally occurring disease in man.

Even more interesting, perhaps, is the fact that Dr. Robert Schwartz of Boston has shown he can produce nephritis in rats by simply injecting them with foreign rat-spleen cells, which presumably reject the host animal and thus reject the kidney, with resulting glomerulonephritis. What interests me in this, of course, is that this all goes back to Dr. William Dameshek's old idea about some forbidden or abnormal clone of antibody-forming cell. Let us suppose that some clone of lymphocytes in your own body began to mutate, began to change, and then recognized your glomeruli as abnormal. It is possible these lymphocytes could act, as do foreign spleen cells in the rat against the glomeruli; and nephritis would result.

Finally, what about treatment for nephritis? I am inclined to agree with most of the contributors to this conference thus far that we have no real evidence that treatment has done much. All of us have seen individual cases which respond dramatically to treatment. Statistically, however, it is difficult to prove that immunosuppressive therapy significantly modifies the course of the disease. The review of our own 68 cases and groups such as the British series gives no real statistical evidence that we have influenced the natural course of the disease. We may have accelerated the cure that was going to occur anyway. Recovery might have occurred in two or three weeks instead of in two or three years, but I do not think we can say we have found any effective therapy.

What is the cause of our therapeutic failure? One might use, perhaps, the example of complex disease. We know that immune complexes are deposited in the glomeruli. They are deposited under certain circumstances in which the concentration of antigen in the serum is a little in excess of the antibody concentration. In "single-shot disease," that is, where only one injection of antigen is given, the disease tapers off as antibody titer increases and exceeds the concentration of antigen.

Suppose one starts treating a patient at this point and uses nothing but immunosuppressants. One might reinstate the situation of antigen excess and make the disease worse. We seem to have no evidence for such a result but I do think it is a possibility. It may explain why we are not helping persons with immunosuppressive therapy per se, especially when we remember that it is not the antibody that may cause the damage.

In fact there is evidence, as I have already mentioned, that antibody in and of itself may actually protect the kidney or the cancer or, in the case of experimental encephalomyelitis, the brain. Thus antibody may have a protective or enhancing effect. It may not necessarily be the villain it has been thought to be.

Where does one go in therapy, then? I do not know, any more than do the rest of us. Dr. Charles Cochrane, of Dr. Dixon's group, has pointed out that if you destroy all the polymorphonuclear leukocytes with Cytoxan (cyclophosphamide), you can have all the antigen-antibody combinations possible, and the disease does not develop. Certainly Cytoxan has been the subject of much interest in the pediatric literature. It may well be important as therapy for nephritis.

We have heard something about the use of anticoagulants. Heparin in experimental animals may prevent the disease, but too much of it must be used. We think heparin prevents or helps prevent rejection of the transplant, and we have some evidence that it may be helpful in nephritis. But again, we are not enthusiastic about the treatment.

Our old friend aspirin has a great effect upon the platelets. It has been shown to prevent the aggregation of platelets. We and others have used this in the treatment of nephritis and the rejection of transplantation. There is suggestive evidence that it may help prevent the deposition of platelets and their effects on subsequent deposition of fibrinogen. None of these procedures, however, has been proved successful but are of interest.

What about the future? It may well be that by investigating factors other than antibody we shall have more precise tools. For instance, let us say we were to eliminate the fraction of complement that is important in setting up the chain reaction. Would this help? There is suggestive evidence that a factor taken from, of all things, cobra venom, may actually split the third component of complement, and that it may prevent some of these immune reactions. This addition splits the third component and leaves 1, 4, and 2 viable. We do not have the total immunosuppresant effect as with other agents.

There is an Alpha 2 globulin which has been isolated from thymus and from blood which will enhance the survival of skin grafts and prevents antibody formation to sheep red cells in the rat. If it can be purified consistently it, too, may have an effective role in preventing immune disease and nephritis.

Finally, the hope of all who are interested in transplantation is that we may be able to produce tolerance. By tolerance I mean the ability of one animal to tolerate viable cells of another animal without the use of immunosuppressive agents. This can be done.

Let us suppose for a moment that a patient with nephritis is rejecting his kidney and, in this fashion, is developing nephritis. If we could produce tolerance for this patient's own kidney as has been done in animals, we might thereby prevent the progress of nephritis. Actually it has been suggested that the production of tolerance to kidney cells may be important in the prevention of experimentally produced nephritis. Although the author of this suggestion stated that he produced such tolerance with isologous cells, which to me is difficult to understand, I think that the concept is interesting and perhaps important from a therapeutic standpoint.

In summary: we have no therapeutic answers, but I think we do have, on the horizon, some fascinating new possibilities which will be applicable not only to glomerulonephritis, but to transplantation, possibly to the so-called autoimmune diseases such as rheumatoid arthritis and a variety of others, and, possibly, even for cancer.

THE RENAL REGULATION OF SODIUM TRANSPORT*

NORMAN BANK

Associate Professor of Medicine
New York University School of Medicine
New York, N. Y.

DURING the past 10 years a surge of renewed interest in the regulation of sodium by the kidney has taken place as a result of the observations of De Wardener et al.[1] These investigators demonstrated that the natriuresis which follows the rapid intravenous infusion of saline in the dog can occur without any rise in the filtered load of sodium and in the presence of large amounts of mineralocorticoid hormones. Their experiments showed unequivocally for the first time that the kidney possesses some other mechanism or mechanisms for changing the rate of sodium and water reabsorption by its tubules in response to acute changes in extracellular fluid volume, the so-called "third factor." Many other laboratories soon confirmed their findings, and it became evident that these other mechanisms are of prime importance in the regulation of homeostasis.

Although there is still much to be learned about the nature of these tubular regulatory mechanisms an increasing body of experimental evidence suggests that at least one of them is mediated by hydrostatic and colloid oncotic pressure gradients across the wall of the peritubular capillaries. For example, Lewy and Windhager[2] found that when hydrostatic pressure is raised in the peritubular capillaries of the rat kidney by partial clamping of one renal vein, the reabsorption of sodium by the proximal tubules of that kidney is markedly inhibited. The inhibition could not be explained by any change in the cross-sectional diameter of the tubules; that is, by the tubular geometry hypothesis of sodium regulation.[3] Lewy and Windhager suggested that constriction of the renal vein had reduced the rate of uptake of the tubular reabsorbate by the peritubular capillaries, and this led to a rise in pressure in the interstitial compartment of the kidney. They postulated that passive back-diffusion of sodium and water into the cell might be increased because of a higher inter-

*Presented at a *Conference on Glomerulonephritis* held by the New York Heart Association at The Waldorf-Astoria, New York, N. Y., January 27, 1970.

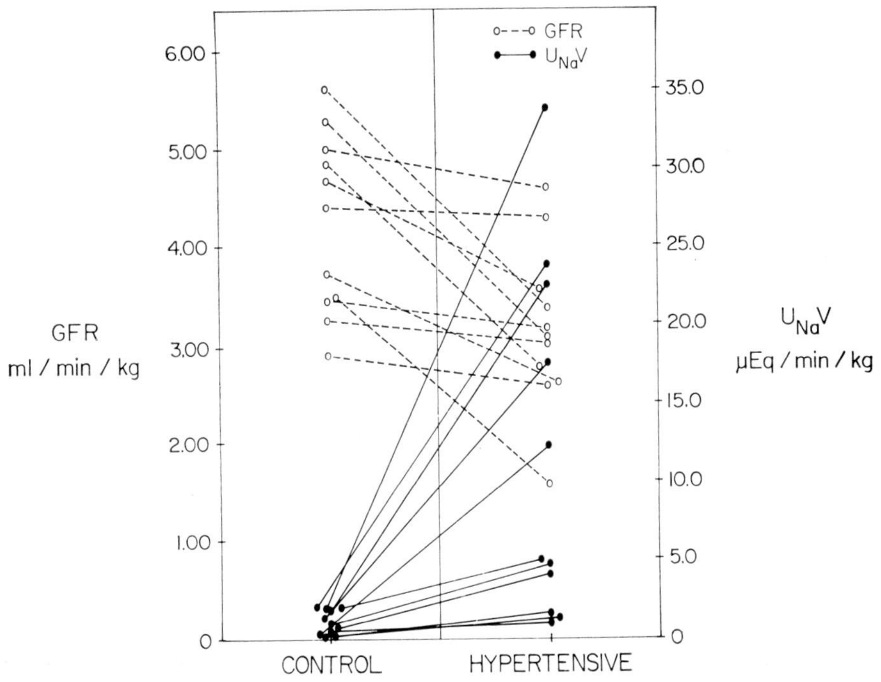

Fig. 1. The effect of acute hypertension on GFR and urinary sodium excretion. Hypertension was produced by bilateral carotid artery ligation.

stitial pressure and that this would account for the reduction in the net reabsorption of sodium.

In our own laboratory, Drs. Koch and Aynedjian[4] were also interested in studying the effect of acute changes in peritubular capillary pressure on sodium transport by the proximal tubules. The protocol which they used in rats was to raise systemic blood pressure acutely to hypertensive levels by ligating both carotid arteries. Figure 1 shows the data on sodium excretion in the urine and GFR. As can be seen, GFR remained relatively constant or fell moderately during the period of hypertension. Sodium excretion, however, increased significantly in all cases; this indicated that tubular reabsorption had been inhibited. Micropuncture measurements of TF/P_{In} ratios at the end of the proximal convolutions on the surface of the kidney, shown in Figure 2, demonstrated a significant fall. When this is considered in concert with the over-all decrease in GFR it seems reasonable to conclude that proximal tubular transport of sodium had been inhibited by the acute hypertension.

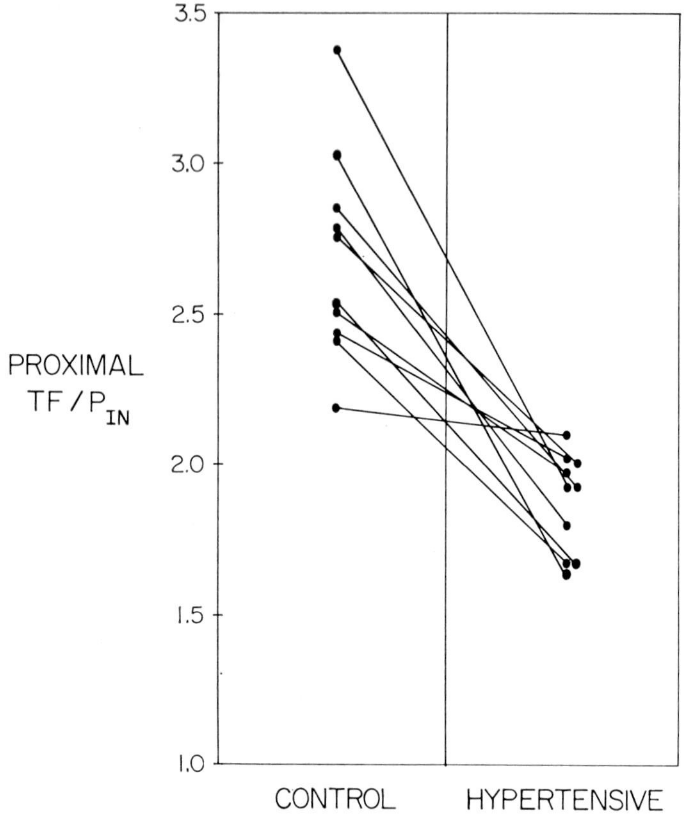

Fig. 2. Tubular fluid/plasma inulin ratios during normotensive and hypertensive periods. Each point represents the average of 3 to 5 observations. The lines connect data from individual rats.

A second, independent, micropuncture technique, the split oil-drop measurement, confirmed that proximal sodium reabsorption had been inhibited. The data indicated that the reabsorptive half-time ($t_{1/2}$) of columns of isotonic saline injected into the proximal lumen increased from a mean control value of approximately 8 sec. to 14 sec. These observations, in addition to demonstrating inhibition of reabsorption, rule out changes in GFR and tubular geometry as possible mechanisms, since the split-drop measurement is independent of these two variables.

In looking for alternative mechanisms to explain the inhibition produced by hypertension we infused large amounts of *d*-aldosterone in another group of animals. This did not prevent the inhibition of prox-

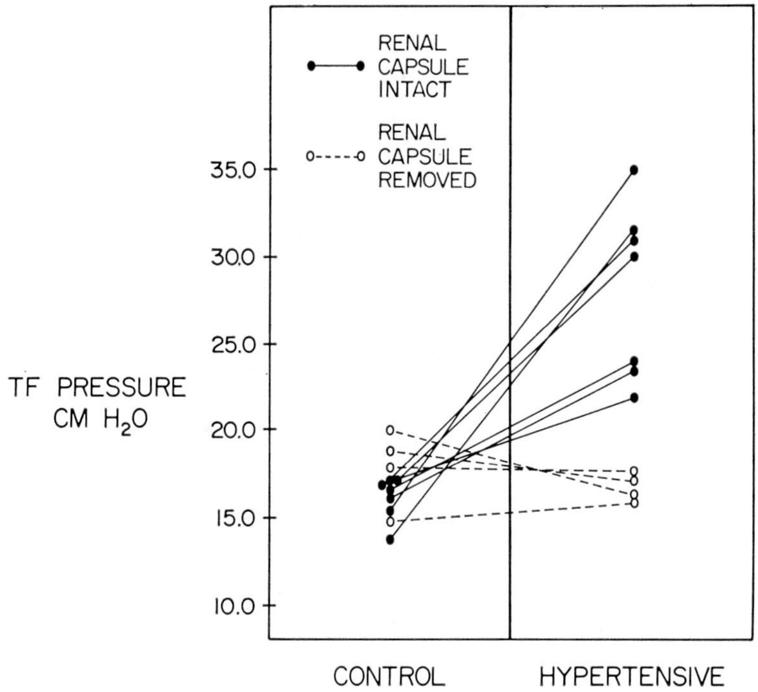

Fig. 3. Hydrostatic pressure in the proximal lumen during normotensive and hypertensive periods. Each point represents the average of 3 to 5 determinations.

imal sodium reabsorption induced by ligation of the carotid arteries. In another group of animals, renal renin content was lowered by oral salt loading for two to three weeks. This also did not prevent the inhibition of proximal sodium reabsorption induced by acute hypertension. It seemed, therefore, that neither aldosterone nor the renin-angiotensin system was involved in the inhibition. Measurement of hydrostatic pressure in the proximal tubules made before and during acute hypertension, shown in Figure 3, demonstrated a definite rise from a mean value of 16 to 28 cm. H_2O. It seems likely that pressure in the adjacent capillaries also became elevated, since the pressures in the tubular lumen and the capillaries usually parallel one another quite closely. This rise in hydrostatic pressure, presumably occurring first in the capillaries and then in the tubular lumen, might have been causally related to the inhibition of sodium transport. In order to test this possibility we partially constricted the aorta above the renal arteries and

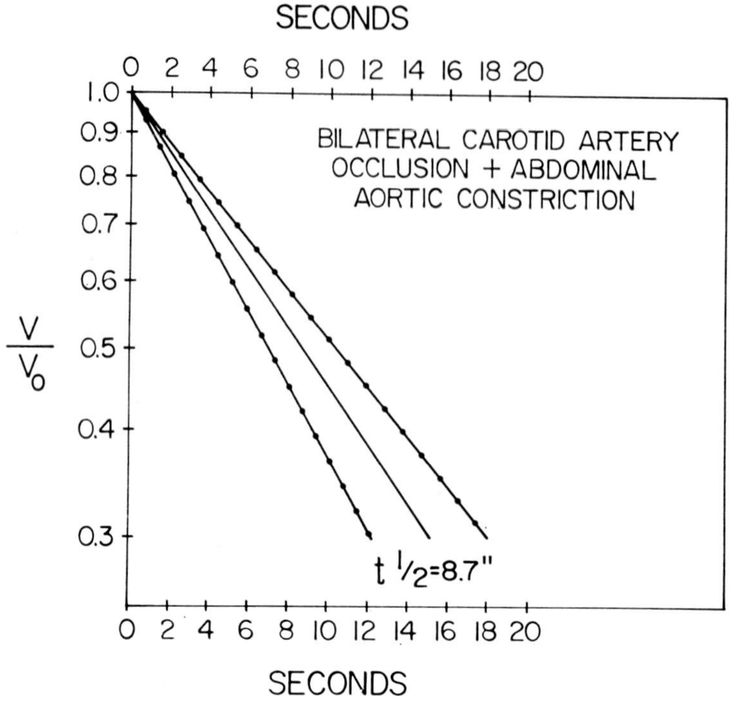

Fig. 4. Split-drop measurements in rats with carotid-artery occlusion and normal renal-perfusion pressure. V is the length of the column of saline at a given time and V_0 is the length at time $= 0$; $t\frac{1}{2}$ corresponds to $V/V_0 = 0.5$. The dotted lines represent standard deviation for the group of observations.

maintained renal perfusion pressure at normal levels at the same time that hypertension was induced in the upper half of the body by ligation of the carotid arteries. The results of split-drop measurements made in these animals are shown in Figure 4. As may be seen, under these experimental conditions, reabsorptive $t_{1/2}$ remained normal. These observations served two purposes. First, they tended to exclude any extrarenal hormone as the causative agent for the inhibition of sodium transport, since aortic constriction should not have prevented a circulating hormone from reaching the kidney. Second, they indicated the importance of renal perfusion pressure per se in the mechanism. We therefore came to a conclusion similar to that reached by Lewy and Windhager[2] and by Earley and his co-workers from clearance experiments in dogs[5, 6] that sodium and water reabsorption in the proximal tubule

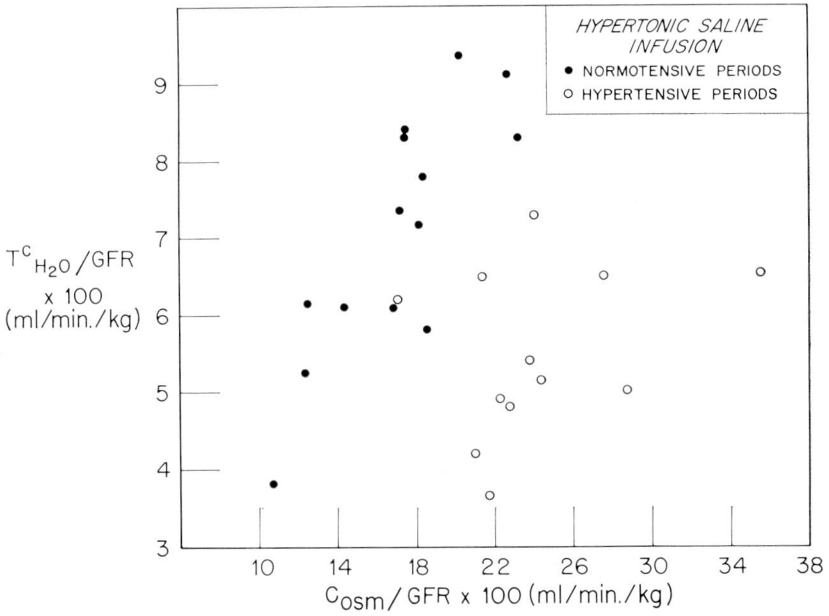

Fig. 5. The effect of acute hypertension induced by epinephrine on solute-free water reabsorption ($T^{C}_{H_2O}$). Normotensive and hypertensive data were obtained in the same rats.

can be influenced markedly by hydrostatic pressure changes in the peritubular capillaries.

More recently we have examined the effect of acute hydrostatic pressure changes in the kidney on sodium reabsorption by the loop of Henle. This was done by measuring solute-free water reabsorption ($T^{C}_{H_2O}$ in rats during hypertonic saline infusion before and during a period of acute hypertension induced by intravenous epinephrine infusion. The results are shown in Figure 5. In the normotensive control periods, $T^{C}_{H_2O}$ rose linearly with increasing rates of osmolar clearance (C_{osm}). In sharp contrast, when blood pressure was elevated by 20 to 50 mm. Hg, $T^{C}_{H_2O}$ fell markedly and sodium excretion increased abruptly. These observations are consistent with the view that sodium transport by the ascending limb of Henle's loop had been inhibited, although other interpretations, such as a washout of renal medullary solutes, are also plausible. In order to determine more certainly whether distal sodium transport had been inhibited, we studied another group of animals in

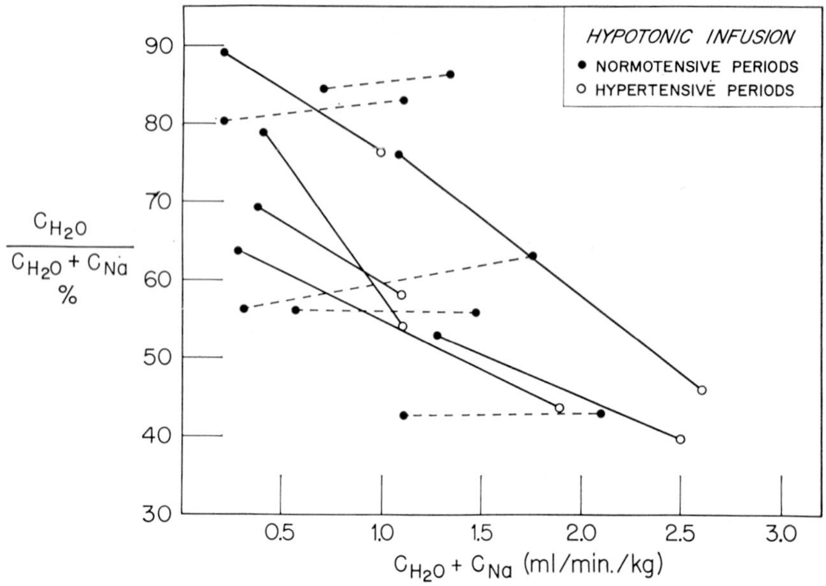

Fig. 6. The effect of acute hypertension on free-water clearance (C_{H_2O}). The values on the abscissa approximate delivery of sodium out of the proximal tubule. The values on the ordinate approximate fractional reabsorption of sodium by the diluting segments of the nephron. Interrupted lines are control normotensive rats in which the rate of infusion was increased progressively.

which endogenous ADH was suppressed and free water clearance (C_{H_2O}) was produced by the infusion of hypotonic mannitrol. The data are shown in Figure 6. The sum of C_{H_2O} and C_{Na}, shown on the abscissa, is taken as a rough approximation of the rate of delivery of sodium from the proximal tubule to the loop of Henle. On the ordinate is the fraction of the delivered sodium reabsorbed by the diluting segment of the nephron to generate free water. In control animals, shown as interrupted lines, the rate of mannitol infusion was increased progressively but blood pressure remained normal. In these control animals, the diluting segment reabsorbed a relatively constant fraction of the sodium delivered to it. In contrast, in every animal in which acute hypertension was produced fractional reabsorption of sodium by the diluting segment fell significantly. These observations cannot be accounted for by changes in medullary solute concentrations, since in the absence of ADH the distal segments of the nephron are thought to be impermeable to water. Therefore, C_{H_2O} is essentially independent of medullary solute concentration. The data strongly suggest that epinephrine infusion had inhibited sodium transport in the distal segments of the nephron responsible for the generation of a dilute urine. In additional control experiments in which renal perfusion pressure was held constant by an aortic clamp, during the infusion of epinephrine, no sodium diuresis occurred; this indicated that epinephrine has no direct effect on sodium transport. We concluded therefore that it was the elevation of renal perfusion pressure which had been responsible for the distal inhibition of sodium transport.

Time does not allow a detailed description of all the other experimental observations which have been made with regard to the role of peritubular physical forces in the regulation of sodium transport, but I shall briefly mention some of them. Windhager and his co-workers[7] perfused the peritubular capillaries of individual nephrons of the rat kidney with dextran solutions of varying concentrations in order to alter colloid oncotic pressure and, simultaneously, they measured sodium reabsorption in the same nephrons. They found a direct correlation between the rate of sodium reabsorption and the colloid oncotic pressure of the perfusing solution. Berliner and his co-workers[8] studied the same problem by injecting solutions of different protein concentration as a bolus into the aortas of rats near the renal arteries, and measuring the protein concentration in the peritubular capillaries and proximal sodium reabsorption. They also found a direct correlation between the colloid oncotic pressure of the peritubular capillary blood and the rate of proximal tubular sodium reabsorption. In our own laboratory[9] we found that the usual inhibition of proximal sodium reabsorption which occurs during rapid infusion of saline can be prevented if hydrostatic pressure is not allowed to rise in the kidney. This suggested that changes in physical forces within the intrarenal blood vessels are largely responsible for the inhibition of proximal sodium transport induced by saline loading.

I should now like to theorize on cellular mechanisms which might explain how changes in physical forces across the peritubular capillary wall could regulate tubular reabsorption. First, it seems likely from a number of observations that the active sodium pump is located along channels made up of infoldings of the basal membrane of the tubular cells, that is, along the basal labyrinth and the lateral interspaces. The anatomy is illustrated in Figure 7, which shows the basal portion of

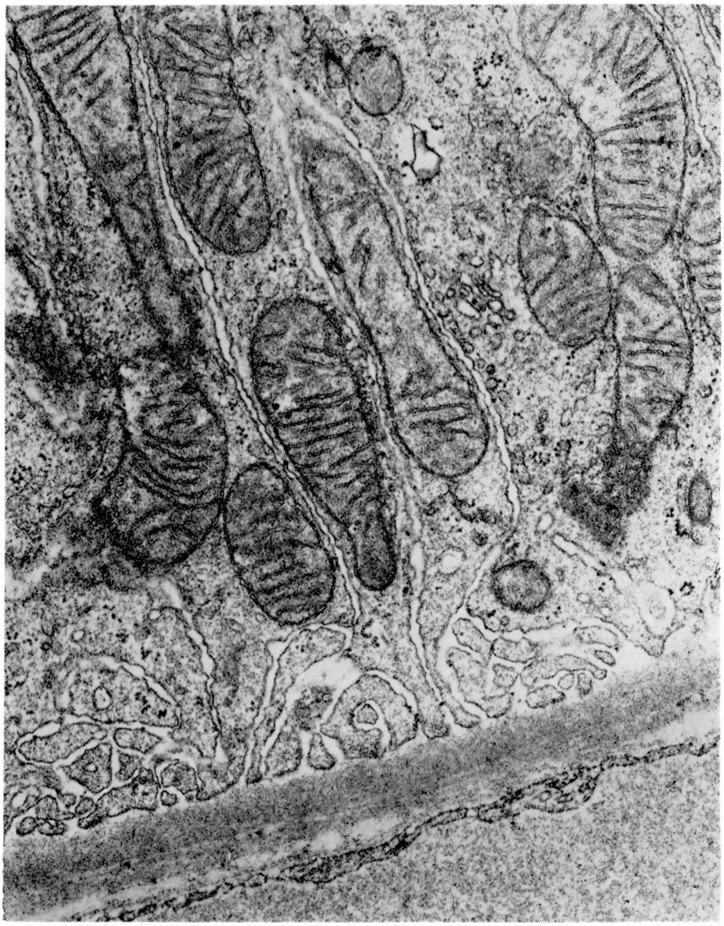

Fig. 7. Electron micrograph of basal portion of rat proximal tubule.

the proximal tubular cells in the rat. Sodium in the tubular lumen probably diffuses passively into the cell down a large electrochemical gradient, and is then actively transported into the lateral interspaces. Diamond and Bossert[10] have proposed a theoretical model based on this anatomy in which active sodium transport creates an osmotic gradient between the interior of the cell and the lateral interspaces. Water is drawn passively into the interspaces, causing flow by convection toward the open ends of the channels facing the basement membrane. At the same time the entering water dissipates the osmotic gradient so that the fluid which

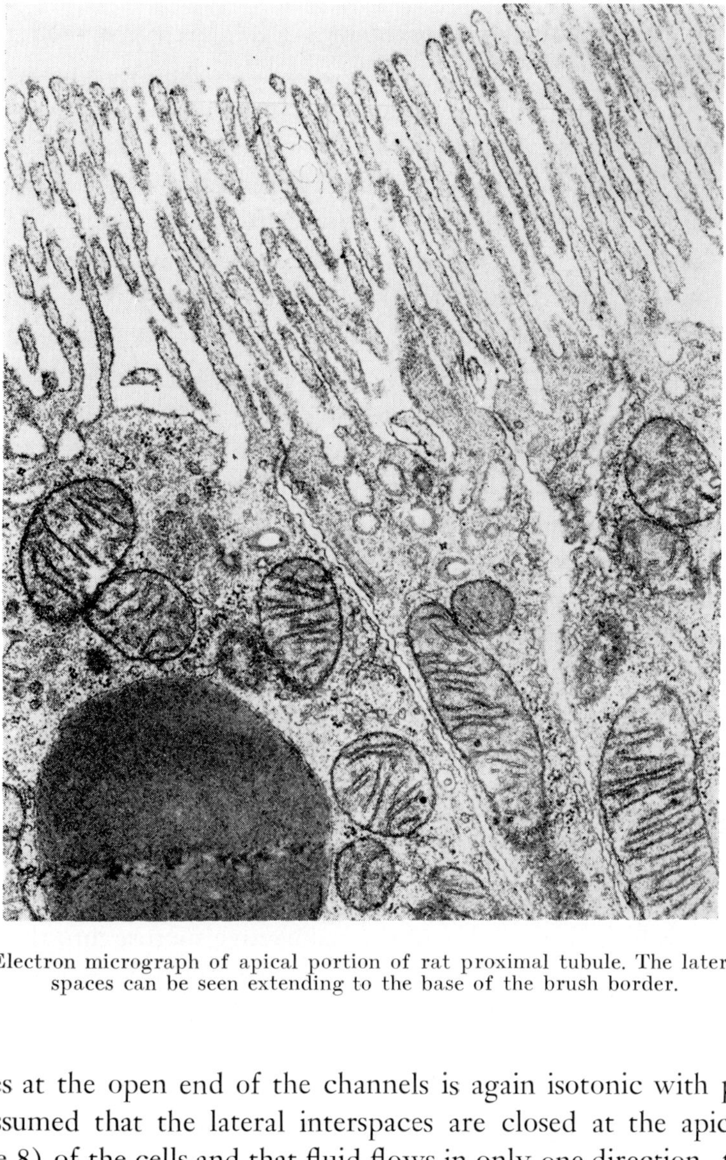

Fig. 8. Electron micrograph of apical portion of rat proximal tubule. The lateral interspaces can be seen extending to the base of the brush border.

emerges at the open end of the channels is again isotonic with plasma. It is assumed that the lateral interspaces are closed at the apical end (Figure 8) of the cells and that fluid flows in only one direction—toward the basement membrane and the peritubular capillaries.

One possible mechanism by which changes in hydrostatic or colloid oncotic pressure in capillaries might affect this transport system is by changing the pressure in the lateral interspaces and the basal labyrinth. For example, if hydrostatic pressure increased or colloid oncotic pressure decreased in the peritubular capillaries the rate of uptake of interstitial fluid by the capillaries would be reduced and pressure might tend to rise in the interstitial compartment. It has been proposed that the higher pressure would distend the interspaces, perhaps causing stagnation of flow and a build-up of higher sodium concentrations.[7] These changes might result in greater passive back-diffusion of sodium into the interior of the cell. Greater back-diffusion might then raise intracellular sodium concentration and thereby reduce the diffusion of sodium from the tubular lumen into the cell. Also, if high concentrations of sodium developed in the lateral interspaces the active transport of sodium might be reduced if the rate of pumping is limited by a concentration gradient.

Although these complex series of events seem reasonable and may eventually prove to be correct other possible mechanisms should also be considered. Several observations suggest the possibility that a generalized increase in permeability of the proximal tubule may be involved in the inhibition of transport which occurs with changes in peritubular forces. For example, it has been found that the reabsorption of several other solutes, such as phosphate[11] and glucose[12] is inhibited by acute saline loading, an experimental condition known to alter peritubular physical forces. Also, Boulpaep[13] has recently reported that the electrical resistance across the proximal tubule falls markedly during saline diuresis; this suggests a shunting of ions from the interstitial compartment into the tubular lumen. In our laboratory we are presently carrying out experiments in which isolated segments of the proximal tubule of the rat are perfused with isotonic saline while the animals are receiving C^{14}-labeled sucrose intravenously. In normotensive nondiuretic animals there is little or no influx of the radioactive sucrose into the tubular lumen. During partial constriction of the renal vein, however, and elevation of peritubular capillary pressure, we have found that a significant influx of C^{14}-sucrose occurs. We interpret these observations to mean that the proximal tubule has become permeable enough to allow influx of an extracellular molecule which normally does not enter. It seems reasonable to expect that smaller molecules and water would also be able to enter the tubular lumen more readily than under normal conditions. In collaboration with Dr. Richard Ames of Roosevelt Hospital, New York City, we are investigating the electron microscopy of the tubules under the same experimental conditions in an attempt to determine the structural pathways for this back-diffusion. Figure 8 is a view of the apical portion of the proximal tubular cells of a normal rat. The lateral interspaces can be seen to extend quite close to the base of the brush border. This seems a possible site for back-flux to occur, although other routes are also feasible.

I am sure that the next few years will be exciting ones in this area, and that much new information will appear about the basic cellular mechanisms by which peritubular physical forces help to regulate the processes of renal transport.

REFERENCES

1. De Wardener, H. E., Mills, I. H., Clapham, W. F. and Hayter, C. J.: Studies on the efferent mechanism of the sodium diuresis which follows the administration of intravenous saline in the dog. *Clin. Sci. 21*:249, 1961.
2. Lewy, J. E. and Windhager, E. E.: Peritubular control of proximal tubular fluid reabsorption in the rat kidney. *Amer. J. Physiol. 214*:943, 1968.
3. Brunner, F. P., Rector, Jr., F. C. and Seldin, D. W.: Mechanism of glomerulotubular balance. II. Regulation of proximal tubular reabsorption by tubular volume, as studied by stopped-flow microperfusion. *J. Clin. Invest. 45*:603, 1966.
4. Koch, K. M., Aynedjian, H. S. and Bank, N.: The effect of acute hypertension on sodium reabsorption by the proximal tubule. *J. Clin. Invest. 44*: 1696, 1968.
5. Earley, L. E. and Friedler, R. M.: The effects of combined renal vasodilation and pressor agents on renal hemodynamics and the tubular reabsorption of sodium. *J. Clin. Invest. 45*:542, 1966.
6. Martino, J. A. and Earley, L. E.: Demonstration of a role of physical factors as determinants of the natriuretic response to volume expansion. *J. Clin. Invest. 46*:1963, 1967.
7. Windhager, E. E., Lewy, J. E. and Spitzer, A.: Intrarenal control of proximal tubular reabsorption of sodium and water. *Nephron 6*:247, 1969.
8. Brenner, B. M., Falchuk, K. H., Keimowitz, R. I. and Berliner, R. W.: The relationship between peritubular capillary protein concentration and fluid reabsorption by the renal proximal tubule. *J. Clin. Invest. 48*:1519, 1969.
9. Bank, N., Koch, K. M., Aynedjian, H. S. and Aras, M.: Effect of changes in renal perfusion pressure on the suppression of proximal tubular sodium reabsorption due to saline loading. *J. Clin. Invest. 48*:271, 1969.
10. Diamond, J. M. and Bossert, W. H. Standing-gradient osmotic flow. A mechanism for coupling of water and solute transport in epithelia. *J. Gen. Physiol. 50*:2061, 1967.
11. Massry, S. G., Coburn, J. W. and Kleeman, C. R.: The influence of extracellular volume expansion on renal phosphate reabsorption in the dog. *J. Clin. Invest. 48*:1237, 1969.
12. Robson, A. M., Srivastava, P. L. and Bricker, N. S. The influence of saline loading on renal glucose reabsorption in the rat. *J. Clin. Invest. 47*:329, 1968.
13. Boulpaep, E. L.: Third Annual Meeting of the Amer. Soc. of Nephrol., December 1-2, 1969, Washington, D. C.

PROTEINURIA IN RENAL DISEASE*

E. Lovell Becker

Professor of Medicine
Cornell University Medical College, New York, N. Y.

More than 150 years ago Richard Bright recognized that patients with disease of the kidney had coagulable urine. In the ensuing years there has been considerable discussion and numerous studies planned to explain the mechanisms whereby protein appears in the urine in normal individuals as well as in patients with renal disease.

In 1924 Wearn and Richards[1] searched for protein in proximal tubular fluid of frogs; an acetic acid-potassium-ferrocyanide precipitate test was used. In 11 samples no protein precipitate was found. Walker, Bott, Oliver, and MacDowell[2] measured protein concentration in 41 samples of glomerular and proximal tubular fluid from the guinea pig and rat. Protein was measured by direct inspection of the flocculation occurring in a capillary tube treated with trichloracetic acid and compared to varying dilutions of normal plasma, which was assumed to contain 7% protein. The results suggested that tubular fluid contained protein in a range of concentrations from zero to more than 200 mg.%. This would exclude the possibility of a grossly porous glomerular filter. Dock[3] inhibited tubular function by perfusing rabbit kidneys with cold serum and found 15 to 22 mg. of protein per 100 ml. of urine. Later proximal tubular albumin was calculated at 7.6 mg.% by measuring the amount of dye labeled in albumin in histological sections of the proximal tubule.[4]

Dirks, Clapp, and Berliner[5] determined the concentrations of albumin and globulin in proximal tubular fluid of five dogs by a quantitative gel-diffusion precipitin technique. Albumin concentrations in 18 samples were in the range of 2 to 8 mg.%, while in another 18 samples no precipitation was noted, and in two samples 10 and 15 mg.% of both albumin and gamma globulin were noted. Further, albumin concentration did not change according to any pattern when plotted as a function of distance along the tubule.

In summarizing these data it is difficult to speculate as to the amount

*Presented at a *Conference on Glomerulonephritis* held by the New York Heart Association at The Waldorf-Astoria, New York, N. Y., January 27, 1970.

of albumin reabsorption or indeed the amount filtered by normal man, but in animals a tubular albumin concentration of less than 1 mg.% would account for all albumin excreted. Since there is so little information in man, i.e. since only urine and plasma may be analyzed, we must consider several different approaches. There are several methods available for evaluation of proteins in the urine and serum: for example, electrophoresis, gel diffusion techniques, chromatography, and immunoprecipitation as well as immunoelectrophoresis.

For proteins ultimately to appear in the urine they must pass the glomerular barrier. This barrier is made up of the glomerular capillaries which contain three distinct layers: the endothelial cell, the basement membrane, and the epithelial cell. Proteins in passing the glomerular capillary traverse the endothelial cell with its attenuated and fenestrated cytoplasm; the basement membrane, which is made up of a less dense endothelial portion and a more dense medial portion; and a third less dense epithelial portion of the basement membrane. The proteins then must find their way through the epithelial cells. In the various disease states these different layers may be altered, but the exact mechanism whereby proteins are able to pass these layers is not understood.

Farquhar and Palade[6] injected ferritin molecules intravenously into normal rats and aminonucleoside nephrotic rats. Since ferritin is about the same size as albumin, and is electron-dense, it is particularly well suited for electron-microscopic studies. These workers noted that the ferritin molecules easily passed through the "pores" in the endothelial cells. The ferritin was noted in the basement membrane in only an occasional normal rat but was readily seen in the basement membrane in nephrotic rats. The epithelial cell allowed ferritin molecules to pass in nephrotic rats by the "slit pores" or through the foot processes. The authors further noted that the epithelial cell-foot processes phagocytosed the ferritin molecules. This degradation of protein may account for split-protein products found in the urine, and it also may account for the total amount of protein found in the urine.

There are several mechanisms or types of proteinuria which are clinically recognizable:[7]

1) The defective glomerular capillary. This is the greatest cause of heavy proteinuria seen in humans. The layer of the glomerular capillary that is defective is not known. Most probably all three layers are involved, particularly the basement membrane.

2) Failure of normal tubular reabsorption. It has been suggested that reabsorption of proteins, particularly small molecular-weight proteins, is a continuing process; however there is no direct evidence in man to support this concept.

3) Proteinuria that arises secondary to abnormally high concentrations of normal plasma proteins. This may be encountered in patients after infusion of salt-poor albumin. When albumin is infused, there is not only albuminuria, but heavier molecular-weight proteins are also found, particularly in patients with nephrotic syndrome. Patients with carcinoma of the bronchus may excrete increased amounts of orosomucoid, a normal plasma protein of low molecular weight.

4) Abnormal proteins present in the plasma may be excreted. This urinary loss may occur because they are of smaller molecular weight, or because a maximum reabsorptive rate for the particular protein has been exceeded, so the increased amounts are no longer transported by the renal tubules. Bence-Jones proteins and hemoglobin are examples of such proteins.

5) Abnormal losses of proteins. This category of proteins may be found in the urine secondary to the exfoliation of cells of the kidney or ureter. There may also be proteins that arise de novo in the kidney. In certain calculous diseases, in rheumatoid arthritis, and in patients with abnormal lymph drainage or chyluria there may be abnormal proteins present.

Persistent and massive proteinuria affects whole-body metabolism: there is an increased rate of protein synthesis above the normal of 0.25 gm./kg./day. With this increased synthesis over long periods of time, patients with massive proteinuria may compensate for their losses so that the serum-protein concentration will be normal. To determine the losses of protein in the urine there are numerous tests available, such as the Buiret reaction, trichloracetic acid, and the sulphosalicylic-acid test. The standard of reference for protein determination is the microkjeldahl, which is probably the best method but admittedly more difficult.

In comparing one patient to another, which is necessary in investigative procedures, one may relate the protein loss to creatinine clearance, height, weight, or body-surface area, but in the cases of marked wasting or edema this may be inaccurate. It has been suggested that the cube of the height would give an index which is more comparable between patients although physiologically meaningless. Protein excretion per 24 hours is the best available method for following patients with renal disease. However, in order to eliminate variations of serum concentration it is well to consider the possibility of a clearance of albumin as a measure of kidney function. To take this one step further: if this is related to the clearance of water or of creatinine, which is closely approximate to the clearance of water, it might be a more exact method whereby functional damage to the glomerular filter can be assessed. While this test is of great value in detecting renal disease and following the actual course of the disease, it is of little value in differential diagnosis.

It is incorrect and misleading to require proteinuria for a diagnosis of renal disease. For example, proteinuria may be absent, intermittent, or in minimal quantities in chronic pyelonephritis, urinary-tract obstruction, renal tubular diseases, medullary cystic disease, and in some stages in the natural course of chronic glomerulonephritis.

Differential clearances of urine protein are of value in understanding mechanisms, pathological changes, and response to therapy. By the use of clearances of various molecular-weight proteins larger than albumin, it is possible to classify the disease process as to the types of proteins excreted. Using an immunochemical-precipitation technique as described by Soothill[8] eight serum proteins were evaluated. By preparing antisera to the various proteins a U/P concentration ratio can be determined. Since only one urine is obtained for all the proteins studied the flow rate cancels out, but we have a ratio of virtual clearance. It is possible to relate the test-protein clearance to a standard of reference (transferrin) and relate this to the molecular weight of the test protein. A plot of these data will allow the construction of a straight line, where slope may be determined and the angle with the intercept determined.[9]

In general, patients with heavy proteinuria may be found to excrete proteins which follow two general patterns. The first is a rather nonselective proteinuria, that is, the heavy molecular-weight globulins are excreted in addition to albumin, so that it can be said that the glomerular membrane is highly permeable to all molecular weights of protein. Patients with this type of excretion pattern respond very poorly, if at all, to steroid or immunosuppressive therapy. In contrast to this group is another group of patients in whom predominantly low molecular-weight proteins are excreted, that is, the glomerular filter is serving as a highly selective membrane. By and large, patients who fall into this category have a good response to steroid or immunosuppressive therapy. To differentiate these two further, the angle made by the slope of the plots mentioned above is obtained and those who have a selectivity of greater than 67° usually respond to steroids, and those with a selectivity of less than 54° do not respond. In some instances, particularly with a small total protein excretion, the log log plot of these proteins does not follow a straight-line pattern, but may have a convex "dog-leg" pattern. This phenomenon is difficult to understand but it is most frequently seen in patients with minimal proteinuria or in normal individuals in whom the urine must be concentrated manifold to have sufficient protein to determine the clearance of the particular protein under investigation. Differential protein clearances allow for classification of glomerulonephritis according to expected responses to therapy but are of little value in determining the etiology. For example, two patients with different etiologies may have the same degree of selective proteinuria. In summary, this test is of value in determining expected response to therapy.

Proteinuria of Tubular Diseases

Proteinuria resulting from tubular disease is composed of proteins of molecular weights less than albumin in the studies reported. As early as 1950 Friburg[10] found a proteinuria from industrial workers exposed to cadmium dust. The proteins present were found to be in the range of 20- to 30,000 molecular weight. Later Butler found a protein in patients with the adult Fanconi syndrome which was also present in several other kidney diseases such as galactosemia, acute tubular necrosis, and nephrocalcinosis.[11] This was referred to as a tubular protein and was found to have a molecular weight in the 42- to 46,000 range.

Tubular proteins have been studied by concentrating the urine approximately 50 times and by pervaporation and freeze-drying of these proteins. However, these techniques resulted in the loss of small amounts of protein, and it is conceivable that the proteins were altered by freezing. For these reasons ultrafiltration is the most popular method, and the one presently being used by most laboratories. Proteins have been studied by gel filtration, which allows for separation based on molecular size. Also, immunoelectrophoresis has been used with various forms of polyvalent antisera. All the proteins studied have been found in normal serum and normal urine. In 1967 Harrison and Blainey[12] made specific antisera to individual tubular proteins. One was an alpha 2 protein of 23 Å molecular size, and the other a 17 Å postgamma protein. They were able to determine the clearances of these proteins; the highest clearances were obtained in the adult Fanconi syndrome. It was determined that the protein clearances were not helpful in the diagnosis of chronic pyelonephritis nor in separating pyelonephritis from glomerulonephritis, but they were helpful in diagnosing and in studying the proteinuria of patients exposed to cadmium.

Certain enzymes which are proteins have shown considerable promise in studying the tubular component of proteinuria. Those enzymes with molecular weight higher than albumin usually are not excreted in the urine unless there is marked increase in glomerular permeability. Enzymes of a lower molecular weight than albumin can be used as indicators of tubular proteinuria. Those most commmonly studied are lysozyme and ribonuclease. In the adult Fanconi syndrome lysozyme clearances are as high as 20% of the creatinine clearances and ribonuclease is even higher.

In summarizing the concepts applicable to proteinuria in man, consider three hypothetical situations.

First, a normal man with a plasma concentration of 40 gm./l. of high-molecular-weight protein and 4 mg./l. of low-molecular-weight protein. Assuming a glomerular-filtration rate of 100 l./24 hr. there would be a glomerular-filtration protein concentration of 2 mg./l. for both proteins and 360 mg./24 hr.

If there is tubular reabsorption of 95% there will be left for excretion 10 mg. of heavy-molecular and 10 mg. of lower-molecular-weight protein.

Now consider a patient with glomerulonephritis in whom the predominant loss is via glomerulus, so there is an increase in proteins in the glomerular filtrate.

Needless to say, we cannot measure directly the situation with the low-molecular-weight or even the high-molecular-weight proteins, but we may assume filtration of about 360,000 mg. of high-molecular-weight proteins and 360 mg. of low-molecular-weight proteins/24 hr.

If there is 95% reabsorption, an unknown factor, 18 gm. of high-molecular-weight protein and 18 mg. of low-molecular-weight protein will remain for excretion.

In patients with "tubular proteinuria" we still have the same filtered load/24 hr. but now, instead of 95% reabsorption, there is only 50% reabsorption. This will leave 180 mg. of the higher-molecular-weight proteins and 180 gm. of low-molecular-weight proteins.

SUMMARY

There are two major and obvious areas where studies of proteinuria must be even further expanded. The handling of proteins by the normal kidney is not understood but techniques are available which will help to investigate this problem. Second, information of the pathological processes pertaining to proteinuria must be obtained.

Newer techniques may help to solve these problems.[13] At the present time micropuncture studies are available, for example in the rat, which have shown fractional absorption along the proximal tubule of such substances as insulin and ribonuclease amounting to 30 to 55% of the injected load. Not only was there a constant fractional absorption of the proteins in the proximal tubule, but smaller amounts were absorbed from the distal convoluted tubule.[14] The isolation and study of transport of small molecular-weight proteins has been employed to differentiate glomerular, tubular, and normal proteinuria. Recently Peterson, Everin, and Berggärd,[15] by use of beta-2 globulin, albumin, and total protein were able to differentiate glomerular and tubular proteinuria from normal proteinuria. In certain cases such as pyelonephritis, however, the information obtained served only to give the extent of one or the other type of proteinuria.

Studies of proteinuria utilizing nonprotein macromolecules have provided much insight into the mechanisms of proteinuria. It is difficult to carry out many studies using proteins normally found in serum because of the limiting factor of tubular reabsorption, particularly in normal individuals. For this reason, only in massive proteinuria do we find sufficient protein in the urine to carry out studies without concentrating the urine many times. With the use of nonprotein macromolecules as polyvinylpyrolidone (PVP) measurement of normal and abnormal glomerular permeability may be undertaken. These nonprotein macromolecules must not be protein-bound, they must be capable of passing the basement membrane and they must not be secreted or reabsorbed by the tubules.

PVP seems to fit these criteria, and further, they may be labeled with radioactive iodine^{125}. This permits studies of not only normals but of patients with renal diseases in all stages of severity. This technique has great promise for the future, and by use of gel-filtration-separation techniques, further information can be gleaned.

This summary of proteinuria in renal disease is meant to outline our present understanding of the problem and review some of the studies which hold promise for the future.

REFERENCES

1. Wearn, J. T. and Richards, A. N.: Observations on the composition of glomerular urine, with particular reference to the problem of reabsorption in the renal tubules. *Amer. J. Physiol. 71*:209, 1924.
2. Walker, A. M., Bott, P. A., Oliver, J. and MacDowell, M. C.: The collection and analysis of fluid from single nephrons of the mammalian kidney. *Amer. J. Physiol. 134*:580, 1941.
3. Dock, W.: Proteinuria and the associated renal changes. *New Eng. J. Med. 227*: 633, 1942.
4. Sellers, A. L., Griggs, N., Marmorston, J. and Goodman, H. C.: Filtration and reabsorption of protein by the kidney. *J. Exp. Med. 100*:1, 1954.
5. Dirks, J. H., Clapp, J. R. and Berliner, R. W.: The protein concentration in the proximal tubule of the dog. *J. Clin. Invest. 43*:916, 1964.
6. Farquhar, M. G. and Palade, G. E.: Glomerular permeability. *J. Exp. Med. 113*:47, 1961.
7. Hardwicke, J. and Soothill, J. F.: Proteinuria. In: *Renal Disease,* Black, D. A. K., ed., 2d ed. London, Oxford, Blackwell, 1967, p. 252.
8. Soothill, J. F.: Studies on proteinuria with special reference to immunochemically determined differential protein clearances. *Guy's Hosp. Rep. 111*:355, 1962.
9. Joachim, G. R., Cameron, J. S., Schwartz, M. and Becker, E. L.: Selectivity of protein excretion in patients with the nephrotic syndrome. *J. Clin. Invest. 43*:2332, 1964.
10. Friburg, L.: Health hazards in the manufacture of alkaline accumulators with special reference to chronic cadmium poisoning. *Acta. Med. Scand.* (Suppl. 240) *138*:1, 1950.
11. Butler, E. A. and Flynn, F. V. The proteinuria of renal tubular disorders. *Lancet 2*:978, 1958.
12. Harrison, J. F. and Blainey, J. D.: Low molecular weight proteinuria in chronic renal disease. *Clin. Sci. 33*:381, 1967.
13. Manuel, Y., Revillard, J. P. and Betuel, H., eds.: *Proteins in Normal and Pathological Urine.* Baltimore, Md. and Manchester, England, Univ. Park Press, 1970.
14. Cortney, M. A., Sawin, L. L. and Weiss, D. D. Renal tubular protein absorption in the rat. *J. Clin. Invest. 49*:1, 1970.
15. Peterson, P. A., Evrin, P. E. and Berggärd I. Differentiation of glomerular, tubular, and normal proteinuria: Determinations of urinary excretion of beta 2 microglobulin, albumin, and total protein. *J. Clin. Invest. 48*:1189, 1969.
16. Hulme, B. and Hardwicke, J. Human glomerular permeability to macromolecules in health and disease. *Clin. Sci. 34*:515, 1968.

MANAGEMENT OF END-STATE NEPHRITIS: BIOCHEMICAL ALTERATIONS*

GEORGE E. SCHREINER

Professor of Medicine
Director, Renal and Electrolyte Division
Georgetown University Medical Center
Washington, D.C.

THE face of uremia is shown in Figure 1. Several years ago, in writing our book on uremia,† we devoted a chapter to "The Search for the Uremic Toxin." As far as I am concerned, the search continues.

I think one of the most exciting concepts that really made modern physiology was the thought of Claude Bernard that we had regulatory mechanisms for our internal environment. As you recall, Dr. Walter B. Cannon coined a word that was not found in dictionaries at that time but that has done a great deal to help us conceptualize the role of the kidney in the body economy and, conversely, the role of the diseased kidney in failing to maintain the body's economy. That word was "homeostasis." It was a new word that became important for many generations of medical students. Now we can look at kidney disease from the standpoint of the biochemical changes coincident with end-stage renal failure.

Let us look at the kidney in its "normal" state (Figure 2). Remember, Homer Smith once said, "We are what we are because we have the kind of kidneys we have." Because we have the kind of kidneys we have, we have a certain amount of freedom in our environmental control. We can go far afield from a source of water. We can maintain widely disparate diets: we have the possibiilty, let us say, of going from the rice diet of the Orient to the pure beef diet of the Argentine pampas, with a whole range of magnitude in terms of nitrogen intake and what it means for the body metabolism. We can go to the moon—to outer space—on a "tube" diet. This sort of freedom really is the gift of our kidneys. We

*Presented at a *Conference on Glomerulonephritis* held by the New York Heart Association at The Waldorf-Astoria, New York, N. Y., January 27, 1970.

†Schreiner, G. E. and Maher, J. F. *Uremia: Biochemistry, Pathogenesis, and Treatment.* Springfield, Ill., Thomas, 1961.

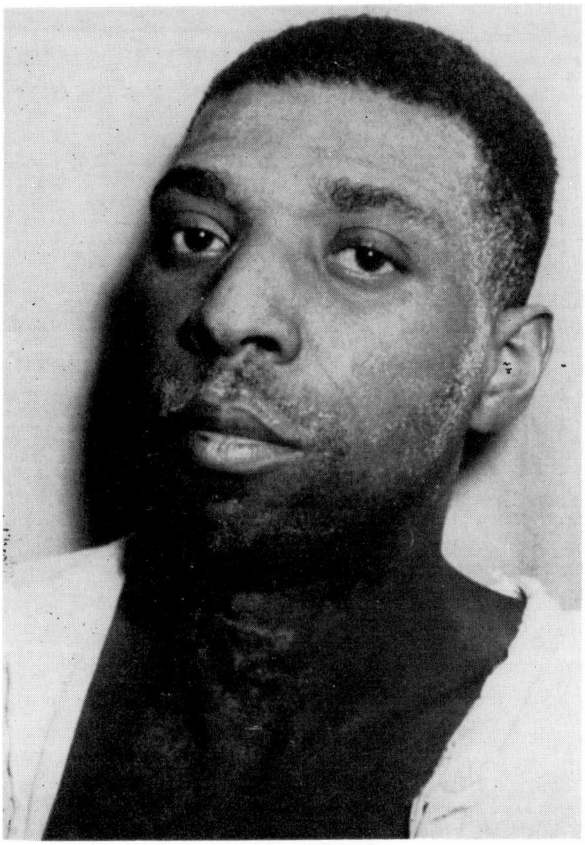

Figure 1

can therefore look at the normal man with a healthy kidney as having both a ceiling and a floor for the intake of certain vital substances.

We have listed in Figure 2 sodium, potassium, protein, water, and "X"—the unknown—to indicate that there is a good deal yet to be learned.

If a person is put on a 30- to 40-gram salt diet, he will retain some of this salt and go into positive balance for a short period of time, until his homeostatic mechanisms come into play. He will then very likely be able to get back into balance on a very high level of salt intake if he has normal kidneys. Conversely, if I put him on a rice diet with 10 mEq. of sodium he will go into negative sodium balance for a few days until his

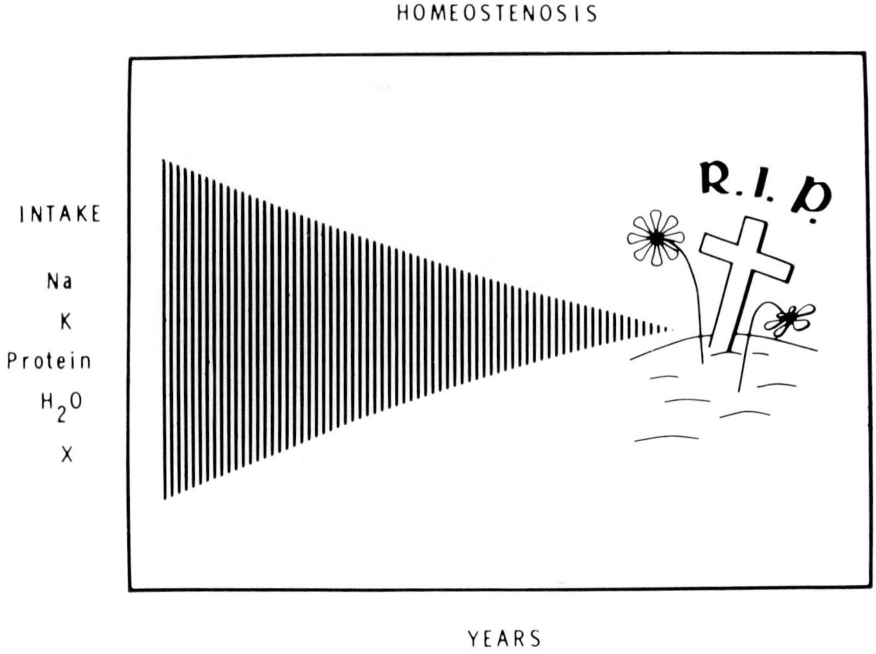

Figure 2

homeostatic mechanisms catch up, and then he will come back into balance at low levels. We have the flexibility of a high ceiling and a low floor with respect to at least these major items that we deal with every day.

What renal disease essentially does is to limit our flexibility very gradually. If a patient is studied quantitatively as the disease progresses, the disorder not only lowers the ceiling, but it also tends to raise the floor irregularly for each of these methods of intake. We know that the patient with a filtration rate of 10 cannot stand a 40-gram salt diet, but what many physicians forget is that neither can they stand the rice diet or the kind of salt restriction that patients with normal kidneys can tolerate. We have therefore, in a very real sense, a loss of freedom and a loss of flexibility in our environmental control.

If Dr. Cannon could coin a word, we too can create a word to describe this biochemical process of end-stage renal failure. We call this gradual narrowing of flexibility "homeostenosis."

This really is the natural history of renal disease. Of course the dis-

TABLE I. SUGGESTED MECHANISMS FOR THE UREMIC SYNDROME

1) A single circulating toxin—as yet unidentified.
2) Combined derivatives of protein—urea, creatinine, uric acid, etc.
3) Inorganic and organic acid retention—including sulphate.
4) Retention of proteolytic enzymes.
5) Absorbed products of intestinal putrefaction.
6) Guanidine and phenol poisoning.
7) Alterations in osmotic pressure.
8) Alterations in choroid plexus with escape of circulating toxins into spinal fluid.

ease does not progress in this regular fashion; it happens in an irregular fashion, so that we have to study each patient as a separate entity. As this stenosis continues the individual is called upon more and more to tighten his environmental control. In the earliest stages of renal failure he no longer feels well on a free-protein diet, but his feeling of well-being increases if his diet is a little under 100 grams of protein. As the blood-urea nitrogen rises he feels better if the protein diet is under 60 grams. As his renal failure progresses, he feels better if it is under 40 grams. Finally, in extreme degrees, we go to the specialized synthetic diet that you have heard described. There comes a time, however, where no flexibility exists and the individual has to move to the substitution techniques. This is the end point. If one does not introduce substitution techniques at this point we lose the patient.

The many suggested mechanisms for the uremic syndrome are listed in Table I. There are persons who believe simply that the syndrome is caused by a single circulating toxin as yet unidentified. There are those who see it in the combined derivatives of proteins, such as urea, creatinine, and uric acid. There are those who see it in inorganic- and organic-acid retention, including sulphates. There are those who seek it in the upsetting of the binding or the actions of the proteolytic enzymes. There are those who talk about absorbed products from an altered intestinal membrane. There are specific poisons, changes in osmotic pressure, and even localized anatomical changes in the choroid plexus, for example, with the escape of circulating toxins into the spinal fluid with resulting cerebral manifestations.

Figure 3 reminds us of one of the greatest fallacies in the study of end-stage renal disease: that this is a disease of old age. Some of the early

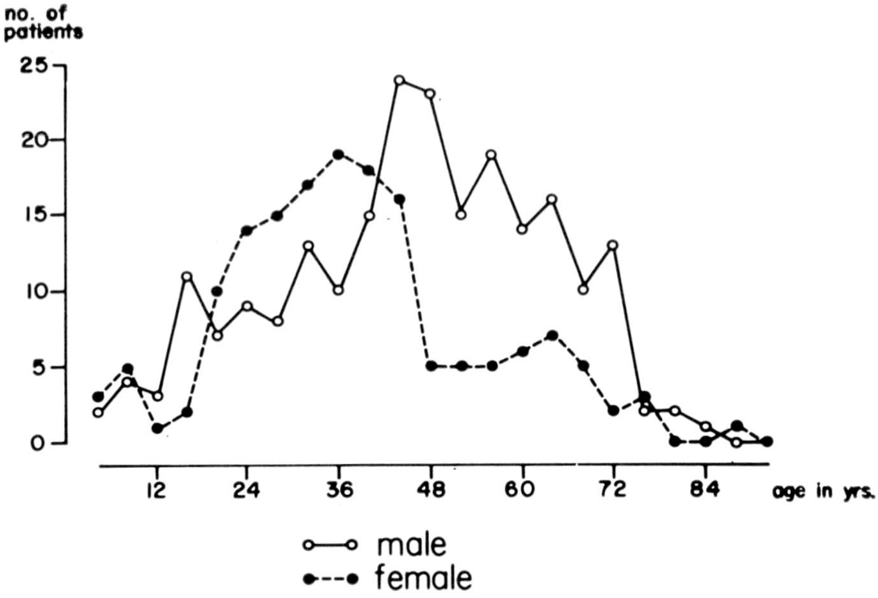

Fig. 3. Age and sex in 380 patients with uremia.

studies done on arteriosclerosis in city and county hospitals suggested that it was an end-stage chronic disease which affected people at the end of their life spans. Actually, in a general hospital and in our own Georgetown University Medical Center, the peak of the death rate occurs in males at the height of their economic productivity and in females during the height of their reproductivity.

A familiar concept which must be understood in terms of interpreting blood chemistries and biochemical changes is the relation of urea-clearance and filtration rate to the blood-urea nitrogen (Figure 4). Many of us now have computer and automated-technology laboratory tests at our disposal and are detecting patients with elevated blood-urea nitrogens. We are forced to try to discuss a laboratory finding. What do we do about interpreting an abnormal laboratory finding when it is presented to us? We must know something about renal physiology if we want to interpret such a finding intelligently.

It is possible, as one lowers the filtration rate resulting from a disease, to have a blood-urea nitrogen within quite normal limits during the time that up to 60 to 70% of the glomeruli are deemed destroyed. I

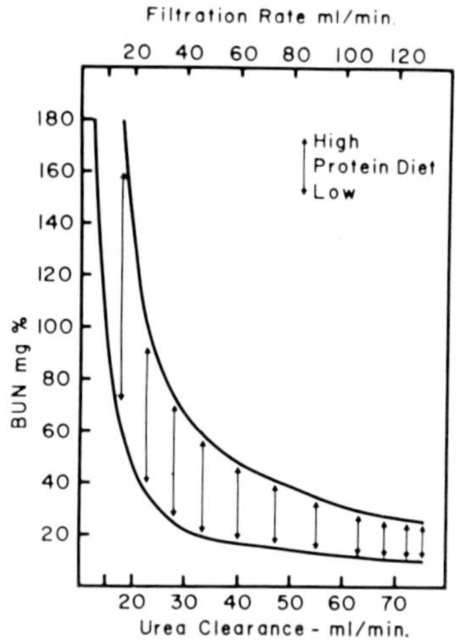

Fig. 4. The relation of urea clearance and filtration rate to BUN on high and low protein diets.

think this is unusual. I think there is almost no other situation caused by a disease that has such characteristics. Imagine what the dermatologists would do if 70% of your skin were destroyed before you came to them, or what the hematologist would think if 70% of your blood were destroyed before you came to him. The kidney is a very silent organ, and one has to approach the renal problem by almost purely intellectual and laboratory techniques in many instances. The correlation between filtration rate and blood urea is altered by the diet of the individual, so that one has to interpret this in the light of whether one is working with a high- or a low-protein diet.

The other important part of this classic curve is that once you get below a certain level of kidney function, the curve rises very steeply, so that very small changes in function, a loss of one or two cubic centimeters per minute in the filtration rate, may result in marked changes in the blood chemistry. Conversely, very minor improvements in the filtration rate may result in marked improvement in the blood chemistry, so that the percentage of change in the blood chemistry is not an index of the percentage of change in kidney function when one is dealing in the pathologic range of azotemia. This is an important primary concept for physicians who are treating patients with end-stage renal failure. A curious phenomenon exists in our series. Up to a certain point there is a

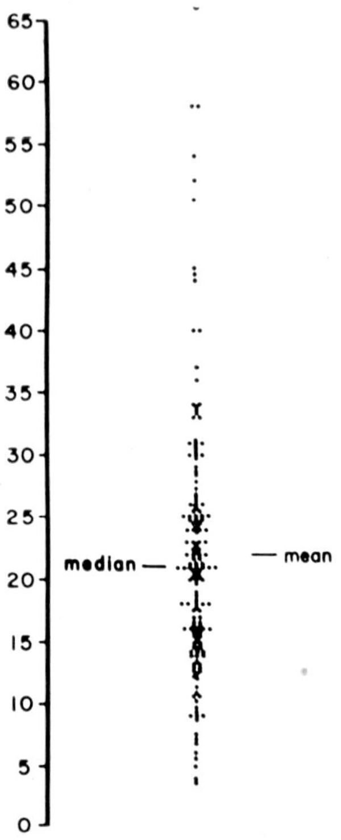

Fig. 5. Highest creatine in 164 dialyzed uremic patients.

relation between azotemia and the death or survival rate, but after this point there is not.

Figure 5 gives you some idea of the median, mean, and range of creatinine in dialized uremic patients; it shows one of the more acceptable parameters of kidney function which is followed closely by nephrologists.

Figure 6 shows another useful technique, which is to study serial changes in the creatinine-BUN ratios. These range in the area of about 10%. When this changes, it can be of diagnostic significance. For example, we found in reviewing all of our cases of acute tubular necrosis and after serial changes in the creatinine-BUN ratio, that we could pick out those whose tubular necrosis was caused by two diseases. We have had carbon tetrachloride and bichloride of mercury poisoning where, in both instances, the toxin had a hepatic effect and tended to cut down quan-

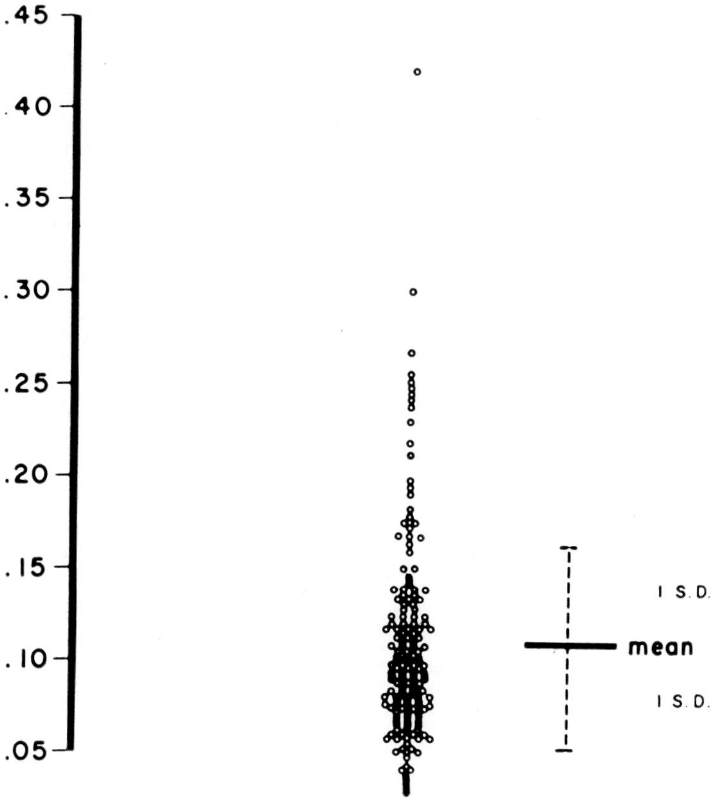

Fig. 6. Creatinine/BUN ratio in 164 dialyzed uremic patients.

titatively the rate of urea synthesis while, of course, the accumulation of creatinine followed as a property of the metabolism of muscle metabolism and the rate of filtration.

Another diagnostic consideration with abnormalities of creatinine-BUN ratios lies in the diagnosis of obstructive uropathy, since a disproportionately high blood urea may be seen in obstruction of the lower urinary tract. Of course these disproportions are seen in individuals who have blood in the GI tract or any other source of rapid tissue breakdown, catabolic hormones, fever, hemolysis of blood, hematomas in the tissues, and so forth.

Table II reviews one of the complications which is of particular interest to cardiologists. Uremic pericarditis is a focal process that leads

Table II. UREMIC PERICARDITIS

Pathology
Focal process begins posteriorly.
Fibrin deposited over denuded areas.
Fibrous adhesions produce compartmentalization.
Inflammatory response in underlying fibrous fatty tissue.
Capillary and fibroblasts invade adhesions.
Granulation tissues subject to rupture and hemorrhage.
Final conversion to resistant scars.

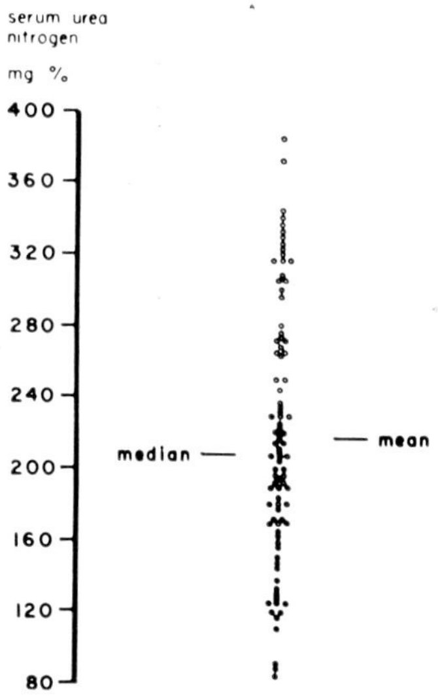

Figure 7

to the deposition of fibrin over denuded areas of the membrane covering the heart.

Figure 7 depicts the biochemical correlation of this. These are the median and mean serum-urea readings in 93 patients where autopsy indicated that the uremic pericarditis was present. In most of our patients, in fact more than 80%, the condition was recognizable in life by either auscultation of a rub, by pain, or by x-ray findings.

Another curious factor of the biochemistry of urea is the duration of the effects of the toxin (Table III). In analyzing such data one comes to believe that uremic toxin fulfills some of the definitions that we have for dialyzable poisons, such as barbiturates. There is a time-dose-cyto-

TABLE III. UREMIC COMA
Time lag in postdialysis awakening

Case	*Diagnosis*	*Days of oliguria*	*Highest BUN*	*Highest creatinine*	*Hours to awaken*
1†	ARI, CRI, RHA	—	190	15	0.2
2	ARI	3	100	30	2
3	ARI, CRI	3	184	21	2
4	ARI	6	178	24	3
5	ARI	10	290	21	4
1*	ARI, CRI	—	165	7	11
6	CRI	—	265	45	14
7	ARI	13	180	20	39
8	ARI, CRI	16	150	40	48
9	ARI	15	138	59	48

*First dialysis—Case 1
†Second dialysis—Case 1
ARI—acute renal insufficiency, CRI—chronic renal insufficiency, RHA—renal hyperchloremic acidosis.

TABLE IV. SIMULTANEOUS BLOOD AND SPINAL FLUID CHEMISTRY

	Urea nitrogen mg.%	*Creatinine mg.%*	*Uric acid mg.%*	*Phosphorus mg.%*	*Ribonuclease units*
	43-yr.-old w. m.—pyelonephritis, uretero-sigmoid anastomoses				
Predialysis					
Blood	170	20	19	—	165
Spinal fluid	115	6.2	2		225
Postdialysis					
Blood	58	8.8	5.4	—	190
Spinal fluid	68	4.4	1.6		190
	31-yr.-old w. m.—polycystic disease and pyelonephritis				
Predialysis					
Blood	285	30	30	—	
Spinal fluid	255	8.4	6.4		
Postdialysis					
Blood	86	12.6	8.0	—	
Spinal fluid					
	21-yr.-old w. f.—acute renal insufficiency				
Postdialysis					
Blood	57	5.3	8.2	4.5	
Spinal fluid	90	5.1	2.2	2.2	

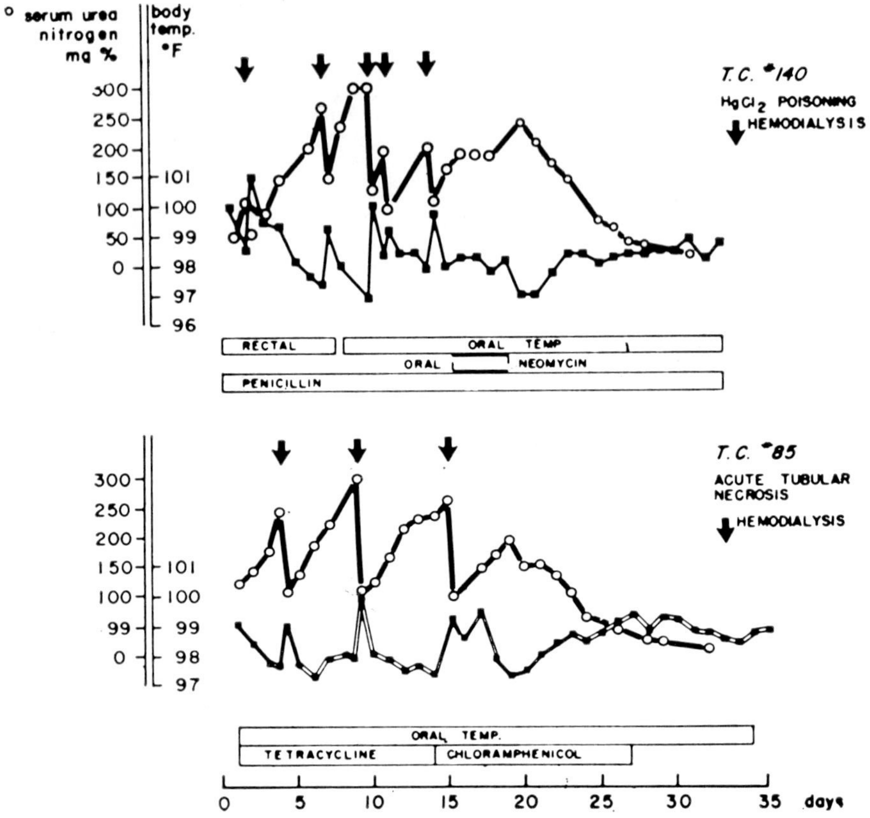

Fig. 8. Uremic hypothermia.

toxic relation. The duration of exposure of the body tissues to the particular toxins with which we are not acquainted has something to do with both the reversibility of the syndrome and the time it takes to heal.

For example, we rated a group of patients with acute renal insufficiency according to their highest BUN and creatinine, and categorized them by the hours it took for their first awakening from deep coma and recognition of the world around them as an objective end point. This did not correlate with any of these things, but it did correlate with the days during which oliguria had been present before they went into uremic coma.

Another interesting phenomenon concerns the behavior of the blood-brain barrier. Table IV shows some blood and spinal-fluid analyses for various biochemical substances. One sees, for example, that urea, which is always lower in spinal fluid than in blood, comes out higher after the removal of the material from the blood by hemodialysis. Indeed, elevated uric acid, which does not pass very freely to even an uremic blood-brain barrier, nevertheless bears a lower ratio in the postdialysis state.

Figure 8 depicts a negative correlation between accumulation of urea and body temperature. This is the uremic hypothermic effect in which the arrows represent dialyses and in which one can see that each time the level of urea is lowered the temperature rises. Each time the blood urea is allowed to accumulate the temperature goes down. This is true both in relation to normal body temperature in many patients and in infectious fevers. It is also true in fevers induced artificially by pyrogens. This would indicate that there is a hypothermic effect from the uremic toxin.

This is just a very brief sampling, obviously, since many of us have spent years in writing books on the biochemistry of uremia, and it is not something that one can cover completely in a short paper. I do want to impress on you a basic principle, however, and that is that progressive renal disease represents a progressive narrowing of flexibility on the part of the subject in terms of his freedom to enjoy wide variations in intake of food and water. With progressive disease, the biochemical relations do not follow a static straight line, but follow a well-known physiological curve which bears such a peculiar relation that very minor changes in the late stages of renal disease result in very large changes in blood chemistry, and very small improvements result in very large improvements in blood chemistry. If we are to interpret intelligently the biochemical findings, we must read behind these numbers into the physiological processes which they represent.

DIETARY MANAGEMENT OF END-STAGE UREMIA*

MILTON E. RUBINI AND JOEL D. KOPPLE†

Departments of Medicine
Wadsworth Veterans Administration Center
University of California at Los Angeles
Los Angeles, Calif.

THE last 10 years have greatly altered the prognosis of the patient with end-stage uremia. It is in this period that chronic hemodialysis and renal homotransplantation have been demonstrated to offer a practical means of salvage of uremic patients otherwise facing an immediately hopeless prognosis. Unfortunately the number of patients that can be offered such treatment is still small. A third contemporary development, improved dietary management of uremia, has received less attention but offers important benefits to the large numbers of uremics that for medical or logistical reasons cannot be handled by either of the more dramatic definitive therapies. Dietary management offers a new dimension of the therapeutic approach to the complex of interrelated symptoms that we call uremia. The essence of this dietary program is to restrict protein intake while allowing adequate quantities of total calories and essential amino acids to maintain nitrogen equilibrium. Wasteful catabolism of tissue protein to toxic nitrogenous metabolites, which in some way aggravates the uremic state, is diminished. It is the purpose of this discussion to review briefly the general principles of dietary management and, especially, the application of such specialized diets in the management of uremia.

The basic tenets in any dietary regimen in uremia are to maintain at maximum the residual renal function and to keep homeostatic stresses within the ability of renal response. The severely damaged kidney cannot adjust output to wide ranges in intake.[1-4] Thus if adequate fluid is withheld, the inability to concentrate limits the conservation of

*Presented at a *Conference on Glomerulonephritis* held by the New York Heart Association at The Waldorf-Astoria, New York, N.Y., January 27, 1970.
†Veterans Administration Research and Education Associate.
This study was supported by Public Health Service Contract 44-68-953 and Training Grant TI AM 5383 from the National Institute of Arthritis and Metabolic Diseases, Bethesda, Md.

water, and dehydration occurs. If adequate salt is withheld, the wasting of salt and subsequent hypovolemia may lead to further diminution of renal function. If excess fluid is proferred, the inability to excrete free water may lead to water intoxication and hyponatremia. Excessive salt loading may aggravate hyperpiesis or lead to hypervolemia and cardiac failure. Because renal excretory function is enhanced with high solute excretion rates and expanded extracellular volume, it seems reasonable to increase salt intake until mildly positive salt balance is induced. Further, an indirect advantage of a high sodium intake is its thirst-provoking effects which encourages the patient to imbibe more fluids.[5] As more sodium is prescribed, fluid turnover accelerates and the renal excretory function may improve.

However, management is not so simple. In some uremic patients small differences in sodium intake will induce either the retention of fluid and hypertension or progressive hypovolemia and decreasing renal function. Such patients must be taught to control their sodium balance by regulating sodium intake according to their blood pressure, presence of edema, and their body weight. Self-regulation of this degree may require the maintenance of meticulous records of daily sodium intake. Our patients are provided with lists of the sodium content of foods and menus, and are periodically asked to keep dietary diaries.

Provided the volume of urine is adequate, potassium is reasonably well tolerated.[6] However, lethal hypokalemia of dietary origin is occasionally seen with gross indiscretions. Resin therapy may offer protection against surges of hyperkalemia.[7-9] Calcium supplements may be useful in the occasional patient with recurrent tetany, as calcium absorption is inhibited by uremia, and in patients with severe hyperphosphatemia, phosphate-binding gels may protect against metastatic calcification.[10, 11] As protein metabolism creates a proton load, the inability to produce urinary ammonia is critical, and progressive acidosis may ensue if the ability to excrete acid is exceeded. Alkaline-ash diets have been recommended, but it is usually simpler and easier to supplement directly with sodium bicarbonate or calcium carbonate.

Because anorexia, abdominal discomfort, nausea, and vomiting are prominent symptoms of uremia, dietary management may be difficult. It is against a background of a high fluid intake, salt loading to edema or unmanageable hypertension, and restriction of food such as dried fruits that are very high in potassium, that protein limitation is recommended. The quantity and character of protein intake in uremia is the focus of this presentation.

"Rich" (high-protein) foods have been recognized for nearly a century to affect the progress of uremia,[12] and in the last 25 years low-protein diets have been uniformly recommended. Red meat was once considered nephrotoxic and more harmful in renal disease than white meat or milk.[13] The idea of avoiding protein was reached empirically and reinforced by the knowledge that the kidney excretes the end products of nitrogen metabolism. Because high-protein diets were associated with a high-blood urea, the rationale of low-protein diets was that less urea was produced and, hence, less "uremic poison," even though early investigators were skeptical of the contention that urea, per se, was toxic. This rationale was further modified by Addis to the concept that excretion of nitrogen placed less metabolic demands upon the kidney in a now somewhat incongruous analogy to the failing heart.[14] Others thought they could demonstrate a direct renal toxicity of excessive protein intake.[15, 16]

It was generally advocated that daily ingestion of protein should be limited to 0.5 to 0.6 gm./kg. of body weight plus an amount equal to urinary protein losses.[13, 17] This level of protein intake was selected because it approximated the minimal protein requirements determined from balance studies in normal young people;[18-20] higher-protein intakes were noted to intensify uremia. The quality of protein recommended for chronically uremic patients received scant consideration even though 40 gr. of randomly selected protein might easily supply inadequate quantities of essential amino acids. The fact that many uremic patients are already debilitated, on occasion catabolic, and often die with progressive inanition seems to have been overlooked or thought to be unimportant because of the poor prognosis of the underlying disease.

Surprisingly little was known about the basal nitrogen requirements of chronically ill patients, and most of the data on nitrogen requirements and equilibrium were based on studies of well persons. The National Academy of Science's recommendation of 0.9 gm. protein/kg. for normal persons is probably liberal, with a generous allowance for incomplete digestion and a low biologic value of a mixed protein intake.[21] There is a suggestion that with protein depletion, the diminished protoplasmic mass is associated with a diminished "labile protein pool."[22, 23] With adaptation to low intakes of protein, protein and amino-acid degradation decreases while synthesis of amino acids into protein is enhanced.[24-28] How low a protein intake can be and yet maintain nitrogen equilibration indefinitely is uncertain. Studies based on European or American normal subjects which utilize proteins of high biologic value suggest a "floor" at around 0.5 gm./kg.[18-20]

With protracted low-protein feeding there appears to be continued adaptation and difficulty in the measurement of small but cumulative losses from the skin over long periods, and the probable loss of small amounts of nitrogen into expired air limits precise quantification of balance.[29-31] In parts of the world where dietary protein intake is restricted and of poor quality, generations of individuals appear to survive, although perhaps not thrive, on intakes of protein that induce negative nitrogen balance in American college students.

Intimately related to the minimum level of protein intake is the coincident caloric intake. Caloric requirements for nitrogen equilibrium increase as protein intake diminishes, and an adequate caloric intake is critical for optimum protein utilization at low levels of protein intake. Even at relatively high levels of caloric intake, further increases in calories may improve nitrogen balance.[32] The nitrogen-sparing action of carbohydrate is also pertinent. Even as little as 50 to 100 gm. of carbohydrate substantially reduces the production of urea during starvation and, hence, "spares" nitrogen.[33] The concept of a urea-sparing effect of certain diets as compared to others has received little attention in the management of uremia, even though retained urea was considered a correlate of uremic symptoms.

Giordano has revolutionized the concepts of dietary requirements in uremia by showing that endogenous urea could be reutilized and synthesized into protein under certain conditions: 1) the subject receives an adequate amount of calories; 2) nitrogen intake is minimized; and 3) essential amino acids are supplied in sufficient quantity.[34, 35] He further suggested that azotemic patients may have a lower nitrogen requirement than normal since they have greater amounts of urea available for amino-acid synthesis. He developed and publicized a diet that met these caloric and nitrogen requirements. Subsequently Giovannetti published data confirming the important clinical value of this diet;[36-38] similar laudatory clinical results were reported by British and American investigators using modifications of this diet.[39-47]

The so-called Giordano-Giovannetti diet, as it is popularly termed, is a 20-gm. protein diet in which the protein is primarily of high biologic value and contains, by extrapolation from Rose's data in normals,[48] the minimum daily requirement of all the essential amino acids. The protein selected is generally that of whole eggs, but meat and potato protein have also been used.[46, 49, 50] As proteins from vegetable and grains have low biologic values, it was initially recommended that these be assiduously avoided except as incidental to low-protein foods chosen for their caloric, mineral, and vitamin contents, and to make the diet more palatable. Wheat-starch foodstuffs and high carbohydrate and fat desserts are major sources of calories essentially free of nitrogen. Emulsified fats and concentrated carbohydrate drinks have also been used.[51, 52]

The therapeutic results with these diets were most encouraging. With the fall of plasma urea nitrogen from over 200 mg./100 ml. to near normal levels over a 1- to 2-month period, uric acid and phosphate also diminished. Red-cell production was reported to have been increased[53] and, most strikingly, anorexia, nausea, vomiting, singultus, pruritus, and drowsiness improved dramatically. Some investigators have even reported prolongation of survival. More important than the length of survival was the quality of life so produced. The disabled, debilitated uremic took a new interest in life as he was able to remain out of the hospital for protracted periods of time, and even to return to work. The ideal candidate for such diets seems to be the individual with sufficient diminution in renal function to cause symptoms, but with the residual clearance above 3 cc./min.

In all studies a group of hard-core patients simply would not accept this degree of dietary restriction. They found the diet monotonous and rebelled within a brief period of time. The very young and the very old seemed to have more trouble adhering to such diets; Italian and British patients seemed to be more willing to undertake such drastic dietary restrictions than Americans. The personality of the investigator, the emphasis and support offered the patients, and to some degree the intellectual and economic background of the patients studied seemed important in their acceptance. While the therapeutic success in some patients was unquestionable, it was less clear whether this drastic restriction to a diet most difficult to prepare and continue was critical. Was it the level of protein intake, the abstinence from nonessential amino acids, or the increased quality of the amino acid mixture that was responsible?

SERUM CHEMISTRY AND UREA CLEARANCES
IN PATIENTS FED THREE LEVELS OF PROTEIN INTAKE*

	20 gm.	*40 gm.*	*1 gm./kg.*	*20 gm. vs. 40 gm.*	*20 gm. vs. 1 gm./kg.*	*40 gm. vs. 1 gm./kg.*
n	20	23	14	Statistical differences†		
Serum urea nitrogen	55.4 ± 4.5	98.8 ± 7.9	134.7 ± 9.0	<0.001	<0.001	<0.01
Serum creatinine	12.4 ± 0.8	14.5 ± 1.2	12.4 ± 0.7	ns	ns	ns
SUN/serum creatinine ratio	4.5 ± 0.4	7.0 ± 0.4	11.2 ± 0.9	<0.001	<0.001	<0.001
Urea clearance	3.1 ± 0.2	3.2 ± 0.3	4.5 ± 0.6	ns	<0.05	ns

The data presented in this table were collected at the time of lowest serum urea nitrogen levels after equilibration had occurred with each diet. When serum-urea nitrogen rose continuously, as it often did with the 1 gm./kg. protein diet, the final chemical determination done prior to termination of this diet are depicted. Urea nitrogen/creatinine ratios are the mean of the individual ratios with each diet.

*Mean ± standard error

†p values

In the past four years we have conducted more than 70 dietary studies of nondialyzed uremic patients. In an initial study outpatients were randomly assigned to either a 20-gm. Giordano-Giovannetti type diet of a 40-gram mixed protein diet which supplied an abundance of essential amino acids.[54] Unexpectedly, patients were observed to improve clinically to an equal degree with both diets. The incidence and severity of neuropathy, hematocrit, and survival rates were also similar. More edema-free weight was gained with the higher-protein intake. Patients prescribed the lower-protein diet disliked it, usually intensely, and frequently consumed closer to 28 to 30 gm. of protein.[55] We became suspicious that protein restriction may be less important than the quality of protein eaten, provided excess protein is not taken.

A more rigidly controlled study was then undertaken in which each patient served as his own control while being fed in random series, three isocaloric diets (20 gm./day, 40 gm./day and 1 gm./kg./day of protein), until azotemia stablized or uremic decompensation occured.[56] Again, patients fared equally well while ingesting either the 20- or the 40-gm. protein diet. In fact, some patients described a greater sense of well-being and of general comfort when they ate 40 gm. of protein than when they took the more restricted diet. Most of the patients fed the 1 gm./kg. protein diet quickly deteriorated and developed

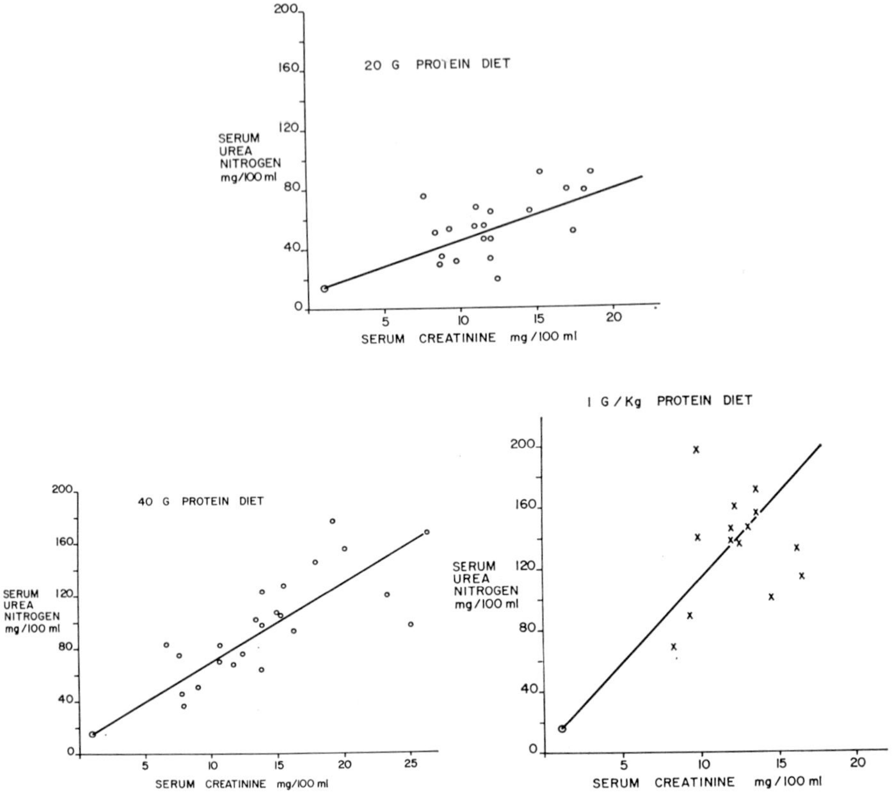

Figs. 1, 2, and 3. The relation of serum creatinine to urea nitrogen for various levels of protein intake is shown. A visually fitted line arbitrarily fixed at the normal value of serum urea nitrogen, 15 mg./100ml., and serum creatinine, 1 mg./100 ml., has been added. Note the slopes of these lines: 0.4, 0.6, and 1.0 increases as daily protein intake increases. All diets were isocaloric. Each symbol depicts a single patient after stabilization on the diet and represents the lowest SUN achieved. As some patients were studied on more than one diet, they are represented in more than one figure; occasionally a patient was studied with the same diet a second time some months later and is plotted separately on each occasion.

anorexia, nausea, vomiting, singultus, muscle cramps, twitching, malaise, and a uremic taste. Azotemia increased rapidly and progressively, and this diet had to be discontinued. Only two patients, with urea clearances of 7 and 10 ml./min. respectively, were able to tolerate this high a protein intake. The table on page 855 depicts serum-urea nitrogen, creatinine, urea nitrogen; creatinine ratios and urea clearances from the total experience with outpatients. Azotemia increased as protein intake increased without change in creatinine. Figures 1 to 3 illustrate the

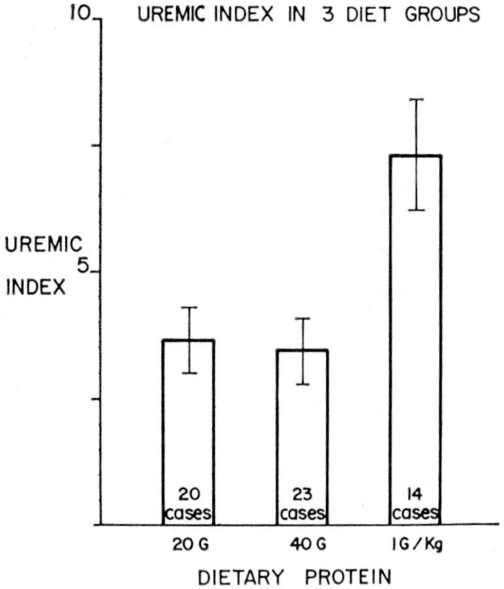

Fig. 4. Mean uremic index ± standard error is depicted for each diet. This semiquantitative rating of 6 uremic signs and symptoms was similar to the 20 gm. and 40 gm. protein diets and much worse with the 1 gm/kg. protein diet. Uremic index was depicted at the time of lowest serum urea nitrogen after equilibration had occurred.

relation between azotemia and renal function for each level of protein intake.

The intensity of uremic signs and symptoms was evaluated semiquantitatively in each patient at 2- to 5-week intervals and rated 0 (normal) to 3 (severely abnormal). Scores for appetite, vomiting, sense of well-being, insomnia, uremic twitching, and uremic taste at the nadir of azotemia are summated into a "uremic" index depicted in Figure 4. Scores of patients fed 20- and 40-gm. protein diets are similar and were radically different from those fed the 1 gm./kg. protein diet. Singultus, muscle cramps and epistaxis were also similar with the 20- and 40-gm. protein diets and distinctly less common than with the 1-gm./kg. protein diet. To control intake further and to examine nitrogen balance, seven patients were fed 0.3 gm./kg. (20 gm.) or 0.6 km./kg. (40 gm.) protein diets under metabolic balance conditions.[57] Serum urea nitrogen: creatinine ratios after stabilization were observed to correlate with protein intake: 3.7 ± 0.43 and 5.6 ± 0.23 (mean ± standard error). These ratios are lower than those obtained in studies of outpatients with these two diets (4.5 and 7.0 respectively) and indicate upward deviation from dietary prescription in the outpatients. When we calculated similar ratios from series of patients with the same residual filtration rates reported by other investigators in the British and American literature, those varied from 4.2 to 5.6 and indicate that dietary adherence in the hands of the most enthusiastic of investigators was partial, and seemed no better than in studies of our outpatients. We find ourselves increasingly opposed to the idea that drastic restriction of protein to 20 gm./day is necessary even were it generally possible. Even under the precisely controlled conditions of a metabolic ward, patients fared equally well with 40 gm. protein/day.

The 20-gm. protein diet induced negative nitrogen balance in each patient. Although in time nitrogen balance became less negative and eventually neutral balance might have been achieved, this would only occur at the expense of hundreds of grams of lost tissue protein. Herndon,[58] Giordano,[59] and Ford[60] have also found that a 20-gm. protein diet, even when primarily of high biological value, is inadequate to maintain nitrogen balance. Several investigators have drawn a different conclusion but their calculations in general have ignored such factors as losses of protein during adaptation and allowances for unmeasured losses in the skin and its appendages, sweat, and expiration.[36, 45, 49] The increased frequency of infection and progressive inanition in uremic patients may be related to the state of protein depletion.

The course of one patient who adhered compulsively to dietary prescription is illustrative:

Case Report

J. S., a 51-year-old Caucasian male, felt well until May 1966, when he developed anorexia, nausea, vomiting, twitching, singultus, malaise, a uremic taste, and fetid breath. These signs and symptoms progressed. Albuminuria and mild hypertension had been noted five years earlier. In October a diagnosis of uremia was made, and the patient was referred to Wadsworth Veterans Administration Hospital. On physical examination, the patient was found to be anxious and mildly depressed. Blood pressure was 150/100. Vibratory sensation was slightly decreased in the left great toe. Physical examination was otherwise unremarkable. Serum creatinine was 8.6 mg./100 ml; urea nitrogen was 83 mg./100 ml.; uric acid was 9.0 mg./100 ml.; hematocrit was 28%; urea clearance

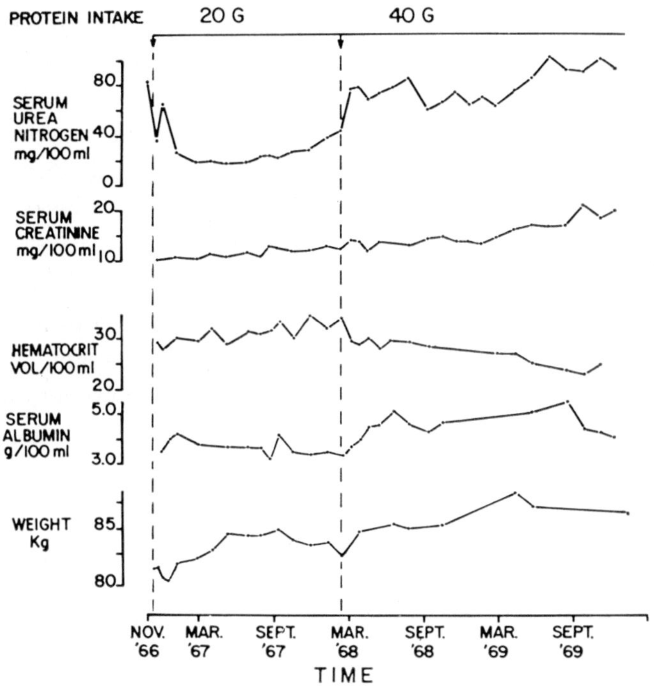

Fig. 5. The course of the serum-urea nitrogen and creatinine, hematocrit, serum albumin, and body weight are depicted in a chronically uremic patient who adhered rigidly to a 20-gm. and a 40-gm. protein diet.

was 3.2 ml./min.; excretion of urinary protein was 1.2 gm./day. Nerve-conduction velocities in the median, ulnar, and common peroneal nerves were normal bilaterally. On November 11, 1966 the patient was started on a high-caloric 20-gm. protein diet containing 2 eggs. Multivitamins, methyldopa, amitriptyline, and sodium restriction were also prescribed. Within one week, there was symptomatic improvement and, by January 1967, the patient's appetite was normal; nausea, vomiting, and uremic taste were gone. Energy and the tolerance of exercise were almost normal and the patient was able to work a 40-hour week. By March he said he felt as well as he had in several years. Figure 5 illustrates several aspects of the clinical course. SUN decreased to a low of 19 mg./100 ml. Serum creatinine initially remained unchanged at 10 to 11 mg./100 ml. and then in August 1967 it began to increase slowly. Hematocrit was unchanged. Serum albumin levels remained low normal, although body weight increased and stabilized. Until early

1968 traces of pitting edema were frequently present in the lower extremities; thereafter he was edema-free. The patient adhered meticulously to a 20- to 21-gm. protein diet although he gradually began to urge the staff to give him greater allowance of protein. In February 1968 he was prescribed a high-caloric 40-gm. mixed protein diet.

SUN increased abruptly to 70 to 80 mg./100 ml.; hematocrit decreased. Serum albumin and body weight increased. The patient stated he "felt better all the way around." He enjoyed his meals immensely and was no longer depressed over being deprived of food. Despite the increasing serum creatinine he continued to feel robust and worked a rigorous 40 hours per week. In May 1968 the patient and his wife toured Europe for one month. In October nerve-conduction velocities were found to be decreased in both common peroneal nerves. Vibratory sensation at that time was mildly decreased in both great toes; pinprick, light touch sensation and reflexes in the extremities were normal.

In February 1969 the patient was transferred to another hospital for training in home hemodialysis. Since he has continued to feel so well and to work full time as of February 1970 he still has not undergone dialysis. Nerve function has slowly deteriorated further. He is generally well, but tires more readily.

Comment. This patient has had an unusual course in that his advanced renal disease has progressed very slowly and he has tolerated renal failure so well. Although his experience in 1966 indicates that a restriction of dietary protein was necessary to alleviate uremic symptoms, this patient seemed to do at least as well with the 40-gm. as with the 20-gm. protein diet. Indeed, with a serum-creatinine concentration of 20 mg./100 ml., he felt well enough to enjoy life and to work full time. The SUN serum-creatinine ratios and dietary-interview data leave no doubt that this man adhered rigidly to his diet. Interestingly, two parameters of nutritional status, serum-albumin levels and body weight, increased with the advent of the 40-gm. protein diet, which suggested that the second diet was indeed nutritionally superior. Hematocrit decreased shortly after starting the 40-gm. protein diet, possibly because of enhanced production of some uremic toxin from the increased protein intake or to progression of the renal disease.

There is now general consensus that patients who have chronic renal failure but are not undergoing dialysis should adhere meticulously to a low protein diet, which provides the minimal daily requirement of all of the essential amino acids. To achieve this degree of dietary adherence requires reorientation of the patient's attitude, self-image, and goals. Frequent periodic interviews with a dietician are useful to reinforce motivation and reeducate patients. Use of dietary diaries provides excellent training and stimulates adherence. In controlled studies, however, we have failed to find a critical advantage of the 20-gm. protein diet over the less restrictive 40-gm. protein diet. In fact, the more restrictive diet is emotionally frustrating, engenders guilt from dietary deviation, and probably induces at least some degree of protein depletion. Further, we are skeptical from the published SUN/serum creatinine ratios whether patients generally adhere to this diet except under the carefully regulated conditions of a metabolic ward.

It must be emphasized that adherence to the 40-gm. protein diet also requires an aggressive approach by the medical team. With less meticulous supervision, patients will ingest more protein, especially of low biological value, and uremic deterioration may then occur. Although the optimal caloric content for these diets has not been determined precisely, it is felt that it should be at least 35 kcal./kg. There are individual variations in caloric requirements and we believe it is preferable to furnish as many calories as patients will tolerate unless obesity threatens. Less than 2,000 kcal./day is associated with increased degradation of protein and, therefore, with increased production of urea and presumably of other toxic nitrogenous metabolites.[61]

The level of renal function at which these protein-restricted diets lose their effectiveness in maintaining patients relatively symptom-free varies from individual to individual. Several of our patients appeared quite robust and energetic, and felt well with urea clearances between 2 and 3 ml./min. Above 3 ml./min. most patients did well but an occasional patient felt poorly despite greater clearances of urea. The clinical response to the dietary treatment appears to be related to age, physical condition, presence of other diseases, and the attitudes and emotional strength of the patient. Despite consistent symptomatic improvement we find that uremic neuropathy not infrequently progresses and, occasionally, signs of pericarditis occured even in patients who felt well and worked full time.

There is no single criterion for determining when dietary treatment no longer is adequate and maintenance dialysis or renal homotransplantation should be inaugurated. We consider deterioration of nerve-con-

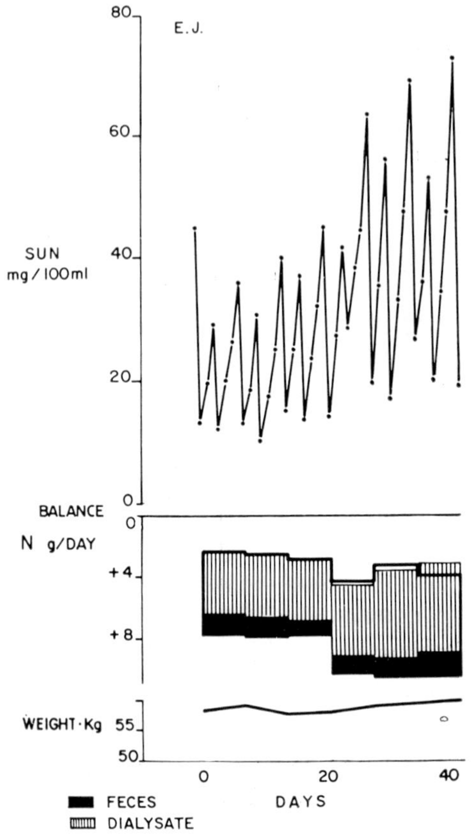

Fig. 6. Serum urea nitrogen, nitrogen balance and dry body weight are depicted in an anephric wasted 39-year-old male undergoing an 11-hour Kiil hemodialysis twice weekly while receiving 0.75 and 1.25 gm. of protein/kg. Diets were isocaloric. The nitrogen balance data are shown with intake plotted downward from the zero line and fecal and dialysate nitrogen plotted upwards. The distance between the zero line and the heavy line indicates positive nitrogen balance corrected for change in body urea content. It is estimated that approximately 1 additional gram of unmeasured nitrogen was lost per day and nitrogen balance is less positive by this amount. With greater protein intake, nitrogen retention and body weight increased, although the patient became progressively more azotemic.

duction velocities or clinically evident sensory or motor neuropathies to be strong indications for maintenance dialysis or renal transplantation even in patients whose uremic symptoms are controlled by diet.

The beneficial results in the nondialyzed uremic has an obvious bearing on the patients who undergo chronic hemodialysis. If dietary management could protract the interval between dialysis or delay the time when a patient could not survive without dialysis, the need for facilities for dialysis might be reduced. Here the problem was more complex, for with chronic dialysis large amounts of accumulated urea, and presumably some of the toxic nitrogenous metabolites associated with uremia, are removed episodically. Concomitantly, a substantial quantity of amino acids are wasted during dialysis.[62, 63] Perhaps the key observation is that patients with chronic dialysis regularly gain weight dramatically after successful transplantation. The effect of hemodialysis itself, with this disruption and distortion of plasma amino-acid concentrations in plasma and tissue, upon dynamics of protein is unknown.

Studies of Ginn suggest that a high caloric diet containing 0.75 gm. of protein/kg. of ideal body weight was optimum for patients undergoing twice-weekly maintenance hemodialysis.[64] Most of the protein ingested, 0.63 gm./kg., was of high biological value. Our own data confirm these observations (Figure 6), but moderate additions of low-quality protein seem to have no deleterious effect while greatly improving morale.[65] We therefore now recommend a high caloric diet containing the same quantity of high-quality protein and 15 gm. of unselected protein.

We have also begun to evaluate a regimen of infrequent hemodialysis combined with the use of a high caloric diet containing an electrodialyzed whey-protein formula. Such a diet provides a protein source of very high biological value. Twenty grams of protein are supplied from electrodialyzed whey and 6 gm. of protein from miscellaneous sources to increase caloric intake and palatability. An additional 20 gm. of protein of high biological value is fed during hemodialysis. Preliminary data on four patients with minimal renal function who are undergoing 11-hour coil hemodialysis at 7- to 14-day intervals indicate that this diet minimizes the development of uremic symptoms while providing adequate protein for neutral to positive nitrogen balance. Patients on this whey diet generally felt as well at 10 to 11 days after dialysis as they do in four days after dialysis when on a more conventional 60-gm. protein diet. Blood-urea concentration is also lower. Dietary resistance may prove a serious limitation to the widespread use of such a diet, and the possibility of the progression of neuropathy or onset of pericarditis, despite the sense of well-being of the patients, has not yet been excluded. At least, this diet may be useful for patients who desire a "vacation" from hemodialysis.

With growing interest in home dialysis, in which a patient can dialize himself daily, dietary modification or restrictions will probably become less important except to insure an adequate intake of calories, vitamins, and high-quality protein. If, on the other hand, the interval of dialysis is fixed at several days, a higher protein intake without concern for the kind of protein taken undoubtedly will exaggerate uremic symptoms, and any nutritional advantages of the increased intake will be a questionable "trade-off." Merely decreasing total protein intake drastically is difficult to enforce, and it generally leads to a precarious state of chronic protein malnutrition.

There remain some apparently inexplicable differences among high-quality proteins. Morrison has recently reported that patients fed 0.7 to 1.0 gm./kg. of milk protein require dialysis much less frequently than do patients who receive similar quantities of protein from meat.[66] Others have substituted lean meat protein for egg protein in protein-restricted diets with untoward results.[45] Josephson reported that infusion of essential amino acid improves nitrogen balance and uremic symptoms.[67] Finally, Giordano has reported that by using a synthetic mixture of essential amino acids he was able to maintain a positive nitrogen balance with intakes substantially lower than can be achieved with protein from naturally occurring foods, including eggs, which supply similar quantities of essential amino acids.[34, 59] Such data are too sketchy for full acceptance of the implication that an amino acid when ingested as part of a protein is different metabolically than when fed or infused as a free chemical entity.

Enthusiasm for diets containing carefully selected protein of high biological value, which supply ample quantities of essential amino acids, has sometimes obscured the importance of nonessential amino acids and implied that the latter are best avoided. Many investigators have suggested the importance of nonessential nitrogen for the maintenance of nitrogen balance.[34, 68] Even proteins of highest biological value contain mostly nonessential amino acids, and no diet composed of natural foods can avoid contributing large quantities of nonessential amino acids to the metabolic pool.[69] Further, we found that feeding large quantities (20 to 25 gm.) of the eight free essential amino acids in roughly the proportions found in egg protein can produce very abnormal plasma levels and severe acidosis in patients with chronic renal failure.

The main problem of these specialized diets continues to be acceptance on the part of the patients. The more rigid the diet the more monotonous and less suitable it is for a practical therapeutic regimen. Advances in food technology may someday abolish this difficulty and make what is preferable for health also satisfying. The uremic patient has often lost much of his ability to enjoy life. He has many adverse symptoms; he faces an uncertain prognosis; his sexual capability has vanished; his income-producing activity is limited. His enjoyment of food is one of his remaining psychic resources. When his gastrointestinal symptoms improve, he seizes the opportunity to enjoy food with great enthusiasm, only to find himself trapped by a stern physician-dietitian authority that tries to keep him on a highly unpalatable diet. The fact that a less restrictive protein diet offers virtually identical symptomatic benefits and may offer biologic advantages as well is helpful. The fact that a patient feels better is a major fortification of dietary prescription, and application of such diets is most effective in the patient whose gastrointestinal symptoms are the most debilitating.

Acknowledgment

Dr. James Shinaberger and Dr. Jack Coburn participated in many of the studies reviewed. The help of Miss Molly Sorensen (dietetics) and Miss Sybil Gordon (laboratory) is acknowledged.

References

1. Kleeman, C. R., Epstein, F. H. and White, C.: The effect of variations in solute excretion and glomerular filtration on water diuresis. *J. Clin. Invest. 35*:749, 1956.
2. Kleeman, C. R., Adams, D. A. and Maxwell, M. H.: An evaluation of maximal water diuresis in chronic renal disease. 1. Normal solute intake. *J. Lab. Clin. Med. 58*:169, 1961.
3. Gonick, H. C., Maxwell, M. H., Rubini, M. E. and Kleeman, C. R.: Functional impairment in chronic renal disease. 1. Studies of sodium-conserving ability. *Nephron 3*:137, 1966.
4. Coleman, A. J., Arias, M., Carter, N. W., Rector, F. C., Jr. and Seldin, D. W.: The mechanism of salt wastage in chronic renal disease. *J. Clin. Invest. 45*:1116, 1966.
5. Gilman, A.: The relation between blood osmotic pressure, fluid distribution, and voluntary water intake. *Amer. J. Physiol. 120*:323, 1937.
6. Leaf, A. and Camara, A. A.: Renal tubular secretion of potassium in man. *J. Clin. Invest. 28*:1526, 1949.
7. Flinn, R. B., Merrill, J. P. and Welzant, W. R.: Treatment of the oliguric patient with a new sodium-exchange resin and sorbitol. *New Eng. J. Med. 264*:111, 1961.
8. Scherr, L., Ogden, D. A., Mead, A. W., Spritz, N. and Rubin, A. L.: Management of hyperkalemia with a cation-exchange resin. *New Eng. J. Med. 264*: 115, 1961.
9. Berlyne, G. M., Janabi, K., Shaw, A. B. and Hocken, A. G.: Treatment of hyperkalaemia with a calcium-resin. *Lancet 1*:169, 1966.
10. Koppel, M. H., Coburn, J. W. and Massry, S. G.: Intestinal Calcium Absorption in Renal Failure: Effect of

Dietary Calcium, Vitamin D, Hemodialysis and Transplantation. Washington, D. C., Amer. Soc. of Nephrol., 1969. Abstracts, p. 36.

11. Parfitt, A. M.: Soft-tissue calcification in uremia. *Arch. Intern. Med. 124*:544, 1969.
12. Mosenthal, H. O. and Richard, A. E.: The interpretation of a positive nitrogen balance in nephritis. *Arch. Intern. Med. 17*:329, 1916.
13. Fishberg, A. M.: *Hypertension and Nephritis.* Philadelphia, Lea & Febiger, 1954, pp. 228-29.
14. Addis, T.: *Glomerular Nephritis, Diagnosis and Treatment.* New York, Macmillan, 1948.
15. Farr, L. E. and Smadel, J. E.: The effect of dietary protein on the course of nephrotoxic nephritis in rats. *J. Exp. Med. 70*:615, 1939.
16. Newburgh, L. H. and Curtis, A. C.: Production of renal injury in the white rat by the protein of the diet. *Arch. Intern. Med. 42*:801, 1928.
17. Merrill, J. P.: The Treatment of Renal Failure, 2d ed. New York, Grune & Stratton, 1956, pp. 217-18.
18. Sherman, H. C., Gillett, L. H. and Osterberg, E.: Protein requirements of maintenance in man and the nutritive efficiency of bread protein. *J. Biol. Chem. 41*:97, 1920.
19. Hegsted, D. M., Tsongas, A. G., Abbott, D. B. and Stare, F. J.: Protein requirements of adults. *J. Lab. Clin. Med. 31*:261, 1946.
20. Bricker, M. L., Shively, R. F., Smith, J. M., Mitchell, H. H. and Hamilton, T. S.: Protein requirement of college women on high cereal diets with observations on adequacy of short balance periods. *J. Nutr. 37*:163, 1949.
21. Recommended Dietary Allowances. Nat. Acad. Sci.-Nat. Res. Council Pub. 1964. Washington, D. C., 1968, p. 19.
22. Waterlow, J. C., Cravioto, J. C. and Stephan, J. M.: Protein malnutrition in man. *Advances Protein Chem. 15*: 131, 1960.
23. Allison, J. B. and Wannemacher, R. W., Jr.: The concept and significance of labile and over-all protein reserves of the body. *Amer. J. Clin. Nutr. 16*: 445, 1965.
24. Gan, J. C. and Jeffay, H.: Origins and metabolism of the intracellular amino acids pools in rat liver and muscle. *Biochem. Biophys. Acta 148*:448, 1967.
25. Harper, A. E.: Diet and plasma amino acids. *Amer J. Clin. Nutr. 21*:358, 1968.
26. Schimke, R. T.: Differential effects of fasting and protein-free diets on levels of urea cycle enzymes in rat liver. *J. Biol. Chem. 237*:1921, 1962.
27. Gaetani, S., Paolucci, A. M., Spadoni, M. A. and Tomassi, G.: Activity of amino acid-activating enzymes in tissues from protein-depleted rats. *J. Nutr. 84*:173, 1964.
28. Mariani, A., Spadoni, M. A. and Tomassi G.: Effect of protein depletion on amino acid-activating enzymes of rat liver. *Nature 4891*:378, 1963.
29. Mitchell, H. H. and Edman, M.: Nutritional significance of the dermal losses of nutrients in man, particularly of nitrogen and minerals. *Amer. J. Clin. Nutr. 10*:163, 1962.
30. Sirbu, E. R., Margen, S. and Calloway, D. H.: Effect of reduced protein intake on nitrogen losses from the human integument. *Amer. J. Clin. Nutr. 20*: 1158, 1967.
31. Costa, G.: Hypothetical pathway of nitrogen metabolism. *Nature 4750*:549, 1960.
32. Munro, H. N.: General Aspects of the Regulation of Protein Metabolism by Diet and by Hormones. In: *Mammalian Protein Metabolism,* vol. 1. New York, Academic Press, 1964, p. 381.
33. Gamble, J. L.: Physiological information gained from studies on the life raft ration. *Harvey Lectures 42*:247, 1947.
34. Giordano, C.: Use of exogenous and endogenous urea for protein synthesis in normal and uremic subjects. *J. Lab. Clin. Med. 62*:231, 1963.
35. Giordano, C., de Pascale, C., Balestrieri, C., Cittadini, D., and Crescenzi, A.: The incorporation of urea-^{15}N into serum proteins of uremic patients on

low nitrogen diets. *J. Clin. Invest. 45:* 1013, 1966.

36. Giovannetti, S. and Maggiore, Q.: A low nitrogen diet with proteins of high biological value for severe chronic uraemia. *Lancet 1:*1000, 1964.
37. Monasterio, G., Giovannetti, S. and Maggiore, Q.: The place of the low protein diet in the treatment of chronic uraemia. *Panminerva Med.* (English ed.) *7:*479, 1965.
38. Giovannetti, S.: Diet in chronic uremia. *Proc. 3d Int. Congr. Nephrol. 3:*230, 1966.
39. Berlyne, G. M.: *Trans. EDTA 1:*173, 1964.
40. Berlyne, G. M., Shaw, A. B. and Nilwarangkur, S.: Dietary treatment of chronic renal failure. Experiences with a modified Giovannetti diet. *Nephron 2:*129, 1965.
41. Shaw, A. B., Bazzard, F. J., Booth, E. M., Nilwarangkur, S. and Berlyne, G. M.: The treatment of chronic renal failure by a modified Giovannetti diet. *Quart. J. Med. 34:*237, 1965.
42. Berlyne, G. M. and Shaw, A. B.: Giordano-Giovannetti diet in terminal renal failure. *Lancet 2:*7, 1965.
43. Berlyne, G. M. and Hocken, A. G.: The Dietary Treatment of Chronic Renal Failure: In: *Nutrition in Renal Disease.* Baltimore, Williams & Wilkins, 1968, p. 38.
44. Berlyne, G. M., Gaan, D. and Ginks, W. R.: Dietary treatment of chronic renal failure. *Amer. J. Clin. Nutr. 21:* 547, 1968.
45. Snyder, D. and Merrill, J. P.: Conservative management of uremic renal failure with a select protein diet. *Trans. Ass. Amer. Physicians 79:*409, 1966.
46. Franklin, S. S.: Gordon, A., Kleeman, C. R. and Maxwell, M. H.: Use of a balanced low-protein diet in chronic renal failure. *J.A.M.A. 202:*477, 1967.
47. Lonergan, E. T. and Lange, K.: Use of a special protein-restricted diet in uremia. *Amer. J. Clin. Nutr. 21:*595, 1968.
48. Rose, W. C.: The amino acid requirements of adult man. *Nutr. Abstr. Rev. 27:*631, 1957.
49. Orlowski, T. and Polec, R.: Potato diet in terminal renal failure. *Proc. EDTA 3:*368, 1966.
50. Kluthe, R.: Contribution to the Dietetic Management of Chronic Renal Failure. In: *Progress in Nephrology.* Proc. 5th Symp. of the Gesellschaft für Nephrologie. Lausanne 21-23. Sept. 1967. G. P.-F. Roch-Ramel, ed. Berlin, Springer, 1969.
51. Parsons, F. M. and Fore, J.: High carbohydrate intake for oral use in acute renal failure. *Lancet 2:*386, 1963.
52. Urdaneta, L. F., Subramanian, V. W. and Griffin, W. O. Jr.: "High liquid glucose" for oral use in renal failure. *Proc. Soc. Exptl. Biol. Med. 122:*974, 1966.
53. Shaw, A. B.: Diet, Anaemia, and Renal Failure. In: *Nutrition in Renal Disease.* Baltimore, Williams & Wilkins, 1968, p. 150.
54. Kopple, J. D., Sorensen, M. K., Coburn, J. W., Gordon, S. and Rubini, M. E.: Controlled comparison of 20-g and 40-g protein diets in the treatment of chronic uremia. *Amer. J. Clin. Nutr. 21:*553, 1968.
55. Sorensen, M. K. and Kopple, J. D.: Assessment of adherence to protein-restricted diets during conservative management of uremia. *Amer. J. Clin. Nutr. 21:*631, 1968.
56. Kopple, J. D., Shinaberger, J. H., Coburn, J. W. Sorensen, M. K. and Rubini, M. E.: Evaluating modified protein diets for uremia. *J. Amer. Diet Ass. 54:*481, 1969.
57. Kopple, J. D., Shinaberger, J. H., Rubini, M. E. and Coburn, J. W.: Unpublished observations.
58. Herndon, R. F., Freeman, S. and Cleveland, A. S.: Protein requirements in chronic renal insufficient patients. A study of the nitrogen minimum. *J. Lab. Clin. Med. 52:*235, 1958.
59. Giordano, C., Esposito, R., de Pascale, C. and de Santo, N. G.: Dietary treatment in renal failure. *Proc. 3d Int. Congr. Nephrol. 3:*214, 1966.
60. Ford, J., Phillips, M. E., Toye, F. E., Luck, V. A. and de Wardener, H. E.: Nitrogen balance in patients with chronic renal failure on diets contain-

ing varying quantities of protein. *Brit. Med. J. 1*:735, 1969.

61. Robson, A. M., Kerr, D. N. S. and Ashcroft, R.: Urea Metabolism in Chronic Uraemia: Effect of Protein Restriction, Anabolic Steroids and Antibiotics. In: *Nutrition in Renal Disease.* Baltimore, Williams & Wilkins, 1968, p. 71.
62. Giordano, C.: Discussion. *Amer. J. Clin. Nutr. 21*:391, 1968.
63. Kopple, J. D., Shinaberger, J. H., Swendseid, M. E., Umezawa, C. Y. and Rubini, M. E.: Amino Acid Metabolism During Hemodialysis. Washington, D.C., American Society Nephrology, 1969. Abstracts, p. 36.
64. Ginn, H. E., Frost, A. and Lacy, W. W.: Nitrogen balance in hemodialysis patients. *Amer. J. Clin. Nutr. 21*:385, 1968.
65. Kopple, J. D., Shinaberger, J. H., Coburn, J. W., Sorensen, M. K. and Rubini, M. E.: Optimal dietary protein treatment during chronic hemodialysis. *Trans. Amer. Soc. Artif. Intern. Organs 15*:302, 1969.
66. Morrison, R., Hegsted, M. and Myers, C.: High biological value protein diets and infrequent hemodialysis. *Fed. Proc. Abstracts 28*:808, 1969.
67. Josephson, B.: Amino acids and uremia. Presented at the 4th Int. Congr. Nephrol., Stockholm, Sweden, 1969, in press.
68. Kies, C. V., Shortridge, L. and Reynolds, M. S.: Effect on nitrogen retention of men of varying the total dietary nitrogen with essential amino acid intake kept constant. *J. Nutr. 85*:260, 1965.
69. Orr, M. L. and Watt, B. K.: *Amino Acid Content of Foods.* Home Economics Research Report No. 4. Washington, D.C., December 1957.
70. Kopple, J. D., Umezawa, C. Y., Rubini, M. E. and Swendseid, M. E.: Unpublished observations.

RENAL TRANSPLANTATION: PRESENT STATUS*

ALBERT L. RUBIN, JOHN C. WHITSELL, ROBERT R. RIGGIO, GABRIEL H. SCHWARTZ, DAVID S. DAVID, AND KURT H. STENZEL

Rogosin Laboratories
Departments of Surgery and Biochemistry
The New York Hospital-Cornell Medical Center
New York, N.Y.

INTRODUCTION

RENAL transplantation has become a recognized form of therapy for end-stage renal disease over the past few years, and more and more centers are now undertaking this procedure. When successful it results in complete restoration of renal function and of health. The procedures are not, however, uniformly successful, and many problems remain in determining the proper management and immunosuppressive therapy for these patients. We have had experience with 120 renal transplants at the New York Hospital since 1963 and have encountered most of the problems inherent in this procedure. We here present some of the methods we have established as a result of this experience.

SELECTION AND CARE OF RECIPIENTS

All patients with end-stage renal disease should be considered for both dialysis and transplantation. The first consideration is to institute adequate dialysis if renal function has deteriorated to the point where the patient is symptomatic. Transplantation is not an emergency procedure and, as will be seen, many studies must be carried out prior to surgery. Transplantation can be considered as a primary procedure if renal function is adequate, along with proper diet and medical management, to keep the patient relatively asymptomatic, and the risks of dialysis and blood transfusion can then be avoided. The patient should

*Presented at a *Conference on Glomerulonephritis* held by the New York Heart Association at The Waldorf Astoria, New York, N. Y., January 27, 1970.

This study was supported in part by the New York State Kidney Disease Institute, the Kidney Foundation of New York, the New York Heart Association, and U.S. Public Health Service Research Grant HE08736 from the National Heart Institute, Bethesda, Md.

be one who can be restored to health by restoration of renal function which, of course, eliminates patients with illnesses other than kidney disease, which are rapidly fatal. The selection of a recipient cannot be completely routinized; each patient must be individually evaluated. Patients in the older group, for instance, with coronary artery disease and atherosclerosis may do better with chronic dialysis. Our criteria are thus quite flexible, and we consider most uremic patients as candidates for transplants.

It is of critical importance to ascertain the status of the lower urinary tract in potential recipients by avoiding cystourethrogram and, if necessary, cystoscopy. Lower urinary tract obstruction must be corrected prior to or at the time of transplant. Usually this is accomplished prior to the transplant. In cases where the bladder is irretrievable, an ileal conduit can be constructed prior to surgery to receive the transplanted ureter. Three of our patients have had ileal conduits and they have had no problems with infections or mechanical abnormalities during a follow-up period of over three years. Nephrectomies may also be done before or during transplant or even after the transplant operation. In 10 patients in whom we elected to leave the kidneys in, posttransplant nephrectomies two to six months later were completely uncomplicated and required only brief hospital admissions. We believe, however, that there are certain definite indications for pretransplant nephrectomies. These include the presence of large polycystic kidneys, infected kidneys (in such cases nephrectomy is combined with ureterectomy if there is ureteral reflux), and severe, persistent hypertension in spite of adequate dialysis. Some patients with rapidly progressive glomerulonephritis with antiglomerular basement membrane antibody might also be nephrectomized in the hope that the antibodies will decrease over a period of months. The evidence for this point, however, is certainly not complete.[1]

Most patients will need some form of maintenance dialysis while awaiting transplant. If the patient has a living related donor and requires only a few dialyses, peritoneal dialysis may be done. Patients who must await cadaver kidneys will usually require hemodialysis, although an occasional patient can be adequately maintained with peritoneal dialysis. Fistulas are preferable for hemodialysis, since they obviate the problems of infection and thrombosis that are more common with arteriovenous shunts. Transfusions represent excellent sources of sen-

TABLE I. EVALUATION OF LIVING RELATED KIDNEY DONORS

History
Physical examination
Social service and psychiatric interview
Urinalysis
Urine culture ×3
Complete blood count
BUN
Creatinine, creatinine clearance
Uric acid
Calcium, phosphorus, sodium, potassium, chloride carbon dioxide combining power
Blood sugar, SGOT, SGPT, bilirubin
Chest x ray
EKG (if indicated)
Blood type, lymphocyte types
IVP
Renal arteriogram

sitization by histocompatibility antigens carried on the surface of white blood cells, and care should be taken to remove these cells from the blood. Buffycoat poor packed cells usually contain white cells, but these can be eliminated by either rapid freezing under controlled conditions or by irradiation. The killed cells are apparently much less immunogenic.

Selection of Donor

For practical purposes there are at present two sources of kidneys: cadaver donors and living related donors. Family members are often anxious to donate a kidney for a child or sibling, and if so they are interviewed by a physician, nurse, and psychiatrist associated with the transplant team. Details of the procedure, as well as the over-all possibilities for success or failure are carefully delineated. Meanwhile major blood-group determination and tissue typing are done. If these appear compatible the donor undergoes a complete history and physical examination plus the studies outlined in Table I. We have not taken any donors under 21, but have set no upper age limit; we have left this to the discretion of the medical-surgical transplant team. The physiological age is, of course, much more important than the chronological one. Several donors have been ruled out for obesity, however, since this sub-

TABLE II. CRITERIA FOR CADAVER-ORGAN TRANSPLANTATION ADOPTED BY THE MEDICAL BOARD OF THE NEW YORK HOSPITAL

A) Consent for removal and transplantation of an organ must be given by: 1) the donor prior to death, or by 2) the next of kin as defined by law.

B) Cause of death must be evident and the damage irreversible.

C) The responsibility for determining brain death for the donor rests with two attending physicians not associated with the medical teams preparing, performing, and maintaining the organ transplant. These physicians will be either an anesthesiologist, a neurologist, or a neurosurgeon. Their joint opinion as to the donor's acceptability on the basis of the evidence of brain death must be recorded in the medical record prior to any operative procedure.

D) The death certificate shall be completed before any transplant procedure is initiated.

E) Subject to the opinion of the examining physicians, the following criteria are proposed to define brain death.

1) Lack of spontaneous respiration for three minutes in the presence of reasonably normal pO_2 and pCO_2 concentrations and this state of respiratory unresponsiveness must be maintained.
2) Fixed pupils, unresponsive to light.
3) The electroencephalogram must be isoelectric at full gain.
4) The patient is in irreversible coma.

F) The patient must not be under the effects of central nervous system depressants or drugs that block neuromuscular function or hypothermia.

G) Individuals dying from, or suspected of dying from criminal violence cannot serve as donors, as such a procedure might prejudice the interest of the state and the defendant, and interfere with the administration of justice.

stantially increases the operative risks. Most of this evaluation can be done in the clinic, but the last procedure, the arteriogram, requires overnight hospitalization. Several donors have been ruled out because of multiple renal arteries on both sides.

Cadaver organs represent different and, in some ways, more complex administrative problems. First, there must be an active cadaver procurement program so that potentially useful kidneys do not go to waste. This includes public as well as professional education and the availability of personnel to remove and transport kidneys. Liaison with the family of the donor should be made, and several months later a letter expressing gratitude and a follow-up of the procedure should be sent. We now use a Belzer[2] perfusion apparatus which allows more time after removing cadaver organs for mobilization of personnel and patients and for typing procedures. Some idea of the kidney's function can also be obtained by its behavior on this apparatus. Before using the perfusion machine, the incidence of acute tubular necrosis after cadaver transplant in our series was close to 80%. This figure dropped to 20%

after the perfusion apparatus was used. Most cadaver donors we utilized died of cerebral causes—trauma, hemorrhage, or primary tumors—and the usual criteria for brain death were applied (Table II). When the donor is declared dead and the family has agreed to the procedure, blood and lymphocyte typing are done. This information is fed into a computer and the names and clinical data of suitable patients are immediately typed out. The recipients are then notified and prepared for surgery. While the kidney is being perfused there is ample time for all these procedures and, in fact, a kidney biopsy may also be done. Cadavers with malignant tumors, other than primary cerebral ones, are not used because of the danger of transplanting malignant cells.

Typing Procedures

It is apparent from skin transplants in mice that graft survival is dependent on the genetic proximity of donor and recipient. The importance of ABO compatibility in human renal grafting is evidenced by the fact that virtually all kidney transplants performed in the presence of ABO incompatibility reject within the first few postoperative hours or days. Consequently, we require ABO compatibility before a donor is considered.

Leukocytes and, in particular, lymphocytes have been used during the past few years to characterize host-specific histocompatibility antigens. Lymphocytes are readily available and have cell-membrane antigens that are closely related to those on kidney cells cultured from biopsy material. Histocompatibility antisera have been obtained from multitransfused individuals, multiparous women, and previously transplanted patients, and the specificities of these sera have been defined. At present approximately 13 antigens are evaluated. White cells are separated from defibrinated blood. In the agglutination assay, microscopically observed clumping of white cells by the antisera identifies the presence of the antigen. In the cytotoxicity assay,[3] after separating the neutrophils and other white-cell types from the lymphocytes, cell death induced by the antisera and complement is measured by the entrance of a nonvital dye into the cells. A very important additional test is the assay of a recent recipient's serum for the presence of preformed circulating antibody to the prospective donor's cells. If a transplant is performed in the presence of such an antibody, the graft undergoes a severe, early (hyperacute) rejection.[4] We do not perform a transplant in the presence of a donor-directed cytotoxic antibody. The development of such an antibody is attributable to multiple white-cell or platelet-containing blood transfusions or previous transplant rejection.[5] Some individuals have antibodies against as many as 90% of potential donors. Suitable donors were eventually found for two such patients in our series, and the results of the transplants have been excellent one year later. The development of cytotoxic donor-directed antibodies after transplantation is associated with a high incidence of severe early rejections and vascular changes in the graft.[5]

Matching of donor and recipient is accomplished by comparing their antigen patterns. An *A* match occurs only in identical twins and in some siblings. In a *B* match no antigens are present in the donor that are not in the recipient. One major incompatibility is termed a *C* match, while two or more major incompatibilities is a *D* match. An *F* match occurs where a preformed, donor-directed antibody is present. Most investigators have noted a correlation between matching grade and length of graft survival, especially in related living-donor transplants. We have also found this to be the case in our related living-donor series. It should be noted, however, that some badly matched patients have done well and a few good matches have had a less than optimum outcome. Since it has been postulated that human genetic information on histocompatibility is contained in two subloci on a single chromosome, analysis of related donor transplants for the number of chromosome differences may explain some unexpected results. Improved immunosuppression and unidentified histocompatibility antigens may also account for these apparent discrepancies. Many investigators feel that tissue typing plays a small role in selection of cadaver-kidney recipients. The ability to perform well-matched cadaver transplants depends in large measure on the availability of a large pool of previously typed and prepared recipients on chronic dialysis, a rapid and accurate method for identifying the best matches and detecting preformed antibodies, and the means for perfusing cadaver kidneys. These features are now present in the New York area.

Surgery

The surgical procedures have been described, and will not be detailed here. In general, the kidney is placed in the recipient pelvic fossa, the renal artery anastamosed end to end to the recipient hypogastric artery, the renal vein anastamosed end to side to the external iliac vein, and the ureter is tunneled into the bladder so that the transplant ureteral orifice is low in the area of the trigone. Usually urine formation begins promptly after establishing the blood supply. When children are transplanted with adult kidneys, the kidney is placed intra-abdominally. The vena cava and right common iliac artery or the aorta are used for revascularization in these instances.

Immunosuppression

Except in the case of isografts, immunosuppression must be used to prevent immunological destruction of the renal graft. All immunosuppressive techniques used clinically are broad spectrum, and they depress all or more host defense mechanisms. Fortunately the immune response to a kidney allograft is much more easily suppressed than are immune responses to infectious agents.

The measures used for immunosuppression include cytotoxic drugs, glucocorticoids, extracorporeal irradiation, graft irradiation, thoracic duct drainage, and antilymphocyte globulin.

The cytotoxic drugs exert their effects by disturbing immune-cell function, especially that of short-lived lymphocytes.[6] These drugs affect sensitization at a time when antigen stimulates the conversion of quiescent, small lymphocytes to active, sensitized cells.[6] Once lymphocytes have become sensitized, the cytotoxic agents now used are ineffective in the therapeutic dose range. These drugs also have a nonspecific anti-inflammatory effect which is probably significant.[6] Azathioprine (Imuran) is the most commonly used cytotoxic agent in renal transplantation. The usual dose is 4 mg./kg. the evening prior to transplantation, 3 mg./kg. the following day, and then 1 to 2 mg./kg./day. Because of its limited therapeutic effect on sensitized lymphocytes, the azathioprine dose is not increased during acute rejection. On the contrary, with the decrease in creatinine clearance present during rejection the dose of azathioprine must often be lowered to prevent leukopenia.

Glucocorticoids constitute the most commonly used immunosuppressive agents. In man the small lymphocytes are relatively resistant to steroids.[6] In addition there has been no convincing evidence that steroids decrease antibody formation in man.[7] It seems likely that steroids exert their main effect on the immune response via their anti-inflammatory action. Steroids impede adherence of inflammatory cells to damaged vascular endothelium, and they stabilize lysosomal membranes.[6, 7] We usually administer 100 mg. prednisolone on the day of transplant, and rapidly taper the dose over the next two weeks. Steroids in doses up to 500 mg. per day constitute the mainstay in the therapy of acute rejection episodes. The most common complications of therapy are infection, poor healing of the wound, gastrointestinal bleeding, psychosis, and osteonecrosis.

Small lymphocytes are very sensitive to radiation but, once sensitized, they become relatively resistant.[6] Thus the efficacy of local radiation to the transplanted kidney during a rejection episode is not proved. In spite of this our therapy for severe rejection is local radiation with a total of 600 rads in divided doses. Recently Persson et al.[8] have demonstrated that extracorporeal irradiation of the blood prior to and during the early days after renal transplantation will decrease the incidence of early rejection and improve renal allograft survival. The usual total preoperative dose given in several treatments is 5,000 to 9,000 rads per blood volume. Another 10,000 to 20,000 rads are given over two to three weeks postoperatively. Persson et al. noted that morbidity and the incidence of leukopenia and infection were less at doses under 40,000 rads than with alternative immunosuppressive regimens.

Decreasing the number of circulating lymphocytes by drainage of the thoracic duct is a relatively safe and effective method of immunosuppressive therapy.[9] A thoracic-duct fistula is created about one week prior to transplantation and over the next few days 10 l. or more of lymph and more than 20×10^9 lymphocytes can be removed. The lymphocytes are separated by centrifugation, and the lymph fluid is reinfused. The major drawbacks of this method are poorly functioning fistulae and infection at the fistula site.

During the past two or three years increasing use has been made of antilymphocyte globulin (ALG) as a clinical immunosuppressant. Studies by Medawar and his colleagues,[10] who used mouse-skin grafting, have shown that antilymphocyte serum and ALG are potent agents in prolonging homograft survival although the mode of action of ALG is somewhat unclear. Among the suggested effects are destruction of lymphocytes, which leads to lymphopenia, sterile activation of lymphocytes, which renders them unresponsive to the foreign graft, blindfolding of lymphocytes, and sequestration of lymphocytes in liver or spleen. Many workers in human transplantation have found that ALG is effective in prolonging renal graft survival, but agreement on this point is not uniform. Starzl and his co-workers[11] have noted decreased serum creatinines, lower steroid requirements, and improved over-all success rates with the use of ALG.

Some of the variations in reported results stem from differing methods of preparation and titration of ALG. There is no currently accepted *in vitro* technique for assaying potency of ALG, although we recently described a method based on opsonization properties of ALG that appears unusually reliable in a mouse system.[12] Most of the ALG we have used has been prepared in horses, by use of spleen as the antigen, although thoracic-duct lymphocytes and thymus cells are preferable if available. After immunization the IgG fraction is separated and assayed by lymphocytotoxicity and lymphoagglutination. Prolongation of skin grafts in nonhuman primates[13] appears to be a promising although costly method for determining the potency of ALG, and methods for utilizing the opsonization test for human material are under investigation.

It is much too early to know if ALG has any effect, in the dosages employed by most centers, on renal-graft survival. We are evaluating three dosage levels: 0.5 to 1 mg./kg., 5 to 10 mg./kg., and 20 to 30 mg./kg. The ALG is given, intravenously and daily for two weeks, and then gradually decreased. Only cadaver recipients are routinely treated. There are certain major operational problems involved in a program such as this: obtaining a constant and reliable source of antigen, maintaining facilities for large animals, serum fractionation, and sterility and pyrogenicity testing. These problems are individually small but they can sometimes reach formidable levels in a transplant-dialysis laboratory.

Our impression of the immunosuppressive efficacy of ALG has been favorable although our experience with this agent has lasted only one year and is therefore too short a period for statistical evaluation. Improvement in our cadaver results coincided with the use of ALG, though other factors such as improved histocompatibility and management of patients may play a role. Side effects attributable to ALG have been relatively minor in our series. Local pain and fever are seen occasionally; thrombocytopenia and urticaria, rarely. Anaphylaxis occurred once and responded to appropriate therapy. We have seen no damage to glomeruli by ALG immune deposits, nor have we demonstrated heterologous ALG by fluorescent staining of biopsies from transplanted kidneys during treatment with ALG. Enhancement of viral infections by ALG may be an occasional problem.

A special problem is the development of antibodies to ALG and the rapid immune clearance of ALG after repeated therapy. We have been interested in developing tolerance to ALG by giving the patient 50 mg./kg. of highly purified, aggregate-free animal IgG. The half-life of ALG, as determined by I^{125} ALG clearance is often doubled by this pretreatment, and approaches control values.[14]

Immunosuppressive agents now in use represent the best available means for prolonging grafts. There are, however, definite risks of poor wound healing and of infection inherent in their use. Less toxic and more specific immunosuppressive techniques are urgently required for prevention and suppression of rejection. Among the techniques we have found most helpful in evaluating new agents are human peripheral lymphocyte cultures,[15] mouse-skin grafting, and dog renal transplants. The first two methods are useful for rapid screening and are convenient for studying the mechanism of action of promising materials. The latter technique offers insight into the suitability of the agent in clinical transplantation. Several promising substances we have recently evaluated are Cinanserin,[15] an antiseritonin agent with no bone marrow toxicity, asparaginase,[16] and an alpha-2 globulin fraction.[17]

The ultimate goal in tissue transplantation is the safe and reliable induction of immune tolerance to graft-specific antigens. Tolerance can be achieved in human patients to certain purified antigens, and a great deal of work is being done to isolate and purify histocompatibility antigens so that they may be similarily used to induce tolerance. The phenomenom of immunologic enhancement offers another approach to the improvement of graft survival. This phenomenon is the suppression of the immune response to a particular antigen by passive administration of antibody specific to that antigen. Both these techniques are still in the investigative stages and much more must be learned before they can be applied to man.

Rejection

Rejection almost always occurs to some degree after kidney transplantation, but fortunately it is usually reversible. There are three clearly recognized types of rejection: hyperacute, acute, and chronic.

Hyperacute rejection is the most fulminant type and is seldom, if ever, reversible. It is undoubtedly due to humoral antibody and can occur within minutes of transplant or can be delayed for several days. Clinically there is a rapid and dramatic decrease in urine volume and creatinine clearance over a period of several hours. Pathologically there is a vasculitis, fibrin deposition in the small blood vessels and glomeruli, polymorphonuclear leukocytes in the glomeruli, and areas of local necrosis and interstitial edema. Treatment with heparin, ALG, steroids, or local irradiation have been uniformly unsuccessful in our hands, and ultimately the kidney must be removed. This is an unusual type of rejection and can be minimized by testing for preformed antibody in the recipient to donor cells. This is done by use of donor lymphocytes, kidney cells, or both. The occurrence of a hyperacute rejection does not indicate that future transplants will be unsuccessful, but preformed antibody must be very carefully sought in these instances.

Acute rejection is the most common form of rejection and appears to be primarily due to cellular immunity. Clinically it is usually manifested by fever, a gradually decreasing volume of urine and creatinine clearance (over several days), proteinuria, round cells in the urine, and elevated serum-alpha-2 globulins. The major pathologic finding is focal infiltration of large round cells with some interstitial edema. Glomeruli and blood vessels are usually affected only minimally. This type of rejection usually responds to increased dosages of glucocorticoids.

Chronic rejection is an indolent phenomenon clinically, with gradually decreasing creatinine clearance and minimal if any systemic manifestations; and it is relatively resistant to increased dosages of glucocorticids. This form of rejection also appears to be caused by circulating antibody, and it is manifested by gradual narrowing and obliteration of small blood vessels.

The question of recurrent glomerulonephritis is of great importance but often difficult to document. The incidence is undoubtedly higher in identical twins[18] and is possibly related to the lower doses or absence of immunosuppression. Some patients clearly have circulating antiglomerular basement-membrane antibodies, and these patients may develop recurrent disease. In our experience this has been unusual. Proteinuria is quite common during acute rejection episodes, and the nephrotic syndrome may develop following rejection.[19]

Complications

Many complications continue to plague transplant procedures, but fortunately most of these can be adequately treated.

During the surgical procedure itself, blood loss may be a problem. This can usually be minimized by adequate preparation of the patient by peritoneal or hemodialysis. Postoperative problems associated with the vascular anastamoses have been rare. We have had three instances of renal vein thrombosis in 120 transplants; one was associated with an unrecognized ureteral stenosis and hydronephrosis. Urologic complications are more common; they consist of leaks from the ureteral implantation site, ureteral stenosis and, occasionally, perinephric abscess formation. A sudden cessation of the flow of urine in the first few postoperative days may be a result of mechanical causes, and these must be promptly investigated. Other common causes of early oliguria are, as previously mentioned, acute tubular necrosis and hyperacute rejection.

In the immediate posttransplant period there is often a profound diuresis. The causes of this are not precisely known, but several factors have been identified. We have found decreased reabsorption of sodium during this period, and similar findings, along with occasional glycosuria, have been reported.[20] Kountz et al.[21] have recently found a decreased extraction ratio for PAH in transplanted kidneys. The corrected renal blood flow was thus higher than normal, and this increased flow persisted for several weeks posttransplant. Several mechanisms have been suggested for the diuresis: it is probably caused by a combination of some proximal tubular dysfunction, possible hyperemia, and increased osmotic load. The clinical fluid and electrolyte problems are handled by determining the urine electrolytes and by replacing losses of both volume and salts. A central venous pressure catheter (CVP) is helpful during the immediate postoperative period to monitor needs for more or less fluid replacement. Patients often require large amounts of colloid during this time to maintain the CVP. This is usually given in the form of 5% plasmanate.

The diuresis gradually subsides over three to four days, and renal function, barring episodes of rejection becomes normal. The incidence of acute renal failure after cadaver transplantation is high if long, warm, ischemic times occur, and these patients must be continued on frequent dialysis.

Infections pose very serious problems, especially if renal function is poor either because of acute tubular necrosis or hyperacute rejection. The combination of immunosuppressive therapy and uremia depress defense mechanisms of the host to dangerous levels. Pseudomonas infections are among the most serious we have encountered, as well as occasional fungal diseases such as cryptococcal meningitis, aspergillosis, and mucormycosis. Abscess formation in the perirenal area can often be treated with drainage, but if the kidney is involved or if there are intrarenal abscesses the kidney must be removed.

Viral infections also occur, the most serious being viral hepatitis. Several patients have had persistant SH antigen, and one patient in our series died of liver failure one year after viral hepatitis. Herpes zoster has occurred but has remained localized. One patient, in fact, developed a typical herpetic lesion two days after transplantation while receiving 100 mg. of prednisolone per day, as well as antilymphocyte globulin and Imuran. This lesion also remained localized and the patient recovered uneventfully. Cytomegalovirus infections are common, but in our experience have been mild and self-limited.

Long-term complications have been few in our experience. There is some evidence that the incidence of malignant disease is increased in patients who receive immunosuppressive drugs. One of our patients developed a tumor involving the brain that appeared pathologically to be a reticulum-cell sarcoma. This occured about eight months post-transplant. The patient was unusual in several respects, however: he had had tuberculosis as a child, and there was an incidental finding of a papillary carcinoma of the renal pelvis in one of his own kidneys, which was removed at the time of transplant.

Nevertheless the incidence of malignant disease must be carefully assessed in long-term kidney-transplant patients.

Results

The object of any medical treatment is to return the patient to a normal life. Successful renal transplantation does this in a much more complete way than hemodialysis. We have seen the anemia of uremia, which persists in chronic hemodialysis, corrected as rapidly as one month after institution of good renal function (creatinine less than 2.5 mg.% and a clearance above 40 cc./min.). The patient thus feels stronger and is able to resume normal activity. Nerve-conduction studies also return to normal after successful renal transplantation. One 16-year-old girl who was completely paralyzed in both lower extremities was up in a walker one month after transplant and was able to walk normally after six months. Dwarfed children below the age of 16 who have good renal function postoperatively have had spurts of growth in spite of doses of glucocorticoids, which are reportedly sufficient to inhibit growth. In eight children whose growth has been closely followed, six grew more than 2 cm. within less than one year after successful renal transplant. The two who did not grow had poorly functioning transplants. The most impressive growth spurt was in a 14-year-old boy who grew 5 cm. within six weeks after transplant. Amennorhea was found in 22 of our 26 females between the ages of 13 and 39 who were on chronic dialysis prior to transplantation. Of 16 who now have excellent renal function after transplant (creatinine less than 1.4 mg. %) 12 have regular menses, which began one to six months posttransplant; the other four have irregular menses. Of the 12 with regular menses, five pregnancies have occurred in four patients, two delivered normally, one required a cesarean section due to the graft obstructing the birth canal, and two are in the third trimester. The children are all normal. Seven of the 26 women who received transplants have married posttransplant. Almost all our transplanted patients, including those with poorly functioning grafts (creatinine 3 to 5 mg.%, clearances 10 to 30 cc./min.), have returned to their jobs, which include that of housewife, intensive care nurse, pharmacist, and taxicab driver. The young people have returned to school. Thus one sees nearly complete rehabilitation in patients with functioning renal grafts.

The over-all incidence of success is now about 80 to 90% with living related donors, and 50 to 60% with cadaver donors. Mortality is less than 10% in most centers.

Summary

Renal transplantation is now an accepted mode of treatment for end-stage renal disease. An interdisciplinary effort is required to extend this therapy to all those who could benefit by it, and regional programs must be evolved. Two major requirements for providing clinical transplantation are: adequate dialysis facilities and the availability of cadaver organs.

REFERENCES

1. Dixon, F. J.: The pathogenesis of glomerulonephritis. *Amer. J. Med. 44*:493-98, 1968.
2. Belzer, F. O., Ashby, B. S., Gulyassy, P. F. and Powell, M.: Successful 17-hour preservation and transplantation of human-cadaver kidney. *New Eng. J. Med. 278*:608-10, 1968.
3. Terasaki, P. I., Vredevoe, D. L. and Porter, K. A.: Serotyping for homotransplantation: V. Evaluation of a matching scheme. *Transplantation 4*: 688-99, 1967.
4. Williams, G. H., Hume, D. M., Hudson, R. P. Jr., Morris, P. J. and Milgrom, F.: Hyperacute renal homograft rejection in man. *New Eng. J. Med. 279*: 611-18 1968.
5. Patel, R. and Terasaki, P. I.: Significance of the positive crossmatch test in kidney transplantation. *New Eng. J. Med. 280*:735-39, 1969.
6. Schwartz, R. S.: Therapeutic strategy in clinical immunology. *New Eng. J. Med. 280*:367-74, 1969.
7. David, D. S., Grieco, M. H. and Cushman, P.: Adrenal glucocorticoids after 20 years: a review of their clinically relevant consequences. *J. Chron. Dis. 22*: 637-711, 1970.
8. Persson, B., Rosengrun, B. Bergentz, S. E. and Hood, B.: Evaluation of preoperative extracorporeal irradiation of the blood in human renal transplantation. *Transplantation 7*:534-44, 1969.
9. Tilney, N. L., Atkinson, J. C. and Murray, J. E.: The immunosuppressive effect of thoracic duct drainage in human kidney transplantation. *Ann. Int. Med. 72*:59-64, 1970.
10. Medawar, P. B., Biological effects of heterologous antilymphocytic antisera, In: *Human Transplantation,* Rappaport, F. and Dausset, J., eds. New York, Grune & Stratton, 1968.
11. Starzl, T. E., Akith, C. G., Terasaki, P. I., Putnam, C. W., Brettschneider, L. and Marchioro, T. L. Heterologous antilymphocyte globulin, histocompatibility matching and human renal homotransplantation. *Surg. Gymec. Obstet. 125*: 1023, 1968.
12. Bull, F. G., Stenzel, K. H. and Rubin, A. L.: Opsonizing antibodies in antilymphocyte serum. *Clin. Res. 18*:423, 1970.
13. Balner, H., Dersjant, H. and Van Bekkum, D. W.: Testing of antihuman lymphocyte sera in chimpanzees and lower primates. *Transplantation 8*:281-90, 1969.
14. Weksler, M. E., Buil, F. G., Schwartz, G. H., Stenzel, K. H. and Rubin, A. L.: Immunologic responses of graft recipients to antilymphocyte globulin: Effect of prior treatment with aggregate-free globulins. *J. Clin. Inv.* In press.
15. Schwartz, G. H., Stenzel, K. H. and Rubin, A. L.: Depression of lymphocyte transformation by drugs *in vitro* effects of a new immunosuppressant, Cinanserin. *Transplantation 8*:704-11, 1969.
16. Schwartz, G. H., Stenzel, K. H. and Rubin, A. L.: Asparaginase effects on human lymphocytes. *Clin. Res. 17*:602, 1969.
17. Riggio, R. R., Schwartz, G. H., Bull, F. G., Stenzel, K. H. and Rubin, A. L.: Alpha-2 globulins in renal graft rejection: Effects on *in vitro* lymphocyte function. *Transplantation 8*:689-94, 1969.
18. Glassock, R. J., Feldman, D., Reynolds, F. S., Dammin, G. J. and Merrill, J. P.: Human renal isografts: A clinical and pathologic analysis. *Medicine 47*:411-54, 1968.
19. Harlan, W. R., Holden, K. R., Willians, G. M. and Hume, D. M.: Proteinuria and nephrotic syndrome associated with chronic rejection of kidney transplants. *New Eng. J. Med. 277*:769-76, 1967.
20. Ogden, D. A., Sitpirja, V. and Holmes, J. H.: Function of the renal homograft in man immediately after transplantation. *Amer. J. Med. 88*:873, 1965.
21. Kountz, S. L., Truex, G., Bailey, L. E. and Belzer, F. O.: Serial hemodynamics after renal allotransplantations in man. *Circulation 41*:217-24, 1970.

CONFERENCE ON GLOMERULONEPHRITIS*

Panel Discussion, Afternoon Session

JEROME LOWENSTEIN, *Moderator*

Assistant Professor of Medicine
New York University School of Medicine
New York, N.Y.

NORMAN BANK, MILTON E. RUBINI, GEORGE E. SCHREINER

DR. JEROME LOWENSTEIN. Dr. Bank, did you want to say something about the possible role of physical factors in the sodium retention and diuresis seen in acute glomerulonephritis?

DR. NORMAN BANK. Yes. There was not enough time during my discussion to relate the newer findings on peritubular control of sodium reabsorption to clinical conditions, but these recent observations may have several clinical implications. For example, as I indicated, the protein concentration in peritubular capillary blood seems to have a great deal to do with the rate of absorption of sodium. In conditions such as congestive heart failure, filtration fraction is usually quite high. That is, renal blood flow is reduced to a greater extent than is glomerular-filtration rate. This means that the concentration of proteins is probably higher in the peritubular capillaries than in normal individuals. It seems possible that the mechanism for retention of sodium in congestive heart failure may be related to the higher concentration of protein in peritubular capillary blood, which would be expected to enhance reabsorption.

In cirrhosis of the liver there is often a reduced renal blood flow. Patients thus afflicted might similarly have elevated protein concentrations or diminished hydrostatic pressure in their peritubular capillaries, which might then tend to enhance the reabsorption of sodium and lead to the formation of edema.

As far as intrinsic renal disease is concerned, one can speculate about the situation in chronic renal disease more readily than in acute renal disease. When there is a reduced number of functioning nephrons in

*Held by the New York Heart Association at The Waldorf-Astoria, New York, N. Y., January 27, 1970.

chronic renal disease, the blood supply to these remaining nephrons is in all probability increased above normal levels. It has been shown that the filtration rate is greatly increased in the remaining nephrons of experimental animals with renal disease. Because of the higher blood supply to these surviving nephrons, the peritubular capillary hydrostatic pressure may be somewhat higher than in normal individuals. A higher peritubular pressure might contribute to the progressive decrease in tubular reabsorption per nephron that occurs in patients with advanced states of renal disease; the decrease allows them to remain in sodium balance despite a greatly reduced over-all glomerular filtration rate.

In acute nephritis the problem is more difficult to explain on the basis of peritubular physical forces for several reasons. One reason is that the data from most studies show that filtration fraction is lower than normal in acute nephritis. That is, glomerular filtration rate is reduced more than is renal blood flow. This would be expected to lower the concentration of proteins in the peritubular capillary blood, which according to the theory would inhibit sodium reabsorption. There might be, however, a reduction in hydrostatic pressure in the peritubular capillaries which could conceivably play a role in leading to the retention of sodium in acute nephritis. Another possibility is that there may be a redistribution of blood flow within the kidney in these patients. If the cortical nephrons get a greatly diminished blood flow, and most of the renal blood flow is going through deeper medullary nephrons, sodium retention might result because the deeper nephrons may normally reabsorb more sodium than the cortical nephrons. Perhaps this might play some role in the formation of edema.

Dr. Lowenstein. Dr. Rubini, alleviation of uremic symptoms by restriction of protein does not prove that some metabolite of protein is the toxin or the source of toxins in the uremic syndrome. Have you been able to produce uremic symptoms in patients with reduced renal function who have not otherwise had uremic symptoms by overloading with protein, by forced feedings, or by feeding proteins of a lower biologic value?

Dr. Milton E. Rubini. I think that this fits into most of our clinical experience. For example, consider the patient who first gets sick after a Christmas or Thanksgiving dinner, i.e., a massive dietary overload. We have not tried to duplicate this situation experimentally.

Dr. Schreiner. Several years ago a private surgeon in Washington was fond of administering protein hydrolysate postoperatively to all patients. Every once in a while he would administer it to someone with chronic renal disease. We were then receiving patients with really fulminating uremia from one hospital in particular. Patients would be referred to us with frost and neurological symptons developing rapidly; they would improve by simply waiting for the elimination of the protein hydrolysate. I think it is possible to produce uremia in patients with renal disease by overloading with protein or protein hydrolysate.

Dr. Rubini asked me to mention the uniform donor card for persons willing to donate organs. The project for this card, which has been a long time aborning, developed as follows.

Many years ago several of the health foundations talked about a uniform donor card. The problem was that we did not have uniform laws, so that we had to start at a grass-roots level. As you know, there has been a Committee on Uniform Legislation of the American Bar Association that has worked with the Committee of the American Medical Association, with many health foundations, and with the Ad Hoc Committee of the National Institutes of Health (NIH). Finally a Uniform Donor Act has been introduced in most state legislatures. It has been the most rapidly moving piece of legislation in the history of the United States. As of now it has been passed by 43* state legislatures, and another five states have testamentary disposition by simple codicils without recording, so that the technique of a card is now legal in 45 states.

The seemingly insurmountable problem was to get several hundred people to agree on the wording for such a card, which was no mean task. We finally succeeded. Wording has now been formulated that suits all the foundations; it has also been approved by the usual group of Harvard law professors, plus the general council for the General Services Administraetion and the NIH.

One and a half million of these cards will be in the hands of practicing physicians. They were reproduced in the March 9 issue of *Modern Medicine*. They will be available through many of the foundations, including the Kidney Foundation, the eye banks, and so forth. All three groups will have these cards. Here is the wording.

"This uniform donor card of .... (name). It is to take effect

*Forty-eight jurisdictions as of July 1970.

on my death. The remarks below indicate. . . ." and then there are three choices with regard to various organs or in entirety. It mentions limitation or special wishes, if any, and then, on the back, it is signed by the donor and two witnesses. There is the donor's signature and date of birth, which is included because some states require that the donor be at least 18 years old; others, 21. Then there are the signatures of the donor and of two witnesses, and a statement that this is a legal document under the Uniform Anatomic Gift Act or similar legislation.

As I said, this card is now valid in 48 states. A bill validating it for the District of Columbia has passed the Senate and is expected to pass the House. Everyone will be seeing it in many different forms over the next year. I urge you to study it in order to be able to answer the questions that patients will ask in requesting it.

If this card is found in the wallet of any person who is dying or dead in any state that has passed the legislation, no other registry and no other legal instrument is necessary.

Dr. Rubini. Let me add as an afterthought that there was a meeting in Los Angeles in December that brought together transplant units from all parts of the country and from Canada.

Several developments are especially interesting. First, the typing system is now countrywide and, with standard antiserum from NIH, we are starting to get the same match classifications from various parts of the country.

Second, methods for preserving organs are improving to the point that in many cases we are now transplanting 6, 8, and 12 hours after death of the donor. We now can go to three days in dogs.

This means that kidneys being "harvested"—and I use the word advisedly—in Los Angeles can be used all over the western states. Even New York is no farther away from the West than a five-hour airplane ride, well within the concept of putting all our patients in a single pool of recipients and, within the next year or so, delivering the best match kidney to wherever that patient may be. There are all sorts of interesting stories about delivering kidneys to patients many hundreds of miles from the site of harvest. This is becoming more and more practical.

We still must make every effort to increase the availability of donor kidneys. We shall then find fertile ground for their utilization by teams that can put them to much better use than was possible two years ago.

Dr. Lowenstein. I might say that we are doing that in the New York area, and that we have quite a large pool that uses machines for preservation. We have flown kidneys from New Jersey by helicopter and they have been put on the machine in New York Hospital. Once when they did not match those of our patients, we sent two to The Mount Sinai Hospital and four to Montefiore Hospital. Many hospitals are showing interest in this development. The next step is to hook up with the West Coast.

DR. SCHREINER. We have a 12-hospital and university network consisting of Johns Hopkins, Maryland, Georgetown, the University of Virginia, the Medical College of Virginia, Duke, Chapel Hill, North Carolina, Bowman Gray, and Emory. We have a single computer that does the matching for the whole dialysis pool. We have done three transplants since the first of the year. One was from Atlanta, one from Richmond, and one from Charlottesville. In the case of the kidneys that came from Atlanta: the donor died at 5:45; his kidneys were on a commercial Delta Airline flight at 6:30; in Washington, D.C., at 7:30; and making urine there at 9:00 o'clock. The big delay in New York City is in getting to La Guardia airport and back by surface transportation.

CONFERENCE PLANNING COMMITTEE

Dr. E. Lovell Becker, *Chairman*

DR. JACOB CHURG
DR. JEROME LOWENSTEIN
DR. JOHN H. LARAGH
DR. KURT H. STENZEL
DR. GERARD M. TURINO

AN ANTHROPOLOGICAL ESSAY BY THOMAS HODGKIN

It is well known that in eras preceding our own, medicine was a learned profession and physicians often were learned men. Before it became customary for constricted schools and constricted teachers to produce narrow pupils, members of the medical profession frequently earned distinction in the humane letters or in the natural sciences.

A splendid example is William Withering. He not only contributed to mineralogy—as Dr. Frederic D. Zeman has shown[1]—but he was botanist enough to recognize that the active component in a witch's recipe was probably the foxglove.

Where are we now? On three occasions I have brought digitalis leaves into an active cardiological department and found that no member of the staff could identify them. Perhaps we should not bewail this; the foxglove is no longer relevant to cardiology and some men will tell you that general education has not much relevance to medicine.

Before the comparatively recent professionalization of anthropology, much if not most of the research in this science was done by physicians. The Founding Fathers were Johann Friederich Blumenbach (1752-1840) and Petrus Camper (1722-1789). A towering 19th-century figure, eminent in anthropology and pathology, and distinguished also in politics and in public health, was Rudolf Virchow (1821-1902). The names of other eminent physician anthropologists would make a long list, which would include the names of Samuel George Morton, Ales Hrdlicka, T. Dale Stewart, T. Mitchell Prudden (a pupil of Virchow and Koch), and many others.

To this roster we must add the name of Thomas Hodgkin (1798-1866), the distinguished morbid anatomist and Quaker philanthropist. On May 21, 1845, Hodgkin read before the Ethnological Society of London an essay *On the Ancient Inhabitants of the Canary Islands.* This work was published in the *Edinburgh New Philosophical Journal,* vol. 39, pp. 372-86, 1845.

The problem was that of the origin of the Guanches, the aboriginal

1. Zeman. F. D.: William Withering as a mineralogist. *Bull. Hist. Med. 24*:530-38, 1950.

occupants of the islands. From a review of available descriptions in the ancient and early modern literature, Hodgkin concluded that the early Canary Islanders were tall, athletic, and vigorous. But measurements which he made on a few fragmented Canarian mummies indicated that the skeletons were small. He solved this contradiction by the simple inference that the Canary Islands had been occupied by different races at different times.

In the introductory section of his essay Hodgkin remarks that he had "occasion to classify a considerable collection of human skulls, including specimens from various parts of the globe. . . ." Neither in this part of his research nor in the part that was specifically concerned with the Canary Islands did he report any observations on pathological conditions. This is somewhat astonishing in the author of the famous *Lectures on the Morbid Anatomy of the Serous and Mucous Membranes.*[2]

Hodgkin's anthropological essay derives from an era in which research in what we now call physical anthropology was to a great extent a province of the anatomist. It is also worthwhile to recall that the earlier pathologists referred to themselves as anatomists—evidence that their concern was with lesions rather than with processes. Hence it is not astonishing that men who had contributed to pathology should also show interest in what we now call physical anthropology.

More recently, in 1925, the Canary Islanders formed the subject of an investigation by the illustrious Earnest A. Hooton[3] of Harvard. Hooton's volume contains a few remarks on pathology. Most interestingly, Hooton observed that cranial fractures in the islanders were usually on the left side, presumably because of blows delivered by right-handed assailants.[3]

S.J.

2. Since this was written, a new bibliographical study of Hodgkin has appeared: Kass, E. H. and Bartlett, A. H.: Thomas Hodgkin, M.D. (1798-1866): An annotated bibliography. *Bull. Hist. Med. 43*:138-75, 1969 (see esp. pp. 160-61).

3. Hooton, E. A.: *The Ancient Inhabitants of the Canary Islands.* Harvard African Studies, vol. 7. Cambridge, Harvard Univ. Press, 1925, 401 pp.

BULLETIN OF
THE NEW YORK ACADEMY
OF MEDICINE

VOL. 46, NO. 11 NOVEMBER 1970

CONTINUING EDUCATION OF THE PRACTICING PHYSICIAN

A STATEMENT BY
THE COMMITTEE ON MEDICAL EDUCATION*
OF
THE NEW YORK ACADEMY OF MEDICINE

It is generally conceded and widely preached that the medical education of the physician should be a continuous process that continues throughout his active lifetime as a practitioner. It has been frequently affirmed that the obtaining of an M.D. degree, licensing by a state, and certification by a specialty board should not be regarded as end points in his training, but rather as permits to proceed on a course of treating patients while learning. This has long been so and, within the past few years, there has been mounting pressure, from within the profession itself, for the establishment of minimum standards for continuing medical education.

In support of this position the large and expanding body of scientific and medical knowledge, changing concepts about the role of the physician in society, the evanescent nature of man's memory, and the practical isolation of many practitioners from professional contact with their peers have been cited. To those should be added some of the characteristics and interests of tomorrow's medical students and trends in

*Approved by the Committee on Medical Education, May 14, 1970.

medical education, which promise to accent the need for continuing education.[1, 2] As described by Dr. D. H. Funkenstein,[1] director, Program for Research in Medical Education, Department of Psychiatry, Harvard Medical School, these include decreased emphasis on scientific attitude; shift to the pragmatic use of science—biological, physical, social, and behavioral—rather than attempting to make the physician a "scientist"; increased interest in a shortened time span between secondary school and career; increased study and interest in social and behavioral sciences; decreased study and interest in biological and physical sciences not directly relevant to clinical problems.

The half-life of a physician's medical knowledge and skills generally is taken to be about 10 years after the end of his formal training.[3] This apparent loss of knowledge is the result of a combination of forgetting plus failure to keep up-to-date with changes and advances in medicine; the factor of forgetting possibly carries a bit more weight.[4]

Granted that the education of the physician should be a continuing process over his lifetime of practice, what should be the nature of this education and what are the available effective procedures? Much money is being spent on programs and gadgets. Ideas and assertions are almost legion, but factual evidence of effectiveness, in terms of resultant improvement in the practice of medicine, is scarce and hard to come by. Following are some findings and observations with examples of programs now widely in use.

The televised Clinical Science Seminars instituted by the New York Academy of Medicine in 1963 and terminated in 1968 failed to draw substantial audiences and, according to one analysis,[5] failed to demonstrate much of a learning effect. In 1968 an advance mailing to 6,000 generalists and internists in the metropolitan area, announcing six weekly one-hour televised lectures, resulted in a confirmed audience of 249 who saw, on the average, two thirds of the programs. Dr. John F. Stokes, reciting the British experience, stated that "The results of our efforts to keep doctors abreast of the times through the medium of television have been somewhat disappointing, and we may do better to concentrate on moulding the attitude of those now entering the profession."[6] A report on an evaluation of the northern California postgraduate medical television programs concluded: "Neither the information level nor the behavior of the target audiences were affected by the programs."[7] Dr. A. T. Hunter,[8] in a report on the medical education television programs (METV) of the Committee on Continuing Education of the Faculty of Medicine of the University of Western Ontario, was a bit more sanguine in his conclusions. He found that "Medical Education Television is seen as being a potentially useful aid to continuing medical education by a large percentage of doctors, but is not seen as fulfilling that potential in its present form." An anonymous comment in the February 1970 issue of the newsletter of the Association of Medical Television Broadcasters, Inc., points out a major problem with this medium: "Although television hardware development has progressed rapidly in the last decade, the educational quality of programming and production innovation has not improved correspondingly. The use of audiovisuals in health sciences is in a state of polished mediocrity."

Dr. David P. Lauler[9] believes that the failure of medical television to date as an isolated entity is to be found in its isolation. "The exploitation of a given medium (television) without leveraging its advantages in juxtaposition to other media doomed the television medium to failure. . . . The major limitation in the production of television or movie material resides in the software aspect."

Dr. Lauler also emphasizes the importance of motivation to the learning process. "No matter how effective the teaching exercise is, unless the learner involves himself in the exercise, all is for naught." As Donald H. Williams[10] has commented, "It is doubtful if salvation cometh from dutiful somnolent passivity in a pew on Christmas and Easter Sundays each year." Taylor and his associates, in their analysis of criteria of physician (specialists) performance[11] found the "number of refresher courses taken during career" to be an "unstable" criterion of little importance. Williamson and McGuire[12] compared the effectiveness of continuing education by means of the consecutive case (simulated) conference with that of the traditional lecture method and found that, after a six-month interval, "overall, no significant change in clinical judgement, as measured by these problems, could be documented for either educational method."

Lewis and Hassanein[13] found that 57% of the 2,090 physicians practicing in Kansas during 1956-1965 participated in courses of continuing education offered by Kansas State University; about 7% took as many as half the course-hours recorded. Pertinent here are the facts that "maternal and perinatal death rates in various areas were unrelated to hours of continuing education in obstetrics and pediatrics taken by local physicians. Similarly, high regional rates for certain operative procedures were not associated with increased use of appropriate postgraduate education."

Motivation also requires that the learner place himself in a learning environment. Vollan (cited by Lewis and Hassanein[13]) found attendance at postgraduate courses to be directly related to the number of years of residency training after graduation. Also, it was found to be highest for those practicing in communities of less than 5,000 people and lowest in metropolitan areas. Apparently New York City fits the pattern.

The annual Graduate Fortnight instituted by the New York Academy of Medicine in 1927 proved to be immensely popular during the 1930's and again on the termination of World War II with young physicians returning from the services and others preparing for board examinations or in need of refresher courses to assume desired positions in civilian life. As the immediate, practical value of the Fortnight became less and less apparent, attendance dropped off, and the Fortnight was shortened to a two-day and then to a one-day session, finally to be dropped and replaced by the televised Clinical Science Seminars, the fate of which has been previously described. Dr. Isidore Sternlieb[14] has described the educational activities of the Bronx County Chapter of the American Academy of General Practice (AAGP) in part as follows:

> In January of 1962, we of the Bronx County Chapter of the American Academy of General Practice sponsored a course in practical psychiatry for physicians under the aegis of the New York State Department of Mental Hygiene and given by the faculty of the Albert Einstein College of Medicine. We invited about 1,400 physician members of the Bronx County Medical Society, which included a little over 100 general practitioners who were members of the AAGP and required certification of continuing education. We enrolled about 60 physicians, 45 of whom were members of the AAGP who required the course credit. Only 15 of the remaining 1,300 doctors took the program. They didn't need certification and apparently were not interested. ——But we never reached a greater percentage of the doctors, except during one year, about two years ago, when Medicaid participation required 50 hours of continuing education of each physician. That year we had a 100 per cent in-

crease in enrollment and these new doctors told me that they had not taken any refresher course since they graduated from medical school 25 to 35 years ago. This spurt in attendance fell off immediately after Medicaid dropped this requirement.

As stated by Torrens and Weinstein,[15] a major impediment to the continuing education of the general practitioner arises from the fact that "the organization and structure of the present-day urban teaching hospital is not geared to the needs of the nonspecialist physician. As a result, the nonspecialist physicians in the communities around urban teaching hospitals are unable to play an effective role in upgrading the quality of medical care delivered by the community physician. In order to change this situation new structures must be devised within the urban teaching hospitals to allow nonspecialist physicians greater access to the skills and resources of the teaching hospital." Referring to physicians in the community about St. Luke's Hospital in New York City, Torrens and Weinstein reported that, when asked why they did not take a more active part in the programs open to them in three teaching hospitals in the area, "almost all of the physicians replied that the programs were of little value to them in their practices. Most of the programs at the three major teaching hospitals were directed toward members of one particular medical specialty or another; they were usually conducted by physicians or researchers who spent most of their time working in a limited area of a particular medical specialty. The nonspecialist physicians from the community felt that it would be necessary for them to have much more background information and training in the particular medical specialty before they could interpret, integrate, and use the information provided by these laboratory-oriented lectures. As a result, they did not attempt to take part in these sessions." Those who did take part in some sort of organized continuing medical education were said to have done so under the auspices of "the New York County Medical Society, The New York Academy of Medicine, various specialized medical-social organizations, or the non-teaching hospitals with which they were affiliated." Torrens and Weinstein recommend that each teaching hospital should establish a single, clearly defined office or department whose sole purpose would be to handle the referral of patients and requests for assistance from the physician in the community. "There should be one single place to which the community physician knows he can turn for assistance with problems of patients in his practice and from which he can obtain information about patients he has referred to the teaching hospital for care."

In spite of the abundance of educational opportunities in New York State, and particularly in New York City, the New York State Committee on Medical Education[16] in 1963 stated that ". . . it is estimated that no more than 25% of practicing physicians participate in continuing education of any kind—even hospital staff meetings—with regularity." The committee went on to suggest "that the situation might eventually become so acute as to require periodic examination for re-licensing in the profession."

Among the reasons advanced by Dimond[17] for poor attendance at postgraduate courses is the fact that practicing physicians represent one of the most "seasoned" of student audiences. "These students will not tolerate useless class-room hours much less pay for them. There must be a high order of user satisfaction to make these students willing to participate." He recommends sabbatical leaves for the private practitioner and the establishment of regional and national graduate medical centers catering and devoting themselves to the needs of the man in practice. "The opening of medical education, spreading medical student and house officer teaching to all regional facilities, will be a key stimulus to bring the practicing physician into that best of environments where one is both teacher and taught."

Three quotations from *Continuing Medical Education*, [18] the publication of the American Medical Association may be helpful at this point.

> 1) If the physician were to have some way of judging the end results of his performance and were to see that there were deficiencies when comparing the outcome of his efforts with the outcome that might be expected, he would then be in a position to ask himself what there is about his performance that yields results that are less than criterion results. To accomplish this goal he would need some way of examining what it is he does, so that he might know precisely what he might better do differently. This is the essence of education: *specific identification of educational needs based on analysis of real situations, with subsequent introduction of specific educational efforts directed toward those needs* [emphasis ours]. To-date, most programs for continuing medical education have not been organized on this basis.

2) The science of the medical disciplines provides the subject matter of medical texts. The science and the art of clinical practice, i.e., the diagnostic and therapeutic process, also find expression in the medical literature but depend for the most part on guided learning through *repetitive* [emphasis ours] clinical experiences in which the physician acquires certain attitudes, skills, and essential information about many subjects. But there is no objective uniformity of the diagnostic-therapeutic process and certainly the physician can never cover every clinical situation in his learning experience. Much depends on transfer of knowledge—*and on the integrity of the physician's problem-solving ability* [emphasis ours].

Existing education systems largely disregard the facts of place and circumstance under which physician and patient come together, of the variability in stage and severity of the disease process, and of the variations in expected outcome as determined by time-process factors of repeated physician-patient contacts.

3) Meeting the continuing education needs of practicing physicians really implies a *constructive approach to the removal of impediments to their efficient performance* [emphasis ours]. Such impediments can be of great diversity and may not be at all a function of the information input to the physicians. Thus, a principle function of the concept of "community medicine," inasmuch as it attempts to mobilize community resources to aid the physician to meet the health requirements of the American people, is identical with the prime function of continuing medical education.

The aim of continuing medical education is to maintain and improve standards of medical care and the health and welfare of the patient. Essential for the success of educational programs are relevance, repetition, active participation, facilitation, and motivation. Essential also is recognition of "the ephemeral nature of factual knowledge and the relative permanency of learning sets, i.e., study habits and skills, as well as attitudes towards and motivation for learning."[19]

Dr. Eisele[20] cites Dr. R. L. Evans as authority for the statement that "There is a consensus that there are 3 basic criteria for continuing medical education: it must be continuous, it must be community-hospital-based, and it must be directly related to the physician's day to day activities in the care of his patients." Eisele goes on to say that "There is no educational tool that equals the internal medical audit in meeting these criteria. The episodic educational exposures provided by refresher courses and by the great variety of educational experiences brought into the hospital from the medical center are useful and highly desirable, but they are merely adjuncts and they are not effective substitutes. When outside programs replace the hospital's own patient-oriented programs, and this is often a great temptation, the medical staff's continuing education is incomplete and inadequate." Dr. Clement R. Brown, Jr.,[21] has described a combined education-treatment program, based upon the medical audit and problem-oriented patient records, that is under way at the Chestnut Hill Hospital in Philadelphia, Pa. A report on the effectiveness of his "bi-cycle" concept had not been published by the time of this writing.

Annually, beginning in 1966, physicians in and about New Haven, Conn., have voluntarily organized a review of internal medicine. From an initial emphasis on preparation for board examinations the course evolved into a comprehensive, clinically oriented review of the field. It has been characterized by a steady enrollment growth (from 26 to 60 physicians over the four years; 20% of the enrollees repeating the course one or more times), high attendance rates (75 to 85%), and low costs (between 25 and 45 cents per lecture hour).[22] The initial 17-hour course grew, over the years, to 26 hours.

Dr. MacLeod[22] considers the growth of this "highly structured yet informal" review course to have been a function of the relevancy of the course material and a sensitivity to the changing needs of the group. "The principles of student participation in planning and administration, and continuous feedback through questionnaires served as the basic framework for the organization of the course." It may also be pertinent that 75 to 85% of the enrollees were out of medical school less than 10 years, that "one third to one half" held positions at Yale or other teaching hospitals and about the same proportion were candidates for the American Board of Internal Medicine examination, Part I.

No continuing medical education program, no matter how well conceived, can help the physician who declines to participate or who is thwarted or frustrated in his efforts to learn. The physician must be motivated, and impediments in the way of his development of professional competence must be removed.

In addition to the AAGP requirement for participation in continuing-education activities as a condition of membership, examples of inducements now being offered to physicians to continue their medical learning beyond the completion of their formal education include such things as The Physician's Recognition Award given by the AMA, the certificate that attests to their doing so, the requirement of the American Board of Family Practice for periodic recertification and the requirement of the Oregon Medical Association (the state medical society) of proof of participation in a minimum number of educational programs for continued membership in the society. Thought is being given to periodic recertification by the American Board of Internal Medicine and the American College of Surgeons. Both the American College of Physicians and the American Psychiatric Association have self-evaluation programs in operation and the American College of Surgeons and the American Academy of Pediatrics are in the process of developing such programs. Self-evaluation programs, however, are not likely to have much effect on the nonmotivated physician.

Summary and Conclusions

There is said to be a shortage of physicians and a crisis in medical care. That there is a shortage of physicians, at least in terms of demand, particularly in the ghettos of large cities and in many rural areas appears to have been documented to the satisfaction of most authorities.[23] That crisis in medical care has arisen directly from this shortage is a moot point. Nevertheless, it now is national policy to improve the quality and quantity of medical care, particularly of that provided for the poor and other especially vulnerable persons, such as the aged and the mentally ill. The continuing medical education of the practicing physician has been incorporated as a major component of the Regional Medical Programs to forward these ends. Continuing medical education, in this concept, involves a good deal more than providing opportunities for the physician to listen to lectures and take refresher courses. Intrinsic are his involvement in the community, his knowledge and use of community facilities and expertise, and the efficiency of his operation. Impending is the additional responsibility for many physicians to make advantageous use, from the standpoint of the community, of a new type of allied health professional, the "physician's assistant."

Postgraduate or continuing education, as it now is being termed, has been with us ever since we have had graduates. All physicians participate, to a varying extent, in one or more of the available forms which range from empiricism through study of and reference to professional journals and texts, peer consultations, in-hospital programs (grand rounds, clinical-pathological conferences, case audits, etc.) to periodic lectures and refresher courses. Many physicians in active practice appear to make considerable use of, and regard highly "consultation with colleagues"[8] and have little use or esteem for refresher courses[3, 8] and hospital staff conferences.[8] No doctor of medicine relies entirely on his own experiences. Empiricism is equated with quackery.

The introduction of audiovisual aids, particularly television and radio, into continuing medical education, as a means of bringing authoritative and useful information to the practicing physician in such a way that he will retain it, does not appear to have had results anywhere near commensurate with the time, effort, and money expended on facilities and program production and distribution. A number of reasons have been advanced for this, but a major defect appears to be inadequacy of the "soft-ware" of both subject matter and method of presentation. More and better evaluative work on the effectiveness of radio and television as practical and acceptable learning aids for the practicing physician needs to be done before we can make a recommendation on their general use for this purpose.

It must be said that deficiencies in evaluation and lack of good evidence for lasting learning effects on participating student-physicians also exist in regard to other programs and courses used and promoted for the continuing medical education of the practicing physician. The well-prepared and motivated physician learns, and applies what he learns, almost regardless of the pedagogic merits of the course or of the teacher. He who is not well grounded and lacks interest learns little and quickly forgets that little, even with the best program and teacher. In between these two extremes there are many physicians whose standards of medical practice might well be affected by the suitability and educational merit of teaching exercises to which they are exposed. Because of this variable, because of the inability to measure accurately and reliably the full extent of a physician's practical knowledge by examinations and because of varying discrepancies of multiple causation between what physicians know about the art and science of medicine and the standard of care received by their patients, the evaluation of continuing medical education programs is a very difficult matter, one which might be made easier by focusing attention on the end point, the care of patients.

In view of the foregoing, the Committee on Medical Education concludes, as has Dimond,[17] that the certificate concept, if judged only on the basis of total number of hours in some kind of postgraduate course, is fallacious in that it implies unwarranted merit to course work. The committee also strongly opposes any mandatory examinations for maintenance of the currency of one's medical license. The available information does not support a positive relation between the results of most such tests and the quality of care provided by practicing physicians for their patients.

The committee finds that, since the public and private hospitals of New York State and, particularly, those of New York City represent, at their best, a concentration of clinical and scientific facilities and talent well above the national average which are not being used to full advantage in many instances,[16] since the motivated physician will and does take advantage of those worthwhile opportunities for learning that are made available to him and, since 35% of the physicians in the metropolitan area are reported to have no hospital connections and only about 25% of practicing physicians are said to make use of their presumed educational opportunities,[16] the prime problems to be overcome in regard to continuing medical education in the New York metropolitan region are: 1) the lack of motivation among physicians; 2) impediments in the path of some physicians to advancing their knowledge and practical skills; and 3) the failure of community hospitals to meet the needs of neighborhood physicians—to become involved in the communities which they presumably serve.

The committee recommends:

1) As a very important incentive to better medical practice, peer-group evaluation of the individual physician in his own working environment. It considers as of at least equal importance measures designed to make that environment as conducive as possible to providing optimal medical care.

2) Active encouragement of group practice and the establishment of community health centers to increase the availability to the practicing physician of the supporting services of allied health personnel, to improve and promote ambulatory care, to expedite more efficient and productive use of the physician's knowledge and skills, to promote

preventive medicine, to help reduce the over-all cost of medical care, and to decrease the likelihood of the development of professional isolation of the community physician.

3) Strengthening all record-keeping procedures in hospitals by improving secretarial services and developing computer techniques, thus increasing the usefulness of such records as instruments of education and facilitating the audit of caring for patients.

4) Establishing programs based on management-type or audit-type procedures whereby both hospital and community physician may participate in mass audit exercises, reviewing each other's charts or record-room charts generally, to indicate features of particular diseases which must be considered and appropriate approaches in their management.

5) Establishing consultative clinics to which community physicians may bring problem cases for review by recognized consultants.

6) Establishing a central mechanism for the more efficient and wider dissemination of information on medical educational opportunities for practicing physicians in the New York metropolitan area.

7) Strengthening community hospital libraries along lines recommended by the Post-graduate Medical Institute of Massachusetts[24] and the National Library of Medicine, and tying them into a computerized library network, with strategically situated terminals, backed by the facilities of the New York Academy of Medicine Library-Medical Research Library of Brooklyn-New York Medical Library Center complex.

8) Expanded study and critical evaluation of audiovisual and other technical aids to continuing medical education and communication.

REFERENCES

1. Smythe, C. McC.: Potential educational services from a national biomedical communications network. Report of a conference. *J. Med. Educ. 44*:1084, 1969.
2. Dennis, J. L.: Medical education: Its responsibility to society. J.A.M.A. 213: 585, 1970.
3. Carmichael, H.: Panel on Existing Self-Evaluation Programs. In: *Congress on Medical Education.* Council on Med. Educ., A.M.A. Chicago, February 6, 1970.
4. Du Bois, A. B., Nemir, Jr., P., Schumacher, C. F. and Hubbard, J. P.: Graduate medical education in basic sciences. *J. Med. Educ. 44*:1035, 1969.
5. Menzel, H., Maurice, R. and McGuinness, A. C.: The effectiveness of the televised clinical science seminars of the New York Academy of Medicine. *Bull. N. Y. Acad. Med. 42*:679, 1966.
6. Stokes, J. F.: A British view of the American scene. *Pharos 30*:89, 1967.
7. Mock, R. L., McCoard, B. F. and Prest-

wood, R.: Northern California postgraduate medical television: An evaluation. *J. Med. Educ. 45*:40, 1970.
8. Hunter, A. T.: *A Report on Project No. 605:, 7-418, Medical Audience Educational Program.* London, Ont., Faculty of Medicine, Univ. Western Ont., 1970.
9. Lauler, D. P.: Communications in medicine. *Mod. Med. 94:* June 29, 1970.
10. Williams, D. H.: A taxonomy of continuing medical education endeavor. *Canad. Med. Ass. J. 96*:1040, 1967.
11. Taylor, C. W., Lewis, E. B., Nelson, E., Loughmiller, G. C. and Price, P. B. Synthesis of multiple criteria of physician performance. *J. Med. Educ. 44*:1063, 1969.
12. Williamson, J. W. and McGuire, C.: Consecutive case conference: An educational evaluation. *J. Med. Educ. 48:* 1068, 1968.
13. Lewis, C. E. and Hassanein, R. S.: Continuing medical education: An epidemiologic evaluation. *New Eng. J. Med. 282*:254, 1970.
14. Sternleib, I.: *Practitioners' Needs and Desires in the Area of Continuing Medical Education.* An Address to the Committee on Medical Education of the New York Academy of Medicine, December 11, 1969.
15. Torrens, P. R. and Weinstein, K. Role of the urban teaching hospital in training of nonaffiliated physicians. *J.A.M.A. 204*:435, 1968.
16. New York State Committee on Medical Education: *Education for the Health Professions.* Albany, N. Y. The Board of Regents, New York State Education Department, 1963.
17. Dimond, E. B.: Changing trends in postgraduate education. *Mod. Med. 83*:1970.
18. Division of Scientific Activities, A.M.A.: *Continuing Medical Education.* Chicago, A.M.A., 1968.
19. Collet, L. V. S. and Dohner, C.: Change in attitude as an index of effectiveness for short courses in continuing medical education. *J. Med. Educ. 45*:237, 1937.
20. Eisele, C. W.: The medical audit in continuing education. *J. Med. Educ. 44:* 263, 1969.
21. Brown, Jr., C. R.: *Relationship of Patient Care to Continuing Education.* A.M.A. Congress on Medical Education, Chicago, February 9, 1970.
22. MacLeod, G. K.: Continuing medical education: One approach. *J.A.M.A. 212:* 1171, 1970.
23. Fein, R.: *The Doctor Shortage, An Economic Diagnosis.* Washington, D.C., Brookings Inst., 1967.
24. Stearns, N. S. and Ratcliff, W. W.: A core medical library for practitioners in community hospitals. *New Eng. J. Med. 280*:474, 1969.

A CRITIQUE OF THE CONFLICT BETWEEN MISSION-ORIENTED AND CLINICAL RESEARCH*

LOUIS M. ROUSSELOT

Assistant Secretary of Defense, Health and Environment
U.S. Department of Defense, Washington, D.C.

TODAY we honor a distinguished faculty member of the University of Indiana: Harris B. Shumacker, Jr., professor of surgery of the Indiana University Medical Center. This meeting, as we all know, is jointly sponsored by the Indiana Chapter of the American College of Surgeons and Indiana University. Dr. Shumacker has served them both long and well. His contributions to both and to his great love–surgery –are innumerable and cannot be recounted now. Thinker, investigator, teacher, and master surgeon, all are elements of this versatile and complete man. Surgical research has been one of his most ardent pursuits.

How fortunate is my fate to join and participate with you in this *Festschrift*. These many years it has been my good fortune to follow, closely and from afar, the exploits of Harris Shumacker. The subject of my address, "Mission-Oriented and Clinical Research," has a strong exponent in Dr. Shumacker.

So applicable, to quote from another famous Hoosier, James Whitcomb Riley, are these lines:

> High-spirited from boyhood, with a most inquirin' turn—
> He wanted to learn ever'thing on earth they was to learn;
> He's ast more plaguy questions in a mortal-minute here
> Than his grandpap in Paradise could answer in a year![1]

Or, to continue on another pathway:

> I come upon it suddenly, alone—
> A little pathway winding in the weeds
> That fringe the roadside; and with dreams my own
> I wander as it leads.
> Full wistfully along the slender way
> Through summer tan of freckled shade and shine,
> I take the path that leads me as it may—
> Its every choice is mine.[2]

---

*Presented as the first Harris B. Schumacker, Jr., oration at the joint meeting of the Indiana Chapter of the American College of Surgeons and the Indiana State University, Terre Haute, Ind., April 17, 1970.

Statistical data were supplied by Col. Robert Joy, M.C., U.S.A., of the Department of Defense Research and Engineering, Medical Training Offices of the United States Army, Navy, and Air Force.

My path in this essay is a timely one, albeit controversial both in national and university circles.

The Conflict Between Mission-Oriented and Clinical Research

A current shibboleth in many councils, including Congress, the Department of Defense, and even among some educators, is the subject of mission-oriented research. The connotations thus leveled do our military medical departments a great disservice.

In these days of austerity budgets, medical research in civilian as well as federal medical areas has felt the stress, along with many other worthwhile endeavors all high on the nation's priority scale. Your own Indiana University Clinical Research Center and its director, Dr. C. Conrad Johnston, can aptly attest to this. The hatchet has fallen, though not too severely, on our so-called "mission-oriented" research, but we have had the door virtually closed on our clinical research programs.

At this juncture I wish to make crystal clear my support of President Richard Nixon's priorities in federal spending and in his attempt to control inflation, that arch villain eroding all our national priorities, of which medical research must accept its just share.

The thesis of my presentation is the delineation of mission-oriented medical research vs. clinical research, their relative importance to one another, our mission and, in turn, the practice of medicine.

What is mission-oriented research? The mission of the medical departments of the armed forces can be stated quite simply. Primarily it is to provide the necessary medical support to the armed forces so that they may effectively implement national policies. These policies, of course, are set by the president with the advice and counsel of the National Security Council and State Department. In no wise are they directed by the Department of Defense. The second part of our mission requires the provision of necessary health services to all others eligible for such services. In the case of our active-duty personnel, about 2.5 to 3.5 million of our citizens are involved. Our eligible dependents, retirees, and their spouses and dependents add another 6 to 6.5 million. The magnitude of this task is apparent when one realizes we are discussing about 5% of our national population. Also implicit in this dual mission is the goal of returning the invalidated soldier to duty as quickly as possible. Of paramount importance and common to both portions of the mission is the need to provide medical care of the highest quality.

As you know, the largest fraction of our armed forces is made up of noncareer personnel. Our military men are inducted involuntarily via the draft or they volunteer with or without the pressure and threat of the draft. Many are your sons and nephews or sons of close friends and acquaintances; they are not numbers or nameless faces. They are the prime youth of our country, and they are giving themselves in support of our national security. We owe to them, the nation's committed ones, care of the most superior type in all fields of medicine and surgery. I shall not belabor the fact of our equally great obligation to the career and retired members of our armed forces.

What is high-quality medical care and wherein does medical research play a role, be it mission-aligned or patient-oriented clinical research? Many have attempted to define high-quality care. This cannot be accomplished in one terse sentence. It requires the application of many criteria, including preventive medicine, the quality of the environment, diet, and the application of our knowledge of immunization. It includes the entire health-care delivery system from the solo practitioner to that highly complex structure, the hospital, be it a community or teaching hospital. It means early recognition and prompt treatment of abnormal states and diseases. It requires the use of a host of the accumulated, proved, scientific medical information, and all the expertise of the clinician. Scientific facts and advances used in this process evolve from research.

The pioneering efforts of the American College of Surgeons date back to 1913. Along with other members of the Joint Commission on the Accreditation of Hospitals, the college has developed a whole series of requirements to promote a high quality of medical and hospital care.

A physician's store of knowledge is acquired primarily in premedical and medical school years. With this base the doctor, to deliver high-quality care, must have access to continuing education and must be assisted by a health team with equally high-quality basic education. The doctor is similar to the engineer in that he must be aware of the increasing likelihood of obsolescence in his particular field. It has been estimated that graduate engineers will have to be retrained four times during their earning years in order to keep up with the technology explosion!

An essential part of continuing education and the rendition of quality care for the military physician, as for his civilian counterpart, is to work in a milieu including many creative minds. Creative minds in medicine are best nurtured in a questioning and probing environment. "Not so long ago many medical schools did not approve of, and in fact opposed encouraging their students to engage in research. Now it is encouraged, expected, and in some schools even required."[3]

Our military health-care system is vast. As mentioned before, it is responsible for the delivery of health and medical services to an eligible population of approximately 10 million men, women, and children on a worldwide basis. The spectrum of care varies from the management of trauma and disease in times of conflict to the most sophisticated care in our large teaching hospitals and routine screening in satellite dispensaries. It encompasses the broadest aspects of preventive medicine with great emphasis on environmental quality control. Because of the global nature of our responsibilities, tropical disease looms large in our patient-care spectrum, and trauma patients fill many of our beds by virtue of the Vietnam involvement. Finally, we should not forget the great toll of injuries caused in the United States by autos and scooters. This part of our environment seems beyond our control. This great pool of patients, all of whom are beneficiaries of our system, makes an ideal setting for the teaching of health-manpower personnel at all levels. Mission-oriented and clinical research both permeate this vast teaching sphere but with varying emphasis.

An effective national-defense posture must include a force with a strong comprehensive program in medicine, medical research, and all the allied health sciences.

With our worldwide commitments on and under the sea, on land, in the air—ranging from arctic to tropical climates—and with esoteric diseases encountered in remote areas, our forces are exposed to a wide range of hostile environments. This is further augmented by the destructive effects of modern weapons, both nuclear and conventional.

Mission-oriented medical research, then, is medical research in problem areas peculiar to the hostile environments just reviewed. Admittedly, high priority should be given to research programs which are clearly oriented to the military mission. Experience has shown that basic research and applied research, including clinical research, are interdependent. Basic research requires the cumulative knowledge of many disciplines,[4] concepts, and techniques. The transference of a basic scientific discovery to a practical application has often been unexpected though direct. The late Alfred Blalock, great surgeon, educator, and investigator, in his discerning essay "The Nature of Discovery,"[5] aptly discoursed in the same vein. He distinguished four general categories by which discoveries were made. These four included: 1) those made by chance or accident; 2) those made by intention or design; 3) those made by intuition, imagination, or hunch; and 4) those made by combinations of two or all of the foregoing methods.

Sir Alexander Fleming's accidental discovery of penicillin resulted from a chance observation. In a routine culture plate of staphylococci Fleming observed that a contaminating mold exercised an inhibiting effect on bacterial growth. This basic discovery was made by chance. Subsequently Sir Howard W. Florey and Dr. Ernst B. Chain purified and standardized a potent antibiotic: penicillin. The latter was a discovery by design or intention. Blalock gave many examples of discovery by chance, design, or hunch, and I commend his paper to you.

With this in mind it is clear that no sharp line can be drawn between basic and applied research. An arbitrary division between these two compartments is unrealistic. Clinical research is in essence applied research; it is thus vitally important in the delivery of high-quality medical care. This form of applied research is severely circumscribed by two factors. First, it must ultimately be carried out on man and, second, the research must be conducted by physicians. Legal, humane, and professional considerations dictate that a physician be in charge.

The basic education of a military medical officer is in the hands of the civilian medical schools. This educational period is aimed at providing a basis for the practice of bedside medicine, and although some schools now encourage some research exposure, it does not stamp the embryo M.D., on his graduation, as an investigator. To proceed a step further: the truly effective military physician must be highly skilled in the arts of the medical profession and well versed in those of the military profession. To become well versed in the responsibilities of the military profession requires a period at least equal to the time necessary to complete most residency-training programs.

Facilities for biomedical research and development are superb and numerous throughout all three services. These serve to familiarize military personnel with medical and biological problems relating to all phases of national defense. This is essential to ensure that we shall have a sufficent supply of officers with the necessary expertise in these problems. In their later years such physicians will serve as policy makers and as chiefs of mission-oriented research laboratories.

Further emphasizing this policy is the quotation of Dr. Keith Cannan of the National Research Council, who, in speaking to the Armed Forces' Epidemiological Board, said:

> The major responsibility for the support of medical research in the nation lies with the National Institutes of Health. Its deliberate policy is to extend support to proposals spontaneously submitted by investigators, and so is neither in a position to, nor does it attempt to organize programs directed toward the solution of specific problems of operating agencies. Such problems can only be visualized investigatively, and attacked by the particular agency whose mission is challenged by the problem concerned.[6]

Our medical services cannot wait for civilian research, or for research funded by the National Institutes of Health, to find the answers which a military situation demands now. Crash programs hastily conceived and developed are not the answer. They are wasteful, and the results are not always ready when needed.

Each of the three medical services has a galaxy of research institutes or laboratories, some close to teaching hospitals in this country, while others are situated in remote foreign areas. There are 26 such institutes in the continental United States and seven subordinate units dispersed worldwide. Major institutes based in the United States include the Walter Reed Army Institute of Research; the Armed Forces Institute of Pathology; and the Brooke Army Hospital Burn Unit. For the navy there are such noteworthy institutions as the Naval Research and Radiobiology Laboratories at Bethesda, Md., the Frozen Blood Study Group in Chelsea, Mass., and the Submarine and Hyperbaric Unit at New London, Conn.

The Air Force School of Aerospace Medicine in San Antonio and the Aerospace Medical Research Laboratories at Wright-Patterson Air Force Base have outstanding study groups in physiology and in environmental simulators. The basic studies emanating therefrom have made supersonic and manned flight to outer space successful under extremely hostile conditions.

Overseas research laboratories are situated in Vietnam, Malaysia,

Panama, Thailand, Germany, Egypt, Ethiopia, and Taiwan.

This total research effort is manned by 5,788 military and civilian workers. These include physicians, scientists, and technicians. Our institutes are primarily involved in pure mission-oriented research in precise categorical areas. As listed in the FY 1970 budget, their areas of research include: 1) communicable and infectious disease; 2) tropical medicine; 3) malaria–therapeutic development; 4) combat surgery; 5) medical materiel including protective clothing; 6) nutrition and food research; 7) environmental medicine; 8) aviation medicine; 9) deep-sea medicine; 10) radiobiology; 11) toxicology; 12) internal medicine; and others.

The fiscal support of these projects is derived from the total Department of Defense Research and Engineering (DDR&E) budget. This is primarily directed toward the development and testing of planes, missiles, and other forms of military hardware. Biomedical research is funded at approximately $95 million, and constitutes only a small fraction, or 1.4%, of that total DDR&E effort (approximately $7.2 billion). Two thirds of these medical research monies are "spent-in-house" appropriations and one third are extramural grants. These sums are specifically allocated for mission-oriented medical research.

Current projects, easily identifiable and justified toward this objective would include, for the army: 1) therapy of burn casualties; 2) development of antimeningococcus vaccine; and 3) new antimalarial compounds.

For the navy: 1) physiological studies of saturation diving; 2) development of cold-water suits for naval aviators; and 3) radiation effects in nuclear submarines.

For the air force: 1) laser safety and crew protection in air-force operations; 2) toxic hazards of propellants and materials; 3) biodynamics-design criteria for emergency-escape systems; and 4) physiological endpoints in acceleration.

I now approach the crux of my discussion. Less clearly delineated, organized, and supported by adequate funding and personnel is the position of clinical research in our medical system. Our difficulty is the rigid limitation of funds for clinical research. Under existing legislation we are currently probing means whereby funding may be made available to support clinical research as a most important segment of medical research; it should parallel our mission-oriented research. Medical research on diseases or on hostile environments which affect or may affect our military forces, such as the projects enumerated earlier, fall into this category.

Since the mission of our Medical Corps is to render medical care of the highest quality to the sick and injured of a population of 10 million, both in and out of uniform, wherein is the dichotomy, if we acknowledge the role and equal importance of clinical research toward the attainment of this goal?

This broad concept has implications which pervade the entire structure of our military medical-care system. To provide the highest quality of medical care, the military services must be attractive to qualified professional scientific and technical personnel, who must be afforded every opportunity to attain professional excellence and recognition. This attainment must embrace not only the narrow field of military or so-called mission-oriented medicine, but also clinical medicine. The precursor and keystone of the best in clinical medicine is clinical research. As Owen Wangensteen has so aptly stated, "All progress in medicine can emerge only through research."

To proceed a step further: inherent in our medical system are training programs which must meet the certifying requirements of the specialty boards. All the certifying specialty boards attest to the importance of clinical and laboratory investigation as an integral part of an approved specialty-residency program. The report of the Institute of Defense Analysis, dated August 1962, and the Task Force Report of the American Academy of Orthopaedic Surgery gave added support to this philosophy.

The interdependence of mission-oriented and clinical research, and the possibilities of serendipities in either direction needs little emphasis to an audience such as this.

Must research in shock be done only in a special research-study unit in Vietnam? Actually this type of research may be very self-limiting and self-defeating. Does not a study of shock in a stateside hospital offer equal and possibly broader potential benefit? Weekend casualties of the motor car are an ever-increasing pool for investigation. Clinical research in a teaching hospital within the United States would additionally encompass septic shock and cardiac shock, both of nontraumatic origin.

Missile-fuel propellants developed by NASA chemists resulted in the syntheses of a group of chemicals known as the methyl-hydrazines.

A spin-off from the complex chemical syntheses was the discovery of procarbazine. Procarbazine, along with vincristine, prednisone, and nitrogen mustard, has produced a chemical combination successful in controlling the dread cancer known as Hodgkin's disease in 80% of the cases so treated.

In the research and development of synthetic-plastic-inlay protheses for large bony defects of the mandible, must only high-velocity missile wounds be studied? Must facial-bone defects resulting from highway accidents be ignored? Is such a wound as the latter less worthwhile as a basis for study?

Must we discontinue training immunologists and surgeons as part of specialist teams in organ transplantations? Scientists of our naval medical department have done pioneer and epochal work in freeze drying and preservation of cancellous bone and bone-marrow tissue. Must the potential benefits of marrow transplants or the propagation of lymphocyte-cell lines in treatment of leukemias and infections be lost? There are a number of tropical diseases as well as protozoan and virus diseases which are susceptible only to cellular immunity and may be susceptible to lymphocyte treatment.

Our air-force medical department has developed a superb intraservice computerized tumor registry. The Department of Defense has a unique capability in this area, and in fact has initiated a feasibility study on the early expansion of this pilot project. This envisions a triservice program that encompasses 250 of our army, navy, and air-force hospitals worldwide. The potentials to both civilian medicine and our military patients of this form of clinical research are almost limitless. Can we afford to neglect it?

By stifling the support of clinical research we throttle the attraction to and the development within the armed forces medical departments of imaginative and creative individuals as part of our medical, dental, and scientific staffs.

To reiterate, then: our mission is not only to care for active-duty personnel for mission-oriented diseases or trauma, but to render optimum care for the whole man, his dependents, retirees, and their dependents.

At present most of the meager support of our clinical research resides in the funds previously referred to as Department of Defense Research and Engineering funds. This support is now threatened. Because the conduct of both types of investigations are so vital to our mission and to the maintenance of the highest professional and technical standards, to deny it to our medical personnel would directly reduce the quality of medical care. Inevitably the sequel would be a gradual deterioration of our highly effective armed-forces medical services.

We believe this misconception between mission-oriented and clinical research should be corrected, and the importance of clinical research be recognized and supported.

In closing, with a fond salute to Harris B. Schumacker, I shall again draw upon Indiana's poet laureate:[7]

Then ho! and hey! and whoop-hooray!
Though winters clouds be looming,
Remember a November day
Is merrier than Mildest May
With all her blossoms blooming.
While birds in scattered flight are blown
Aloft and lost in dusky mist,
And truant boys scut home alone
'Neath skies of gold and amethyst:
While twilight falls, and echo calls
Across the haunted atmosphere,
With low, sweet laughs at intervals—
So reigns the rapture of the year.

Then ho! and hey! and whoop-hoorany!
Though winter clouds be looming,
Remember a November day
Is merrier than mildest May
With all her blossoms blooming.

REFERENCES

1. Riley, J. W.: How John Quit the Farm. In: *Riley's Songs of Cheer*. New York, Grosset & Dunlap, 1883 (reprinted 1905), p. 59.
2. Riley, J. W.: A Country Pathway. Ibid., p. 117.
3. Gregersen, M. I.: *New Wine and Old Bottles*. Carnegie Review No. 11. New York, April 1967.
4. Cannan, R. K.: *Final Report on Review of Medical and Biological Programs within the Department of Defense*. Washington, D.C., Inst. for Defense Analysis, 1962, p. 23.
5. Blalock, A.: The nature of discovery. *Trans. Amer. Surg. Ass. 5*:1, 1956.
6. Cannan, R. K.: Op. cit., p. 21.
7. Riley, J. W.: The Rapture of the Year. In: *Riley's Songs of Cheer*. New York, Grosset & Dunlap, 1905, p. 19.

THE USE OF AMNIOCENTESIS FOR PRENATAL GENETIC COUNSELING*

Melvin Gertner,† Lillian Y. F. Hsu, Joan Martin, Kurt Hirshhorn‡

Department of Pediatrics
Division of Medical Genetics
The Mount Sinai School of Medicine, New York, N. Y.

Transabdominal amniocentesis for prenatal detection of genetic disorders has become a useful adjunct in genetic counseling. An increasing number of biochemical disorders can be diagnosed by examination of amniotic fluid or by studying the metabolism of fibroblasts cultured from the fetal cells.[1, 2] The sex of the fetus can be determined by examination of the cells for sex chromatin bodies. Karyotyping the cultured fibroblasts from these cells provides a means of detecting chromosomal abberrations.[1-3]

Various techniques have found applicability in the in utero detection of heritable biochemical disorders. It has become possible to diagnose some of these disorders directly from the amniotic fluid supernatant by noting the accumulation of abnormal metabolites.[4] Other enzyme deficiencies may be detected by direct assay from amniotic-fluid cells or the fibroblasts cultured from these cells. Still others may be diagnosed by the finding of abnormal metabolism of these cells as a result of the specific enzyme deficiency. Table I lists the metabolic disorders which have been diagnosed in utero and describes the abnormal findings in these cases.

There are a number of other disorders in which the involved enzyme has been detected in amniotic-fluid cultures from normal fetuses. It is therefore likely that an affected fetus could be diagnosed by demonstrating an absence of the specific enzyme. Table II identifies these disorders and the associated enzymes.

---

*Presented at a meeting of the Section on Pediatrics, February 12, 1970.

†Postdoctoral trainee of the U.S. Public Health Service (HD 00210).

‡Career Scientist of the New York City Health Research Council (I-513).

This study was supported in part by Research Grant HD 02552 of the National Institute of Child Health and Human Development, Bethesda, Md.

TABLE I. METABOLIC DISORDERS DETECTED IN UTERO

Disorder	*Abnormal findings*	*Reference*
Hurler's Syndrome	Abnormal accumulation of labeled sulfate by cultured fibroblasts or elevation of heparitin sulfate in amniotic fluid	4, 5
Pompe's disease	Absence of α1-4 gluocosidase	6
Lesch-Nyhan syndrome	Decreased incorporation of labeled hypoxanthine by cultured cells or deficient IMP pyrophosphorylase	7, 8, 9
Galactosemia	Absence of galactose-1-phosphate uridyl transferase	10
Lysosomal acid phosphatase deficiency	Decreased acid phosphatase in lysosomes of fetal cells and cultured fibroblasts	11
Tay-Sachs' disease	Absence of hexosaminidase A	12
Adrenogenital syndrome	Elevated pregnanetriol level in amniotic fluid which is reduced by intrauterine injection of hydrocortisone	13
Metachromatic leukodystrophy	Absence of aryl sulfatase A	2

TABLE II. ENZYMES DETECTED IN AMNIOTIC-FLUID CELLS OF NORMAL FETUSES AND THE METABOLIC DISORDERS CAUSED BY DEFICIENCY OF THESE ENZYMES*

Disorder	*Deficient enzyme*
Maple-syrup urine disease	2-keto-isocaproate decarboxylase
Homocystinuria	Cystathionine synthetase
Gaucher's disease	Glucocerebrosidase
G-6-PD deficiency	Glucose-6-phosphate dehydrogenase
Hyperammonemia	Ornithine transcarbamylase
Refsum's disease	Phytanic acid α-hydroxylase
Sphingomyelinosis	Sphingomyelinase
Orotic aciduria	Orotidylic pyrophosphorylase and orotidylic decarboxylase
Acatalasemia	Catalase
Citrullinemia	Argininosuccinate synthetase
Generalized gangliosidosis	Absence of β-galactosidose A,B,C

*Reviewed by Nadler, 1969.[10]

TABLE III. PATIENTS CLASSIFIED AS HIGH-RISK GROUP

Indication for amniocentesis	*No. of patients*
Previous child with Down's syndrome	7
Advanced maternal age (40+)	7
Drug users	7
Two relatives with Down's syndrome	1
Previous child with Duchenne's muscular dystrophy	2
Previous child with X-linked cerebral sclerosis	1
Previous child with familial dysautonomia	2
Family history of Tay-Sachs disease	2
Previous child with Pompe's disease	1

TABLE IV. RESULT OF STUDIES OF AMNIOTIC FLUID OBSERVED FROM HIGH-RISK GROUP

Indication for amniocentesis	*Result*
Child with Down's syndrome	4 normal karyotypes, 1 trisomy 21
Advanced maternal age	5 normal karyotypes, 1 47, XXY karotype, 1 no growth
Drug users	6 normal karyotypes, 1 no growth
2 relatives with Down's syndrome	Normal karyotype
Child with Duchenne's muscular dystrophy	Negative sex chromatin 46, XY karyotype
Child with Pompe's disease	Normal level of α 1, 4 glucosidase
Family history of Tay-Sachs disease	Normal levels of hexosaminidase A
Child with familial dysautonomia	No detachable catecholamines
Child with X-linked cerebral sclerosis	Negative sex chromatin

Samples of amniotic fluid obtained from 50 women by transabdominal amniocentesis were examined in this investigation. Of the samples examined, 20 were obtained from women whose pregnancies either were being terminated for psychiatric reasons or were being monitored for erythroblastosis. The remaining 30 specimens were obtained from women who were at an increased risk of producing abnormal offspring. In this high-risk group, the punctures were done between the 14th and 18th weeks of pregnancy. In the other patients the gestational age varied from 14 to 30 weeks. No fetal or maternal complications are known to have resulted from the procedures.

The indications for amniocentesis in the group with high-risk pregnancies are summarized in Table III.

The fluid was centrifuged and the supernatant removed for biochemical studies. The cells were resuspended in 5 ml. of McCoy's medium with 30% fetal serum, glutamine, penicillin, and streptomycin. This suspension was then placed in a Falcon flask and incubated overnight in 10% CO_2 in air for cell attachment. The medium was changed the next day and once a week thereafter.

With this technique, sufficient numbers of dividing cells for chromosomal analysis were obtained in three to 36 days in 90% of the cases. The majority of successful analyses were obtained between the 14th and 18th days.

For chromosome studies the cells were synchronized by trypsinization 24 to 48 hours before harvesting. They were then suspended in nutrient medium, replanted in Falcon flasks, and treated with Velban (12 to 16 hours). The next day the attached cells were removed by trypsinization and both these cells and those floating free in the medium were harvested by a method previously described.[14]

The results of the studies which have been completed to date are shown in Table IV. In all 25 pregnancies which have come to term, the prenatal diagnosis has been confirmed and there have been no congenital anomalies which could be attributed to the amniocentesis.

Comment should be made about several of the high-risk patients referred to in Table IV. Unfortunately a child with Down's syndrome was born to the woman in the older age group whose cells did not grow. The patient at risk for X-linked cerebral sclerosis elected to continue her pregnancy in spite of the 50% risk and delivered a normal male. The woman whose previous child had Pompe's disease delivered a normal infant, now a year and a half old. In this family cultivated skin fibroblasts were also studied histochemically; positive metachromatic staining was found in both parents and in their affected child. Skin fibroblasts cultured from their present offspring showed no metachromatic staining, which indicated that he may not even be a carrier of the disease. No catecholamines were detected in any of the amniotic fluids; this indicated that this cannot be used as an in utero diagnostic test for dysautonomia. Three women in the high-risk group elected to have therapeutic abortions on the basis of the prenatal studies. A patient whose daughter has Down's syndrome was found to be carrying a female with an extra chromosome in the G group, and she underwent abortion. The aborted fetus had some of the stigmata of Down's syndrome, i.e., mongoloid slant of the eyes with epicanthal folds, redundant skin folds of the back of the neck, and clinodactyly.

The 47-year-old patient who had one mentally retarded 10-year-old son was carrying a fetus with 47 chromosomes; the extra chromosome was a C-group chromosome. The sex constitution was XY, but the cells were positive for sex chromatin bodies which indicated that the fetus was a male with Klinefelter's syndrome. At termination of the pregnancy the abortus was found to be a male.

The patient who had one son with Duchenne's muscular dystrophy was found to be carrying a male fetus with a 46, XY chromosome distribution, and cells which were negative for sex chromatin bodies. She requested termination of her pregnancy because of the 50% risk of bearing another affected son.

Conclusion

Data concerning the use of transabdominal amniocentesis for prenatal genetic counseling have been presented. The study, and others cited, have shown that in high-risk pregnancies this procedure, performed early in the second trimester of pregnancy, can make it possible to provide antepartum prediction of a fetus affected with a genetic disorder. Reliable intrauterine detection of some biochemical disorders will require the study of a much larger number of normal and affected pregnancies, but work in this field is rapidly progressing. The recent report[13] of the treatment of a fetus affected with adrenogenital syndrome by intrauterine injection of hydrocortisone is encouraging. Increasing numbers of disorders have become detectable prenatally; additional studies will not only lead to the possibility of eliminating, by therapeutic abortion, a significant proportion of individuals affected with genetic disease, but may also lead to rational approaches of prenatal therapy.

Acknowledgment

We thank Dr. S. Cherry and Dr. T. Kerenyi of the Department of Obstetrics and Gynecology at The Mount Sinai School of Medicine for performing the amniocenteses.

REFERENCES

1. Nadler, H. L.: Antenatal detection of hereditary disorders. *Pediatrics 42*:912-18, 1968.
2. Nadler, H. L. and Gerbie, A. B.: Role of amniocentesis in the intrauterine detection of genetic disorders. *New Eng. J. Med. 282*:596-99, 1970.
3. Jacobson, C. B. and Barter, R. H.: Intrauterine diagnosis and management of genetic defects. *Amer. J. Obstet. Gynec. 99*:795-807, 1967.
4. Matalon, R., Dorfman, A., Nadler, H. L. et al. A chemical method for the antenatal diagnosis of mucopolysaccharidoses. *Lancet 1*:83-84, 1970.
5. Fratantoni, J. C., Newfeld, E. F., Uhlendorf, B. W. et al.: Intrauterine diagnosis of the Hurler and Hunger syndromes. *New Eng. J. Med. 280*:686-88, 1969.
6. Nadler, H. L. and Messina, A. M.: *In utero* detection of type II glycogenosis (Pompe's disease). *Lancet 2*:1277-78, 1969.
7. Berman, P. H., Balis, M. E. and Dancis, J.: A method for the prenatal diagnosis of congenital hyperuricemia. *J. Pediat. 75*:488-91, 1969.
8. DeMars, R., Sarto, G., Felix J. S. et al.: Lesch-Nyham mutation: Prenatal detection with amniotic fluid cells. *Science 164*:1303-05, 1969.
9. Fujimoto, W. Y., Seegmiller, J. E., Uhlendorf, B. W. et al.: Biochemical diagnosis of an X-linked disease *in utero*. *Lancet 2*:511, 1968.
10. Nadler, H. L.: Prenatal detection of genetic defects. *J. Pediat. 74*:132-43, 1969.
11. Nadler, H. L. and Egan, T. J.: Deficiency of lysosomal acid phosphatase: A new familial metabolic disorder. *New Eng. J. Med. 282*:302-07, 1970.
12. Schneck, L., Valenti, C., Amsterdam, D. et al.: Prenatal diagnosis of Tay-Sachs disease. *Lancet 1*:582-83, 1970.
13. Nichols, J.: Antenatal diagnosis and treatment of the adrenogenital syndrome. *Lancet 1*:83, 1970.
14. Lisgar, F., Gertner, M., Cherry, S. et al.: Prenatal chromosome analysis. *Nature 225*:280-81, 1970.

NASAL RECONSTRUCTION BY SCALPING FLAP IN A CASE OF MALIGNANT MELANOMA OF THE NASAL TIP

ROBERT HOEHN*

Assistant Professor of Surgery
Division of Plastic Surgery
Columbia University College of Physicians and Surgeons
New York, N.Y.

CASE REPORT

IN early 1966 this 74-year-old retired white machinist noticed deepening pigmentation in a nevus at the tip of his nose, slightly to the right, which had been present and unchanged for 35 years. In October 1966 an excision biopsy of this 1.2-cm. lesion by a dermatologist showed malignant melanoma; at the same time deep curettage and electrodesiccation were carried out. Recurrence of melanoma in the scar was proved by biopsy five months later, and the patient was referred for definitive treatment and reconstruction. In view of the patient's vigorous health, his continuing responsibility for looking after his invalid wife, and in the absence of clinical or laboratory evidence of regional or distant metastases, it was felt that a curative procedure was indicated. Moreover, chance for cure existed uniquely in this case since, as Pack, Gerber, and Scharnagel had shown in 1952,[1] distant metastasis from melanoma in this location occurs late rather than early.

Wide local excision was performed on March 28, 1967 (Figure 1), and right radical neck and left suprahyoid dissections were done on April 22, 1967. None of the 69 nodes examined was positive. Because of subsequent biopsy-proved local recurrence (Figure 2) the wide nasal excision was extended across the midline on June 24, 1967. Finally, all that remained were small fragments of the right and left alae with intact cartilage remnants, an intact septal cartilage somewhat reduced in its anteroposterior dimension, and a narrow rim of skin at the glabella (Figure 3). Histologically, the specimen showed

*Now director, Division of Plastic and Reconstructive Surgery, University of Colorado Medical Center, Denver, Colo.

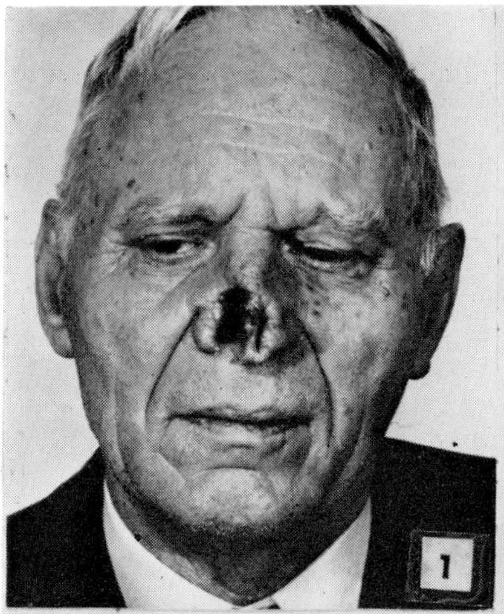

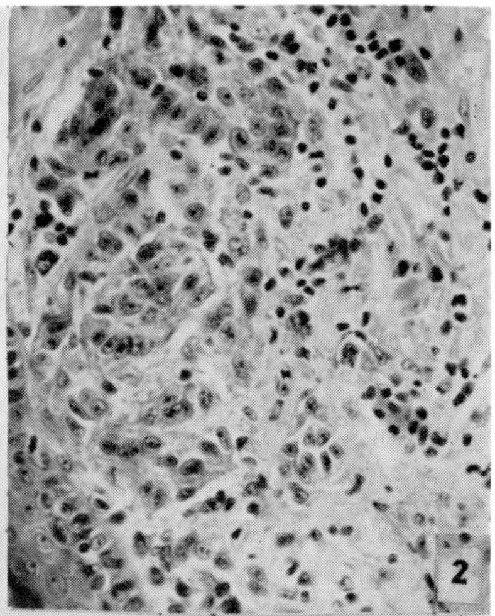

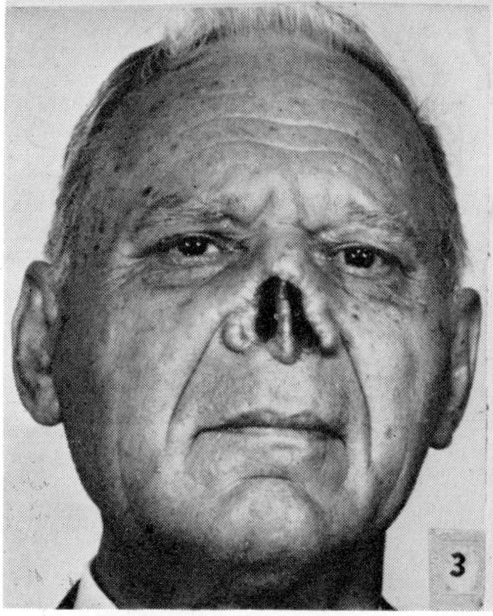

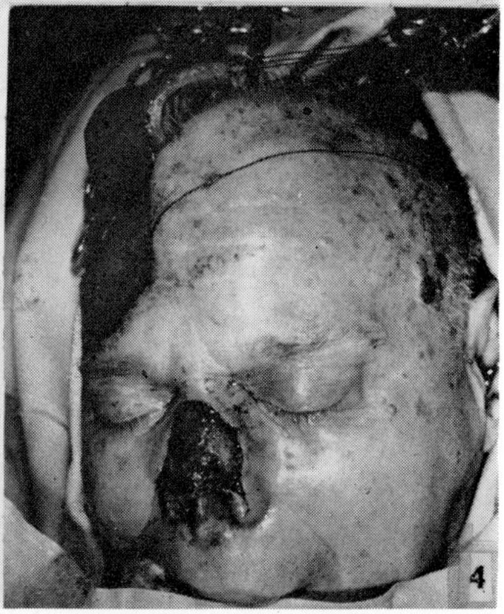

Fig. 1. A 74-year-old machinist; malignant melanoma of nasal tip; wide excision six months after onset and multiple recurrences despite curettage and electrodesiccation by a dermatologist.

Fig. 2. Histological appearance of recurrent tumor before reconstruction.

Fig. 3. Final wide excision of melanoma extending across midline. Note small remnants of alar cartilages and partial resection of septum.

Fig. 4. First-stage nasal reconstruction by scalping flap. Note local hinge flaps turned in for lining of new nose.

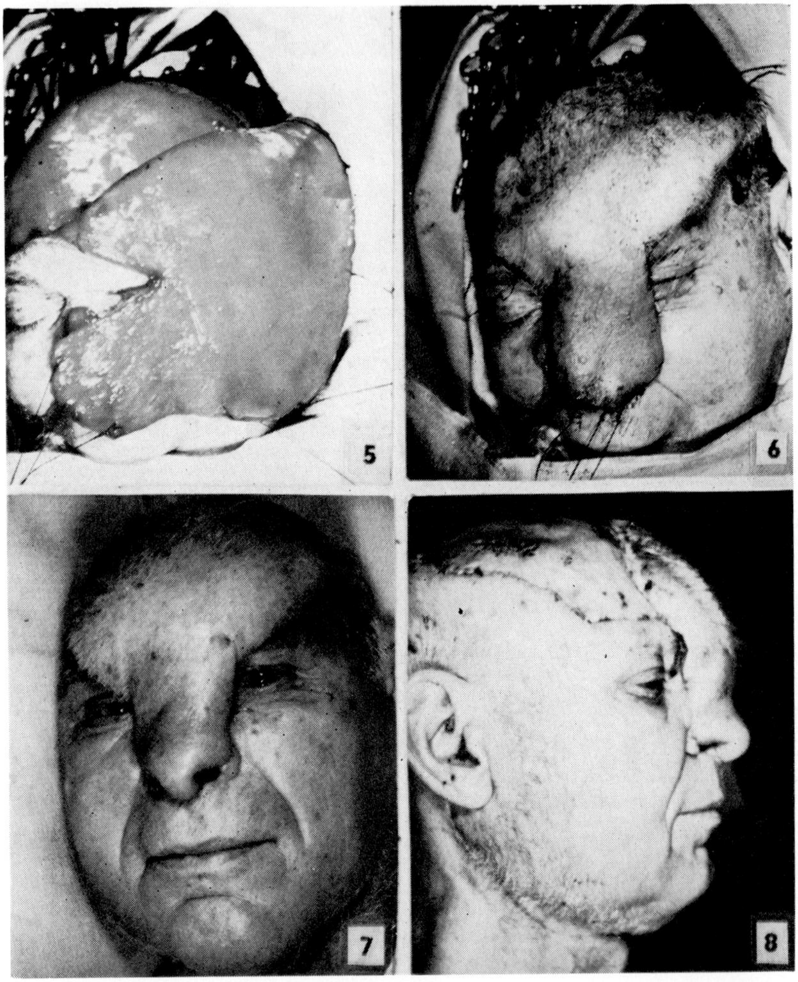

Fig. 5. Reflected scalping flap carrying lateral forehead donor tissue.

Fig. 6. Flap folded upon itself to carry forehead tissue to the nose. Donor defect is temporarily protected by split-thickness skin graft.

Fig. 7. Three weeks after notation of scalping flap (front view). Base of nasal portion being cross-clamped daily on days 17 to 23.

Fig. 8. Three weeks after flap rotation (side view). Note nostril margins folded in and split-thickness skin graft covering flap-donor site.

only cicatricial changes in the skin at the site of previous excision of melanoma.

Since there had been excellent wound healing and no further clinical or pathological evidence of tumor activity, nasal reconstruction by scalping flap was begun on July 25, 1967 (Figures 4, 5, 6). Local hinge flaps were turned in for partial lining of the new nose.

The pedicle was divided after cross-clamping for 10 minutes daily from the 17th to 23rd postoperative days (Figures 8 and 9) and the carrying flap returned to its bed on August 17, 1967. A full-thickness skin graft from the supraclavicular area was placed into the forehead donor defect.

After defatting and a Z-plasty to correct notching of the left alar inset of the flap, the contour of the nose was satisfactory until July 1968, when the patient complained of airway collapse (Figure 10). This was due to inadequate support of soft tissue at the tip. Accordingly, an 8th-rib cortical strut (6 cm. × 1 cm.) was countersunk and wired into the nasal pyramids (Figure 11). An x ray confirmed that it was intact several months later.

The final result (Figures 12, 13, and 14) was characterized by well-supported airways and minor changes in external contours and skin pigmentation that blended with other facial features.

Discussion

Authorities generally agree that malignant melanomas arise from the junctional cell nevus originally described by Traub and Keil in 1940.[2] This is a flat, sometimes slightly elevated, darkly pigmented, hairless lesion of the skin. It is so named because the nevus cells are located at the epidermal junction. Webster, Stevenson, and Stout (1944)[3] found preexisting benign nevi in 65% of their cases of malignant melanoma, but this was not substantiated by Lund and Kraus (1962).[4] Boyd[5] notes that melanomas also originate in melanoblasts of the eye and, less commonly, in mucous membranes of the rectum, nose, or meninges.

For many years Unna's concept that the nevus cell was of epidermal origin (1893)[6] had been accepted. He explained the lack of connection of the nevus cells with the epidermis by the postulate that they drop away from the epidermis to lie below it. Masson (1951)[7] postulated an origin of the nevus cells from the cells of the

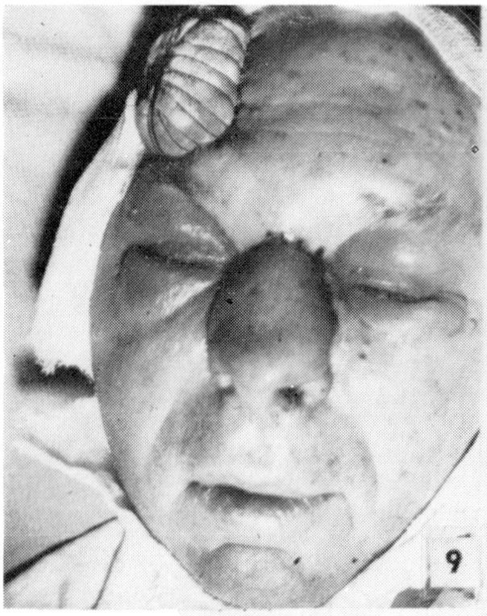

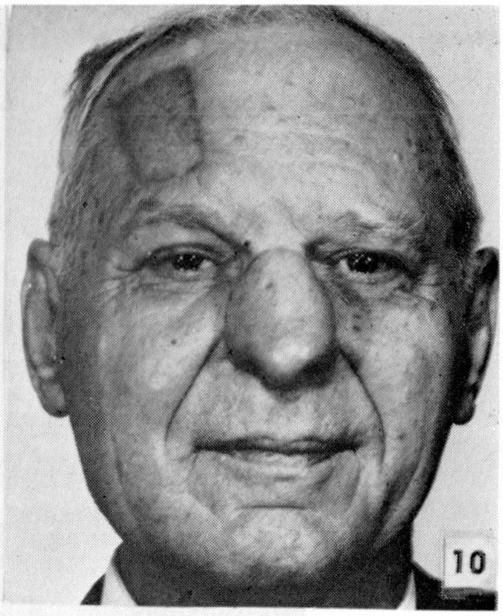

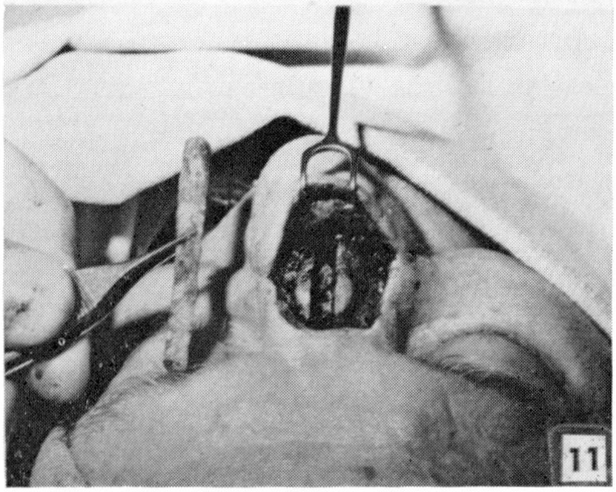

Fig. 9. Carrying portion of flap returned to original location after division at level of glabella. Split graft in lateral-forehead donor site.

Fig. 10. Ten months after scalping flap reconstruction. Satisfactory aesthetic result but patient had partial airway obstruction due to inadequate soft-tissue support at tip.

Fig. 11. Cortical rib graft being countersunk and wired into nasal pyramids to support tip.

sheath of Schwann. Montgomery and Kernohan (1940)[8] studied 460 pigmented nevi and concluded that the nevus cell has multiple origins, the majority from epidermal elements and, in their series, 11% from neuroid cells.

Most of the nevi found on the soles, palms, and genitalia will be of the junctional variety (Pack, Lenson, and Gerber, 1952[9]). Malignant melanomas are found most frequently in these areas and also on

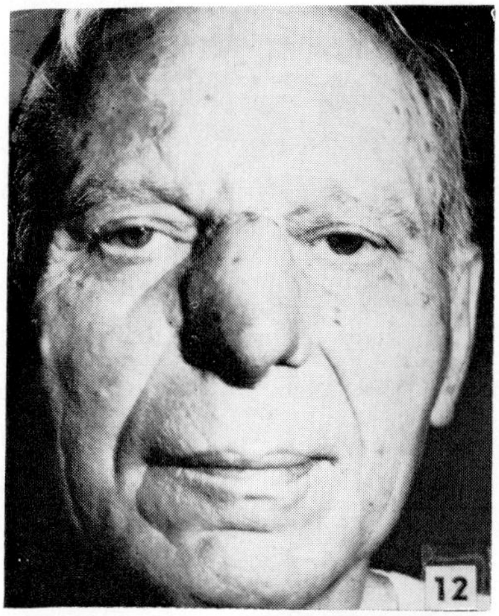

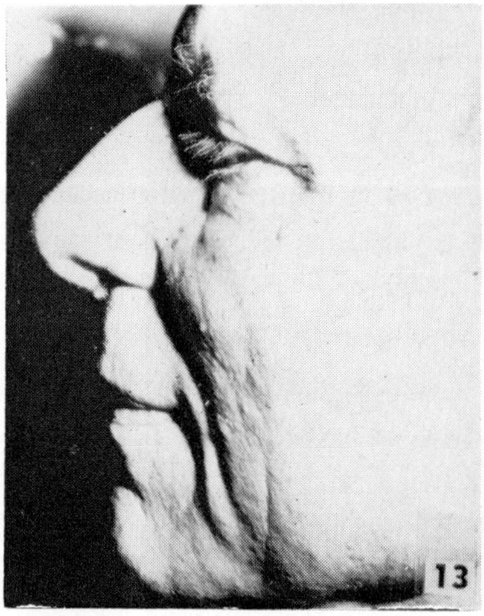

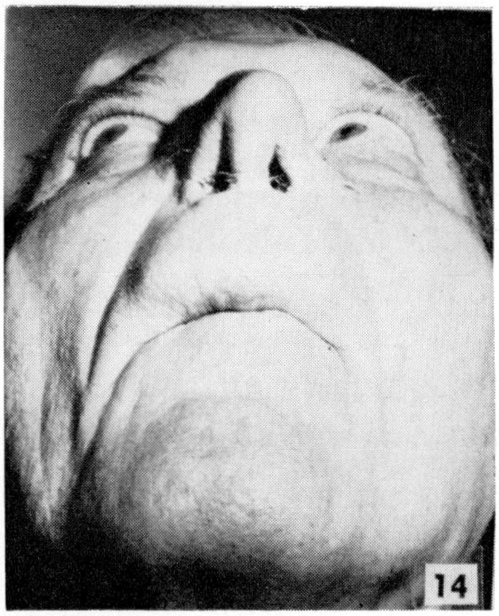

Fig. 12. Final result one year after construction of flap began.

Fig. 13. Final result (side view). External contours and skin pigmentation blend well with facial features and complexion.

Fig. 14. Final result (from below). Note well-supported tip.

the face and neck. The trauma and exposure to solar or other irradiation to which these areas are subject may bear upon the high incidence of melanoma in these sites. Much more rarely the malignancy may arise on the external skin of the nose, as in this patient, or from the mucous membrane of the nasal cavity.

Three clinical types of melanomas are recognized: 1) superficial:

a dark macular lesion located in the upper skin layers; 2) invasive: a firm, nodular, pigmented lesion fixed deeply within the skin; and 3) amelanotic: a nodular, firm lesion, attached to the skin, but without pigmention.

The typical microscopic findings of melanoma include the presence of junctional activity, melanin pigmentation, invasion of surrounding tissues, and abnormal mitotic figures.

This patient demonstrated a classic stage in the evolution of melanoma: the sudden darkening of a pigmented scar of long standing. It is well known that any rapid change in color or size is ominous, especially in a nevus of the face or lower extremities.

Among those conditions from which malignant melanomas must be differentiated are pigmented basal-cell carcinomas, subungual hemorrhage, senile keratosis, benign nevi, dermatofibroma, and sclerosing hemangioma. Current opinion discourages the use of incisional biopsy as a diagnostic procedure for melanoma. Rather, the entire lesion should be excised with a margin of several centimeters, if possible, to avoid dissemination of malignant cells. However, some surgeons feel, as we do, that with large lesions proper incisional biopsy allows a sounder decision about a radical or disfiguring procedure. Frozen-section studies are too unreliable unless the histology is classic.

There has been some disagreement about the treatment of melanoma. Pack, Scharnagel, and Morfit (1945)[10] advocated such radical procedure as amputation of extremities or extensive fascial dissection in continuity with node dissection. Other surgeons classify the lesion (superficial, invasive, or amelanotic) by excision and base their judgment about future management on whether there is regional lymph-node involvement. With all three types of melanoma the primary lesion should be excised widely, allowing a 5- to 7.5-cm. margin if possible and including any underlying fascia (Brown and Byars, 1940[11] and Conway and Jerome, 1954[12]). Whether it is advisable or even possible to dissect the regional lymph nodes with reasonable hope of benefit is of course a question to be judged separately on the basis of the type and location of the lesion and the surgeon's convictions about the efficacy and justification of radical surgery.

Allen in 1949[13] reported on his study of 362 cases of malignant melanoma undertaken in an effort to differentiate the fatal from the nonfatal melanocarcinoma. He gained the impression that there is no distinguishing histological feature which permits this prediction but that, in general, those with a superficial skin melanoma have a quite high survival rate compared with those with a superficial lesion located on a mucosal surface. Although distant metastases usually occur early, when the nose is the primary site of the malignancy, metastases occur late. In Pack et al.'s series of 1,190 cases of melanoma (1952[1]), there was a five-year over-all survival rate of 21.4%, with 15.8% for men and 27.4% for women. Webster, Stevenson, and Stout (1944)[3] concluded from a study of 68 cases that 24% had been given inadequate surgical treatment.

At the Memorial Center for Cancer and Allied Diseases in 1963 a 20-year series of 825 patients was analyzed for survival figures by McNeer and Das Gupta (Converse, 1964[14]). Three groups emerged:

1) Those with melanoma confined to the primary site with histologically negative nodes: 71% survived for five years and 62% survived for 10 years.

2) Those with melanoma involving only the regional lymph nodes: 19% survived for five years and 12% survived for 10 years.

3) Those with histologically proved distant metastases: no patient survived for five years,

Procedure of Choice

For defects of the nose which are too large for reconstruction by a local or a composite graft, some sort of forehead flap is the method of choice because of its proximity to the nose, its similarity in color and texture, and its excellent blood supply. The scalping-flap technique of Converse (1942)[15] was chosen for this particular case. The natural objection to a forehead flap is the secondary scarring in a visible area. There are several techniques for minimizing this defect:

1) The Kazanjian midline flap[16] leaves only a single verticle closure in the rent between the two intact frontalis muscles. The ultimate scar can be almost invisible.

2) If the donor site is chosen far to the side of the forehead, the defect is less visible in the full-face view.

3) "Blush-area" skin (postauricular or supraclavicular), as opposed to a skin graft from other body areas, blends well with the forehead in covering the secondary defect.

4) Care must be exerted to preserve the frontalis muscle because its

damage can result in a noticeable absence of expression of the forehead.

For the sake of completeness it should be mentioned that pedicle flaps from a distance may also be used for nasal reconstruction. The classic example is the Tagliacozzi[17] arm-to-nose pedicle. However, this is not only inconvenient but cannot compare in color and texture match to the forehead skin.

In planning any forehead flap it is useful to use the "design in reverse" technique, by which a pattern of the amount of tissue required is designed from a piece of semirigid cloth or plastic material held over the defect. This is transferred to the donor site on the forehead and the carrying portion of the flap is designed on the scalp. The template is cut to correspond exactly to the size and configuration of the combined forehead and scalp flap. With the template fixed at the estimated point of rotation of the flap, the pattern is brought down over the nasal defect and adjustments made in its size and shape until there is no tension on the flap and there is adequate material over the nose for reconstruction. The template is then autoclaved at the time of operation and the process reestimated for accuracy prior to the first incision. This maneuver was carried out in this case.

The scalping flap is an extension by Converse (1942)[15] of Gillies' "up and down" mid-forehead flap (1935).[18] The advantage is in the concealment of most of the incisions within the scalp and the placement of the donor defect in the relatively inconspicuous far side of the forehead. If care is taken to preserve both frontalis muscles, and if a full-thickness supraclavicular graft is applied to the forehead defect, both expression and skin coverage remain normal.

This patient was fully rehabilitated and once again assumed the complete care of his invalid wife. A quiet man, he paid us the compliment of discarding the gauze dressing which for so many months he wore to conceal his nasal defect. According to a neighbor, the patient died quietly at home of natural causes on October 4, 1969.

REFERENCES

1. Pack, G. T., Gerber, D. M. and Scharnagel, I. M.: End results in the treatment of malignant melanoma. A report of 1190 cases. *Ann. Surg. 136*:905-11, 1952.
2. Traub, E. F. and Keil, H.: The "common mole": Its clinicopathologic relations and the question of malignant degeneration. *Arch. Derm. Syph. 41*:214-52, 1940.
3. Webster, J. P., Stevenson, T. W. and Stout, A. P.: Symposium on reparative surgery: The surgical treatment of malignant malanomas of the skin. *Skin*

Clin. North. Amer., April 1944, pp. 319-39.

4. Lund, H. Z. and Kraus, J. M.: *Melanotic Tumors of the Skin.* Washington, D.C., Armed Forces Inst. Path., Section 1, Fascicle 3, 1962, pp. 47-61.
5. Boyd, W.: *A Textbook of Pathology,* 8th ed. Philadelphia, Lea & Febiger, 1970, pp. 1421-22.
6. Unna, P. G. Naevi und naevocardinome. *Berlin Klin. Wchnschr. 30*:14-16, 1893.
7. Masson, P.: My conception of cellular nevi. *Cancer 4*:9-38, 1951.
8. Montgomery, H. and Kernohan, J. W.: Pigmented nevi with special studies regarding a possible neuro-epithelial origin of the nevus cell. *J. Invest. Derm. 3*:465-91, 1940.
9. Pack, G. T., Lenson, N. and Gerber, D. M.: Regional distribution of moles and melanomas. *Arch. Surg. 68*:862-70, 1952.
10. Pack, G. T., Scharnagel, I. and Morfit, M.: The principle of excision for primary and metastatic melanoma of the skin. *Surgery 17*:849-66, 1945.
11. Brown, J. B. and Byars, L. T.: Malignant melanoma, with report of 4 and 7 year cures. *Surg. Gyn. Obstet. 17*:409-15, 1940.
12. Conway, H. and Jerome, A. P.: Nevi and melanoma of the face. *Plast. Reconstr. Surg. 14*:200-23, 1954.
13. Allen, A. C.: A reorientation on the histogenesis and clinical significance of cutaneous nevi and melanoma. *Cancer 2*:28-56, 1949.
14. Converse, J. M.: *Reconstructive Plastic Surgery.* Philadelphia, Saunders, 1964, vol. 1, p. 317.
15. Converse, J. M.: A new forehead flap for nasal reconstruction. *Proc. Roy. Soc. Med. 35*:811-12, 1942.
16. Karanjian, V. H.: The repair of nasal defects with the median forehead flap: Primary closure of the forehead wound. *Surg. Gyn. Obstet. 83*:37-49, 1946.
17. Tagliacozzi, G.: *De Curtorum Chirurgia per Insitionem,* 1597.
18. Gillies, H.: Experiences with tubed pedical flaps. *Surg. Gyn. Obstet. 60*:291-303, 1935.

APPLICATION OF ELECTROTHERAPY TO NONCARDIAC THORACIC DISORDERS

David Charles Schechter

Clinical Assistant Professor of Surgery
Section of Cardiovascular and Thoracic Surgery
New York Medical College
New York, N. Y.

Electricity has been used therapeutically for several centuries. With much justification, modern endeavors have focused chiefly on the application of electricity in cardiac disorders. A resurgent interest has been manifesting itself of late in directing the products of greatly improved technology to the electrical treatment of diseases of other organs. Whether this contemporary preoccupation with electrotherapy will eventually yield as rich a bounty as the now-familiar artificial pacemakers, defibrillators, monitors, cardiovertors, and other such devices remains to be seen. In any event efforts to that end will depend partly on an awareness of previous accomplishments. The purpose of this essay is to review briefly such antecedents as they pertain to noncardiac ailments of the chest.

Bronchopneumonic Derangements

The Reverend John Wesley is probably due a meed of recognition for being the first therapist to employ electricity willfully on himself to treat an intrathoracic complaint. The evangelist was stricken with acute bronchopneumonia, which did not clear with cathartic draughts. Finally on Sunday, March 23, 1783, he submitted to the remedy that he had used so often on his flock:[1]

> Finding still some remains of the fever with a load and tightness across my breast and a continual tendency to the cramp, I procured a friend to electrify me thoroughly, both through the legs and the breast several times in the day. God so blessed this that I had no more fever or cramp and no more load or tightness across my breast. In the evening I ventured to preach three-quarters of an hour and found no ill effect at all.

If physicians were at loggerheads about the efficacy of electricity in the multitudinous conditions where it was assayed, there was at least one regarding which there seemed to be no divergent opinions—namely, that it was salubrious for difficulties of breathing. This was displayed most dramatically in respiratory resuscitation, but was also operative in various parenchymal diseases.

There are numerous articles that date to the 18th century on the use of electricity in the management of asthma; however, none is as noteworthy as the one written in 1816 by Philip.[2] This gentleman distinguished between "habitual asthma," in which electricity was salutary, and "spasmodic asthma," in which it was not. He likewise performed a "double-blind study" in rough version:

> I wished to try, if the impression on the mind in the employment of galvanism, had any share in the relief obtained from it. I found, that by scratching the skin with the sharp end of a wire, I could produce a sensation so similar to that excited by galvanism, that those who had most frequently been subjected to this influence were deceived by it. By these means, and arranging the trough, pieces of metal, &c. as usual, I deceived several who had formerly received relief from galvanism, and also several who had not yet used it. All of them said that they experienced no relief from what I did. Without allowing them to rise, I substituted for this process the real application of galvanism, merely by immersing in the trough one end of the wire with which I had scratched the nape of the neck, the wire at the pit of the stomach having been all the time applied as usual by the patient himself. Before the application of the galvanism had been continued as long as the previous process, they all said they were relieved.

Philip envisioned a small battery that was to be *worn by the patient himself* so as to circumvent delay in substituting treatment:

> As it often happened that a very small galvanic power, that of not more than from four to six four-inch double plates, relieved the dyspnoea, may we not hope, that a galvanic apparatus may be constructed, which can be worn by the patient, or sufficient power to prevent its recurrence in some of the cases, in which the occasional use of the remedy does not produce a radical cure?

It is understood, of course, that "asthma" was employed as a generic designation for a multitude of conditions with the hallmark of impaired breathing. This circumstance, plus discordance about the etiopathogenesis of genuine bronchial asthma, fostered muddled thinking regarding when and how electrification should be undertaken. Sometimes galvanic corsets were used on the chest, while at other times the whole patient was exposed to a faradic current. Most often the vagus—that omnipresent *bête noire* of thoracic diseases in the 19th century—was attacked. William Neftel[3] told of some patients relieved by this last maneuver:

> Mr. P., aet. 43, commenced to be asthmatic in his ninth year, after whooping cough. The symptoms at first slight, increased every year in severity and frequently, until they assumed the true character of asthma, appearing in paroxysms, between which the patient had no difficulty of breathing. There were especially some circumstances, which would always call forth an attack, for instance: some articles of diet, and especially a late dinner. Sexual intercourse would invariably be followed by an attack, and so also would the least cold. There were some places, or houses, where he could never remain over night, without suffering from asthma, while in others, on the contrary, he felt free from it. In this case the galvanization of the pneumogastric (anelectrotonus) was followed immediately by a beneficial effect. Since the first treatment, which was occasionally repeated, the patient has not had a single attack during the remainder of the winter, although he was out every day, even in the most inclement weather.
>
> Mrs. C., aet. 30, sent to me by Dr. Marion Sims, December 9th, 1968. She has been affected with severe asthma from her childhood, and different kinds of treatment have been used without any benefit. Galvanization of the vagus (catelectrotonus) has immediately relieved her from an attack, and she remains still free from asthma, after having been treated fifteen times.
>
> Mr. J., aet. 35, suffered from severe asthma, for which he had been treated by many excellent physicians. Dr. Elsberg sent him to me September 21st, 1869, during an intense attack, which had already lasted for a fortnight, entirely depriving him of sleep. After the first application of the galvanic current, by means of which I endeavored to produce a condition of anelec-

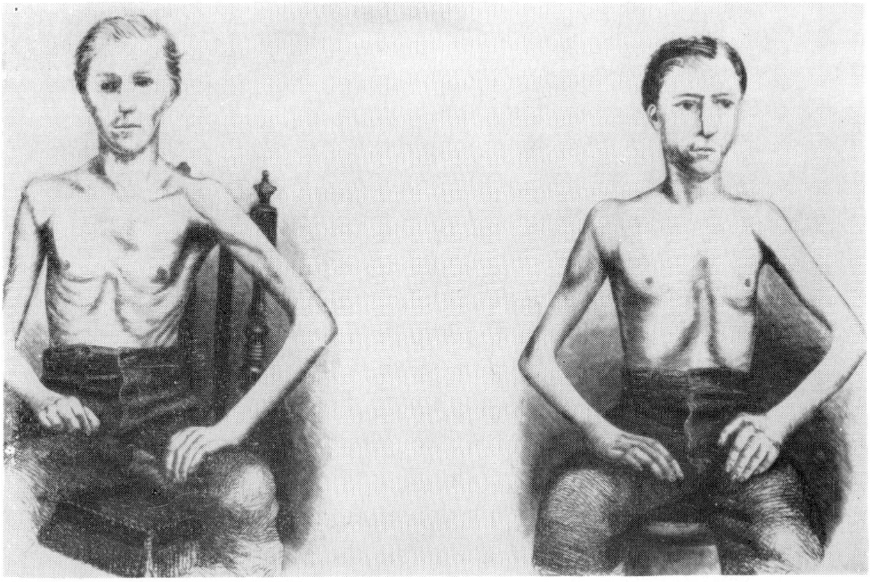

Fig. 1. Portrayal of a tubercular before and after J. Seiler's "galvanization by influence." The electrodes were placed adjacent to but not directly on the chest.

trotonus of the vagus, he slept very comfortably the whole night, and the paroxysm disappeared.

Wilheim Erb,[4] himself an electrotherapist of no mean repute, sounded unusually subdued in his appraisal:

> Nervous asthma occupies the foremost position with regard to electrical treatment. On account of the uncertainty of our views concerning the real nature and site of asthma, no slight difficulties arise with regard to the choice of the location and the form of the application of electrical currents. . . . We are therefore restricted to a purely empirical method of treatment. From the observations hitherto made, it follows that undoubted results can be attained in bronchial asthma by the use of electricity. . . . But numerous further observations are necessary before we can decide upon the value and the special indications of the individual plans of treatment.

Evidently this cautious outlook was not shared everywhere. Asthma continued to be treated by electricity well into the present century; the results were usually eyed with glowing approbation.[5-15]

Another parenchymal disorder which was treated electrically was tuberculosis. Of course the schemes used to treat tuberculosis in those days involved no end of trumpery, such as the king's touch. That John Wesley,[16] Elisha Perkins,[17] and their colleagues should have listed "consumption" among the variegated conditions which they vouched having cured by electricity was not unforeseen. But it is rather astonishing to find in the same company someone such as William Nisbet,[18] an acknowledged authority on tuberculosis. At least he admitted that electrotherapy was just mitigatory and should preferably be confined to scrofulous tumors. The patient was to be placed on an insulating stool, and Franklinic sparks shot on the protruberances until slight inflammation resulted. "The application should be made daily for the space of five or six minutes at a time; and where the swelling is not far advanced we have many instances of its success."

In 1860 J. Seiler[19] published a monograph regarding the adjunctive use of electricity to promote dilatation of the thoracic cavity in kyphoscoliosis, tuberculosis, laryngitides, and many other intractable ailments. His method, called "galvanization by influence," consisted of passing a current across two electrodes placed adjacent to but not directly on the patient's body. A large series of cases supported by spirometric data and mensurations of chest circumference testified to good results. Seiler speculated that electricity acted deeply—on the elastic fibers of the tracheobronchial tree—in addition to its more obvious effects in ameliorating the tone of the respiratory muscles.

The system of "electromuscular gymnastics," advocated in 1866 by A. Bastings,[20] met with greater acceptability. Not unreasonably, the rationale here was that stronger tonus of the thoracic musculature would better enable consumptives to grapple with their handicapped breathing.

> This is not done with a view to directly affect the tuberculous deposit at all; but, by strengthening the muscles of the chest, to so improve the respiratory power that more air can be inspired, and so benefit result to the the healthy portion of the lung, and indirectly, through better oxygenation of the blood, to a certain extent on the diseased portion and on the whole system.

Several score patients were treated in this way. One physician[21] used it on a group of children who "presented the appearance of debility,

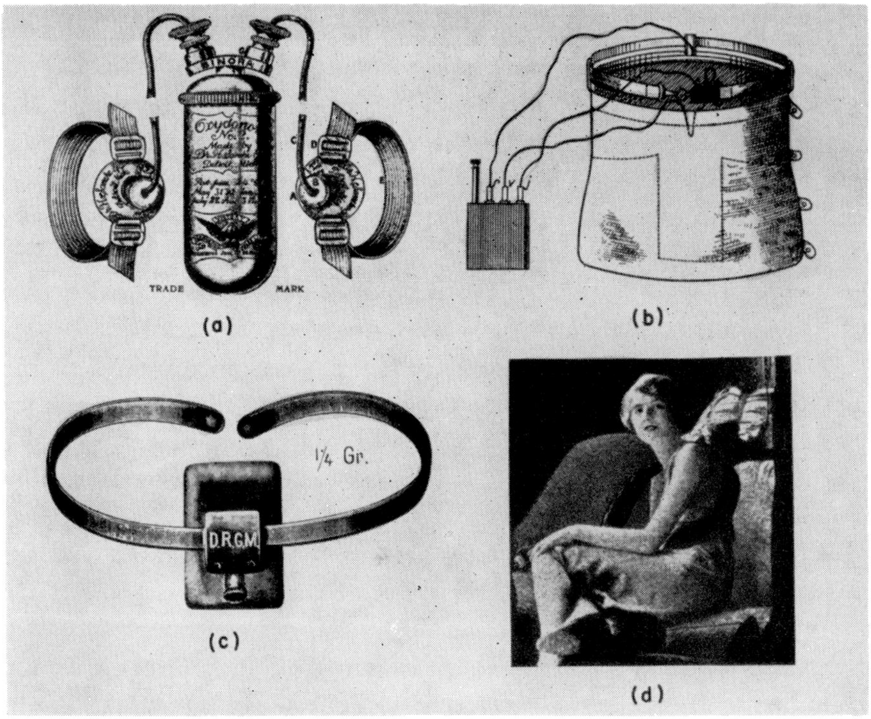

Fig. 2. Quasi-medical electric trumpery for the treatment of thoracic disorders. It was blantantly foisted on the profession and laity alike. (*a*) Hercules Sanche's "Oxydonor," based on the mysterious vehicle of electrical "diaduction," by which panacean agency oxygen molecules were propelled into the bloodstream. (*b*) M. Joly's "Faradic Corset" (*Presse méd. 36*:740, 1934). Actuated by both inspiration and expiration, this garment was alleged to bring about "conditioning . . . and tonification (of all abdominal muscles) . . . and provoke ionization phenomena capable of reequilibrating the nervous organo-vegetative system." (*c*) H. Aub's "Autoelectrode." Strapped around the thorax, it enabled electricity to be administered irrespective of whether the patient was "standing, lying down or sitting." (*d*) Gaylord Wilshire's "I-on-a-co." Plugged into an ordinary household socket and sported bandoleer-fashion, it invested the chest in an electromagnetic field. The flamboyant inventor of this cure-all became very rich.

languor, and lack of force so frequently found among the poorer classes." The results were "wonderful." Not only were the children's chest muscles greatly increased in size after a number of applications, but their "breathing was deeper, their appetites better, and they were more cheerful and lively."

There were skeptics, however. Leaving it to his readers to guess whether he had either Seiler or Hastings in mind, one deprecator[9] stated dryly:

> In lung diseases medical literature is, if possible, more barren of information. I can find nothing trustworthy at all on the subject. It is true, that there are some astounding assertions made by one man, with regard to the cures he has made of a great number of cases of phthisis, even when in advanced stages; but I regret to say, they do not bear the stamp of truth, and for that reason I forbear even recording the name of the author. As far as my own experience goes, I do not believe, that disease affecting the lung structure itself, is at all influenced by any form of electricity applied to the pneumogastrics; however, at the same time, I must say that I do not feel qualified to give that as positive opinion; but, judging from the provings of the current on the healthy nerve, and what little clinical experience I have had in these diseases, I am strongly impressed with the idea, that it is not homaeopathic to diseases of nutrition, affecting parenchyma of the lung.

Even more strongly worded reprobations did not dissuade physicians from using electricity to try to manage a dreadful disease for which there was little else to offer. The idea of fortifying the respiratory muscles was part and parcel of the regimen for consumptives anyway. Such individuals were instructed to pursue calisthenics or singing lessons for that purpose, and the program of electromuscular gymnastics constituted a convenient alternative for those who were not predisposed to athletics or tonality!

Besides electrogymnastics, stimulation of the phrenic nerve was frequently practiced in tubercular patients, both for the sake of augmenting the girth of the torso and also to aid the absorption of pleural effusions by exercising the diaphragm. There was scant evidence to show that the low intensity of electricity ordinarily used was able to penetrate the lung substance. However, any doubts in this respect were dispelled when high-frequency currents came into vogue. (An experimenter[22] interposed a light bulb between two wires embedded in the parietal pleura of a dog. When a high-frequency current was applied to the exterior of the chest, the bulb became incandescent!) One can find, as recently as 50 years ago, comments of the following sort.[12]

> The patient, clad in a thin undershirt, is seated on a low revolving stool in a convenient position near the apparatus. . . . The indifferent electrode, which is applied to the abdomen,

should be connected with the pole of the lower potential. The active electrode consists of a wire brush and is connected with the pole of higher potential and is brought near to the thorax. Care should be taken that the brush does not touch the thorax because the thermal action of the current will cause great pain and often superficial burns. The applications may be applied daily or if necessary only every second day, and the sessions may last from ten to fifteen minutes. The remedial action of the current is supposed to relieve the pain, to antagonize the muscular atrophy, to cause a revulsion in the skin and by reflex irritation to excite the respiration.

During the treatment the patient inhales ozone and ozone is presumed to form in the alveoli of the lungs, through the passage of current. The ozone acts as an oxidizer and therefore is a powerful germicide.

In addition to all this the current activates the circulation and nutrition in the lungs and therefore increases the general resistive power. The treatment should be directed to that portion of the skin directly over the lesion as well as to the entire thorax. The first application may increase the body temperature and the local symptoms. In this case the intensity of the current may be regarded as too great and should be reduced.

Lesions of the Great Vessels and of the Esophagus

In bygone eras when the interior of the thorax was closed to the surgeon many diseases of the great vessels and of the esophagus were irremediable. Some hardy physicians undertook trials with electricity in various conditions affecting those organs. Every now and then the issue was gratifying.

Peripheral aneurysms were often treated by electrocoagulating their contents but nobody dared to tackle thoracic aneurysms in similar fashion until 1846. In that year Luigi Ciniselli described his "cure" of an aneurysm of the descending thoracic aorta by galvanopuncturing the mass across the chest wall. In 1870 he published a monograph[23] that summarized his experience in 23 cases. Six patients recovered, 16 died, and the result in the last was unstated. Of the six persons reported cured, one had a relapse at three months, another at 17 months, a third at four months, but was reoperated on and was still well eight months

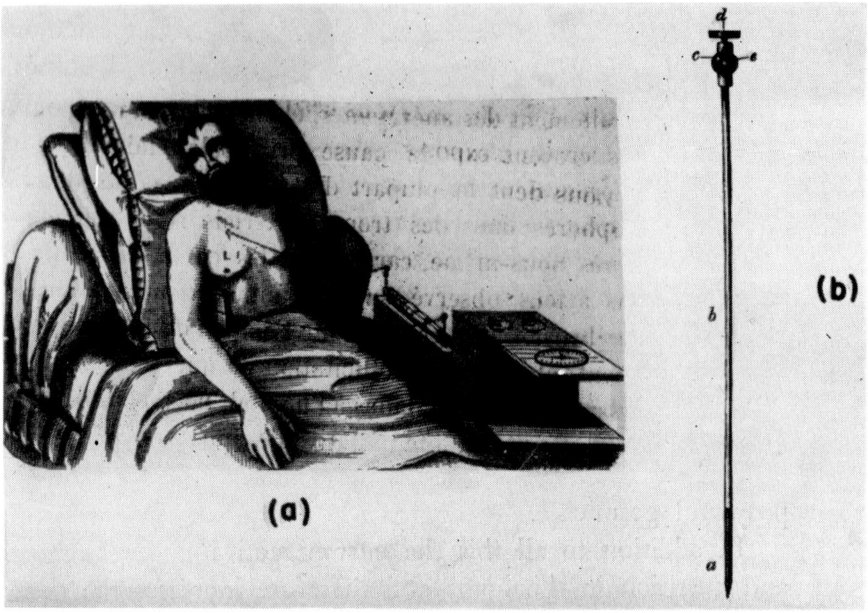

Fig. 3. The palliation of thoracic aortic aneurysms by electropuncture. (*a*) The technique illustrated. (*b*) A needle used for that purpose.

later. The remaining three patients were well between four and one-half and nine months postoperative.

It would perhaps be helpful to the reader, who may be aghast at the thought of passing needles percutaneously into thoracic aortic aneurysms, to be reminded of the standard regimen of management for those lesions in that epoch. In essence, it consisted of a starvation diet and a motionless existence:

> Absolute bed rest . . . if possible in a perfectly horizontal posture, should be maintained for months . . . .
>
> In regard to drugs . . . gentle laxatives are admissible; perhaps digitalis, if the pulse be too rapid. Iodide of potassium might be tried; also cold or compression; if need be, leeches might be applied.

The appalling situations with which surgeons were called on to deal can best be understood by perusing the case histories *in extenso*. The following passage, from John Duncan's report[24] in 1866, is illustrative:

> The tumour grew faster than ever, and by the 10th of No-

> vember had acquired a bulk truly enormous. So high did it reach in the neck, that as he sat, stooping from weakness, his chin rested upon it; and he asked me one day if it might not push back his head by its increase. It covered half of the sternum and of each clavicle, and from side to side over its highest part it measured thirteen inches. It was no longer smoothly hemispherical. Nodulated eminences has arisen here and there. Now one and now another had rapidly increased, reddening the skin, and threatening to burst, but hitherto they had failed to do so. At length, however, there came at the upper part a small vesicle, the size of a pea, perhaps from friction of the coverings. It was smeared with lard, and the softest lamb's-wool was placed between the clothing and the skin. Thus treated, it shrivelled and disappeared in a day or two; but, on the 15th of November, another of the same size filled with bloody serum arose lower down, where the skin was extremely thin. As this tightened and puckered with the pulsation, it seemed as if every moment it would give vent to a gush of blood. It burst in a day or two, but exposed simply the raw surface of the skin as after a blister. This surface then took on a slow ulcerative action, deepening little but gaining in superficies, while one or two new vesicles formed around it, which either dried up again to its extent. Matters progressed thus, while the patient's strength rapidly failed, till, on the 2d of December, a very slight oozing of blood took place, which was stopped by applying the perchloride of iron solution. It was evident, however, that, if nothing were done, the patient could live but a day or two at furthest, for bleeding from some point of the extensive ulceration must speedily recur. What was to be done had of course been anxiously and often thought over and discussed. . . . It was determined as a last resource to apply galvano-puncture. . . .

An editorial[25] in the *British Medical Journal* endorsed the procedure in no uncertain terms, and even gave detailed instructions on how it was to be accomplished.

As mentioned, fascinating stories are embodied in the pertinent case reports.[7a, 7b, 11, 26-36] They are well worth reading.

With regard to the esophagus, it is eminently clear from close examination of the records that, when successful treatment was docu-

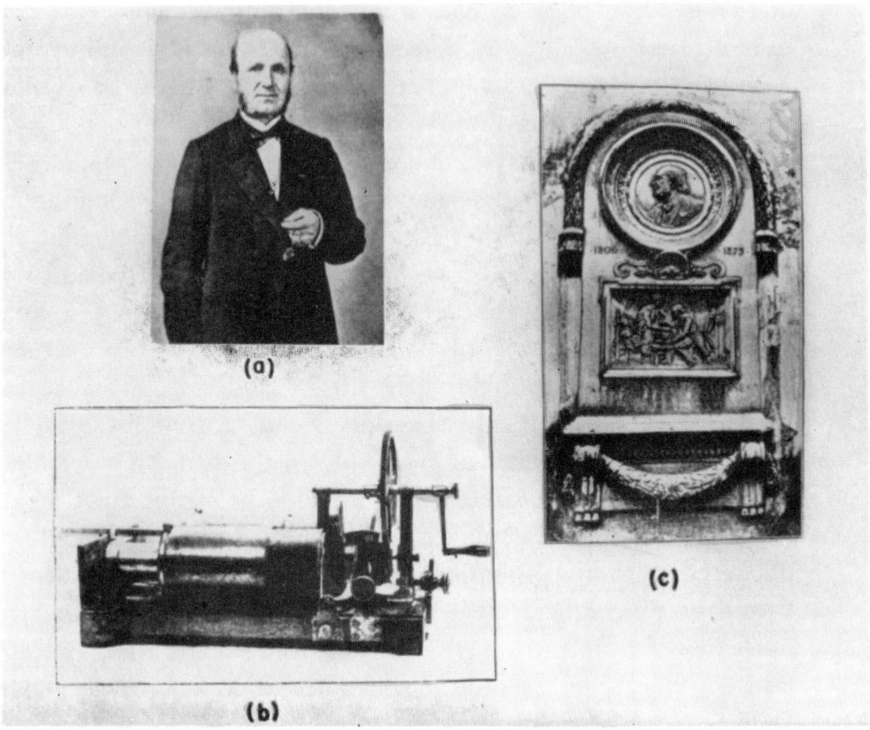

Fig. 4. Guillaume Duchenne, the peer of 19th century electrotherapists, conducted outstanding investigations in myology and neurology. He set the performance of electrophrenic stimulation on a rational basis. Although he treated angina pectoris and dysrhythmias with electricity, he averred that the heart itself was excited indirectly by this medium, via "reflexogenic zones" in the chest wall. (*b*) The actual induction-coil instrument designed by Duchenne and used clinically by him. (*c*) Tablet at the Salpêtrière Hospital, Paris, commemorating Duchenne, who is also honored by a statue at Boulogne.

mented, the condition in question was predominantly functional in nature. One such case of neurasthenic phagodynia was relieved in 1779 by Duncan[37] over a six-week period by directing electrostatic sparks to the throat on alternative days. Dysphagia, either psychosomatic or frankly neurogenic, has been treated until quite recently by electricity passed through suitably insulated esophageal mandrins.[6, 11, 38, 39]

Sporadically, organic "esophagism" was also treated by electricity. The goal here was to lyse simultaneously a cicatrix or mass while a relaxing spasm was superimposed on the obstruction. A sample of this type of enterprise was the narrative rendered by John Butler[9] of how an esophageal stricture was overcome.

Artificial Respiration by Electrophrenic Stimulation

In 1756 Leopoldo Caldani[40] excited the phrenic nerve of a dog with a discharge from an electrostatic induction machine and noticed jerking motions of the chest wall. He passed over the possible clinical utility of this phenomenon. Christoph Hufeland[41] in 1783 proposed the application of electricity to the phrenic nerve in asphyxia of newly born infants; one pole was directed toward the cervical vertebrae and the other placed on the epigastrium. The same notion occurred to Johann Bernstein,[42] Ludwig Froriep,[43] and Guilelmus Herder,[44] but it is questionable whether any of them actually put the plan into practice.

The actual performance of electrophrenic stimulation appears to have had for its fountainhead an experiment done in 1818 by Andrew Ure.[45] He transacted with a condemned criminal to purchase his body. This was removed after it had hung on the gallows for about one hour. After a series of preliminary tests in which it was ascertained that the muscles of the torso and extremities were susceptible to electrification, small incisions were made in the neck and beneath the fifth costal cartilage. On applying wires of a voltaic battery to these areas,

> . . . The result was prodigious: one saw instantly reestablished in the cadaver the movements of a strong and laborious respiration; the chest rose and fell, the abdomen advanced and then collapsed, and the diaphragm widened and contracted as in natural respiration.

Ure repined that vital structures had been damaged during the preliminary tentatives:

> We are inclined to believe that, without prior injury to the spinal cord and blood vessels of the neck, had we first activated the pulmonary organs, there is probability that we would have been able to restore life.

For this reason, and because of the more difficult access of the nerve in the neck, he recommended excitation of the phrenic mechanism by the intercostal approach.

Clinical corroboration was soon forthcoming.[46] The case was that of an inebriated man who had fallen into water and had been immersed six or seven minutes. He was then carried half a mile, the stomach-pump used, and ordinary means of restoration exhausted. A Dr. Ferguson, surgeon to the Westmeath Dispensary, exposed the diaphragm below the seventh rib, and applied a battery of 50 pairs. Spasmodic action of the diaphragm commenced at once and, shortly after, regular respiration. The man was saved.

Leroy D'Étoilles[47] advocated phrenic stimulation by electropuncture:

> When the battery is ready, the rescuer takes specially-prepared pins, slender, 6 to 7 millimeters long, and ending in discs equipped with rings or hooks. They are meant to make the galvanic fluid penetrate under the skin, across the fibers of the principal respiratory muscle. The pins are inserted to the sheath between the seventh and eighth ribs. One of the conductors is connected to one of the pins, the rescuer takes the other pole in his hand, and every two seconds he touches with a finger the head of the other pin placed on the opposite side of the chest. If one should not have pins in readiness, punctures not exceeding skin thickness may be made with a lancet, a pocket-knife, or the tips of scissors, so that the transmission of the galvanic fluid should take place. The punctures should be made as has been stated above, between the seventh and eighth ribs, on the lateral aspects of the chest, on a line corresponding to the epigastrium. The ends of the wires of the battery conductors are placed in contact intermittently with one of the small wounds, in the same manner as has been described for the needles.

Electrophrenic stimulation was accorded a niche in the arsenal for resuscitation; but seldom was justice done to its worth by discussion. The following passage, which deals with the management of poisoning, is from a contemporary textbook;[5] it typifies the measure of attention paid to phrenic stimulation:

> The great peril besetting the patient is the fatal indulgence of sleep; and this danger was averted under the old form of treatment by many expedients which were of necessity rough and cruel. Modern science supplies us with more effective and desirable means in the stimulating powers of electricity.
>
> The electric current must be applied by placing the negative electrode at the nape of the neck, and the positive electrode at the pit of the stomach; if this does not act with sufficient

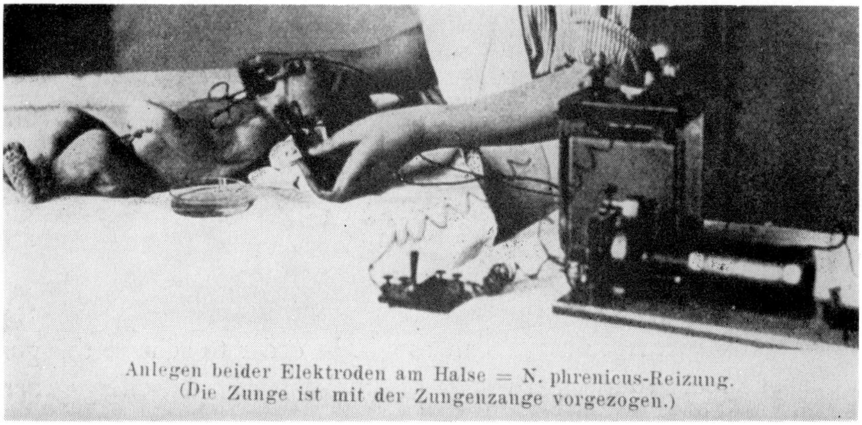

Fig. 5. Electrophrenic stimulation for resuscitation of the newborn, as practiced in 1927 by Fritz Israel. Note the hand switch to control the rate of stimuli administered. The alliterative remark in parentheses refers to traction on the tongue to facilitate assisted breathing.

> power, insert a needle between the eighth and ninth ribs on either side, so as to reach the diaphragm, and then allow the current to pass. The current must not be applied too strongly, or otherwise we may defeat the object we have in view.

Perhaps no single physician deserves more credit than the ever-enthusiasic Guillaume Duchenne de Boulogne[48] in conscripting votaries for the cause of electrotherapy in resuscitation. A vocal and convincing individual, his appeals were reinforced by an impressive series of successes. His most enduring and valuable contribution, however, was to have placed on a solid foundation the system of electrophrenic stimulation as a means of effective artificial respiration. Before technological advances made available the "iron lung" and many mechanical ventilators, a few dozen lives were saved by the expedience of electrophrenic stimulation. Duchenne's preoccupation with the method was an outgrowth of studies on the physiology of the diaphragm.

The topic, as elaborated upon in Duchenne's classic monograph, is in language which has a modern ring, although penned more than 100 years ago.

> Certain toxic agents (carbon monoxide, opium, chloroform, dipththeritic intoxication, etc.), certain serious fevers, such as cholera, can greatly perturb respiration, either because the

nervous centers do not send the quantity of influx necessary to accomplish the acts of breathing, or because the organs which preside over these different acts have lost their excitability to varying degrees and become, so to speak, paralyzed. One sees, in those cases, the respiratory movements more or less slowing, and sometimes even ceasing completely and suddenly; then asphyxia is imminent.

One of the first indications to fulfill, simultaneous with administering medication appropriate to the specific intoxication, is to purvey air to the respiratory tract, in quantity sufficient to reestablish and sustain homeostasis. In order to achieve this goal, one seeks to awaken respiratory movements by exciting general sensibility, or by mechanically and physically introducing air into the lungs.

It is electric excitation, either by cutaneous faradization or by faradization of the phrenic nerves, which answers best to these diverse requirements. . . . When cutaneous faradization has not been able to reanimate contractions of the inspiratory muscles, even if asphyxia is so advanced that one believes to already see the apparent signs of death, it is possible to still hope of recalling life ready to escape by mechanically introducing air into the respiratory tract.

It is in this situation that I counsel having immediate recourse to faradization of the phrenic nerves which, in making the diaphragm contract, enlarges concomitantly the vertical diameter of the lungs and the transverse diameter in their inferior portion, as demonstrated by my electrophysiologic experiments. It is assuredly the best means of imitating natural respiration.

Successful cases of respiratory resuscitation by a staccato of faradic discharges to the phrenic nerve were reported in 1856 by Hugo Von Ziemssen.[6] In one, a 27-year-old domestic was found in her bed one morning, asphyxiated by charcoal fumes. Counter-irritation of the skin proved unavailing in inducing respiration. When Von Ziemssen was called in, the pulse and breathing were almost imperceptible, the skin was pale, the limbs were cold, and rales in the trachea were conspicuous. Upon rhythmically faradizing the phrenic nerves, the chest was seen to expand, the girl began to cough, the cheeks showed a faint flush, and the digits became warmer. Faradization was continued, with

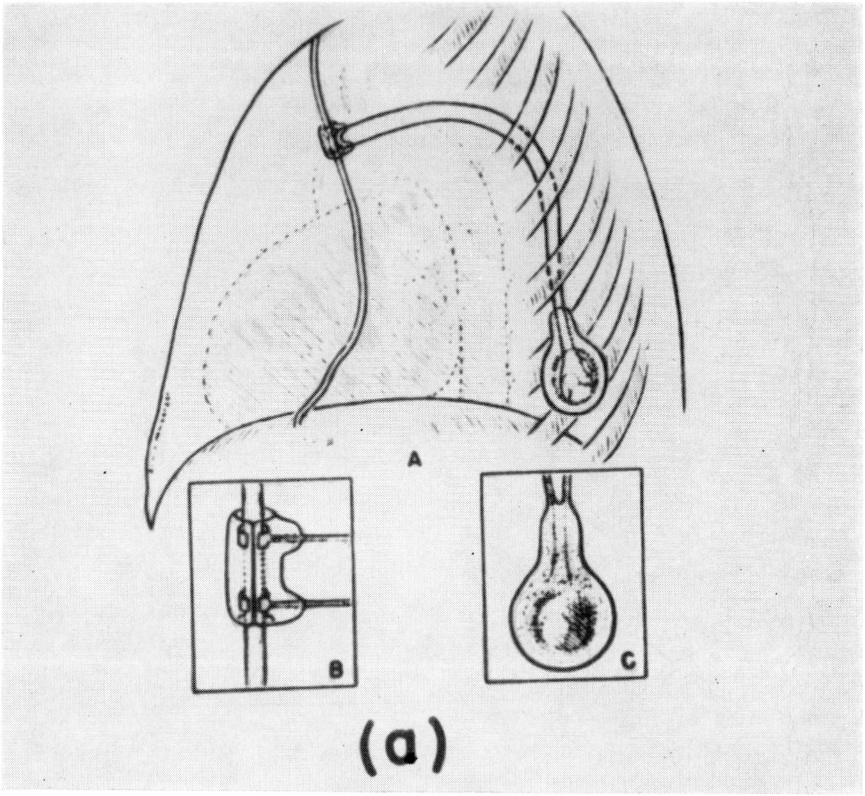

6(*a*) legend see 6(*b*)

brief pauses, for two hours, when respiration was fairly reestablished. Eleven hours afterward respiration was regular, and the patient was quite well the next day.

Rhythmic electrophrenic stimulation became an accepted mode of combating depressed or arrested breathing. In 1873 one writer[7] gave a précis of noteworthy case histories recorded since Von Ziemssen's initial account.

Thereafter the customary technique of performing electrophrenic stimulation was as given in this set of instructions:[8]

> 1) Let an assistant put the head, shoulders, and arms of the patient in a fixed position, while another stands ready to assist the expiratory movements by pressure.
>
> 2) Graduate the current to a strength sufficient to produce

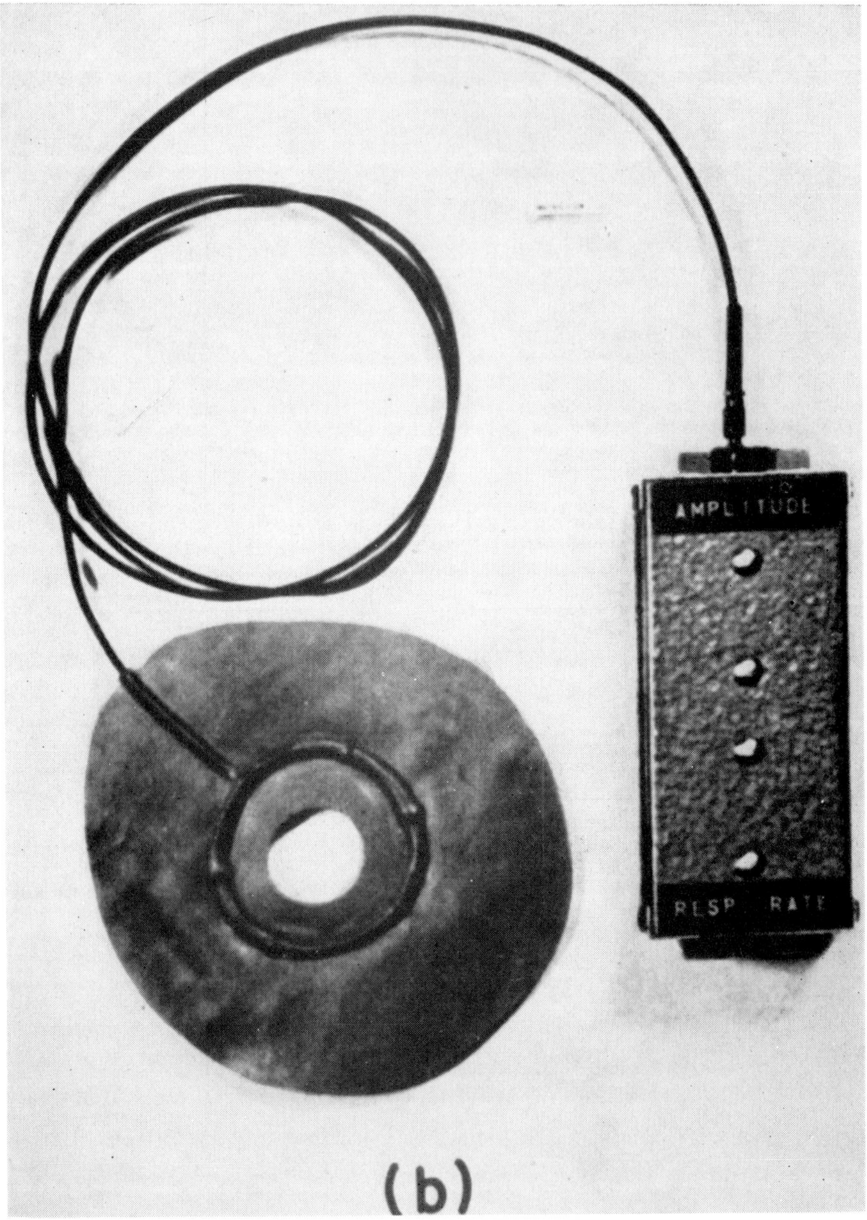

6(*b*)

Fig. 6. Radiofrequency inductive technique for long-term electrophrenic stimulation in chronic respiratory insufficiency. (*a*) The receiver and (*b*) transmitting coil and transistorized pulser employed clinically by William Glenn, Alexander Mauro, and their associates. Reproduced by permission from: van Heeckeren, D. W. and Glenn, W. W. L.: Electrophrenic respiration by radiofrequency. *J. Thorac. Cardiov. Surg. 52:* 655-65, 1966.

vigorous contractions of the muscles of the ball of the thumb, and then press the sponge electrodes (which should be of large size and well moistened) firmly over the phrenic nerves at the outer borders of the sternocleidomastoid muscles and at the lower end of the scaleni muscles.

3) Interrupt the current (either by removing one of the electrodes, or by an interrupter), about three times a minute, while the assistant presses firmly on the abdomen, pausing occasionally to observe the effect.

4) If after a number of interruptions no inspiratory movements appear, increase the strength of the current.

In some cases it is sufficient to put one electrode over the phrenic nerve and the other in the seventh intercostal space.

Large electrodes are used so as to affect the other muscles which have a share in inspiration (scalenus-anticus and sterno-cleido-mastoid) simultaneously with the phrenic nerve. The object of holding the arms and shoulders in a fixed position is to prevent the interference which may arise from the contractions of the muscles of the arms, at the same time to obtain the co-operation of the serratus and pectoral muscles.

Paradoxically, the inception of resuscitative maneuvers such as cardiac massage, mechanically assisted breathing, analeptic injections, and cardiac needling supplanted rather than complemented electrophrenic stimulation. True, there were sporadic reminders of it, such as Fritz Israel's excellent article[49] in 1927 on repetitive excitation of the phrenic nerve to salvage asphyxiated newborn infants. But the technique was seldom resorted to by the profession at large.

Prolonged rhythmic phrenic stimulation by electronic means started to be explored in 1948 by Stanley Sarnoff, Esther Hardenbergh, and James Whittenberger.[50-54] Long-term stimulation by radiofrequency transmission has been perfected and used by William Glenn and his colleagues in several cases of chronic respiratory insufficiency.[55, 56] Also, trials have been made of electrophrenic stimulation enjoined to a cause other than artificial respiration: excitation of the nerve in a diaphragmatic pedicle bound to the heart of aorta has sustained blood pressure at a satisfactory level when harmonized electrically with ventricular systole; this preparation has thereby fulfilled the function of an "auxiliary myocardium."[57, 58]

REFERENCES

1. Hill, A. W.: *John Wesley Among the Physicians.* London, Epworth, 1958.
2. Philip, A. P. W.: On the effects of galvanism in restoring the due action of the lungs. *Philos. Trans. 1*:22, 1817.
3. Neftel, W. B.: *Galvano-Therapeutics.* New York, Appleton, 1871.
4. Erb, W.: *Handbook of Electro-Therapeutics.* New York, Wood, 1883.
5. Lawrance, R. M.: *On the Application and Effect of Electricity and Galvanism in the Treatment of Cancerous, Nervous, Rheumatic, and other Affections.* London, Renshaw, 1853.
6. Ziemssen, H. Von: *Die Electricität in der Medicin.* Berlin, Hirschwald, 1857.

7a. Althaus, J.: *A Treatise on Medical Electricity.* London, Longmans, Green, 1873, 3d ed.

7b. Idem.: *The Value of Electrical Treatment,* 3d ed. London, Longmans, Green, 1899.

8. Beard, G. M. and Rockwell, A. D.; *On the Medical and Surgical Uses of Electricity,* 8th ed. New York, Wood, 1891.
9. Butler, J.: *A Text-Book of Electro-Therapeutics and Electro-Surgery.* New York, Boeric & Tafel, 1878.
10. Jellinek, S.: *Medizinische Anwendungen der Elektrizität.* München, Oldenbourg, 1906.
11. Jones H. L.: *Medical Electricity,* 7th ed. Philadelphia, Blakiston, 1918.
12. Jacoby, G. W. and Jacoby, J. R.: *Electricity in Medicine.* Philadelphia, Blakiston, 1919.
13. Webb, J. G.: *Electro-Therapy: Its Rationale and Indications.* Philadelphia, Blakiston, 1920.
14. Turrell, W. J.: *The Principles of Electrotherapy and their Practical Application.* London, Frowde, Hodder & Stoughton, 1922.
15. Die Elektrogalvanische Heilkunde. Lindau, Germany, Wohlmuth, 1953.
16. Wesley, J.: *The Desideratum; or, Electricity Made Plain and Useful.* By a lover of Mankind and of Common Sense. London, N.P., 1759.
17. Steiner, W. R.: Dr. Elisha Perkins of Plainfield, Conn., and his metallic tractors. *Bull. Soc. Med. Hist.* (Chicago) *3*:79, 1923.
18. Nisbet, W.: *Inquiry into the History, Nature, Cause and Different Modes of Treatment Pursued in the Cure of Scrofula, Pulmonary Consumption and Cancer.* London, Johnson, 1800.
19. Seiler, J.: *De la Galvanisation par Influence.* Baillière, Paris, 1860.
20. Bastings, A.: *Réforme Médicale sous le Double Rapport Scientifique et Pratique.* Paris, Baillière, 1883.
21. Vaust, H.: Sitzung der Gesellschaft für Medicin und Naturwissenschaften zu Brüsell, vom 2 Mai 1864. *Medicin. 38*: 599, 1864.
22. Maragliano, cit. by Larat, J.: *Traité Pratique d'Électricité Médicale.* Paris, Vigot, 1910.
23. Ciniselli, L.: *Sugli aneurismi dell'aorta toracica finora trattati colla elettropuntura.* Milano, Brancadoro, 1870. Also: *Annali Universali di Med. 214*:292, 1870.
24. Duncan, J.: On the galvano-puncture of aneurisms. *Edinburgh Med. J. 11*: 920, 1866.
25. Editorial: The electro-puncture treatment of aneurism. *Brit. Med. J., 2*:516, 667, 1873.
26. Tripier, A.: *Manuel D'Électrothérapie.* Paris, Baillière, 1861. Also: *Application de l'Électricité à la medicine et à la chirurgie."* Paris, Baillière, 1874.
27. Duncan, J.: On the treatment of aneurism by electrolysis, with an account of an investigation into the action of galvanism on blood and on albuminous fluids by (Dr.) Thomas R. Fraser. *Edinburgh Med. J., 13*:101, 1868.
28. Decristoforis, M.: Aneurisma dell' aorta trattato coll' elettro-puntura, etc. *Edinburgh Med. J. 16*:537, 1870.
29. Browne, C.: Intra-thoracic aneurism treated by electrolysis. *Lancet 2*:266, 1873.
30. Bastian, H. C.: Clinical lecture on a case of aneurism of the arch of the aorta treated by galvano-puncture. *Brit. Med. J. 2*:594, 623, 1873.
31. Communications: Treatment of aortic

aneurism by galvano-puncture. *Brit. Med. J. 2*:293, 382, 1873.
32. Fischer, F.: Ein Fall von Aortenaneurysma, behandelt mit der Galvanopunctur nach Ciniselli. *Berlin Klin. Wochensch. 45*:607, 1875.
33. Bowditch, H. I.: Thoracic aneurism treated by electrolysis, with remarks thereupon. *Boston Med. Surg. J. 94*:57, 1876.
34. Dujardin-Beaumetz, G.: Note sur un cas d'anéverysme de la crosse de l'aorte traité par l'électro-puncture. *L'Union Med. 136*:761, 826, 1877.
35. Communication: Electro-puncture in aortic aneurysm. *Brit. Med. J., 1*:1276, 1890.
36. Delherm, L. and Laquerrière, A.: *Electrologie.* Paris, Maloine, 1928.
37. Duncan, A., cit. by Mauduyt, M.: Mémoire sur les différentes manières d'administrer l'électricité, et observations sur les effets qu'elles ont produits. *J. Méd. 65*:416, 1785.
38. Lewandowski, R.: *Elektrodiagnostik und Elektrotherapie.* Wien, Urban & Schwarzenberg, 1892.
39. Larat, J.: *Traité Pratique d'Électricité Médicale.* Paris, Vigot, 1910.
40. Caldani, L.M. A.: *Institutiones Physiologicae.* Venice, Pezzana, 1786.
41. Hufeland, C. W.: *De usu vis electricae in asphyxia experimentis illustrato,* Inauguraldissert. Gottingae, 1873. Also: *Encyclopädisches Wörterbuch der medicinischen Wissenschaften.* Berlin, Boike, 1829, vol. 3, pp. 536, 545. Also: Cit. by Eysselsteijn, G. van: *Die Methoden der künstlichen Atmung.* Berlin, Springer, 1912.
42. Bernstein, J. G.: *Praktisches Handbuch für Wundäzte nach alphabetischer Ordnung in vier Teilen.* Leipzig, Schwickert, 1786.
43. Froriep, L.: *Dissertatio de methodo neonatis asphyctis succurrendi,* Inaugualdissert. Univ. Gottingen, 1801.
44. Herder, G.: *Beiträge zur Erweiterung der Geburtshilfe.* Leipzig, Maukianis, 1803.
45. Ure, A.: Experiments made on the body of a criminal immediately after execution, with physiological and philosophical observations. *J. Sciences Arts 12*:1, 1818. Also: *Ann. Chimie Physique 14*:350, 1828. Also: *Bibl. Britt. 10*:128, 1829.
46. Ferguson, cit. by Althaus[7a, 7b] and by Beard and Rockwell.[8]
47. D'Étoilles, J. Leroy: Instructions sur l'asphyxie. *J. Soc. Naufrages 4,* 1840.
48. Duchenne, G. *De l'Électrisation Localisée et de son Application à la Pathologie et à le Thérapeutique,* 3d ed. Paris, Baillière, 1872.
49. Israel, F.: Ueber die Wiederbelebung scheintoter Neugeborener mit Hilfe des elektrischen Stromes. *Zeit. Geburt U. Gynäk. 91*:602, 1927.
50. Sarnoff, S. J., Hardenbergh, E. and Whittenberger, J. L.: Electrophrenic respiration. *Science 108*:482, 1948.
51. Sarnoff, S. J., Hardenbergh, E. and Whittenberger, J. L.: Electrophrenic respiration. *Amer. J. Physiol. 155*:1, 1948.
52. Whittenberger, J. L., Sarnoff, S. J. and Hardenbergh, E.: Electrophrenic stimulation. II. Its use in man. *J. Clin. Invest. 28*:124, 1949.
53. Sarnoff, S. J., Whittenberger, J. L. and Hardenbergh, E.: Electrophrenic respiration. III. Mechanism of the inhibition of spontaneous respiration. *Amer. J. Physiol. 155*:203, 1948.
54. Sarnoff, S. J., Maloney, J. V., Sarnoff, L. C., Ferris, B. G. and Whittenberger, J. L.: Electrophrenic respiration in acute bulbar poliomyelitis. *J.A.M.A. 143*:1383, 1950.
55. Glenn, W. W. L., Hageman, J. H., Mauro, A., Eisenberg, L., Flanigan, S. and Harvard, M.: Electrical stimulation of excitable tissue by radiofrequency transmission. *Ann. Surg. 160*:338, 1964.
56. Anagnostopoulos, C. E. and Glenn, W. W. L.: Electronic pacemakers of the heart, gastrointestinal tract, phrenic nerve, bladder, and carotid sinus: Current status. *Surgery 60*:480, 1966.
57. Kantrowitz, A. and McKinnon, W. M. P.: The experimental use of the diaphragm as an auxiliary myocardium. *Surg. Forum 10*:266, 1959.
58. Nakamura, K. and Glenn, W. W. L.: Graft of the diaphragm as a functioning substitute for the myocardium. *J. Surg. Res. 4*:435, 1964.

UTILIZING COMPUTERS IN EVALUATING HEALTH DATA*

JOHN C. DUFFY

Medical Director
International Business Machines Corporation
Armonk, N. Y.

BEFORE discussing some of the specific methods we have developed for utilizing computers in the evaluation of occupational health data and medical information acquired through a voluntary health-screening examination program, I shall describe some of the general principles of the applications of computers in any field.

The computer is devised for the purpose of increasing man's productivity by enabling him to produce more per unit of time and to increase the quality of his production. However, the computer, if it is to be utilized effectively, requires careful and intelligent planning.

Instead of speaking of the computer as a single item, I shall discuss the data-processing system of which the computer is an integral component. A data-processing system is a series of planned actions and operations performed upon specific information, arranged to achieve a desired result. The procedures and devices that constitute the data-processing system may range from pencil-and-paper calculations to complete machine operations, but the procedures are basically the same. The computer performs four basic operations: input, storage, processing, and output. First, it is necessary to defiine the task to be done and the output which is required. Having defined these requirements, it is necessary to gather the pertinent information and then develop a set of instructions for the processing, referred to as a program. The program tells the computer where to find the information, how to arrange it, what calculations to perform, how to arrive at the final answer, and what to do with it.

There are several ways of putting information into the computer, from the conventional punch cards to direct input into the computer through various devices. After the information has been entered into

*Presented at a combined meeting of the Section on Occupational Medicine and the New York State Society of Industrial Medicine, Inc., October 22, 1969.

the computer it is acted upon by the program. The program is initially entered into computer storage and awaits the information to be processed. Computer storage is also used for gathering information to be acted upon through the arithmetic-and-logic features of the processor before the results are assembled in the desired format as output. Various storage units are also used for maintaining the histories of patients. The arithmetic-and-logic functions are performed in the heart of the computer, the processing unit, at microsecond speeds. Finally, after the computational work has been completed, the output can be received in several forms. This may range from voluminous results printed at speeds of more than 1,100 lines a minute to a specific answer automatically printed out by a typewriter or displayed on a cathode-ray tube.

As physicians discussing utilization of computers in the analysis of health data, we should be aware that all the computer's information is stored and that its work is done by a code made up only of 0's and 1's: the binary system. In many instances our medical information is presented in a fashion which is not immediately convertible into such digital form. Therefore such analog information must have special programs and equipment for conversion into digits.

With this brief background in the processing of electronic data, I shall describe three areas in which we utilize our accumulated data. First, in an occupational health program it is necessary to have certain health information for administrative purposes. Second, it is necessary to acquire information about the nature and types of health problems that arise from the environment of the work. These health problems might be caused either by environmental exposures or by mechanical injuries. In conjunction with the accumulation of such data one can acquire other health information on an epidemiological basis. A third application is in the area of preventive medicine through early detection of potential disease by periodic multiphasic screening examinations. In our company we call this approach a Voluntary Health Screening Examination Program.

Before I describe the functions of the medical department may I express the belief that, as physicians in occupational medicine, we should be aware of the application of the processing of electronic data in the field of industrial hygiene—an important function of the medical program of our company. Computers may be applied to the direct monitoring and recording of data in such broad and diverse areas as monitoring the general air of a work space or specific physical stresses such as ionizing radiation and noise. Computers may be used for monitoring stack emission, waste line, or water pollution. As with the automated clinical laboratories, computers may receive input from colorimeters, spectrophotometers, chromatographs, or other analytical devices. The computer may be used for the specification and design of engineering control for potential health hazards. For example, a mathematical model may be designed to compute the optimum specifications for exhaust from a stack based on parameters and ranges for the emission rate, exhaust rate, temperatures, wind velocities, stack diameter and height, diffusion coefficients, and acceptable downwind concentrations. Epidemiological studies of biological data and environmental data may be correlated and compared with a control group to assess the risk of potential exposure. There may be an assessment of a stressful situation, as when employees work at a series of tasks in which the exposure to noise varies while the tasks are neither serial in nature nor constant in time. Epidemiological studies of small groups that have similar occupational exposures and a high prevalence of a particular disease process, when compared to a controlled group has the potential of leading to a previously unrecognized disease caused by an occupational exposure.

Before proceeding to a description of the applications of electronic data processing in our medical department a brief discussion of the computerized Personnel Data System would be appropriate. This system, commonly called PDS, maintains current information about all employees within the domestic company. Similar systems are operational for subsidiary companies within the World Trade Corporation. The Personnel Data System maintains basic biographical data about each employee. It also maintains information as to job assignment, education, and duration of employment, as well as other administrative items, including confidential medical data. The medical data is divided into three coded forms: first, the code for employees with specific handicaps and the identification of the handicap; second, coded information on medical restrictions; and, finally, the International Classification of Diseases Adapted codes for specific diagnoses.

I shall now describe briefly the operations of our medical department. Each employee has an assigned medical-record location. Within plants, laboratories, or headquarters, this location may be near his place of employment. For our operations in sales and service, where there may be many small offices, a medical-record location is assigned at the regional headquarters and all medical procedures and policies are administered from this regional office. Within plants, laboratories, and headquarters we separate our operations into two phases. There may be one or more first-aid stations staffed by registered nurses. The greatest volume of our calls are handled through these stations; the nurses operate under signed standing orders provided by the responsible physician. There will be a central medical unit staffed with the appropriate number of physicians, nurses, technicians, and clerical personnel.

For administrative purposes, we evaluate within the first-aid stations the staff requirements, the purpose of particular visits, and the number of visits. Therefore it is necessary to determine what should be recorded. For our purposes we require this basic information: the identification of the employee, his division, the location within the division, the employee's department, and the identity of the first-aid station which he has visited. In addition we separate our recording into three general categories: industrial injury or illness, nonindustrial injury, and nonindustrial illness. Having determined the general classification of what is to be recorded, we must select the method of recording the information or the input into our system. The particular type of input is dependent upon the data-processing equipment which is available, the work load, and the personal choice at the locations. The recording method calls for one data-processing card for each visit. The information entered on these cards is either completely handwritten, or handwritten and mark-sensed in combinations; it may be completely mark-sensed, or punched directly into the card by using a device known as the porta-punch. In any event, identical information is recorded by each location. After processing of the information for administrative purposes, each location may determine its personnel requirements related to the numbers of visits, types of visits, and the times when visits occur in each individual first-aid station.

From the first-aid stations and from the information accumulated on the industrial injury and illness card, we are able to evaluate the frequency of specific types of health problems that arise within a particular department. We may also analyze all of the recorded data from a suspected hazardous area to determine what is actually happening to employees. Each location has the ability to make an individual breakdown according to its specific requirements. There are significant differences between manufacturing facilities within the same operating division. For example, we range in potential exposure from chemical to mechanical operations. In conjunction with the accumulation and review of industrial injury and illness data, we can manipulate the nonoccupational health information in the same manner. We do not routinely correlate this information but may do so if there is the suspicion of some job-oriented problem. For example, if we suspect that we are treating more respiratory problems in one first-aid station, we can compare the incidence of respiratory complaints from this area in order to determine if there is a statistically significant greater incidence than among a similar control group. Further analysis can be made for individual departments. If the results are significant, then a detailed study of processes, changes in processes, or the addition of new materials may be evaluated in an attempt to isolate and define whether this observed increase in incidence of disease is related to the occupation.

Within the medical department we use a medical-visit card which records the reason for all visits to this facility. From this source we obtain a measurement of the total activity by type of visit. This enables us to evaluate the utilization of our professional resources and also to audit each location for compliance with policy. The medical-visit card has 17 major groups of primary reasons for the employees' visits; it also has space to indicate secondary purposes of the visits. This secondary category may be used at the option of each medical department for specific studies.

The medical summary card provides a method for entering the basic medical information into the Personnel Data System for notifying the Personnel Department of job restrictions on new employees at each location. As I have indicated previously, this information is categorized in three groups. First, there is the handicap code, which defines handicaps that permit comparisons with those of other companies and of government agencies. It also permits an evaluation and audit of compliance with policy by individual location. This information is available to medical and to personnel managers only. The purpose of making this available to the personnel manager is to enable him to comply with the provisions of most states' second-injury laws. Second, medical-restriction codes are comprised of seven categories with 54 specific recommendations as to restrictions required for the particular individual. Information accumulated in this fashion provides management with an estimate of the mobility of its employees at that particular location and is important at the time of major product change or technological innovation. The information concerning the individual employee who may be considered for reassignment is available to managers. Third, the International Classification of Diseases Adapted codes are entered; these provide a statistical profile of the scope and nature of the health problems within the population of any location. This profile varies according to the size and age of the plant and its population. It indicates to the managing physician where he should place the greatest emphasis in his medical program. This information is available to the medical department only.

We do accumulate other information. Base-line hearing data is acquired for all new employees. For those employees who have repeated exposure to noise in excess of 85 decibles in the broad band, periodic audiometric examinations are performed. The purpose is to identify susceptible individuals, provide protective devices, record any change over time and, if necessary because of changes in the audiogram, to reassign the employee. At the present time we are engaged in an analysis of these data for specific locations. Our purpose is to evaluate present procedures and to establish better data upon which to base the frequency that these examinations are performed.

When an employee has been absent for more than 10 working days he is required to visit the medical department and present a certificate concerning his illness. We should accumulate this information after any absence, but practically this is not feasible. This 10-day medical certificate provides the basic information about the employee, his division, location, and department. It records the number of working days, the total number of days of absence, the days of hospitalization, if any, and the diagnosis of the disorder that caused the absence; it also shows what surgical procedure, if any, had been performed. This information is coded according to the International Classification of Diseases Adapted. We have had this capability of coding and analyzing data on absences but have implemented it on a corporate basis only within the past few months. It is our intent to relate the findings to the results of our multiphasic health-screening examination program. Our purpose in accumulating these data is to be able to analyze our absences by diagnoses, age groups, and sex, and to correlate the reasons for absence with the diagnostic information in the data bank which has been accumulated as a result of the multiphasic screening. Finally, we wish to compare the patterns of absence and illness between participants and nonparticipants in the multiphasic-screening examination.

In September 1968 our corporation initiated a multiphasic-screening examination program for employees age 41 and over, with eligibility for examination during the month of birth. The frequency of this examination is related to the age of the participating employee. The examination is voluntary; however, we have recorded a participation in excess of 80% of the eligible employees; we now have more than 26,000 records in our data bank at the conclusion of one year of operation.

As I previously mentioned, the Personnel Data System contains pertinent information about all employees. From this system we obtain each month a list from the computer of eligible individuals by location of medical responsibility. This eligibility list is sent to the location, which extends an invitation to the employee to participate in the program. The medical-responsibility location also receives computer-prepared cards for each individual for three specific items: first, the automated chemistries which identify the specimen and is used during the processing; second, an x-ray identification card, which provides for the collection in coded form of the radiologist's findings, as well as his evaluation of the quality of the x-ray film; and, finally, a card for the electrocardiogram that permits the cardiologist to record his interpretation in coded form; the codes are compatible with the computer program.

If the employee accepts the examination he is given an appointment to report to the medical department in a fasting state. He completes a questionnaire, which consists of 167 mark-sensed questions. A medical-data sheet with pertinent information such as height, weight, blood pressure, hearing, and vision is completed by the nurse. This too is a mark-sensed sheet. Blood is drawn, a standard 14 × 17 chest x ray is taken, and an electrocardiogram is recorded on tape. This recording consists of the analog signals of the vectorcardiogram as well as a strip chart. All this information is sent to a central medical-data center, which is located in White Plains, N.Y. The questionnaire and the medical-data sheet are processed through an optical reading device with a punch-card output which serves as the form for entering the information into the computer. The blood serum with the identifying card is sent to the automated chemistry laboratory. The computer is used in the control process of this laboratory. The computer checks the standards at the beginning of processing, corrects for drift in the system by using the results of every 10th specimen, which is also a known standard. The computer calculates the mean and standards for pooled serum on a daily basis to confirm the laboratory's capability to reproduce results accurately. The computer also calculates the mean run each day for each chemistry and compares these results with the accumulated laboratory mean for each chemistry.

The electrocardiogram results are received from 25 major locations on tape. As I have indicated, this is a recording of the analog signals of the vector-cardiogram. There is an interface with the computer, which performs an analog-to-digital conversion, and the computer performs an analysis of the digital equivalent. We have made a provision that our cardiologists review all abnormal and borderline interpretations of the computer and have made it possible to replace the computer interpretation by the cardiologist's interpretation if there is a difference. The cardiologist also checks every 20th electrocardiogram interpreted as normal by the computer. There is a high correlation of agreement in this quality-control procedure. The x rays are interpreted by a radiologist and the coded interpretations is entered into the system. Those interpretations not subject to codification are transcribed, key-punched, and the English-language statement is entered into the computer.

All this information is correlated in the computer and, where appropriate, compared to preassigned expected ranges for specific observations or tests. The output from the computer is a printed medical report for each individual examination and is accompanied by a computer-generated medical-disposition card. All the information, including the printed results and disposition cards, are returned to the medical-record location where the employee is informed of the results. The employee is also informed that this is not a complete examination and is referred to his personal physician. Ninety per cent of the participants indicate that they wish to have the results forwarded to their attending physicians. Subsequent to the review with the employee the medical-disposition card for his examination is completed; the card indicates what diagnoses or observations were made during the examination. These diagnoses and observations are coded by the use of the International Classification of Disease Adapted (ICDA). The disposition card, with its information, is returned to the Medical Data Center and is entered into the employee's record in the computer. The cycle is now complete.

With multiphasic screening in existence for a year and with the results of 26,000 examinations in the data bank we must ask: "What is being done with the medical data that has been acquired?" I believe it would be impossible to approach a systematic analysis of so many data without the use of computers. We determined that it was most feasible to enter the information into disc storage rather than on tapes or other storage devices. Disc storage permits more rapid access to any individual participant's data by allowing us to go directly, rather than sequentially, to that portion of the file containing the individual's record or to those portions of the file where specific data are stored for each participant. This is particularly useful when it is necessary to alter or to add to the record.

One of the major problems in any medical study is the retrieval of information. Originally we determined on a rather empirical basis the types and specifics of the medical information and procedures which were to be included in this multiphasic-screening examination. The chief tool for the retrieval of information used in the Voluntary Health Screening Examination Program is a large-scale computer-information-retrieval program which we call the "bridging" program. This computer program is a flexible, parameter-controlled system used to select, filter, edit, and present data from the master data file and the Personnel Data System. This system offers us a high degree of versatility in the filtering and output of data. It provides access to any or all of the files, in any order, for any combination of filtering or output. In addition, the bridging system is equipped with an option for random selection, a highly desirable feature for sampling studies. Also, it can handle multiple-sequential searches during the same computer run. Another retrieval program, "Matrix," can generate various kinds of cross-tabulations from the many variables in the file.

We have developed our approach to the analysis of this quantity of health data by using statistical evaluation of our results. First, to address the questionnaire. There are some simple problems for which analysis would be a dull and lengthy assignment. For example: which questions are consistently answered "Yes" or "No"? A more difficult correlation is a question of which two or more questions are consistently answered in the same manner and, finally: are there clusters of questions which are answered in similar fashion? The medical-data sheet must also be analyzed in the same manner as the questionnaire.

Initially we addressed most of our analytical efforts to the laboratory and electrocardiography, with some effort in the field of radiology. In the laboratory we have used expected ranges for the various chemistries based upon published material; however, we realize that we shall require redefinition of the expected range for each chemistry. Based upon the information now available, the expected ranges of the various chemistries appear to vary with age and probably with sex. In analyzing the information we must also consider geography and race. In the early phases of this program we recognized the need to acquire additional information concerning these factors. For example, for the first 9,842 examinations we see that the mean for glucose as computed and plotted by the computer is 101 mgm.% for the employees examined within our own medical departments in the United States. We observed more difficulties in collecting specimens when using fee-for-service physicians. Therefore we performed an analysis of the results from one of our regional offices, but excluded those examinations performed in our own department. In this instance we observed a mean of 95 mgm.%, as computed by the computer. Through the use of such techniques we have been able to upgrade the quality of specimen collection and to minimize variations. Another observation has been that there is a gradually advancing mean that depends upon age. These data continue to be refined further, and similar studies are under way for each of the other chemistries. Additionally, as with the questionnaire, we are in the process of determining which tests consistently show a low productivity in producing significant clinical findings.

A review of 1,200 records on patients in the data bank shows that we had 1,287 employees with reported ICDA diagnosis of cardiovascular disease. We further refined this information to those diagnostic codes for ischemic heart disease. Of the 1,287 diagnostic classifications, 414 were within this code. We further refined the information as to the incidence by age groups and as to whether it had been previously known to the employees.

We are embarking upon further studies. First, a reevaluation of all these employees to determine any change in status over a specified period of time; we then plan to compare this new information with the results of previous examinations. We are including information as to what the employee has done to alleviate the condition during the interim between examinations. Second, we are matching this group with a control group that satisfies specified criteria as to age, sex, physical, and historical information but that does not have electrocardiographic evidence of coronary-artery disease. These two groups are the basis for proposed additional studies. One study is to establish those factors that are similar and those that are different between the two groups. This may permit us to evaluate the possibility or probability for a particular individual to develop coronary-artery disease. We recognize that there is a great deal of published material in this area, and we believe that the published information provides a sound basis for writing the necessary programs which can apply to the investigation of other clinical conditions. Another long-term study is intended to determine the clinical similarities and differences between these two groups.

In the field of radiology we are evaluating findings and the types of findings by the specific x-ray diagnostic statement which has been entered into the computer. This is not a particular problem when it is a simple tabulation of numeric coded responses. However, it is necessary to take a different approach when a diagnostic statement in English has been entered. For this contingency we have developed a program which enables us to search our file for specific statements or combinations of statements in English and to perform analyses of this information.

The medical-disposition card provides the ICDA diagnosis, indicates the source of primary information for this diagnosis, whether the diagnosis was previously known and the advice given to the participant. When we have received these disposition cards we shall be able to correlate actual information within the data bank against the clinical judgment of the physicians. Through this we should be able to determine the particular value of some of our procedures.

In conclusion: I am convinced that we in occupational medicine have an exceptional opportunity to evaluate much information about the health of the working population. There is potential for a significant contribution to individual health, to community health, and to the fund of general medical information. It is necessary that we give critical thought to the systematic accumulation and recording of the data and our methods of storage and retrieval. Only through such detailed thought shall we have the data in a form suitable for statistical analysis and evaluation. I have described briefly the collection of data and the methods for storage, processing, output, and retrieval used in our medical program. We use such techniques for administrative purposes, to determine the nature and types of the health problems that arise out of the work environment. Our system has the capability of acquiring nonoccupational health information on an epidemiological basis. Finally, I have described briefly a multiphasic screening-examination program, outlined some of the steps required for the evaluation of data and procedures, as well as some areas that may have a potential for statistical prediction of the probability of developing certain diseases. This effort would be impractical without our ability to use high-speed electronic data processing equipment.

INFIBULATION, POPULATION CONTROL, AND THE MEDICAL PROFESSION*

GERHART S. SCHWARZ

Chief, Radiology Services
Bird S. Coler Hospital

Professor of Radiology
New York Medical College

New York, N. Y.

THE term infibulation as used in this presentation refers to the practice of drawing a ring or similar device through the prepuce or otherwise occluding it for the principal purpose of making coition impossible. In its wider sense, infibulation refers also to a variety of methods of occluding the female genital tract, but these will not be considered here.†

At this point it seems appropriate to explain how I, as a radiologist, became interested in this subject. It occurred during my previous work as radiologist at the Squier Urologic Clinic of the Columbia Presbyterian Medical Center where I had the pleasure of associating with Dr. John Lattimer and many other urologists. My radiological activities were confined almost exclusively to urology during those four stimulating years, and I owe the urologists a great debt for many a radiologic inspiration.

The immediate occasion for concern was my performing cineroentgen studies of the bladder and urethra regularly on children and my noticing that a high dose of radiation was delivered to their gonads. In an attempt to design a gonadal radiation shield, I reviewed all United States patents for genital protectors and found among them to my

---

*Presented at a meeting of the Section on Historical Medicine, January 28, 1970.

†Female infibulation is a widespread custom affecting probably many million women in Central Africa. It is a surgical operation usually performed on girls at the age of seven or eight in which the labia are freshened and approximated to one another until they grow together thereby forming an impenetrable bridge [except for a small opening left for discharges]. Its purpose is to insure premarital chastity. Prior to the wedding night it is opened again by a midwifelike surgeon. Infibulation of this type is the mark of upper class breeding, a means of becoming eligible for marriage. With the advent of the African female student at European Universities quite a number of infibulated women have been seen by European gynecologists recently.[1] The custom is most prevalent today in East Africa and Africa south of the Nile cataracts, among Nubians, Bedschas, Gallas, Somalis, Harraris, and Danakils. It is also performed in Malaysia from 10 to 15 years of age. It is said to have been carried into Africa by the Arabs.[2] Though declared illegal in Sudan 20 years ago, infibulation continues to be practiced widely there today.[3]

amazement a large number of devices for the prevention of masturbation. Infibulation represents only a small segment of the material that I have collected since then.

The subject of this discussion may be divided into the history of infibulation and the history of population control, with the purpose of trying to find out where and when these two met and joined forces. It is best to consider first the physical anthropology of infibulation.

Male infibulation may be looked upon as the extreme opposite of circumcision. The ritualistic overlay which is associated with circumcision ceremonies has obscured the physical biological aspects of this custom. Infibulation originated probably in Central Africa, for Egyptians practiced it as early as 3000 B.C. It is widely accepted in Malaysia, New Guinea, Ceylon, and the southern portion of India. Members of the races who inhabit these areas possess—by our standards—an unusually long foreskin, which ends in a narrow tubelike extension. This may be classed as a mild phimosis, a muzzle that makes intercourse painful, disagreeable, or at least less desirable than it would be otherwise. Circumcision serves here to facilitate cohabitation and procreation and is generally performed at the age of 14 as part of a virility ceremony.

Conversely, the members of the European races who inhabit the northern shores of the Mediterranean Sea are born with a short prepuce which rarely covers the glans completely. Among them a desire developed to have the preputium longer than nature had provided and to have it cover the glans. In the Etrusco-Greek civilization a code of modesty and morality thus developed which prescribed that the glans penis had to be covered at all times when a person appeared naked in public. In that culture athletes who performed publicly and disrobed customarily wore a leather band which was either wound around the tip of the prepuce or extended through two preputial perforations. When drawn tight it caused the prepuce to cover the glans completely, thus serving the rules of propriety. In contemporary literature this device is generally referred to as *kynodesme*. The ancient Greeks used this word as a jocular term because of its meaning "dog chain." The proper word for it was *angtera*, i.e., fastener—a term which was later applied to the metallic fibula. It is reasonable to assume that the English word anchor (e.g., ship's anchor) possesses the same root. Its scientific Latin terms is *ligatura praeputialis* or *praeputii*.

An example is a bronze statuette of an Etruscan boxer 9 cm. high, now owned by the British Museum.[4] Here the leather string serves not only to occlude the prepuce but also to secure the penis to the fighter's loin. Another illustration of the Greco-Etruscan custom is found on the back of an Etruscan mirror (Figure 1) now housed in the Museo Gregoriano in Rome. It depicts Atalanta and Peleus* The preputial ligature of Peleus can be seen quite clearly.[5]

There are many paintings and incised† pictures on Greek vases and Etruscan mirrors that depict the use of the *kynodesme*. Suffice it to mention here two more examples, one of which illustrates the manner in which the *angtera* was applied. It appears on a kylix-crater (a large drinking vessel corresponding in size to a small contemporary punch bowl) found in Capua in 1878 and now housed in the vase collection of the Berlin Antiquarium.[6]

The other is the Ficoroni Cysta,‡ which is considered the finest specimen of its kind. Here, the fight between Amykos and Polydeukes (Pollux) is shown with both combatants wearing the *angtera*[7] (Figure 2).

A life-sized statue depicting Anacreon is a more controversial relic representing a man wearing a preputial ligature. It is housed in the Nye Carlsberg Collection of the Glypthothek in Copenhagen. The actual ligature does not show, only its effect.§

The Romans, who succeeded the Etruscans, applied their engineering

*According to Greek mythology Atalanta of Arcadia was a princess who would give her hand in marriage only to the man who would conquer her in physical combat. Peleus, the father of Achilles, did not win the battle; another suitor, Meilanion (Hippomenes, according to another version), won the race with her by dropping three golden apples along the course. Atalanta could not resist the temptation to stop and pick them up, proving thereby that the weakness of woman is not always physical. There is controversy among archeologists as to the identity of the male figure; some believe it represents Pelias, a son of Poseidon. The specimen is slightly damaged and only the first three letters "Pel" are clearly legible. The motif of the legend is not unique. The story of Brunnhilde in the Niebelungen saga is similar. Further, Achilles, according to the Iliad, fought and killed Penthesilea, the queen of the Amazons, despite the fact that he was in love with her.

†Incised: archeological term for engraved (eingeritzt).

‡The cysta is an Etruscan toilet vessel dated ca. 400 B.C., a cylindrical vessel of the size and shape of a modern umbrella stand. It was found near Lugano in 1745, purchased by a Mr. Ficoroni and donated to the Kirchnerian Museum of Rome (Museo del Collegio Romano). It is now listed as in the Museo Guilia of Rome. According to the story, Pollux (one of the Argonauts) wanted to replenish the water supply of his ship Argo on the Bithynian Coast but Amykos, the king of the Bebrythians, would not let the sailors have it until Pollux tied him to a tree.

§Anacreon, born in the 6th century B.C. in Theos, Asia Minor, is Greece's best known poet and singer of love songs, most of which have been preserved and translated into modern languages.

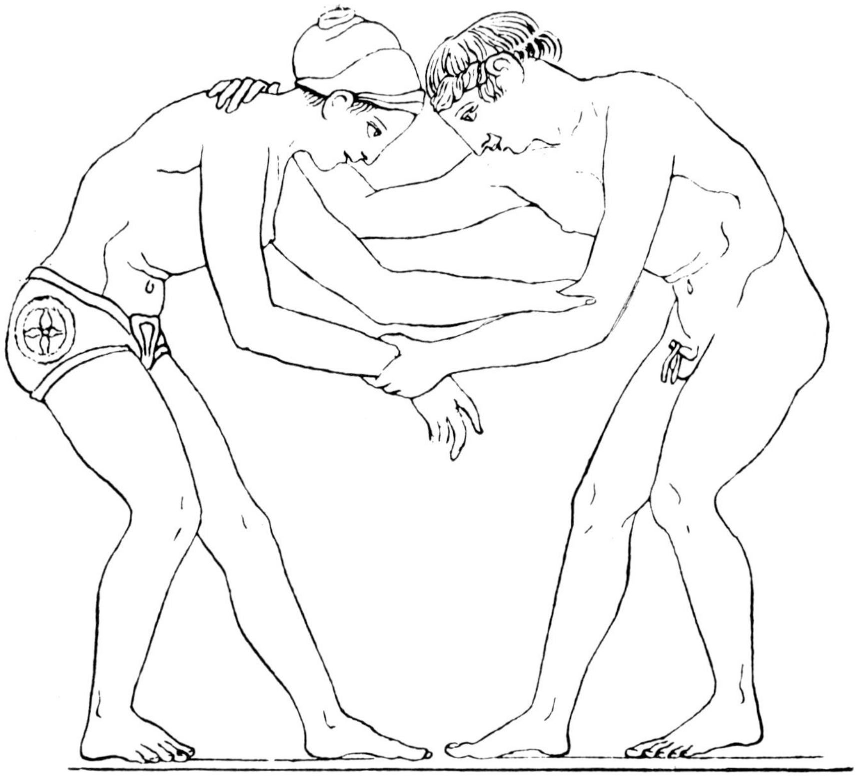

Fig. 1. Etruscan mirror depicting fight between Atalanta and Peleus. Reproduced from Stieda, L.: Die Infibulation bei Griechen and Römern. *Anat. Hefte 9,* 1902.

talents to this practice and devised the true fibula. The Latin term fibula connotes any closing device such as a clasp, clamp, clip, safety pin, brooch, or ring. Infibulation was commonly accomplished by inserting a metal ring, usually made of silver, through two perforations in the prepuce. Its ends were welded together by a *faber* or silversmith. If it was attached in this manner it could not be removed by its wearer; the penis was permanently locked, thus preventing any sexual activity. According to Celsus[8] its two main purposes were: 1) "to preserve the voice" and 2) *valetudinis causa.* Aulus Aurelius Cornelius Celsus, the best known Roman writer on medical subjects and proponent of Hippocratic medicine, though not a physician himself,[9] did not doubt that the change of voice could be delayed by infibulation. In the 19th century such a notion was ridiculed as "unscientific." Yet contemporary statistics show that the onset of puberty and menarche has advanced in

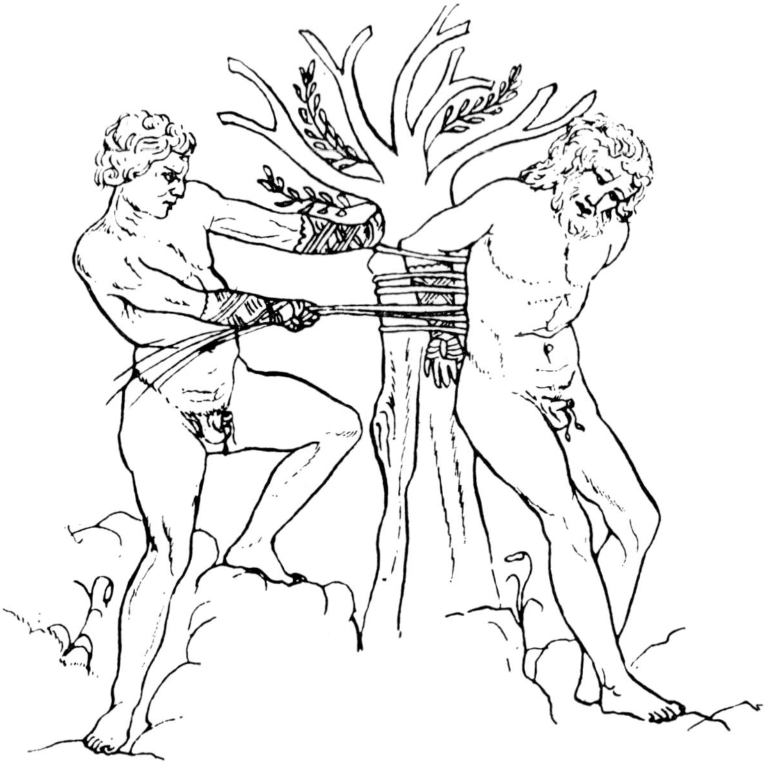

Fig. 2. Picture on the Ficoroni Cysta. Fight between Amykos and Polydeukes, both wearing *knyodesme*. Reproduced from Stieda, L.: Die Infibulation bei Griechen and Römern. *Anat. Hefte 9,* 1902.

the Western world by up to two years in the past 50 years. This is attributed in part to improved nutrition and in part to the constant exposure of our children to sexually stimulating pictures in advertisements, motion pictures, and television.[10] It is now being argued that sexual maturation is governed by a neurohormonal mechanism. Celsus may have been right after all.

As to the second reason (*valetudo*) more questions may be raised. Valetudo means health as well as morality. As far as health is concerned, Celsus may have been referring to masturbation. As far as morality is concerned more information is available. Indeed in the middle period of the Roman Empire, police prefects in some cities decreed that in order to prevent lewdness only infibulated actors and cither players (*citharoidei*) might appear in public.

Another form of temporary voluntary infibulation developed among

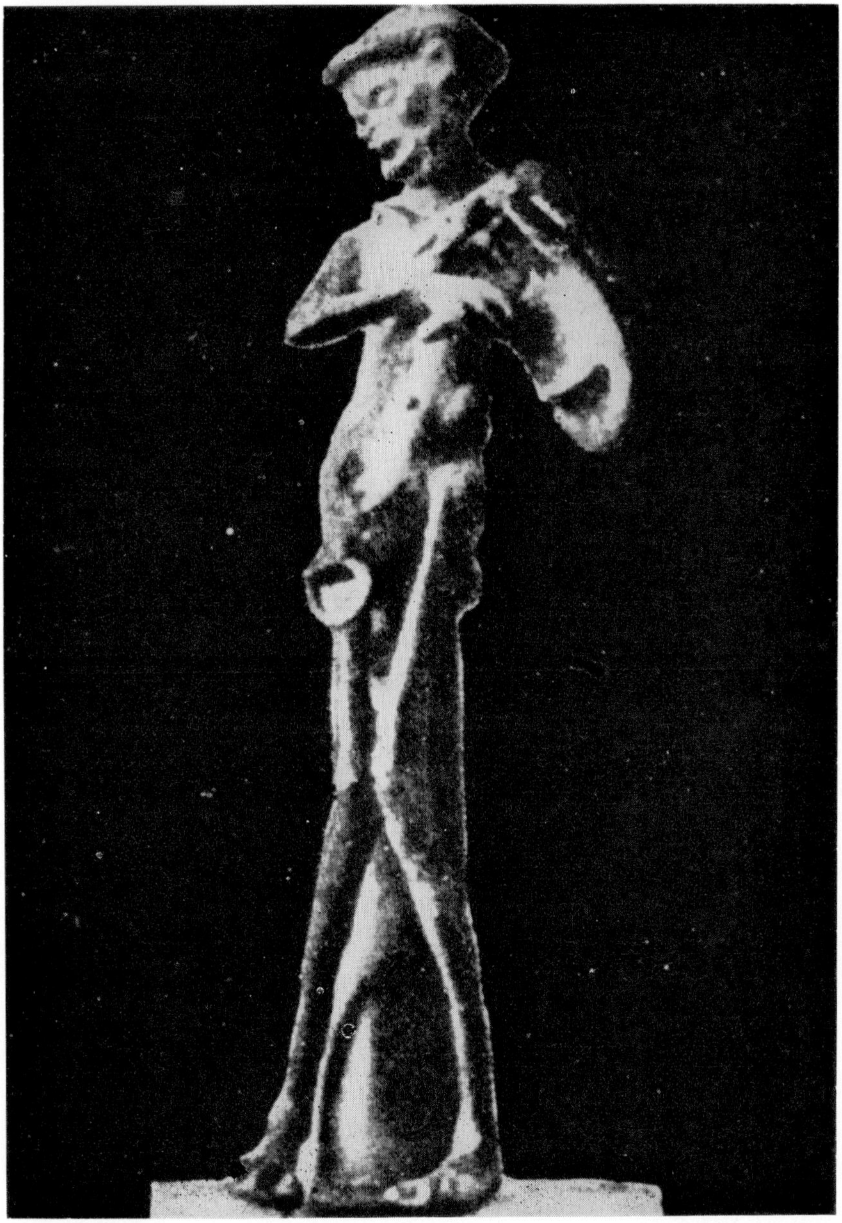

Fig. 3. Bronze statuette of an infibulated Roman cither player. Reproduced from *Bilderlexikon der Erotik,* vol. 1. Vienna, Leipzig, Kulturforschung, 1928.

athletes of the late Roman Empire. A richly decorated copper sleeve was placed over the penis and fastened to it by means of a cross pin which was drawn through two perforations in the prepuce. In this connection, the misfortune of Menophil (a Jewish performer) was commented upon in epigrams by five different Roman writers. Being circumcised, he had to attach his fibula by means of a clamp but, to his embarrassment, lost it during his performance.

An infibulated Roman cither player is shown in Figure 3. It is a bronze statue 10 cm. high which is preserved in the Kirchnerian Museum* at Rome. Line drawings of it have been published by Winckelmann,[4] Stieda,[7] and Hovorka.[11] The ring perforating the prepuce or the tip of the penis is slightly lighter in color than the rest of the statue. Another statuette has been overlooked by the Viennese archeologist and anatomist Hovorka[11] but described by Stieda.[7] It is a bronze statuette 9 cm. high of a man with African features. It is located in what was once known as the Royal and Imperial Court Museum of Vienna.† Here the ring is of the same color as the body of the statue. The origin of the statue is unknown.

Almost complete historical darkness covers the period that followed the fall of the Roman Empire. The intense religious convictions of the Middle Ages made references to the human body less frequent, and infibulation disappeared as a topic of writers except (according to unconfirmed information) in the Jesuit literature, where it was said to have been discussed as an instrument of morality.

With the advent of the Renaissance, however, it again became possible to depict the human body in detail. Moreover, the study of the ancient Greek and Roman culture was resumed, and it is not surprising that infibulation became evident again, as for instance in some of Michelangelo's paintings.[20]

Figure 5 shows a stone relief by K. Buchholtzen on the external wall of the Kaiserhaus in Hildesheim, Germany, dated 1580. The man depicted here is obviously infibulated.[13] The next pictorial presentation of infibulation appeared in England in 1650.[14] In his book‡ John Bulwer§ presents an illustration of an infibulated man as well as one with a pre-

*Now the Museo Preistorico ed Etnografico, L. Pigorini.

†Now the Austrian State Museum of Art and History.

‡The title of the 3d edition of *Anthropometamorphosis* was changed to *Man Transformed or The Artificial Changeling.*

§The author's pseudonym of Chirosophus, M.D., stands for John Bulwer, a London physician who invented a hand language for deaf-mutes.

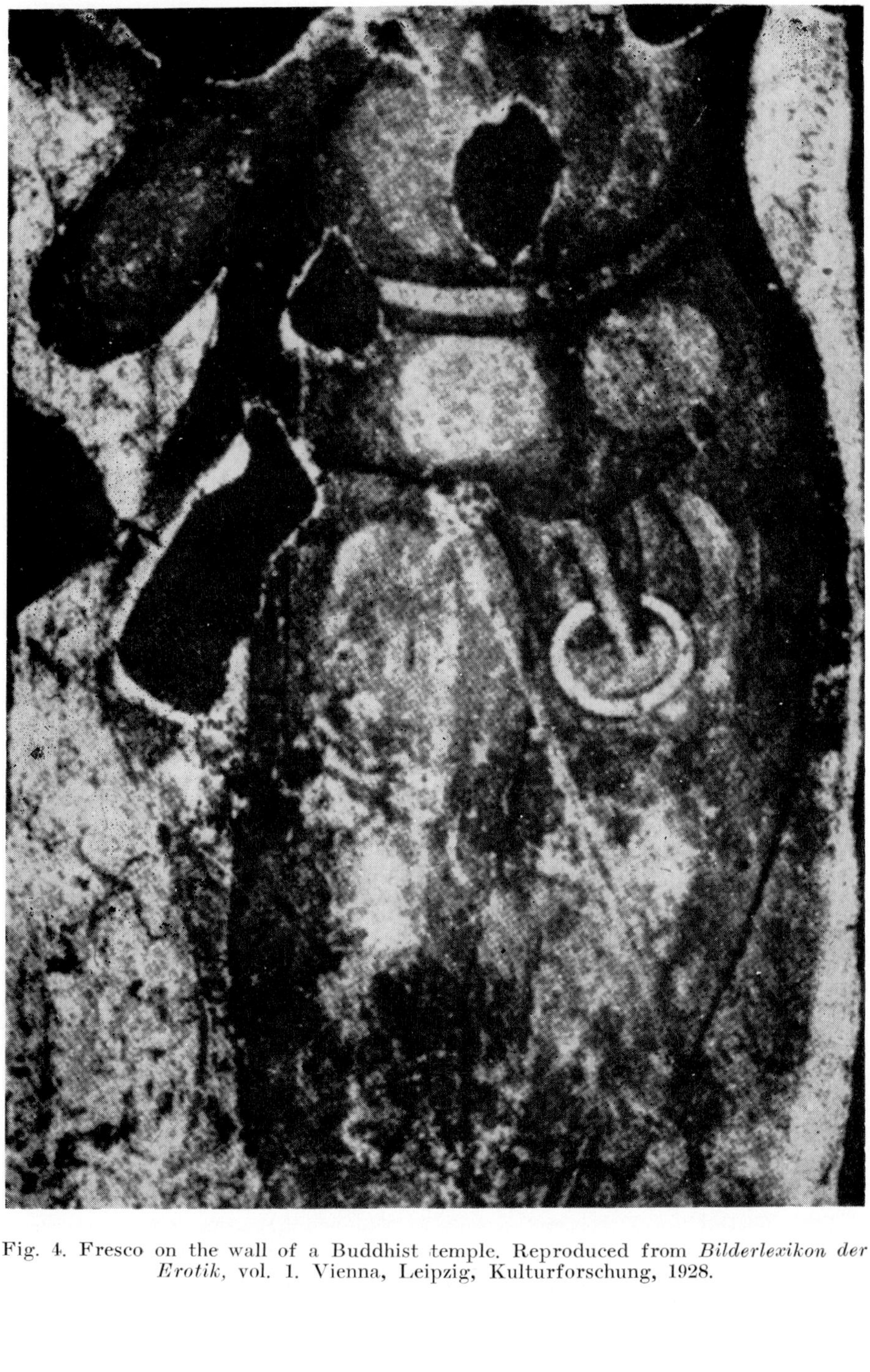

Fig. 4. Fresco on the wall of a Buddhist temple. Reproduced from *Bilderlexikon der Erotik*, vol. 1. Vienna, Leipzig, Kulturforschung, 1928.

putial ligature. However, he misunderstood the method which he describes as "buttoning up the prepuce with a brass or silver button on both sides of the glans, a kind of rationall invention. . . ." He mistook, most likely, the *ampallang* of the Dayaks or the *kambi* of the Alfurs, inhabitants of northern Celebes, for a method of infibulation. In actuality, this instrument serves the opposite purpose, namely, to increase sexual pleasure for the woman. A Dayak woman of Borneo may obtain a divorce if her husband refuses to undergo the operation. Several buttonlike ampallangs and kambis were depicted by Hovorka.[11]

Continental Europe was now emerging gradually from the shadow of the Inquisition. In the first half of the 18th century nearly every textbook on surgery and many other medical treatises contained a chapter entitled: Circumcision, Recutitio, and Infibulation. These three operations are placed in the same category not without reason. Though circumcision was rarely performed because of the psychological aftermath of the Inquisition, recutitio, i.e., restoring a foreskin or enlarging an existing but small one, was in great demand because its lack labeled the person so afflicted as an heretic or a Jew or a Mohammedan. Only 100 years earlier, this had been a matter of life and death.*[20] An example of the juxtaposition of these three operations is the book of Schurigius (Martin Schurig), 1720.[16] In his chapter dealing with these three procedures he describes in great detail the technique of applying the fibula. He attaches no value judgment to the operation, and the off-hand manner in which he discusses it suggests that it was more common than one would have expected it to be.

The same practice of treating circumcision, recutitio, and infibulation in one subchapter is evident in the most popular textbook on surgery of its time. In it Dionis,[18] personal physician to Louis XIV, chief surgeon to the dauphiness and to the duchess of Burgundy, describes the operation in sufficient detail to enable the intelligent reader to perform it. His book went through 11 editions and was translated into 74 languages, including Japanese.

He does not endorse infibulation unequivocally but recommends it

*The Inquisition was abolished officially by Napoleon as late as 1808.[15] However, it had ebbed considerably by the 18th century. The Inquisition was not the only institution, however, which imposed the death penalty for circumcision. In 168 B.C. the Seleucid Emperor Antiochus did likewise in an attempt to hellenize the Jews under his rule. Jewish athletes of that period underwent an operation called *"epispasmos"* (a form of stretching) reminiscent of recutitio.[20]

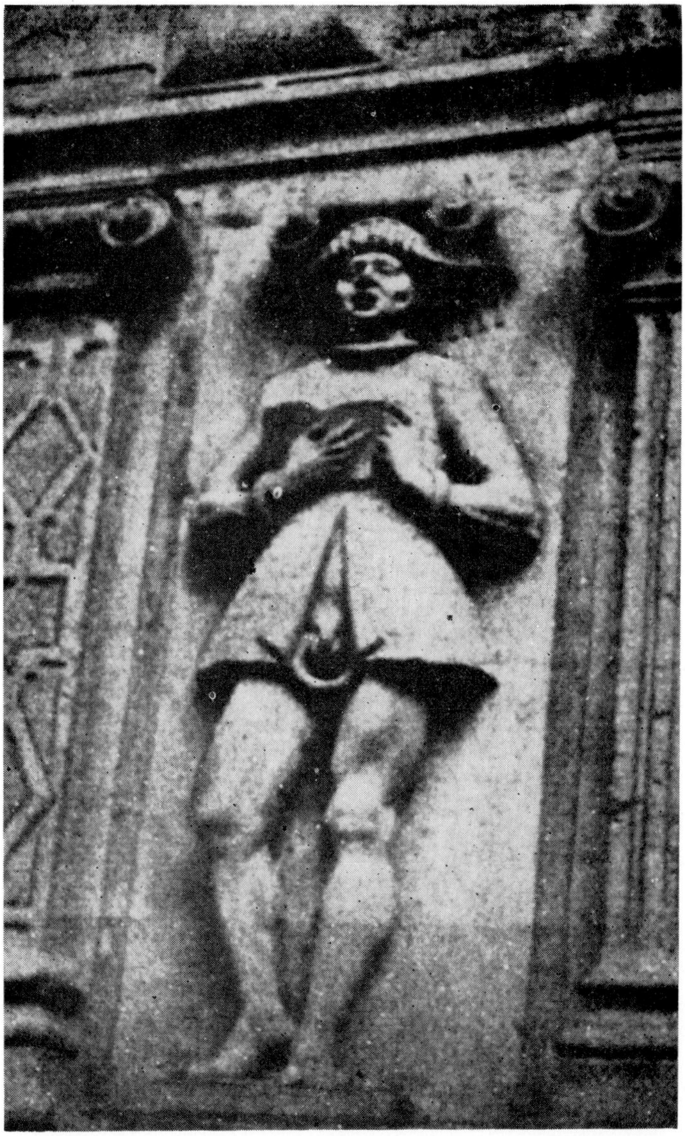

Fig. 5. Stone relief by K. Buchholtzen on the external wall of the Kaiserhaus in Hildesheim, Germany, dated ca. 1580. Reproduced from *Bilderlexikon der Erotik,* vol. 4, 1931. Vienna, Leipzig, Kulturforschung, 1928.

only for countries that have a hot climate: "These operations are not necessary in northern and temperate zones as they are in regions with a hot climate . . . where the fires of passion carry men early toward the embraces of love." As for the purpose of infibulation he may be regarded as the first physician who applied it to a demographic concept: ". . . it is maintained that this buckle prevents consort with women until the age of 25, which is the time of removal; the powers of these young men cannot dissipate and are preserved for the generation of strong children who will serve well the republic."

The term republic denotes "*res publica*" or "the state" but it remains as a portent of future events.* The concept of a republic as a system of society was just emerging as a conversational topic and the revolution was soon to knock at the door of France; this event would have a profound influence on the philosophy of population control.

Let us now turn to the history of population control, a vastly more complex event which can be discussed here only in the briefest manner.

Man interfered with the balance of nature unintentionally before he had any knowledge about the connection between intercourse and pregnancy. Circumcision and incision were practiced to facilitate copulation—as stated at the onset of this essay—and may be regarded as factors which have increased the birth rate in the Central African Belt beyond nature's equilibrium for the past 3,000 to 5,000 years.†

As soon as adequate biologic knowledge of the origin of pregnancy was available, society entered the stage of *intentional* population policy. Once such thinking was established, two trends developed: a desire to increase, and a desire to decrease the numbers of a given tribe, society, country, or empire. The history of population control oscillates between these two extremes. In the Bible we have the Lord's promise to Abraham, to multiply his seed "as the stars of heaven," as well as the well-known example of the Pharoah's ordering that all newborn males of the Hebrews be put away. Likewise, the Bible reports that in honor of the gods the Canaanites sacrificed some of their children in a fire. Infanticide was

*In the official English translation the term "commonwealth" was used.

†There still exist tribes in New Guinea which practice circumcision but are ignorant of the cause of pregnancy, which is ascribed to friendly spirits invading the woman. Since child marriage is customary there, menstruation occurs only under "pathological" conditions, i.e., a missed pregnancy, and is regarded as "the curse," the woman so afflicted is segregated. One might regard such a society as one which enjoys maximum and nearly total utilization of its generative powers.

a widespread practice which was still in force in China only a few decades ago. In ancient Greece, on the other hand, Lykurgos arranged for personal meetings between young men and women in order to induce them to marry. His intention was to increase the population. In ancient Greece and Sparta governments offered various inducements for having a large number of children and laws were passed ordering impotent husbands to solicit the services of healthy males to impregnate their wives.[63] In Sparta citizens with large families were exempt from military service and taxes.

Positive and negative legislation, i.e., laws designed to increase or to decrease population, coexisted in many countries. According to Demosthenes, Athenian law forbade marriage for men less than 18 and women less than 15 years of age. Spartans abandoned or cast out weak and malformed children on Mt. Taigetos. Sparta provides a classical example of legislation which tried to achieve quality and quantity at the same time by rewarding prolific families while eliminating sick children. Legislation in ancient Rome was designed largely to increase population but it fluctuated so greatly that a categorical statement about the attitude of the Roman Empire in regard to population control cannot be made. Women who had many children were rewarded by permission to wear a special dress. Pregnant women stood under legal protection and were protected against arrest and torture up to 40 days postpartum. Land of newly occupied countries was given only to Roman citizens who had more than four children.

In the middle ages the philosophy of Christianity influenced legislation in most European countries; however, its effect on birth rate is difficult to judge because of the lack of statistics, whereas in the preceding Roman Empire population statistics had been well developed. A more definite evaluation can be made of modern times therefore and it appears that since the start of mercantilism France was in the forefront of the effort to increase the birth rate. It was argued that the country with the largest number of citizens could export the largest amount of goods and collect the largest sum of money. In France a secondary motive was introduced later, namely, that of military competition with Germany, a motive that has not faded from the mind of its people until this very day. In general, since 1675 the French method consisted of tax relief and actual monetary awards for prolific families, but aristocrats were given higher awards than commoners.

A major change in methodology occurred through registration of births and deaths; this started with England (1537), France (1539), and Germany (1501 to 1595)[63] and depended on the principality that enacted such laws. It remained for the 17th century, however, to start a compilation and comparison of the birth rate with the death rate. In 1662 John Graunt, an English cloth merchant, created a new science by publishing a book entitled *Medicinal Statistics or Natural and Political Observations upon the Bills of Mortality Chiefly with Reference to the Government, Religion, Health, Air and Disease*,[17] London, 1662.

Sixty years later the medical profession entered the field of population control. Johann C. Kundmann, a Leipzig physician, reported in 1737 that the infant mortality in Breslau of 1722 was 43%.[72] The idea that the death rate could be favorably influenced by the finding and recording of the causes of death grew rapidly throughout Europe, and physicians were engaged to improve conditions accordingly. It was found that the infant mortality varied between 20 and 55% depending on the country; Sweden had the lowest rate and Austria and Italy the highest. Many governments took to the building of hospitals, orphan homes, and regulation of midwifery after this statistical fact came to light. Hygienic living was advocated and influenced by government edicts, particularly through Empress Maria Theresa and her successor, Joseph II. One of the most active proponents of government-imposed health measures was Johann Peter Frank (1745-1821), who advocated the creation of a "medical police" in 1779, for which he is justly called the father of public health.[19] However, this very Dr. Frank warned in his book of the dangers of unlimited population increase, which would produce "dissention, shortages and increase in misery with the effect that in a short period of time the useless heap of humanity would be annihilated by the stronger ones." He thus became one of the precursors of Malthus. It is to the credit of the medical profession that this proposal, which contained an objective, somber warning of the consequences of overpopulation, originated from a physician.

In 1784 the same Dr. Frank remarked in the second edition of his *Medical Police* that the spectacular growth in the number of physicians, hospitals, and orphan homes had done little to improve the situation. The training of physicians had become so poor "that doctors have done more damage to the populace than all the diseases together."

Other factors also began to favor reduction of the population. The philosophy of free trade initiated by Richard Cobden dispossessed the farmer in England and nearly abolished agriculture in Great Britain. Previously one of the major reasons for having many children in a family was the fact that they represented unpaid labor, which enabled the farmer to prosper. With the decline of agriculture this motive faded from society.

The proletarian who hired himself out to the manufacturer or mine owner lost the incentive for a large family as soon as child labor was restricted. In France and most of continental Europe the Napoleonic code, which prescribed that all sons of a farmer should inherit an equal share of his land, led to a subdivision of farms to a point at which farming could no longer sustain a large family.

The French Revolution favored a planned national economy. This became a new factor in the evaluation of the significance of the birth rate of a nation. The entire civilized world now began to fear the threat of the teeming hungry masses that assumed power. Referring to the threat of a French Revolution, Prince Kaunitz (1711-1794) warned Emperor Joseph II with the words: "An entire people in arms is in majesty equal to the Emperor."[21]

It is not surprising, therefore, that a man would appear at that time whose teaching has a decisive influence on mankind even today. He was Thomas Robert Malthus (1766-1834). Malthus developed the thesis that population increases geometrically while food and other means of subsistence increase arithmetically.[22,63] People would thus outstrip their own supply of food.* He believed that socialism would cause a rapid increase of the population and disturb the balance of nature. He was fatalistic toward the misery of the people and indifferent to the role of disease and held that eradication of one disease (such as smallpox by vaccination) would only make place for another plague. He had given up the ministry to become professor of economics at Haileybury College but his earlier training was reflected in the remedies he advised: moral sexual abstinence and repeal of the poor laws.

His theory found an echo in his counterpart at Oxford. Here, Nassau William Senior (1790-1864), professor of political economics from 1825 to 1847, asserted that when a group of people multiplies N times, the

*Malthus mentions as his spiritual predecessors: J. Steuart (*An Inquiry into the Principles of Political Economy,* 1767); Montesquieu; Benjamin Franklin; Arthur Young; and Townsend.

product of its labors increases only N-X times.[23, 63] He coined the term "law of diminishing returns" for it, which is still with us.

Europe, now placed in a philosophical pincer movement emanating simultaneously from Oxford and Cambridge, reacted predictably. It embraced Malthusianism.

In 1827, however, a physician arose who believed that morality cannot be trusted to produce sexual abstinence, particularly in the lower classes where it was lacking most but needed more urgently than elsewhere. He proposed a more reliable mechanical means, a special form of infibulation, which would be made obligatory, and inspected regularly by the state for the purpose of punishing those who broke its seal. His essay is probably the most curious document ever issued by a physician on behalf of population control.[24]

Figure 6 shows the first two pages of his 48-page pamphlet, *Von der Übervölkerung in Mittel-Europa und deren Folgen auf die Staaten und ihre Civilisation*, "Submitted in reverence to the Royal Prussian High State Ministry by the author." Dr. Karl A. Weinhold was Regierungsrath and Hofrath, recipient of decorations, professor of medicine and surgery at the University at Halle-Wittenberg, and member and honorary member of many societies. He does not mention Malthus but received his inspiration from an article by Hoffmann[25] which deals with the fear of overpopulation of Central Europe.

Instead of using a ring closed by a jeweler or secured by a padlock so that its wearer cannot remove it, Weinhold preferred soldering the ends of a wire together by means of a state seal. The official nature of the act, the seal of the government, and the fact that it would be impossible for the wearer to close the wire had he secretly opened it, emphasize the involvement of the state in population control. A new metal seal could be affixed only by the government as the only possessor of the mold or template. An illegal or unauthorized opening of the seal would be apparent immediately, therefore, and could be detected at periodic inspections. Inspection and control of infibulation were assigned to a judicio-medical authority. Likewise, punishment for secret opening of the metallic lock would be under the jurisdiction of an office in the lower courts.

". . . Opening of the infibulation, secretly and by force, which is likely to be undertaken by individuals of the age of 14-17 years, will be punished by flogging, regardless of the person. Opening by persons 18-24 years of age, however, will be punished by use of the treadmill which should be suited best to divert excessive sensual forces from the genital organs to the work-evading arms and legs. And those of the age of 25-30, especially those who repeat the offense, shall be punished by jailing on water and bread so as to ensure once and for all that society will not be caused to sink into poverty by the illegal lust of frivolous and sloven men. What crimes would thereby be prevented!!!"

Weinhold demanded that the following persons should be infibulated: 1) all beggars and all other impoverished persons living outside of matrimony; 2) all who suffered from long-lasting illness and therefore were not able to work, and who were already receiving alms from the community; 3) all male servants, journeymen, and apprentices in the cities and in the country; 4) all unmarried military personnel of the lower ranks; 5) since equality before the law has to be in effect in a free state, the genteel and often very unruly youth of the exalted classes cannot be exempt from punishment if they overstep the borders of morality, but will have to submit—with some modifications—to the same law.

Weinhold was opposed almost immediately by Siemerling[26] and Warhold,[27] and nothing has been uncovered in the literature that would indicate that Weinhold's proposal met with a favorable reception. It is proper, however, to continue the study of history beyond this event and trace the attitude of the medical profession toward infibulation as well as population control until the present time.

After about 1780 the medical profession accepted infibulation in slowly increasing degrees as a remedy and preventive for masturbation in boys.* To understand the spirit of the times it is well to contemplate Figure 7, from a copper engraving by Penzel that served as frontispiece to a book, *On Children's Immorality and Self-Pollution*, by a school expert.[29] It shows a father having his son swear, on the hand of the skeleton whose arm is extended toward the boy, that he would never indulge in self-abuse because it meant certain death. Below, it, a poem

*Broca, a Paris physician, used infibulation also on masturbating girls.[28] A five-year-old girl was so treated after a chastity belt made by Mr. Charrière had failed. The author felt that such belts are effective in boys only, girls succeed in circumventing them by inserting foreign bodies. Surveillance by mothers, chastity belts, and infibulation combined were thought to be effective in girls, however. In the discussion several physicians were doubtful and recommended clitoridectomy instead.

Von der

Uebervölkerung

in

Mittel-Europa,

und deren Folgen

auf

die Staaten und ihre Civilisation.

Von

C. A. Weinhold,

der Philosophie, Medicin und Chirurgie Doctor,
Königl. Preuſs. Regierungs- und Medicinalrathe, Ritter des rothen Adlerordens dritter Klasse, ordentlichem Professor der Medicin und Chirurgie an der Universität zu Halle-Wittenberg, der Kaiserlichen Akademie der Naturforscher, so wie einiger andern gelehrten Gesellschaften Mitgliede und Ehrenmitgliede.

Halle,

bei Eduard Anton.

1827.

Fig. 6. Two front pages of pamphlet by Weinhold, C. R. Halle, Anton, 1827 (see p. 981).

Dem

Königlich Preussischen

Hohen

Staats-Ministerium,

ehrfurchtsvoll überreicht

vom

Verfasser.

by von Canitz* is printed which in free English translation reads:

When vile desire casts its spell
Then through this picture filled with hell
Look at the dead bones with dismay
So that your lust may fade away.

---

*Friedrich Rudolf Ludwig von Canitz, German poet and diplomat (1654-1669). His poems were published posthumously in 1719.

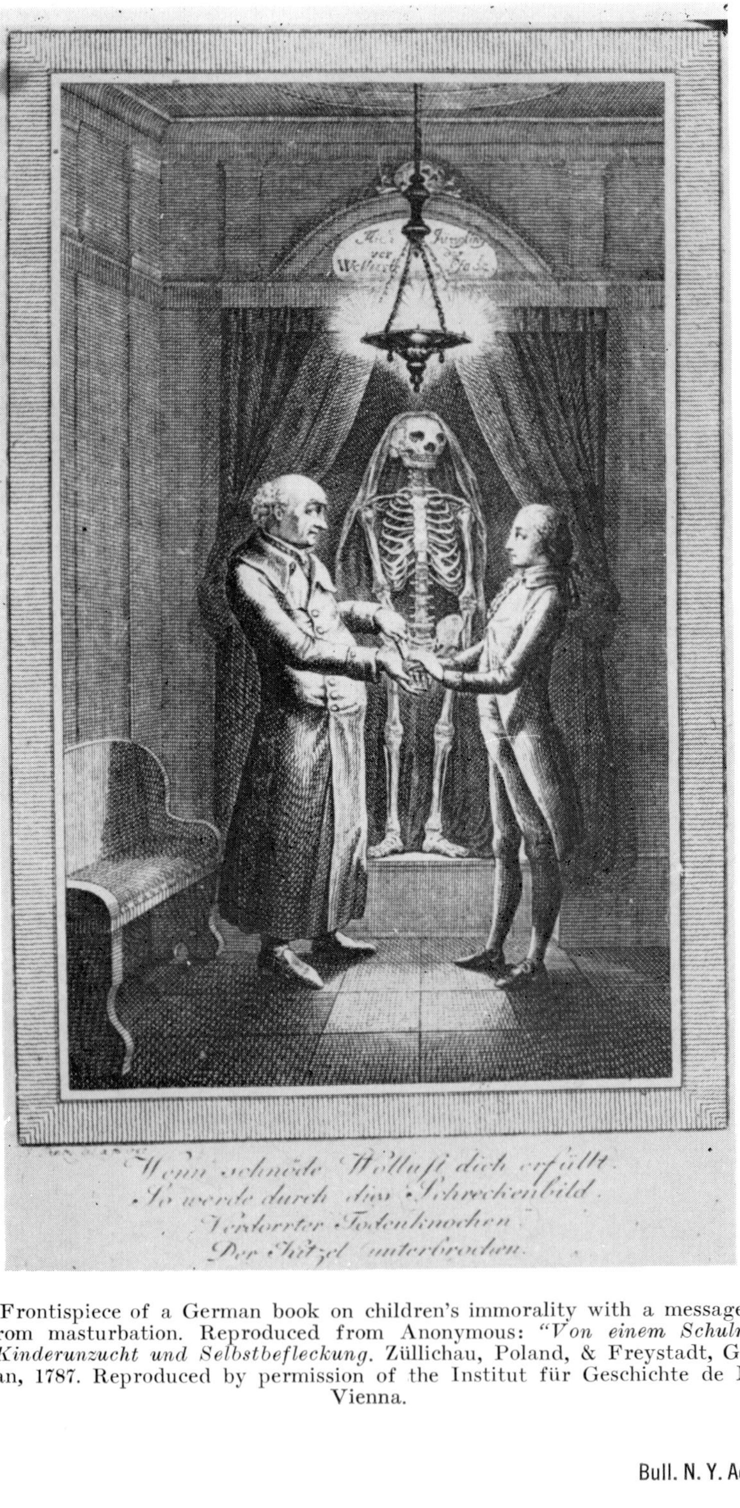

Fig. 7. Frontispiece of a German book on children's immorality with a message to abstain from masturbation. Reproduced from Anonymous: *"Von einem Schulmanne"; Ueber Kinderunzucht und Selbstbefleckung.* Züllichau, Poland, & Freystadt, Germany, Fromman, 1787. Reproduced by permission of the Institut für Geschichte de Medizin, Vienna.

This was the spirit of the times, and no physician of the 18th century would have denied that masturbation, unless stopped early, had lethal consequences. The most enthusiastic endorsement of infibulation as a preventive came, however, from a teacher. J. H. Campe edited, and mostly wrote himself, a 17-volume work dedicated to a reform of the educational system of Braunschweig.[30] In it he extols infibulation, which according to him already had been recommended to the public as "the most reliable preventative" by a Dr. Börner of Leipzig. Campe was introduced to this method by a bachelor colleague who was of robust build and in excellent health. When Campe congratulated him on his good fortune he showed him that he was infibulated: "I have worn my ring now for 15 years and have all reason to thank God that he had me find this means to secure my innocence, health and peace of mind."

Campe went on to say that he had a number of his own students infibulated by a surgeon without any adverse effect. According to Campe the usefulness of the method is threefold: 1) it makes self-abuse impossible, 2) it causes an erection to be painful, thereby suppressing lewd emotions, and 3) it is a reliable protection against involuntary seminal losses during sleep. Campe described a modification of the ring, designed to avoid pressure upon the glans (Figure 8). He concludes this chapter as follows: "What I regret is that this most certain remedy is applied only to half of our youth, namely boys, but not to children of the opposite sex."

His recommendation found an immediate echo in at least two physicians. Samuel Gottlieb Vogel, *Hofrat en Hoogleerar te Rostock*, according to the Dutch edition of his work, recommends it "in desperate cases." Though he disclaims personal experience with it, he praises it highly and prefers rings made from whale bone or tortoise shell to metal ones. He discusses several medical objections which had been raised and dismisses them with the words: "These unhappy people must be treated with the same attention as those patients who are in the highest peril. And indeed, aren't they? A victim of the black plague hardly is in as great a danger as such an onanist. . . . What little significance have they (the minor side reactions) compared to the disaster which is being prevented thereby?. . . . I ardently wish that more of those to whom Onanism has become an unfortunate habit from which nothing can drive them away would decide to accept this operation for their own sake as well as for the salvation of others!"[31a, 31b]

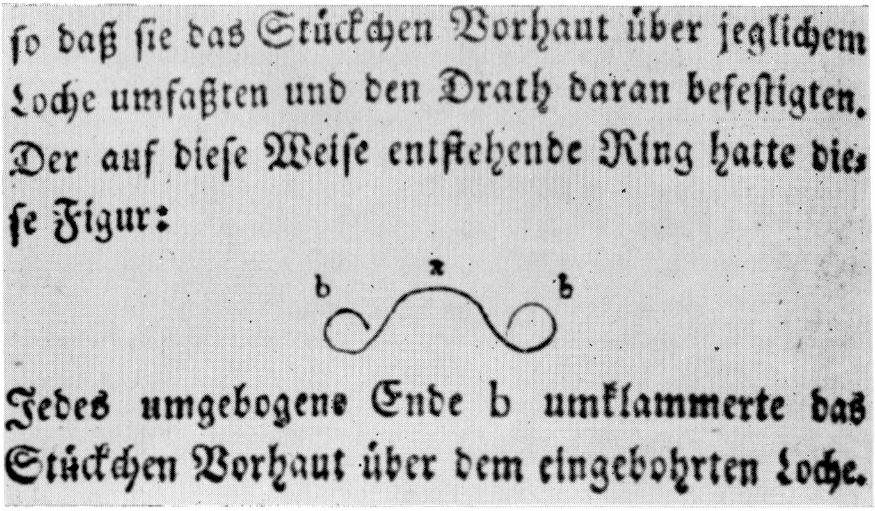
so daß sie das Stückchen Vorhaut über jeglichem Loche umfaßten und den Drath daran befestigten. Der auf diese Weise entstehende Ring hatte diese Figur:

Jedes umgebogene Ende b umklammerte das Stückchen Vorhaut über dem eingebohrten Loche.

Fig. 8. Campe's modification of the device for infibulation intended to avoid irritation. Reproduced from Campe, J. H.: *Allgemeine Revision des gesammten Schul und Erziehungswesens von einer Gesellschaft praktischer Erzieher*, vol. 16. Wolfenbüttel, Schulbuchhandlung, 1786.

Three years later J. C. Jaeger[32] also endorsed it: "It is still today both practical and useful for those young persons . . . since it occasions but little pain, can be done in a few moments and meets with the most excellent results."

In the first quarter of the 19th century public condemnation of the evil habit had risen to such a crescendo that German students formed associations, very much like the modern Alcoholics Anonymous, in which they openly forswore the degrading vice. Offenders were called before the executive committee to defend themselves. These societies, which also advocated a purification of the German race and claimed that masturbation was but a consequence of "French influences" (i.e., the former French occupation and the Francophilia of the ruling circles of that time), flourished between 1817 and 1821. Thereafter they were dissolved by various German governments as subversive but German physicians continued to extol the good that these organizations had done for the youth of Germany. Dr. Heinrich Robbi was one of their advocates[33] yet he did not fully endorse infibulation because "it produced a cure in rare cases only."[34] He preferred chastity belts and other mechanical devices,[35] and listed addresses where they could be bought. Others were more specific in their rejection of infibulation. An anonymous "practical Pedagogue," for instance, stated that several of his students succeeded in circumventing their infibulation by stretching its preputial bed and achieving ejaculation with partial erection so that he had to resort to encasing their organs in tubes attached to linen pants which prevented access by their hands.[36] The author claims to have invented this device but it had been described previously by the French orthopedist G. Jalade-Lafond.[37] A more medical argument against the operation was used by Marx, who reported scirrhous degeneration of the prepuce following infibulation.[38] Rust similarly reported a patient of Dr. Dupuytren* who suffered cicatricial contractions after infibulation.[39]

The height of the infibulation mania was reached toward the end of the 19th century when the solitary vice, as it was now called, was more severely condemned than ever before. Under the cloak of scientific enlightenment and rational detachment physicians the world over had fallen victims to the emotional appeal of Victorianism. To tolerate masturbation in a patient had become worse than performing an illegal abortion nowadays. It was not only a disease that had to be treated vigorously but also a crime that had to be punished by making the treatment painful, humiliating, and vindictive. Numerous treatments were added to infibulation by the highest medical authorities of that era, methods which possessed ethnographic significance. Among them were cauterization of the verumontanum, neurectomy, excision of the spermatic cord, castration for males, cauterization of the labia, clitoridectomy,† and "ovariotomy" (i.e., ovariectomy) for females.[40, 41, 47, 56, 58, 69] Since most of these measures led to permanent sterility, they assumed demographic importance. Infertility was considered a small price to pay for cure of the evil; it was not so much the welfare of the patient but that of the nation that was at stake. Victorian and Edwardian physicians felt that the vice was sapping the strength of the state. Lallenmand‡

*Baron Guillaume Dupuytren, 1778-1835, a surgeon known for his description of the scirrhous contraction of the palmar aponeurosis now named after him. It so happens that this Dupuytren's contracture of the hand is often associated with a similar contracture of the penis (Peyronie's disease) which is entirely unrelated to infibulation.

†It is probably no coincidence that the two most imperialistic countries (England and Austria) revived the same operation at the same time.[40, 41]

‡Claude François Lallemand (1790-1853), French surgeon, best known for his discovery of what are now called Bence-Jones protein bodies.

wrote: "... It is a menace to the future societies; therefore, it is urgently necessary for us to try and extirpate this public calamity."[44] Rohleder referred to it as the "most widespread people's pestilence *(Volksseuche)*."[51]

Though it is doubtful that these operations were performed often enough to have affected the birth rate in the Western world, another new feature of the Victorian masturbator's medical management did reach the proportions of population control: the patient was now being dissuaded from marrying. Marriage, once regarded as a most acceptable remedy, was now considered immoral and medically contraindicated. Many cases were cited in which the habit persisted even after marriage. Patients afflicted by this weakness were now warned that their children might suffer life-long debilities unless a premarital cure was achieved. It is not surprising therefore that they submitted to infibulation quite willingly as one of the less drastic methods available.

In 1876 Yellowlees, physician superintendent of the Glasgow Royal Asylum, played host to a quarterly meeting of the Medico-Psychological Association.[42] There he presented 12 patients which had been infibulated by him with "most excellent results." The first patient so operated upon had been wired for 18 days at the time of presentation. His mental state had improved so greatly that he now was able to work in the carpenter shop. "The moral effect of it in the house was excellent, and one man was seen weeping over his in anticipation," states the reporter. In the ensuing discussion two other physicians commented favorably upon this presentation.

Sixteen years later Dr. Yellowlees had another opportunity to express himself on the virtues of infibulation. He had become a contributor to Tuke's *Dictionary of Psychological Medicine* and was placed in charge of a five-column entry on masturbation.[43] Here he wrote: "When honest efforts fail and the patient declares in pitiful despair that he cannot forsake the vice . . . some direct operative interference may be of much service [He continues here with a description of his method of infibulation] . . . and a moral as well as a material victory has been gained." "To prescribe sexual intercourse as a certain cure for masturbation is wrong, both morally and medically. . . . The duty of parents as to warning their children against secret vice is delicate and difficult . . . but this risk seems small compared with the danger of allowing a child to contract, for want of warning, a habit so baneful and degrading."

Victorianism did not stop at the borders of the British Isles. Continental Europe displayed the same sentiment. In France it was Fournier who praised infibulation in successive editions of his book until at least 1893.[45] In Nothnagel's *Handbuch der Medizin* Fürbringer stated in 1895 that in Germany and Austria[46] "purely medical measures are not very successful though the physician faces yet many a thankful task here . . . such as (e.g.) perforation of the prepuce with introduction of a ring." He also recommends partial circumcision and the wearing of mittens and shackles at night but concludes that all these measures, including cages placed around the genitals, could be circumvented and that sanitaria with strictest supervision are the best treatment for "the little sinners." Since he believes that masturbation is the result of *excessive* sexuality he feels that marriage is contraindicted since it would lead to additional excesses. Unless the young man or woman is cured, marriage should not be contemplated. Further, to respond to requests by patients for help or advice in such matters as finding a marital partner "lies clearly outside the province of the physician." Supervision in schools is essential and corporal punishment is an "indispensible precondition for effective prophylaxis."

As in the case of Yellowlees, Fürbringer contributed an article on onanism to a German medical encyclopedia in which he expressed the same sentiment until 1911; by then he had added to the armamentarium also clitoridectomy for girls.[47]

The most representative work of those times is Rohleder's book: *Die Masturbation*. In his first three editions (up to and including 1912[51]) he endorses infibulation for difficult cases. At that time he still considered it a disease though he discounted exaggerated fears of its consequences and presented statistics showing that it is more widely practiced than generally realized. In the same year Moll[48] failed to mention infibulation though he described external penis rings, so called spermatorrhea rings, which awaken the patient at night by means of sharp points if tumescence of the penis should occur. This is, however, a purely voluntary instrument worn by those who want to be cured. Such rings were sold in most drugstores at the turn of the century; some were wired to set off an electric alarm at the moment of temptation.[55, 70] An autobiographical account of such a ring worn at night appeared recently. The ring was largely ineffectual "and sex won" according to the author.[49] The year 1912 probably marks the turning point in the history of infibulation, as far as Europe is concerned, for in his next edition (1921), Rohleder reversed his attitude completely. He states now: "All in all, clitoridectomy of the female, like infibulation of the male, remain operations no longer to be used."[50]

As the lights went out over Europe in 1914 the ghost of infibulation was put to rest. The medical profession turned to treating war wounds and checking epidemics instead. After the end of World War I, society refused to return to its old ways of life, and infibulation became extinct in Europe. An exception is a case reported by a German physician as late as 1929 in which a patient sought medical help for removing his own infibulation prior to his contemplated marriage. He claimed that he had been infibulated by a French physician several years previously for therapeutic reasons (see photograph).[57]

In the United States the popularity of this procedure commenced later and ended later. It was mentioned by physicians of this country mainly in the second half of the 19th century. In 1854 R. T. Trall, M.D., recommended a ligature for treating masturbation[52] and nocturnal emissions. In 1878 Bauer[53] reported a case in which dementia was cured by infibulation. It was necessary, however, to apply a second ring on the eighth postoperative day because the first one had been placed incorrectly and permitted the patient to relapse partially into his pernicious habit. References appeared in American medical journals to an occasional cure of epilepsy by infibulation,[54] but in general there was a preference for more complicated mechanical devices. Warren, for instance, favored such apparatus because according to him infibulation tended to cause balanitis.[59]

A definite endorsement of infibulation was expressed, however, by Winter[60] in a paper read before the Washington Obstetrical and Gynecological Society on February 7, 1902. When this author in his speech turned finally to the ultimate treatment "after muffling of hands and putting children to bed spreadeagle style had failed," he stated: "pierce the prepuce with a silver needle, the ends of which should be tied together."

Probably one of the last instances in which the procedure was recommended in the United States occurred in 1920. The title plate of this book is so remarkable that it is reproduced herewith (Figure 9). This publication is noteworthy for its exceedingly strong condemnation of masturbation, more reminiscent of the late Victorian period of Europe than that of the Roaring Twenties:[61]

NATURE'S SECRETS REVEALED

Scientific Knowlege of

The Laws of Sex Life and Heredity

or

EUGENICS

Vital Information for the Married and Marriageable of All Ages; a Word at the Right Time to the Boy, Girl, Young Man, Young Woman, Husband, Wife, Father and Mother; Also Timely Help, Counsel and Instruction for Every Member of Every Home

Together with Important Hints on

SOCIAL PURITY, HEREDITY, PHYSICAL MANHOOD AND WOMANHOOD

By Noted Specialists

Embracing the Story of Life and How to Tell It; Also a Department on Ethics of the Unmarried

By

PROF. T. W. SHANNON, A. M.

International Lecturer, Author of Self-Knowledge, Personal Help for Parents, Personal Help for Men, Personal Help for Young Women, Personal Help for Boys and Personal Help for Girls, etc.

Introduced by

BISHOP SAMUEL FALLOWS, D. D., LL. D.

Medical Department by

W. J. TRUITT, M. D.

Formerly Associate Professor of Obstetrics, National Medical College, Chicago, Assisted by Celebrated Specialists

---

PROFUSELY ILLUSTRATED

Published by

THE S. A. MULLIKIN COMPANY

Mullikin Building, Marietta, Ohio

1920

Fig. 9. Title page of an American health book for adolescents and newlyweds in which infibulation is recommended. Reproduced from Shannon, T. W.: *Nature's Secrets Revealed: Scientific Knowledge of the Laws of Sex Life and Heredity, or Eugenics.* Marietta, Ohio, Mullikin, 1920.

Chapter XV

Self-Pollution

By far the worst form of venereal indulgence is self-pollution or onanism or masturbation. And it is incomparably the worst for several important reasons:

It is wholly unnatural, and in every respect, does violence to nature . . . and causes the most ruinous irritation, exhaustion and debility to the system. . . . Children forming those ruinous habits when very young, become early victims and fall prematurely into the grave.

When Everything Else Fails, Then What?

When everything else fails we have no hesitation in recommending surgical treatment. This is of various kinds, from repeated blistering to that ancient operation . . . called infibulation.

Probably this marks the historical end of the method in the United States.

Let us now return to population control and examine its history after Dr. Weinhold's proposal and trace it briefly to the present time with special reference to the role played by physicians and those active in related fields.

Theory and practice rarely agree. At the time when all sociological factors favored a reduction of the birth rate, when the intellectual elite of France, England, and Germany clamored for birth control, and when even governments began to fear the ever-multiplying masses of discontented people, the population of Europe increased with great rapidity. There can be no question that the medical profession was largely responsible for this paradox. Though the birth rate fell and emigration to the United States rose, the total population of Europe continued to increase. According to Sundbärg its total increase was nearly 1% per year in 1830 and 0.6% per year in 1860. This is attributable to improved living conditions in the cities, for which physicians were largely responsible. Better infant care, improved obstetrical practice, the discovery of bacteria, better nutrition, and attention to hygiene, etc., began to have their effect toward the end of the 19th century. No wonder that an occasional Malthusian voice openly opposed the physician. Möser, for instance, wrote, "One should not take the pleasure of generation from the people but rather stop the doctor's handiwork" (as quoted by S. Peller).[63]

Some governments were *also* in favor of malthusianism. Prince von Oettingen, the cabinet minister, stated in the second Bavarian Chamber that laws to reduce the propagation of the lower classes by such means as hard-to-obtain marriage licenses, high marriage fees, higher minimum age of consent, etc. are necessary "in order to close the gates to the revolution."

Finally, in 1870 the Malthusian League was founded. This event may be looked upon as the most ironical development in the history of population control. This league was handicapped from the start because it had to confine itself largely to advocating birth control, i.e., contraception, since abortion, infanticide, and the withholding of medical care from the aged were morally and legally unacceptable. It so happened, however, that the birth rate had been dropping all along and little propaganda was needed to cause it to decline further. On the other hand, an even more ironical detour occurred when Germany invaded France only a year later and became victorious. By 1873 the entire Western world was in a panic. Forgotten were all the pious pronouncements of the malthusians; a new breeding craze set in no sooner than the Malthusian League had been founded.

In the forefront, as was to be expected, stood France, which had become the victim of what was thought to be Germany's biological vitality. Again it was a physician who rose to the occasion. The French physician Lombard presented a paper at a Medical Congress in Lyons in 1873 in which he demanded that married couples must not be permitted to sleep in separate beds.[63] In his opinion the entire future of France was at stake.

France has continued along the lines of this thinking. World War I confirmed her worst fears. As if she anticipated this disaster, she passed several laws in 1911, 1913, and 1914 to encourage the founding of large families. Monetary subsidies to pregnant women and to nursing mothers, reduced railroad fares to members of large families, low interest loans, tax reduction, and higher wages according to the number of children in the family, etc. were enacted. Since 1920 France has awarded bronze medals to families with five children, silver medals to families with eight, and gold medals to families with 10 living children. Likewise in 1920 a law for the suppression of abortion and contraception was passed.

The disastrous effect of World War II has convinced France now more than ever of the wisdom of these measures. At present a monetary subsidy makes it possible for any family with five or more children to live without working. The peak of positive population control was probably reached in Germany during Hitler's reign, however. There unmarried mothers received honorable government citations for their contribution to the German people, and their children were made children of the German Reich, thereby removing from them the stigma of illegitimacy.

Across the Atlantic, as well as across the Pacific Ocean, similar developments took place. For instance, New Zealand, which feels itself endangered by a possible Japanese invasion, rewards mothers for every child they bear. One week after delivery the mailman brings a check made out to the mother and handed over to the mother, not to the husband; this weekly allowance continues until the child reaches the age of five. Rich and poor alike receive these grants.

Of greater interest is the development of population control in the United States. The year 1873 marks the passage of the Comstock bill. This bill forbade not only the distribution of pornographic material by mail but also of any text or picture which would provide information on contraception or abortion. According to S. Peller[63] 23 states forbade information on contraception by 1930, 14 went so far as to prohibit even statements about where such information was available and, in 22 states, the possession of the means of contraception was punishable.

The medical and paramedical professions, however, never relented. It was a slow, uphill fight. Marie Stopes, a British paleobotanist, founded the first birth-control clinic of the British Empire in Manchester, England, in 1921.

Margaret Sanger,* a former nurse, wrote many treatises on birth control and was arrested several times in this country but was never convicted. The Margaret Sanger Clinic still exists in New York City. My own teacher, Professor Alfred Labhard, chairman of the Department of Gynecology and Obstetrics at the University of Basle, was a relentless and fearless preacher of birth control. Professor Alan Frank Guttmacher, a graduate of Johns Hopkins University and director of

*M. Sanger, born in Corning, New York in 1883, graduated from a nurses' training school in 1915. She was founder and editor of *Woman Rebel,* later *Birth Control Review,* and author of *My Fight for Birth Control,* 1931, and of *Margaret Sanger: An Autobiography,* 1938.

the Department of Gynecology and Obstetrics at The Mount Sinai Hospital, has popularized the concept of family planning and has created an international organization that started in New York City, called the Planned Parenthood of America Association.

And now a brief comment on where we stand today. We have moved deliberately from the physician to the medical student. We feel that birth control together with many other aspects of population control will be ours to guide and implement *only* if we involve ourselves in this subject deeply and earnestly. This will best be accomplished if we expose the medical student to demographic thinking, just as I was influenced by Professor Labhard in my own student days. This step has now been undertaken on a grand scale.

From March 23 to 26, 1969, The Institute on Medical Education and Family Planning convened in Washington, D.C., under the auspices of the Association of American Medical Colleges and the Division of International Medical Education. This meeting was supported by the Agency for International Development, The Rockefeller Foundation, and the Pan American Health Organization. Its proceedings were reprinted in a special supplementary issue of the *Journal of Medical Education*[62] and represent a milestone in the history of family planning. In his introduction Dr. Robert J. Glaser, chairman of the Executive Council and Assembly of the Association of American Medical Colleges stated: "Since the dire predictions of Malthus, the importance of the population issue has been alternately ignored and widely debated. Today the situation seems crystal clear: barring a nuclear holocaust, there is no alternative to famine in some parts of the world. . . . Today it [family planning] is almost universally accepted, tacitly or officially. . . . We believe the Institute will have a wide impact in this country and abroad in helping to focus attention on aspects of family planning that should be the particular concern of those responsible for the education of tomorrow's physicians."

This special issue contains more than 50 separate entries such as articles, reports, statistics, methods, experiences, discussions, and resolutions pertaining to the United States as well as many foreign countries.

I believe that the medical profession has arrived at a conscious commitment to population control. Whether it will persistently favor an increase or a decrease in population or will fluctuate between the two extremes only the future will tell. One thing is certain, however: very few physicians of the future will escape confrontation with this problem.

ACKNOWLEDGMENTS

For their help in providing me with essential material thanks are expressed to the staff of the Library of the New York Academy of Medicine, as well as to Miss Cecile E. Kramer, Miss Eva H. Eckert, and Mr. Philip J. Weimerskirck of the Medical Library of the Columbia-Presbyterian Medical Center; Mr. Adolph Placzek, director of the Avery Library for Art and Architecture at Columbia University; Professor Erna Lesky, chairman of the Institute for History of Medicine, University of Vienna; and Mrs. Gina Buika, director of the Medical Library, New York Medical College, Center for Chronic Disease, Bird S. Coler Hospital.

CITED REFERENCES

1. Stiegler, R.: Personal communication, 1969.
2. Eulenburg, A., ed. *Real-Enzyklopädie der gesamten Heilkunde.* Vienna, Leipzig, Urban und Schwarzenberg, 1896, 3d. ed., vol. 11, esp. pp. 538-39.
3. Huber, A.: Die weibliche Beschneidung: Tropenmed. *Parasit. 20:*1-9, 1969.
4. Winckelmann, J. J.: *Monumenti antichi inediti spiegati ed illustrati,* 2d ed. Rome, C. Mondacchini, 1821. As quoted by Dingwall,[65] p. 61, and by Stieda,[7] p. 308.
5. Gerhard, E.: *Etruskische Spiegel,* Part II (esp. pp. 212, 213, plate CCXXIV). Berlin, Reimer, 1843. As quoted by Stieda,[7] p. 307.
6. Klein, W. K.: Krater aus Kapua. *Arch. Ztg. 37:*31-33, plate 4, 1879. As quoted by Stieda,[7] p. 307.
7. Stieda, L.: Die Infibulation bei Griechen und Römern. *Anat. Hefte 19:*240-09, 1902.
8. Celsus, A. C.: *De Medicina.* Daremberg, L., ed. Leipzig, Teubner, 1859, vol. 7, chap. 15: p. 385.
9. Kelly, E. C.: *Encyclopedia of Medical Sources.* Baltimore, Williams & Wilkins, 1948.
10. Tanner, J. M.: Age at Onset of Puberty and the Trend Toward Earlier Maturation. In: *Endocrine and Genetic Diseases of Childhood.* Gardiner, L. I., ed. Philadelphia, Saunders, 1969.
11. Hovorka, O.: Verstümmelungen des männlichen Gliedes bei einigen Völkern des Alterthums und der Jetztzeit, mit besondered Berücksichtigung der sogenannten Infibulation und Kynodesme. *Mitt. Anth. Gesellschaft* (Wien) *24:* 133-34, 1894.
12. *Bilderlexikon der Erotik.* Institut f. Sexualforschung, Vienna. Vienna, Leipzig, Kulturforschung, 1928, vol. 1, plate 147, p. 489.
13. Ibid, vol. 4: p. 318, 1931.
14. Cognomento Chirosophus, J. B.: *Anthropometamorphosis,* etc. London, Hunt, 1653, pp. 353, 381.
15. Coulton, G. G.: The Inquisition. In: *Encyclopedia Americana 15:*147-48. New York, Chicago, Washington, 1955.
16. Schurigius, M.: Spermatologia. Frankfurt am Main, Beck, 1720.
17. Jones, H. W.: Public Health: In: *Encyclopedia Americana 22:* 758-763 (p. 759 re. Graunt). New York, Chicago, Washington, D.C., 1955.
18. Dionis, Pierre: *Cours d'Operations de Chirurgie,* 4th ed. Paris. Severin, 1740.

19. Frank, J. P.: *System einer vollständigen medizinischen Polizei,* new ed. Mannheim, Schwan & Götz, 1804, vol. 2.
20 Edwardes, A.: *Erotica Judaica; A Sexual History of the Jews.* New York.
21. Büchmann, G.: *Geflügelte Worte.* Berlin, Haude & Spenersche Buchhandlung, Max Paschke, 1919, p. 313.
22. Malthus, T. R.: Essay on the Principles of Population, 1798: In: *Encyclopedia Americana 18:*171. New York, Chicago, Washington, 1955.
23. Senior, N. W.: *Outline of the Science of Political Economics,* 1836.
24. Weinhold, K. A.: *Von der Übervolkerung in Mittel-Europa und deren Folgen auf die Staaten und ihre Civilisation.* Halle, Eduard Anton, 1827.
25. Hoffmann: Über die Besorgnis, das der Menschen zu viel werden könnten. In: *Neue Monatsschrift fuer Deutschland.* Buchholz, F., ed. 1827, pp. 198-220.
26. Siemerling, F.: *Gegen die Infibulation als ein von Prof. Weinhold vorgeschlagenes Mittel, die Übervölkerung zu hindern.* Stralsund, 1827. As quoted by Dingwall,[65] p. 56.
27. Wahrhold, E.: *Die Weinhold'sche Übervölkerung betreffend.* Halle, 1827. As quoted by Rust,[39] p. 587.
28. Broca, M.: Masturbation invéterée: Infibulation. *Bull. Soc. Chir. Paris 5:*10-15, 1865.
29. Anonymous (attr. to Schummel) *"Von einem Schulmanne": Über Kinderunzucht und Selbstbefleckung.* Züllichau, Poland & Freystadt, Germany, Frommann, 1787.
30. Campe, J. H.: *Allgemeine Revision des gesammten Schul-und Erziehungswesens von einer Gesellschaft praktischer Erzieher.* Wolfenbüttel, Scholbüchhandlung, Germany, 1786, vol. 16, pp. 218-25.
31a. Vogel, S. G.: Unterricht für Eltern, Erzieher und Kinderaufseher, etc. Stendal, 1786, pp. 132-40. As quoted by Rust,[39] p. 587, and by Dingwall,[65] p. 51.
31b. *Onderwys for Onders, Opvoeders en Opzieners von Kinderen,* etc. Haarlem, Loosjes, 1790, pp. 126-139.
32. Jaeger, J. C.: Grundriss der Wund-Arzneykunst: 124. Frankfurt am Main, 1789, p. 124. As quoted by Dingwall,[65] p. 51.
33. Robbi, Heinrich: *Die Veranlassung zur Selbstchwächung bei der männlichen und weiblichen Jugend und ihre traurigen Folgen.* Dresden & Leipzig, Arnoldische Buchhandlung, 1827, pp. III-IV.
34. Ibid, p. 57.
35. Ibid, p. 53, footnote.
36. Anonymus: *Von einem praktischen Pädagogen: Über die Behandlung der Unarten, Fehler und Vergehungen der Jugend, Sowohl im älterlichen Hause als in der Schule, nebst der Beschreibung eines durch Erfahrung begründeten neu erfundenen, mechanischen Heilmittels gegen die Onanie oder Selbstbefleckung.* Graudenz (now Grudziadz, Poland), Röthe, 1829.
37. Jalade-Lafond, G.: *Considérations sur la Confection de Corsets et de Ceintures, Propres à s'opposer à la Pernicieuse Habitude de L'Onanisme.* Paris, Méquignon-Marvis, 1818.
38. Marx: Infibulation suivie de la dégéneration squirreuse due prépuce. *Report Gen. d'Anat. Physiol., Path.* (Paris 4): 114, 1827. As quoted by Dingwall,[65] p. 54.
39. Rust, J. N.: *Theoretisch-praktisches Handbuch der Chirurgie.* Berlin, Enslin, and Vienna, Gerold, 1833, vol. 9, pp. 584-87.
40. Braun, G.: Die Amputation der Clitoris und Nymphen; ein Beitrag zur Behandlung des Vaginismus. *Wein. Med. Wschr. 15:*1325-28, 1865.
41. Brown, I.: *On the Curability of Certain Forms of Insanity, Epilepsie and Hysteria in Females.* London, Hardwicke, 1866.
42. Quarterly Meeting of the Medico-Psychological Association held at Glasgow, 1876. *J. Ment. Sci. 22:*336-37, 1876 (Yellowlees).
43. Tuke, D. H., ed. *A Dictionary of Psychological Medicine.* London, Churchill, 1892, vol. 2, pp. 784-86.
44. Lallemand, C. F.: *Des Pertes Seminales Involontaires.* Paris, Bechet, 1838-1842, 3 vols.

45. Fournier, H.: De L'Onanisme. Paris, Baillière, 1893.
46. Fürbringer, P.: *Die Störungen der Geschlechtsfunktionen des Mannes.* Vienna, Hölder, 1895.
47. Eulenburg, A., ed.: Real-Enzyklopädie der gesamten Heilkunde, 4th ed. Vienna, Leipzig, Urban & Schwarzenberg, 1911, vol. 11, pp. 51-63.
48. Moll A., ed.: *Handbuch der Sexualwissenschaften.* Leipzig, Vogel, 1912, vol. 16, pp. 627-721.
49. Blackburn, T.: *A Clip of Steel.* London, MacGibbon & Kee, 1969.
50. Rohleder, H.: *Die Masturbation,* 4th ed. Berlin, Kornfeld, 1921, esp. p. 356.
51. Rohleder, H.: *Die Masturbation,* 3d ed. Berlin, Fischer, 1912.
52. Trall, R. T.: *Home-Treatment for Sexual Abuses, A Practical Tractise.* New York, Fowlers & Wells, 1854.
53. Bauer, L.: Dementia brought on by excessive self-abuse—cure by infibulation. *St. Louis Clin. Record 4*:271-73, 1878.
54. Bauer, L.: Infibulation as a remedy for epilepsy and seminal losses. *St. Louis Clin. Rec. 6*:163-65, 1879.
55. Mayes, J. A.: Spermatorrhea treated by the lately invented rings. *Charleston Med. J. Review 9*:351-53, 1854.
56. Eyer, A.: Clitoridectomy for the cure of certain cases of masturbation in young girls. *Int. Med. Mag.: 3*:259-262, 1894-1895.
57. Levy-Lenz: Ein Fall von Infibulation bei einem infantilen. *Med. Klinik* (Berlin) *25*:1619-1620, 1929.
58. Haynes, T.: Surgical treatment of hopeless cases of masturbation and nocturnal emissions. *Boston Med. Surg. J. 109*:130, 1883.
59. Warren, C. E.: Genocatachresia. *St. Louis Med. Surg. J. 63*:73-77 and 206-207, 1892.
60. Winter, J. T.: Self-abuse in infancy and childhood. *Amer. J. Obst. v. 5*:828-34, 1902.
61. Shannon, T. W.: *Nature's Secrets Revealed: Scientific Knowledge of the Laws of Sex Life and Heredity, or Eugenics.* Marietta, Ohio, Mullikin, 1920.
62. Family planning and medical education. *J. Med. Educ. 44*:1-246, 1969.

GENERAL REFERENCES

Most of the sources listed below have been referred to in the text in regard to specific points; therefore they are numbered consecutively as are other references.

63. Peller, S.: *Fehlgeburt und Bevölkerungsfrage.* Stuttgart-Leipzig, Hippokrates, 1930.
64. Hirschfeld, M. ed.: *Sittengeschichte der jüngsten Zeit.* Geburtenregelung in der Nachkriegszeit. Leipzig & Vienna. Sexualwissenschaft Schneider, 1931-32, vol. 2, pp. 317-57.
65. Dingwall, E. J.: *Male Infibulation.* London, John Bale & Danielsson, 1925.
66. Elster, L.: Bevölkerungslehre und Bevölkerungspolitik. In: *Lehr-und Handwörterbuch der Staatswissenschaften,* 2d ed. Frankenstein, ed. Jena, Fischer, 1899, vol. 2: 704-73.
67. Spitz, R. A.: Authority and masturbation; Some remarks on a bibliographical investigation. *Yearbook Psychoan. 9*: 113-45, 1953.
68. Hare, E. H.: Masturbatory insanity. *J. Ment. Sci. 108*:1-25, 1962.
69. Graham, H.: *Eternal Eve; The History of Gynecology and Obstetrics.* Garden City, Doubleday, 1951. (Re ovariotomy: pp. 520-22).
70. Milton, J. L.: *On the Pathology and Treatment of Spermatorrhea.* London, Renshaw, 1887.
71. Thompson, L.: A Self-Regulating System of Human Population Control. *Trans. N.Y. Acad. Sci. 32*:262-70, 1970.
72. Kundmann, J. C.: *Raroria naturae et artis item in re medica; Saltenheiten der Natur und Kunst.* Breslau & Leipzig, Hubert, 1737.

NEW YORK HEART ASSOCIATION

ABSTRACTS OF PAPERS PRESENTED AT THE SCIENTIFIC SESSION ON RESEARCH, HELD AT HEART HOUSE, NEW YORK, N. Y., APRIL 28, 1970

*Hypersensitivity Reactions of the Heart: An Experimental Model**

ROBERTO LEVI

Department of Pharmacology
Cornell University Medical College
New York, N. Y.

Electrocardiographic changes are relatively common in the immediate type of hypersensitivity reaction. Signs of altered generation and conduction of the cardiac impulse leading to arrhythmias have been reported. Ischemic changes, sometimes complicated by myocardial infarction, have also been reported.

An experimental model was developed to examine pathophysiological mechanisms involved, in the hope that this would lead to a therapeutic approach. Hearts of guinea pigs were passively sensitized *in vitro* by coronary perfusion with appropriate amounts of rabbit antiovalbumin. The hearts were then challenged with ovalbumin. Coronary effluents were collected and assayed for histamine content.

Sinus or nodal tachycardia and atrioventricular dissociation were invariably observed. Degree and duration of cardiac impairment correlated with the amounts of histamine concomitantly released by the heart. Electrocardiographic changes were always reversible, with the exception of few cases in which there was an irreversible reduction of the coronary flow. The cardiac effects of histamine released during the crisis of acute hypersensitivity could be reproduced on the sinus and atrioventricular nodes by the addition of histamine to the coronary circulation of nonsensitized hearts. Here too the effects were clearly correlated with the concentration of histamine.

This experimental model may prove to be a useful investigative tool in the treatment of cardiac arrhythmias caused by hypersensitivity reactions. *(Supported by the New York Heart Association.)*

*Dr. Levi's paper was selected by the Committee on the Scientific Session on Research of the New York Heart Association, to receive the Association's first annual J. Murray Steele Award, established in honor of the late J. Murray Steele, M.D., a director of the New York Heart Association, 1951-1964, for the best presentation before the Scientific Session on Research.

The Hypoxic Mammalian Heart: Metabolism and Hemodynamic Performance

C. Apstein, R. Gmeiner, and N. Brachfeld

Department of Medicine
Cornell University Medical College and the Institute for Muscle Disease
New York, N. Y.

The metabolic and hemodynamic properties of the hypoxic myocardium probably play an important role in ischemic heart disease, especially in patients with an acute myocardial infarction where the peri-infarction tissue may be hypoxic; the ultimate fate of this hypoxic tissue and its contractile ability may significantly influence the morbidity, mortality, and complications which follow an infarction. For these reasons the biochemical and hemodynamic performance of isolated working rat hearts was studied under aerobic and hypoxic conditions with 5.5 mM. glucose or 5.5 mM. glucose + 0.4 mM. palmitate as substrate.

Peak aortic systolic pressure was higher ($p < 0.01$) when palmitate was present for both aerobic and hypoxic perfusions. Under aerobic conditions, the presence of palmitate decreased the uptake of glucose by 15% and the production of lactate by 41%. With hypoxia, there was a mean increase of glycolysis of 100%; nevertheless, the presence of palmitate decreased glucose uptake by 48% and lactate production by 36%. Total palmitate uptake was reduced 44% by hypoxia, and its oxidation to CO_2 was decreased by 80%. Incorporation of palmitate into tissue lipid was increased by 90%, primarily into the triglyceride fraction. The presence of palmitate decreased the utilization of carbohydrate under both aerobic and hypoxic conditions, but this effect was much greater under conditions of reduced oxygen availability.

The site of inhibition also varied with the amount of oxygen available. Under aerobic conditions, glycogenolysis was markedly reduced, but the uptake of glucose was only slightly inhibited; with hypoxia the converse situation obtained, and the uptake of glucose was markedly inhibited by the presence of palmitate, but there was no inhibition of glycogen breakdown.

The presence of palmitate decreased the hypoxic stimulation of glycolysis (Pasteur effect) and improved hemodynamic performance. This phenomenon may have therapeutic implications in protecting the hypoxic heart against lactic acidosis without diminishing the energy available for contraction. *(This abstract is based on work supported by the National Institutes of Health Contract PH-43-67-1439 and Grant HE-06216, by the New York Heart Association and by the Muscular Dystrophy Association of America, Inc.)*

Myocardial Inceptive Excitability Threshold

D. A. Bloomfield and N. Kasirajan

Cardiopulmonary Laboratory
Maimonides Medical Center
Brooklyn, N. Y.

In contrast to the slow rise in excitability threshold in the first weeks of myocardial pacing, the threshold at the inception of pacing (I.T.) was found to fall rapidly. The I.T. was measured by use of a special stimulator with an accuracy of 0.01 mAmp. in patients undergoing placement of pacing catheters. Measurements were performed in sinus rhythm, acute or chronic heart block in a supine, awake, and fasting state. In all instances threshold levels fell over the course of 200 to 300 sec. of pacing to stable, reproducible base levels less than 50% of the initial values. Variation in prepacing rhythm, pacing rate, reversal of polarity, or duration of stimulus did not influence the trend of the falling I.T., and the phenomenon was repeatable with the stimulating electrode in different myocardial sites.

Similarly, while the difference between stable base threshold and the energy required to recapture pacing from subthreshold levels (R.T.) was only 0.02 mAmp, the difference at inception of pacing was usually greater than 0.2 mAmp. R.T. at inception was in the order of twice I.T. but fell, with the same time course at I.T. The paradoxical responses of facilitated excitation were not due to mechanical damage to cellular membrane, as a 10-min. interruption in pacing allowed the I.T. to rise toward its initial level. Also, typical falls in I.T. could be elicited from catheters in position for hours without pacing. Similar falls were not excluded by high-energy stimuli delivered during the refractory phase in sequential-pacing experiments in animals. The response was considered due to electrically induced local changes in transmembrane ion gradients.

Clinical Experience and Hemodynamics with Synchronous Unidirectional Intraaortic Balloon Pumping in Medically Refractory Cardiogenic Shock

D. Bregman, D. C. Kripke, and R. H. Goetz

Department of Surgery
Albert Einstein College of Medicine
New York, N. Y.

Although the over-all mortality of myocardial infarction has improved, patients in whom cardiogenic shock supervenes still face an 85% to 100% mortality from progressive pump failure. Intra-aortic balloon pumping (IABP) currently appears to be the most effective mechanical heart assist through its ease of application and its effectiveness in decreasing left-ventricular work and increasing coronary blood flow. We have developed a dual-chambered balloon in which a spherical distal balloon initially inflates and occludes the aorta. This is sequentially followed by the inflation of a cylindrical proximal balloon in the same diastolic interval, which pumps blood entirely toward the aortic root. We have clearly shown in dogs that this unidirectional system results in a 50% greater increase in coronary blood flow over and above that obtained with an omnidirectional single-chambered balloon of equal displacement.

Our clinical experience to date includes three patients in medically refractory cardiogenic shock for an average of 44 hours prior to assist, with a systolic B.P. below 80 mm. Hg and an average cardiac index of 1.01 $1/M^2$. One has been discharged and is well; one was successfully assisted for 15 hours but extended his infarct and succumbed; the third was assisted for 16 hours, became hemodynamically stable, but subsequently died 42 hours postassist. In our comatose patients the sensorium cleared rapidly, central venous pressure fell promptly (average 10 cm. of H_2O), and the average hemolysis was 3.2 mg%. The maximum dp./dt. rose significantly (average 83%) while the presystolic ejection time decreased (average 36%), which suggested a definite improvement in ventricular performance. All hemodynamic data are stored in a memory bank for instantaneous recall, which permits a prospective assessment of the clinical course and of the proper time to initiate and terminate assistance in a patient under study.

Use of the dual-chambered balloon holds promise for reducing the mortality rate of refractory cardiogenic shock which complicates myocardial infarction.

Left Ventricular Volume and Function in Congenital Heart Disease

WILLIAM J. DEELY AND AARON R. LEVIN

Department of Pediatrics
Cornell University Medical College-The New York Hospital
New York, N. Y.

Left ventricular end-diastolic (EDV) and end-systolic (ESV) volumes were measured in 6 normal children and 70 patients with congenital cardiac defects by use of biplane angiocardiography. The diagnoses included pure shunt lesions at atrial, ventricular, and pulmonary artery level, Fallot's tetralogy, pulmonary and aortic valvular stenosis, and mitral regurgitation. Stroke volume (SV) and ejection fraction (EF) were derived from measured volumes. Myocardial contractility index (MCI) was determined from left ventricular stroke work and EDV index. Patients with left-to-right shunts had above-normal EDV, ESV, and SV, which were greatest in ventricular defects and patent ductus. Fallot's tetralogy and mitral regurgitation also showed elevated values. Patients with semilunar valve stenosis fell within the normal range, though aortic stenosis tended to have longer volumes. Elevation of EF was present in shunt lesions but normal in all others except for Fallot's tetralogy, in which it was reduced. An inverse relation between ESV and EF existed for all entities, but for aortic stenosis, in which marked elevation was present, MCI was below normal. ESV, EDV, EF, and MCI were directly related to the severity of aortic stenosis. No correlation was found between age and any index measured. Cardiac rate was inversely related to EDV and SV in all but shunt-lesion patients. No correlation was noted between end-diastolic pressure (EDP) and volume measurements, though patients with aortic stenosis tended to have high EDP compared to Fallot's tetralogy, in which EDP was low.

Direct and Indirect Assessment of Left Ventricular Function in Coronary Artery Disease

B. DIAMANT AND M. SHAPIRO

Department of Medicine

R. FLEMING AND H. BALTAXE

Department of Radiology
Cornell University Medical College
New York, N. Y.

Left-ventricular (LV) performance is influenced by the extent of coronary artery disease (CAD). To evaluate the relation of indirect to direct measurement of LV function, 50 patients who had undergone LV and selective coronary angiography were subjected to left-ventricular end-diastolic pressure (LVEDP) correlated with indirect pre-ejection period (PEP) and left-ventricular ejection time (LVET). PEP and LVET were obtained from simultaneously recorded phonocardiogram, electrocardiogram, and external carotid pulse, and expressed in percentage of rate-corrected normal. Significant CAD was deemed present with $>$ 50% of lumen compromised. Patients were divided into groups: I, 3-vessel disease, 22 patients; II, 2-vessel disease, 12 patients; III, 1-vessel disease, 6 patients; IV, 0-vessel disease, 12 patients. LVEDP of Group I was significantly higher than that of III and IV ($p < 0.005$). PEP of Group I was significantly longer than that of III and IV ($p < 0.025$). LVET of Group I was significantly shorter than that of III and IV ($p < 0.05$). Correlation coefficient for PEP and LVEDP was +0.57 ($p < 0.001$). Presence and extent of CAD were found to influence direct and indirect assays of left ventricular function. *(Supported by USPHS Contract 43-67-1439, Myocardial Infarction Research Unit.)*

Noradrenergic Mediation of Cerebrovascular Spasm and Hypocapnic Vasoconstriction

R. A. R. Fraser, B. M. Stein, R. E. Barrett, and J. L. Pool

Department of Neurological Surgery
Columbia University College of Physicians and Surgeons
New York, N. Y.

Previous investigations in our laboratory, that have utilized the catecholamine fluorescent technique have demonstrated the presence of an abundant noradrenergic periarterial fiber plexus in intracranial vessels of monkey and of man. Our study of experimental vascular spasm in monkeys has revealed a marked depletion of this catecholamine fluorescence after repeated spasm. This has suggested the possibility of noradrenergic mediation of cerebrovascular spasm. This hypothesis was tested in 26 normal and 2 sympathectomized monkeys, using catecholamines and their releasing and blocking agents. The effects of these agents on hypocapnic induced vascoconstriction were also studied. Fluorescent histochemical examination of the vessels was undertaken at the conclusion of each experiment after photographic documentation of changes in vessel caliber.

Data acquired from this study indicate that blood applied to the adventitia of the normal vessel consistently results in spasm. A reduction of arterial pCO_2 also results in severe constriction of the vessels. Alpha adrenergic blocking agents in the subarachnoid space 1) produce dilatation of blood-induced spastic vessels, 2) render a normal vessel incapable of spasm, and 3) result in arterial dilatation above normal caliber. Hypocapnic arterial constriction is removed by alpha-adrenergic blockade. The periarterial noradrenergic fiber plexus is depleted of its catecholamines by repeated spasm, catecholamine-releasing agents, and by surgical sympathectomy. The latter procedure, however, does not modify the ease of subsequent induction of spasm.

These data suggest that vascular spasm of the intracranial vessels is mediated at the noradrenergic receptor, and that blood contains an alpha adrenergic substance capable of acting at the receptor site. Alpha adrenergic blockade removes or prevents the appearance of blood-induced spasm. Further, it is postulated that the periarterial nerve fibers exert a significant tonic, constrictive effect on the cerebral vessels as their pharmacological removal or blockade results in a dilated vessel. Finally, adrenergic blockade of hypocapnic-induced vasoconstriction implies that CO_2-induced changes in cerebrovascular tone may be mediated through the noradrenergic system. *(Supported by a grant from the New York Heart Association and by an NIH Special Fellowship to Dr. Fraser [F112203-01] and NIH Grant 1-T01-NB-05618-02.)*

Hemodynamic Studies in Heroin-Induced Acute Pulmonary Edema

K. Gopinathan, D. Saroja, J. Richard Spears, Arthur Gelb, and George Emmanuel

Department of Medicine
State University of New York Downstate Medical Center, Brooklyn, N. Y.

Pulmonary edema has been recognized to occur during acute heroin overdose, but its mechanism has not been previously studied. Six young addicts with clinical and radiographic signs of pulmonary edema induced by heroin underwent cardiac catheterisation within 24 hours of onset of symptoms. The pulmonary capillary pressure was normal in all patients. The average pulmonary artery pressure was 32/13 mm. Hg (range 23/11 to 54/19). The level of pulmonary hypertension was proportional to the severity of the subject's hypoxemia; breathing 100% oxygen lowered the pulmonary artery pressure to the average value of 22/8 mm. Hg. Cardiac index and stroke-volume index were elevated to an average of 4.46 1/min./M^2 and 54 ml./beat/M^2 respectively. Pulmonary capillary blood volume, estimated from two-level diffusion capacity measurements, averaged twice the normal value (145 ml.) Arterial-oxygen tension averaged 62 mm. Hg during breathing of air and increased to 477 mm. Hg during 100% breathing of oxygen.

It is postulated that, in the absence of pulmonary-capillary hypertension, hypoxic vasoconstriction of pulmonary arterioles may be a mechanism of production of acute pulmonary edema. *(Supported by USPHS Grant HE-11840.)*

Fructose Absorption and Metabolism

Matthew J. Guy and Julius J. Deren

Maimonides Medical Center, Brooklyn, N. Y.

Fructose absorption was studied *in vitro* by employing rat intestinal rings incubated in a Krebs-Ringer buffer that contained C^{14}-fructose and measuring $C^{14}O_2$ production or radioactivity accumulation in the intestinal rings.

Over a 30-minute incubation, production of $C^{14}O_2$ increased linearly with the concentration of fructose substrate from 10^{-6} to 10^{-3}M. but this leveled off from 10^{-3} to 5 × 10^{-3}-M. Phlorizin (10^{-4}M.), 3-0-methylglucose (10^{-2}M.), and galactose (10^{-2}M.) did not depress the rate of $C^{14}O_2$ production. However, glucose (10^{-2}M.) cut $C^{14}O_2$ production by 50%.

The rate of entry of radioactivity into gut segments was linear over the initial 10 minutes when correction was made for the extracellular space by using H^3-methoxyinulin. Varying fructose concentrations from 10^{-5} to 5 × 10^{-2}M. elicited no saturation kinetics in the initial rate of uptake; adding 5 × 10^{-4}M. phlorizin or 10^{-2}M. glucose did not effect initial rates of uptake.

At 1 mM. fructose enters less than half as fast as glucose, galactose, or 3-0-methylglucose but more than twice as fast as sorbose. Adding 5 × 10^{-4}M. phlorizin retards the uptake of glucose, galactose, and 3-0-methylglucose to approximately the rate of sorbose entry while leaving the rate of the entry of fructose constant at double this common baseline rate for all other hexoses tested where the glucose-hexose carrier mechanism is rendered inoperative by phlorizin.

Some mechanism, perhaps carrier mediation, apparently augments passive diffusion for the absorption of fructose. This mechanism seems independant of the well-known glucose-galactose-hexose carrier system. Future studies must explain our failure to demonstrate saturation kinetics or competitive inhibition if this fructose-transport mechanism is to fit the contemporary carrier model.

Osmotic Effects of THAM

WILLIAM C. HEIRD,* RALPH B. DELL, TREVOR PRICE, AND ROBERT W. WINTERS

Department of Pediatrics
Columbia University College of Physicians and Surgeons, New York, N. Y.

One of the reasons advanced for the alleged superiority of THAM over $NaHCO_3$ for correction of acid-base disorders is that THAM, which lacks sodium and penetrates cells, will not produce osmotically induced redistribution of body water. This assumption has been tested directly in groups of 5 to 6 nephrectomized dogs given hyperosomotic infusions of either THAM or $NaHCO_3$ and in whom TBW (THO space) and plasma Pco_2 were maintained at essentially constant levels. Representative mean rises of ECF volume ($C1^{36}$ space) and plasma osmolality (Osm) one hour after completion of the infusions were as shown in the accompanying table.

*Supported by New York Heart Association Fellowship program.

These results demonstrate: 1) that hyperosmolar THAM produces major changes in ECF volume and osmolality whether it acts as a buffer (Group A) or not (Group B), and 2) that the magnitude of these changes are as great as those seen with an amount of $NaHCO_3$ (Group C), which provides greater buffering than THAM (Group A). Theoretically, these results are not unexpected; THAM at normal blood *p*H of 7.4 is 70% ionized and would be expected to exert 1.7 mOsm. per mM. administered while the total osmotic load of $NaHCO_3$ administered (2 mOsm./mM.) would be expected to decrease since, in buffering, some HCO^-_3 is converted to CO_2 *(Supported by PHS Grant HD-03993.)*

Group	*Infusion*	*ΔOsm.*	*ΔECF*
A	10 mM./kg. THAM (*p*H 8.5)	16.2 mOsm./kg. H_2O	11.3%
B	10 mM./kg. THAM (*p*H 7.3)	19.2 mOsm./kg. H_2O	13.1%
C	10 mM./kg. $NaHCO_3$	14.5 mOsm./kg. H_2O	8.6%
D	None (control)	3.4 mOsm./kg. H_2O	1.25%

Distensibility Characteristics of the Canine Pulmonary Artery in Vivo

CLARITA E. HERRERA AND MILENA L. LEWIS

Department of Medicine
New York Veterans Administration Hospital, New York, N. Y.

Pulmonary vascular compliance remains a point of dispute because significant changes in right ventricular output produce little change in pulmonary blood volume yet at the same time produce only minor changes in pulmonary-artery pressure. Knowledge of the *in vivo* volume-pressure (compliance) characteristics of the separate components of the bed might elucidate the apparent discrepancy. The present study evaluates the compliance of the pulmonary artery of intact anesthetized dogs, and relates it to other hemodynamic parameters.

In 9 dogs balloon catheters were introduced into one branch of the main pulmonary artery (MPA). Cardiac output was measured by the indicator dilution technique. Pulmonary-artery volume (PAV) and total pulmonary blood volume (PBV) were calculated from transit time of a radioactive indicator measured by appropriately collimated detectors over the heart-and-lung fields. Measurements were made during a control period and repeated during occlusion of one branch of the MPA, electrically induced hind-limb exercise, and exercise with unilateral occlusion.

Occlusion of one PA branch resulted in an average increase in flow through the opposite lung of 86%. PAV in the unoccluded bed rose markedly in 8 of the 9 animals (m = + 69%). Average compliance of the arteries was 18% of initial volume/mm. Hg PPA (0.43 ml./ml. H_2O pressure). PAV varied directly with the PPA_{diast} ($r = 0.609$, $p < 0.01$). The data suggests decreasing compliance with increasing volume, but the trend is not statistically significant. Following unilateral PA occlusion the postarterial volume (PBV-PAV) in the opposite lung rose in 10 studies, fell in five and remained unchanged in 3. The postarterial volume varied inversely with PPA_{diast} and compliance appeared to decrease with PPA_{diast} but the trend was not statistically significant.

The present study confirms PA distensibility shown in isolated lungs. The data suggests that resistance to outflow from the arterial vessels is determined by vascular elements downstream whose distensibility determines the diastolic pressure in the PA, and whose volume is a significant portion of the total lung-blood volume.

The Mechanism of Oxygen-Induced Hypoventilation

CLEMENT E. MARKS, JR., AND ROBERTA M. GOLDRING

Department of Medicine
New York University School of Medicine, New York, N. Y.

The present study investigates the mechanism of oxygen-induced hypoventilation (OIHV) in patients with respiratory insufficiency. Previous studies have not related this phenomenon to degree of hypoxemia, reduced CO_2-responsiveness, or altered ventilatory mechanics.

Sixteen patients with obstructive pulmonary disease, alveolar-hypoventilation syndrome, obesity, or interstitial fibrosis were studied. The magnitude of OIHV was expressed as change in P_aCO_2 from air control during 15 min. of breathing 100% O_2. Ventilatory response to CO_2 ($\Delta Ve/\Delta P_aCO_2$) was measured during breathing 5% CO_2-in-air and 5% CO_2-in-95% O_2.

Control P_aO_2 for all patients ranged from 31 to 95 mm. Hg, P_aCO_2 from 35 to 72 mm. Hg, and maximum breathing capacity from 20 to 125% predicted. Although OIHV was observed in all patients with $P_aO_2 < 50$ mm. Hg, $P_aCO_2 > 70$ mm. Hg, and maximum breathing capacity < 43% predicted, some patients with less severe respiratory insufficiency demonstrated OIHV.

The CO_2-in-air response was not reduced in all patients with OIHV; however, the CO_2-in-O_2 response was less than 0.4 l./min./mm. Hg in all patients who demonstrated this phenomenon.

Statistically significant correlation ($p < 0.001$) was demonstrated between the degree of OIHV and the ratio:

$$\frac{CO_2\text{-in-}O_2 \text{ response}}{CO_2\text{-in-air response}}$$

OIHV occurred in all patients in whom the CO_2 drive that remained when hypoxemia was removed was less than 66% of the total drive as expressed by the ratio. In 4 patients restudied, improvement in the degree of OIHV related to an increase in this ratio.

The present study indicates that OIHV is related to the proportional contribution of hypoxemic drive to total ventilatory drive regardless of the degree of hypoxemia, magnitude of over-all drive, or etiology of respiratory insufficiency. *(Supported by Research Grant 8-0154-24 of the New York Heart Association.)*

Physiologic Predictors of Death in Acute Myocardial Infarction

S. S. Scheidt and S. J. Fillmore

Department of Medicine
Cornell University Medical College
New York, N. Y.

Since the advent of the specialized monitoring unit most deaths in hospitalized patients with acute infarction have resulted from refractory heart failure or shock. Current supportive treatment is often unsatisfactory and the mortality of cardiogenic shock is approximately 80%. Criteria are needed for the selection of patients at high risk in whom unconventional therapy such as mechanical circulatory support may be evaluated.

Ninety-eight studies have been performed in 35 patients from 5 to 239 hours after acute infarction. Hemodynamic measurements were well correlated with clinical findings. Mean cardiac index was 2.6 l./min./M.^{2} in patients with uncomplicated infarction (Clinical Class I), 2.4 l./min./M.^{2} in patients with congestive failure after infarction (Class II), and 1.0 l./min./M.^{2} in patients with shock following infarction. Corresponding stroke-volume indices were 33 ml./beat/M.^{2} in patients without complications; 30 ml./beat/M.^{2} in the presence of congestive failure, and 10 ml./beat/M.^{2} in the presence of cardiogenic shock. Mean left-ventricular end-diastolic pressure was 12 mm. Hg in Class I patients, 20 mm. Hg in Class II patients, and 22 mm. Hg in patients with shock. Hemodynamic measurements provided objective assessment of prognosis after myocardial infarction. Mean heart rate was significantly higher ($p < 0.005$), and cardiac index, stroke-volume index, cardiac and stroke work were significantly lower ($p < 0.005$) for each in patients who died as compared with those who survived. There was no significant difference in central blood volume, pulmonary arterial or left-ventricular end diastolic pressures between the two groups.

Analysis of data obtained during the initial physiologic study after admission to hospital for acute infarction indicates that certain measurements are predictive of death. Thus, cardiac work exceeded 3.0 kg.-m./min. in all survivors but was above this value in only 1 of the patients who eventually died. Similarly, stroke work was above 30 gm.-m./beat in all but 1 survivor and below this value in all but 2 of those who died. Only 6 of the 14 patients who died were in shock at the time of the initial study. Time of death varied from 5 hours to 2 months (median 30 hours) after the first physiologic measurements.

Cardiac and stroke work are derived from several variables and appear to be useful in identifying high-risk patients who may be candidates for unconventional therapy. *(Supported by USPHS Contract 43-67-1439, Myocardial Infarction Research Unit.)*

Oxygen Consumption of the Lung in Granulomatous Disease

J. S. Schwartz and P. R. B. Caldwell

Department of Medicine
Columbia University College of Physicians and Surgeons

T. S. Cottrell

Department of Pathology
New York Medical College

New York, N. Y.

Studies in man with granulomatous pulmonary disorders have suggested that the diseased lung may utilize as much as 10% of the oxygen consumed by the body. Moreover, studies in dogs with induced pulmonary granulomas have given similar estimates when the dogs breathed room air, but smaller values when they breathed an hypoxic mixture. Since these *in vivo* estimates entailed a number of assumptions, we have examined the *in vitro* behavior of granulomatous lung tissue from rabbits prepared by intravenous injections of complete Freund's adjuvant after the method of Moore and Schoenberg *(Brit. J. Exper. Path. 45*:488, 1964). At the height of the disease the rabbits were sacrificed, the pulmonary artery was rinsed with saline, and adjacent aliquots of the lung were taken for pathologic and metabolic study. Morphometric measurement showed that, on the average, 92% of the lung consisted of granulomata. Chopped tissue slices were suspended in Krebs Ringer solution equilibrated with oxygen tension over a range of 10 to 240 mm. Hg and the oxygen consumed was measured by use of a Yellow Springs Instrument Oxygen Monitor System. The aliquot was then analyzed for soluble protein content. At an oxygen tension of 150 mm. Hg, the specimens from 10 diseased rabbits utilized, on the average, 9.4 ± 1.6 μl. O_2/mg. protein/hr. compared to a value of 6.3 ± 0.6 in 10 controls ($DF = 18$; $t = 5.8$; $p < 0.001$). The larger respiratory rate of the granulomatous tissue, coupled with the fact that the abnormal lungs were four times heavier than the controls, support the observations in men and dogs that the oxygen utilized by diseased lung may be appreciably increased. Also, at oxygen tensions below 100 mm. Hg the *in vitro* respiratory rate of lung tissue fell linearly with reduction in equilibrating tension. While this behavior resembles that seen in diseased dogs *in vivo,* the mechanism of the fall in respiration in both systems remain unexplained. *(Supported by USPHS HE-05741, HE-02001, and HE-5443.)*

The Reversibility of Postischemic Myocardial Contractile Failure by High-Energy Phosphates

ANILKUMAR SHAH

Cardiology Section
New York Veterans Administration Hospital

Department of Medicine
New York University College of Medicine

SARKIS J. KECHEJIAN

Department of Medicine
New York University College of Medicine

VINCENT J. FISCHER

Cardiology Section
New York Veterans Administration Hospital

State University of New York Downstate Medical Center
Brooklyn

New York, N. Y.

The effects of ATP and ADP infusion on contractile force development by normal and postischemic myocardium were studied. The preparation was the isometrically contracting *in situ* feline right ventricular papillary muscle perfused with oxygenated Tyrode solution that contained 4% low MW dextran, by Langendorff technique at 23° to 27° C. Hearts were paced at regular rates. After obtaining control contractile force at optimal muscle-length coronary flow was stopped for 20 to 30 minutes. Contractile force fell and arrhythmia usually occurred. Resumption of perfusion with Tyrode solution resulted in rise in contractile force to 30 to 60% of control. After a steady state was reached, 0.5 mM. ATP in Tyrode solution was infused for 3 to 5 minutes. The contractile force increased to 60 to 100% of control. When 0.5 mM. ADP was infused through muscles in postischemic state, contractile force increased only to 30 to 40% of control. If 0.5 mM. ATP was then infused through the same muscles, contractile force increased to 60 to 90% of control.

Fluorodinitrobenzene (FDNB) inhibits intracellular resynthesis of ATP from creatine phosphate and ADP. When 0.38 mM. FDNB in glucose-deficient Tyrode solution was infused, contractile force showed a gradual fall to the point of cardiac standstill. If perfusion with Tyrode solution was resumed when contractile force had decreased to 50% of control, force continued to fall slowly or remained stable. Infusion of 0.5 mM. ATP in Tyrode solution without glucose resulted in increase in contractile force to 70 to 100% of control. When ADP was infused to the FDNB-treated preparation, contractile force either decreased further to 18 to 20% of control or increased slightly.

In the postischemic papillary muscle ATP appears to be capable of entering the cell and of providing energy for contraction. The manner by which it enters is uncertain at present, as is the existence of a possible secondary action upon the membrane transport system. *(Supported by the U.S. Veterans Administration and the New York Heart Association.)*

Muramidase Excretion in Nephrotic Syndrome

RAYMOND L. SHERMAN* AND E. LOVELL BECKER

Department of Medicine
Columbia University College of Physicians and Surgeons, New York, N. Y.

Muramidase excretion has been used as an indicator of low-molecular-weight protein excretion in renal disease. In this study 31 patients with nephrotic syndrome secondary to lipoid nephrosis, membranous, and proliferative glomerulonephritis were studied. Muramidase determinations were performed on both serum and urine of all patients. Muramidase excretion differed in the three groups of patients. Five patients with lipoid nephrosis, all with normal renal function, had little or no muramidase in the urine and the serum levels were normal. Five of 9 patients with membranous glomerulonephritis had increased urine muramidase concentrations, 4 of these had abnormally high serum values; all 5 patients had impaired renal function. Eight of 16 patients with proliferative glomerulonephritis had elevated muramidase concentrations in urine, and 4 of these had high serum concentrations. Six of these patients had serum creatinine concentrations above 1.3 mg.%.

It is concluded from these observations: 1) that the serum concentrations of muramidase increase with impairment of renal function, and that a direct correlation can be established between serum concentrations of muramidase and creatinine; 2) that there is no correlation between serum concentration and urinary excretion which suggests that defective tubular reabsorption of low-molecular-weight proteins is causing the appearance of muramidase in the urine; 3) that muramidase concentration in the urine is independent of total excretion of protein since several patients with massive proteinuria excreted only trace amounts of muramidase.

In summary: poor correlation between muramidase concentration in serum and urinary-excretion rate seems to favor the concept that reduced tubular reabsorption is the cause for increased muramidase excretion. *(Supported in part by grant 5 RO1 AM05009 from the National Institutes of Health.)*

*Fellow of the New York Heart Association.

In Vivo *Hemodynamic Comparison of Mitral Valve Prostheses*

M. J. SILVERSTEIN AND R. W. M. FRATER

Department of Surgery

E. L. YELLIN

Departments of Surgery and Physiology
Albert Einstein College of Medicine, New York, N. Y.

Analysis of the hemodynamic performance of the natural mitral valve and five low-profile mitral prostheses has been undertaken by use of our technique of rapid valve exchange. Sixteen experiments in five dogs were performed over a wide range of flow rates. A-V pressure gradients were recorded simultaneously with the instantaneous mitral flow obtained with an intracardiac electromagnetic flow probe sutured supravalvularly.

In addition to the standard calculation of effective orifice areas, we have also selected parameters and techniques of data analysis which emphasize the dynamic characteristics of the valve-fluid system, i.e., the timing between gradient and flow events including the timing and contribution from atrial contraction. The valves performed as shown in the table below.

Several other observations are worth noting. Atrial contraction before the peak of early diastolic filling adds little to the filling volume; after the peak it adds as much as 25 to 30% more volume. All the valves responded to augmented filling due to atrial contraction in the same manner as the natural valve. Each valve permitted a filling volume sufficient to maintain the cardiac output. The filling volume was limited by the time of atrial contraction and the magnitude and rate of change of the pressure gradient. The inertia of the blood as it flows from the pulmonary veins through the atrium and into the ventricle allows the flow to continue after the gradient has reversed. The observation in both the natural and prosthetic valve that flow starts immediately upon reversal of the gradient can best be explained by the inertia of pulmonary inflow, and an actively relaxing ventricle.

EFFECTIVE ORIFICE AREA AS A PER CENT OF THE EFFECTIVE AREA OF THE ECCENTRIC MONOCUSP VALVE— BASED ON PEAK AND TEMPORAL-MEAN PRESSURES AND FLOWS

	Peak values	*Mean values*	*Average of peak and mean*
Eccentric monocusp	100	100	100
Capetown	83	62	73
Kay-Shiley	74	67	71
Cross-Jones	88	74	81
Wada	80	74	77

Hypoxemia-Induced Pulmonary Edema

J. RICHARD SPEARS, K. GOPINATHAN, D. SAROJA, JACKSON H. STUCKEY, AND GEORGE EMMANUEL

Department of Medicine
State University of New York Downstate Medical Center, Brooklyn, N. Y.

The role of acute hypoxemia in the production of pulmonary edema was studied in seven dogs under pentobarbital anesthesia. Extravascular lung-water volumes were calculated from indicator dilution measurements of labeled red cells, albumin, and water during air breathing and during one hour of 5% oxygen breathing. Serial blood samples were analyzed for whole-blood histamine and plasma-serotonin levels. Pulmonary arterial, pulmonary-artery wedge, left atrial and systemic pressures, pulmonary vascular resistance, pulmonary compliance, and airway resistance were determined throughout the experiments. Wet/dry lung-weight ratios and histological findings were compared.

The volume of extravascular lung water increased by at least 50% in three dogs and did not change in four. Pulmonary artery pressure increased in all dogs from an average of 35/15 to 57/23 mm. Hg; the largest increase in extravascular lung water was observed in the dog with the highest elevation of pulmonary artery pressure. Pulmonary-capillary pressure remained unchanged. Pulmonary vascular resistance averaged 215 dynes•sec•cm.$^{-5}$ during air breathing and 222 dynes•sec•cm.$^{-5}$ during hypoxemia. Histamine and serotonin levels decreased during hypoxemia from 0.029 to 0.022 μg./ml. and from 0.12 to 0.09 μg./ml. respectively. In the absence of pulmonary capillary hypertension, hypoxic vasoconstriction of pulmonary arterioles may be a mechanism of production of acute pulmonary edema. *(Supported by USPHS Grant HE-11840.)*

Thyrotoxicosis and Reversal of the Electron Transport in Cardiac Mitochondria

ENDRE M. TARJAN AND SHIN-ICHI KIMATA

Cornell University Medical College
New York, N. Y.

Harvard Medical School
Boston, Mass.

Rabbit-ventricle mitochondria (Mc) isolated and assayed identically, exhibited two alternative "succinate-linked" kinetic characteristics: I) ATP-dependent electron-transport reversal and respiratory control (RC) by ATP; II) no ATP requirement for rapid reversal of electron transport and no RC by ATP. The controlled and active state QO_2's in II were 50 to 100% higher than in I. One minute of preincubation of Mc yielded these kinetic conversions:

$$\text{(I)} \underset{\text{50 }\mu\text{M oxaloacetate, or 2.5 mM L-malate}}{\overset{\text{200 }\mu\text{M pyruvate, or 40 }\mu\text{M octanoate, or 2.5 mM CSA}}{\rightleftharpoons}} \text{(II)}$$

These and other results strongly suggest that under specific conditions the "substrate-level" events can greatly affect the apparent coupling of oxidative phosphorylation, and that oxaloacetate may regulate not only the oxidation of succinate and the reduction of mitochondrial pyridine nucleotides (as evidenced by other workers), but it can affect the state-4 rate as well as the respiratory control by ATP (phosphate potential).

Kinetics (II) were most readily obtained after *in vivo* thyroxine treatment (20 μg. T_4 injected per 100 gm. body weight per day for four days). As the recent evidence for loose coupling by *in vivo* administered T_4 rests mainly on respiratory measurements performed under conditions closely similar to those here employed, the aforementioned effect represents a mechanism that may resolve the current controversy in the literature pertinent to the effect of *in vivo* thyroxine on oxidative phosphorylation. *(Supported by USPHS Research Grant 5 RO1 HEO 4413-08.)*

Kinetics of Lidocaine in Blood

THOMAS TUTTLE

Department of Medicine

ARTHUR HAYES

Departments of Medicine and Pharmacology
Cornell University Medical College
New York, N. Y.

The pharmacodynamics of lidocaine depend on the method of administration. Previous studies with constant infusion suggest that blood levels reach a plateau after 30 to 60 min. Twelve patients in sinus rhythm were infused with lidocaine for 24 hours at a rate of 30 μg./kg./min. Blood samples were assayed at frequent intervals during infusion and for 12 hours thereafter. Mean blood concentration approached a constant level only after 8 to 12 hours. Blood level after discontinuation of infusion fell exponentially with t½ of 105 min. The rate of cumulation after onset of infusion and this metabolic decay are the same. Single IV doses of 0.5, 1.0, and 2.0 mg./kg. were given to 40 patients. Three exponentials comprise the decay curve. The first, t½ = 8.5 min., reflects distribution out of intravascular compartment. The second, t½ = 30 min., represents redistribution to total body water and some fat depots. This was conformed by the calculated volume of distribution. The third segment, t½ = 120 min., agrees with the metabolic half-life observed after infusion. Although antiarrhythmic action may persist for 10 to 30 min. after a single dose, the duration of activity does not correlate with "therapeutic" blood levels of 2 to 5 μg./ml. reported from infusion studies. This discrepancy reflects the lack of a steady-state equilibrium after a single injection. *(Supported by USPHS Contract 43-67-1439, Myocardial Infarction Research Unit.)*

Magnesium-Ion Inhibition of Renovascular Constriction

ANDRE VALCIN, AMBRISH MATHUR, HOWARD GOLDSON, ALAN RASHKIN, AND BERNARD S. LEVOWITZ

Department of Surgery
The Jewish Hospital and Medical Center of Brooklyn
Brooklyn, N. Y.

Previous experiments had demonstrated magnesium-ion (MG^{++}) inhibition of kalemic and catecholamine-induced vasoconstriction of the mesenteric artery. The effectiveness of this cationic blockade prompted a study of renovascular responses to regional infusions of Mg^{++} in the presence of local and generalized peripheral vasoconstriction. Noncannulating flow probes were placed about the renal arteries, and the ureters were individually catheterized in 30 dogs. Bolus or continuous infusions of Mg^{++} (50% $MgSO_4 \cdot 7H_2$) – 4 mEq. $Mg.^{++}$/ml.) were delivered via the renal artery while the other kidney served as a control. Simultaneous injections of graded amounts of Mg^{++} and epinephrine, norepinephrine and neosynephrine were made to evaluate cation inhibition of renal vasoconstriction. Bilateral renal blood flows, urine volumes, and sodium excretions were measured during the selective infusion of Mg^{++} before and after hemorrhage and intravenous catecholamines. In a representative study 1.5, 3.5, and 6 mEq. of Mg^{++} neutralized renal-artery constriction by 1.6 μg. of neosynephrine, norepinephrine, and epinephrine respectively. Arterial infusion of Mg^{++} (0.8 mEq./min.) upon completion of the surgical preparation produced an increase in blood flow, urine volume, and natriuresis by mean factors of 1.4, 9, and 12 respectively compared with controls. Before or after intravenous catecholamines and hemorrhage Mg^{++} infusion prevented or reversed the depression of renal function noted in the untreated kidney; neutralization ceased within 10 min. of discontinuing the infusion. Our findings suggest that regional instillation of Mg^{++} neutralizes or reverses sympathetic renal vasoconstriction of pharmacologic or endogenous origin. The cation blockade appears to be rapid in onset, of brief duration and concentration dependent. *(Supported by Grant FR-00503 from USPHS, and a grant from G. D. Searle & Co.)*

Vasodilator Effect of Papaverine and Phosphodiesterase Activity

Y. Vulliemoz, M. Verosky, L. Triner,* and G. G. Nahas

Department of Anesthesiology
Columbia University College of Physicians and Surgeons
New York, N. Y.

We have reported evidence that indicates that the adenyl cyclase (AC)-phosphodiesterase (PDE) system which regulates intracellular cyclic-AMP participates in the regulation of uterine muscle tone and contractility. These experiments were designed to investigate the role of this system in the regulation of vascular smooth-muscle tone and contractility. AC and PDE activity was assayed in rabbit aorta and the vascular responses to drugs which act on these enzymes were studied. It was first shown that papaverine (P) inhibits PDE activity. This inhibitory action of P (K_i about 10^{-5} M.) is more than 10 times greater than that of theophylline (T). T and P decreased aorta-strip contraction caused by epinephrine (E), norepinephrine, and phenylephrine. When the effect of T or P was simulated by the addition of dibutyryl cyclic-AMP (2×10^{-3} M.), the contractile response was decreased by approximately 90%. These results support the concept that intracellular cyclic-AMP participates in the regulation of vascular tone and reactivity: higher levels decrease and lower levels seem to increase the contractility. The effect of P seems to be related to the inhibition of PDE, which results in an increased level of cyclic-AMP in the cell. This mechanism of action of papaverine was studied in other systems regulated by cyclic-AMP. In striated muscle P (5×10^{-4} M.) decreased glycogen content to the same extent as E (10^{-5} M.): from a control concentration of 5.96 μg./mg. dry weight to 3.31 μg. and 3.37 μg., respectively. Both drugs when combined produced an additive effect; they decreased muscle glycogen to 1.86 μg./mg. dry weight. In adipose tissue papaverine (10^{-4} M.) increased E (10^{-5} M.)-induced lipolysis (from 6.21 to 8.15 glycerol μm./gm. of tissue). These results and the direct measurements of PDE activity demonstrate the inhibitory action of P on this enzyme. The vasodilatory effect of papaverine appears to be exerted through this mechanism. *(Supported in part by the Bob and Dolores Hope Gift for the Study of Shock.)*

*A senior investigator of the New York Heart Association.

HOSPITALS DEPICTED IN OLD MAPS AND PANORAMAS (II)

In a previous essay[1] attention was called to types of medical and historical information that might be obtained from old city maps and old panoramic views. It was suggested that works of that character might contain some of the origins of modern medical cartography. It was shown also that in a decorative late 16th-century view of Bergen, Norway there are clear pictures of two small hospitals, one designated *Hospital von den Teutschen* (German Hospital), the other being a municipal hospital (*Spittal der Stat*). The picture on which this discussion was based was drawn by Hieronymus Scholeus and engraved by Frans Hogenberg; it was published by Georg Braun in the fourth volume (1594) of his six-volume collection, *Civitates Orbis Terrarum*, which was issued seriatim in Cologne from 1576 to 1618.[2]

In the same discussion attention was called to an essay by Professor V. Møller-Christensen,[3] who remarked that in Scandinavia it had been customary for lepers to be treated in special hospitals that were named for St. Jørgen (St. George);[4] these were usually situated outside the walls of cities.[5]

The statements of Prof. Møller-Christensen prompted a reexamination of Georg Braun's *Civitates Orbis Terrarum* with the purpose of ascertaining what could be discovered about hospitals. A number of observations immediately presented themselves.

The map of Visby (V.39),[6] a portion of which is reproduced in

1. Jarcho, S.: Hospitals depicted in old maps and panoramas (I). *Bull. N.Y. Acad. Med. 46*:737-41, 1970.
2. For modern versions and excerpts see: *a*) Skelton, R. A., editor: *Civitates Orbis Terrarum.* Kassel & Basel, Barenreiter, 1965. *b*) Oehme, R., editor: *Alte Europäische Städte-Bilder.* Stuttgart, Tauchnitz, 1954. *c*) Braun, G.: *Alte Deutsche Städtebilder; 12 Farbige Blätter.* Stuttgart, Asmus, 1955. *d*) Braun, G.: *Old European Cities; Twenty-four 16th Century Maps and Texts.* With an interpretation by Arthur Hibbert and a description by R. Oehme. London, Thames & Hudson, 1955.
3. Møller-Christensen, V.: *Ten Lepers from Naestved in Denmark.* Copenhagen, Danish Science Press, 1953.
4. Haeser, H.: *Geschichte christlicher Kranken-Pflege und Pflegerschaften.* Berlin, Hertz, 1857, pp. 31-32.
   Much additional information will be found in Virchow's famous essay on leprosy. Virchow, R.: Zur Geschichte des Aussatzes, besonders in Deutschland. *Arch. path. Anat. Physiol. 18:* 138-62, 273-329, 1860; *19*:43-93, 1861; *20*:166-98, 459-512, 1861 (see esp. *18:* 144 ff).
5. See also Sederholm, E.: History of Leprosy in Sweden. *Lepra 8* (suppl.): 341-66, 1909 (esp. pp. 342 ff.).
6. Maps in Braun's *Civitatis Orbis Terrarum* will be cited by book and number, e.g. V. 39 signifies Book V, map No. 39.

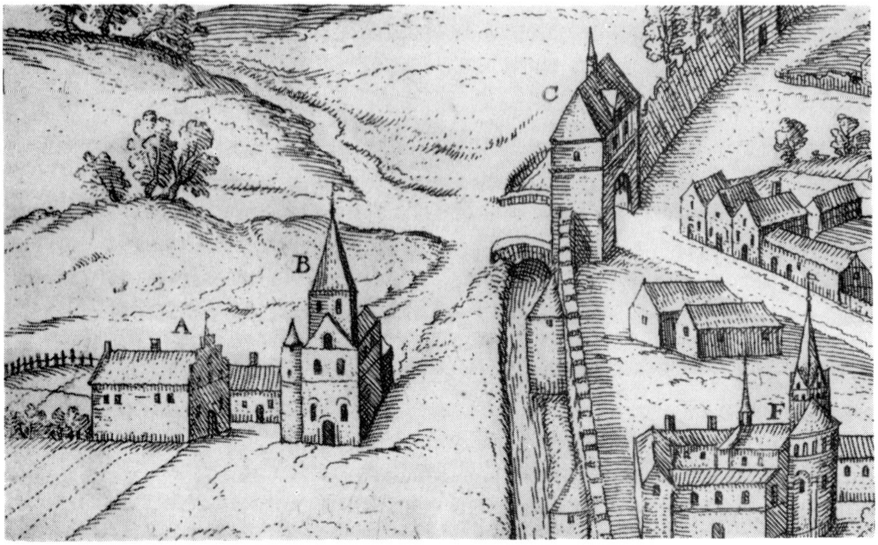

Fig. 1. Visby. *A:* Public hospital. *B:* Church of St. George. *C:* North Gate of city. Braun V. 39.

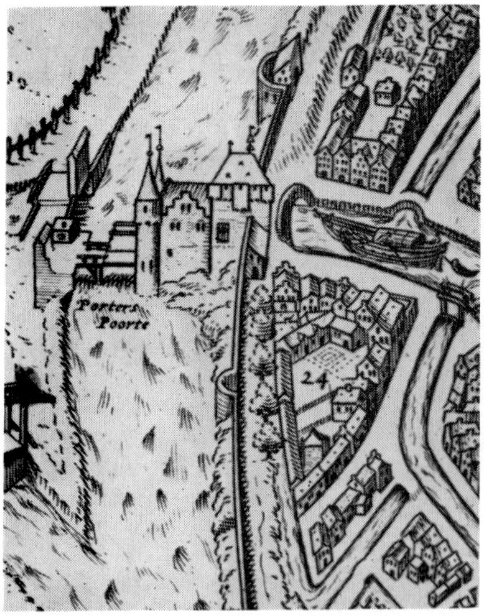

Fig. 2. Gouda. No. 24 originally used by nuns, later used by lepers; the buildings are just inside the city wall. Braun IV. 14.

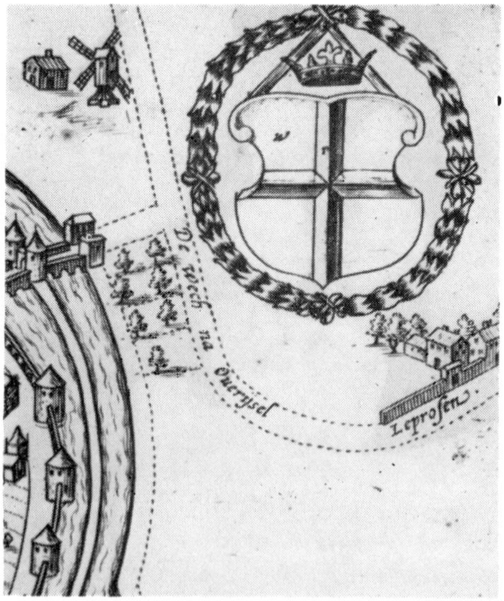

Fig. 3. Amersfoort. A group of buildings marked *Leprosen* is situated outside the city. Braun IV. 15.

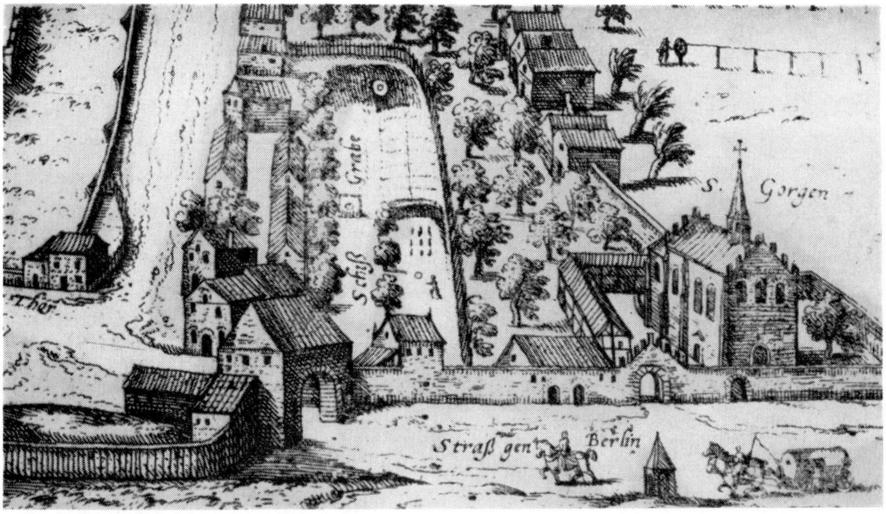

Fig. 4. Stettin. Note *S. Gorgen* at the edge of the city, on the road to Berlin. Braun IV. 41.

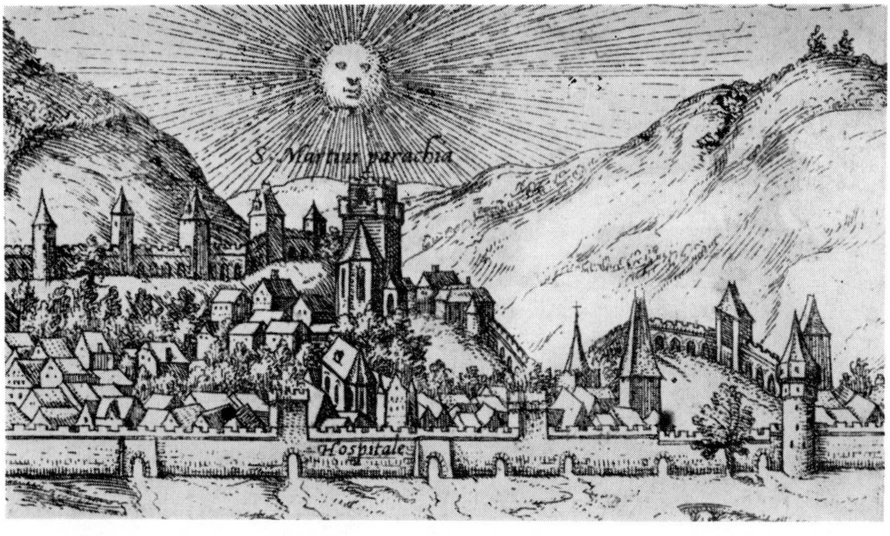

Fig. 5. Ober Wesell. *Hospitale* immediately within city wall. Braun IV. 24.

Figure 1, shows a Templum S. Georgii and a Nosocomium Publicum in close proximity; both are outside the city walls. The map of Colding (Kolding, Denmark; V. 32), not reproduced in the accompanying illustrations, shows a Sanct Jorgens Hoff and a hospital; both are at the extreme periphery of the city.

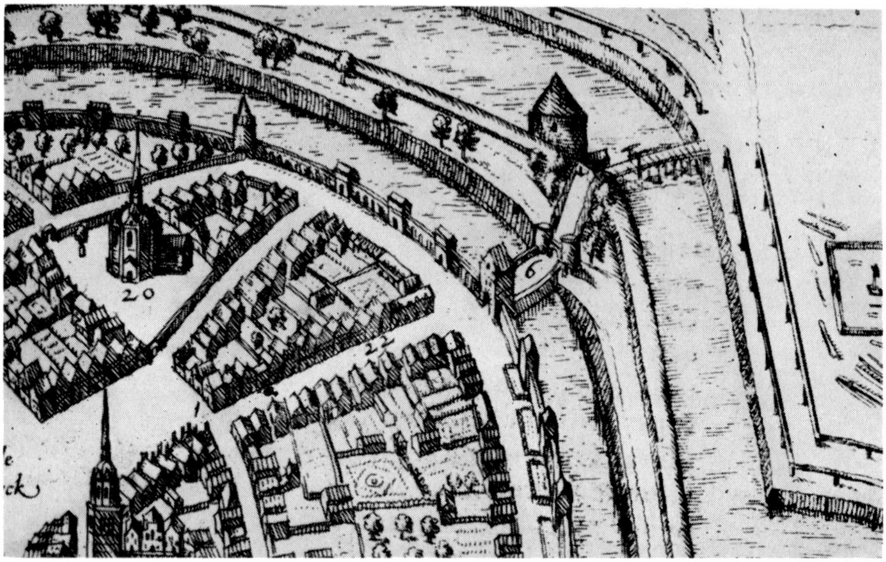

Fig. 6. Hamburg. No. 6 designates the *Hospital porta,* which leads to No. 22, the hospital. Braun IV. 36.

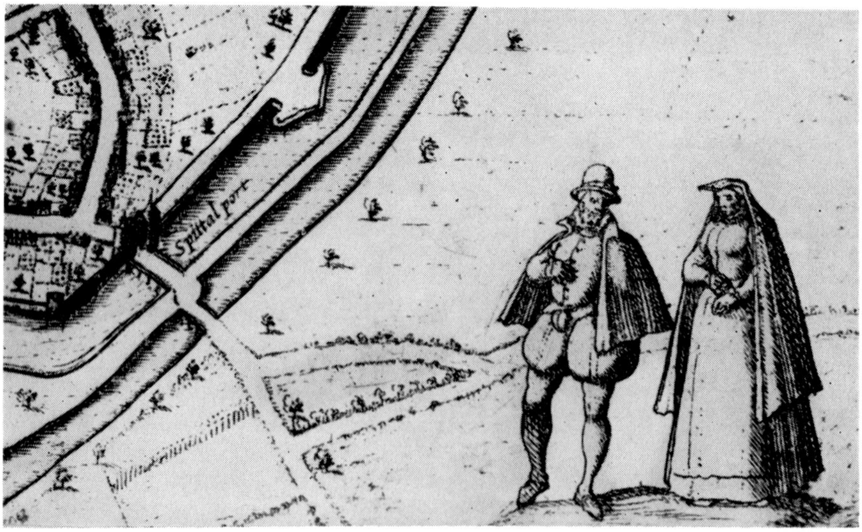

Fig. 7. Zutphen. Note *Spittal port.* Braun IV. 16.

The map of Gouda[7] (see Figure 2) depicts a building formerly inhabited by nuns and now used by "leprosen"; it is situated immediately within the walls of the city. On the map of Amersfoort,[8] a portion of which is shown in Figure 3, in the extreme upper right corner there is a building marked Leprosen, situated just beyond the city, on the road to Overijssel. The extreme lower right corner of the map of Stettin[9] (see Figure 4) shows a building marked S. Gorgen, situated outside the walls, on the road to Berlin. Hospitals situated well beyond the city and depicted at the borders of the map appear also at Ekelenford[10] and Weimar;[11] there is nothing to indicate that these were leprosaria. In the map of Ober Wesell[12] (Figure 5) a hospital or hospice is shown just within the city wall.

Perhaps because hospitals were so often situated either a short distance beyond city walls or just within them, the gateways are sometimes named after the hospitals. For example on the map of Hamburg[13] (Figure 6) one gate is named *Hospital porta.* Perhaps for the same reason a gate at Zutphen[14] is marked *Spittal port* (Figure 7) and one at Lille[15] is designated *la porte de malade.*

These small facts suggest that old maps and panoramas may contain much information that is significant to the physician and to the medical historian. The present study has shown how often urban hospitals were situated peripherally. It might be desirable to continue the investigation by studying their location with respect to prevailing winds, to altitude, and to bodies of water. In many instances corroborative information could be derived from the local and regional medical geographies that were published in increasing numbers during the 18th century. An investigation conducted in this way might reveal the extent to which the Hippocratic treatise *Airs, Waters, Places* was influential in the choice of sites for hospitals.

ACKNOWLEDGMENTS

I thank Mrs. Maude Cole of the New York Public Library and Mrs. Richard North for assistance in the preparation of this essay.

All the illustrations are presented by courtesy of the Rare Book Division, the New York Public Library (Astor, Lenox, and Tilden Foundations).

S. J.

7. Braun IV. 14
8. Braun IV. 15
9. Braun IV. 41
10. Braun V. 31
11. Braun III. 42
12. Braun IV. 24
13. Braun IV. 36
14. Braun IV. 16
15. Braun III. 19

GOVERNMENT AND WELFARE IN NINETEENTH CENTURY ENGLAND

The provision for the education of the people is more clearly within the power and the duty of an enlightened government, on the ground, not simply of moral obligation, but of improving the national industry, increasing, consequently, the national wealth, and of elevating generally the character of the people, and so advancing the general improvement, and promoting public happiness and order. But it is vain to look to any government for any thing like a paternal superintendence of its people. On a large scale it is not practicable. Those who govern can scarcely be expected to have virtue, and disinterestedness, and wisdom, sufficient for such a task; and those who are governed would not willingly submit to their injunctions or regulations. Any compulsory influence would be unavailing. But, then, it is the duty of every just government to afford to every one of its subjects, as far as depends on itself, the means of subsistence; and institutions or regulations, by which the right and opportunity for a man to exert his talents in a way not morally injurious to another, are taken away, or abridged, in any degree interfered with, seem wholly wrong and unjust. It would be invidious in me, because perhaps out of place, to point out in any way how the institutions of this country so interfere, if interfere they do; but, as I have said before, the condition of a large portion of the population,—I speak of those in the rural district,—being prevented the opportunity of applying the labor by which they might secure not only a subsistence, but the comforts of life, forebodes nothing but evil, and may, with strong reason, engage the anxious inquiries of those who have any power in the case, either of alleviation or remedy.

The population is increasing throughout the kingdom with amazing rapidity; and, strange as it may seem, the fact is beyond a doubt, that the increase is always greater among the wretched poor, whom extreme misery has made entirely reckless of consequences, than among that class whose circumstances are comparatively comfortable, and who have learnt that their comfort can be secured only by a wholesome and wise providence. The complaint is universal and continual, that the population is too numerous; but this does not prevent their increase.

Few will be bold enough to hazard the question, Who is here who has not a right to be here? nor, like a party of shipwrecked sailors in a boat, to propose the decision by lot, as to which of the party shall be thrown overboard. But the great question must be met—not, How are the surplus population to be got rid of? but, How shall they be sustained? The insular character of Great Britain necessarily and absolutely limits its capacity of providing for its population from its own soil, although that capacity is yet far from being reached. Idleness begets idleness; beggary produces and perpetuates beggary; crime engenders crime. Sickness and neglect—a sad relief, alas! to the benevolent mind—may do something towards checking this rapid accumulation; for it is stated in the commissioners' returns, and has been asserted recently in the House of Peers, by a distinguished nobleman, that, in England and Scotland, fifty thousand individuals perish annually by disease, arising from the wretchedness of their habitations, owing to imperfect ventilation, and the want of sufficient drainage. This, however, is a small number to be set against the annual increase. Emigration may somewhat alleviate the evil; transportation contributes its small share. It is a curious fact, however, that disease seems scarcely to produce any sensible impression on the population, and that the losses occasioned by severe and wide-spread epidemics are rapidly filled up and obliterated. The effect of the extraordinary improvements already made, and daily being made, in machinery, in the manufacturing districts, is to diminish the amount of human labor employed, and throw more destitute hands into the labor market. What, then, under these circumstances, is to be done, is a question to the great moment of which I have already alluded. It is not, in such a case, for men to wrap themselves up in their own selfishness and indifference, and say, "Let things take care of themselves."

I was conversing with a friend on this subject, a gentleman of great intelligence, and not wanting in benevolence; and his remark was, that an increase of production would do little for the lower classes, for they would get no more; with the price of bread, their wages, if lower be possible, were likely to be reduced; the advantages of such increased products would, of course, go into the hands of the land-holders and farmers, or the large manufacturers and mill-owners; and that, for his part, he saw no ultimate remedy but starvation; that is, such an actual reduction of the means of living, that multitudes should gradually perish from want, and so thin off the surplus population. He said this, too, with all the coolness and indifference with which he would speak of brushing off the flies from the dinner-table. "Good God!" I said within myself, "has it come to this, that familiarity with want and misery can render the heart of man capable of contemplating such a result with calmness, and that human life on earth should come to be deemed utterly worthless? If there be any humanity, or any religion, left in the world, they must be roused to prevent such a catastrophe."

Whatever anxiety, however, the prospect may excite in a benevolent mind, there is no room for despair. It is not consistent with the nature of my present undertaking, to discuss this subject, in its various bearings and aspects, in this place. If life and health are spared me, I shall do it in another form. The people do not so much demand charity, as work. They do not so much require to be supported, as to be allowed to support themselves. The remarkable experiment, already referred to, of Mrs. Gilbert, a sagacious and benevolent woman, at Eastbourne, in Sussex county, who has four hundred tenants, on small allotments, and of whom not more than three have failed to pay their rent punctually, and who, on these small allotments, do, in many cases, all that is necessary, and in all, much for the support of their families, should command attention. There remains, as I have before stated, an immense amount of land, which might be cultivated and rendered productive. These considerations present the strongest inducements to an improved agriculture. More land should be brought into cultivation; that which is cultivated should be better cultivated. The laborers should have every encouragement and opportunity to help themselves. The interest of the farmers cannot be separated from that of the laborers; the interests of one class from that of another. Embarked in the same vessel, they must succeed or suffer, they must sink or swim, together.

I have been, again and again, told that a material change has taken place in the condition of the farm laborers, within the last fifty years, or even a much less time. The practice of forming large farms, by uniting small ones, has tended to remove the laborer farther from the intercourse and superintendence of his employer. Being engagd in large numbers, individual interest and character have been lost sight of; and, cottages on the estates having been suffered to fall into decay, and not being renewed, the laborers have been driven into villages, with a great restriction of their comforts, and exposed to the temptations incident to such localities. The large establishments have lost that patriarchal character which used to belong to them, men are employed much more by the day, and the week, than by the year, as formerly; and are used, and thrown aside, as occasion may require, like mere implements upon the farm. These strong personalities, so favorable in their influence upon the lower classes, and not without most valuable moral effects upon the higher, have almost ceased to exist. . . .

From Colman, Henry: *European Agriculture and Rural Economy, from Personal Observation.* Boston, Phelps, 1844-47, vol. 1, part 2, pp. 136-40.

FRIENDS OF THE RARE BOOK ROOM

OF THE NEW YORK ACADEMY OF MEDICINE

It is the hope of the Academy that every Fellow will visit the Rare Book Room and become a "Friend." If you are already a "Friend," please tell another Fellow what the Rare Book Room offers.

* * *

A Recent Acquisition

William Clowes. A Rightful frvtefvll and Approoved Treatise, for the artificiall Cure of that Malady called in Latin Struma, and in English, the Evill, cured by Kinges and Queenes of England . . . London, 1602. A copy of the rare first edition of this work on scrofula and its supposed cure by the royal touch.

* * *

Annual Member	$10.00	Contributing Member	$100.00
Sustaining Member	25.00	Life Member	500.00

Tax deductible

* * *

Please make check payable to:

FRIENDS OF THE RARE BOOK ROOM

Mail to: CHARLES C. MORCHAND, *treasurer*

111 East 88th Street, New York, N. Y. 10028

OFFICERS AND STAFF OF THE ACADEMY: 1970

JOHN L. POOL, *President*

Vice Presidents

ARTHUR A. FISCHL — EDWARD E. FISCHEL — ALBERT C. SANTY

JAMES E. THOMPSON, *Treasurer*

HANS H. ZINSSER, *Recording Secretary*

Trustees

GORDON M. BRUCE
HOWARD REID CRAIG
JOSE M. FERRER, JR.
MILTON J. GOODFRIEND
WILLIAM J. GRACE
LOUIS M. HELLMAN
ROBERT L. LEVY
JOHN L. MADDEN
AUBRE DE L. MAYNARD
JOHN P. WEST

Council

The President — The Vice Presidents — The Trustees
The Treasurer — The Recording Secretary

Chairmen of the Standing Committees on:

Admission
Library
Medical Education
Public Health
Medicine in Society

JAMES E. MCCORMACK, *Director*

THOMAS BASLER, *Librarian*

Executive Secretaries of the Standing Committees

ARTHUR J. LEWIS, *Public Health*

ROBERT S. GOODHART, *Medical Education*

MARVIN LIEBERMAN, *Medicine in Society*

SAUL JARCHO, *Publications*

Business Manager

ROBERT BRERETON

Library Consultants

JANET DOE — CURT PROSKAUER

Legal Counsel

DAVIS POLK AND WARDWELL

EDITORIAL BOARD

CHARLES A. RAGAN, JR., *Chairman*
RALPH W. GAUSE
FRANK L. HORSFALL, JR.
J. LAWRENCE POOL
ROBERT J. SLATER
FRANK C. SPENCER
STUART S. STEVENSON
FREDERICK G. ZAK

SAUL JARCHO, *Editor in Chief*

THE NEW YORK ACADEMY OF MEDICINE

JOHN L. POOL, M.D., *President* JAMES E. MCCORMACK, M.D., *Director*

COMMITTEE ON MEDICINE IN SOCIETY

John M. Cotton, M.D., *Chairman*

John W. V. Cordice, Jr., M.D.
Chairman, 1970 Annual Health Conference

Norton S. Brown, M.D.
Duncan W. Clark, M.D.
William Cooper, M.D.*
Edwin F. Dailey, M.D.
Murray Dworetzky, M.D.
William W. Field, M.D.
Alfred M. Freedman, M.D.
Maxwell L. Gelfand, M.D.
Carl Goldmark, Jr., M.D.
Irving Graef, M.D.
Sidney M. Greenberg, M.D.
August H. Groeschel, M.D.
Carlo E. Grossi, M.D.
Harold D. Harvey, M.D.
Philip E. Henig, M.D.
Arthur I. Holleb, M.D.
John L. S. Holloman, Jr., M.D.
Louis Leiter, M.D.
Mack Lipkin, M.D.
David Lyall, M.D.
Henry B. Makover, M.D.
Rowland L. Mindlin, M.D.
Marvin E. Perkins, M.D.
S. David Pomrinse, M.D.
Joseph Post, M.D.
Willard C. Rappleye, M.D.
J. Beall Rodgers, M.D.
Leonard S. Rosenfeld, M.D.
Frank A. Seixas, M.D.
Carl H. Smith, M.D.
Samuel Standard, M.D.*
Milton Terris, M.D.
Edward Tolstoi, M.D.
George M. Wheatley, M.D.
Herbert B. Wilcox, Jr., M.D.
Byard Williams, M.D.

MARVIN LIEBERMAN, Ph.D., *Executive Secretary*

---

*Deceased.

BULLETIN OF
THE NEW YORK ACADEMY
OF MEDICINE

VOL. 46, NO. 12 DECEMBER 1970

COMMUNITY PARTICIPATION AND NATIONAL HEALTH POLICY*

JOHN W. V. CORDICE, JR.

Secretary
Queens Clinical Society
Jamaica, N. Y.

By now it should be fully evident to all that the true spirit and tradition of this nation demands that those inalienable rights of life, liberty, and the pursuit of happiness guaranteed to all citizens include the right to the possibilities of sustained and vigorous good health. Robust good health is an undeniable essential upon which the other inalienable rights are built. If this be so—and it is so—a national health policy must exist with laws providing guarantees for all citizens. To date this policy is nonexistent. Its absence is deplorable and must be remedied. There are those amongst us who, although agreeing with the foregoing, still do not feel that there is truly a crisis in health care in this nation at present; or who feel that, at most, better financing of the present system will achieve what is needed in health care. I submit that the overwhelming weight of evidence to date proves these persons to be sadly mistaken.

*Presented at the 1970 Health Conference of the New York Academy of Medicine, *Community Participation for Equity and Excellence in Health Care,* held at the Academy April 23 and 24, 1970.

I ask you to picture our proud nation with its present technology and capabilities wallowing in its own garbage and excreta, breathing pollutants of all kinds, eating garbage, witnessing an increasing venereal-disease rate, pandemic drug abuse, pandemic neuropsychiatric disease, pandemic alcoholism and malnutrition, pandemic home and automobile accidents, and an infant mortality rate about 15th among the nations of the world—a nation where the poor and the near-poor are denied the possibility of having what those who have access to health care recognize as grossly inadequate, poorly coordinated, and blatantly expensive. This is a pathetic commentary on our proud and wealthy nation.

Changes in our health-care system so vitally necessary will require imagination, innovation, and acceptance of challenges and hazards of change when these are directed toward betterment for all. Undoubtedly there are many exciting and perhaps daring innovations which must be developed—in manpower, organization, administration, and financing—to achieve this end. In opinions expressed on the medical establishment we are frequently admonished to remain "realistic" in our national goals for health-care planning. I submit that ingenuity and imagination should be emphasized in health-care planning, and that these are not necessarily the antithesis of practicability and realism.

Further, I ask, is it realistic to put men on the moon? Is the development of supersonic aircraft realistic? Is transplantation of the human heart and other organs realistic? Is development of a multiple, independently targeted reentry missile realistic? If these highly imaginative achievements are considered justifiable despite their great cost, because of their significant relation to the national interest, then I submit that there can be no more important implementation of the national interest than to attend comprehensively to the health-care needs of the citizens of this nation. No matter what wide-ranging directions we may take in efforts to solve our health problems, it is axiomatic that the person most vitally affected, namely, the consumer, must be heard, and must become part of this process.

Again, we are all aware that there are those who feel that no significant input by the consumer is necessary because the expert and dedicated professional, the sociologist, the social worker, the community worker, consultants in various areas of expertise, administrators, politicians and, last but not least, philanthropists and boards of trustees, have the moral and ethical fiber never to be laggard in their duty to the citizens to whose welfare they are dedicated. Nonetheless, may I remind you of those many institutions and organizations, steeped in the loftiest of traditions, tax-free, their charters fairly dripping with sweetness and dedication to the public good, often with slogans of piety and wisdom emblazoned in their hallowed halls, often engraved on their ivy-covered walls, sometimes in Latin, Greek, Hebrew, or English—and with all this, they fail in many respects to act relevantly and with impact on the needs of society today.

New systems, therefore, must be evolved; systems that are responsive and that will remain responsive and relevant to the needs and interests of the citizens served. To my mind, the best guarantee in any system that such a system will remain responsive to these needs and interests is valid participation by the people served, both in policy making and in the delivery of services. It is our hope that as a result of our deliberations here we may begin to describe what valid or meaningful participation is and how it may be achieved—and that our discussion will set the climate for the achievement of a national health policy and the means to its implementation.

ROLE OF THE COMMUNITY IN DEVELOPING IMPROVED HEALTH CARE*

HERMAN BADILLO†

Former Borough President of the Bronx, New York, N. Y.

HERE in the city of New York the question of the role of the community in developing improved health care is coming into a new and crucial period, but I am concerned that not enough people in the community realize this. The new Health and Hospital Corporation will be taking title to the 18 municipal hospitals on July 1 [1970] and assuming responsibility for their operation. We members of this corporation were sworn in by the mayor about two months ago, and we have had several meetings, but we have not heard from the community. I think that Dr. Arthur Logan and I—Dr. Logan represents Manhattan, while I represent the Bronx—have probably received the most response from the community, but even that has been a minimal response. This is sad, for the new Health and Hospital Corporation has 15 members, and it already has become a political structure. Five members are appointed by the City Council (the council, of course, has decided there should be one from each borough); five members are appointed by the mayor, also on the basis of one for each borough; and there are five city officials. Of the 15 members there are only two blacks and one Puerto Rican, although of course most of the population in the city hospitals is black and Puerto Rican. There is, so far as I know, no community person—I think I am supposed to be the community person on the panel, at least I was the only person now on the board who opposed the creation of the Health and Hospital Corporation. But no one in that group has been involved over the years in developing health care at the community level. The two blacks are doctors and of course they are interested in the community, but they cannot be called community representatives. Already there is a feeling that this board is supposed to be like the boards of the voluntary hospitals which merely approve the actions of their presidents. I am a member of the

*Presented in a panel, Role of the Community in Developing Improved Health Care, as part of the 1970 Health Conference of the New York Academy of Medicine, *Community Participation for Equity and Excellence in Health Care,* held at the Academy April 23 and 24, 1970.

†Newly elected Member of Congress, House of Representatives, 21st District, New York, N. Y.

board of several hospitals; and these boards are composed of judges, distinguished persons, and fund-raisers who meet once a month. Generally their activity is only to ratify whatever the president and the executive director have done.

I tell you this because I am concerned that what is happening here is that we are continuing the process of government by mysterious committees that has begun in many other areas of the New York City government. For example, we should consider New York City's experience with the Metropolitan Transportation Authority (MTA). You may remember that recently the mayor was very upset because the MTA suddenly increased the subway fare from 20 to 30 cents. But because he said it was a seperate corporation nothing could be done. What he did not say, however, was that the MTA had been organized with his support and that he had voluntarily relinquished his authority to regulate the subway fare. Moreover, although the mayor criticized the action of the MTA in increasing the fare, he did join in the proposals put forward by others to return the authority for the operation of the subways to the city of New York.

It is clear that there is a new approach to local government by which public officials create a corporation to take the responsibility from their shoulders and then, if something goes wrong, they blame the corporation. That is a good idea from the point of view of the public official, but not of the city or of its citizens.

The new Health and Hospital Corporation was created, in my opinion, to take the responsibility for hospitals away from the mayor, particularly responsibility for financing health care. The structure of the corporation provides that the city will bind itself to give $175 million a year for health care. But $175 million this year is not $175 million five years from now; and any public official who could make an arrangement under which he committed himself to a basic amount permanently would feel that he had made a good bargain. The community must insist that even if there is a corporation the City of New York and the State of New York must commit themselves to give whatever amount is required to provide adequate health care—whether it is $175 million, $275 million, or $375 million.

The citizens of the city of New York must realize, further, that the creation of this new hospital corporation provides an opportunity to define the roles which the community might play in providing health care. We now have an opportunity to review and revise the entire structure and the operation of municipal hospitals. No longer is it mandated by law that in the operation of municipal hospitals there be advisory boards of the sort we have today. The advisory boards of Lincoln Hospital and Metropolitan Hospital and Harlem Hospital, for example, could be made up of community people with real responsibility. All of these areas have been opened up for discussion, and it is important that those who are concerned about health care, particularly about community participation in health care, recognize that the next six months in the city of New York are going to be crucial if we are to move toward increased community responsibility and authority over health care. I should like to see--as a result of this conference or of further discussions–the formation of community groups with spokesmen sufficiently concerned to request that they meet with members of the new corporation, and who will request that community groups have greater authority in the operation of municipal hospitals.

I am calling upon you to take the initiative in this respect now. I am telling you that the corporation is in existence, that the board is in existence, that you should begin to request that committees be set up by the board of directors of this corporation to take into account the needs of the community. Because if you do not, it is not going to happen. And then, a year from now, you will complain that the community has not been taken into account and the fault will have been your own, because you did not take action to insure that community participation would in fact take place.

You will have an opportunity very soon, when the mayor announces the budget for health care for fiscal year July 1, 1970 to June 30, 1971. There will be public hearings at the forthcoming meeting of the Board of Estimate; at that forum you will have an opportunity to come and speak and say what you think ought to be done in health care in the city of New York for the next year. At that forum you can ask for increased powers, and if additional funds are required to make these powers effective, you can ask for them at that time.

Accordingly, I am glad that I have had the opportunity to come here, because we still have time. If you begin to work in the next month, I think that the role of communities in the city of New York can become a symbol of what the role of communities could be throughout the nation. Whether that community role becomes a reality depends upon what you do in the next month and in the year to come.

DISCUSSION OF THE DIVISION OF THE ROLE OF THE COMMUNITY IN DEVELOPING IMPROVED HEALTH CARE*

EDGAR CAHN

Director
Citizens Advocate Center
Washington, D.C.

AFTER listening to a member of my own profession, the legal profession, speak about our health system, I am more convinced than ever that certain criticisms which my wife and I have leveled at the legal profession are equally applicable to the health professions.

The question is not one of intent, or sincerity, or even effort. The fundamental question is what the system for delivery—either of legal or health services—looks like when you approach it from the perspective of the consumer, the person who is supposed to benefit from those services, who consumes them, who depends upon them.

In a piece which my wife and I wrote about the legal profession we found it necessary to admit that the product which we, the legal profession, were selling—quality legal services—was virtually unusable for the purpose for which it was sold (to produce effective remedies and clear guides, or rules, indicating the limits of permissible behavior). The production and distribution system that we had been attempting to expand through decentralized neighborhood legal-service programs or "retail outlets" was basically obsolete; and the manpower supply was sharply curtailed by unnecessary, nonfunctional, protectivist, guild restrictions. In consequence we concluded that, by any test that *Consumer Reports* might impose, the product merchandised by the legal system would be placed in the Unacceptable category. Those tests might be said to include: simplicity and speed of operation, availability, dependability, cost, risk involved in use, uniformity of quality, and satisfaction (both monetary and psychological) with the product.

The same questions, from the same vantage point, that of the con-

*Presented in a panel, Role of the Community in Developing Improved Health Care, as part of the 1970 Health Conference of the New York Academy of Medicine, *Community Participation for Equity and Excellence in Health Care,* held at the Academy April 23 and 24, 1970.

sumer, must be asked about the medical system. Moreover, the medical system must be viewed not merely as a system for producing medical services (a brand name monopoly) any more than the legal system must be viewed as a system for producing legal services. The market for one is health, just as the market for the other is justice. And both the medical and legal professions must be judged in terms of their capacities to meet the minimally egalitarian needs for health and justice of a democratic society.

The consumer has not fared very well from either system. This is somewhat predictable; the history of consumer representation suggests that the consumer does not do a very good job of looking out for himself. We all do fairly well for ourselves as producers, but we do not do so well as consumers—either of material objects, such as appliances and cars, or of social goods such as medical and legal services. It may simply be a facet of human nature: that we are lazy or otherwise remiss in protecting ourselves as consumers. I simply report that the only way in which consumer interests appear to have been adequately represented is when people have been paid to protect the consumer's interest and when they have been protected while representing the consumer from being coopted, compromised, or rendered impotent.

The legal profession is, in this sense, unique. It is the only profession where it is not only permissible, but in fact mandatory for a lawyer to fight for a client. That function is built into the legal system; in fact, the role of the advocate is the cornerstone of our legal system.

But I put it to you that if a teacher fights for the quality of education received by students, or if a doctor challenges the quality of health care of patients, he will not be similarly protected or insulated. Yet I submit that the only way in which we are going to see the equitable delivery of health services in a manner that adequately protects consumer interests (not just in the planning process, or through retroactive ratification of a plan, but as part of the ongoing planning, operation, and revision of health-care systems) is to bring into being a network of paid consumer-advocate roles—advocates for the patient viewed as the consumer of the products produced and merchandised by the entire health industry.

The alternative to fashioning some such formalized and protected advocate role to insure accountability is disturbingly clear. We see it in its extreme form in the case of the American Indian—where a bureaucracy charged with the care of the American Indian has now reached a ratio of one bureaucrat to every 18 Indians, and on one of the largest Indian reservations has reached a ratio of one helping official to every single Indian family. Average expenditures on that reservation average over $8,000 per year for each Indian family. But the median annual income of a family on that reservation—a family of five—is less than $2,000.

That bureaucracy, charged with the care of the Indian, simply provides a microcosm of the greatest domestic growth industry in this country today: that charged with the care of the poor. And we shall go the same way in the ghetto, the migrant camp, and the Appalachian hollow that we have on the reservation: the proliferating of officials but not ensuring benefits to the ultimate beneficiary, the consumer. This is not a matter of sincerity or intentions. It is a matter of results—ultimately, of accountability. By accountability I mean the ability to compel performance of the kind specified and desired to ensure results.

Law—viewed as a body of rights enforceable in courts—represents one such mode of accountability. And there is gradually emerging a body of doctrines, rights, and laws which establish certain levels of accountability, certain minimal standards of performance for the providers of medical services. Some of these stem from the Constitution, others from the statutes, regulations, and guidelines that govern the terms on which federal funds are made available for medical care. Some guidelines must be extrapolated from other fields of law—but increasingly we shall hear about the right to equality of treatment, the right to certain specified kinds of services, the right to confidentiality, the right to eligibility, and the right to knowledge of one's condition. Such a body of law must emerge so that the law can provide a forum of last resort for those deprived of access to medical treatment. But I hardly propose that the way to assure accountability in the health-care system is to superimpose one delivery system which fails to produce justice for the consumer on top of another delivery system which fails to provide health for the consumer.

Instead I suggest that within the health-care system itself there must begin to emerge advocate roles that are protected and insulated—whether in the form of client advisory groups, or peer-group review, or through participation in policy making, in hiring and firing, or through all the approaches to accountability that are now being tried in other fields.

There must be a way whereby a doctor who criticizes a hospital administrator's decision or policy—or a health advocate who criticizes a policy—is not subject to being silenced by retaliation. The only way in which the health-care system is going to be forced to serve the public is to expand the role of the advocate at all levels—to make the administrators, the professionals, the medical schools, the health-insurance companies, the physicians, the nurses, the medical technicians, and the entire production and distribution system directly accountable to the ultimate consumer.

I must say in all candor that I see too few doctors or medical students who are willing to speak out on issues. Partly this is a direct consequence of your own professional and scientific orientation by which a desire for certainty, for empirical evidence of a scientifically sound nature and of sufficient quantity to justify a generalization is viewed as the prerequisite of a diagnosis. But only two years ago there were disturbingly few doctors who were willing, in the absence of such a body of scientific knowledge, to stand up and say that hunger existed on a widespread basis in this county. The six doctors who went down to Mississippi to investigate conditions there several years ago are to be cited for their courage. Some who spoke out subsequently were threatened with the withdrawal of their hospital privileges. Others were subjected even more subtly to the sanctions that come from the professional disapproval of their fellow doctors that can take less dramatic but more devastating forms. At the time when *Hunger, U.S.A.** was first published, there were few doctors who would speak out, and virtually no studies dealing with the extent of hunger and malnutrition among the poor. To be sure there were plenty of studies about obesity and vitamin deficiencies among members of the middle class. But because little research on malnutrition had been done by the medical profession the profession chose, by and large, to take the position that it could offer no opinion about the extent of hunger and malnutrition in this country. There were some who did speak out. But because the case had not yet been proved beyond reasonable doubt it was not yet considered respectable to speak out. Yet there

***Hunger, U.S.A.* A report by the Citizens' Board of Inquiry into Hunger and Malnutrition in the United States. Boston, Beacon, 1968.

is a duty to speak from inadequate data sometimes; there is a duty to speak from less than perfect knowledge, particularly when we know that if we remain silent the decision will be made by default. It is the duty of the profession—a duty which will never be discharged by external compulsion and resort to the courts—to speak out on the health needs of this society, not just on crisis care but health in the broadest sense of the word.

It is fashionable these days to talk about pollution. To me, pollution means that those who are producing goods of one sort or another are creating certain kinds of damage or waste for which they do not have to pay. They are making profits while society at large, or some segment of society, bears part of the cost which should instead be borne by the polluting enterprise. Pollution means that producers are not bearing the true costs of the profits they are making. My profession and yours are, in this sense, polluters of our society. My profession produces quality products for a few—justice for the few—and by its method of production, the method it preserves and perpetuates chooses to produce a kind of social pollution called injustice, lack of justice, or absence of justice for the many. Scarcity is now taking the product of legal redress out of the reach not only of the poor but also of the middle class—so that law becomes an instrument of injustice —a polluter of any larger atmosphere of social justice which we might seek to preserve, restore, or attain.

The same thing is true of the medical field—where the producer does not bear the cost of the profits he is making, whether those profits come from overpricing of prescription drugs or from overpricing caused by the fee-for-service system and the built-in incentives for overuse of hospitalization. The result is inflation. The price tag for health care goes up but the product remains the same and the availability of supply does not expand substantially, even though the profits do. I call that pollution also, for the result is the absence or lack of high-quality health services, the extensive care, preventive care, comprehensive care to which everyone should have a right in this society.

If this situation is to change, then more persons within the profession must speak out—both against the form of social pollution resulting from the absence of total health care and about the profession's own responsibility for these conditions.

Finally, I must say that when we talk about consumer participation more is at stake than the improvement of health services.

There are those here who bear the scars of attempts to expand citizen participation in various social service systems: in education, welfare, law, and medicine. And I shall not deny that extending the democratic process to the operation of the health system is fraught with danger, controversy, and the possibility of error.

But the values of such participation must be acknowledged explicitly. There are unique benefits that can be derived only from consumer participation:

First: one involves simply the mobilization of additional resources, manpower, support, and participation, to do a job that cannot possibly be done by a profession that is minuscule in number.

Second and equally important: consumer participation provides a source of knowledge, of unique insight and feedback about the failure or inadequacy of the present health-care delivery system.

Third: to the extent that health itself depends upon one's sense of dignity and of control over one's own destiny, to the extent that health is a psychological as well as a physical condition, then involvement of consumers may well determine whether treatment is actually used and, if used, whether it is actually effective. I am reminded of talks I have had with Indians on the reservations who say that they are forced to make a choice between the white man's medicine and their own people's medicine—that to benefit from the services offered by the Public Health Service they were forced to reject and abandon the traditions of their people—that concept of health which sees the individual's health as bound up with the welfare of his family, his community, and with the moral order of the universe. Consumer participation as an assertion of dignity is thus an end in itself—a form of health.

Fourth and last: I say that consumer participation is the only way in which the members of this society will be able to live under today's shortages and unfilled needs while working constructively for a better future.

People do not live happily with privation but they can reconcile themselves to scarcities if they have a say in choosing between *x* and *y*, if the scarcity they must endure is at least partially of their own choosing.

In the 1930's we saw the industrial order placed in jeopardy from strikes, sabotage, and unrest until this country began to recognize the principle of collective bargaining—the necessity of providing means whereby people could sit down at a bargaining table where they could be fully and fairly represented and where they could have some faith that the process was a fair one and that they had got the best out of it that was possible for the time being.

Today we are in the process of negotiating not simply the terms of a contract governing wages, hours, and working conditions but of the entire social compact which encompasses dignity, opportunity, justice, equality, and health. Consumer participation is the counterpart of the collective bargaining process. A willingness to abide by the terms of this social compact will depend upon whether those who negotiated that contract are viewed as genuine representatives who have a parity of bargaining power and who fight hard for the best terms they can get. Contracts negotiated by phony leaders, by puppets, by Uncle Toms are as unlikely to win support from the poor as sweetheart contracts and company unions are to inspire workers.

We know what happens in the industrial order when people do not feel bound by the terms of a contract: a wildcat strike. In our major cities, we also see what happens when the terms of a social contract are imposed unilaterally and insensitively: a wildcat strike not on the industrial level but on the entire social level. We call it a riot.

Consumer participationreal, meaningful, genuine—is the only guarantee, frail as it may be, that people will be willing to endure the terms of a social contract and to have sufficient faith in the system to work within its limits. This is what is ultimately at stake in our discussion today.

DISCUSSION OF THE ROLE OF THE COMMUNITY IN DEVELOPING IMPROVED HEALTH CARE*

Theodore O. Cron

President
American Patients Association
Washington, D.C.

First, let us understand how *we* use this term community. For most people in health services, community means local people. This is the original, limited idea of community that came with the poverty programs: "Community Action Programs," or CAP's, as they are called. These are communities *seriatum*, which are no threat. But doctors, hospital administrators, and government officials find it difficult to take the next big step in logic: community also means public – public in specific municipalities and public in the general, national sense. Therefore, as an opening statement, let me say that the American Patients Association differs markedly from the American Medical Association and the American Hospital Association in that we can absorb and comprehend both the *micro-* and the *macro*-meanings of community: the neighborhood and the nation.

Second, to speak on the subject of this panel: the role of the community is to alter *fundamentally* the health policies of government. In other words, it is as important to give ideas, support, and muscle to Councilman Edward Sadowsky and Administrator Gordon Chase here in New York City as it is to work with Senators Russell Long and Ralph Yarborough in Washington and, yes, with Secretary Robert H. Finch also.

Those of us with some labor union background know well enough that the local has a better chance of winning a good contract if the international gets the right word to the head of the industry committee. And every medical society in the United States – in spite of all its bunting and incantations for the good old local values – will ante up each year for the war chest of the American Medical Political Action Committee,

*Presented in a panel, Role of the Community in Developing Improved Health Care, as part of the 1970 Health Conference of the New York Academy of Medicine, *Community Participation for Equity and Excellence in Health Care*, held at the Academy April 23 and 24, 1970.

which operates at both ends of Pennsylvania Avenue in Washington. So our Association is concerned with changing the policies of governments — local, state, and federal. We believe that this is the *primary role of the community* in developing improved health care.

Third, if we are to affect policy changes, what should our priorities be? We say unequivocally that the first change that must be made is the policy of access. At every level of our society, we must extend the protections of the Fourteenth Amendment to health care.

I understand very well that this invites potentially the same kind of turmoil in health that still occurs in education. As a former employee of the U.S. Office of Education in 1964 and 1965, I know what is on the horizon. But the practices of discrimination, of segregation, and of division that run through our health agencies must be changed, otherwise all other changes and developments will be little more than loose bandages on a flowing wound.

Right now — today, even as we meet here in comfort — there are Americans who cannot receive necessary health care because they can not overcome the barriers of discrimination. I am talking about rich blacks and poor Jews, rich Mexican-Americans and unemployed Poles. I am saying that health, at this point in time, is possibly our most segregated public service; hence it is the service most in violation of federal law and of basic, human justice. And that is where policy must change.

Fourth, let me say that I am over 30 and, therefore, do not qualify as an idealist. The American Patients Association is concerned with equal protection in health for the most pragmatic, dollar-wise, "strict-constructionist" reasons. It is impossible to plan public services and facilities if discrimination is practiced. We object, *as taxpayers,* to any health-planning council that does not affirm equal access and equal availability of health service to every citizen in a given area, local or national. The illegalities of discrimination are, first of all, an incurred debt, added to overhead; someone is going to sue — and win. In our view it is as simple as that. Then again, the poor black child you wish to ignore today may grow up and marry the banker's daughter tomorrow; so you may as well count *all* babies into your plans at the very beginning. And our economy is still flexible enough to make rich people poor and poor people rich.

But more to the point: if there is to be a means test, it should be applied to the *providers* of care, not to the patient. In other words, we must ask the health provider, "Can you afford to give good medical service to anyone who walks in the door?" Today, however, we are more inclined to ask the patient, "Do you think you have enough money or insurance to walk through this or that medical door?" What is the community's role, then? To ask the right questions of the right people.

Fifth and last: we must have some idea of the ultimate objectives of community participation in health policy and planning. Our Association does not pick its issues ad hoc. I hope my explanation of the equal-protection issue has already implied that. Obviously we emphasize equal protection because we demand better logic in health planning—logic which cannot work in a segregated system.

Another objective is to make the consumer of health service recognized as participating in care—not just receiving it during a crisis.

Oddly enough, the drug industry, with whom I have had my differences, understands this very well. Their product development and sales programs lean with increasing emphasis on patient self-diagnosis and prescribing. It is an old story in the patent-medicine field. But it has been happening in the field of prescription drugs as well.

Every physician present knows that *doctors* have *not* prescribed the oral contraceptive; they have merely ratified the self-prescribing of 8 million women. Every physician here also knows that doctors are not responsible for the use of 10 billion tranquilizers a year; they have again merely given the stamp of approval—a prescription—to what their patients have requested. But these are extreme examples of patients practicing medicine.

What we should understand is that the future role of the lay public will be to carry the major responsibility for preventive medicine, for the maintenance of neighborhood health, and for a revived, modernized concept of family medicine. Doctors and hospitals will continue to practice "crisis medicine" because other kinds of medicine do not require seven years of higher education, staff privileges, board certification, and Medicaid vendor numbers, nor do they command high income either.

Let us be candid: we are not going to expand our present inventory of medical-education plant and personnel in the next three to five years; in fact, this inventory is contracting right now. We are not going to turn medical practice around to de-emphasize crisis, disease-oriented medicine; no physician in his right mind would replace his present, disease-treatment $25 office fees with a health-maintenance practice of $5 office fees. (The only people who say this must happen are fee-for-service lawyers whom even *I* cannot afford!) And, as in education, we are not going to become friendly egalitarians overnight.

Hence the role of patients—of the community—is to educate and involve the average citizen in preventive medicine and health maintenance as never before; also, to stop fighting crisis medicine and accept it for what it actually can do—save lives in a crisis; and, third, to press, through every legal means possible, for the extension to the field of health of the equal protection clause of the Fourteenth Amendment.

DISCUSSION OF THE ROLE OF THE COMMUNITY IN DEVELOPING IMPROVED HEALTH CARE*

LLOYD WESCOTT

President, Hunterdon Medical Center
Member, Special Committee on Provision of Health Services
American Hospital Association
Rosemont, N. J.

THE discussion so far has concerned itself mainly with the lack of adequate health services in cities, with special emphasis on those in the ghetto areas. May I point out to you, however, that lack of adequate health care is just as great in many rural areas, rich and poor alike, as it is in the cities. This rural problem may be harder to solve than that in the cities because of the wide distribution of the population involved.

Recently a *New York Times* story told of a new rural hospital in Iowa, unable to open because there were no doctors. Last winter I visited a comparatively well-to-do county of dairy farmers and small cities and towns. They had about five hospital beds per 1,000, more than they needed, of course, distributed among six small hospitals, but they had a desperate shortage of doctors. One community, with a 50-bed hospital, had a total staff of two general practitioners and one surgeon. They provided all inpatient care, delivered the babies, manned the emergency room, handled the office and house calls for about 15,000 people, and were working themselves into an early grave.

Situations like this are going to be very hard to deal with because they will probably require a complete reorganization of the present system. So, in supplying health services to America, we have not only the problems of the central cities or of Appalachia, but also of prosperous rural communities and small towns.

The topic of this panel is the involvement of communities in health programs. Certainly, to accomplish any significant and rapid

*Presented in a panel, Role of the Community in Developing Improved Health Care, as part of the 1970 Health Conference of the New York Academy of Medicine, *Community Participation for Equity and Excellence in Health Care,* held at the Academy April 23 and 24, 1970.

social change, it is necessary to involve the community in a very real way. This is particularly true in the field of health. Let me tell, briefly, how we, in Hunterdon County, N. J., managed to involve the community and develop a comparatively outstanding health service. We involved the community not on the basis of some preconceived theory but simply because there was no other way to get the job done.

Our project, the Hunterdon Medical Center, started in 1947. At that time we had a community of about 45,000 people, basically rural and basically agricultural. The towns were small, and there were only two significant industries. The population was far from homogeneous. The farmers ranged from those whose farms had been in the family for generations to first-generation Polish and Jewish immigrants, largely in the poultry business. One section of the county, toward New York, had a wealthy suburban population. On the opposite side of the county was a small town that was reported to have had the highest percentage of its population on relief during the depression years of any muncipality in the state. As with any such grouping of people, there were strong regional and social differences, and strong antipathies between communities.

After World War II we realized that we had a serious lack of medical services. We had no hospital. During the war we had actually peddled our patients from one neighboring hospital to another to find beds. We had a number of family doctors, but they were mostly well along in age and desperately in need of assistance. There were no specialists of any kind in the county.

Those interested in solving the problem brought it to the attention of the county Board of Agriculture, which was the only county-wide organization, and I, as a dairy farmer, became involved and ended up as chairman of the Study Committee. We determined, without much effort, that we did indeed need better medical services. We believed that our principal need was a hospital and that we could have a reasonably good one if we tried.

The county Board of Agriculture then appropriated the money to hire a consultant. It is interesting to note, in passing, that our consultant was Dr. E. H. L. Corwin, who was then secretary of the Committee on Public Health of the New York Academy of Medicine. Dr. Corwin told us that we obviously did need a hospital, but pointed out that we needed more than just a hospital—we also needed better medical care. He outlined for us a community health center which would form the nucleus for countywide health services. He proposed a full-time staff of specialists; he urged involvement of the primary physician or family doctor in the closest possible way; and he arranged for us an affiliation with New York University School of Medicine.

There we had our plan; the question was how to implement it. We presumed the building would cost $2,000,000, $800,000 of which we hoped to get through a Hill-Burton grant. This left us $1,200,000 to raise. We called in fund raisers, and they told us that it was hopeless, that we could not possibly raise more than $650,000 in our community. We decided against giving up our grandiose scheme by cutting back our plans to a 30- or 40-bed institution, which conceivably we might have built with $650,000 of our own money and a smaller Hill-Burton grant. We decided then to act as our own fund-raising organization and, at this point, we began to involve the community in a very real way. We defied many of the hard-and-fast rules of conventional fund-raising. We told our people that there were approximately 10,000 families, which meant that we would have to raise an average of $120 per family. We did make clear that some families could give nothing, some could give less, and that others would have to give more. But just this simple statement brought the whole challenge within the comprehension of every family in the county. Most fund raisers will tell you that at least 65% of the money should be in hand before the fund drive is opened if it is to be a success. We decided to start with just two gifts—our one big industrial gift of $50,000 and our big personal gift of $25,000—just to get people's minds shifted out of low gear, away from the usual Red Cross drive.

We stated further that during the drive only money contributed by the trustees would be spent, and that their own contributions would be held in escrow and would be returned in case of failure. Predicating the fund drive on the possibility of failure hardly seemed practical. The simple fact of the matter was, however, that the drive became a direct challenge to every person in the community, and resulted in one of the most extraordinary exhibitions of community support that I have ever known. By the time we had raised $1,200,000 we had received actual cash gifts from more than 80% of the families in the community. In the cornerstone are the names of 10,000 donors, hand-inscribed in India ink on 100% rag paper by the inmates of the State Reformatory for Women who, incidentally, also had raised money for the medical center.

To the people of Hunterdon this is "our hospital." We have all the volunteers we can possibly use, in every capacity. We are able to mount an annual fund drive, now by mail, and raise over $150,000 a year from about 1,500 donors.

The center has continued to grow. Ten years after it opened we embarked upon an expansion program which cost considerably more than the original building. Our original staff of eight full-time specialists has now grown to 26, and we have been able to attract nearly enough family doctors to serve the community.

In spite of our success we must admit there were two areas in our county that we failed to involve to this degree. One, quite distant from the center of the county where the hospital is located, is a mill town containing the industry that had given the original gift of $50,000. This was an old corporation that had been very paternalistic to its employees over the years. Most of the employees felt that the company had taken care of their obligations and, while many gave, the giving was purely nominal; a real identification with the hospital has never developed. The other community that failed to respond was our poorest community, mentioned earlier. Historically it had related to a larger city—the state capitol, which was almost as close to them as was the location of the hospital. Again, we obtained many small gifts, but no considerable amount of money and, again, this community has not felt close to the center. To solve these problems the medical center is now undertaking, in effect, to extend itself into both of these communities. In one we open, this July, a health center staffed by full-time primary physicians tied directly to the medical center. We hope to open a similar unit in the other town next year. It is our belief that these centers will grow and, as the county grows, eventually will become satellite hospitals. Actually we may develop a third health center in a third corner of the county in the expectation that it also will grow into a satellite hospital in the future. We are convinced that we can develop a sense of community involvement in these satellites which, in turn, will tie the communities to the parent institution.

As you can see, we did manage to secure a remarkable degree of community participation. The reasons are threefold, I think.

First, the need was clear to everyone. The need affected the lives and well-being of all families. Second, the challenge we offered was hopeful and exciting—it was not a bargain-basement challenge. Third, I think we convinced everyone that without the support of virtually all, the center could never come into being. When it did, it would be *their* hospital.

The result of this kind of involvement is not only that it enables the people in a community to raise money to build a building but also that the center will be used, that those who gave will think of it as theirs, and turn to it in time of need, as to a friend.

Let me repeat that our success in achieving this degree of community involvement came about because of the need to solve our own particular problem in our own community and not because of some theory of social action. When I am called on to recount our experience it is difficult to say how it might relate to the problems of another community.

However, there does seem to me to be an element common to the failure of so many health-service organizations, of most welfare programs and, to an increasing degree, of our educational system: they fail to benefit the people they were designed to serve. This element, I believe, is what I have heard called the "come-and-get-it" attitude, or what I call the "let-them-eat-cake" syndrome.

In most northern states, particularly mine—New Jersey—the monthly welfare allotments are reasonable. The taxpayer feels he is paying all that he should, and he is dismayed to find that welfare clients become alienated, rejected, and pauperized. He feels that he must cling to the concept that every welfare recipient is ipso facto incompetent or lazy or worse. He is confident that a caseworker can teach a mother on welfare how to raise her children and cope with the problems of daily living in the ghetto. Thus our society develops elaborate theories of social work, spends millions of dollars and, when the system fails to work, fails to try to find out what we are doing wrong. We say it is the recipient's fault.

The same thing is true in education in the inner cities. We develop increasingly complex theories of education, provide reasonably adequate buildings, pay our teachers reasonable wages, and we give them tenure. The teachers can increase their earning powers by going to college and learn still more pedagogical theory. Yet children graduate from high school virtually unable to read. Again, we do not ask what we are doing that is wrong. We say it is the children's fault.

Just so in medicine. Our nation's scientific knowledge is unsurpassed. We certainly spend more per capita on health care than any nation in the world. The doctors and nurses who staff our city hospital wards and outpatient clinics are certainly highly skilled, but the medical care that reaches vast sections of our population is woefully inadequate. We talk of heart transplants, hyperbaric chambers, and new, obscure modalities of treatment, yet hundreds of thousands of our people are conceived, born, and grow to adulthood without even minimal health care.

Yes: in welfare, in education, and in health care, we say "here it is; come and get it." If persons do not respond it is their fault, not ours. We seem convinced that a lot of cake will cure serious malnutrition.

What can we do about it—we, here, today? Most of us are involved in some way with the delivery of health-care services, either as professionals or as members of citizen boards. We represent the responsible establishment. It makes no difference if we are long-standing members or newcomers, we may be black or white or young or old, we are now the establishment, and the responsibility is ours. What can we do?

First, we must recognize that there is no specific social theory that will provide the answers, and that if a program fails to work, we—not they—are usually at fault. We must recognize that every community presents a different situation needing a different solution. For example, merely placing a few minority representatives on a rigid self-congratulatory governing board may only increase tensions. In some communities the professions are anxious to seek change; in others, they resist. In some, the community is largely black and urban; in others, largely white and rural. Some persons are prosperous; some poor. Some areas need no new buildings; others find this a priority.

So let us not generalize about things, let us not waste time striking out against the past, or against each other, or against this profession or that. Some doctors are indifferent and interested only in money, but far more stand ready to serve. They cannot join with us, however, if we insist that they are our enemy. Let us recognize that community problems must be solved at the community level, in relation to community resources and attitudes. The nation is now fully alerted to the problem, and there will be new programs and more money. It is up to us to make full use of them in our communities.

COMMUNITY PARTICIPATION FOR EQUITY AND EXCELLENCE IN HEALTH CARE*

General Discussion I

SIDNEY M. GREENBERG, *chairman*

Clinical Associate Professor of Medicine
Cornell University Medical College
New York, N. Y.

DR. EDGAR CAHN. There is a simple question that we are up against: the question of money. A promise of more equality of health care may have been implied by the new legislation, but if the increase in funds allotted is going to be swallowed up in profits and in increased fees and salaries of professionals, we shall end up again with the same dual medical-care system we had before except that higher costs will exist for the middle class and the poor. How is the medical profession going to deal with the issue of rising costs?

MR. THEODORE O. CRON. Two things come to mind. One is that the present systems we have now, private insurance and Medicare, constitute a patchwork. If we begin to expand health care to cover everyone who needs it, including health-maintenance services for every citizen, as I believe we should, then everyone must participate in some way in the financing. There should be not only a payroll tax but, more important, a tax on all citizens. This is basically what we are doing now for our other major public service, education. And this is probably the way we shall go in health. There will be a division of the country into rateable and taxable health districts, and this will provide the financial foundation for our national health system.

We must concentrate our attention more on health maintenance rather than entirely on acute and episodic illness.

DR. CAHN. There is another crucial question. We are all now participating financially under the Elementary and Secondary Education Act to help improve education, particularly for children from poverty

*The 1970 Health Conference of the New York Academy of Medicine, held at the Academy April 23 and 24, 1970.

areas. And the studies of where that money has gone indicate that it is going to pay the cost of overhead for state education departments. I believe it will take more money to provide adequate medical care, but I have enormous faith in the capacity of the affluent to take the lion's share of what is supposed to assure equal medical services for all.

COMMENT FROM THE AUDIENCE. Let us address ourselves to the accountability of the medical profession.

MR. CRON. We have asked the Bureau of Health Insurance of the Social Security Administration to tell us what the customary and prevailing fees are that are being paid to physicians by the federal government under Titles 18 and 19. The reply: This is privileged information. Insurance companies have it, and we really have no authority under law to release such information. One of our principal aims is to obtain inspection of those books.

COMMENT. In the community we are talking about community control of the school system, community control of the police department, and community control of our health services. We want to control our health services because the health services have failed the poor people of this country.

MRS. ELIZABETH T. WILSON, *chairman of the Board of Directors, Neighborhood Family Health Center, Philadelphia, Pa.*, and *temporary, appointed fiscal officer of the National Consumer Organization.* Philadelphia is the city of brotherly love and, I hope, of sisterly affection. I hope that the panel is in great sympathy with what is being said, because in the very near future you may be called upon to back up your words. My concern in this over-all, complex situation is the syphoning off from communities by the power structure, by the delegate agencies, from each community a substantial amount of funds in the form of overhead expenditures. I fail to understand how one hospital or one delegated agency can receive such a large amount for signing checks.

MR. IRVING BLUMBERG, *member of the Mayor's Organizational Task Force on Health Planning in New York City and cochairman of the New York Citizens Committee against Mental Illness.* It would be appropriate to mention that the present composition of the Mayor's Organizational Task Force on Health Planning was itself a product of a two-year struggle between the City of New York and consumers, and between the community groups and certain restrictive forces that are interested primarily in hospital power and hospital administration.

We do have in the mayor's Task Force a balanced representation of the interests of the people of the City of New York. It is not accidental that in the Declaration of Independence rights are listed in the following sequence: life, liberty, and the pursuit of happiness. And of course our concern with health comes under that first right.

MR. OLLIE NEAL, JR. I represent the Lee County Cooperative Clinic of Marianna, Arkansas. From my own experience I have found that in order to represent the views of any group of people effectively, you must somehow be a part of that people. What I am saying is that if any person who is in a position to establish any kind of community project is not a part of that community that person will not represent effectively the views of that community.

You know, the whole theory in the past, as expounded by the American Medical Association and other sources, has been that the patient should accept passively whatever services are provided. And we feel, in Lee County, that this ought not be the case in the operation of our clinic.

DR. SIDNEY M. GREENBERG. It is quite evident what the feelings are for the need for community policy making, planning, participation, and control of health services. And as Mr. Lowell G. Norling has said, the community can play an enormously important role in the education of the health professionals in regard to the nature of health services. Anyone who is practicing medicine is well aware of the fact that unless one has the cooperation of the patient and the physician in working together for a common goal, one is not going to get very far in a therapeutic function.

The same thing happens in the community. As much as the community wants control of policy, it must have the cooperation of physicians and all other kinds of auxiliary personnel to make a program meaningful. I get the feeling from the discussion that a question is being asked by people in the community: What are you, as professionals, going to do about this? I should like some discussion about that. What are the professionals going to do about helping the community and its organizations to obtain their goals?

MR. EDDIE C. THOMPKINS, *Childrens Memorial Hospital, Chicago, Ill.* The funds that were appropriated under the Office of Economic Opportunity will generally expire in about two years. Many of the programs cannot generate income. Much of community participation depends upon federal funds. Should the program not be funded federally, then many of the health centers will probably revert to city administrations. My question is: How can communities develop their own self-sufficiency in financing and managing health programs?

MR. HERMAN BADILLO. I think the problem is that the municipality is fully aware of what might happen, and it is trying to escape the problem by passing it on to an intangible body. As a result there will be less of an opportunity for the communities to finance the programs they need. If the communities are going to be in a position to define their future they will have to begin to see their position now. We must begin to define what precisely is meant by community control, and what exactly is the authority of the community groups. For example, in the area of accountability, it would seem to me that it would be a legitimate thing for community groups and community boards of municipal hospitals to act, for many hospitals were established years ago when the ethnic distribution of their surrounding neighborhoods was entirely different than what it is now. Today, for example, there are areas in the south Bronx where there is greater need for prenatal or maternal care. This need did not exist in the same magnitude years ago when the area was a Jewish neighborhood and when families were smaller. Another illustration of accountability has to do with the affiliation contracts in the City of New York, under which medical schools enter into agreements with the city to decide how they are going to operate hospitals. The schools take the attitude that they have the sole power of decision.

But since the schools are using public funds the community should have a part in those decisions. On many occasions in the work of the New York City Board of Estimate hospitals have presented applications for money from Washington, D.C. in which they would seek to establish a particular health service in the City of New York. Upon examination I have found that the reason was that someone had gone to Washington, spoken to an assistant secretary of health, and found that there was money available—for example, for psychiatric services—and that money was brought into the area.

The money was available because someone knew someone else, not because of the need or because it had the highest priority. It seems to me that there should be a diagnosis of the community in the same way that there is a diagnosis of a patient and, based upon the needs of the community, the funds available should be used to meet them.

At the present time community groups are not in a position of management at all. Right now in the hospital field the authority is totally with the medical schools and the hospitals. You must first get the community groups involved to make decisions in programs under way now, and you can then push for more funds.

COMMENT. Community health councils all across the country have been serving in advisory and policy-making positions now for over three years. Soon they will be managing those health centers and programs without federal funds. I do not see any developments nationally whereby these community groups will be able to manage these programs. I do not see any training programs for management skills. We need training programs to enable us to operate after federal funding has expired.

RUBY McDONALD, *Health Council, Detroit Model Neighborhood, Detroit, Mich.* To you I am nobody. To the big shots in Washington, I am nobody. But *we* are somebody. This is what I have to say to you, to Washington, and to everyone else concerned about health. In order for the United States—not Detroit, not Ohio, not Washington, not New York—to have a feasible, complete, and comprehensive health service, it is graduation time. Not just for a poor man who struggles for a dime, a dollar, and a little bit of health treatment, but for you. Come into our communities. Some of you doctors and nurses should work right along with us. And when we get through designing this health package together, let us take it to Washington and tell the authorities: this is what the people need, because we know what we need.

MR. ZARON W. BURNETT, *senior director, Community Action and Training (TNFHC), Trenton, N. J.* One of the big things I think we need very desperately is the conviction and the dedication of the medical profession. In my city we cannot get medical people full time. Why? We have been in operation now for almost a year. We do not have one full-time physician, and we have been trying to recruit for a year. There is something definitely wrong. And we know there are over 20,000 people in the city that need this care, and there is not one doctor.

MRS. RUTH ADKINS, *chairman, East Harlem Health Council, New York, N. Y.* I suggest to the New York Academy of Medicine that the next time it holds a conference it obtain the participation of the United Federation of Teachers and of social workers to get community people to come, to sit down with the doctors and discuss their problems. Also we need to involve the public-relations persons and the community-relations persons of all the hospitals, because they need to be educated, too, about what is going on in the community. We are tired of being told that we are exerting too much pressure, that we want too much. I am accustomed to seeing most of you at meetings, but I should like to see something more powerful come out of this one.

MISS ANA DUMOIS, *Mayor's Organizational Task Force for Comprehensive Health Planning, New York, N. Y.* Dr. Greenberg asked: What is the role of the professional in this whole question of community participation? As a professional who has been working with community groups, I should like to raise a few questions which I think we have to answer. We have heard about the very young, dedicated, radical, younger professionals: medical students, doctors, and social workers. When we speak about community concerns I wonder whether we mean a transfer of power from the health establishment, from the senior doctors, to community control, or whether we really mean a transfer of power from the establishment, from the senior doctors to the younger generation of professionals, the ones that know the rhetoric and the ones who exercise community control. I have been very concerned that many of us want to be controlled by the community only if we can make sure that the community group is going to agree with us. The minute community groups do not agree with us we professionals begin to question whether that group is really representative. Right here in New York City you professional people may be called within a very short time to go to the assistance of one of the first really community-controlled health projects in this nation: one that was favored by the professionals, the young social workers, militant, radical doctors until the group in that community who created the program became sophisticated enough to disagree with them. As soon as that group began to disagree with the professionals and gave specific instructions to them to do something, the professionals rebelled. Do we want to transfer power to the community groups, or do we want to transfer power to the younger professionals in order that they may develop the kind of system that will be the same kind we have now, unresponsive to the community?

DISCUSSION OF THE ROLE OF THE HEALTH PROFESSION IN ACHIEVING EFFECTIVE CONSUMER PARTICIPATION*

THOMAS E. BRYANT

Director, Office of Health Affairs
Office of Economic Opportunity
Washington, D.C.

FROM the beginning of our efforts at the Office of Economic Opportunity (OEO) to bring better health care to poor Americans, participation by the consumer has ranked high among our goals.

The original Economic Opportunity Act included the now famous phrase, "maximum feasible participation of the poor." This phrase was never formally defined. And I, for one, am glad that it was not. Because the concept was left flexible, it has grown and evolved. Indeed, in scores of communities across the nation it is constantly being defined and redefined as health professionals and neighborhood residents try to learn how best to work together toward common goals.

The need for positive participation by the consumer is stated specifically and simply in the Neighborhood Health Center program legislation. This law stipulates that local projects must be designed "to assure that . . . services are made readily accessible to the residents . . . (and) are furnished in a manner most responsive to their needs and with their participation. . . ."

The Neighborhood Health Center guidelines elaborate this provision, stating that the councils "shall participate in such activities as the development and review of applications for OEO assistance . . . the selection of the project director, the location and hours of center services. . . ." etc.

Let me share briefly with you some of the critical roles that consumers have played, especially in our neighborhood health centers. In 50-odd communities where these centers are being developed with OEO

*Presented in a panel, Role of the Health Profession in Achieving Effective Consumer Participation, as part of the 1970 Health Conference of the New York Academy of Medicine, *Community Participation for Equity and Excellence in Health Care,* held at the Academy April 23 and 24, 1970.

aid there are now individuals and families whose futures have been changed by the gift of health. But the value of the centers has been proved not only in the high quality of health services they have provided. They have meant a new way of life for many through job opportunities. And they have held out new hope for the future for poor residents who have become involved in decisions that affect the lives of their families and neighbors as they share in the responsibility of operating a health center.

These new projects prepare and employ neighborhood aides as outreach workers trained in basic health and social service skills. This not only brings jobs into the community but helps to meet critical health-manpower shortages and to make the efforts of health professionals more efficient and more effective. These workers, known and trusted in the areas where they live, explain the workings of the centers to their neighbors and build bridges between them and the staff of the projects.

They offer a variety of services to poor people, both in their homes and at the center. Their services include information on nutrition, personal and domestic hygiene, and a helping hand to guide patients through the often frustrating paper work.

The aides also advise the staff about problems which too often do not surface in the ordinary medical encounter. They know about the problems that an ill patient's family and neighborhood may pose for him. They identify needs often unnoticed: of the elderly and the blind, forgotten in back alley rooms, and of the physically or mentally ill.

In addition to providing employment at the centers where health care is provided, local projects seek effective mechanisms to involve users of services in planning and operations.

Neighborhood residents participate on health councils and boards. These groups are working out their roles and functions through day-by-day discussion and debate.

Another highly noteworthy development is the growth of new nonprofit neighborhood health corporations to sponsor projects. These corporations, which include on their boards poor persons, health professionals, and members of other interested groups are coming into existence at an increasing rate. They are assuming broader, shared responsibilities for program development, direction, and monitoring.

These new alliances for health, involving all community groups concerned with the provision of better services, hold tremendous potential for the future organization and administration of local health services. These corporations are seeking both new methods of community control and better ways of ensuring that the quality of their services is a source of community satisfaction and community pride.

Consumer participation will also be a vital component of efforts to involve the nation's hospitals in the development of innovative methods of providing health services to low-income groups. Hospitals are showing a growing interest in aspects of the comprehensive neighborhood-health-service concept, which encourages a higher priority to quality programs of ambulatory care. In this way hospitals can upgrade their services and make them more responsive to community needs and desires. OEO grants are being made available to help selected hospitals to plan reorganized outpatient departments and related facilities. These projects, aimed at identifying the most effective ways of restructuring services to eliminate fragmented and impersonal procedures, also seek methods of involving poor persons in planning and evaluating services. They, too, offer new jobs and new careers for neighborhood people.

This brief summary indicates there are many different paths along which the goals of better health care and consumer participation have led us. We have sought to establish effective partnerships—between federal and local authorities and between consumers and professionals.

In this effort we have tried hard at OEO to ask the right questions, to be good listeners, and to respond appropriately. These are not easy tasks, but much has been learned and important gains have been made.

Tensions inevitably arise when health professionals and poor people, not accustomed to talking to one another and working together, sit down and grapple with issues that affect in vital ways the future well-being of themselves and their children. But there is nothing to fear, we have found, from open constructive dialogue, frank and searing as it may be at times. Rather, it is a sign of a more honest relation and greater maturity—a sign that vital issues too long ignored are at last being met.

As health professionals and community groups join together and turn increasingly to better techniques, we begin to see a clearer hope of breaking the cycle of illness and poverty blocking the path upward for so many Americans. Overall, the OEO experience supports the faith that the consumers and health professionals of this nation have the wisdom and strength to design and develop health-care systems that will further the dignity and well-being of us all.

DISCUSSION OF THE ROLE OF THE HEALTH PROFESSION IN ACHIEVING EFFECTIVE CONSUMER PARTICIPATION*

ROBERT C. LONG

Trustee
American Medical Association
Chicago, Ill.

Chairman
Committee on Health Care of the Poor
Louisville, Ky.

THE first step on the part of the health profession in achieving effective consumer participation in the provision of health care is to realize and accept the concept that health is a community affair. This concept implies, indeed it insists, that the responsibility for health no longer rests solely with health professionals.

To implement the concept that health is a community responsibility requires planning. While it is a new and often frustrating experience for both nonprofessional and professional community leaders alike, it is none the less essential. Planning should conserve critical resources through a system of priorities, should prevent duplication, and it may provide a rich communitywide educational experience as diverse elements join in an attempt to bring better health to the community.

No one plays a more important role in community planning than the consumer. It is the consumer who best knows the health needs of his area and who, in working in partnership with physicians and others, establishes priorities and works toward providing better health care to the community.

Within this context what other roles should organized medicine play, both at the community level and nationally?

First, a definition of the term organized medicine may be helpful. By this term is meant the county medical societies, the state medical associations, and the American Medical Association (AMA); the latter is a federation of county and state societies which serves both the public

*Presented in a Panel on the Role of the Health Profession in Achieving Effective Consumer Participation, as part of the 1970 Health Conference of the New York Academy of Medicine, *Community Participation for Equity and Excellence in Health Care,* held at the Academy April 23 and 24, 1970.

interest and the physician's interest throughout the entire country.

Nationally the AMA has played a strong role in advocating the provision of better medical care for all, especially to the poor, and it is in this area that the crisis is so grave.

I have been privileged to act as chairman of the AMA's Committee on Health Care of the Poor, and our first published report* is before you. It affirms some of the basic concepts of health care and emphasizes that consumer participation is essential, and it sets forth programs for action throughout all levels of organized medicine.

Recently the AMA, in testifying before Congress, urged greater funding for health activities of the Office of Economic Opportunity (OEO). In other testimony it strongly advocated increased funding for medical schools and increased funding for student loans so that a larger number of men and women from minority groups could enter medical school.

In addition, the AMA has recently entered into partnership with Temple University, Philadelphia, Pa., in the field of research and development of models of health-care delivery.

There are other activities in which the AMA is engaged but I believe that I have made my point: the AMA is deeply committed and actively involved in programs designed to improve the health of the poor.† Furthermore, AMA policy clearly states the important and essential role of consumer participation.

While much can be done by a national organization, the most meaningful, effective action is at the local, i.e., community level insofar as health-care delivery is concerned.

Here the consumer joins with representatives of the county medical society, community hospitals or a university medical center, local government, the communications media and other organizations to plan and implement programs which will result in the delivery of better medical care for that community. Effective consumer participation at the decision-making level is the sine qua non of the success of such community activities.

---

*Committee on Health Care of the Poor: *A Report on the Health Care of the Poor.* Chicago, AMA, 1970.

†Since this 1970 Health Conference of the New York Academy of Medicine, the AMA has donated $50,000 to a ghetto community in Chicago, Ill., for the purpose of improving the accessibility and availability of health care in that area.

DISCUSSION OF THE ROLE OF THE HEALTH PROFESSION IN ACHIEVING EFFECTIVE CONSUMER PARTICIPATION*

PAUL LOWINGER

Associate Professor
Lafayette Clinic
Wayne State University
Detroit, Mich.

I WISH to make a personal statement about community control. I want to share some of my own personal embarrassment and anxiety about this matter because this is the appropriate place to discuss it. For the last fifteen years I have been part of Lafayette Clinic, which is the Department of Psychiatry at Wayne University in Detroit. I have been aware through those years that as a teacher, researcher, and clinician I was doing an excellent job with residents and medical students. But one day I started looking at data on how my institution functions, and I discovered that we really have a very narrow perspective of service. One less charitable than myself might describe us as economically biased and racist in our approach to the selection of patients. Of course, I ought not to say anything like that about my own institution. We are located in an inner-city model-neighborhood area. I discovered that although the model-neighborhood area is only 38% white, and although we are in the center of this depressed area 82% of our patients are white; 47% of the people, who number 117,000, earn less than $3,000 a year, but that this is true of only 17% of our patients. Remember, ours is a public institution and we take only persons who cannot afford private care. Forty-four per cent of patients in model neighborhoods have eight grades or less of school, but this is true of only 15% of our patients; and so on. Perhaps the most shocking statistic is that of the 109 patients in this survey[1] only one was more than 60 years of age. It is not just the poor, the black, and the undereducated that we

*Presented in a panel, Role of the Health Profession in Achieving Effective Consumer Participation, as part of the 1970 Health Conference of the New York Academy of Medicine, *Community Participation for Equity and Excellence in Health Care,* held at the Academy April 23 and 24, 1970.

are not treating, but also the aged, who are screened out by all kinds of institutional acts: not deliberately, not consciously, of course.

What is community control? It was summarized by a conference on ghetto medicine[2] and in a recent article by Rick Kunnes,[3] who is well known as the leader of the New York demonstration against the American Medical Association in 1969. This article speaks of the policy-making decisions formulated by members of a board who control personnel. service, money, and management. These persons control the planning of new facilities, their size, location, and whether they are going to be established in store fronts or glass-and-steel offices. Community control includes a directive for job training, so that persons of the community can become health workers and so that services are free to the consumer, are decentralized, and concentrate on prevention.

This is not a concept that should be limited to the Office of Economic Opportunity or to government clinics. It should apply to all health institutions: Jewish hospitals, Catholic hospitals, Protestant hospitals, medical-school hospitals, boards of health, and academies of medicine. Until this idea begins to be implemented, we are going to remain in a severe health crisis. Everyone knows that the health-care crisis is worsening; both the consumer and the statistics know this. Community control is going to come about, but it is not going to come about as a result of planning by professionals, paraprofessionals, well-meaning liberals, and a few radicals. It is going to result from revolutionary, creative, and innovative action taken by persons in relation to their institutions. It will take grass-roots activity, and it will be resisted and fought by the present boards of hospitals and other institutions.

It will also be fought by many health professionals, so where do *I* fit in? Why do I talk about it? Because I am undertaking the establishment of a new program for combatting drug abuse in the state of Michigan.[4] One of my first responsibilities is going to be the creation of a new community mental-health facility which, like all state facilities, is going to be imposed on the community without any clear-cut control or planning related to local needs and wishes.

So this is a very embarrassing position. Does anyone want to help? I think what is going to happen, not just in my facility, but in all facilities, is that the community is actively going to develop techniques for assuming responsibility. And that will happen in a variety of ways. One kind of outside control will be that of unions traditionally concerned with wages, hours, and working conditions. But unions traditionally are not meeting the needs of the new breed of health workers, which include a number of professionals. The established unions are going to give way to groups like the new League of Revolutionary Black Workers, which is much more concerned with control of facilities. This is in a Michigan tradition: recall the sitdown strikes of the 1930's in the Flint auto plants.

Communities are not going to tolerate institutions that do not take direction in fundamental ways from persons who live in the community. This has been exemplified several times recently. One of the precipitating causes of the black rebellion in Newark, N.J., was a projected land grab by a medical school, a project that was changed after the smoke cleared and a new agreement was written. It was not entirely accidental that a small clinic was burnt to the ground in Watts, Los Angeles, in 1965. There are many other examples of this kind of pressure on health institutions in New York, California, Kansas, and elsewhere.

Health professionals who are concerned about community control should realize that they are technical persons offering services. Institutions taken over by coalitions of community and health workers experience a good deal of shifting of personnel. There will be transitional leaderships. Programs will change markedly. I think such changes are in store for institutions like the one I am going to head and like the ones you are involved in, and these changes we must anticipate if we want community control in the true sense.

From my viewpoint the health-care crisis and its causes are part of the national crisis that exists in every part of American life. But the health-care crisis is so acute that community control of health facilities seems to be one of the few techniques we have left to get us out of the morass in which we find ourselves. I see elements of community control as rationalizing the chaotic system. I think there is going to be a period of social change, and I think we are all going to be involved in it. It is going to come from communities that are going to make and realize demands. This has occurred in some of the health institutions related to Columbia University, at Lincoln Hospital in the Bronx, New York City, and in San Francisco General Hospital, where there was a strike of health workers recently. We are not just dealing with federal guidelines and institutional practices. We are dealing with increasing health consciousness and a radicalization of persons on issues of health comparable to their political activism on schools, employment, and on the police.

I conclude by reading a statement from a great American physician who speaks of our time.

> For one to be a revolutionary doctor or to be a revolutionary at all, there must be a revolution. Isolated individual endeavor, for all its purity of ideas, is of no use, and the desire to sacrifice an entire lifetime to the noblest of ideas serves no purpose if one works alone, solitarily, in some corner of America, fighting against adverse governments and social conditions which prevent progress. . . . And now we have come to the nucleus of the problem we have before us at this time. Today one finally has the right and even the duty to be, above all things, a revolutionary doctor, that is to say a man who utilizes the technical knowledge of his profession in the service of the revolution and the people. But now the old questions reappear: How does one actually carry out a work of social welfare? How does one unite individual endeavor with the needs of society? We must review again each of our lives, what we did and thought as doctors, or in any function of public health, before the revolution. We must do this with profound critical zeal and arrive finally at the conclusion that almost everything we thought and felt in that past period ought to be deposited in an archive, and a new type of human being created. If each of us expands his maximum effort towards the perfection of that new human type, it will be much easier for the people to create him and let him be the example. . . .[5]

REFERENCES

1. Kish, K. and Lowinger, P.: *Do University Programs in Psychiatry Serve the Inner City.* A Demographic Analysis. Annual meeting of the National Medical Association, Atlanta, August, 1970.
2. Norman, J., ed.: *Medicine in the Ghetto.* New York, Appleton-Century-Crofts, 1969.
3. Kunnes, R., Community control of community health. *New Phy. 19*:28-33, 1970.
4. Rensberger, B.: Psychiatrist fired at addict care center. *Detroit Free Press,* May 7, 1970.
5. Guevara, C.: On Revolutionary Medicine. In: *Vencermos! The Speeches and Writings of Che Guevara.* Gerassi, J., ed. Simon and Schuster, New York, 1968.

DISCUSSION OF THE ROLE OF THE HEALTH PROFESSION IN ACHIEVING EFFECTIVE CONSUMER PARTICIPATION*

P. Walton Purdom

President-elect
American Public Health Association

Professor and Director
Environmental Engineering and Sciences
Drexel Institute of Technology
Philadelphia, Pa.

Some people have asked me what this button is on my lapel. The question astonished me because the button is an Earth Week symbol. I had thought that almost everyone knew what was happening this week, yet I have received this inquiry. I use this incident as an illustration because the movement is a student movement; it is primarily a movement of young people. But I observe reactions occurring around the country: "they picked the wrong subject," "they didn't select the one with the right priority," or else "they are not going to follow through on it and achieve anything effective." In some 30 years of experience in this field, I have never seen any person or group alert the American people to the problems of the environment as much as these students have done in the last three months. They are to be commended.

In the Philadelphia area, the role of the professional with respect to the students for Earth Week was this: the students invited some of us—doctors, lawyers, engineers, and others—at the colleges to meet with them in sessions over a period of two or three weeks in order to discuss with them the technical aspects of environmental problems; then they carried on from there. They did not ask us whether we felt they should have a big meeting in Fairmount Park or anything like that. They did not ask us what to do. They asked us what the problems and the technical aspects were. This was our role in Earth Week and I think it was a very proper role. This shows that there are persons who con-

*Presented in a panel, Role of the Health Profession in Achieving Effective Consumer Participation, as part of the 1970 Health Conference of the New York Academy of Medicine, *Community Participation for Equity and Excellence in Health Care,* held at the Academy April 23 and 24, 1970.

sider the problems in health too important to be left to the professionals. These issues are political issues: they are in the political arena. Since I have become an officer of the American Public Health Association (APHA), some persons have written to me and this is what they have said: "We have been working in the environment field for many years. It has always been run by professionals. Now we are getting a lot of interest by people who are not professionals, and could I do something about this, so that the field reverts to the professionals." This is what the people who wrote have been working for all their lives, and they just do not realize it. They have been trying to get people interested in health and environment. Now the people are interested and the professionals do not know what to do about it. The professional should welcome such participation by persons who are concerned and should serve as an advisor.

Another role for the professional is participation in a professional organization. I shall give an illustration from the APHA and its recent reorganization. Some of you are familiar with this; but for those of you who may not be, I shall review the subject briefly. A conference known as CAFOR* was held over a period of days at Harriman House in order to consider the nature of the association, its responsibilities and role in the search for means to meet the health needs of the people, and the way in which the association should relate to other organizations, especially to consumers, in the fulfillment of the purposes of the association.

At the annual meeting immediately prior to the conference, the governing council directed that a list of persons in attendance be expanded to include some consumer participants; this was done. The additional persons invited had been active in some way in local health activities in neighborhoods and had a variety of characteristics. These guests participated in all sessions, both workshops and plenary sessions on the same basis as the professional members of APHA. The results showed the wisdom of the governing council in making this decision. The consumers continually reminded us of the necessity to keep the health of the people as our foremost concern whenever guild interest or professional idealism tended to divert us from the reality of the health needs of the people.

*Conference on Association Functions, Organization, and Relationships.

Unquestionably CAFOR decided that the APHA should continue to be a professional organization primarily. However, provision was made to encourage persons interested in the health of people to participate as full members. In addition to adopting substantial changes which would make the policy-formulating bodies of the association more representative, the requirement of fellowship—which is a professional recognition—was eliminated as a prerequisite for election to office. It was recognized that this in itself was not enough to make the APHA acutely aware of the views of consumers on matters of health. Other mechanisms seemed necessary. These cannot be established by the APHA alone, but require involvement of the consumer in decisions that affect their relation to the association.

As a step in this direction, it was suggested to the local arrangements committee that a substantial number of consumers be invited to attend the annual meeting in Philadelphia. Also, Community Health, Inc. arranged that a few consumer representatives from various parts of the country should attend. These consumer guests were extended every privilege of participation, including the privilege of the floor in meetings of the Governing Council. At times the air was charged with tension. Occasionally the remarks were highly emotional, but the result was that our resolutions were concerned with the realities of life as experienced by those who need the help and the services that the professionals can provide.

The matter cannot be left to rest here. The APHA has determined that it must follow up on the implementation of its proposals for a better way of life. Accordingly an Action Board was created to implement the technically based recommendations formulated by the Professional Development Board. Frequently when we discuss health matters as professionals, particularly those who may be specially interested in the medical role, we seem to overlook the relation between environmental conditions and the health of the individual. Most likely the relation is emphasized by the consumers who are present, because they know environmental problems from personal experience and consider them important.

Another type of participation can take place in organizations composed of citizens. Health professionals may be invited to participate in such organizations. I am thinking of groups like housing associations, clean-air councils, health councils, and others of this type. Sometimes the health professionals feel uncomfortable in such groups because the zeal of the group tends to exaggerate some of the technical facts. The professional has to learn to overcome this feeling and to help such groups by interpreting technical information in their areas of interest. One organization I might mention is the Delaware Valley Citizens Council for Clean Air. This is supported by the Tuberculosis and Respiratory Disease Organizations in some 11 counties and three states in the Philadelphia area. Laymen and persons interested in health and professionals —such as engineers, lawyers, and doctors—come together and work for cleaner air. They had a strong impact on the standards that have been adopted. In Pennsylvania they have prevailed on the Air Pollution Commission to alter its position in the interest of more stringent standards aimed at better protection of health.

In all the kinds of situations that I have mentioned there is a problem of communication. It seems incumbent on the professional to attack this problem, to be the one who makes the conscious effort to interpret technical information in layman's language and to help the consumer understand the political process, and the parliamentary procedures and the manner of using them. Unfortunately, poor communication and failure to identify common interests make the consumer and professional appear to be antagonists. This results from misunderstanding on superficial issues. We need each other—the political strength of the consumer and the technical knowledge of the professional of the problem and its solution—in order that we can both bring about the social action and social change that are necessary for a desirable quality of life.

DISCUSSION OF THE ROLE OF THE HEALTH PROFESSION IN ACHIEVING EFFECTIVE COMMUNITY PARTICIPATION*

STEPHEN R. SMITH

Vice President, Region II
Student American Medical Association
Boston University School of Medicine
Boston, Mass.

FEW here today would deny the right of a person to have some say in the type of health care he receives and for which he pays. The concept that consumer participation is a desired, needed, and necessary facet of proper health-care delivery will no doubt go unchallenged. Problems and disagreements will arise when the discussion centers around what kind of participation and its degree. If the consumer is to be the initiating force, should he be involved in the earliest stages, and should he be part of an advisory council or actually control the operations? These questions will be discussed at length by others. What I wish to discuss now is exactly who is speaking for the consumer.

All too often in political movements or other associations the leader emerges in such a way, perhaps, as not to reflect genuinely the constituency he supposedly represents. In fact, the only reason I am here "representing" student opinion is that I have a bigger voice with a matching ego than most other students who are probably equally qualified. My point is that those so-called consumers we so glibly speak about may not be representative of the real health-care recipients.

For instance, there would be no sense in having a wealthy woman from Westchester County on the board of a city hospital which she has never seen and in which she will never be treated, despite her very real and sincere interest in helping. In order really to know what the needs and feelings of a community are, one must be a member of that community. There is too great a chance that such an outsider will be

*Presented in a panel, Role of the Health Profession in Achieving Effective Community Participation, as part of the 1970 Health Conference of the New York Academy of Medicine, *Community Participation for Equity and Excellence in Health Care,* held at the Academy April 23 and 24, 1970.

so caught up in her own cultural background that she will perceive all she sees in that distorted fashion. The result may well represent too much of her and too little of the community actually served.

The ideal we can all hope for is that suddenly, from the grass roots of the community, will arise a group of citizens clear in their intentions, lucid in their speech, and determined in their efforts to bring the proper health-care systems to their community. Impossible? No indeed, but rare, to be sure. If such a thing did occur, it could be expected that the establishment would reel back in disbelief, regroup its facilities, and then not react at all.

Such a truly community-inspired program is the Northeast Neighborhood Association in New York City on the lower East Side. But, as I said, such a case is rare. The more likely situation is for the health profession itself to assume a leading role in initiating a new health program. We cannot and should not wait for spontaneous community action. As is true with most aspects of life in any poverty-stricken area the populace is dispirited, alienated, and unconvinced that it is part of society. An impetus is needed to break this cycle. Once a single link is broken many alternatives may appear, and it is here that a health program becomes relevant in the entire scheme of general social change. A health clinic that involves the community, responds to it, and is manipulated by it can serve as a catalyst for further action and involvement. Where is the consumer in such a project—is he the person who is being directly served by the clinic? The function of the health services is not only to act on the people but to involve them, to extract from them. The physician, therefore, must act more than as a mere health professional, he must be a human being reacting with another human being, helping him to help himself. Each patient is the consumer, it is *he* who is sick, it is he who knows the sickness that also infects his community. It is impossible to concern ourselves only with microorganisms and the like; starvation, unemployment, rat-infested homes, and racism are also health problems, for they make a society sick. There is no escaping this fact. If we are to talk about responding to the consumer we are obligated to respond as men, not just as health professionals. Our challenge lies in curing society; it is not just a case of lead poisoning in a three-year-old tenement dweller. But we can take the first step in our roles as health professionals.

Ours is a crucial role: we must have the sensitivity to be able to relate as fellow human beings to one another. We must not concern ourselves so much with meeting requirements to establish community boards, etc. A board meets outside of the doors of the examining rooms everyday in the city hospital. How do you act toward these board members everyday? This is where it can all begin. Get that poor, miserable, unemployed black patient to give a damn about the state in which he finds himself. The best way to do that is to express concern yourself. Ask him about the long waits, the red tape, the lack of transportation, the discontinuous care, the poor hours. Tell him what he can do about it and follow it up by use of those mechanisms that exist everywhere for the asking.

Get a trailer, load it with supplies, and drive it down to Second Street. Talk to the patients as you treat them, and there is your consumer participation. Be willing to respond and change. The health clinic also must be dynamic; it must respond to the needs of those it serves. True consumer participation cannot be an hour once a week, it must be an ongoing thing with constant feedback and interaction. Any one of us could do that, except me. Why? Because I am a student. I am learning my profession on human guinea pigs, and the people out there know it. Let us be honest: we derive much egotistic satisfaction out of going into communities to help, but students cannot provide health care. We are there to learn: you are there to treat. But, just as you must not be satisfied in healing the body alone, we must not be satisfied with learning alone. The role of the student must be that of the primary catalyst, the prime mover in involving the consumer with the health profession. It is a natural role for the idealistic, energy-filled champion of social justice. The student must convince the patient that the profession is receptive to its consumers and can be manipulated by them. The student must seek out potential leaders who express the true sentiments of the community and then involve these leaders intimately in the system. If the health system is to respond to the consumers and serve them well, it must utilize them, possibly as ancillary personnel, especially as family-health workers who can explain the importance of health to the people. This is one of the few effective ways of gaining the confidence of the community: by making its inhabitants aware of their health problems and of bringing them to the clinic. And remember, health problems extend far in scope: these very people may emerge as leaders in movements toward general social change.

Thus we see that consumer participation cannot be a lightly used phrase. All attempts must be made to engage the interest of the real consumer, the one we meet each and every day of our lives in our work. We must act toward our patients in a human way, with reactions and feelings and interest. We must realize that health is an inseparable part of all social problems, and that persons in the community involved in matters other than health can act just as well to express the community's health needs. Likewise, when community citizens are engaged in the health-care system, they must be encouraged to deal with the ills of all society. We must realize that students are traditionally in the forefront of social change, and that health students must be utilized in this role.

If we could act in our lives as I have suggested, then we could rest assured that the resulting consumer participation would be the cure we all are seeking.

DISCUSSION OF THE ROLE OF THE HEALTH PROFESSION IN ACHIEVING EFFECTIVE CONSUMER PARTICIPATION*

REV. WALTER WALDRON

Holy Cross Cathedral
President, Association of Boston Urban Priests
Vice President, South End Community Health Center
Boston, Mass.

I FIND myself in a somewhat difficult, perhaps contradictory, position in that I find myself in many areas of disagreement with my fellow panelists. I find that, supposedly as a man of faith, I do not have too much faith in the ability of the Office of Economic Opportunity (OEO) even to continue in existence, let alone to continue funding worthwhile programs. I take issue with the fact that the American Medical Association is not a powerful organization, especially after the John Knowles incident.

And I am very much concerned that we have made such a ballyhoo about the environmental problem. This problem is important; it is central, but I question the motivation of this country in stressing it. I think, perhaps, a strong part of the motivation is to make us forget we never solved the problems of housing and education in the 1960's. As OEO sinks quietly into the sea and the housing crisis continues to grow, it is hoped that we shall not even notice it.

Finally, I question that it is not important to work in the small corners of America. I find that if there is going to be reform or revolution or radicalization, or what have you—if it is not done by persons in the corners of America, it is not going to be done. And that is where I stand. I propose to speak on the corner of America where I am, and of the little experience that I have had there. I do not know much about national programs, I am not a member of national federations, etc. I just know from my own experience of helping with the formation of a community-controlled clinic.

*Presented in a Panel on the Role of the Health Profession in Achieving Effective Consumer Participation, as part of the 1970 Health Conference of the New York Academy of Medicine, *Community Participation for Equity and Excellence in Health Care,* held at the Academy April 23 and 24, 1970.

Regarding the issue of community involvement and health improvement: there are two political realities and one health-care reality that must be realized first.

Persons in low-income areas in cities are very distrustful of institutions—of city hall, welfare, churches, or hospitals. Expressed altruistic intentions of these institutions are subject to suspicion based on past performance. In city hospitals there are long waits, lack of personnel from the area where the hospital is located, the taking by the hospital of valuable land, shoddy treatment of persons, etc. Society's institutions are just not trusted in the core city.

Second, because of the ineffectiveness of society's dealing with conditions in poor areas of cities, in housing, education, police brutality, etc., the word "community control" is more than a slogan. It is a growing insight that people are intuiting as necessary if conditions can ever really change. In this area, health has had, indeed, a very low rating because poor education and lack of housing which, day in and day out, affect the lives of persons directly, have been the main object of attack and concern, and they still are. Yet in this area of health there is now an increasing awareness that the community can and should control its own health-care systems. The medical professsion can provide the medical assistance; the hospitals, the back-up resources; and the community, the control of programs, policies, personnel, and finances.

The health-care reality is that proper care is inadequate in cities today. I think everyone has said that so far. It is hardly necessary to mention the fact that in crowded parts of the city there are very few doctors and in some sections not one. The only possible recourse persons have is the local hospital, already overcrowded and outmoded. Yet persons do not use the hospital except in what they consider a dire emergency because of the absurd waits and shoddy treatment that many of them have already received there. Among Puerto Ricans, who now form a larger and larger percentage of inner-city residents, there is a definite mistrust of hospital institutions, and this accounts in part for their subsequent poor health.

It is in the light of these three realities—institutional mistrust, community control, and inadequate care—that a new kind of medicine is to be practiced in the cities. I say this because of my own experience in helping to form a community-controlled clinic in the South End of Boston. Such an operation, run and operated by an elected board of persons, not professionals, just community persons, can adequately meet the health needs of individuals and the community in any given area.

First, the days of the general practitioner are over. In the city such physicians have been nonexistent for a very long time and yet nothing has been done to fill the vacuum that they left.

The general practitioner was able to engender a feeling of trust in a client that outpatient departments of hospitals are too impersonal to achieve. A community-controlled clinic can bring back that element of trust. There is a growing concern that a patient should see the same doctor at every turn. A patient is far more apt to come to see such a doctor for small ailments and for the crucial preventive medicine that he ordinarily would not seek at a hospital. Terrifying statistics on tuberculosis, infant mortality, anemia, parasites, and the death rate in cities are largely attributable to the lack of preventive medicine there.

Second, a clinic such as ours provides more quickly the resources and technical ability of a back-up hospital. So there is the combination of a family doctor and the latest and most complicated medical practice in one package. The patient is well served in this procedure, and the back-up hospital has to meet the qualifications of the clinic. In other words, the hospital has now to answer to the persons it serves. For example: Boston City Hospital is our back-up facility for pediatric care. Yet when we established an obstetric-gynecological component, we completely rejected the unit at City Hospital because of its barbaric conditions and the poor attitude of some of the staff; we chose instead Boston Lying-In Hospital. We are able to do this because we are autonomous even though some of our funding is from City Hospital. Our expressed desire is that our patients get the best available care; moreover we feel that, at the same time, we can act as an advocate for the community in changing conditions in hospitals that we judge second-rate. This particular action of ours will certainly hurt the hospital, for many of its patients are from this area. The community's ability to choose a different back-up hospital for its different services will help ensure that a hospital will meet its responsibility, especially to the sick and poor.

Third, a community-determined clinic is able to overcome the aversion that persons have to look for good health care, an aversion created by their experience with hospitals. Any such clinic will rely heavily on outreach work. This means the hiring of community persons to reach other persons in the community, to help them understand the need for good medical health care, to provide them with help in getting this care by, for instance, good transportation systems. This outreach work is not a luxury in the city but a necessity. For many, medical care and hospitals are frightening experiences. The presence of an efficient medical facility is hardly enough to ensure its use by persons who live near it. However, when community persons are employed by the clinic, when it is known that friends and neighbors help run the clinic, then health care is more of a personal responsibility and less something to be avoided.

Fourth, the value of community concern about health is not to be undervalued. A community health clinic is a tangible vehicle of education. When there are so many important issues that face an inner city, health, in fact, receives little attention. And interest in health is surely raised when the program for health care and the style of its delivery is determined by persons in the community itself. This is nothing more than the democratic process at work.

Fifth, much as the community needs education in proper medicine, so do the medical professionals need education in community. There is a vast difference between the patient and the doctor—economically, culturally, academically, in style of living, usually in race, and perhaps in language. These factors, though not strictly medical, very much determine the relation between the giver and the receiver of medical assistance. The sensitivity of the "professional" staff can be more assured if it is hired by the community and knows that it is responsible to persons who live in the area. Medicine must learn that social conditions and environment, such as crowded living conditions, no heat, no hot-lunch program at school contribute to bad health.

These, then, are some of the major positive results that come from community-determined clinics: 1) the advantages of a family doctor; 2) the expertise of hospital back-up services; 3) health care reaching those farthest from it; 4) a new community attitude toward health; 5) a new medical attitude toward the community; and 6) a program that gives persons charge of their own destiny because they have charge of their own institutions.

What I say to the hospital professional is that this type of arrangement is a threat to the hospital system if the system becomes defensive about itself.

If the name of the game is "Power, power, who has the power" then it is a threat.

If the hospital is afraid that some of its departments will come under too close scrutiny and judgment from nonprofessionals, then it is a threat.

If the belief in medical circles is that persons in the community concerned about health are not sophisticated enough to provide decent health care, then it is a threat.

If hospitals are unwilling to be competitors in a free market in which the consumer in the city for the first time has the true freedom to choose the facility and the doctor he wishes, then it is a threat.

In an endeavor such as this, the initiative can come from either the hospital or the residents of the community. Wherever it comes from, under the political and social realities existing today, there must be one goal, one vision, one dream—a cooperative effort between the hospitals and the community—a dream and a goal that are determinative of all actions and strategy; and *that* is the proper health care of individuals and the community itself. The elected community board has its own responsibilities which it has a moral obligation to fulfill. The medical profession, as a service industry, must assist the community in meeting its responsibility.

I conclude by mentioning some of the ways in which the medical profession can in fact assist.

1) Open up your pocketbooks! Last year, Boston City Hospital turned back $2,000,000 of unused funds to the city government. Obviously, there is not only something wrong with the medical practice, but also with the accounting procedure. Open up your pocketbooks and give fiscal responsiblity to the community clinics. If it is true that it is the hand that rocks the cradle that rules the world, then it is the man that writes his own check who controls his own life. And this is what we are seeking.

2) Let the community decide what medical services it needs and can administer. There should be no funds from government or hospitals so earmarked that a community may have to choose a service it does not consider a priority in its area. We know what we need most! With the cooperation and assistance of the hospitals, we can provide it.

3) All doctors whom the community hires should be given staff positions in the back-up hospital.

4) The medical profession should provide facilities for training programs for persons the clinic wishes to add to the staff in paramedical positions.

5) A community clinic is not a training ground for medical students in universities. We want the best in health care now! We do not need university volunteers unless, for every volunteer, a corresponding position is opened in the university for a student from the community. If the university is getting benefit from the community, then fair is fair, and the community should use the university for its benefit. And I say this not only about the health porfession but also about education and social work.

COMMUNITY PARTICIPATION FOR EQUITY AND EXCELLENCE IN HEALTH CARE*

General Discussion II

JOHN L. S. HOLLOMAN, *chairman*

Chairman, Physicians Forum
Member, Regional Advisory Group
New York Metropolitan Regional Medical Program
New York, N. Y.

MR. OLLY NEAL, JR. My comments and my question will be directed primarily to Dr. Robert C. Long of the American Medical Association (AMA). I have read most of a report on health care of the poor prepared by the Committee on Health Care of the Poor of the American Medical Association. I am from Lee County, Ark., a county with a population of 23,000. It is very rural; it is also very poor. Seventy-five per cent of the population earns less than the poverty index established by the Office of Economic Opportunity guidelines for rural areas. Fifty per cent of those persons earn less than $2,000 a year. Does the national office have any kind of influence on local groups such as the Lee County Medical Society? Dr. Blumenthal has not been admitted to the Lee Medical Society; consequently he cannot use the facilities of or refer patients to, the hospital in the county. And I am wondering, since our county has only four other doctors for the 23,000 patients, two of whom are semiretired and working half time, if the AMA feels that these doctors can handle the health care for 23,000 patients, and if it does not feel that they can, then why is it that the county group is not encouraged to work with other physicians and groups working to provide health-care delivery in that county?

DR. ROBERT C. LONG. The question is very appropriate, and I shall answer it as directly and as honestly as I know how. The American Medical Association can urge, advocate, plead, persuade, and set examples for state and county medical societies. Each state and county medical society is an autonomous organization and may take what the

*The 1970 Health Conference of the New York Academy of Medicine, held at the Academy April 23 and 24, 1970.

AMA says and say "Yes, that makes good sense, I think we shall do something about it," or they can say, "Well, that does not apply to us." So we are taking first steps. It is a slow process, as I have tried to indicate. We do not have coercive power over our country and state medical societies. Second, three doctors for 23,000 people are obviously not nearly enough. I am sure you also do not have adequate facilities.

Comment from the Audience. My question is also directed to Dr. Long. You said in your remarks that the AMA believes that health is a community affair, and then a few minutes later you said that you saw the medical profession and the AMA as taking a leadership role. And I wonder if you see the inherent paternalism in that kind of statement, and what the AMA is prepared to do about that problem.

Dr. Long. Within a community there are many people who must play leadership roles. One of those persons—the most important, I think, from the viewpoint of this audience—is the consumer, the person living in the urban ghetto who has become a leader of that community and goes to other segments of the community to get better medical care for that area. I am talking about a partnership, a gathering together of the resources of a community to provide better medical care.

Comment: Mr. Chairman, a caption on a book states, "Medical Care to the Poor." I do not think we are talking about medical care to the poor. And I ask that it be resolved that such a caption be deleted from any over-all program. What we wish is medical care for all the people, not just for the poor.

Comment. Is this emphasis on local-community services and the avowed lack of power that the AMA has in dealing with its constituent state and local medical societies a way of sidestepping the whole issue of responsibility on the part of the organized segment of the medical profession, as opposed to the disorganized segment?

Dr. Long. Absolutely not. We are committed, we are involved, and we shall go forward—we are not sidestepping any responsibility.

Comment. I think that our discussions all day today have had a dichotomy which is extremely dangerous in that it has had the community over here and everybody else over there. The community by implication has been poor, black, or Puerto Rican—a minority group, whatever word you want to use. And the implication is that everybody else here is not a member of the community and should not participate or be concerned about participation. This implies that we have the consumers over here and professionals or providers over there. The implication seems to be that providers are never consumers. I grant that some consumers, or maybe many consumers, are never providers. But I doubt that professionals never receive or consume health care. I suggest here that perhaps the doctors, the American Public Health Association, and the students ought to consider these questions: "What kind of health care do I want as a consumer?" "What kind of health care do I want for my five-year old child?" "How can I apply my professional, technical expertise to get what I want as a consumer?" The fact is that we are all intermittent consumers of health care.

DISCUSSION OF THE "HOW" OF COMMUNITY PARTICIPATION IN DELIVERING HEALTH CARE*

MIGUEL F. BARRAGAN

Field Representative
Southwest Council of La Raza
Phoenix, Ariz.

I SHALL try this morning to do the unfair and the impossible: something I do not necessarily relish. I refer to addressing you of the medical profession in behalf of more than 10 million Mexican Americans, Cubans, Puerto Ricans—Spanish-surnamed citizens, few of whom I see in your midst.

Because health is not an immediate priority among the millions of poorly educated, poorly fed and poorly housed Spanish-surnamed Americans, my words do not present a magic solution to the medical crisis in our country, but rather a harsh challenge to those of you in the medical pyramid who wield some power, to change and become relevant.

Minorities throughout this country, especially Spanish-surnamed Americans who insecurely straddle two languages and cultures, are becoming increasingly aware that most institutions and agencies operate within a rigid framework of professional colonizers; that not only health, but the educational and welfare systems, are so stubbornly locked between an economic and political base controlled by professionals that they constitute a power package resisting change and meaningful participation of low-income consumers—the colonized.

Consider the accompanying diagram.

The participation by citizens in delivering health care is still largely a slogan in our country. The poor in our barrios and ghettos, powerless victims of America's institutional and systematic violence, have lost faith. "Maximum feasible participation of the poor" has not gone beyond the point of rhetoric and intellectual exploitation.

---

*Presented in a panel, The "How" of Community Participation in Delivering Health Care, as part of the 1970 Health Conference of the New York Academy of Medicine, *Community Participation for Equity and Excellence in Health Care,* held at the Academy April 23 and 24, 1970.

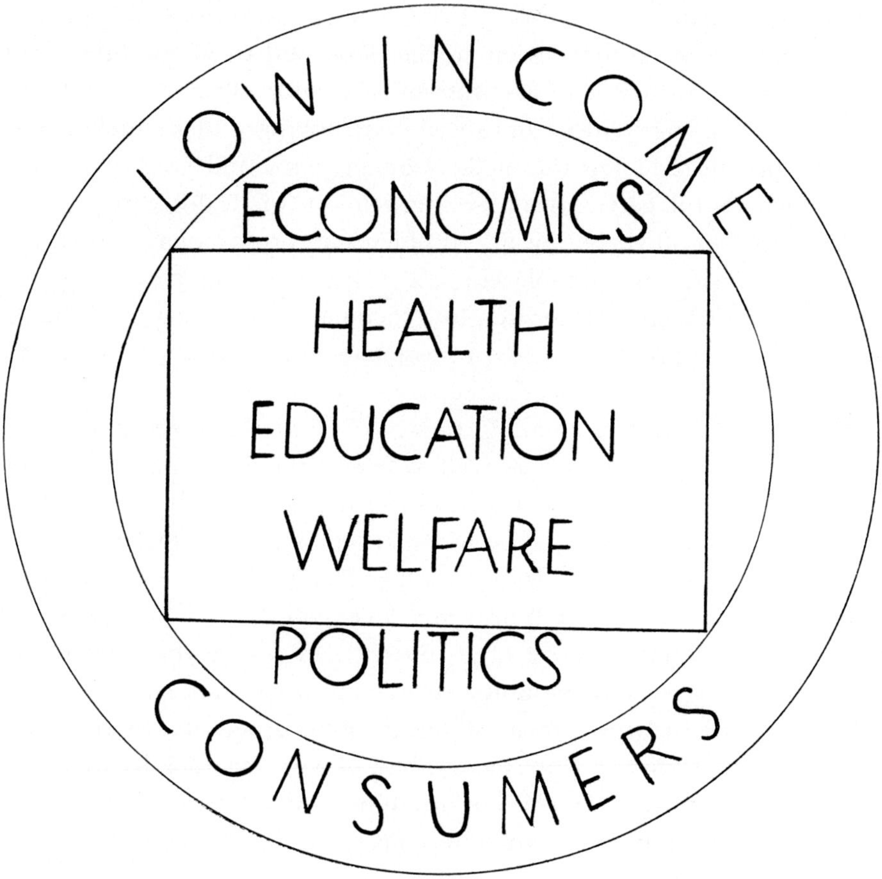

Before meaningful participation can be a reality for the low-income consumers, they must understand clearly the relation of the medical-industrial complex to the high cost of health services in which some of you are so deeply entrenched. They must penetrate the institutional rhetoric and dissolve the syndrome of medical professionalism which directly affects the availability and quality of medical care. Only in this manner can innovative health programs truly be designed and negotiated by low-income consumers who consider health no longer a privilege but a right.

In organizing the barrios, I often advise the poor to have three agendas of reform: 1) to change themselves; 2) to change professionals; and 3) to change institutions.

There is no doubt that educated persons, as well as illiterates, change as they try to change their world. If the medical institutions and agencies change so as to be more relevant to the poor, and if, in the process of altering the performance of institutions, the poor change through the process of social engagement and social confrontation, then much can be accomplished in reducing the medical bureaucracy and in allowing the poor a meaningful participation in the delivery of health care.

America can solve her health problems if professionals, especially those in authority, are humble enough to listen and aggressive enough to bring about change. Minorities, low-income consumers, are providing this wonderful opportunity to professionals and institutions in every walk of life.

Much of the creative thinking today is coming from the poor, who are talking of confrontation as well as innovation, negotiation as well as substitute models which will better meet the needs of the community.

Spanish-surnamed Americans across the nation from Delano, Calif., to the east side of Chicago, from Colonias Del Valle in southern Texas to Spanish Harlem in New York, are developing a new slogan: *De la pobreza al poder* (from poverty to power). Be aware that the barrios are implementing new community efforts and organizational techniques to build power to negotiate in all institutions, especially those which provide health services. Low-income consumers are establishing nonprofit community development corporations to attack the socioeconomic problems of malnutrition, unemployment, irrelevant education, and inadequate housing, all of which often cause poor health. From these nonprofit corporations under community control, the creative thinking of low-income consumers has begun to emerge in the form of proposals and programs which clearly spell out health needs as well as specific involvement in the areas of: 1) research; 2) training; and 3) participation of the indigent in all phases of education, prevention, outpatient services, hospitalization, rehabilitation activities, and other related health services. The sophisticated low-income consumer has begun to challenge the professionals in health care, government, and private foundations to break down the barriers to high-quality health services. For instance, in many cities that I service in the Southwest, consumers are requesting the transformation of county hospitals into communitywide health facilities. They are fed up with the stigma of county hospitals and the double standard of health care. Assisted by some socially conscious doctors and nurses, the poor are requesting health centers and neighborhood clinics under their own control. Finally, innovative solutions are being proposed by the indigent, who request insurance, health plans, or vendor-payment systems whereby they will be allowed to purchase medical care, hospital care, and prescriptions through the hospitals and pharmacies of their own choice.

In conclusion, I present a final challenge to those of you who have the authority and power to change the medical institution and health agencies of our country. May you have the courage to stand up and be criticized because you are willing to be different, to be controversial, in bringing about those changes which will benefit millions of Americans in desperate need of medical care and high-quality health service.

I have great hope and admiration for those young medical students, doctors, and nurses who are now attempting to make the medical profession more relevant. Like some of their predecessors, these persons do not feel threatened, but rather challenged by the innovations and demands of the poor. Amid social limitations and institutional frustrations, they are examining their own thinking, their own attitudes, and their value system, if not for the physical health of the powerless minorities, at least for the social well-being of our nation.

DISCUSSION OF THE "HOW" OF COMMUNITY PARTICIPATION IN DELIVERING HEALTH CARE*

JOHN W. HATCH

Director of Community Health Action
Tufts-Delta Health Center
Mound Bayou, Miss.

Assistant Professor of Preventive Medicine
Tufts University School of Medicine
Boston, Mass.

THE Tufts-Delta Health Center is located in Bolivar County, Miss., 100 miles south of Memphis and 20 miles east of the Mississippi River. Since 1967 the center has been providing services to a population of about 16,000 people living in 10 small towns and scattered rural locations situated in a 500-square-mile service area. Eighty per cent of the population is black and, within this group, 85% is poor. The population curve is skewed: the median age is 15 years, while the average age of heads of households is 54 years. Migration is selective as to age, sex, and education; a disproportionately large number of younger, better-educated males elect to migrate to large metropolitan areas north of Mississippi.

The first contacts with this community began in the fall of 1965. At that time a final decision as to the location of Tufts' rural health center had not been made. While this area's characteristics were within the frame of factors considered essential for a workable operation, we felt it essential to determine the level of community receptivity to the type of project we proposed. It is easy to assume that persons who are poor and often sick would readily embrace a project focused on bringing relief to one dimension of their multiphasic needs. Many are now beginning to realize that needs and priorities are influenced by the total life situation of the group providing the assessment. Rural Mississippi is no less complex in terms of conflicting values and social forces than the urban ghetto is proving to be.

*Presented in a panel, The "How" of Community Participation in Delivering Health Care, as part of the 1970 Health Conference of the New York Academy of Medicine, *Community Participation for Equity and Excellence in Health Care*, held at the Academy April 23 and 24, 1970.

The first contacts within the target area were with persons likely to use the service. Although I was born and raised in the rural south, I had become urbanized and felt it essential to take steps to become attuned to the people with whom I wished to communicate. I elected to spend several months living with poor families residing in the area. I worked as a farm laborer and shared in the social life of the community in which I lived. Experiencing diarrhea in a crowded rural home without toilet facilities is considerably more impressionable than reviewing data on the high rate of intestinal disorder, its probable cause, and the statistical fact that 90% of the housing is dilapidated and without plumbing. It is likewise easy to assume that the conditions that appall outsiders are not so difficult for local people who have long experienced neglect, a harsh environment, and injustice. Most people, local or outsiders, are uncomfortable in 105° F. heat coupled with dust, high humidity, and hard work. Black men and women of the area, after more than 300 years of conditioning, had not accepted as just the tendency of local merchants' policy of requiring blacks to wait until all whites were served. Much of the conversation of my neighborhood centered around the life styles and eccentricities of white folks and black gatekeepers. While neither group was very much trusted or respected, they were almost always approached with caution and treated deferentially. A group of men discussing a serious local issue, upon being approached by a white person, would shift the conversation to a trivial topic. Expressions and positions would not change and it was never necessary for each person to turn around to know that "the Man"* was approaching. My contacts with white storekeepers, labor supervisors, the welfare office, and with professional blacks were usually directed by them as though my mental development was that of a not-very-bright eight-year-old child.

Behavior within the safety of the family, of an extended group of friends, of the church, and of other poor persons' organizations was quite different. Persons addressed as Mary and John during the day became Mr. and Mrs. Deacon, Mr. Chairman, Exalted Rulers, and Worshipful Masters within the context of that part of the social system controlled by themselves. These organizations and associations tended to enforce values of the poor black community. An elaborate system of

*"The Man" is an expression used by black people when referring to the person supervising them or to a white man.

sanctions, rewards, limits, and controls so vital to the group's survival and vitality were generally invisible to white people.

I had wondered if the movement had made much difference in the relations between blacks and whites in rural areas; it had not. I wondered whether poor blacks and middle-class blacks were significantly closer together; they were not. Was the extended family generally intact? Yes. Were local organizations and associations able to sustain their importance in the lives of persons? Yes. I am not suggesting that one who has viable options to leave can react as deeply as those who do not, but I do feel that sharing living conditions does provide feelings and insights that cannot be obtained from a distance.

Would the target population regard us with suspicion and mistrust? Most assuredly. Our coming to the area did not pose a threat to the black poor of the general service area, although some persons in the all-black town of Mound Bayou did express concern that the presence of white people might end the relative degree of freedom the town enjoyed from enforcement of laws by whites and racist-inspired terrorism often experienced by blacks in many parts of Mississippi.

Efforts toward gaining entry were aimed toward those most likely to be threatened by the proposed project: medical practitioners, those with proprietary interest in medically related enterprises, those who viewed the project as a threat to their positions of power and prestige. The array of objectors included white conservatives who had visions of an integrated hippie movement. Others saw the program as an attack on the free-enterprise system and a camouflage for activism in civil rights. Some gatekeeper blacks were concerned at the implications of an operation they perceived as being black-oriented functioning outside their sphere of control. Several black militants questioned the appropriateness of a "white" institution that proposed to provide services in a predominately black community. Others felt all such programs amounted to pacification and only tended to delay the day of confrontation. We certainly could not assure the varied interested groups that the center would operate within a frame acceptable to them. We did listen and answer questions honestly. Our accessibility and willingness to talk probably defused several potentially explosive situations.

The poor were involved and became supportive of our efforts to secure community approval. A number of house visits were made, and individuals and families volunteered case material supportive of the project. Public meetings were well attended. More than 300 letters of support flowed into the office of Tufts Medical School. Gaining entry, at least in our situation, was quite different from gaining support or community participation as generally understood.

When the stressful phase of gaining entry was past we began intensive orientation contacts with the population we had contracted to serve. A locally recruited staff of 12 and the professionals of the center made home visits with a view toward getting acquainted and of providing some idea of the project's goals to our hosts and hostesses. We learned a great deal. Beyond the statement that doctors and nurses were coming, persons found it difficult to relate to other dimensions of the program. From home visits or, rather, from information based on questions and concerns emerging from the home-visiting experience, we moved to both small-group and mass meetings. The small-group meetings were most valuable in providing insight into interest and friendship groups. A person surrounded by his peers on his home ground proved to be much more comfortable asking questions and expressing concern than in one-to-one contacts. Mass meetings proved excellent for dissemination of information but were obviously limited as tools for two-way communication. During the first three months of our presence in the community clinical services were not available. Our credibility greatly increased with the beginning of these services. We had, however, responded to individual and family crises from the beginning. As dialogue increased between members of the staff and of the center with several communities, special concerns began to emerge: the range included water, housing, food, clothing, pest control, and disabled elderly persons. Each community was encouraged to select temporary committees to begin work on issues of their choice and to act as contact persons between the community and the center. Our staff asked the community also to consider representation in terms of other unique interests and needs of persons at different stages and situations in their lives. Clusters essential to representativeness were identified as 1) youth: one male, one female; 2) female head of household under 31: one male, one female; 3) one person over 65 living on welfare; 4) the head of a household living on the plantation; 5) the head of a household with teen-age children: one male, one female; and 6) three community leaders without regard to income.

The ad hoc committees began to schedule informational meetings geared to the special concerns of their community. We soon found out that the number one priority was not health as traditionally viewed. Food—that is, the lack of it—was the most pressing problem in the fall and winter of 1967. Could we help this community to find answers to this most basic of human needs? Members of the staff were mobilized to help persons apply under existing programs, and they were encouraged to assume advocacy in selected cases. For whatever reasons, existing programs aimed toward avoiding malnutrition were not working. This concern over food eventually led to the development of a cooperative farm owned, staffed, and administered by displaced tenant farmers and sharecroppers. Considerable support for the project was provided by the staff of the center, but from day one it was the community's project. The cooperative has succeeded in providing nutritious food to more than 5,000 persons annually. The community justly feels proud of its accomplishment. The cooperative is now moving toward becoming a self-sustaining food-producing and food-processing enterprise. Providing the level of support needed by the cooperative during its first year of life did slow down the development of other priorities of the center. The cooperative now operates 600 acres of vegetable-crop land, and it now uses the most modern equipment available. This was made possible through hard work coupled with support from the Ford Foundation and from the Office of Economic Opportunity.

By leaps and bounds interest in center-related programs increased. Several communities moved to the point where more formal structure was needed to carry out the variety of functions they had undertaken. One community was given assistance and support in establishing a water supply; this required substantial amounts of legal and engineering service. Clean-up projects, emergency-clothing centers, cooperative purchasing of fuel, and home repair were among the projects under way. Until about a year after the opening day there had not been a formally organized citizens group responsible for areawide planning. The need for such an organization had never been in doubt. We simply did not possess the knowledge to do this earlier. We had observed councils without accountability to their constituencies that rapidly became more like clubs than bodies of delegates. Moreover, we were serving a 500-square-mile rural area. Persons did not generally know others beyond their own negihborhoods. The single common organizational structure known to the residents of the area was that of the Baptist Church. It seemed sensible to follow this model. This accounts for the relatively high level of autonomy accorded the local communities. Each community—by this time eight were formally organized—was asked to participate in the formation of an areawide council that would become responsible for the major planning, action, and monitoring for the several communities. During this period there was a flurry of action in the local communities and limited interaction among some of the associations. Conflicting demands emerged from several directions. The local association selected three people to sit on the council's planning committee. Each delegation included one member of each sex and one member under 30. Planning sessions were held once weekly on Sunday afternoons for a period of three months. Members of the center's staff, assigned to development work, were required to attend and were charged with responsibility for strengthening the flow of information between the local associations and the council's planning groups. A major part of this role was defined as providing support to the delegates at both levels of involvement. Goals of the council were formulated at a number of sessions involved with various aspects of the functioning of the center and with community priorities. This period of informal association provided the group with the opportunity to identify its natural leaders and was the setting for considerable testing of the center's staff. There was considerable dissatisfaction at the staff's inability to provide answers to issues accorded highest priority by representatives of the community. We were often reminded of our desire to deal with root causes and were asked why we talked about comprehensive community health if in fact we did not have the means of effectively dealing with real problems.

After considerable effort it was agreed that the center could provide only a part of the needs considered essential by the community for basic change. At one especially stimulating meeting a delegate sensed the mood of the group and challenged those present "to do their own thing" as the only sure means of attaining the broad-based goals envisioned by the planning committee. This led to questioning the desirability of a council for the area focused primarily on health-related concerns, and eventually it led to the decision to form an organization capable of dealing with the broader-based agenda. The structural form eventually adopted was that of a nonprofit development corporation with a form strongly suggestive of that of a Baptist Church convention. The body presently represents two health and civic associations and is incorporated as the North Bolivar County Health and Civic Improvement Association. In addition to the more traditional health and related concerns the council has developed a legal services program, is now in the process of becoming the sponsoring agency for a low-cost housing development, and is pursuing the possibility of an association with the National Federation of Settlements as a possible means of strengthening its 10 neighborhood services and community centers. Today's agenda includes discussion around potentially self-sustaining ventures and the desirability of diversified funding.

In a real sense the center is now the junior partner in a broad-based program that may best be described as community development. We see this as the appropriate relation between a service agency and its host community.

We are still asked to provide more services and input than we can manage, but I feel the community is aware that we shall continue to do our best. Several other institutions of higher learning, national health and welfare agencies, and private industries are now involved in the region. Long-denied change seems about to come to the Delta.

In summary, I should like to point out the major understandings gained from the project that seems to have broader application:

1) Becoming attuned to the cultural life of the community is an essential requirement for successful participation in it.

2) All communities have strengths that may not be visible to the casual observer. To build, these strengths must be discovered and enhanced.

3) Most poor communities view outside efforts toward intervention with considerable suspicion. Based on their past experiences, this is a rational view.

4) Most poor people do not view problems within the narrow frame in which they are placed by institutionalized planning and will likely appear apathetic or will attempt to use the available resources on a scale beyond the intent of its custodians of first resort, the professionals.

5) The most appropriate function of such an agency is that of an ally or junior partner that provides its service with quality but is strongly supportive and involved in the community's plans for development.

6) A service agency can play a catalytic role in the development of resources essential for basic social and economic change.

DISCUSSION OF THE "HOW" OF COMMUNITY PARTICIPATION IN DELIVERING HEALTH CARE*

Olly Neal, Jr.

Business Administrator
Lee County Cooperative Clinic
Marianna, Ark.

Before I begin my discussion I should like to make one comment: I have heard the words professional and professionalism tossed about during these sessions quite frequently, and I wonder whether a professional is one who has the necessary training and knowledge only in a particular field. I wonder if a professional should not also have some ability to apply that knowledge in his profession. This question came to me because in one of the round-table discussions and in one of the sessions here I have heard the frequent comment that we professionals are interested in doing something helpful in working with the poor but that the poor just are not interested and we just cannot reach them. My response is very simple: I wonder just how professional we are.

I shall try to tell you briefly something about the development and operation of the Lee County Cooperative Clinic and then, perhaps, I shall tell you something about what I think its implications are.

The topic of this discussion is "the 'how' of community participation in health care delivery." As I see community participation in the delivery of health care, it comes out just a little bit differently. I choose to talk just a little about "the 'how' of community control of health-care delivery." Because, you see, I agree with what John W. Hatch and some of the other good people have said at this conference: that participation is not very meaningful if it is merely an opportunity to present advice that is very likely to be rejected. Somebody spoke here about a group or a government organization that made a decision on a problem after having discussed it with an advisory group but did not—that is, was not courteous enough—to bring the advisory group in to their decision

*Presented in a panel, The "How" of Community Participation in Delivering Health Care, as part of the 1970 Health Conference of the New York Academy of Medicine, *Community Participation for Equity and Excellence in Health Care,* held at the Academy April 23 and 24, 1970.

making. I think the advisory group was really, as the speaker described it, just *nothing*. I have a term for it, but I do not think it is proper for this audience.

Lee County, Ark., is located in the east-central area of the state on the Mississippi River. It is a county of 23,000 population; has a number of very small towns; Marianna, the county seat, is the largest with a population of 5,000.

Sixty per cent of the population of the county, 23,000, is black, and 75% of that population earns an income that places it below the established poverty index for rural income. And 25% of the population are members of families that earn less than 1,000 dollars per year.

It has been suggested to us that Lee County is one of the 10 poorest counties in the nation. We have not documented this.The economy of the county is basically plantation-oriented. I shall cite one instance that I know you will find almost unbelievable. Members of commercial organizations of the county, particularly druggists and the one black funeral director (I can speak about him because I know him personally) still find it necessary to pass along a portion of their earnings to the plantation owner. You may not understand exactly what I mean. If a family that lives on a plantation finds that it must go to the drug store to get a prescription filled, the druggist, after filling the prescription, passes along to the owner of the plantation a percentage of the charge for that prescription. When the funeral director takes a body from that plantation he passes along to the plantation owner 20% of his burial fees, although he swears he is not doing it now. That is what I mean by plantation economy. As we indicated, there is a high incidence of poverty in Lee County; more than 75% of all families earn less than 3,000 dollars a year. The natural result of this is a high incidence of hunger and malnutrition, which are followed by poor health.

Health care for the poor has been almost nonexistent, so that the county's residents have developed an attitude of defeat, or *had* developed an attitude of defeat. It is from this kind of situation, and from this attitude of defeat that the Lee County Cooperative Clinic developed.

A few years ago the Office of Economic Opportunity (OEO) started to develop programs designed to increase the economic opportunities of the poor. But I think that many of the OEO programs are really designed as pacifiers. In its attempt at pacification (the neighboring county had had riots and that sort of thing) OEO sponsored in part the development of neighborhood action councils in the county to give the people an opportunity to express themselves and to direct their attention to the things they thought were important in their communities. Some time after the development of these neighborhood action councils, the Volunteers In Service To America (VISTA) that included a volunteer doctor (I think he is the first and only one) came into Lee County. Now the fact that the poor found it difficult to get a doctor (there are four doctors in Lee County, two of them semi-retired because of age, which makes three doctors for the 23,000 persons), caused the volunteer to be warmly received.

When the volunteer doctor came into Lee County and attempted to address himself to the needs of the poor he moved in such a way as not to suggest that he had all the answers. He started to make house calls. This was with good reason, for the owner of the house our doctor rented as residence would not allow black people to come into that house, even though the owner was not living there. So our doctor found it necessary to practice from the back seat of his automobile. As he went around the county he asked questions such as: "How can I be useful? How can I be helpful? How can I best meet your expectations and fulfill your hopes?" The county people, unsophisticated though they were, knew or believed that it would be necessary for him to have some sort of office facility, so that he could see more persons than he could in automobile trips throughout a very large county. From this developed the idea of an outpatient clinic. Now, recognizing that Dr. Daniel Blumenthal, our volunteer doctor, could not possibly provide health care for the approximately 17,500 persons (that is how many fall below the poverty index in Lee County and therefore are eligible for his services), it was concluded that some kind of medical assistants would be needed to help carry the load. To develop the idea we used in part the model provided at Mound Bayou, Miss. We worked closely with the St. Jude Hospital in Memphis, Tenn., and used their ideas and assistance in training. We call our paramedical people "health aides."

It was believed that these health aides could do several things. First, they could provide a kind of follow-up service that the doctor could not undertake because of the sheer magnitude of the problem. Second, they could serve as translators between doctor and patient. They could serve as go-betweens to bridge the gap between polished professional and crude patient. For when a white man comes into our area he looks like all other white men, and white men tell us, "Boy—you get over there and wait." Since Dan Blumenthal is white he really needed someone to assist him in communicating. And if his work was to be effective he needed someone to communicate with those for whom he wished to provide a service. He needed someone to tell them where he was, so to speak. This, then, was the reason for our developing the idea of training and developing health aides.

All the health aides are from the community served. They were trained in part by Dr. Hatch's facility in Mound Bayou, in part by the staff at St. Jude Research Hospital in Memphis, and in part by our own doctors and nurses.

At present our staff includes one doctor, two nurses, and a laboratory technician who are from VISTA. We have four health aides, one bus driver, one receptionist, and one business administrator (myself). The latter seven are from the community. We are entirely subject to the will of our board of governors; to make certain that this is the case the president and the secretary of the governing board sign all our checks. So that if we decide that we do not like the way something is going we can either reach an agreement with the governing board or move on.

In addition to signing all checks that dispense clinic funds the governing board members assume responsibility for the development and operation of the clinic. They selected and arranged for a building to house our clinic; they decided the days and hours of operations; they hired the staff, including myself; they selected a bus and are presently determining the route that the bus will take in an effort to solve the problem of transportation for patients; they provide for an effective transfer of information between the clinic and the community; they have raised funds; and they have recruited volunteers. All these things have really determined the basic operation of the clinic.

We operate on a budget of approximately $60,000 for an eight-month period; of this sum, $40,000 dollars comes from the OEO's Emergency Food and Medical Services, and $20,000 from community-volunteered goods and services.

Our health aides make many initial contacts in the community. Because they live in the community and because they are known as community people many problems come to them before they would come to the attention of the doctor.

Our county's residents operate on a crisis basis for health care. That is, they see the doctor only when there is no other alternative. Either they see him to sign death certificates or for other such things. As our health aides and I are part of the community we find that we learn of cases of illness early in their inception. We think that we can eventually move toward something very close to preventive health care, which of course will involve a great deal of work in the area of nutrition. We are presently working on a plan to provide a nutritional program.

All of these things, let me remind you, are not done on my initiative; they are not done by my deciding this is what we need in our county. These things are brought to the attention of the board, and we move only when the board decides the move is a good one.

Now I know that you are thinking, "Well, normally you can take a board of that particular character and mold it around to your own way of thinking." We know this to be true, too. However, because of our feeling that communities must learn to control their own destinies we have made every effort, and we shall continue to make every effort, to have that board make decisions independently of its thinking toward me. I have been able to do this effectively, I believe, for two reasons. One is that I was born and raised in the county; the board members knew my mother and father; they knew me when I was a baby, so they do not have to look up to me. The second reason is that I encourage them to make decisions of their own. It is my belief that the next administrator will not have to push the board; he will have to follow their dictation, so to speak, because they will have become sophisticated and more aware of their responsibilities, their duties, and their capabilities.

It is our opinion that the delivery of medical care must meet the needs of the community served and must address itself to its aspirations. The community must control nonmedical decisions that are made. Meaningful communication must be established in some way between the health professionals and the community served. Doctors must recogize that they are not gods. While we all appreciate you and look to you for help, those of us who are working in the community have many ideas as to what a community is. And on many occasions we have ideas that are ahead of your own. Many of you have spent most of your years in the sterile atmosphere of a medical school, and you do not know much about what is going on out there in the streets of the nation.

Some effective means must be developed by which the complaints and recommendations of patients can reach the health professionals and will be acted upon by persons in a position to effect changes. And we see that the way this can be done is through real community control of the delivery system. The community people must somehow serve as a part of the staff of any health-care delivery facility. This, in my opinion, is the only effective way to make certain that there is a true interpretation of the thought and attitudes on both sides.

Any do-gooder liberal group seeking to provide health care in some less fortunate area must not avoid the action-oriented people. You must deal with them.

At this conference a situation in New York City has been discussed in which decisions were made and implemented in the Gouverneur area without contact with the advisory board. If anyone still thinks a community is going to remain passive because one is doing good work he is sadly mistaken. We are capable of survival under any conditions. You must know this because we have managed to survive in the United States this long. So when you tell me you are going to offer me 15 cents, and I know I need a dollar, I am going to tell you to take your 15 cents, and go to hell because if I need a dollar I am going for a dollar. So do not think that because one is doing good work, that in itself ought to be considered the complete solution of the problem: one must address oneself to the attitudes, aspirations, and desires of the persons for whom one proposes to do this good work.

The Lee County Cooperative Clinic has been very controversial in our area. The whole ideal of providing free medical care for those who are incapable of paying for it has met with a great amount of resistance among local officials. As I have said, the majority of persons in the area look favorably on the project, as indicated by their participation in clinic activities. The local medical society has rejected our activities completely. The local druggists have indicated that they found us distasteful. However, when we have suggested to them that we should like to purchase drugs from them by way of a charge account they have been quite willing to accept this because it made good economic sense and did not concern their personal likes and dislikes.

Our doctor at this time cannot refer patients to or use the facilities of the local county hospital. The local hospital is supported by local tax funds and was built with money from the Hill-Burton Fund. We have had indications from the chairman of the hospital board that as long as any doctor works with us he will not be able to use the facility.

Let me now describe a few things we have in mind that indicate that the administrator is not exactly on top of the situation. As I have said earlier, black people represent 62% of the population in Lee County. We have had a sleeping community. It is my intention to do more than operate an outpatient clinic in Lee County because all the indications are that if we sit back and try to administer a clinic in the sterile atmosphere of that little cubicle called our office we shall find our efforts futile. It is my belief that we must deal with the whole range of social, political, and economic problems in that county.

Some of you who are a little more conservative and have operated on a fee-for-service basis all of your professional lives may be a little adverse to some of our ideas. We are going to set up cooperatives, and I am not talking about what I am going to do personally, because my knowledge of the kind of cooperatives that will be applicable in our area is not broad. But people who do have the knowledge, the people in the county, will set up and operate these cooperatives. I am talking about farm cooperatives, something that may be very foreign to many of you who have never ventured away from your two-acre suburban lawns. Some of my black brothers and sisters also may have forgotten. But we want to set up farm cooperatives, and we want to set up a cooperative for groceries. It will probably not equal some of the supermarkets you have here in New York. But we are going to provide for the needs of our people. And we are going to do this because we recognize that the racism that exists in America must be met in such fashion. We shall move toward those things that will make us independent of those of you who feel that we should come to you hat in hand.

I moved from Arkansas to Chicago for a few years in the belief that I should find the promised land. After spending a few years there I decided I had better go back home. All you professionals here are much smoother, you are much more subtle, you tell us all good things, and you move around us. You cannot communicate with angry, aroused persons, as at Gouverneur, because they talk too loud, and you do not want to talk to them. You do not call me boy, you call me Mr. Neal, but you are still misleading me.

I am not going to talk about a statistic, but I am sure most of you were here when a very liberal gentleman refused to give any meaningful answer to a question I asked. That is racism too. You can call it what you want to, but it is not meaningful communication.

As I have said, we have one doctor who will be departing from our clinic June 30. If any of you are interested in working with our program, you may talk to us, although I should remind you that our community controls our program, and that if you feel that you have all the ideas, then you must realize that, while we are desperate, we are not begging.

THE MEDICAL-SERVICES ASSOCIATE: A NEW HEALTH CAREER FOR THE IMPROVEMENT OF HEALTH-CARE DELIVERY*

STANLEY S. BERGEN†

Chief of Community Medicine
The Brooklyn-Cumberland Medical Center

Associate Professor of Medicine
State University of New York Downstate Medical Center

HAROLD NIERENBERG

Dean, Adult, Evening, and Continuing Education
Long Island University

ARNOLD M. LEWIS

Project Director, Medical Services Associate
The Brooklyn-Cumberland Medical Center

DOMINICK FIRRIOLO

Professor of Biology
Long Island University

Brooklyn, N. Y.

INTRODUCTION

THE need for reorientation of health-care priorities in the United States has brought into sharp focus the gap that has developed in the training of health manpower. Now that we have come to realize the lack of personal health services available to our citizens we have accepted the fact that we have insufficient health manpower to deliver these services. There is no doubt that Abraham Flexner[1] provided the United States with an important service with his exposé of the inferior facilities available for the training of physicians in the early 1900's. However, poor subsequent planning has led to the development of a large differential between production and need as the attrition of physicians during the subsequent 60 years has been paralleled by a relative decrease in the number of physician graduates available to serve the

*Presented in a panel, Absence of a National Health Policy on Training and Utilization of Manpower, as part of the 1970 Health Conference of the New York Academy of Medicine, *Community Participation for Equity and Excellence in Health Care,* held at the Academy April 23 and 24, 1970.

†Now senior vice president, Health and Hospital Corporation of Southern New York, New York, N. Y.

population. Despite recent attempts to expand and supplement existing educational facilities it seems evident that adequate numbers of physicians will not become available in the foreseeable future.[2]

At a time when health care was a privilege, the obvious gaps in the delivery of health services to many segments of our population were tolerated. The physician was established, along with a few other health professionals, as the only acceptable vehicle for the delivery of health care. While most of the population still looks to the physician as the "healer" and thus the ultimate source of medical care, we must ask if he is in fact the most economic and the only qualified person to provide medical services to all the sick.

In a recent editorial in the *New England Journal of Medicine* Dr. Victor Fuchs and his associates[3] have called attention to the fact that the health-care industry is beset by a very specific problem: that of a top-heavy executive or upperclass and a large group in the lower classes of employment within the industry. There is a shortage of personnel at the so-called middle-management level. This shortage is emphasized by the fact that only those in the higher categories are either licensed or given the status of direct deliverers of health care to the people. In comparing this situation with 19 other industries, Dr. Fuchs emphasizes its disastrous effects on the development of the industry, on its costs, and on many of the parameters of service the health industry is called upon to deliver. Of the many solutions suggested to remedy this situation, one of the most feasible seems to be the expansion of health-care delivery by the development of new categories of "middle-medical personnel": those individuals trained to work under the direction of a physician and to assume a portion of his duties.

Background

During the last 10 years we have witnessed the awakening of great interest in the development of the allied health professions.[4, 5] Individuals previously in so-called dead-end jobs in health and other industries have been recruited into training programs for multiple specific job categories. Many of these programs are institutionally based but others combine academic resources such as community colleges or baccalaureate programs with hospital and medical-center facilities. The degree of training and the time committed to academic education obviously bears a relation to the level of attainment. The greater the degree of technical content the more limited the mobility of the program. Attempts have been made to develop reentry points for those who wish advancement and core-health curricula are being developed with the intent of providing a basic fund of knowledge applicable to many career opportunities. It is estimated that 125 such career categories are now available, and this may rise to more than 200 within the next five to 10 years.[6] Despite these basic and important approaches to the problem, such programs have merely succeeded in broadening the basic manpower pool. Our ability to deliver personal health services to the consumer, the patient, has not been expanded to a great degree. New categories of professionals must be developed, trained, and provided direct contact with patients, with responsibilities that will enable them to provide primary medical care if we are to improve the health-care delivery of the system.

Long Island University, Brooklyn Center, a private liberal arts university, and the Brooklyn-Cumberland Medical Center, an 850-bed voluntary-municipal hospital complex in the downtown area of Brooklyn, joined in early 1969 to develop a program for the training of medical-services associates. Precedent for this cooperative venture is based on the fact that both institutions cooperate at present in the training of baccalaureate-degree nurses and cytotechnologists while also conducting a number of graduate-degree programs in the medical sciences. The two institutions are located in the Fort Greene, Bedford Stuyvesant area of Brooklyn, and are thus acutely aware of the lack of health resources in the inner city that surrounds them. This area has the second highest rate of prematurity and prenatal deaths in the city; the highest rate of lead poisoning, the lowest rate of dental care, and high rates of narcotics addiction and alcoholism. There is an acute lack of neighborhood health-care personnel; delivery of care is provided primarily through the facilities of the Medical Center. The practicing physician is vanishing since economic deprivation, fear of attack or robbery, and other environmental problems have discouraged new physicians from coming into the neighborhood and have led to the rapid attrition of physicians prevously practicing in these communities.

The Program

The Medical-Services Associate Program is similar to the two-year course now provided at Duke University Medical Center, which trains assistants to work with physicians in hospitals and the rural areas of North Carolina.[7] These physician's assistants have proved extremely useful in the delivery of personal health services. The goal of our program is to recruit residents from the inner-city areas of Brooklyn in the hope that they will remain in the area and aid in the upgrading of its health resources. The medical-services associate will undergo a two-year training program including the study of didactic courses in the basic concepts of the human anatomy, physiology, pathology, pharmacology, English, mathematics, sociology, psychology, medical ethics, and medical terminology. Each participant is exposed to approximately one year of clinical experience by working in the medical-care areas of the Brooklyn-Cumberland Medical Center. Each will be taught to take the routine parts of medical histories, perform routine physical examinations, participate in and assist with procedures performed by physicians, assist at operations, review patients' charts for routine procedures, and spot-check developments of disease processes on each patient assigned to their care. The medical-services associate will not be placed in a competitive relation with the nurse. This program is an attempt to create a new professional. There is no desire to compete with or weaken existing professions, nor is there any attempt to displace present paramedical personnel. Although the medical-services associate will be similar to the nurse in some aspects of his background training and basic course preparation, he will not be utilized in any area which might displace a nurse from her customary and traditional activities. The medical-services associate will be a professional who will work closely with the physician and be under his direct supervision and thus be his responsibility. We hope to lighten the load of the physician by eliminating the need for him to perform routine duties. The physician is thus released for those activities for which his expertise is best suited. Dr. E. Harvey Estes, director of the Duke program, who reported in a recent article in the *Journal of the American Geriatrics Society*[8] estimates that the physician's assistant, who works in conjunction with and under the direction of the practicing physician, can increase the productivity of that physician from 30 to 50%.

The Community as a Resource

The main purposes of our program are: 1) to recruit minority group individuals into a new profession; 2) to upgrade those individuals now in dead-end, low-level jobs in the health industry, and 3) to provide a viable entry point for career-ladder training, now so woefully lacking. We envision this profession as one that will not only increase the personal status of the individual graduate within his community but that, we hope, will upgrade and provide good medical care to more people. The Department of Community Medicine at the Brooklyn-Cumberland Medical Center, in its attempts to develop a delivery-care system for the Fort Greene-Bedford Stuyvesant area of Brooklyn, has been frustrated in its ability to provide adequate professional manpower to assure that these programs succeed. Thus it becomes apparent that indigenous citizens might provide the best resource for permanent health-care professionals.

From the inception of the program, community involvement has been extensive. Two significant community groups were kept intimately informed of the developments of the protocol and grant requests. These included the Community Board of the Department of Community Medicine and the Fort Greene Coordinating Council. Attempts at recruitment of community people into the program were all conducted through community agencies such as the local poverty programs. The Central Brooklyn Model Cities Program was involved in recruitment and participated actively in this endeavor. Support from Model Cities has been extensive both in the form of personnel and finances. Although basic minimum standards for participants within the program were established by Long Island University to meet the academic requirements of that institution, community representatives joined with our staff in attempting to seek out and identify those individuals who might be best motivated to deliver health care to their fellow citizens. Candidates who expressed a desire to upgrade themselves in the health-care field, those who exhibited academic and personal qualities, and those who indicated motivation and a capacity for success received prime consideration. Thus we did not adhere to traditional techniques in the choosing of candidates for the program. We believed that such methods tend to exclude more often than include candidates that could benefit from career training. Where appropriate school or armed-forces records were reviewed, however, we depended primarily upon a personal interview for evidence of motivation and psychological adaptability to the health-care field. All candidates were subjected to a basic college entrance examination prior to these interviews, which were conducted by a joint committee that consisted of two faculty members and a student from Long Island University, and two physicians and a nurse from the Brooklyn-Cumberland Medical Center. These individuals were joined by eight community representatives, four from the Central Brooklyn Model Cities Program and four from the Fort Greene Coordinating Council. Interviews were conducted by a panel discussion method with groups of candidates interviewed jointly. Individual scores for the interviews were tabulated and compared at the end of the interview.

Current Status

The initial class consists of 17 males and 6 females. This includes nine ex-military corpsmen, three practical nurses, and one registered nurse who was trained overseas. Twenty are from minority groups. The program has been in operation three months, and we find the esprit de corps of the students to be extremely high. The personal rewards to the faculty have been far beyond those anticipated. We find that the students are extremely well motivated and a very engaging group of individuals with whom to work. They are very interested in the health-care field, and the application of their energies and their academic powers is exceedingly rewarding to observe. If success could be measured by interest and enthusiasm alone this class would certainly be first in that category.

Ongoing evaluation of the program and approval of changes in the curriculum depend on an Evaluation and Curriculum Committee. The staff, with the assistance of members of this committee, has developed an integrated program of training that includes academic courses and clinical work concomitantly. Contact with the patient has been encouraged early in the training period. This committee consists of members of the faculty of Long Island University, members of the professional staff of the Medical Center, a dean of the local community college, the dean of Adult, Evening, and Continuing Education at the Long Island University, two members of the staff of a public health hospital, two members of a medical school faculty, students enrolled in the program, and community citizens. We included community individuals on the Evaluation and Curriculum Committee so that we might teach our students not only the scientific and academic aspects of health care but also those social and economic factors needed for the full appreciation of the problems faced by the patient as he attempts to secure adequate health care.

At present the program awards certificates; however, in the near future we expect to grant degrees. The Long Island University Faculty Committee on Curriculum and Innovative Programs has supported our program enthusiastically and has requested formal proposals leading to the award of a two-year associate degree and a four-year baccalaureate degree. This would provide the student with reentry and the ability to prepare himself for specialization and administration.

The Need for a National Policy

No one can argue the need for increasing the national supply of health manpower. However, if this is to be accomplished we must recognize the potential of many professionals to provide health-care services. When one realizes that some areas of our country have a ratio of one physician to 4,000[9] patients compared to a national average of 1:666[10] the need for additional personnel becomes evident. Unfortunately, not only total numbers but distribution is a problem. Changes must be made in our orientation toward licensure as the sine qua non for the health professions. We must break away from the guild system and relate programs of training and delivery to the concept of the participation of a team and the utilization of the skills of many.

There must be a national emphasis on the development of "middle-medical personnel." Job descriptions and analyses must be developed to outline the duties and responsibilities of such categories of health professionals. Training programs must be created in an academic setting so that mobility is encouraged while dead-end technical training and specific job categories are limited or incorporated into new broader-based programs. High schools, community colleges, and universities must be encouraged to cooperate with each other in such endeavors. A national policy must be developed by the appropriate governmental and voluntary health agencies to outline and standardize training programs, academic requirements, and institutional accreditation procedures.

The individual candidate must be provided core-curriculum training and the opportunity to reenter the training system at a later date with the objective of promotion without loss of credit or need for new and different prerequisites.

Allied health professionals must be utilized not in addition to but instead of the physician wherever and whenever such delegation of authority is feasible, based upon the principles of good medical-care practice. It may now be the time for all of us to admit that the elusive term "high-quality care" is an impractical goal and a phantom of the imagination. The scientific success of medical research has not been translated into an equal improvement in the nation's health. Greater emphasis on the delivery of basic health care and the practice of prevention might better serve the health needs of all. The medical-services associate potentially can help us attain this important goal.

Conclusion

We realize the need to create a qualified graduate in whom we can develop high ethical principles and attitudes toward health care. The graduate of any such program must learn to respect the sanctity and dignity of his individual patients: the consumers. The medical-services associate can provide primary health care to large segments of the inner-city population and, under the supervision and direction of a physician, he can be successful in delivery of ambulatory care and in providing needed manpower resources within the hospital and other health-care institutions. The horizons are unlimited, however. Only by joining the resources of the community with academic and professional institutions shall we be able to succeed in this endeavor.

REFERENCES

1. Flexner, A.: *Medical Education in the United States and Canada,* Bulletin No. 4. New York Carnegie Foundation for the Advancement of Teaching, 1910.
2. Moore, F. J.: Information technologies and health care. *Arch. Intern. Med. 125:* 351-55, 1970.
3. Fuchs, V. R., Rand, E. H. and Garrett, B.: The health manpower gap reexamined. Editorial. *New Eng. J. Med. 282:*338-39, 1970.
4. Perry, J. W.: Career mobility in allied health education. *J.A.M.A.210:*107-10, 1969.
5. Lenzer, A.: New health careers for the poor. *Amer. J. Public Health 60:*45-50, 1970.
6. *Education for the Allied Health Professions.* United States Department of Health, Education, and Welfare. Public Health Service No. 1600, April 1967.
7. Estes, E. H., Jr. and Howard, D. R.: Potential for newer classes of personnel: Experience of the Duke physician's assistant program. *J. Med. Educ. 45:* 149-55, 1970.
8. Estes, E. H., Jr.: Advantages and Limitations of Medical Assistants. *J. Amer. Geriat. Soc. 16:*1083-87, 1968.
9. *Health Manpower Perspective 1967.* United States Department of Health, Education, and Welfare. Public Health Service No. 1667, 1967.
10. *Source Book of Health Insurance Data.* New York, Health Insurance Institute, 1969.

TRAINING OF ALLIED HEALTH PROFESSIONALS AND PHYSICIANS' ASSISTANTS*

MICHAEL M. DACSO

Dean, Institute of Health Sciences
Hunter College of the City University of New York
Professor, Rehabilitation Medicine and Community Medicine
The Mount Sinai School of Medicine
New York, N. Y.

THE shortage and maldistribution of health manpower has been plaguing not only this country but, one might say, the rest of the world also with increased intensity. The difficulties in making adequate health services available have been a matter of deep concern both to those who were responsible for providing such services as well as to the recipients. The conventional and, for a long time, the only suggestion to remedy this chronic health problem was to produce an increasing number of doctors. In the last few years, however, it has become increasingly evident that for a variety of reasons we shall not be able in the foreseeable future to produce a sufficient number of physicians. Further, it is now recognized that an increased production of physicians alone will not solve this complex problem. After some initial resistance it is now generally accepted that the physician alone, without the cooperation of a score of specially trained health professionals, is in no position to cope with the multiple and diverse demands of the ever-broadening health-delivery system. The physician's training qualifies him for the task of preventing and curing diseases and of restoring the disabled but, as a rule, he lacks competence to carry out many of the strictly technical and administrative responsibilities. If, however, in the absence of other solutions he tries to be a clinician and, at the same time, to perform such technical and administrative chores, his efficiency as a clinician will suffer. A situation will inevitably develop from which he will emerge as an ineffective clinician, constantly overworked and

*Presented in a panel, Absence of a National Health Policy on Training and Utilization of Manpower, as part of the 1970 Health Conference of the New York Academy of Medicine, *Community Participation for Equity and Excellence in Health Care,* held at the Academy April 23 and 24, 1970.

frustrated; one whose patients will not benefit from his clinical knowledge.

In the last three or four decades a large number of new health professions have developed that have made the delivery of health services more effective and more widely available. A score of new health professionals have become an essential part of everyday medical practice. In spite of the indispensable contributions of these specialists, *the need for a generalized type of assistant to the physician has become increasingly felt:* a carefully selected person whose education, training, and practical experience would qualify him to relieve the physician of many of his duties and chores, for which independent *clinical* judgment is not needed. Those who have the responsibility of making medical services universally available are quite enthusiastic about this new member of the health team. However difficulties created by this new development are not to be overlooked. One of the major problems is the acceptance of such an assistant by the medical profession. It seems that after the initial guarded reaction a majority of those physicians who have become familiar with the potentials and capabilities of the physician's assistant (PA) have developed a realistically pragmatic attitude and have increasingly demanded the training of this supporting health professional. Organized medicine, from the American Medical Association to the local county medical societies, has on many occasions expressed its support. From the scattered information available it seems that patients have also been receptive to physicians' assistants in actual clinical situations and in private and institutional environments. With only a handful of teaching programs at present in operation, there are only a few PA's in service. Therefore, at this point of development, there are no operational problems which would materially interfere with the functioning of the PA. However the history of the development of health professionals, not excluding the physician, tells us that as soon as a new health specialist enters the practicing phase, inevitable difficulties in adjustment arise. These difficulties manifest themselves on several levels, the more important being the new professional's relation to the already established members of the health team—namely, the doctors, registered nurses, technicians, etc. Acceptance of the PA by patients and their families is another question that invites examination. Some of these issues have already been resolved; others, however, still await a solution.

It is of primary importance to define the operational limitations of

A NUMERICAL REPRESENTATION (0–4+) OF AMOUNT OF KNOWLEDGE, SKILL, AND CAPACITY FOR INDEPENDENT ACTION AS THESE RELATE TO FOUR LEVELS OF EDUCATION FOR PERSONNEL IN THE HEALTH OCCUPATIONS*

Level of education	*Knowledge*	*Skill*	*Capacity for independent action*
I Doctorate	4+	4+	4+
II Bachelor's and Master's Degrees	4+	4+	2+
III 2-year College Associate Degree	2+	4+	1+
IV Vocational or technical training	1+	4+	0

*Reproduced by permission from: National Research Council. Ad hoc Committee on Allied Health Personnel. *Allied Health Personnel.* Washington, D.C., National Academy of Science, 1969.

the PA, *who cannot and should not, under any circumstances, act as an independent practitioner.* The PA must be considered an extension of the physician and, as such, must always remain under his immediate supervision. At no time, except in an unanticipated emergency, where a delay might threaten a person's life, should he be allowed to act independently. Even in such a situation a medical doctor should be summoned after the immediate emergency has been met. Essential as his services may be *the PA is not a substitute for a physician. Only a medical doctor can substitute for another physician.*

Even a cursory review of the functioning of a PA indicates that we are dealing with an ancillary medical activity on different levels of technical and theoretical competence. Therefore it is suggested that the education of the PA should also be carried out on more than one level. Not unlike the other major health professionals, the PA should be given his training and education within the combined framework of a college and medical school in a regular four-year baccalaureate course. Community colleges could produce a useful assistant of limited operational scope in two years. Such an aide could perform many of the technical chores in the care of patients. At present some of these important routine activities fall between the doctor and the nurse, and more often than not they remain undone. More sophisticated responsibility for care of the patient requires a thorough basic and clinical education, the type only a four-year college curriculum can provide. See accompanying table.

H. I. Greenfield, an economist, in a talk on health manpower problems, said:

We need schools to provide the whole continuum of degrees—doctor of medicine (MD), master of science in medicine (MSM), bachelor of science in medicine (BSM), and associate of arts in medicine (AAM), as well as new types of related health degrees. The new educational spectrum should include senior medical colleges, junior medical colleges, schools of allied health professions, and community colleges. On the secondary level, vocational schools fit into the picture by their preparation of licensed practical nurses and other health workers in which the job requirements are similar. Corresponding to these new medical workers should be new types of medical facilities where they will work—and here is where the division of clinical facilities fits: neighborhood ambulatory clinics and diagnostic centers (for medical, dental, and mental problems), hospital satellites, and comprehensive medical service centers.*

As the number of new programs grows it is important that the courses be designed to allow the students free upward and lateral mobility. An open road must be kept open for those who, in the course of their studies, show sufficient interest and talent to qualify for admission to medical school.

Present experience indicates that a majority of the applicants for courses as PA's have had some previous experience in health services. The greatest interest is shown by individuals with previous experience in the medical services of the armed forces. To a great extent, because of the efforts of an ad hoc committee of the National Academy of Sciences, an intensive campaign is now underway to facilitate the entry of the returning veteran into the civilian health-service systems. While for a variety of moral and technical reasons these men and women should receive high priority, it would be a rather impractical policy to restrict these training programs to returning veterans exclusively. Nurses after appropriate retraining may have great potential for extended clinical responsibility.

It is anticipated that some applicants not accepted by medical schools may want to become physicians' assistants as a second-best solution to fulfilling their interest in the healing sciences. In this connection a word of warning has been sounded by a medical educator who suggested that special precautions be taken with these students, lest they quickly try to become *independent* health practitioners.

**J.A.M.A. 205*:1542-44, 1968.

This raises another important and so far largely unresolved problem: What type of licensing and accreditation should be provided for this health professional? With the anticipated growth in the number of these professionals an answer to this and other important legal and administrative problems can no longer be postponed. Beyond the strictly legal responsibilities to the patients, their relatives, and the community, the ethical commitments must also be carefully spelled out within the framework of the ancient and revered code accepted by the medical profession.

Last but not least: a few words are in order about the utilization of this new member of the health professions. As has been repeatedly emphasized, the PA cannot be allowed to practice without the immediate supervision of a licensed physician, who is legally and morally responsible for all his professional activities. Such vital restriction determines the PA's role in the health-delivery system. Hospitals, ambulatory services, community health centers, health departments, and other institutions that provide health care are all in great need of such specially trained assistants. Private physicians in some instances already utilize the services of such well-trained assistants. The anticipated spread of group practice will also require greater numbers of such skilled persons. Thus, from this sketchy overview, it is clear that, as the concept of this new health professional becomes more generally known, there will be a growing demand for his services. In anticipation of this development and in response to the existing need, efforts should be exerted to organize both academically and clinically high-level educational opportunities for these new health professionals.

One of the major benefits expected from the introduction of the PA into the spectrum of the health professions will be the increased availability of direct medical services in rural and urban localities. However, at this early stage of development, a word of warning is not entirely out of order. Any idea of using the PA as a means of providing second-rate medicine, sometimes referred to as "poor man's medicine," should be unconditionally discouraged. If there is a place for these new health professionals in the present medical system, they should be used in the care of all patients regardless of their financial or social status.

SOCIAL POLICY AND GUILD POLICY IN HEALTH MANPOWER*

Tom Levin

Assistant Professor of Community Health
Assistant Professor of Psychiatry
Director, Health Careers Program
Albert Einstein College of Medicine
New York, N. Y.

The public, health consumers, health professionals and health providers have been encouraged to believe that the present administration has developed a strategy which will respond effectively to our urgent needs for additional health manpower. That strategy, the military-corpsman retraining program, is probably the most seductive current health-manpower concept in America. It is certainly opportune and appropriate to encourage young veterans to enter the health field. Unfortunately, however, as a significant contribution to our health manpower needs, the corpsman strategy is a fake!

The corpsman strategy is a hoax because it must fail for corpsman and consumer unless it is accompanied by a meaningful reform of the morass that exists in the over-all national supply, training, utilization, and accreditation of health personnel.

Of the putative 30,000 corpsmen returning to civilian life annually, 70% have expressed interest in continuing a career in the health field.[1] It should be noted that this "interest" is quickly dissipated as the returning corpsmen try to fit into the medieval salary and job structure of the civilian health system. While some programs have reported significant success in "retraining" military corpsmen for new roles such as physician assistants, in the future such programs face many obstacles. Legislative acceptance of amendments to educational statutes and professional-practices acts designed to encourage programs for assistants to physicians has been discouraging. The recent American Medical Association demurrer on the title "physician assistant" reflected fear that such a title may be construed as "assistant physician."[2] On the other

*Presented in a panel, Absence of a National Health Policy on Training and Utilization of Manpower, as part of the 1970 Health Conference of the New York Academy of Medicine, *Community Participation for Equity and Excellence in Health Care,* held at the Academy, April 23 and 24, 1970.

hand many representatives of the nursing profession have expressed fear that the physician assistant may be utilized to fill supervisory and specialty-nursing positions. The military corpsman, who in actual practice has frequently functioned as a physician's surrogate and a nurse, is caught between two guild-jurisdiction fiefdoms. Further, corpsmen have shown reluctance to accept career goals within the traditional hierarchy of hospital nursing and have complained of restrictions of function and limited opportunities for advancement. A recent survey of discharged corpsmen in Texas yielded an important "straw in the wind." Of the corpsmen surveyed only two expressed interest in remaining in the health field—and then only if they could train to become physicians.

Even if one accepts discharged military corpsmen as an important source of recruits to the health system, many of us will experience great difficulty in responding to a health-manpower strategy that is tied to an expanding American military foreign policy. The American health system needs a comprehensive and rational system of health-manpower education rather than relying upon temporary expedients and on the by-products of military policy.

Present health-manpower policy in the United States does not reflect forceful initiative by government agencies to fulfill their roles as guardians of public and consumer interests. Rather, municipal, federal, and state policy is implemented by procedures of licensure, certification, and accreditation which reflect at the best a compromise between special-interest groups and the providers of health services. The ultimate beneficiary of the training and utilization of health manpower, i.e., the consumer, has little or no role in determining policies of health manpower. The truthfulness of G. B. Shaw's observation that professions are a conspiracy against the public is nowhere more evident than in the area of health-manpower policy.

This "conspiracy" in the health field is carried out with the active connivance of service providers, guilds, and educational institutions through a series of "smoke-filled-back-room" agreements which establish self-validating and self-servicing procedures.

The various health-professional associations determined *internally* (i.e., without public participation) their requirements for membership in their guilds. Guild membership thus becomes the basis for establishing qualifications for professional competence. After formal and informal negotiations between various guilds and providers these so-called standards of competence are transformed into governmental regulations, enforced by licensure boards selected almost exclusively from professionals nominated by the guilds or acceptable to them.[3] These boards then set educational requirements which become the basis of the educational programs of the health-professional schools. Health providers collaborate actively in this perverted process by setting employment qualifications which conform to guild-membership requirements, and to the derivatives of these requirements as expressed in governmental regulations. As a consequence we now have a most absurd system of education and training, directed primarily toward the fulfillment of guild requirements rather than toward the needs of patients.

Some of you may recall a recent example of the absurdity of guild dominance over public interest. The fiasco occurred at the Harlem Hospital School of Nursing in New York in October 1968 when, as the result of a remarkable guild-oriented approach to social analysis, the Harlem Hospital School of Nursing was disaccredited.[4] This action was initiated by the National League for Nursing primarily because 30% of the graduation class failed to pass the New York State examination for acceptance as R.N.'s This, in face of the fact that 70% of the graduates of Harlem Hospital School of Nursing (largely drawing its students from and serving ghetto neighborhoods deprived of education and health care) had passed the same examination. The guild response of removing the credentials of an institution which provides young black women from a ghetto neighborhood with a career of service in an area of medical famine, I submit, is unconscionable social irresponsibility.

The relevance of the program in health education itself is determined then by the success of the students in meeting the requirements originally set by these same guilds. Schools in the health professions regularly present their success in terms of the number of candidates passing guild-determined, governmental evaluation procedures. Service facilities are rated on the basis of the number of guild-acceptable professionals on the staff. Service institutions cooperate by passively accepting internship and field-placement requirements which put guild expectations for training above the interests of the consumer. Public accountability for health services has been completely subverted by a special-interest group conspiracy.

Involvement of the consumer only becomes desirable to the guilds when this systematized absurdity results in inadequate quality and quantity of health personnel. Then the consumer is asked to participate by paying (through higher taxes and hospital bills) for the repairs necessary to maintain this destructive system.

A number of strategies must be developed to achieve a greater responsiveness to the needs of the consumer in manpower policy. First, however, alternatives to control by guilds will require forceful utilization of public funds by governmental agencies as a lever to establish more relevant educational programs, staffing patterns, and community participation in health-educational and manpower decision-making.

Further, we must recognize that a mere increase in the number of physicians, nurses, physician assistants, medical technologists, social workers, inhalation therapists (or any other of the hundreds of different classifications of health workers) will not solve our problem. Almost 100 separate craft guilds in the health field spawn an incredible number of proliferating job titles,[5] descriptions, and classifications that frequently overlap, contradict, and impede function. Reading a list of presently utilized titles in the health field will existentially demonstrate the absurdity of such divisiveness and fragmentation. Education of health workers today increasingly emphasizes technical competence within a narrow sphere. We must reverse this trend and address instead the generic nature of health education rather than its narrow guild specialization. If a comprehensive and unified health service is our goal we must direct ourselves to educating health workers who will be responsive to the common elements in their function.

For the last few years the Albert Einstein College of Medicine Health Careers Program has analyzed health tasks, guilds, and job classifications.[6] We have found that the existing job descriptions fall within three generic areas of health skills. While this classification seems simplistic, I believe it is necessary step toward integrating the present atomized educational system.

The first generic cluster derives from those activities and skills involved in ministering to a patient's bodily needs. This area, which might be described as "laying on the hands," we have designated "direct patient-care" skills. The second generic-skill area, which involves primarily social and emotional interaction with individuals or groups, we have designated as the "social and interpersonal" area. The third generic skill area, characterized by the use of an intervening technical instrumentation between patient and practitioner, we designated as the "technical-health" specialties.

In addition to reorganizing health-career education around generic clusters we must also articulate the levels of the complexity of skills in the health occupations into an incremental system. An incremental program recognizes that each level of achieved expertise, knowledge, and skill has applicability as a prerequisite to a further level of increased complexity. While we give lip service to this concept, for all intents and purposes we operate a closed system. As an example, very few nurses ever become physicians yet there is hardly a more useful preparation for medical education and practice! The blame cannot be laid entirely upon the American Medical Association; rather, I think, the "uncle Tom" vocational role of the American nursing profession should be examined.

Another major area of reform in health education concerns the question of relevance. That has become a charged word over the last years. Without exploring the larger sociological issues, relevance for health-career education must creatively utilize reality contacts with the needs of patients in order to build a curriculum that prepares for responsiveness to the patient as a whole man. Relevance in the curriculum means that we must not educate people the way we train dogs. Health students should not learn tricks of narrow application of skills. Rather they must learn how to learn continuously. They must learn how to build on experience. They must learn how to deal with the integration of materials. To save time, I shall forego a discussion of the vertical versus the horizontal concept of curriculum. I shall simply note that in this country, not only in health, but in all areas, the horizontal concept of curriculum has led to education within sterile boxes of academic expertise, with a consequent growing dissatisfaction among students with limitations of the practitioner.

We shall also have to deal with the whole question of experience in developing relevant education. Experience as an educational component in the health field has quite rightly earned a most odious reputation. This experience—field placement for the social worker, internship in medicine, and the infamous experience of diploma schools of nursing—has shown that without adequate control, field placement becomes a coolie system for the exploitation of entry-level professionals.

We know that some diploma schools have in the past been misused and perverted by an avaricious health establishment to such a degree that they could best be described as vocational "plantations" which provided young girls to serve the health establishments. But that does not necessarily mean, to follow the analogy, that it is the activity itself that was disreputable. Rather, it was the exploitative economic and social relation between the health system and its students that turned the hospital administrator into a plantation manager and the nurse educator into a field boss. To develop relevance in health education we need field experience–but it must be provided with social dignity and economic justice. Students should receive payment and recognition for the services they perform comparable to the health workers performing similar tasks.

We must also develop an approach to education for health skills that prepares health workers to respond to the unique and special needs of the communities they serve. We cannot continue to develop abstract health-education and health-service standards and requirements. We cannot follow recommended job-staffing patterns without recognizing that there is no such thing as a national model. The American Nurses Association, the American Medical Association, or the Council on Medical Education cannot develop a national standard of job functions that applies equally to suburban Great Neck and Lincoln Hospital in the South Bronx. The populations of each area have different needs that must be recognized.

Health students, most importantly, must be educated to the relevance of social needs generally and particularly to the issue of the social direction of our service-delivery system. Philosophically and practically, it is not possible to respond productively to problems of health manpower today without considering both the delivery models of the services and new concepts of the scope and direction of health services. A totally new orientation is necessary to recognize that in the past the practice of medicine as we know it has been essentially that of the garbage collectors of health and social-policy failure. Medicine, which directed its attention to pathology, was a discipline which focused upon the failure of the health system. Every time we have to deal with the corrective procedures that have traditionally been attributed to medicine, we are responding to the failure of community preventive-health practice. We must reverse this nonsensical state of affairs and recognize that the tasks that most physicians perform today (though important and meaningful to us) are performed because we have failed in our social task of maintaining and preserving health.

All illness and health impairment represents a failure to fulfill our social task successfully. Some critics have balked at this omnibus view of the capability and responsibility of the health profession; they have pointed to such problems as birth defects as unavoidable. Although for many years we shall have to concern ourselves with such problems, they nonetheless reflect failure to develop the social priority of health as a universal human right! Adequate money for research, adequate programs of prenatal care, adequate nutrition, and proper environment would markedly reduce the number of birth defects. Reordering our national social priorities would reduce the need of health scientists and practitioners to address themselves to a reparative rather than a preventive discipline.

We must recognize as a corollary to this view of health practice that health is not a privilege to be accorded by impudent presidents of the American Medical Association. Health is no longer a commodity to be bartered, bought, and sold by guild practitioners in an individual-enterprise system. Health is a right, a born right, and an ongoing right of every human being. As a first step to achieve that right in America, the fee-for-service system must go.

For the health educator the implications are obvious. Education for health workers should be appropriate to their tasks. Health-education institutions must educate a different kind of person for service to the community than for a free-enterprise system. Health in the future will not be the sole responsibility of the professional. Health will be a shared responsibility with the community. The health practitioner of the future will no longer relate to the community he serves the way the medieval nobleman related to his fiefdom, a privileged enclave in which he had absolute power. The health consumer today rejects the role of serf under the professional nobleman. The professional must *serve* the consumer, and must be helped through his education to recognize his service role.

Communities today are demanding the major responsibility for the planning of health services as well as a primary role in the management and administration of service facilities. As a concommitant to this demand, communities are becoming more concerned with the whole question of health-manpower supply—including the selection of people who enter the health field—educational policy, and the utilization of health workers.

To achieve new social goals requires new approaches and a new organization of the institutions that educate health workers. As a beginning, I would propose the immediate and complete abolition of colleges of medicine (which are vocational elitist establishments) and the establishment in their place of comprehensive universities of health. We should also phase out independent community colleges in the health field (which are the new trade schools for the poor) and independent guild-specialty schools (such as schools of nursing, social work, etc.). All of these educational institutions should be subsumed under a health university, with undergraduate and graduate divisions. In such a health university, all health students will recognize the commonalty of their education, their skills, and their tasks, and will work together toward a health-service delivery system which will reflect the comradeship, the mutual respect, and the dedication to the patient that we as health professionals must make the mandate of our life work.

REFERENCES

1. From battlefield to civilian health careers. *Med. World News 11:*41, 1970.
2. Meeting keys on manpower needs. *Amer. Med. News,* Jan. 12, 1970, p. 13.
3. U.S. Department of Health, Education, and Welfare, Public Health Service, National Center for Health Statistics. *State Licensing of Health Occupations.* Washington, D.C., Govt. Print. Off., 1968, pp. 7-9.
4. *New York Times,* October 18, 1967.
5. *Encyclopedia of Associations,* 5th ed. Detroit, Gale Res. Co. 1968, vol. 1.
6. Levin, T. and Russell, T., eds. *Transitional Report: Albert Einstein College of Medicine-Lincoln Hospital Health Careers Program,* 2 vols. New York, Albert Einstein Coll. of Med., 1968. Mimeo.

CAN WE AVOID A $100 BILLION MISUNDERSTANDING?*

HOWARD ENNES

Second Vice President, Corporate Relations
The Equitable Life Assurance Society of the United States
New York, N. Y.

THE title I have given to these comments—Can We Avoid a $100 Billion Misunderstanding?—is meant to be neither facetious nor frivolous. We are dealing with a serious matter, and the time for rhetoric and recrimination is past. This is a time for action—responsible, accountable, cooperative action that will actually move us toward the solution of an exceedingly complex social problem. In all humility and candor, I am concerned that many of us fail to understand the brutal realities that are involved in bringing high-quality health care to all—a goal toward which all here sincerely strive.

I am concerned that we may find ourselves engaged in an "oversell" operation that makes more promises than can be fulfilled and sets up expectations that cannot be realized.

At the rate we are spending we may anticipate that our present annual $60 billion health expenditure may easily hit $100 billion by 1975—and it would be a tragic misunderstanding indeed if we then found little improvement in the actual delivery of health care and in services for maintaining health.

Yet without rather heroic efforts here and now, we can expect just that—a $100 billion misunderstanding. In my view—as we discuss here a national health policy in matters of financing—we must begin by understanding that better health care will cost a great deal of money, manpower, facilities, and other resources.

However, I am not sure that really good health care—accessible and acceptable to those who need care and to those who deliver care—necessarily must cost much more than we now are actually spending. I say this because we are wasting money today with our archaic "nonsystem"

*Presented in a panel, Absence of a National Health Policy in Matters of Financing, as part of the 1970 Health Conference of the New York Academy of Medicine, *Community Participation for Equity and Excellence in Health Care,* held at the Academy April 23 and 24, 1970.

and because of our insistence on thinking in terms of medical illness rather than about *health*. And much of the real and human costs do not show up on the audit sheets—the costs in wastage of time, in inconvenience, in loss of productivity, and in the toll of human dignity exacted by our professional practices and two-class charity methods.

We must understand also that dollars are by no means the only answer. The more likely result of more money alone will be more inflation—as certainly Medicare has taught us—and more of the same in uneven quality and inequitable availability.

We must understand the absolute necessity of a basic restructuring of the apparatus the nation now has to provide medical care and treatment of sickness; in essence, we must understand the necessity for an evolutionary transformation of what we have into a health-maintenance system.

This will not be easy. In today's language it is a "heavy" idea and a "tough" assignment. It will require some basic changes in the nature and structure of institutions, in attitudes and practices of professionals, in perceptions and values of politicians and, of equal importance, in the attitudes, expectations, and responsibilities of individuals, including the so-called consumer and community and business leadership.

What all this understanding requires is a commitment on the part of each of us, and of the professions, and businesses, and community organizations, a commitment to work together in a creative and mutually supportive partnership. If ever there was a problem that calls for wholehearted cooperation in the public interest this is it.

I shall now outline for you how we in private insurance feel this country should move in order to make high-quality health care for all a reality. To do so I must share with you a bit of history to remind you of a basic fact: that there is no simple answer to the health-care problem, and that certainly the answer is not to be found in financing or insurance mechanisms alone. In important respects we face a basic problem of structure and system. Unless something is done about the *way* health care is delivered to people, changing how it is paid for will do little good. Health care is an organizational problem, a problem of priorities, of integration, and of utilization of resources. *It is not a dollar problem alone.*

It is important that we in the insurance business realize that we must accept an important share of responsibility in solving this huge social problem. I am glad to report that we are beginning to do so, and that is where a bit of history comes in.

About a year ago the Health Insurance Association of America concluded that the time had come to take a fresh and fundamental look at the total health-care situation. So we did the usual thing—we set up some committees. But this time there was a difference. Our committees were told to travel around the country and find out what the situation really is. They were told to try to predict the course events were likely to take in the next decade. We felt that if we could get a good picture of the needs of the health-care delivery system, then we could consider constructively what insurance companies could do to foster better organization of health care. Perhaps then we could determine how to cope with costs and reshape our financing mechanisms to accommodate and facilitate the necessary changes.

In wide-ranging discussions with many kinds of authorities our study group found that a paramount issue is the shortage of medical and allied manpower, and that improvement in management of facilities and systems and better use of personnel appear to be major needs both with respect to controlling costs and to improving quality. With regard both to costs and to facilitating access to health care, our tendency to depend on care in hospitals was seen as a most serious problem.

The various forms of medical practice came in for extensive discussion. Throughout there was strong emphasis on the need for ambulatory care and on new methods of organizing care: principally group practice. There was stress on the idea of neighborhood health centers, with use of teams of family physicians, community health aides, and other allied health workers to provide comprehensive care.

It seems clear that the number of solo practitioners will gradually diminish. Even today it is common for physicians in the same speciality to practice as a group. There are also multispeciality group practices, some very large. Considerable opinion exists that the combination of prepayment with multispeciality group practice offers the possibility of significantly improving the delivery of health care; that it can encourage the more expeditious use of less costly forms of care; and that, over-all, it can minimize the inevitable increases in the cost of care.

Most experts accordingly believe that while the financing of health care will continue to be a third-party function, the methods of compensation of practitioners may be expected to change. Per capita and per diem payments may become routine for all types of providers of care.

To this sampling of the findings of the Health Insurance Association study, may I add two more general points.

First, we can expect increasingly to hear more from the consumer, particularly in the cities: he wants a greater share of the decision making in health care, even though larger issues of strategy and the use of resources must be developed at the national level.

The other major fact is that everywhere there is recognition that the poor and the minorities do not share satisfactorily in access to health services and medical technology. To bring all our people into the mainstream of high-quality health care should be a paramount national goal.

Of course the information developed in our study is not new. But the intensity with which these ideas are being put forward, and the degree to which they are shared, is important.

We in the health-insurance business are highly sensitive to the implications of these findings because of our experience in serving as intermediaries for Medicare and Medicaid, and because of our extensive involvement in community health planning over the past three years. Consequently our business is taking a new look at itself and at the nation's needs. In the past we have been largely concerned with health care only as financial intermediaries. Here is the big change in our posture: we now seek to formulate broadening programs in the whole field of health—including financing—that will serve the public interest constructively.

You may be interested to know that from its study-group's work the Health Insurance Association has come up with four basic objectives for our nation's health-care delivery systems of the 1970's: not merely financing, but health-care *delivery* systems. In our view, health-care delivery systems for the 1970's, in essence: 1) should be responsive and relevant: 2) should integrate and interrelate with other social and environmental systems: 3) should reflect consumer and professional interests: and 4) should be organized to provide high-quality health care for all.*

Last fall these objectives and supporting documentation and recommendations were put before the board of the Health Insurance Associa-

*Health Insurance Association of America: *Health Care Delivery in the 1970's.* Chicago, Health Ins. Assoc. of America, 1969.

tion of America. In accepting this report the board urgently recommended to its 313 member companies that they:

1) Continue to inform themselves of evolving developments in health-care delivery.

2) Become more involved in health-care delivery developments and exert their influence to bring about soundly conceived changes in present systems.

3) Formulate programs for, and exert leadership to achieve, a pluralistic system of health economics for this nation which will assure all citizens access to needed health services on an equal basis and regardless of the personal means for payment—making maximum use of private health insurance but recognizing that some use of government funds is necessary for persons of limited income.

I can report, also, as a direct response to this last point, that our association now is in the process of bringing forward an affirmative action program concerning both the organization of delivery of health care and its financing. The action program was approved in principle in February by the Board of the Health Insurance Association of America. A special meeting of member companies is being called to consider and approve the broad plan.

Our proposals follow six main lines. Five of the six deal with the organization and delivery of health care. The sixth spells out the ways and means of offering the entire population insured plans which would emphasize ambulatory and preventive services, and would foster effectiveness and economy of care.

Obviously I am not in a position to spell out details of a program still not yet officially adopted, but I can outline briefly what is involved.

A principal priority is to stress the urgency of increasing the present supply of health manpower and of improving the distribution of it. We believe that federal training and scholarship programs should be materially expanded and consolidated. Further, there should be direct incentives for health practitioners to serve in areas of critical need, including the inner cities and rural areas.

A second thrust of our proposal aims to promote development of ambulatory-care services and centers, including ambulatory and preventive-care benefits in all health insurance plans. It seems to me that we are in general agreement that the nation urgently needs: 1) to improve access to health care for all; 2) to encourage better organization and economy of use of manpower, facilities, and funds; and 3) to enhance the quality and effectiveness of health care. These needs could be met substantially by making "walk-in, one-stop" ambulatory health-care services accessible in every community throughout America.

It is a worthy goal, and one we could reach. It will take money, of course, for facilities, for services, for manpower development, and for planning, but it will also take the will to break away from our obsession with inpatient care, with technological glamor, and a return to more of the individualization and "tender loving care" that has marked American medicine in the past.
and cost-finding.

Needless to say, this is not to deny the pressing need for better organization and management and planning. These, in fact, are the instruments which can restore the human qualities and individualism we seek. And that is why I urge most strongly that comprehensive health planning be strengthened. In my view—and it is shared by the insurance industry, I can assure you—comprehensive health planning is essential if the nation is to use its large but not unlimited resources for the greatest good of both present and future generations.

Planning is needed to identify unmet needs and to establish a rational order for meeting them. Planning also is needed to avoid unnecessary and costly duplication of facilities and services, and to help control operating costs while encouraging new approaches to the effective delivery of health care. Hence one of our proposals for action underscores the importance of community health planning and proposes additional funding. We also assign additional responsibilities and authorities to local planning agencies so they can effectively guide and promote better health-care delivery systems.

Our fourth program for action proposes that we tackle the problem of improving cost and quality controls along several routes: we should preclude federal loans, grants, or contracts unless the project is deemed truly necessary by the community planning process: establish priorities reflecting efficiency incentives and modern management techniques; provide for payment of actual charges for professional services related to prevailing levels and guided by a peer-review mechanism; and reimburse institutions for federal programs only on a "controlled charges" basis that involve review committees and standard systems of accounts

As a sort of footnote to these comments, especially with respect to planning, it does seem to us that at national level we need to apply some of the same concepts of comprehensive health planning that we recommend for the states and localities.

Frankly, we think we need something analogous to the Council of Economic Advisors—perhaps a Council on Health Care—at the very top level of our government. There should be input from providers, third-party groups and, of course, consumers. This council might well be able to help provide some badly needed national coordination and accountability in the setting of objectives and priorities for the delivery of health care, and it could help focus attention on the health aspects of our living environment.

The final major part of the pending Health Insurance Association of America program deals with financing policy. It seeks to make comprehensive private health insurance available to *everyone*. Let me repeat that: to provide access to a decent level of health care for all, and to provide the financial leverage to achieve an essential evolutionary restructuring of delivery systems, comprehensive health insurance should be made available to all. I believe that this national goal can be achieved by starting with and building on voluntary insurance plans now serving in varying degrees about 85% of all Americans, and by providing health insurance paid for by public funds for those who have not yet achieved economic independence.

Specifically, we feel it is crucial that ambulatory and preventive-care benefits should be incorporated in all health-insurance plans. We must give intensive and extensive attention to the fostering of new forms of organization and delivery of care, with particular attention to the various forms of group-medical practice, both fee-for-service and capitation types.

We propose utilizing revised tax incentives for both employers and individuals, and the use of federal-state subsidies for the poor and the near-poor, with graded payments for the near-poor. The subsidized program would function through a pool, or several pools, of private insurers. This pool also would provide for uninsurables.

The program would establish progressive benefit standards with emphasis on ambulatory and preventive services. These standards would become effective in three stages—1972, 1976, 1979—in order to accommodate the practical problems of insurers, the processes of collective bargaining, and the development of needed health-care services and facilities. Employer-employee plans and individual policies would provide comprehensive coverage in virtually all cases—about as fast as can reasonably be expected.

I think we could get a program like this in motion that would, by 1976—the nation's bicentennial anniversary—meet the challenge of health for all our people. I should like to see the nation pledged to improve significantly by that date the availability, acceptability, accessibility, and adequacy of health care for all, with an assured method of financing that is fair and equitable for all.

I think we must begin to think and organize our resources in terms not merely of episodic medical care and hospital and medical insurance, but of health promotion and maintenance. Indeed, perhaps we should start thinking as, reputedly, the Chinese have for centuries: pay the physician to keep us well.

I believe that comprehensive and interrelated programs can be built from present strengths and demonstrated capabilities by combining the flexibility, innovativeness, and managerial skills of the private sector—and the superior scientific and technical competencies of our health and medical professions—with the unique fiscal and legislative capacities of the public sector, supported by the informed participation of the community.

One of the central problems blocking development of more effective health-care delivery systems is the rather elementary and thus overlooked fact that our health-care economy today lacks the marketplace balance provided by competition. Somehow, I think, we must get the incentive of "building a better mousetrap" into the picture. Perhaps the growing interest of consumers, and their active participation might provide some of the incentive, and so foster competition among a variety of different systems of delivery, each trying to meet community and individual needs with economy and quality. Certainly, we can all agree that health care cannot be a monopoly.

I believe further that out of this cooperative endeavor can arise a new partnership of great potential for the health and well-being of the nation, and that health care for all can be made a reality in this decade by undertaking a comprehensive nationwide effort that will begin at once with an integrated series of developmental and financing programs.

Perhaps we might sum it up this way: in the delivery of health care, human well-being, not cost, is the first priority. Nevertheless, runaway cost inflation undermines the capacity of even this affluent nation to provide a decent level of health care for all of its population.

Perhaps the issue is this: Do we have the capacity in this country to use our acknowledged scientific and technical skills and resources to guarantee the right of access to health care to all—access not only through dollars but access to services and facilities capable of delivering high-quality health care? This is a challenge worthy of the best in each of us, individually and collectively.

MISSING LINKS IN ACHIEVING EFFECTIVE SERVICES*

DAVID FRENCH

Professor and Chairman
Department of Community Medicine
Boston University School of Medicine
Boston, Mass.

IT is finally becoming acknowledged and accepted that America's health-delivery system is in a state demanding immediate renovation. Fragmentation and disorganization of the medical system have led to inefficiency, duplication of effort, and wasted money, services, and time. Those who suffer most are the consumers. They are being denied a basic right—good health—because the health-care delivery system remains incapable of providing and insuring that right. In my opinion the problem of health care will be relieved when the consumer assumes a new position in which he directly influences health-care policy at every level in order to produce changes in the system. In addition, a second precursor of effective medical-care delivery is public financing.

England and Wales of the United Kingdom and Sweden offer ready proof that a public-health policy can provide a successful method of insuring good health within a country. Contrary to popular belief, the United States does not provide the world's most effective health care. Osler Peterson et al. introduced evidence to the contrary in 1967 in an article published in the *Lancet* entitled What is Value for Money in Medical Care. Peterson and his associates compared health statistics and policies in England and Wales, Sweden, and the United States, and noted that all are healthy and affluent industrial countries. Despite that similarity their development of health services has led to striking differences in the provision and utilization of medical care. Where the United States relies on free enterprise to provide health care, the two European countries observed in the study have national-health policies. In the

*Presented in a panel, Absence of a National Health Policy in Matters of Financing, as part of the 1970 Health Conference of the New York Academy of Medicine, *Community Participation for Equity and Excellence in Health Care,* held at the Academy April 23 and 24, 1970.

United States the percentage of the gross national product (GNP) invested in health expenditures, as observed and reported by those men, has been increasing steadily, while in England and Wales relative expenses supported by the national health mechanism have been stable. Health expenses in all of these countries are reasonably similar, although the percentage of the GNP distributed in 1963 to allay health needs in the United States is somewhat higher than in England, Wales, and Sweden. There are, however, more significant distinctions between the United States and those nations with national health policies. Statistics reveal that the United States has 136.9 physicians for every 100,000 Americans; Sweden has 105.5 physicians per 100,000 people; and the United Kingdom occupies a position between the two. Average annual doctor-patient contact is notably higher in the United States than in either Sweden or the United Kingdom. It must be noted, however, that the reporting of such statistics is probably less widespread and accurate in the United States.

It is my contention that the United States has the lowest standards for health care of all three countries. For example, maternal-mortality rates from 1963 to 1965 placed the United States in the 12th position in a list of 20 industrial western nations, whereas Sweden placed first with the lowest maternal-death rate. In a 1965 survey of male life expectancy at birth, the United States ranked 18th with the lowest expectancy rate, while the United Kingdom ranked 10th and Sweden boasted the highest life-expectancy rate. In 1967 the United States placed 14th with the highest infant mortality rate while the United Kingdom again placed 10th and Sweden first.

It is true that the technical problems involved in statistical comparisons of different nations present problems in both continuity and accuracy. However, Peterson's study certainly indicates a significant difference in the health-delivery systems of those countries that invest the same percentage of their GNP in health care.

The factors that account for the differences in quality and effectiveness of health-care delivery in the United Kingdom, Sweden, and the United States must relate to the major distinctions in the over-all health systems of these countries. Financing is an integral component of health delivery, and I want to emphasize here that the governments of England, Wales, and Sweden finance a national-health policy whereas the United States lacks such a program. An indirect relation between the quality of health care received and the cost of care delivered is strongly indicated. Perhaps the relative failure of the United States originates in the lack of genuine incentive for improvement which characterizes much of its medical profession. Because health care is bound by few restraints, the quality of care delivered is determined almost exclusively by the competency, motivation, and concern of the individual health-care deliverer.

It is an oversimplified and shortsighted viewpoint which holds that the inability of individual consumers to meet the cost of medical care is the primary factor that obstructs effective health delivery. There are other methods and concerns which should not be ignored. For instance, there have been many legislative attempts at generating national health-insurance mechanisms. They have been concerned almost exclusively with payment. The American Medical Association Medi-Credit System is a foremost example. But in the first year of Medicaid and Medicare, the rate of increase in physicians' fees tripled, and the rate of increase in hospital fees multiplied five times. It seems obvious that the increase was the result of the unrestricted and unplanned allocation of money to a medical-care system without attempting to make the necessary basic changes in its organizational, delivery, and manpower components.

One major change for improving health delivery could be the replacement of the solo practitioner by group practice. In comparison with the knowledge, skill, and technical resources available from a team of physicians, the solo practitioner is considerably less effective. Physicians who work together in an organized fashion can share their knowledge and technical skills to improve the health care delivered to their patients. The merger would be advantageous to physicians as well as consumers because financial benefits would result from the savings accumulated through shared expenses and overhead.

An in-depth analysis of the present state and the future needs of our health system is a prerequisite to the development of a national health insurance policy. One important consideration is human nature, which might serve as an ally in this effort since we can provide financial rewards as incentives for change. An appeal to the average American's desire for money and its material benefits is perhaps the most effective way of inducing significant change in a relatively short period of time within a system as complex as health delivery.

Group practice could encourage the spread of family-oriented care. By focusing on the health-related resources and problems of the family group, we would be able to treat the social and psychological elements of disease as well as its basic biological components. Dealing with the family unit could hasten achievement of the ultimate goal of medicine, prevention of disease, by advancing early and thorough diagnosis.

A third modification demanded of the health system is comprehensive care, which must be a primary component of a national health-insurance program. Groups of doctors that service families would decrease the present fragmentation of effort and reduce expenses for physicians and consumers. Comprehensive care means that the individual components of medical care are interrelated to provide coordination, economy, and efficiency.

Often unconsidered in national-health financing is the relation of the community to individual and family medical problems. Intimate participation of community members should exist at all economic and social levels. Community people belong on the hospital boards and in neighborhood councils to influence health-care policy to meet community needs. The major policy decisions to determine the focus of a care program intended to meet the needs of a specific community can, and should, only be made with the full participation of the community to be served. Only in this manner can services be tailored to meet the special needs of that community.

A community-oriented national-health program that offers family-care delivery by teams of physicians could do much to alleviate fragmentation and costly disorganization. In its efforts to design an efficient health-insurance policy, the Technical Committee of the Committee for National Health Insurance stresses comprehensive care and service. Its program states: "The administrative arrangements and the finances of the National Health Insurance program should be designed to encourage the organization of professional, technical, and supporting personnel and health teams and groups capable of providing comprehensive per capita payments as an alternative to the prevailing fee-for-service method of payment!"

The late Dr. Richard Weinerman explained in a position paper the way the goals of rational and comprehensive delivery of medical care could be achieved. Progress toward a rational health-delivery system is inhibited rather than advanced when changes are imposed by rigid legislation and strict administrative procedures. Instead, advancement can result only through the initiative of motivated consumers and deliverers of health care. Dr. Weinerman explains: "This requires a program for planned progress through the stated goals. It demands also a pervasive flexibility which can allow the changed social and scientific determinants of health and medical care to lead to modification of program goals as well as the means."

Government financing should be aimed at increasing efficiency and economy within the medical system. Dr. Weinerman presents several means of achieving that objective:

1. The avoidence of duplication and waste through coordinated services;
2. The reduction of high costs of professional service through the encouragement of group or team practice and the expanded use of supportive personnel;
3. The elimination of unnecessary costs of hospitalization through improved availability of less expensive ambulatory and long-term institutional and home care services;
4. Reduction of high costs of specialty services, major surgery and expensive laboratory and x-ray procedures, appliances and devices, and use of drugs through achievement of economies and the utilization of available resources;
5. Avoidance of uncontrolled fee-for-service and cost-reimbursement methods of payment to providers of service;
6. Improved efficiency and lower operational unit cost through continuous educational and in-service training opportunities for providers, consumers, and policy makers in the national program;
7. Elimination of the costly process of making initial eligibility determinations and querying status before the payment of bills.

To stimulate physicians' cooperation in achieving the goals outlined by Dr. Weinerman, financial incentives should be introduced to encourage doctors to adopt capitation-payment arrangements under group auspicies. Doctors should be convinced that accepting and promoting this change will produce additional savings through increased efficiency, payment of bonuses, or other financial support. Health personnel that functions as a team, delivers comprehensive family care, and uses allied health personnel would be rewarded because their efficiency would improve, thus increasing their financial realization. Direct rewards could also be provided for establishing liaisons with back-up hospitals, specialty resources, and facilities for long-term care.

The next phase toward financial savings lies in planning and coordinating regional primary-care units and eliminating duplicate facilities, costly services, and supplies. Finally, incentives must be directed toward cost reimbursement to physicians, control over potential health risks, early detection of disease, and techniques of family-health maintenance, in relation to local social-welfare and associated community services.

Because the amount of money expended for the delivery of health care in past years has steadily increased, and since traditional measuring devices indicate little or no improvement, it is obvious that changes are essential. Perhaps we have been measuring the wrong symptoms or conditions and are directed toward goals which are no longer desirable. Instead of relying on traditional goals, we must begin to direct our resources toward earlier diagnosis and, finally, toward prevention of disease. The effectiveness of these methods will be measured by the improvement of the quality of life for those afflicted by chronic and degenerative diseases.

Today we are presented with a unique opportunity to improve America's health-delivery system. Health is and will remain a politically safe issue at a time when the country is polarized in many other areas. Now is the time for direct action to achieve the realistic dream of a universally effective health-delivery system in the United States.

MISSING LINKS IN ACHIEVING EFFECTIVE SERVICES*

BENNETT J. McCARTHY

President
Michigan Hospital Service

Member, American Hospital Association,
Council on Financing

Detroit, Mich.

WE are discussing the absence of national health policy. The importance here given to the topic is highly instructive and encouraging. It shows an awareness of one of our major difficulties and it responds directly to one of the most common criticisms of the health field. When observers speak about a nonsystem of health care, and they do so increasingly these days, this absence of policy is really the basic issue. When we speak of fragmentation or lack of coordination and cooperation among the elements of the health-care system, we are recognizing among other things that national policy is absent, and when we see that even within the private sector there is no agreement on the nature of our problems or on the extent to which we should even publicly acknowledge that they exist, we may well wonder how far we are from the day when generally accepted principles and guidelines can and will be realized.

I am not at all certain that we should fragmentize further by categorizing and separating the areas in which we can see the effect of such absence of policy. Obviously we must better be concerned with solving the problem on a broad, all-inclusive front. However, to the extent that today's financial picture sheds light on the nature of the challenge and offers some examples of how greater coordination may be achieved, a specific discussion of these aspects may be appropriate.

At the outset I suggest that, important as the financial issues may be, the ultimate values to the system as a whole are dependent upon the improvements we can afford in the delivery mechanisms themselves. In

*Presented in a panel, Absence of a National Health Policy in Matters of Financing, as part of the 1970 Health Conference of the New York Academy of Medicine, *Community Participation for Equity and Excellence in Health Care,* held at the Academy April 23 and 24, 1970.

making this comment, I realize I am reiterating what previous speakers have said. Our most critical task, it seems to me, must be to move our thinking away from the concept of episodic health care. We must aim instead for comprehensive care, and we must mold our institutions and the ease of access to them accordingly. It is far easier, for example, to underwrite a new benefit for home health care than to develop enough agencies to provide the service. And it is much easier to provide an in-patient hospital benefit under a typical Blue Cross or insurance-company program than to guarantee the availability of enough beds in the right place at the right time.

My feelings on this issue determine to some degree my thoughts on national health insurance. I believe that if we move quickly enough toward the kind of coordination that is needed to equate resources and public expectations, the private sector can do the job. At least we must try. If our attempt should fail, then a national program to improve matters might be the only solution. Conversely, a national program to perpetuate things as they are or merely to substitute one financial mechanism for another would not be the answer. In any event, the people will be served one way or another. Their collective will invariably seems to put a pragmatic end to disputes of this kind.

The current financial picture of voluntary hospitals on which I shall concentrate illustrates three elements of our situation very clearly. First, the economic uniqueness of health care; second, some effects of the absence of national health policy; and, third, the several methods by which we may hope to overcome this lack.

In some ways it may seem superfluous to dwell on the economic peculiarity of hospitals. Surely educated observers recognize that the normal market forces do not have ordinary relevance to a hospital's financial performance, and that supply and demand either operate enigmatically or not at all with regard to the financing of hospitals. However, a brief review of some essentials may be useful.

In health care, demand is not affected by changes in price to the same extent as with other commodities or services. In truth, demand under some circumstances in the field of health care may not be affected at all by change in price. Higher hospital charges, for example, will not reduce utilization to the same degree that a rise in the price of a television set may reduce the demand for the television set. Similarly, significant increases in supply, most notably the unnecessary and unplanned addition of hospital beds, for example, in a given geographic area will not ease pressure on price or automatically bring supply and demand into better balance. New beds needed will tend to be filled. Precise measurement of productivity or of cost effectiveness is extremely difficult. The relevance of personal income to health expenditures is also very difficult to determine precisely. The additional elements of prepayment and insurance tend to create configurations of use that are far different from what we might expect in the absence of these elements. And, finally, decisions to buy health care or not to buy health care are only rarely left in the hands of consumers; they are almost invariably made by professionals.

The process of enumerating these special economic characteristics at least has the happy effect of reminding us that unique problems demand unique solutions, Logically, however, we must examine the problems before suggesting solutions, and it is here that we begin to see some effects of the absence of a national health policy and some very visible symptoms of changing perspective on the part of both provider and public.

The financial pressures on hospitals have been growing steadily for years in terms of capital requirements as well as in the more publicized squeeze on operating costs. The latter factor is surely familiar to you and may be, in any event, less directly related to questions of policy. But in the area of plant capital investment, new factors have been combining to create a progressively more difficult situation. Many facilities are reaching a point where obsolescence is a critical element in cost. Others are located inappropriately with respect to the needs of people. A more rapid consumption of capital, an accelerated rate of obsolescence, and increased capital needs have been part of the price of technological and scientific progress. Some sources of investment funds, most notably public construction funds and private philanthropy, are becoming far less dependable.

Philanthropy in particular may decline drastically if income-tax reform removes much of the motivation for such gifts, or if other newer sources are developed. The repercussions of such a change are staggering if we consider that as recently as 1967 philanthropy was the largest single source, public or private, of capital funds for hospital construction.

In the light of these developments it is only logical that hospitals should have become more articulate in expressing their financial needs. It is natural that hospitals would increasingly question the traditional limitations on reimbursement methods, and they are doing so. These needs were formalized about a year ago in the American Hospital Association's *Statement on the Financial Requirements of Health Care Institutions and Services*. In that statement, the primary intent was the expression of the need for a broader spectrum of allowable elements in the program of reimbursement. Several of the hospital's financial needs, particularly plant-capital accumulation and bad-debt or charity losses, have not traditionally been reimbursable items. Their inclusion will represent a distinctive departure from past practice.

Perhaps the most illustrative example of this new approach is in the area of plant-capital accumulation. In the hospital's view, third parties such as Blue Cross, government, and others that are working on a contractual basis should assume an appropriate share of the cost of the maintenance and expansion of plant and equipment and for the amortization of capital indebtedness. In the area of expansion, as well as in the area of construction of entirely new facilities, or replacement of existing facilities entirely, the payment mechanism should share in the cost of projects approved by planning agencies. Keep in mind that proviso with respect to planning agencies because I shall return to it in a moment for a further comment.

That new methods of payment hold new potential for easing the capital needs of hospitals is obvious. In terms of timing, they come hand in hand with increased calls for new approaches to cost reimbursement itself. For example, there is widespread interest today in prospective, rather than in retrospective, reimbursement for basic patient care, and for incentive payments based on cost performance or on progressive changes in administrative policy.

Naturally there are many problems to be solved in working out these mechanisms. The mechanisms themselves can become far more complex and the documentation more voluminous. Agreement must be reached on many factors that affect the amounts involved, just as a ball player's performance in one year will go a long way toward determining what his salary will be in the next. We must agree, for example, on the method of depreciation to be used, if any, the amount of expense for equipment that is necessary or desirable, and the handling of capital debts at the start of the program. And the strengthening of community-oriented planning agencies where they exist, or their development where they do not, is an absolute must.

We must assume that the mechanisms can be developed because the innovations we can achieve through this kind of dialogue are indispensable to progress. In Michigan we have begun a project called Experiment 12, in which we are testing some new methods of payment in a pilot group of a dozen hospitals or so, in a specific endeavor to ensure a more stable and more adequate flow of working capital to our hospitals. The program is still new, so we do not yet have conclusive results. In addition, we have set up a board-level task force to study our entire reimbursement program in light of the new American Hospital Association's statement on financial requirements. In both of these efforts we are looking particularly for answers that will help us deal with the financing problems in those areas where we have less than normal precedents to guide us—those economic peculiarities of hospitals, if you will, and their behavior under today's pressures. Clearly, the nonprofit nature of our hospital system limits the ways in which we can attract capital through motivations generally available to a profit-making enterprise. Enterprise and creativity will be needed to find workable substitutes. In developing and implementing new mechanisms we come full cycle back to the need for policy, specifically for coordination and planning. These factors become key substitutes for direct market influences. Planning becomes the technique by which our innovations are shaped and directed toward optimum use of our health-care resources. Coordination becomes the technique by which we can consolidate our efforts and apply universally the innovations and improvements that our new teamwork helps us to achieve.

In this context it becomes clear that planning and coordination have very specific economic functions to play in making the existing system, with modifications, work more effectively. As we integrate these two concepts with changes in reimbursement, we begin to understand their significance. We see one element—the hospitals—analyzing and articulating various needs. The hospitals develop proposals, but they understand well that this is a mere exercise if Blue Cross and government, for instance, are not listening. Blue Cross and government, in their turn, must not only listen but must respond progressively, with new ideas of their own.

In truth, it is imperative for this cooperative process to be duplicated everywhere in our society. In no other way can a uniform kind of national policy be developed. And in no other way can we take advantage of a systemwide basis of individual talents and resources which are currently rendered feeble by the absence of coordination and national policy.

The concept of planning has the same goals. It continually strives to make individual decisions compatible with the over-all welfare of the community and the health-care system. What is interesting here is that we have known about the need for planning for so long, and yet it has only recently emerged as an integral part of specifically financial considerations. Let me quote to you from a comprehensive report on hospital care in the United States. "Hospital trustees and administrators frequently plan their activities and develop their services without regard to broad community, state and national needs. It must be borne in mind that the individual hospital is only one unit of a large, complex and interrelated program which should cover the entire community in which it operates." That report was written 20 years ago, in 1947. In all that time we should have accomplished much more than we have. We should ask ourselves if it must take so long for a new idea to reach respectability, for what was true then is still true today.

The thing that is different now is the time frame. We have less time than we had a generation ago. And the number of alternatives is diminishing. We must also recognize that coordination applies not only to persons and institutions but to ideas as well. Ours is an enormously complex system. As we come to new understandings of cost, productivity, planning, effectiveness, and reimbursement, we must blend our new insights into all our efforts, as quickly and unselfishly as possible. If we succeed, we can yet achieve a health-care system worthy of its reputation for excellence. We can make real the conviction of health care as a right for all, and we can do it without destroying the voluntary approach which has served so many so well for so long.

COMMUNITY PARTICIPATION FOR EQUITY AND EXCELLENCE IN HEALTH CARE*

General Discussion III

MILTON TERRIS, *chairman*

Professor and Chairman
Department of Community and Preventive Medicine
New York Medical College
New York, N. Y.

DR. MILTON TERRIS. Two points are now to be discussed: 1) the belief that the well-to-do know what high-quality medical care is, and that they obtain it; and 2) that paramedical personnel will care for the poor, and that internists and pediatricians will care for the rich.

DR. TOM LEVIN. I think that anyone who feels that the rich receive high-quality medical care is being deceived as much as the rich are. I think that a close examination of the care that all the people in the United States receive, no matter what their economic level is, will show that it varies greatly. We do not really know what goes on inside a doctor's office. The few studies that have been done show that much of the care delivered in the United States irrespective of economic level is not high-quality care. With reference to the second point under discussion, on the use of paramedical personnel, I think the experience in the state of Washington with the Medex program has proved just the opposite of what has been stated. All economic levels have availed themselves of the Medex program. In fact, in the state of Washington patients are now calling doctors' offices and asking for appointments with Medex personnel instead of doctors when they know that their illness can be treated by Medex.

DR. MICHAEL M. DACSO. Instead of becoming a poor man's medicine there is again a danger of its becoming medical-center medicine. We are going to have considerable problems with sending practitioners out in the underprivileged areas.

MRS. DOROTHY NAYER, of the *American Journal of Nursing*, New York, N. Y. May I commend Dr. Levin for his new approach to the

*The 1970 Health Conference of the New York Academy of Medicine, held at the Academy April 23 and 24, 1970.

education of health professionals. One of the things that you have discussed here in the last two days is a great deal of upward mobility and vertical mobility, integrated programs, and so on. But I have heard very little discussion of financing for individuals in such training programs: stipends, not only scholarships and loans, which we know the federal government is not supporting very well, but actual free education beyond the high school level including stipends for students and day-care centers for mothers who can then go to school because their children are taken care of. In these areas we are not doing very well. And I wondered if anybody wanted to comment on that. I think that the point you raised on financing health-professional education is a subject for a conference in itself.

Comment from the Audience. I am wondering why the people whom Dr. Bergen caucused with about his program and Dr. Levin have not thought of the upgrading of registered nurses, who are true doctors' assistants, who many times have saved doctors from charges of negligence when the doctors have not been present. We nurses are the true doctors' assistants, but doctors refuse to accept us except as glorified maids. Everybody knows that up to 20 years ago we were on the household-help list in Washington, and the doctors in the American Medical Association still refuse to accept the registered nurse as anything but household help. We should be given the chance to be upgraded, not necessarily to the grade of an M.D.

Dr. Milton Terris. The truth of the matter is that in the United States the medical profession is practically limited to men. There is very serious discrimination against women, as you know, in the medical profession, and this is now being extended to physicians' assistants, or whatever they are to be called. Let the panel answer.

Dr. Levin. I have four parts to my answer. In the first place, if you recall my presentation, we have four nurses in our program. Second, we think that taking only nurses into this new program would be robbing Peter to pay Paul. We are trying to develop a new profession, a new group of persons who can deliver health care because we feel more manpower is needed. And to use nurses for this purpose would only take them away from their current use. Third, we do want to attract men in this capacity, because men are the wage earners, men have not been attracted to nursing as a career profession, and we believe they should be attracted into health-care fields. Fourth, we believe that the nursing profession itself is very undecided as to where it wants to go. Last January the board of trustees of the American Medical Association announced, just as Mrs. Valentine has, that nurses should be used as physicians' assistants. The next day the American Nursing Association said in righteous indignation that nurses themselves do not want to be physicians' assistants. These problems have all added to the complexity of the situation and have made us seek other solutions.

I should like to make another point. I do not know what you mean by physicians' assistants. Such assistants do not exist. There is neither licensure for it, nor discipline for it nor, in my view, is there a place for it in the present health-care delivery system. However, I suggest that there is a direct patient-care continum of increased complexity of skill and responsibility. I take very unkindly to nurses who state that they are being discriminated against by physicians. There are six different types of nurses. Nurses, in establishing their own class, race, and guild hierarchy, have boxed themselves out of the full continuum of health services.

We plan to train corpsman for a role we call health corpsmen. I have refused to train them to become physicians' assistants because there is no such category. I have insisted that these corpsmen get nursing credentials all along the line, in an escalated way, and I hope that we shall be able to work together to break down the guild barrier that exists against them.

Concluding Remarks

COMMUNITY HEALTH AND COMMUNITY PARTICIPATION*

SHIRLEY CHISHOLM

Member of Congress
U.S. House of Representatives
12th District
Brooklyn, N. Y.

WHETHER one is discussing community health services, urban planning, social work, or urban renewal the events of the last decade have made the need for deeper examination of at least one factor—community participation—increasingly important.

The phrase community participation has been used in various ways —to mask attempts to control services to the community by small cliques of its residents; as a sincere but often misunderstood rallying cry by young idealists; as a wedge onto various boards that might serve as launching pads for individual success by middle-class opportunists.

It was almost 30 years ago that Congress first incorporated the concept into legislation with the passage of the first housing act. That act contained a requirement that local urban-renewal agencies have a citizen's advisory committee composed of residents of the affected areas. In almost all cases the committees were composed of handpicked, malleable, well-to-do citizens who could be counted on not to create too many problems.

Initially the local community boards authorized under the Economic Opportunity Act of 1964 seemed headed in the same direction, even though there were stipulations that such boards have a certain set number of certifiably "poor" residents. However, in those instances where the "representatives of the poor" were not handpicked, they were given little or no training that would have helped them to cope with the boards' more experienced members, thus virtually ensuring that they would be ineffectual.

*Presented at the 1970 Health Conference of the New York Academy of Medicine, *Community Participation for Equity and Excellence in Health Care,* held at the Academy, April 23 and 24, 1970.

It is my feeling that what the president and Congress perceived as goals for the Office of Economic Opportunity (OEO) was the closing of the gap in affluence between the lower and the middle-income brackets. Therefore I am forced to conclude that the war on poverty as such was a failure.

The underlying concept of the war was to be that ill-fated bit of jargon "maximum feasible participation." It is my contention that this phrase was intended to mean some participation in implementation, but no participation in planning.

I cannot be certain that cavalier treatment of the "poor," of their "representatives," and of their legitimate interests was intentional. However, in the final analysis it really does not matter—the results were the same.

Common sense dictates that the only way for the poor to cease to exist as a group trapped in poverty is to obtain sufficient economic and political organizational strength to attain their goals. OEO was not intended to help them to accomplish that except in the most limited sense.

Yet in quite another manner, a manner most definitely unexpected by the architects, the antipoverty program succeeded. It succeeded in pointing up to black Americans that we have struggled too hard in fighting prejudice and too little in attempting to organize; that we have failed far too long to recognize the importance of collective action along ethnic lines, perhaps better known now as Black Power.

The antipoverty program has succeeded in forcing the black and the poor to begin to develop almost every possible type of economic self-help organization. But it has also succeeded in making eminently clear that we cannot do that and ignore the political arena. In fact, we now know that we must involve ourselves deeply in every level of American politics. The question of community participation is a question of politics in the most fundamental sense.

Therefore it is important to remember that the OEO experience began in the twilight of the civil rights movement. Some of the consequences are clear. Though many people who were in the movement solely because of personal opportunism switched their initiative to the war on poverty as the movement waned, it is equally true that there were many true representatives of the interests of the poor who did likewise. This latter group took with them skills and the results of lessons in power relations that they had learned the hard way, as well as the deep-seated convictions that had brought them into the movement in the first place. They were and are convinced that change is not only possible but inevitable. They became and remain ardent and effective proselytizers in the community. When they say maximum feasible participation they mean it literally. Their actions and activities may often rankle the professional, who is engaged in service activities in the community. However, to my way of thinking, their role is at least equally as important as that of the professional.

They have helped the community confront teachers, school boards, lawyers, planners, city councilmen, mayors, doctors, welfare workers, and others, including OEO officials. They have been harassed, harangued, beaten, arrested, jailed, and subjected to defamations of their characters.

They have been called outside agitators—often while living in the community; they have been called Communists—sometimes while voting straight Republican. They have been called opportunists—while living hand-to-mouth on subsistence diets. This and more has happened to them because they believe that we can create a reality that is firmly based upon the democratic theory.

What has often been overlooked in all of the hullabaloo is the fact they too have often been professional planners, social workers, teachers, doctors, or lawyers. Another factor that the so-called professionals have tried to overlook or to ignore is the legitimacy of the demands that they are making—demands that are predicated on the inadequacy and the irrelevancy of the institutions that could and should be serving the people more effectively.

One of the things that has always irritated me most is the attitude that far too many "professionals" take toward the people they supposedly serve. This is especially true of those who claim to serve the black, brown, and poor communities. It is an attitude that is intended to let those being served know that they are considered inferior and, as such, it is reprehensible to me and to those who are being served.

Persons with specialized skills in medicine, planning, education, social work, and other disciplines will always be needed by their society; therefore there is no need to attempt to make people who do not share in certain specialized skills more dependent than is necessary. In fact to do so is inherently dysfunctional to the society and to the individual.

You represent the third group of professionals engaged in providing services to the community that I have had the pleasure of addressing this month. Like your group, the other two conferences, one consisting of professional planners and the other of social workers, had finally got around to discussing the issue of community participation.

One of the things that I tried to make unequivocally clear to both of the prior groups is that it is no longer an issue whether the community can or cannot, or should not, or even will or will not participate in the planning and implementation of the delivery services to itself. The issue now before us is: How can the community best participate in the planning and implementation of those services that most crucially and directly affect its life and well-being?

In speaking to the American Society of Planning officials earlier this month, I said that certain aspects of the OEO experiment, those involving community organizers especially, made it clear that planners could share enough of their own expertise and knowledge with the community groups with whom they were working to enable those groups to become involved in actuality as well as in theory. I think that, within certain limitations, this would apply to community health specialists also.

In my summary that morning, I pointed out that the communities would expect to receive accountability and responsibility from those directly responsible for the providing of services, that is, from the professionals. I hope those of you here today will remain mindful of that factor. It is extremely important.

The second conference that I addressed this month was a gathering of social workers who were involved in discussing their roles as agents of change in society. At that time I contended that the major contributing factor responsible for the conditions forced upon the trapped urban poor was the lack of power. I then went on to note that when I use the word "power" it means books as well as bullets, and knowledge as well as knives; the kind of power that I speak of is based primarily in knowing what is happening to you, why it is happening, and what alternatives are available to help you in preventing it from happening. That type of power is as applicable to the group as it is to the individual.

I think it is important for every professional involved in providing services to the community to understand this because while it may be easier for you, personally, to concentrate on helping the individual patient or client it is also infinitely slower in terms of real change and, as such, potentially more dangerous socially.

The issue here today may be community participation, but your over-all goal is the health and well-being of the community. On April 10th, when I addressed the Planners Conference, I noted that for the black and brown urban dweller the real issue is survival, not progress. My feelings have not changed—that is just as true today as it will be tomorrow or a year from now.

COMMUNITY PARTICIPATION FOR EQUITY AND EXCELLENCE IN HEALTH CARE*

General Discussion IV

JOHN W. V. CORDICE, JR., *chairman*

Secretary, Queens Clinical Society
Jamaica, N. Y.

DR. JOHN W. V. CORDICE, JR. A resolution has been submitted by a caucus of the National Consumer Committee held at noon today. This resolution recommends that the Academy establish and support a consumer-participation community enabled to function effectively by the provision of staff, funding as required, and representation in the governing-board processes of the New York Academy of Medicine. [The resolution was moved and adopted, with 12 persons abstaining.]

We now shall hear representatives of the various committees of the various round tables.

MRS. EDNA A. PHILLIPS, *secretary of the Comprehensive Health Center, Atlanta, Ga.* A poem comes to my mind, and I briefly paraphrase it. It says: If you can't be a tree, be a bush; if you can't be a road, be a trail; if you can't be the sun, be the stars; but be the best of whatever you are. And I think that we, as consumers, and you as physicians and nurses, and you of the staff of the New York Academy of Medicine, shall all have to change, and none of us likes change. I think we must make concessions and work together, which is not easy, as I found from my experiences in Atlanta in trying to obtain many things. The problems confronting us have not arisen in one year; it took many years for them to arise, and it will take years to solve them. The needs are immediate.

One day in Atlanta I went into a home and found a man dying. He did die before we got him to the hospital, and was ill because of privation and the lack of health care. It is frightening to realize that in a city as big as Atlanta persons are going without health care. But I

*The 1970 Health Conference of the New York Academy of Medicine, held at the Academy April 23 and 24, 1970.

am thankful for the opportunity for being here, and I hope that we can all pull together and work for the right solution for everyone: the poor, the middle class, and the affluent, all of whom should have the same medical care.

MR. OLLY NEAL, JR. I shall not try to summarize all that went on in round-table discussions; instead I shall cite the recommendations that were made there. It was stated that this conference will be useless unless action is taken by the Academy to stimulate training in management of the participants so that they can operate their own programs. Medical and nursing schools should have all students spend at least three months in communities for first-hand understanding of the total health problem. Comprehensive health care should be urged. Copies of the proceedings of this conference should be sent to all county and medical societies in the country, with a letter urging new approaches to the old problems. Consumer advocates should be hired to determine which departments can best implement resolutions made at the conference urging them to do so. Community organizations should be contacted to support any such resolutions. A consumer advisory council should be established to develop pressure. Militant actions taken to make health facilities and comprehensive health care responsive to the needs of the public should be supported.

MRS. BESSIE DAVIS, *Reynolds Memorial Hospital, Winston-Salem, N. C.* One of the most important things left for us to do is to define the term community. The "community" should be defined so that when we talk we shall all mean the same thing. Who is the community, and what is "community control"? Persons should be talked *with* in the community, rather than talked *at* and *for*. Another question is: How can we make the medical profession more responsive to the poor? We felt this should be discussed in greater detail, and that some common basis should be developed for future mutual discussion.

ACKNOWLEDGMENTS

Dr. John W. V. Cordice, Jr., was chairman of the 1970 Annual Health Conference Committee of the Academy's Committee on Medicine in Society. The members of the conference committee included: Drs. Irving Graef, Sidney M. Greenberg, August H. Groeschel, John L. S. Holloman, Jr., Milton Terris. Mrs. Barbara Dworetzky served as Conference Coordinator. Mrs. Cynthia Taylor, secretary to the Committee, and Mrs. Linda L. Stennett also assisted.

We acknowledge with thanks the assistance of the following in planning meetings for this conference: Clive C. Bernard, M.D., *South Ozone Park, N. Y.;* Marilyn Darling, *Harlem CORE, New York, N. Y.;* Mrs. Marion Day, *Sydenham Hospital, New York, N. Y.;* Carlton E. Ford, M.D., *New York, N. Y.;* Rev. Wendel Foster, *Bronx, N. Y.;* Thomas M. Gocke, M.D., *director of Community Medicine, Catholic Medical Center of Brooklyn, N. Y.;* Mrs. Patricia Leo, *American Public Health Association, New York, N. Y.;* Preston M. Lewis, *Committee on Health Priorities for Harlem, New York, N. Y.;* Vaughn C. Mason, M.D., *New York, N. Y.;* Mrs. Lillian Roberts, *District Council 37, American Federation of State, County, and Muncipal Employees, AFL-CIO, New York, N. Y.;* Isaiah Robinson, *Board of Education of the City of New York, New York, N. Y.;* and Victor Solomon, *Harlem CORE, New York, N. Y.*

The conference was supported in part by the New York Metropolitan Regional Medical Program, the Commonwealth Fund, and the National Center for Health Services Research and Development, Department of Health, Education, and Welfare, Rockville, Md.

MARVIN LIEBERMAN, Ph.D.
Executive Secretary,
Committee on Medicine in Society

DEMOGRAPHY IN EARLY AMERICA

It has long been obvious that a separation exists between clinical medicine and public health. Whatever the historical origins of this diastasis, one result has been that the study of demography becomes constantly more remote from the interests of the practitioner and has come to be claimed by the hygienist, the economist, the government official, and the specialist in insurance. Concomitantly the physician has run the risk of losing contact with a body of knowledge that is capable of broadening and deepening his outlook.

The development of demographic thought and action in the North American colonies and in the United States from 1600 to 1800 is the subject of an attractive volume[1] recently issued by James Cassedy, Ph.D., a medical historian attached to the History of Medicine Division of the National Library of Medicine.

The author has ingeniously combined a chronological and a topical approach. Introductory chapters are devoted to the social, economic, and political forces which affected the early stages of American demography. In addition to these there are chapters on population theory, insurance, and medical statistics. These difficult subjects are set forth against the background of American life; thereby they are endowed with meaning. The style is simple and lucid throughout.

In his chapter on colonial Massachusetts Dr. Cassedy points out that while the inhabitants of Virginia collected vital statistics chiefly in order to fulfill their obligations to the Virginia Company, the New Englanders were motivated by a recognition of their own needs and aspirations. The histories written by William Bradford and John Winthrop may be regarded as incidental records of vital data. The preservation of systematic demographic information by the Puritans represented an effort to discover the will of God and hence was instituted at an early date. From its onset the mechanism was civil, not ecclesiastical, and was operated by government officials. The Massachusetts Bay system was followed elsewhere in New England and was influential also in the Cromwellian Commonwealth.

1. Cassedy, J. H.: *Demography in Early America; Beginnings of the Statistical Mind, 1600-1800.* Cambridge, Harvard Univ. Press, 1969, 357 pp.

In discussing the famous early demographers William Petty (1623-1687) and John Graunt (1620-1674), Dr. Cassedy mentions the skepticism which mercantilists expressed with respect to the value of colonization. Petty feared impoverishment of the home country through emigration. Others feared that England was erecting a dangerous transatlantic competitor in New England, whereas Virginia and the West Indies could be commended for raising products which gave employment to Englishmen at home. The 20th century "brain drain" to America can be seen to have had a historical precedent of sorts.

The story of the demographic developments that took place in the colonies is surprisingly interesting. For a long time the colonies had nothing resembling the famous bills of mortality that were issued in London; printing was scarce and the laws did not require compilation and publication. Early in the 18th century the newspapers began to fill the gap. The earliest journalistic efforts were sporadic and discontinuous, like some of the newspapers themselves. More continuous and successful were the reports of Benjamin Franklin in the *The Pennsylvania Gazette* and the annual statements of Christ-Church Parish in Philadelphia. Statistics were called to practical use in the inoculation controversy, which involved Cotton Mather, Zabdiel Boylston, and William Douglass. The important contributions of Douglass to statistics are explained and adequate reference is made to the demographic information presented in his well-known history.

Like many another learned author, Dr. Cassedy leads the reader to look into collateral topics which are valuable and fascinating. One of these is Edmund Halley's contribution to demography. Probably through Henri Justell, secretary of the Royal Society, the eminent astronomer had learned of certain tables of vital statistics that had been prepared by one Caspar Neumann (1648-1715), a studious clergyman of Breslau. Neumann's observations covered the five years from 1687 to 1691. Whereas earlier tabulations had been prepared in other cities, apparently Neumann's were the first which systematically recorded the ages of the deceased. By means of this collection Halley was able to calculate the probable duration of life, the details being set forth in his essay *An estimate of the degrees of the mortality of mankind, drawn from the curious tables of the births and funerals at the city of Breslaw, with an attempt to ascertain the price of annuities upon lives.* This paper, which Halley published in the 17th volume of the *Philosophical*

Transactions, and amplified by a supplement elsewhere in the same volume, is the basic document in the history of life insurance. Halley's contribution was well known to Benjamin Franklin and to Alexander Hamilton.

In the final chapter of his impressive book Dr. Cassedy deals with medical statistics. He describes the deficiencies in the American bills of mortality, which were prepared by laymen and which were obscured by inadequacies of terminology. Although William Cullen had taught many American physicians and had given them a system of nosology, Benjamin Rush had turned many away from nosology and this fact can be accounted harmful to the recording of reliable statistics. The influence of Holyoke, Currie, and Ramsay acted in the opposite direction, as did the occurrence of epidemic outbreaks. At the end of the period stood Noah Webster, whose epidemiological studies Dr. Cassedy justly characterizes as "a bold and original attempt to correlate disease and environment."

S. J.

GENERAL INDEX

Volume 46, 1969

A

Abortion laws: The present status of, the New York Academy of Medicine, 281
Abscesses of the liver: The danger of moving the patient, J. B. Morgagni, 71
Absence of a national health policy in matters of financing, Discussion of, D. French, 1129
Absence of a national health policy in matters of financing, Discussion of, B. J. McCarthy, 1135
Abstracts, proceedings of the eighth meeting of the career scientists of the Health Research Council of the City of New York, 457
Abstracts, Scientific session on research, New York Heart Association, The, 997
Academy Medal, Presentation of the, to Harry Eagle, M.D., A. Gilman, 666
Academy Plaque, Presentation of the, to James Burns Amberson, M.D., D. W. Richards, 663
Agricultural laborers in England, The condition of, H. Colman, 293
Albuminuria upon vision, The effects of, H. D. Noyes, 197
Altschuller, Gregory I. The origins of modern scientific thinking, 611
Amberson, James Burns, M.D., Presentation of the Academy Plaque to, D. W. Richards, 663
Angrist, Alfred. The new role of the autopsy in the community hospital, 523
Anthropological essay by Thomas Hodgkin, An, S. Jarcho, 889
Aristotle, A few comments by, 70
Assuring stable and effective financing of local health services: Role of inter-governmental grants in aid, J. F. Kelly, 718
Astérix the Gaul, S. Jarcho, 62
Asthma, Current concepts of the pathogenesis and management of, M. H. Grieco, 597
Autopsy in the community hospital, The new role of the, A. Angrist, 523

B

Badeau, John S. Diplomacy and medicine, 303
Badillo, Herman. Role of the community in developing improved health care, 1028
Baedeker, The doctor travels with, B. Gebhard, 469
Baedeker's description of New York, Medical and nonmedical items in, S. Jarcho, 479
Bank, Norman. The renal regulation of sodium transport, 818
Barragan, Miguel F. Discussion of the "how" of community participation in delivering health care, 1080
Battered child syndrome, The: Parental motivation, clinical aspects, G. V. Laury, 676
Becker, E. Lovell. Introduction (Conference on Glomerulonephritis), 747
Becker, E. Lovell. Proteinuria in renal disease, 830
Bergen, Stanley S., Nierenberg, Harold, Lewis, Arnold M., and Firriolo, Dominick. The medical-services associate: A new health career for the improvement of health care delivery, 1099
Boehme, Diethelm H. Resistance to salmonella infections in inbred mouse strains, 499
Brooks, Angie. Opening statement (Symposium on medicine and diplomacy in the tropics), 299
Bryant, Thomas E. Discussion of the role of the health professions in achieving effective consumer participation, 1054
Bryce, J. Lord Bryce on intellectual productivity, 290
Buchanan, F. H. Disease in Nepal, 484

C

Cahill, Kevin M. Introduction (Symposium on Medicine and Diplomacy in the Tropics), 300

Cahn, Edgar. Discussion of the role of the community in developing improved health care, 1031
Can we avoid a $100 billion misunderstanding?, H. Ennes, 1120
Career scientists of the Health Research Council of the City of New York, Proceedings of the eighth meeting of the, 451
Carey, George W. Urban ecology, geography, and health problems, 73
Carey, Hugh L. A war we can win: Health as a vector of foreign policy, 334
Carp, Louis. Mozart: His tragic life and controversial death, 267
Chelsea physic garden, The, S. Jarcho, 189
Chisholm, Shirley. Community health and community participation, 1144
Churg, Jacob. Pathology of glomerulonephritis, 761
Climatic treatment of hypochondriasis, T. M. Madden, 482
Clinical medicine, On: With notes from the diary of a part-time researcher, A. Vogl, 39
Closing morning discussion (Conference on Glomerulonephritis), D. P. Earle, D. S. Baldwin, and C. M. Edelmann, Jr., 797
Cobliner, W. Godfrey. Teen-age out-of-wedlock pregnancy, 438
Colman, Henry. Government and welfare in nineteenth-century England, 1018
Colman, Henry. The condition of agricultural laborers in England, 293
Committee on Public Health of the New York Academy of Medicine, The. Methadone management of heroin addiction, 391
Community health and community participation, S. Chisholm, 1144
Community participation and a national health policy, J. W. V. Cordice, Jr., 1025
Computers in evaluating health data, Utilizing, J. C. Duffy, 952
Conferences (see also Symposia):
1970 health conference, The. The New York Academy of Medicine, "Community Participation for Equity and Excellence in Health Care," 1025
Glomerulonephritis. The New York Heart Association, 747
Conley, John. Treatment of malignant tumors of the salivary glands, 511
Controlled Dangerous Substances Act of 1969 (S.3246), Statement on the, the New York Academy of Medicine, 509
Cordice, John W. V., Jr., chairman. Discussion IV (1970 health conference), 1149
Cordice, John W. V., Jr. Community participation and a national health policy, 1025
Cranefield, Paul F. and Federn, Walter. Paulus Zacchias on mental deficiency and on deafness, 3
Cron, Theodore O. Discussion of the role of the community in developing improved health care, 1038

D

Dacso, Michael M. Training of allied health professionals and physicians' assistants, 1107
Dammin, Gustave J. Medical research activities overseas, 351
Daniel Drake on geographic variations of disease, 486
Defunct and dying diseases, B. Straus, 686
Demography in early America, S. Jarcho, 1152
Diplomacy and medicine, J. S. Badeau, 303
Discussion of absence of a national health policy in matters of financing, D. French, 1129
Discussion of absence of a national health policy in matters of financing, B. J. McCarthy, 1135
Discussion of the "how" of community participation in delivering health care, M. F. Barragan, 1080
Discussion of the "how" of community participation in delivering health care, J. W. Hatch, 1085
Discussion of the "how" of community participation in delivering health care, Olly Neal, Jr., 1091
Discussion of paper by James F. Kelly: "Assuring stable and effective financing of local health services: Role of intergovernmental grants in aid," A. Willcox, 732
Discussion of paper by Dr. George A. Silver: "American Medicine: Technology outruns social usefulness," M. Lipkin, 161

Discussion of the role of the community in developing improved health care, E. Cahn, 1031
Discussion of the role of the community in developing improved health care, T. O. Cron, 1038
Discussion of the role of the community in developing improved health care, L. Wescott, 1042
Discussion of the role of the health professional in achieving effective consumer participation, R. G. Long, 1057
Discussion of the role of the health professional in achieving effective consumer participation, P. Lowinger, 1059
Discussion of the role of the health professions in achieving effective consumer participation, T. E. Bryant, 1054
Discussion of the role of the health profession in achieving effective community participation, S. R. Smith, 1067
Discussion of the role of the health profession in achieving effective consumer participation, W. Waldron, 1071
Disease in Nepal, F. H. Buchanan, 484
Drake, Daniel. Geographic variations of disease, 486
Drug Abuse and Drug Dependence, Prevention, Treatment, and Rehabilitation Act of 1970 (S. 3562), Statement on the, The New York Academy of Medicine, 642
Duffy, John C. Utilizing computers in evaluating health data, 952

E

Eagle, Harry, M.D., Presentation of the Academy Medal to, A. Gilman, 666
Earle, David P., Baldwin, David S., and Edelmann, Chester M., Jr. Closing morning discussion (Conference on Glomerulonephritis), 797
Earle, David P. Glomerulonephritis: Clinical aspects, 749
Education of the practicing physician, Continuing, the New York Academy of Medicine, 893
Effects of the American revolution, B. Rush, 558
Electrotherapy to noncardiac disorders, Application of, D. C. Schechter, 932
Empyema or hydrothorax in the ninety-fifth doge of Venice, S. Jarcho, 378
Ennes, Howard. Can we avoid a $100 billion misunderstanding?, 1120
Evolution and delivery of medical programs in developing lands, The, E. E. Swanstrom, 324

F

Farah, Abdulrahim Abby. Health problems and goals of a recipient nation, 313
Feldman, Louis L. Group practice development: A service of the department of health, New York City, 113
French, David. Discussion of absence of a national health policy in matters of financing, 1129

G

Gall, F. J. The phrenologist discusses friendship, 646
Gebhard, Bruno. The doctor travels with Karl Baedeker, 469
General discussion I (1970 health conference), J. W. V. Cordice, Jr., chairman, 1149
General discussion II (1970 health conference), J. L. S. Holloman, chairman, 1977
General discussion III (1970 health conference), M. Terris, chairman, 1141
General Discussion IV (1970 health conference), J. W. V. Cordice, Jr., chairman, 1149
Geographic variations of disease, Daniel Drake on, 486
Gertner, Melvin, Hsu, Lillian Y. F., Martin, Joan, and Hirschhorn, Kurt. The use of amniocentesis for prenatal genetic counseling, 916
Gilman, Alfred. Presentation of the Academy Medal to Harry Eagle, M.D., 666
Glomerulonephritis: Clinical aspects, D. P. Earle, 749
Glomerulonephritis, Conference on, the New York Heart Association, 747
Glomerulonephritis, Pathology of, J. Churg, 761

Glomerulonephritis: Pediatric aspects, W. W. McCrory, 789
Goodrich, Charles H., Olendzki, Margaret, and Deuschle, K. W. Mount Sinai's approach to the East Harlem community, 97
Government and welfare in nineteenth-century England, H. Colman, 1018
Greenberg, Sidney M., chairman. Discussion I (1970 health conference), 1048
Grieco, M. H. Current concepts of the pathogenesis and management of asthma, 597
Group practice development: A service of the department of health, New York City, L. L. Feldman, 113

H

Hand, Bernard R., Malm, James R., Bowman, Jr., Frederick O., and Sullivan, Stuart F. The effects of anesthesia and cardiac bypass on pulmonary compliance in man, 22
Harris, E. Smallpox in New York City, 1868-1870, 199
Hatch, John W. Discussion of the "how" of community participation in delivering health care, 1084
Health problems and goals of a recipient nation, A. A. Farah, 313
Helwich on difficulty of respiration, Christianus (Augsburg, 1722), 34
Hemolytic anemia, Disease associated autoimmune, A. Sawitsky and P. B. Ozaeta, Jr., 411
Hemolytic anemia, Drug-associated, R. Zalusky, 427
Hemolytic disorders, Hereditary, E. R. Jaffe, 397
Hodgkin, Unpublished papers of Thomas, Wilks, S., 67
Hoehn, Robert. Nasal reconstruction by scalping flap in a case of malignant melanoma of the nasal tip, 922
Holloman, John L. S., Jr., chairman. Discussion II (1970 health conference), 1077
Hospitals depicted in old maps and panoramas (I), S. Jarcho, 737
Hospitals depicted in old maps and panoramas (II), S. Jarcho, 1013

I

Immunologic mechanisms in several forms of human glomerular diseases, Evidence for, R. T. McCluskey, 769
India office records, The: A source for historians of psychiatry, S. Jarcho, 124
Infibulation, population control, and the medical profession, G. S. Schwarz, 964
Intellectual productivity, Lord Bryce on, J. Bryce, 290
Introduction (Conference on Glomerulonephritis), E. L. Becker, 747
Introduction (Symposium on Medicine and Diplomacy in the Tropics), K. M. Cahill, 300

J

Jackdaw series on the history of medicine and science, The, S. Jarcho, 386
Jaffé, Ernst R. Hereditary hemolytic disorders, 397
Jarcho, Saul. An anthropological essay by Thomas Hodgkin, 889
Jarcho, Saul. Astérix the Gaul, 62
Jarcho, Saul. Christianus Helwich on difficulty of respiration (Augsburg, 1722), 34
Jarcho, Saul. Demography in early America, 1152
Jarcho, Saul. Empyema or hydrothorax in the ninety-fifth doge of Venice, 378
Jarcho, Saul. Hospitals depicted in old maps and panoramas (I), 737
Jarcho, Saul. Hospitals depicted in old maps and panoramas (II), 1013
Jarcho, Saul. Lepers, pariahs, and churches, 287
Jarcho, Saul. Medical and nonmedical items in Baedeker's description of New York, 479
Jarcho, Saul. The anthropological writings of Theophil Mitchell Prudden, 194
Jarcho, Saul. The Chelsea physic garden, 189
Jarcho, Saul. The India office records: A source for historians of psychiatry, 124
Jarcho, Saul. The *Jackdaw* series on the history of medicine and science, 386
Jarcho, Saul. Tollund man and other bog burials, 554
Jarcho, Saul. The mouth as an instrument holder, 643

K

Kelly, James F. Assuring stable and effective financing of local health services: Role of intergovernmental grants in aid, 718

L

Laury, Gabriel V. Battered child syndrome, The: Parental motivation, clinical aspects, 676

Lepers, pariahs, and churches, S. Jarcho, 287

Levin, Tom. Social policy and guild policy in health manpower, 1112

Lipkin, Mack, Discussion of paper by Dr. A. Silver: "American Medicine: Technology outruns social usefulness," 161

Long, Robert G. Discussion of the role of the health professional in achieving effective consumer participation, 1057

Lowenstein, Jerome, Bank, Norman, Rubini, Milton E., and Schreiner, George E. Panel discussion, afternoon session, (Conference on Glomeruulonephritis), 884

Lowinger, Paul. Discussion of the role of the health professional in achieving effective consumer participation, 1059

Lythcott, George I. Observations on America's international medical programs, 361

M

Madden, Thomas M. Climatic treatment of hypochondriasis, 482

Madness and poetry: A note on Collins, Cowper, and Smart, W. B. Ober, 203

Malignant tumors of the salivary glands, Treatment of, J. Conley, 511

Medical and nonmedical items in Baedeker's description of New York, S. Jarcho, 479

Medical research activities overseas, G. J. Dammin, 351

Medical-services associate: A new health career for the improvement of health care delivery, S. S. Bergen, H. Nierenberg, A. M. Lewis, and D. Firriolo, 1099

Medicine, American: Technology outruns social usefulness, Discussion of paper by Dr. George A. Silver, M. Lipkin, 161

Medicine, American: Technology outruns social usefulness, G. A. Silver, 148

Mental deficiency and on deafness, Paulus Zacchias on, P. F. Cranefield and W. Federn, 3

Merrill, John P. An overview of nephritis, 806

Methadone management of heroin addiction, Statement by the New York Academy of Medicine on, 61

Methadone management of heroin addiction, a report by the Committee on Public Health of the New York Academy of Medicine, 391

Michaelis, L. S. The problem of pain in paraplegia and tetraplegia, 88

Mission-oriented and clinical research, A critique of the conflict between, L. M. Rousselot, 906

Morgagni, J. B. Abscesses of the Liver: The danger of moving the patient, 71

Mount Sinai's approach to the East Harlem Community, C. H. Goodrich, M. Olendzki, and K. W. Deuschle, 97

Mouth as an instrument holder, The, S. Jarcho, 643

Mozart: His tragic life and controversial death, L. Carp, 267

Mc

McCarthy, Bennett J. Discussion of absence of a national health policy in matters of financing, 1135

McCluskey, Robert T. Evidence for immunologic mechanisms in several forms of human glomerular diseases, 769

McCrory, Wallace W. Glomerulonephritis: Pediatric aspects, 789

McLaughlin, Mary C. Two health problems: One solution, 454

N

Nasal reconstruction by scalping flap in a case of malignant melanoma of the nasal tip, R. Hoehn, 922

Neal, Olly Jr. The "How" of community participation in delivering health care, 1091
Needed: A health consumers' organization, G. Williams, 532
Nepal, Disease in, F. H. Buchanan, 484
Nephritis, Management of end-state: Biochemical alterations, G. E. Schreiner, 838
Nephritis, overview of, J. P. Merrill, 806
New York Academy of Medicine, The. Continuing education of the practicing physician, 893
New York Academy of Medicine, The. Statement on the Controlled Dangerous Substances Act of 1969 (S.3246), 509
New York Academy of Medicine, The. Statement on the Drug Abuse and Drug Dependence, Prevention, Treatment, and Rehabilitation Act of 1970 (S. 3562), 642
New York Academy of Medicine, The. The Committee on Public Health. Methadone management of heroin addiction, 391
New York Academy of Medicine, The. The present status of abortion laws, 281
New York Heart Association
Conference on glomerulonephritis, 747
Scientific session on research, 997
Nineteenth century wound management of the parturient uterus and compound fracture: The Semmelweis-Lister priority controversy, O. H. Wagensteen, 565
Noyes, H. D. The effects of albuminuria upon vision, 197
Numismatics, Medical: A denarius commemorating Rome's first doctor, Arcagathus (219 B.C.), A. W. Zorgniotti, 448

O

Ober, William B. Madness and poetry: A note on Collins, Cowper, and Smart, 203
Observations on America's international medical programs, G. I. Lythcott, 361
Officers of sections of the Academy 1970, 673
Opening statement (Symposium on Medicine and Diplomacy in the Tropics), A Brooks, 299
Opinions of the American aborigines, W. Robertson, 742
Origins of modern scientific thinking, The, G. I. Altschuller, 611

P

Panel discussion, afternoon session (Conference on Glomerulonephritis), J. Lowenstein, N. Bank, M. E. Rubini, and G. E. Schreiner, 884.
Paraplegia and tetraplegia, The problem of pain in, L. S. Michaelis, 88
Phrenologist discusses friendship, The, F. J. Gall, 646
Physician and the community, The, L. Soutter, 489
Pool, John L. Responsibility of the New York Academy of Medicine in the community, 649
Pregnancy, Teen-age out-of-wedlock, W. G. Cobliner, 438
Prenatal genetic counseling: The use of amniocentesis for, M. Gertner, L. Y. F. Hsu, J. Martin, and K. Hirschorn, 916
Prudden, The anthropological writings of Theophil Mitchell (1849-1924), S. Jarcho, 194
Pulmonary compliance in man, The effects of anesthesia and cardiac bypass on, B. R. Hand, J. R. Malm, F. O. Bowman, Jr., and S. F. Sullivan, 22
Purdom, P. Walton. Discussion of the role of the health profession in achieving effective consumer participation, 1063

R

Radiation carcinogenesis, S. Warren, 131
Relevance of the Kaiser-Permanente experience to the health services of the eastern United States, The, E. W. Saward, 707
Renal disease, Proteinuria in, E. L. Becker, 830
Renal regulation of sodium transport, The, N. Bank, 818
Renal transplantation: Present status, A. L. Rubin, J. C. Whitsell, R. R. Riggio, G.

H. Schwartz, D. S. David and K. H. Stenzel, 869
Responsibility of the New York Academy of Medicine in the community, J. L. Pool, 649
Richards, Dickinson W. Presentation of the Academy Plaque to James Burns Amberson, M.D., 663
Robertson, William. Opinions of the American aborigines, 742
Rockefeller, Nelson A. Universal health insurance, 657
Role of the community in developing improved health care, H. Badillo, 1027
Role of the health profession in achieving effective consumer participation, P. W. Purdom, 1063
Rousselot, Louis M. Critique of the conflict between mission-oriented and clinical Research, 906
Rubin, Albert L., Whitsell, John C., Riggio, Robert R., Schwartz, Gabriel H., David, David S., and Stenzel, Kurt H. Renal transplantation: Present status, 869
Rubini, Milton E. and Kopple, Joel D., Dietary management of end-stage uremia, 850
Rush, Benjamin. Effects of the American revolution, 558

S

Salmonella infections in inbred mouse strains, Resistance to, D. H. Boehme, 499
Saward, Ernest W. Relevance of the Kaiser-Permanente experience to the health services of the eastern United States, 707
Sawitsky, Arthur and Ozaeta, Panfilo B., Jr. Disease-associated autoimmune hemolytic anemia, 411
Schechter, David Charles. Application of electrotherapy to noncardiac disorders, 932
Schreiner, George E. Management of end state nephritis: Biochemical alterations, 838
Schwartz, Gerhart S. Infibulation, population control, and the medical profession, 964
Sherman, Harry. The use of an authority for hospitals, 183
Silver, George A. American medicine: Technology outruns social usefulness, 148
Smallpox in New York City, 1868-1870, E. Harris et al., 199
Smith, Alan DeForest. Richard Wiseman: His contributions to English surgery, 167
Smith, Stephen R. Discussion of the role of the health profession in achieving effective community participation, 1067
Social policy and guild policy in health manpower, T. Levin, 1112
Soutter, Lamar. The physician and the community, 489
Standing committees and officers of sections of the Academy 1970, 670
Statement on Implementation of the New York State Abortion Law. The Committee of Public Health of the New York Academy of Medicine, 674
Straus, Bernard. Defunt and dying diseases, 686
Swanstrom, Edward E. The evolution and delivery of medical programs in developing lands, 324
Symposia (see also Conferences):
Medicine and diplomacy in the tropics, 299
Hemolytic anemia, 397

T

Terris, Milton, chairman. Discussion III (1970 health conference), 1141
Tollund man and other bog burials, S. Jarcho, 554
Training of allied health professionals and physician's assistants, M. M. Dacso, 1107
Tropical Disease Center, The, Symposia sponsored by
Medicine and diplomacy in the tropics, 299
Two health problems: One solution, M. C. McLaughlin, 454

U

Universal health insurance, N. A. Rockefeller, 657

Urban ecology, geography, and health problems, G. W. Carey, 73
Uremia, dietary management of end-stage, M. E. Rubini and J. D. Kopple, 850
Use of an authority for hospitals, The, H. Sherman, 183

V

Vogl, Alfred. On clinical medicine: With notes from the diary of a part-time researcher, 39

W

Waldron, Walter, Discussion of the role of the health profession in achieving effective consumer participation, 1071
Wangensteen, Owen H. Nineteenth century wound management of the parturient uterus and compound fracture: The Semmelweis Lister priority controversy, 565
Warren, Shields. Radiation carcinogenesis, 131
War we can win, A.: Health as a vector of foreign policy, H. L. Carey, 334
Wescott, Lloyd. Discussion of the role of the community in developing improved health care, 1042
Wilks, S. Unpublished papers of Thomas Hodgkin, 67
Willcox, Alanson. Discussion of the paper by James F. Kelly: "Assuring stable and effective financing of local health services: Role of intergovernmental grants in aid," 732
Williams, Greer. Needed: A health consumers' organization, 532
Wiseman, Richard: His contributions to English surgery, A. D. F. Smith, 167

Z

Zacchias on mental deficiency and on deafness, Paulus, P. F. Cranefield and W. Federn, 3
Zalusky, Ralph. Drug-associated hemolytic anemia, 427
Zorgniotti, Adrian W. Medical numismatics: A denarius commemorating Rome's first doctor, Arcagathus (219 B.C.), 448

AUTHOR INDEX

Volume 46, 1970

A

Altschuller, G. I., 611
Angrist, A., 523
Apstein, C., 998
Aristotle, 70

B

Badeau, J. S., 303
Badillo, H., 1028
Baldwin, D. S., 797
Baltaxe, H., 1000
Bank, N., 818, 884
Barragan, M. F., 1080
Beck, C., 460
Becker, E. L., 747, 830, 1008
Bergen, S. S., 1099
Bitensky, M. W., 457
Bloomfield, D. A., 998
Boehme, D. H., 499
Bowman, Jr., F. O., 22
Brachfeld, N., 998
Bregman, D., 999
Brooks, A., 299
Bryant, T. E., 1054
Bryce, J., 920
Buchanan, F. H., 484

C

Cahill, K. M., 300
Cahn, E., 1031
Caldwell, P. R. B., 1006
Carey, G. W., 73
Carey, H. L., 334
Carp, L., 267
Carroll, H. J., 458
Chisholm, S., 1144
Churg, J., 761
Cobliner, W. G., 438
Cohen, B. D., 458
Colman, H., 293, 1018
Committee on Public Health, The, 391
Conley, J., 511
Cordice, J. W. V., Jr., 1025, 1149
Cottrell, T. S., 1006
Cranefield, P. F., 3
Cron, T. O., 1038

D

Dammin, G. J., 351
Dacso, M. M., 1107
David, D. S., 869
Deely, W. J., 1000
Dell, R. B., 1003
Deren, J. J., 1002
Detwiler, P., 460
Deuschle, K. W., 97
Diamant, B., 1000
Dipiazza, M., 460
Doerfler, W., 459
Duffy, J. C., 952

E

Earle, D. P., 749, 797
Edelmann, C. M., Jr., 797
Emmanuel, G., 1002, 1009
Ennes, H., 1150

F

Farah, A. A., 313
Federn, W., 3
Feldman, L. L., 113
Fillmore, S. J., 1005
Fischer, V. J., 1007
Fleming, R., 1000
Fraser, R. A. R., 1001
Frater, R. M. W., 1008
French, D., 1129

G

Gall, F. J., 646
Gebhard, B., 469
Gelb, A., 1002
Gertner, M., 916
Gilman, A., 666
Gmeiner, R., 998
Goldring, R. M., 1004
Goetz, R. H., 999
Goff, J. A., 462
Goldson, H., 1011
Goodrich, C. H., 97
Gopinathan, K., 1002, 1009
Grayzel, A. I., 460
Greenberg, S. M., 1048
Greene, E. L., 462
Grieco, M. H., 597
Guy, M. J., 1002

H

Halac, E., Jr., 460
Hand, B. R., 22
Harris, E., 199
Hatch, J. W., 1084
Hayes, A., 1010
Heird, W. C., 1003
Herrera, C. E., 1003
Herson, J. H., 462
Hirschhorn, K., 916
Hoehn, R., 922
Holloman, J. L. S., Jr. 1077
Hsieh, H. S., 461
Hsu, L. Y. F., 916

J

Jaffe, E. R., 397, 461
Jameson, J., 462
Jarcho, S., 34, 62, 124, 189, 194, 287, 378, 386, 479, 554, 643, 737, 889, 1013

K

Kasirajan, N., 998
Kelly, J. F., 718
Kimata, S., 1010
Kleinschmidt, A. K., 459
Kopple, J. D., 850
Kripke, D. C., 999

L

Langner, T. S., 462
Laury, G. V., 676
Levere, R. D., 458
Levi, R., 997
Levin, A. R., 1000
Levin, T., 1112
Levowitz, B. S., 1011
Lewis, M. L., 1003

Lipkin, M., 161
Long, R. G., 1057
Lowenstein, J., 884
Lowinger, P., 1059
Lythcott, G. I., 361

M

Madden, T. M., 482
Malm, J. R., 22
Marks, C. E. Jr., 1004
Martin, J., 916
Mathur, A., 1011
McCarthy, B. J., 1135
McCluskey, R. T., 769
McCrory, W. W., 789
McLaughlin, M. C., 454
Merrill, J. P., 806
Michaelis, L. S., 88
Morgagni, J. B., 71

N

Nahas, G. G., 1012
Neal, O., Jr., 1091
New York Academy of Medicine, The, 281, 391, 509, 642, 674, 893
Noyes, H. D., 197

O

Ober, W. B., 203
Olendzki, M., 97
Ozaeta, P. B., Jr., 411

P

Pool, J. L., 649, 1001
Price, T., 1003
Purdom, P. W., 1063

R

Rashkin, A., 1011
Richards, D. W., 663
Richards, D. W., 663
Riggio, R. R., 869
Robertson, W., 742
Rockefeller, N. A., 657
Rousselot, L. M., 906
Rubin, A. L., 869
Rubini, M. E., 850, 884
Rush, B., 558
Russell, V., 457

S

Saroja, D., 1002, 1009
Saward, E. W., 707
Sawitsky, A., 411
Saxena, B. B., 462
Schechter, D. C., 932
Scheidt, S. S., 1005
Schreiner, G. E., 838, 884
Schwartz, G. H., 869
Schwartz, J. S., 1006
Schwarz, G. S., 964
Shah, A., 1007
Shapiro, M., 1000
Sherman, H., 183
Sherman, R. L., 1008
Silver, G. A., 148
Silverstein, M. J., 1008
Smith, A. De F., 167
Smith, S. R., 1067
Soutter, L., 489
Spears, J. R., 1002, 1009
Stein, B. M., 1001
Stenzel, K. H., 869
Stuckey, J. H., 1009
Straus, B., 686
Sullivan, S. F., 22
Swanstrom, E. E., 324

T

Tarjan, E. M., 1010
Terris, M., 1141
Triner, L., 1012
Tuttle, T., 1010

V

Valcin, A., 1011
Verosky, M., 1012
Vogl, A., 39
Vulliemoz, Y., 1012

W

Waldron, W., 1071
Wangensteen, O. H., 565
Warren, S., 131
Wescott, L., 1042
Whitsell, J. C., 869
Wilks, S., 67
Winters, R. W., 1003
Willcox, A., 732
Williams, G., 532

Y

Yellin, E. L., 1008

Z

Zalusky, R., 427
Zorgniotti, A. W., 448